MANUAL OF
CLINICAL
IMMUNOLOGY

MANUAL OF
CLINICAL
IMMUNOLOGY

EDITED BY

NOEL R. ROSE

Professor and Chairman, Department of Immunology and Microbiology,
Wayne State University School of Medicine, Detroit, Michigan

HERMAN FRIEDMAN

Head, Department of Microbiology and Immunology, Albert Einstein Medical Center,
Philadelphia, Pennsylvania

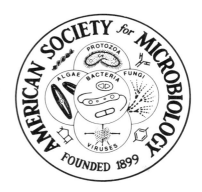

AMERICAN SOCIETY
FOR MICROBIOLOGY

Washington, D.C. 1976

Library of Congress Cataloging in Publication Data

Main entry under title:

Manual of clinical immunology.

    A joint effort of the members of the American Society for Microbiology and the American Association of Immunologists, and companion volume to the Manual of clinical microbiology.
    Includes indexes.
    1. Immunodiagnosis—Handbooks, manuals, etc.
    2. Immunology—Handbooks, manuals, etc. I. Rose, Noel R. II. Friedman, Herman, 1931–   III. American Society for Microbiology.
[DNLM; 1. Immunologic technics. QY25 M294]

RB46.5.M36   616.07'9   76-17595
ISBN 0-914826-09-3 (Cloth binding)
ISBN 0-914826-10-7 (Flexible binding)

EDITORIAL BOARD

LIST OF CONTRIBUTORS

Leslie Abelson
National Cancer Institute, Bethesda, Maryland 20014

N. Franklin Adkinson, Jr.
The Johns Hopkins University School of Medicine at The Good Samaritan Hospital, Baltimore, Maryland 21239

Vincent Agnello
New England Medical Center Hospital, Boston, Massachusetts 02111

William L. Albritton
Center for Disease Control, Atlanta, Georgia 30333

A. D. Alexander
Chicago College of Osteopathic Medicine, Chicago, Illinois 60615

D. Bernard Amos
Duke University Medical Center, Durham, North Carolina 27710

Warren A. Andiman
Yale University School of Medicine, New Haven, Connecticut 06510

Malcolm S. Artenstein*
Walter Reed Army Institute of Research, Washington, D.C. 20012

A. Balows
Center for Disease Control, Atlanta, Georgia 30333

Lewellys F. Barker
Bureau of Biologics, Bethesda, Maryland 20014

Ann Bartlett
WHO Collaborating Laboratory, Nuffield Institute of Comparative Medicine, Zoological Society of London, London NW1, England

Irene Batty
Wellcome Research Laboratories, Beckenham, Kent, England

Joseph A. Bellanti
Georgetown University School of Medicine, Washington, D.C. 20007

Dennis Bidwell
WHO Collaborating Laboratory, Nuffield Institute of Comparative Medicine, Zoological Society of London, London NW1, England

Pierluigi E. Bigazzi
Wayne State University School of Medicine, Detroit, Michigan 48201

Francis L. Black
University of Connecticut Health Center, Farmington, Connecticut 06032

Carl H. Blank
Center for Disease Control, Atlanta, Georgia 30333

Philip M. Blatt
University of North Carolina School of Medicine, Chapel Hill, North Carolina 27514

Kurt J. Bloch
Massachusetts General Hospital and Harvard Medical School, Boston, Massachusetts 02115

Brenda L. Brandt
Walter Reed Army Institute of Research, Washington, D.C. 20012

William E. Braun
Cleveland Clinic, Cleveland, Ohio 44106

* Deceased.

Philip A. Brunell
University of Texas Health Science Center at San Antonio, San Antonio, Texas 78284

Joseph J. Cavallaro
Center for Disease Control, Atlanta, Georgia 30333

Max A. Chernesky
McMaster University, Hamilton, Ontario, Canada L8S4J9

Leonard Chess
Sidney Farber Cancer Center, Harvard Medical School, Boston, Massachusetts 02115

Jens Erik Clausen
Gentofte University Hospital, Hellerup, Denmark

Martin J. Cline
University of California School of Medicine, San Francisco, California 94122

Robert D. Collins
Vanderbilt University School of Medicine, Nashville, Tennessee 37232

J. Colombani
Hôpital St-Louis, Paris, France

Monique Colombani
Hôpital St-Louis, Paris, France

John P. Craig
State University of New York, Downstate Medical Center, Brooklyn, New York 11203

Jean Dausset
Hôpital Saint-Louis, Paris, France

Hugo L. David
Center for Disease Control, Atlanta, Georgia 30333

John R. David
Robert B. Brigham Hospital, Boston, Massachusetts 02115

Neil C. Davis
University of Cincinnati Medical School, Cincinnati, Ohio 45219

J. A. Demetriou
BioSciences Laboratories, Van Nuys, California 91405

Sharad D. Deodhar
Cleveland Clinic Foundation, Cleveland, Ohio 44106

Wallis E. DeWitt
Center for Disease Control, Atlanta, Georgia 30333

Jules L. Dienstag
National Institute of Allergy and Infectious Diseases, Bethesda, Maryland 20014

Richard C. Dimond
Walter Reed Army Institute of Research, Washington, D.C. 20012

F. J. Dixon
Scripps Clinic and Research Foundation, La Jolla, California 92037

Walter R. Dowdle
Center for Disease Control, Atlanta, Georgia 30333

D. C. Dumonde
The Mathilda and Terence Kennedy Institute of Rheumatology, Bute Gardens Hammersmith, London W6 7DW, England

Bo Dupont
Memorial Sloan-Kettering Cancer Center, New York, New York 10021

Lois B. Epstein
Cancer Research Institute, University of California School of Medicine, San Francisco, California 94143

John L. Fahey
UCLA School of Medicine, The Center for Health Sciences, Los Angeles, California 90024

Daryl S. Fair
University of California, Irvine, California 92664

John C. Feeley
Center for Disease Control, Atlanta, Georgia 30333

Euripedes Ferreira
Duke University Medical Center, Durham, North Carolina 27710

Jordan N. Fink
Medical College of Wisconsin, and Wood Veterans Administration Hospital, Milwaukee, Wisconsin 53193

J. M. Flexner
Vanderbilt University School of Medicine, Nashville, Tennessee 37232

Rolf Freter
The University of Michigan Medical School, Ann Arbor, Michigan 48104

H. Hugh Fudenberg
Medical University of South Carolina, Charleston, South Carolina 29401

Henry Gewurz
Rush Medical College, Chicago, Illinois 60612

Thomas J. Gill III
University of Pittsburgh School of Medicine, Pittsburgh, Pennsylvania 15261

Gerald J. Gleich
Mayo Clinic and Mayo Foundation, Rochester, Minnesota 55901

A. D. Glick
Vanderbilt University School of Medicine, Nashville, Tennessee 37232

David W. Golde
University of California School of Medicine, San Francisco, California 94122

Sidney H. Golub
University of California, Los Angeles, Los Angeles, California 90024

Morris A. Gordon
New York State Department of Health, Albany, New York 12201

Gale A. Granger
University of California, Irvine, California 92664

L. J. Greenberg
University of Minnesota Medical School, Minneapolis, Minnesota 55455

Edgar Haber
Harvard Medical School, Massachusetts General Hospital, Boston, Massachusetts 02114

Edith A. Hambie
Center for Disease Control, Atlanta, Georgia 30333

John A. Hansen
Memorial Sloan-Kettering Cancer Center, New York, New York 10021

Pierre Henkart
National Cancer Institute, Bethesda, Maryland 20014

Kenneth L. Herrmann
Center for Disease Control, Atlanta, Georgia 30333

Arnold H. Hicks
Center for Disease Control, Atlanta Georgia 30333

Monto Ho
University of Cincinnati Medical School, Cincinnati, Ohio 45219

Richard Hong
University of Wisconsin Hospitals, Center for Health Sciences, University of Wisconsin, Madison, Wisconsin 53706

Y. H. Inami
University of Hawaii, Honolulu, Hawaii 96822

Michael A. S. Jewett
Memorial Sloan-Kettering Cancer Center, New York, New York 10021

A. H. Johnson
Duke University Medical Center, Durham, North Carolina 27710

Wallis L. Jones
Center for Disease Control, Atlanta, Georgia 30333

Robert E. Jordon
Mayo Clinic, Mayo Medical School, Rochester, Minnesota 55901

John B. Josimovich
University of Pittsburgh School of Medicine and Magee-Womens Hospital, Pittsburgh, Pennsylvania 15213

I. G. Kagan
Center for Disease Control, Atlanta, Georgia 30333

Albert Z. Kapikian
National Institute of Allergy and Infectious Diseases, Bethesda, Maryland 20014

Leo Kaufman
Center for Disease Control, Atlanta, Georgia 30333

William Kaufmann
New York State Department of Health, Albany, New York 12201

Donald E. Kayhoe
National Institute of Allergy and Infectious Diseases, Bethesda, Maryland 20014

Pierre W. Keitges
University of Kansas Medical School, Kansas City, Kansas 66112

D. S. Kellogg
Center for Disease Control, Atlanta, Georgia 30333

George E. Kenny
University of Washington, School of Public Health and Community Medicine, Seattle, Washington 98195

George C. Klein
Center for Disease Control, Atlanta, Georgia 30333

Shaul Kochwa
Mount Sinai School of Medicine, City University of New York, New York, New York 10036

Jukka Koistinen
Medical University of South Carolina, Charleston, South Carolina 29401

Manjula S. Kumar
Cleveland Clinic Foundation, Cleveland, Ohio 44106

Herbert Z. Kupchik
Mallory Institute of Pathology, Boston City Hospital, Boston, Massachusetts 02118

Robert A. Kyle
Mayo Clinic, Rochester, Minnesota 55901

P. Reed Larsen
Harvard Medical School, Peter Bent Brigham Hospital, Boston, Massachusetts 02115

Sandra A. Larsen
Center for Disease Control, Atlanta, Georgia 30333

J. H. Leech
Vanderbilt University School of Medicine, Nashville, Tennessee 37232

Bernard B. Levine
New York University School of Medicine, New York, New York 10016

M. J. Levitt
University of Pittsburgh School of Medicine, Pittsburgh, Pennsylvania 15261

John E. Lewis
Loma Linda University, Loma Linda, California 92354

Lawrence M. Lichtenstein
Johns Hopkins University School of Medicine, and The Good Samaritan Hospital, Baltimore, Maryland 21239

James Lightbody
Wayne State University School of Medicine, Detroit, Michigan 48201

Robert L. Lundak
University of California, Irvine, California 92664

Norman B. McCullough
Michigan State University, East Lansing, Michigan 48824

James E. McGuigan
University of Florida College of Medicine, Gainesville, Florida 32610

K. Robert McIntire
National Cancer Institute, Bethesda, Maryland 20014

J. Ross Mackenzie
Methodist Hospital, Indianapolis, Indiana 46202

El Sheikh Mahgoub
New York State Department of Health, Albany, New York, 12201

R. N. Maini
The Mathilda and Terence Kennedy Institute of Rheumatology, Bute Gardens Hammersmith, London W6 7DW, England

Charles R. Manclark
Bureau of Biologics, Food and Drug Administration, Bethesda, Maryland 20014

Dean Mann
National Cancer Institute, Bethesda, Maryland 20014

George Miller
Yale University School of Medicine, New Haven, Connecticut 06510

Thomas P. Monath
Center for Disease Control, Atlanta Georgia 30333

Maurice A. Mufson
Veterans Administration Hospital, Chicago, Illinois 60680

Frederick A. Murphy
Center for Disease Control, Atlanta, Georgia 30333

Robert M. Nakamura
Scripps Clinic and Research Foundation, La Jolla, California 92037

Howard R. Nankin
University of Pittsburgh School of Medicine and Montefiore Hospital, Pittsburgh, Pennsylvania 15213

Erwin Neter
State University of New York at Buffalo and Children's Hospital, Buffalo, New York 14222

L. Norman
Center for Disease Control, Atlanta, Georgia 30333

Philip S. Norman
The Johns Hopkins University School of Medicine at The Good Samaritan Hospital, Baltimore, Maryland 21239

James O'Leary
University of Minnesota Medical School, Minneapolis, Minnesota 55455

Joost J. Oppenheim
National Institute of Dental Research, Bethesda, Maryland 20014

Dan F. Palmer
Center for Disease Control, Atlanta, Georgia 30333

C. Peebles
Scripps Clinic and Research Foundation, La Jolla, California 92037

Stephen M. Peters
Georgetown University School of Medicine, Washington, D. C. 20007

Lawrence D. Petz
Institutes of Medical Sciences, Pacific Medical Center, and University of California, San Francisco, California 94122

Yosef H. Pilch
Department of Surgery, Harbor General Hospital, Torrance, California 90509

Rao Pillarisetty
Veterans Administration Hospital, San Francisco, California 94121

William Pollack
Ortho Research Institute of Medical Sciences, Raritan, New Jersey 08869

Pamela Pool
Duke University Medical Center, Durham, North Carolina 27710

Knud Poulsen
The University Institute for Experimental Medicine, 71 Norre Alle, DK-2100 Copenhagen, Denmark

Anne-Marie Prieur
Hôpital Necker, Paris, France

Robert H. Purcell
National Institute of Allergy and Infectious Diseases, Bethesda, Maryland 20014

Bruce S. Rabin
University of Pittsburgh School of Medicine, Pittsburgh, Pennsylvania 15261

William E. Rawls
McMaster University, Hamilton, Ontario, Canada L8S4J9

Nancy Reinsmoen
University of Minnesota Medical School, Minneapolis, Minnesota 55455

Alice M. Reiss
Ortho Research Institute of Medical Sciences, Raritan, New Jersey 08869

Gustavo Reynoso
State University of New York (Syracuse) and Wilson Memorial Hospital, Johnson City, New Jersey 03790

Harold R. Roberts
University of North Carolina School of Medicine, Chapel Hill, North Carolina 27514

Ross E. Rocklin
Robert B. Brigham Hospital, Boston, Massachusetts 02115

Marek Rola-Pleszczynski
Georgetown University School of Medicine, Washington, D.C. 20007

Noel R. Rose
Wayne State University School of Medicine, Detroit, Michigan 48201

Richard E. Rosenfield
Mount Sinai School of Medicine, City University of New York, New York, New York 10036

Gordon Ross
Cornell University Medical College, 10021

Naomi F. Rothfield
University of Connecticut School of Medicine, Farmington, Connecticut 06032

Philip K. Russell
Walter Reed Army Hospital, Washington, D. C. 20012

Julius Schachter
University of California, San Francisco, San Francisco, California 94143

Bilha Schecter
National Institute of Dental Research, Bethesda, Maryland 20014

Stuart Schlossman
Sidney Farber Cancer Center, Harvard Medical School, Boston, Massachusetts 02115

Nathalie J. Schmidt
State of California Department of Health, Berkeley, California 94704

K. W. Schmitt
University of Pittsburgh School of Medicine, Pittsburgh, Pennsylvania 19261

Robert S. Schwartz
New England Medical Center Hospital, School of Medicine, Tufts University, Boston, Massachusetts 02115

Merle J. Selin
Center for Disease Control, Atlanta, Georgia 30333

Sidney Shulman
New York Medical College, New York, New York 10029

Reuben P. Siraganian
National Institute of Dental Research, Bethesda, Maryland 20014

Merrill J. Snyder
University of Maryland, School of Medicine, Baltimore, Maryland 21201

Lynn E. Spitler
University of California, San Francisco, San Francisco, California 94143

John A. Stewart
Center for Disease Control, Atlanta, Georgia 30333

Thomas P. Stossel
Children's Hospital Medical Center, Sidney Farber Cancer Center, and Harvard Medical School, Boston, Massachusetts 02115

Lisbeth A. Suyehira
Rush Medical College, Chicago, Illinois 60612

Arne Svejgaard
State University Hospital of Copenhagen, DK-2100 Copenhagen 0, Denmark

Norman Talal
Veterans Administration Hospital, San Francisco, California 94121

Eng M. Tan
Scripps Clinic and Research Foundation, La Jolla, California 92037

Marilyn Taylor
Children's Hospital Medical Center, Sidney Farber Cancer Center, and Harvard Medical School, Boston, Massachusetts 02115

Mary C. Territo
University of California School of Medicine, San Francisco, California 94122

A. N. Theofilopoulos
Scripps Clinic and Research Foundation, La Jolla, California 92037

John S. Thompson
University of Iowa College of Medicine and Veterans Administration Hospital, Iowa City, Iowa 52240

Baldwin H. Tom
Northwestern University Medical School, Chicago, Illinois 60611

Franklin H. Top, Jr.
Walter Reed Army Medical Center, Washington, D.C. 20012

G. Torrigiani
World Health Organization, 1211 Geneva, 27 Switzerland

Edmund C. Tramont
Walter Reed Army Institute of Research, Washington, D.C. 20012

Philip Troen
  University of Pittsburgh School of Medicine and Montefiore Hospital, Pittsburgh, Pennsylvania 15213

J. William Vinson
  School of Public Health, Harvard University, Boston, Massachusetts 02115

Alistair Voller
  London School of Hygiene and Tropical Medicine, and WHO Collaborating Laboratory, Nuffield Institute of Comparative Medicine, Zoological Society of London, London, England

T. A. Waldmann
  National Cancer Institute, Bethesda, Maryland 20014

J. A. Waldron
  Vanderbilt University School of Medicine, Nashville, Tennessee 37232

J. L. Waner
  Harvard School of Public Health, Boston, Massachusetts 02115

Peter A. Ward
  University of Connecticut Health Center, Farmington, Connecticut 06032

Thomas H. Weller
  Harvard School of Public Health, Boston, Massachusetts 02115

Geraldine L. Wiggins
  Center for Disease Control, Atlanta, Georgia 30333

Curtis B. Wilson
  Scripps Clinic and Research Foundation, La Jolla, California 02037

Sten Winblad
  University of Lund, Malmö General Hospital, Malmö, Sweden

Robert J. Winchester
  The Rockefeller University, New York, New York 10021

R. A. Wolstencroft
  The Mathilda and Terence Kennedy Institute of Rheumatology, Bute Gardens Hammersmith, London W6 7DW, England

Ronald M. Wood
  State of California Department of Health, Berkeley, California 94704

John W. Yunginger
  Mayo Clinic and Mayo Foundation, Rochester, Minnesota 55901

Edmond J. Yunis
  University of Minnesota Medical School, Minneapolis, Minnesota 55455

Norman Zamcheck
  Mallory Institute of Pathology, Boston City Hospital, Boston, Massachusetts 02118

Wendell D. Zollinger
  Walter Reed Army Institute of Research, Washington, D.C. 20012

PREFACE

This *Manual* represents a joint effort by members of the American Society for Microbiology (ASM) and the American Association of Immunologists (AAI) to provide medical scientists and physicians interested in clinical immunology with a guide to the rapidly growing field of laboratory immunology. The *Manual of Clinical Immunology* developed as a natural extension of the *Manual of Clinical Microbiology*, now in its second edition as a highly successful publication of the ASM. The first edition of the *Manual of Clinical Microbiology* devoted approximately one hundred pages to various serological tests. The second edition, published in 1974, had very little enlargement of the section on immunological diagnosis, since it was felt that coverage of more than the barest essentials of this rapidly evolving field would require a marked increase in the number of pages. Thus, a companion *Manual of Clinical Immunology* was conceived to deal exclusively with applications of immunology for detection and analysis of a wide variety of diseases, not only those induced by microorganisms.

This *Manual* is directed mainly to laboratory directors and technologists who are responsible for the performance of immunological tests in the clinical laboratory, as well as to graduate students, medical students, post-doctoral trainees, residents, fellows, and clinicians. It is anticipated that the *Manual* will provide authoritative information about the best methods for conducting specific immunological tests. Clinical interpretations of each procedure are also provided, along with a discussion of pitfalls and problems in performing the various analyses.

The organization of the *Manual* is generally similar to that of the *Manual of Clinical Microbiology* in that there are sections dealing with different aspects of immunology with sufficient breadth and background to provide the necessary foundations for clinical studies. The subject matter encompasses laboratory tests designed to measure both humoral and cellular immunological responses of patients but excludes the description of immunological reactions devoted exclusively to identification of microorganisms such as bacteria and viruses. These procedures are covered in the *Manual of Clinical Microbiology*. Thus the emphasis of this *Manual* is on currently used laboratory procedures which aid in the diagnosis not only of diseases caused by microorganisms, but also other pathological conditions such as autoimmunity, immediate and delayed hypersensitivity states, and malignancy. Analyses using antibodies as specific biochemical reagents are also described. Tests conducted directly on patients are included only if they seem pertinent to laboratory examinations or to the broad area of immunological diseases.

The methodologies described in this *Manual* are presented in a manner to be understandable to laboratory personnel in appropriate positions in academic, community, and general hospitals. Descriptions of laboratory tests are given in sufficient detail that a skilled technologist can perform the procedures without going to other references. Step-by-step methods are given wherever possible. In those areas where a number of different techniques are available, the procedures employed by the authors are described in detail. However, brief discussion is included of other methods, pointing out how and why these methods may differ. All authors have been instructed to keep their descriptions of methods as brief as possible, but to indicate the initial ingredients needed for a test rather than merely describing commercially available reagents or kits. Furthermore, when necessary or available, a number of different vendors or sources for reagents are given. The authors have been requested to point out those vendors or sources of reagents they have used personally.

An early organizational decision taken by the editors and editorial board was that the *Manual* should not provide exhaustive reviews of the literature of clinical immunology. References and citations are used mainly for illustrative purposes. In general, each chapter lists only major reference articles and reviews.

The editors wish to thank the more than one hundred authors for the high quality of their chapters and for accepting the peer review procedure established for the *Manual*. The editors are greatly indebted to the section editors who undertook a very heavy commitment of time and effort. The cooperation of a liasion committee of the AAI, consisting of Dr. Mart Mannik as Chairman, Dr. Robert Schwartz, and Dr. John Fahey, is also appreciated, as are the contributions of the Council of the AAI and the Publications Board of ASM in supporting this endeavor. Mr. Robert A. Day, Managing Editor, and the ASM Publications Office staff are to be commended for their patience and co-operation.

It was anticipated by the two sponsoring societies that this *Manual* will fill an important need of various medical specialties and laboratories, including those involved in immunological studies outside the narrower sphere of infec-tious diseases. Revised editions may well be required every few years, especially since the technology used in immunological laboratories is changing at a very rapid pace.

Noel R. Rose, M.D., Ph.D.
Herman Friedman, Ph.D.
April 1976

INTRODUCTION

Clinical Laboratory Immunology: Review and Preview

NOEL R. ROSE AND HERMAN FRIEDMAN

It is the purpose of this *Manual*, as indicated in the Preface, to present information concerning the specific method and rationale for the performance of a wide range of immunological tests that are directly related to patient care. Laboratories devoted to clinical immunology are being established at a very rapid rate in many hospital and medical centers. Historically, many of these laboratories evolved from a serology service as a section of a clinical microbiology laboratory. However, developments in immunology during the last decades have resulted in specialized procedures that are unrelated to microbiology. For example, laboratories devoted to specific clinical applications of immunology, such as tissue typing or tests for autoantibodies, are sometimes administratively part of some other laboratory division or a clinical department outside of the traditional pathology laboratory setting. Many of these specialized laboratories are maintaining their identity and even increasing their scope of operations. It is apparent that clinical immunology is not only a rapidly growing component of laboratory medicine but also an essential ingredient of many areas of clinical medicine. Therefore, some of the traditions associated with other clinical laboratories are either missing or not appropriate. There are very few guidelines at present concerning the establishment of a comprehensive clinical immunology laboratory. Thus, those investigators who wish to do so often have to strike out in new directions.

Historically, laboratory immunology was one of the first clinical laboratory specialties established in medical centers, hospitals, and universities. Long before clinical chemistry became a separate discipline and before anatomical or surgical pathology evolved into important specialties, laboratories were established to carry out the immunological diagnosis of infectious diseases. By the end of the last century, many bacteriologists were offering their services to physicians in providing serological tests for identifying and quantitating bacterial antibodies in patients' sera. They performed Widal tests for typhoid antibodies and a battery of other agglutination tests for monitoring development of an immunological response to pathogenic microorganisms. The complement fixation test, initially employed by Wassermann and his colleagues to detect antibody in patients who were infected with *Treponema pallidum*, was widely performed early in this century. Within a short time such complement fixation tests for syphilis became the "work horse" of laboratory immunology. Complement fixation was adapted to the detection of serum antibodies to a wide variety of microorganisms, especially rickettsiae, fungi, and viruses, as well as protozoa and helminths.

Until the modern era of immunology started in the 1960s, most of the work of the serology laboratory continued to deal largely with antimicrobial immunity. Once it was recognized that immunological phenomena are involved in diverse human diseases, as well as in transplantation rejection and tumor progression, clinical immunology laboratories evolved rapidly. Immunofluorescence was introduced in the 1950s, along with other antibody- or antigen-tagging methods using radioisotopes or enzymes. The development of indirect or passive agglutination procedures, including latex fixation and hemagglutination, and a wide variety of techniques designed to measure or quantitate cell-mediated immunity in vitro followed in short order. The application of these newer immunological techniques has extended immunology very far indeed from the early days of testing for antibodies to microorganisms. For example, serological and mixed leukocyte reactions for transplantation immunology have provided methods necessary not only for matching prospective donors and recipients for organ grafting, but also for giving important new information concerning immunogenetic relationships and immunological competence. These and similar tests are also being presently exploited for detection of tumor immunity. Precise measurement of immunological capabilities of patients with malignancy as well as patients suspected of having autoimmunity, congenital or acquired immunodeficiency, or even long-standing viral infections is now becoming widely practiced.

A major question often asked by those who wish to establish a clinical immunology laboratory is: "What type of tests should we perform?" There is no general answer to this question until an institution decides what type of patient population must be served in terms of immunological diagnosis.

The scope of a clinical immunology laboratory is generally based not so much on the availability of laboratory tests but more on the type of patient care that a specific institution offers. For example, in a general medical center dealing with a diverse patient population, it is important for a laboratory to have capabilities in the area of antimicrobial immunity as well as many tests dealing with immunopathology, including autoimmune and hypersensitivity diseases. An institution that does not have an organ transplantation program does not need tissue typing or ancillary services considered mandatory for a larger or specialized center. Similarly, a general medical center with no pediatric unit would not need the same type of clinical immunology services offered in a modern children's hospital where congenital immunodeficiency diseases are prevalent. Since many physicians in general hospitals examine and treat patients with malignancy, it seems likely that the newer developments in laboratory immunology related to cancer will have to become widely available. Similarly, many immunological disorders, including immediate and delayed hypersensitivity reactions and diseases with autoantibodies such as rheumatoid arthritis or lupus erythematosus, are not rare in general medical centers, and it is essential to have available not only the techniques for detecting immunoglobulin factors which correlate with such diseases but also personnel who can properly interpret the laboratory results.

The format utilized in this *Manual* can provide a general guide in selecting the most appropriate tests. Equally important, any laboratory that offers immunological services should certainly have available trained supervisory and technical personnel who can utilize the technologies effectively. It is essential for such personnel to understand the nature of tests performed rather than to merely follow "packaged" instructions. This seems to be especially important for those medical centers where some aspects of clinical laboratory immunology have become the province of clinical chemistry or clinical pathology departments. For example, immunoelectrophoresis and gel diffusion tests for serum proteins certainly can be performed by persons with little or no training in immunology. However, when problems arise, do such personnel really understand the basic mechanisms involved? Do they know that a precipitin band occurs only under conditions of optimum molecular ratios of antigen and antibody, and that some classes of antibody molecules are superior to others in producing precipitation but may be less efficient in agglutination or complement fixation reactions? Do they understand that a precipitate does not represent a static one-step reaction but is continuing reaction that is dependent upon temperature? Do they recognize that most of the reagents involved, such as agar and buffers, influence the precipitin reaction? There are many test procedures where interaction between antigen and antibody is not visualized directly but by the binding of a radioisotope. Immunoassays, especially those based on inhibition by small molecules, are commonly performed in radioisotope laboratories; these tests involve very sensitive immunological reactions. Do the people who perform these tests know why it is important to follow certain practices? For example, do they know why a test serum should not be permitted to run down the side of the solid-state immunoassay tube?

It seems apparent from the discussion above that the rapid evolution of a variety of newer immunological techniques and procedures in the clinical laboratory will result in a pluralistic system. Organizations such as the World Health Organization and the International Union of Immunological Societies have directed attention to clinical immunology as a major medical specialty and suggested the different types of laboratory services which should be available in medical schools and hospitals. However, there is no consensus at present as to where such procedures should be carried out. Until there is a "settling out" in this field, it is difficult to state categorically the best arrangement or organization for a clinical immunology laboratory. However, all scientists would agree that only techniques which have been well standardized and are properly controlled should be offered as a service to physicians and their patients. It is likely that within the next few years, and certainly before future editions of this *Manual* appear, there must be further developments in research, education, and standardization so that clinical laboratory immunology will join the ranks of other laboratory specialties in providing improved health services.

GENERAL REFERENCES IN CLINICAL LABORATORY IMMUNOLOGY

1. Bellanti, J. A. 1971. Immunology. W. B. Saunders Co., Philadelphia.
2. Bennett, C. W. 1968. Serology. Charles C Thomas Co., Springfield, Ill.
3. Billingham, R., and W. Silvers. 1971. The im-

munobiology of transplantation. Prentice-Hall, Inc., Englewood Cliffs, N.J.

4. Bloom, B. R., and P. R. Glade (ed.). 1971. In vitro methods in cell-mediated immunity. Academic Press Inc., New York.

5. Burnet, F. M. 1972. Auto-immunity and autoimmune disease. F. A. Davis Co., Philadelphia.

6. Campbell, D. H., J. S. Garvey, N. E. Cremer, and D. H. Sussdorf. 1970. Methods in immunology. W. A. Benjamin, Inc., New York.

7. Freedman, S. O. 1971. Clinical immunology. Harper & Row, New York.

8. Friedman, A., and J. E. Prier (ed.). 1973. Rubella. Charles C Thomas, Springfield, Ill.

9. Fudenberg, H. H., J. R. L. Pink, D. C. Stites, and A. Wang. 1972. Basic immunogenetics. Oxford Univ. Press, New York.

10. Gell, P. G. H., R. R. A. Coombs, and P. J. Lachmann. 1975. Clinical aspects of immunology, 3rd edition. Blackwell Scientific Publications, Oxford, England.

11. Grabar, P., and P. Burtin (ed.). 1964. Immunoelectrophoretic analysis. Elsevier Publishing Co., Amsterdam.

12. Habel, K., and N. P. Salzman (ed.). 1969. Fundamental techniques in virology. Academic Press Inc., New York.

13. Hildemann, W. H. 1970. Immunogenetics. Holden-Day, San Francisco, Calif.

14. Hsiung, G. D. 1973. Diagnostic virology. Yale Univ. Press, New Haven, Conn.

15. Kabat, E. A. 1961. Experimental immunochemistry, 2nd edition. Charles C Thomas, Springfield, Ill.

16. Katz, D. H., and B. Benacerraf. 1976. The role of products of the histocompatibility gene complex in immune responses. Academic Press Inc., New York.

17. Kwapinski, J. E. (ed.) 1972. Research in immunochemistry and immunobiology, vol. 1 and 2. University Park Press, Baltimore.

18. McCluskey, R. T., and S. Cohen (ed.). 1974. Mechanisms of cell-mediated immunity. John Wiley and Sons, New York.

19. Nairn, R. C. 1969. Fluorescent protein tracing. The Williams & Wilkins Co., Baltimore.

20. Nelson, D. S. 1976. Immunobiology of the macrophage. Academic Press Inc., New York.

21. Nowotny, A. 1969. Basic exercises in immunochemistry. Springer-Verlag, New York.

22. Park, B. H., and R. A. Good. 1975. Principles of modern immunobiology: basic and clinical. Lea & Febiger, Philadelphia.

23. Pearsall, N. N., and R. S. Weiser. 1970. The macrophage. Lea and Febiger, Philadelphia.

24. Prier, J. E., and H. Friedman (ed.). 1973. Australia antigen. University Park Press, Baltimore.

25. Rapp, H. J., and T. Borsos. 1970. Molecular basis of complement action. Appleton-Century-Crofts, New York.

26. Roitt, I. 1974. Essential immunology. Blackwell Scientific Publications, Oxford, England.

27. Rose, N. R., and P. Bigazzi (ed.). 1973. Methods in immunodiagnosis. John Wiley and Sons, New York.

28. Rose, N. R., F. Milgrom, and C. J. van Oss (ed.). 1973. Principles of immunology. Macmillan Publishing Co., Inc., New York.

29. Samter, M., D. W. Talmage, B. Rose, W. B. Sherman, and J. H. Vaughn (ed.). 1971. Immunological diseases, vol. I, 2nd edition. Little, Brown and Co., Boston.

30. Van Furth, R. (ed) 1970. Mononuclear phagocytes. F. A. Davis Co., Philadelphia.

31. Weir, D. M. 1973. Handbook of experimental immunology, 2nd edition. Blackwell Scientific Publishing Co., London.

32. Williams, C. A., and M. W. Chase (ed.). 1967–1971. Methods in immunology and immunochemistry, vol. 1–3. Academic Press Inc., New York.

33. Zmjewski, C. M. 1968. Immunohematology. Appleton-Century-Crofts, New York.

CONTENTS

Section C
IMMUNOASSAYS

Section D
BACTERIAL, MYCOTIC, AND PARASITIC IMMUNOLOGY

Section E
VIRAL, RICKETTSIAL, AND CHLAMYDIAL IMMUNOLOGY

Section F
IMMUNOHEMATOLOGY

Section G
LABORATORY EXAMINATION OF PATIENTS WITH ALLERGIC AND IMMUNODEFICIENCY DISEASES

Section H
AUTOIMMUNE DISEASES

Section I
TUMOR IMMUNOLOGY

Section J
TRANSPLANTATION IMMUNOLGY

Section K

LICENSURE AND CERTIFICATION PROGRAMS IN CLINICAL IMMUNOLOGY LABORATORIES

Section A

TESTS FOR HUMORAL COMPONENTS OF THE IMMUNOLOGICAL RESPONSE

Chapter 1

Introduction

JOHN L. FAHEY

Introduction of new physicochemical techniques, such as ultracentrifugation and electrophoresis, and new immunochemical methods, such as gel diffusion, radial precipitation, immunoelectrophoresis, and radioimmunoassays, led to important discoveries in biology and medicine. Innovative scientists modified the original procedures so that they would be suitable for clinical application. Better understanding of many diseases resulted. This has been an exciting and fruitful era as many parameters of normal and abnormal immune function have been defined in terms of serum immunoglobulin and complement. Quantitative and qualitative tests of immunoglobulins and complement components in serum (and other body fluids) are now essential resources in the armamentarium of the clinical immunologist.

Immunoglobulin structure is presented succinctly in the first few pages of chapter 99 (Kyle). This subject is not reviewed again here, but that section may be advantageously consulted in connection with the presentations that follow.

General familiarity with the make-up of the immunoglobulin family is assumed, as well as knowledge of the fact that myeloma proteins and macroglobulins contain both heavy and light chains, whereas Bence Jones proteins are composed only of light chains. Another essential concept is that each class of heavy (γ, α, μ, δ, ϵ) and light (κ, λ) chains has a unique composition and configuration; this allows the production of large quantities of specific antisera which can be used to identify and quantify individual classes of immunoglobulin.

Immunoglobulin assessment in body fluids routinely involves three laboratory techniques: serum (zone) electrophoresis, immunoelectrophoresis, and quantitation of major immunoglobulin classes.

Serum electrophoresis provides an overview of the five major electrophoretic groups of serum proteins. Quantitative measurements are important. Low serum gamma globulin level has a different significance when the serum albumin is also low (as in nephrotic syndrome) than when albumin is normal, as occurs in many immune deficiency syndromes. Zone electrophoresis also provides ready qualitative assessment of serum or urine abnormalities. This is particularly valuable for the detection of myeloma proteins and Waldenström macroglobulins (and Bence Jones proteins) as discrete bands discernible in addition to the usual serum or urine protein peaks.

Immunoelectrophoresis permits ready identification of the major classes of normal immunoglobulin and of myeloma proteins and other anomalous proteins (e.g., Bence Jones protein, heavy-chain disease) which cannot be done by zone electrophoresis. It is not, however, a good quantitative technique.

Quantitation of specific immunoglobulins by radial diffusion or other methods allows precise definition of the amounts of each immunoglobulin class. These are important since all classes may not be equally affected by disease. Furthermore, disease progression or therapeutic benefits may be assessed by sequential quantitative determinations.

These three measurements are sufficient to meet most needs for evaluation of immunoglobulins in body fluids. In some cases, however, such as heavy-chain disease, additional physicochemical techniques such as exclusion (Sephadex) chromatography, ion-exchange chromatography, or special electrophoretic procedures may be needed. Furthermore, antisera to immunoglobulin subclasses, e.g., IgG1, -2, -3, or -4, or to Gm or InV groups may be of assistance.

Results of analytic tests may differ between laboratories as a consequence of variations in technique and in the antisera employed as reagents. Reference samples of human serum with agreed-upon immunoglobulin content (such as those provided by the World Health Organization) help to standardize data expression. Reference kits containing known myeloma protein, Waldenström macroglobulins, Bence Jones proteins, and hypogammaglobulinemia sera permit laboratories to test their own effectiveness regularly. Testing of unknown serum and urine samples provided by qualified reference centers can further enhance the performance of these important tests.

Chapter 2

Quantitation of Immunoglobulins

NEIL C. DAVIS AND MONTO HO

INTRODUCTION

Clinical laboratories presently include total serum protein (TSP) determinations and serum electrophoresis (SE) as routine screening procedures for patient sera. It is the general view that, whenever the γ or β region is increased or decreased on the SE scan, further examination by immunoelectrophoretic analysis (IEP) and/or quantitation of immunoglobulins G, A, and M (IgG, IgA, and IgM) is indicated. Excluded from routine testing are IgD, which has no known clinical significance, and also IgE, which requires different methodology. Indeed, quantitation of the first three immunoglobulins is usually performed in all patients with suspected immunoglobulin abnormalities (8).

Many methods for quantitative assessment of the immunoglobulins have been described. Three of these are currently of greatest value:

1. Radial immunodiffusion (RID) with limited diffusion (14) or with timed diffusion (7).

2. Automated immune precipitation (AIP; 10, 11, 17).

3. Electroimmunoassay (EIA), also called rocket technique (6, 12, 13).

RID is the most widely used method for quantitation of the serum immunoglobulins (and other serum proteins) and is the accepted method for standardization of reference sera. Consequently, it is also the method to which other methods are compared. This probably results both from its having been historically the earliest of the modern methods and, even more, from its apparent simplicity and lack of need for sophisticated or expensive laboratory equipment. However, in a survey to assess its accuracy as performed in a number of laboratories (24), results were widely variable. Variability was also observed in the results of immunoglobulin measurement by commercially available plates (9). Many of the difficulties could be attributed to differences in the antisera and reference sera employed (see below), differences which would introduce similar variability in other quantitative methods (AIP, EIA). These latter methods have not yet been evaluated by comparable surveys. Berne (3) has published an excellent critique of timed diffusion as opposed to limit diffusion of the antigen. His conclusion is that, despite the greater incubation time and antibody requirement, limit diffusion is the better choice to obviate variables (time, temperature, etc.) affecting timed diffusion and to obtain highest accuracy.

When patient load is relatively low, i.e., less than 20 determinations per day, RID will probably remain the method of choice. EIA, has now been adapted for quantitation of the immunoglobulins, but has a limitation with regard to capacity, e.g., now eight wells per plate, which may outweigh the time saved over the limit diffusion RID method. If the load is 12 serum specimens per day or less, it is a very satisfactory alternative to RID. For clinical laboratories with a high patient load (i.e., 20 to 40 serum specimens for immunoglobulin quantitation per day) and with the capital and technical staff, additional experience may demonstrate that AIP is the method of choice. Unlike the other two methods, the AIP reaction takes place in a fluid medium rather than a gel, and no diffusion of the antigen or antibody is required. Therefore, antigens which aggregate or have polymeric forms (e.g., IgA and IgM) present no difficulty. All three methods have approximately the same limit of detection.

Although only the quantitation of the immunoglobulins is dealt with here, it should be explicitly understood that any clinical interpretation will depend on also having available the total serum protein value and either SE or IEP patterns. Quantitation alone, for example, might not reveal the early stages of myeloma in a patient, but properly applied IEP would.

By the tests suggested here (i.e., TSP, SE, and IEP, combined with a method of quantitation), immunoglobulin abnormalities such as immunodeficiencies and monoclonal or polyclonal gammopathies can be detected. Immune deficiencies are associated with a wide variety of diseases and with genetic, environmental, and nutritional conditions (2, 18). Although in-depth discussion is beyond the scope of this chapter, the clinical analyst has an essential role in defining both the immune deficiencies and the hypergammaglobulinemias (8).

STANDARDIZATION

Standardization and quality control will be covered in detail in another section of this *Manual*. To minimize variations between results obtained with different reagents and in separate laboratories, the Immunology Branch of the World Health Organization has prepared reference standards for serum immunoglobulin quantitation. Contents of immunoglobulin are expressed in International Units (IU) on a provisional basis until sufficient data are available to express the immunoglobulin content reliably in terms of milligrams per milliliter. Meanwhile, a vial of batch 67/95 (a preparation related to the International Reference Preparation 67/86) can be obtained by writing: Director, Immunoglobulin Reference Center, 6715 Electronic Drive, Springfield, Va. 22151. Directions are included for preparation of a working standard. Also, the preparation of a working standard serum and of high and low internal standard sera and their use in quality control have been described elsewhere (16).

ANTISERA

Antisera are available from several commercial sources, but they usually differ in titer and monospecificity, and they may not recognize all the antibody combining sites of the antigen, particularly in the case of the immunoglobulins which exhibit marked microheterogeneity. Also, different batches from the same supplier may vary. These factors have been suggested (1) as contributing to the lack of agreement of values obtained with commercially available RID plates. Therefore, each antiserum must be carefully standardized. To correlate results obtained by RID, AIP, and EIA, the same antisera should be used.

The immunoglobulin portion of the antiserum can be used to avoid a high background. The antibody-containing gamma globulin fraction of antiserum is readily obtained by the method of Steinbuch and Audran (21) and can be used on volumes of from 10 to 1,000 ml with about an 80% recovery. The method is as follows. Adjust 100 ml of antiserum (antiplasma) to pH 5.5 to 6.0 with 1 N acetic acid. Slowly add 6 ml of octanoic acid (dropwise) to the well-stirred antiserum (mag mix) at room temperature. Continue stirring for 30 min after addition is complete. Centrifuge at 5 C for 15 min at an RCF of 27,000, and filter the supernatant fluid through a moistened Whatman 3 MM paper. Store in small portions at −70 C. The use of 1:10,000 Merthiolate in sera, antisera, and buffers as a preservative rather than the commonly used sodium azide avoids the possibility of explosions from build-up of the latter in copper or lead plumbing systems.

RADIAL IMMUNODIFFUSION

Principles

One of two immune reactants (usually antibody) is added and uniformly distributed in a layer of agar, or agarose gel, followed by introduction of the other reactant (usually antigen) into wells punched in the gel. The antigen diffuses radially into the gel-antibody mixture, forming a visible ring of precipitate at a point dependent on antigen-antibody stoichiometry. As more antigen diffuses out, the precipitin ring dissolves in antigen excess and reappears at a greater distance from the well. This increase in the diameter of the precipitin ring continues with time until the antigen, or antibody, completely reacts.

Certain quantitative relationships exist between the ring diameter and the concentration of the antigen, both while the ring is expanding (7) and after it stops enlarging (14). In the latter case, limit diffusion, a plot of diameter squared (D^2) versus concentration is linear. In the former case (i.e., when the ring diameters are still growing), the plot is approximately linear when the logarithm of antigen concentration is plotted versus the ring diameter. In practice, when quick results are required, timed diffusion might be used, and later, to improve the accuracy, the values could be rechecked after limit diffusion has been reached. However, limit diffusion can be done only if the correct antibody concentration is used (i.e., the concentration should be low enough to give measurable rings at low antigen concentration but high enough to be in antibody excess at high antigen concentrations). Most commercially available immunoplates are designed for the timed diffusion method and cannot be used for limit diffusion *unless it is specifically stated by the manufacturer*.

Preparation of plates

If commercial plates are used, directions continue below under Serum testing. The method described here is primarily designed for limit diffusion.

Equipment.

WPIC Agar Gel Plates, 6.2 × 8.1 cm (2½ × 3¼ inches); Madison Engineering Co., Columbia, Md.

Fast-flow (large-orifice) 10-ml serological pipettes.

Suction flask with rubber tubing and Pasteur pipette.

Water bath, 56 C.

Humidity chamber (two taped window-glass plates, 12 × 12 inches, separated by a 0.5-inch-thick Plexiglas frame and containing a moistened sheet of Whatman 3 MM paper).

Leveling board with adjustable leg height.

Dissecting microscope with measuring reticule with 0.1-mm divisions or other measuring devices.

Template for cutting wells. Glue a sheet of 0.25-inch Plexiglas to the lid of one of the plates. With a drill press and a 0.09-inch drill bit, drill 32 holes as shown in Fig. 1.

Well punch. Use a blunt-end #14 or #16 syringe needle set in a small Plexiglas handle (#14, outer diameter 0.083 inch and inner diameter; #16, outer diameter 0.065 inch and inner diameter 0.047 inch); Small Parts, Inc., Miami, Fla.

Reagents.

Glycine buffer (0.1 M, pH 7.0, with 1:10,000 Merthiolate as preservative).

Agarose (Special Noble Agar can also be used).

Sera

Reference serum or working standard serum.

Internal control serum (high level and low level for each immunoglobulin).

Patient sera.

Antisera

Anti-IgG (γ chain specific).

Anti-IgA (α chain specific).

Anti-IgM (μ chain specific).

Preparation of reagents.

Glycine buffer, 0.1 M, pH 7.0; 0.04 M in EDTA

For each liter of buffer add 7.5 g of glycine to about 600 ml of distilled water; add 100 ml of 0.4 M EDTA (see below) and 100 ml of 1:1,000 Merthiolate. Adjust to pH 7.0 ± 0.05 with 1 N NaOH, make to 1 liter, and recheck pH.

EDTA 0.4 M

Add 152 g of EDTA (ethylenedinitrilotetraacetic acid) tetrasodium salt (molecular weight 380.20) and 148.9 g of EDTA disodium salt dihydrate (molecular weight 372.21) to 900 ml of distilled water, and stir with a magnetic stirrer until dissolved. Make to 1 liter (pH = 7.8).

Agarose, 2%

Place water in a flat pan, cover bottom of pan with boiling beads, and bring water to a boil. In a 2-liter Erlenmeyer flask, add 40 g of agarose moistened with 300 ml of cold glycine buffer, and then add the remaining 1,700 ml of heated buffer to the flask. Place the flask in a boiling-water bath and heat with stirring until a clear solution results. Avoid boiling the agarose solution. While still hot, pour the agarose solution into 20-ml test tubes (approximately 12 ml/tube), allow to cool, and then stopper tightly to avoid evaporation. Store at 5 C.

It should be pointed out that phosphate buffer, Special Noble Agar, and 3¼ × 4 inch glass slides can also be used for the RID system. This is described in detail in an excellent procedural guide available from the U.S. Department of Health, Education, and Welfare (16). The agarose-EDTA system has been used in our laboratory for some time for two reasons: (i) to avoid the known cation-exchange properties of agar toward proteins with a cathodal migration at pH 7 to 8.6 and (ii) to prevent the alteration of some serum components, specifically the complement components.

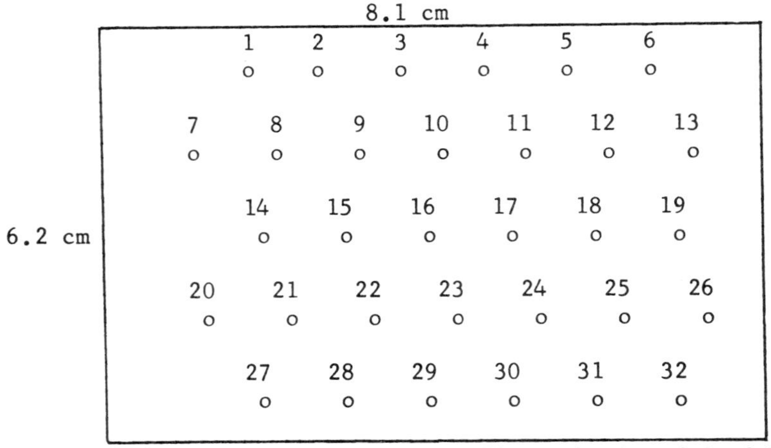

FIG. 1. *Template for cutting wells in an RID immunoplate. The template is made by gluing a ¼-inch-thick layer of Plexiglas to the lid of a 2½ by 3¼ inch immunoplate and drilling holes (0.09 inch) with a drill press to accept a blunt-end #14 syringe needle punch. Wells and rows are 1 cm apart and 1.5 cm from any edge of the plate.*

Preparation of diffusion plates. Large enough volumes of antiserum should be used to avoid repeated determination of proper dilution. The method described here employs diluted sera to conserve antisera and is primarily designed for limit diffusion. A method employing undiluted sera for timed diffusion is described in detail elsewhere (16).

1. Label three of the $2^{1}/_{2} \times 3^{1}/_{4}$ inch agar gel plates 1:5, 1:10, and 1:20.

2. Pipette 2 ml, 1 ml, and 0.50 ml, respectively, of antiserum into test tubes labeled 1:5, 1:10, and 1:20, and place them in a 56 C water bath.

3. Melt 35 to 40 ml of the 2% agarose in a boiling-water bath and transfer it to the 56 C water bath. When the agarose solution has cooled to 56 to 60 C, pull the agarose solution into a wide-orifice 10-ml serological pipette and let drain. Repeat two or three times to warm the pipette, and then pipette 8 ml, 9 ml, and 9.5 ml of agarose, respectively, into the tubes labeled 1:5, 1:10, and 1:20. Mix the contents of each thoroughly while the tubes remain in the 56 C water bath.

4. With separate wide-orifice 10-ml serological pipettes, warmed as above, transfer the contents of each tube to the corresponding agar gel plates placed on a level surface. Remove any air bubbles with a warm wire or needle. The resultant agarose bed is 2 mm thick.

5. Cover plates and allow to cool to room temperature for 20 to 30 min.

6. Using the template shown in Fig. 1 and a #14 or #16 well punch, cut 32 holes. Holes made with a #14 needle hold 4 μliters.

7. Remove the agarose plugs from wells by suction with a Pasteur pipette. Replace covers on plates and set aside. Plates prepared in this manner can be stored at 5 C for 2 weeks, or longer if wrapped in Saran to prevent evaporation.

Serum testing

Evaluation of diffusion plates for suitability. These considerations apply equally to commercially obtained plates or those prepared in the laboratory.

1. Dilute the reference serum or working standard serum with saline: 1:50 for IgG, 1:10 for IgA, and 1:2 for IgM.

2. The reference serum or working standard, diluted as above (100%), and further 75, 50, 25, and 12.5% dilutions of this standard should be used to fill the first five holes of rows 2 and 4 (Fig. 1). Fill wells 6 and 7 of rows 2 and 4 with high internal standard and low internal standard, respectively, diluted as in step 1 above.

3. Incubate the plates in a humidity chamber at 37 C for 20 to 24 h (20 to 48 h for IgM). If timed diffusion measurements are desired, a shorter time and different temperature can be employed (16).

4. At the chosen time, measure the ring diameters by turning the plate upside down on a support which permits light from a high-intensity lamp to strike the plate obliquely from underneath. Measure the ring diameters with a device permitting accurate measurement to 0.1 mm and record them. If rings are slightly oval rather than round, take the average of two measurements made at right angles to each other. If rings are large or faint, with poorly defined edges, antiserum is too dilute. If rings are too small, it is too concentrated. Compute the average of duplicate determinations and record them. Compute the square of the diameters (D^2, square millimeters).

5. For limit diffusion, plot on arithmetic graph paper (2-cycle semilog paper if timed diffusion is used): percentage of reference standard (working standard) on the ordinate and disk diameter squared (D^2) in square millimeters on the abscissa (Fig. 2).

6. With a ruler draw a best straight line. Only that portion of the line that is linear or near linear can be used. Do not extend above or below the linear portion. If the line encompasses the range of concentrations of interest, it can be used. If not, a different time or temperature may have to be used.

7. Estimate the highest dilution of antisera which will give rings of about 7 mm with the high internal standard or undiluted working standard. Rings of approximately 4 mm should be obtained for the 12.5% working standard. Ring diameters smaller than 3.5 mm usually cannot be read accurately.

8. For low-level plates choose an antiserum dilution that will give a ring size of about 7 mm for the 25% working standard.

9. The above procedure from 3 through 8 may have to be repeated with intermediate dilutions of antisera to achieve optimal results.

Quantitation of patient sera.

1. Before use, plates should be allowed to warm to room temperature for 20 to 30 min.

2. In a test tube rack align working standard serum dilutions, diluted internal control sera, and nine patient sera (diluted as in step 1 above or as directed for commercial plates) if duplicates are to be run. If only single determinations are made, each plate will accommodate 25 patients.

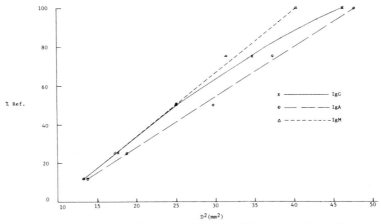

FIG. 2. *Standard reference curve for RID (limit diffusion). The square of the diameters (D^2) is plotted on arithmetic graph paper versus the percentage of reference serum. The best straight line should not be extended above or below points. Values for unknowns are transformed into IU/ml of mg% by reading off percentage of reference serum and converting from Table 1.*

3. Using an ultra-micropipetting device (obtainable from many commercial sources) or capillary tubes or Pasteur pipettes without a rubber bulb, add a constant volume of the specimens to the well. Care must be taken to fill wells to the level of the agarose bed if capillary pipettes are used. Avoid air bubbles or spilling of sera outside of wells.

4. Place standards and unknowns randomly (and in duplicate) throughout the plate. If a plate like that shown in Fig. 1 is used, then fill wells 7 through 11 and 20 through 24 with working standard dilutions. Fill wells 12 and 25 with high internal control serum and wells 13 and 26 with low internal control serum. Fill wells 1 through 6, 14 through 19, and 27 through 32 with the patient sera.

5. After all specimens are added, incubate the slides at 37 C in a humidity chamber or, for most commercial plates, at room temperature, e.g., humidity chamber or plastic bag. After appropriate diffusion time, read disk diameters and plot the reference curves as described.

6. From the reference curve, using the average disk diameter of each patient serum, determine the percentage of reference serum and convert to concentration from the standard table (Table 1).

7. If a myeloma serum is obtained with a concentration of one or more of the immunoglobulins that exceeds the capacity of the immunoglobulin plate (i.e., ring diameter larger than 7 mm), the serum should be diluted until the ring diameter falls within reference limits. Also, if such sera are quite viscous, separate dilutions will give greater accuracy than serial dilutions.

8. Control sera which read outside usual lim-

TABLE 1. *Conversion of percentage of reference serum to concentration of immunoglobulins*[a]

Percentage of reference	IgG		IgA		IgM	
	mg/100 ml	IU/ml	mg/100 ml	IU/ml	mg/100 ml	IU/ml
100	2,550	298	530	315	250	286
75	1,913	223	397	237	188	214
50	1,275	149	265	158	125	143
25	638	74	133	79	63	71
12.5	319	37	66	39	31	36

[a] Shown in abbreviated form. Actual table should show steps of 1%. See Rowe, Grob, and Anderson (20).

its indicate that the run may not be valid.

Sources of error.

1. Spilling of antigen or standard solutions outside of wells.

2. Rings too small or too large and diffuse because of antibody or antigen excess.

3. Wells not filled completely or containing air bubbles.

4. Damage to wells, resulting in distorted precipitin rings.

5. Plates stored too long with resultant evaporation or distortion of agarose bed.

6. Uneven thickness of agarose gel due to improper level when pouring plates.

7. Lifting of agarose gel when removing plugs with Pasteur pipette, allowing sample to leak out of bottom of well.

AUTOMATED IMMUNE PRECIPITATION

Principle

When antibodies react with antigens in dilute solutions, soluble complexes are formed which can be detected by light scattering techniques. The antigen-antibody reaction follows the law of mass action, and, under the right conditions, the amount of complexes formed is a function of both antigen and antibody concentration. If the antibody concentration is kept constant, the number of complexes formed varies in direct proportion to the concentration of the antigen. Consequently, the concentration of the antigen can be determined by measuring the amount of light scattered by the complexes at right angles to the incident beam of light. If the light scatter of an unknown serum sample is compared with the light scatter of dilutions of a reference serum of known antigen concentration, then its antigen concentration can be determined quantitatively (11, 17).

Procedure

Equipment.

Technicon Auto Analyzer II continuous-flow system (Technicon Corp., Tarrytown, N.Y.). Modules common to single- and dual-channel operation:
1. Sampler IV with microprobe and timer assembly (Technicon Part No. 171-BB093-03).
2. Cam 50 per hour, 1:1 (Technicon Part No. 127-1144P01).
3. Proportioning Pump III.
4. Fluoronephelometer with: flowcell (Technicon Part No. 013-B008-01), 355-nm narrow pass primary filter (Technicon Part No. 518-7000-01), and neutral density filters (as required).
   0.6 E (Technicon Part No. 518-7040-01)
   0.3 E (Technicon Part No. 518-7041-01)
Additional modules required for single-channel operation:
1. Manifold (Technicon Part No. 013-A005-01).
2. Single-pen AutoAnalyzer II Recorder (chart speed, 1 inch per min).
Additional modules required for dual-channel operation:
1. Dual Floating Probe (Technicon Part No. 171-B191-01).
2. Manifold (Technicon Part No. 013-A005-01).
3. Single-pen AutoAnalyzer II Recorder (chart speed, 1 inch per min). A two-pen AutoAnalyzer II Recorder (chart speed, 1 inch per min) can be used in lieu of two single-pen recorders.
4. Fluoronephelometer with: flowcell (Technicon Part No. 013-B008-01), 355-nm narrow pass primary filter (Technicon Part

No. 518-7000-01), and neutral density filters (as required).
   0.6 E (Technicon Part No. 518-7040-01)
   0.3 E (Technicon Part No. 518-7041-01)
Included in the purchase price of this system is a recommended 1-week training course in the use of the instrument at the Technicon facility in Tarrytown, N.Y. A manual for operation is also available (TJ-0170) from Technicon Corp.

It is assumed in the procedure described below that the investigator has been trained in the use and care of the equipment as provided in the training course and manual. The method described here presents a simplified modification which obviates certain technical difficulties such as clogging of the probes, connecting pins, etc. A flow diagram of the manifold modification is shown in Fig. 3.

Reagents.

Saline solution: NaCl (reagent grade), 45 g, is added to 5 liters of distilled water and thoroughly mixed. Before use, the solution is filtered through a 0.2-μm filter. At the beginning of each working day, 1 ml of Tween 20 per liter of saline is added, and the solution is thoroughly mixed.
Wash solution: NaOH, 1.0 M. Add 40 g of reagent-grade NaOH to 800 ml of distilled water with thorough mixing. After cooling to room temperature, make to 1 liter.
Antisera.
Sera:
Reference serum or working standard serum.
Internal control serum.
Patient sera.
Instead of using undiluted sera and achieving the appropriate final dilution for each antigen by the prescribed method, sera are manually diluted 1:100, and further dilution is obtained by selecting the correct size (ml/min) sample tubing in the proportioning pump. When the serum sample is mixed with the antiserum (0.32 ml/min), the final dilution can be calculated:

$$\frac{\text{sample (ml/min)} + 0.32}{\text{sample (ml/min)}}$$

$$\times\ 100 = \text{final dilution}$$

Dilution of sera should be done on the day of quantitation since diluted sera are not stable.

Determination of appropriate antiserum dilution.

Start-up procedure

1. Turn on all modules and allow electronic stabilization for 30 min.
2. Pump the saline-Tween solution through

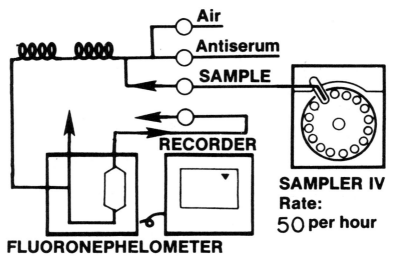

FIG. 3. *Flow diagram for automated analysis of serum immunoglobulins. Sera are manually prediluted 1:100. The sample line for IgG is 0.03 ml/min, for IgA 0.05 ml/min, and for IgM 0.16 ml/min. Antisera line is 0.32 ml/min.*

all lines during the warm-up period.

3. Check that the proper pump tubes are connected for antiserum (0.32 ml/min), for antigen sample (0.03 ml/min for IgG, orn/red; 0.05 ml/min for IgA, orn/blu; 0.16 ml/min for IgM, orn/orn). All pump tubes must be flow-rated and are available from Technicon Corp. or other commercial sources.

4. Prepare a working concentration of the respective antiserum by diluting it with saline-Tween solution. If commercial antisera are used, the correct dilution will be on the package insert; if the proper dilution is not indicated, or if using noncommercial antisera, choose an arbitrary trial dilution such as 1:10. A volume of 5 ml of diluted antisera is sufficient to establish the reference curve with seven dilutions of reference serum.

5. Prepare the reference serum or working standard dilutions. First dilute 1:100 with the saline solution using a 10-ml volumetric flask and a 0.1-ml volumetric pipette. Make 2 ml of each of the following dilutions of the 1:100 dilution (100%): 10, 20, 30, 40, 60, and 80%. Make 4 ml of 50% dilution since more of this is needed. Dilutions of sera are made fresh each day and are only stable for 1 day.

6. Load the sample tray as follows: position 1, 10%; 2, 20%; 3, 30%; 4, 40%; 5, 50%; 6, 60%; and 7, 80%. Place end of run pin adjacent to cup 7. Each cup should be filled to the mark (2 ml), as uneven filling may cause uneven aspiration of sample.

7. Turn the fluoronephelometer FUNCTION switch to position NO DAMP, and set the recorder chart drive switch to position ON.

8. With saline solution flowing through the system, use the BASE LINE control to adjust the recorder to 5% base line (saline base line on the recorder chart paper).

9. Remove the antiserum line probe from the saline solution vessel and place the probe into the flask of diluted antiserum. Allow the system to operate, aspirating antiserum.

10. After the antiserum has been pumped for at least 2 min, remove the sample line probe from the saline solution vessel and place the probe into the 50% dilution cup. Allow the system to aspirate the 50% dilution for 2 min and then place the sample line probe into the sampler arm. Wait 2 min more and push the sampler ON switch.

11. When the antiserum causes deflection of the pen, readjust the BASE LINE control until the pen is positioned at 5% on the recorder chart paper. This adjustment corrects the base line for antiserum light scatter (antiserum blank base line).

12. When the antigen-antibody complexes further deflect the pen (for about 2 min), adjust the STANDARD CALIBRATION control until the recorder pen is positioned approximately at 30 chart divisions (30%) on the recorder chart paper.

13. The pen should return to 5% base line after reference antigen-antibody complexes clear the flow cell.

14. After all samples have been aspirated, shut off the sampler. Allow antiserum to flow through the system for an additional 5 min; then place the antiserum probe into the wash receptacle. When read out is finished on re-

corder, set the recorder chart drive switch to position OFF. If, as sometimes happens, the base line becomes erratic or ragged during a run (e.g., determination of IgM), the flow cell can be cleaned between runs by using a 50-ml syringe to force the 1.0 M NaOH wash solution through the isolated flow cell by disconnecting at the "in" connection. Follow with equal volumes of distilled water and saline solution before reconnecting. Wash with saline solution for 30 min before starting another run.

Shutdown procedure

After completion of a run, turn off the fluoronephelometer. Clean the system by pumping 1.0 M NaOH wash solution through the antiserum and sample lines for 30 min followed by 30 min of distilled water. If the system has become dirty as evidenced by an erratic or "jumpy" base line, the wash solution may be left in the machine overnight. The following morning before starting the regular run, rinse the system with distilled water (30 min) followed by saline solution (30 min).

Evaluation

The peak height in chart divisions above the 5% baseline is recorded for each sample and plotted on arithmetic graph paper versus the percentage of reference serum (Fig. 4). Two criteria can be used in assessing the acceptability of the antiserum dilution. First, in Fig. 4 the areas of antibody excess and antigen excess are indicated. Only the linear portion of the line showing no antigen excess can be used for accurate quantitation. Measurement in antibody excess can be used, but, because of depressed values and the lower slope of this portion, re-

sults are less accurate. If linearity is evident between the 10% and the 60% of reference serum values, the antiserum dilution is acceptable. By proper dilution of antisera, accuracy in the low or high concentration ranges can be selectively maximized.

The second criterion is the shape of the peak on the recorder chart (Fig. 5). A blunted or double peak indicates antigen excess, meaning that the antiserum dilution is too high. Antibody excess cannot be assessed from the shape of the peak but can be seen in the standard reference curve by the lowered slope.

Quantitation of patient sera. Once the correct antiserum dilution has been established for each immunoglobulin, patient sera can be assayed. The above dilutions of the reference serum and internal standards are included in

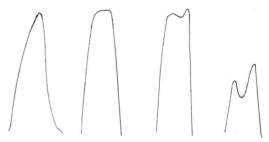

FIG. 5. *Shapes of AIP peaks on recorder chart. The first rounded peak reflects correct antigen-antibody stoichiometry or antibody excess; the blunted or biphasic peaks show antigen excess and cannot be used for quantitation. Samples should be diluted and rerun or antibody concentration increased if seen in determination of correct antiserum dilution.*

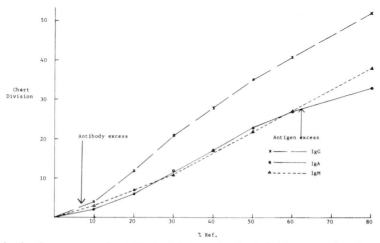

FIG. 4. *Standard reference curve for AIP. Peak heights in chart divisions are plotted versus percentage of reference serum. Unknowns are converted to IU/ml or mg% by use of Table 1.*

every run, and a standard reference curve is plotted.

Proceed exactly as for determination of antiserum dilution but with the following changes:

1 through 5. Same as above.

6. After reference serum dilutions in cups 1 through 7, place saline in cup 8, 1:100 dilutions of the high and low internal standards in cups 9 and 10, and the 1:100 dilutions of patient serum in cups 11 through 40. Place the end of run pin adjacent to the last patient serum cup.

7 through 14. Same as above.

15. Blank run. Since serum samples have inherent light scattering properties, a blank must be determined for each sample and subtracted from the chart value for that sample. The blank is determined by repeating the above procedure under exactly the same conditions of the run (i.e., STANDARD CALIBRATION setting, Damping and Neutral density filter) but with saline running through the antiserum line instead of antiserum. Only one blank run (Blank 1) is needed for determination of the three immunoglobulins in each set of patient sera. Blanks for the other immunoglobulin run (Blank 2) can be calculated by the formula:

Blank 1

$$\times \frac{\text{STANDARD CALIBRATION setting 2}}{\text{STANDARD CALIBRATION setting 1}}$$

$$\times \frac{\text{Sample volume 2}}{\text{Sample volume 1}} = \text{Blank 2}$$

The blank run should be made on the run using the highest serum volume and the highest SC setting. This is usually the case for the IgM run when IgG, IgA, and IgM are being determined. IgA runs usually have significant blanks, but IgG runs do not. Lipemic sera or sera with high triglyceride concentration may give blanks so high that quantitation is impossible. These sera must be diluted further or quantitated by a different method such as IEP.

The shutdown procedure is the same as above.

Plotting of data. The peak heights (minus blanks) of reference serum are plotted on arithmetic graph paper versus the percentage of reference serum (Fig. 4). From the reference curve, using peak heights (minus blanks) of patient sera, determine the percentage of reference serum and convert to mg/100 ml or IU/ml from Table 1.

Sources of error.

1. Inaccurate dilution of patient sera or reference serum.

2. Use of peaks that show antigen excess.

3. Particulate matter in reagents or sera (whole blood cells, fibrin, dust, etc.).

4. Lipemic serum (high blank).

5. Incomplete clotting of serum samples.

6. Incorrect reading of chart divisions for peak height or failure to subtract blank.

7. Cups not filled equally.

8. Variable aspiration of sample. Probe "hanging up" on side of cup.

9. Clogging of probes, connecting pins, or sample lines.

ELECTROIMMUNOASSAY: LAURELL ROCKET TECHNIQUE

Principle

This is another rapid quantitative immunoglobulin method, requiring 4 to 5 h. Laurell (12, 13) combined IEP and RID to achieve the equivalent of limit diffusion in a much shorter time (hours as compared to days) by moving the antigen by electrophoresis into an agarose gel containing antibodies rather than relying on the slow process of diffusion. In 1965 he described crossed electrophoresis, and in 1966 he described the quantitative method first called rocket immunoelectrophoresis but more recently called electroimmunoassay (EIA). An almost identical method was developed independently at the same time by Merrill et al. (15). Modifications of the Laurell technique for quantitative purposes were made by Clark and Freeman (6). There are several ways in which this versatile method can be and has been used. For example, the rocket method may be particularly useful for measurement of IgG in cerebrospinal fluid. EIA is described in detail in an excellent manual (1) and in a review article with some 505 references (22).

Basically, test conditions are used so that antibodies will not move in the gel during electrophoresis, but antigen molecules will because of differing electrophoretic mobilities. Initially, as the antigen molecules migrate, there is antigen excess and the small soluble complexes formed with the antibody molecules continue to migrate at a slower rate in the antibody-containing gel. As electrophoresis continues, conditions are reached whereby the size of the antigen-antibody complexes causes precipitation. The precipitate no longer moves and is passed by unbound antigen or smaller complexes until all the antigen (or antibody) is consumed. At this point, a pointed "rocket" is formed which will not move even on continued electrophoresis.

The area or, more commonly, height of the rocket is quantitatively related to the concentration of the antigen in the sample applied:

$$\text{area} = K \times \frac{\text{antigen}}{\text{antibody}}$$

At first, quantitation of the immunoglobulins by EIA obviously presented difficulties since they have very similar or identical electrophoretic mobilities to the antibody (usually IgG) in the gel and formed precipitates on both anodic and cathodic sides of the application wells. Several methods have been developed to modify the antigen or antibody chemically in order to alter their mobilities. Two methods will be described: (i) carbamylation of the antibody (4, 5) and (ii) copolymerization of antigens with glutaraldehyde (19). The methods described here are for a "micro" version of EIA in which plastic plates containing the immunogel are used. This approach offers many simplifications of the technique, conserves antisera, and is a method being used on commercially available plates (ICL Scientific, Fountain Valley, Calif.). Quantitative crossed immunoelectrophoresis is not described here because it is technically much more difficult and offers little or no advantage for routine quantitation of patient serum immunoglobulins. The "macro" method using glass slides and/or molds to cast gels and also detailed instructions for crossed immunoelectrophoresis have been described (1).

Procedure

Equipment.

Electrophoresis apparatus: Several commercial firms offer appropriate electrophoresis systems. That used here is obtainable from ICL Scientific. The type of equipment developed by Laurell and his group is available from Dansk Laboratorieudstyr A/S, Copenhagen, Denmark. Built-in water cooling systems are almost mandatory to dissipate the heat generated during the electrophoresis if high voltage (8 to 10 V/cm in the gel) is used. For low-voltage electrophoresis (1 to 3 V/cm in the gel) cooling may not be necessary. The electrophoresis apparatus should hold the plates in a horizontal position to avoid skewed precipitates. The entire apparatus should be covered (Plexiglas) to avoid changes in temperature and humidity.

Power supply: Any power supply with rectified current and stabilized voltage with a total output variable from 0 to 250 V (0 to 100 mA) will suffice. A switch to reverse polarity of the system after each run is very convenient to avoid pH changes in the buffer reservoirs.

Voltmeter: A voltmeter (0 to 20 V/cm) is useful to check actual potential drop in the gel and to avoid anode/cathode confusion.

Wicks: The design of the equipment will more or less dictate the type of wick used. Laurell used agarose wicks, but this requires a specially built apparatus. Cotton, paper, or sponge wicks can be used. For cotton wicks, surgical lint folded to give 1 to 2 mm of thickness is appropriate. Good contact between the gel and wicks must be assured. Paper wicks can be cut from filter paper such as Whatman 3 MM. They cannot be reused, whereas the cotton wick, after washing, can. Both paper and cotton wicks are sources of relatively high resistance, and the distance between the buffer and the gel should be kept as short as possible. Sponge wicks are convenient; they can be placed directly in the buffer vessels and the immunoplates can be placed gel side down directly on the sponge. A small weight placed on the upper plastic side of the plate assures good contact.

Gel puncher: The punch described for RID is used. The design of a very convenient gel puncher that cuts and removes the agarose plug in one operation has been described (23).

Template: Glue a bar of ¹/₄-inch Plexiglas to the top of a lid of the type of gel plate being used. Using the method described under RID, drill eight holes as shown in Fig. 6. A very convenient gel plate with imprinted numbers (1 through 8) and anode/cathode markers is available from ICL Scientific.

Leveling board.

Water bath (45 to 55 C): The gelling temperature of 1% agarose varies somewhat from one manufacturer to another, but a high enough temperature should be used to maintain a gel consistency that pipettes and spreads easily and produces a film of uniform thickness.

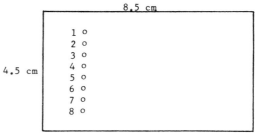

FIG. 6. *Template for EIA immunoplates. A bar of ¹/₄-inch Plexiglas is glued to the lid of the plate, and eight 0.09-inch holes are drilled 1.5 cm from short edge and 0.5 cm from long edge of plate, 0.4 cm apart. The line of holes should be exactly parallel to the short edge. Wells are cut with a blunt-end #14 syringe needle punch. A second set of holes can be made in the same way 3 cm above the first set to increase capacity for number of samples per plate.*

Reagents.

Sera

Reference serum or working standard serum.
Internal control serum.
Patient sera.

Antisera.

Buffer: Many different buffer systems have been used in various types of electrophoresis to achieve different effects such as better resolution, distinctness of precipitin lines, etc. (for detailed discussions, see 22). The two buffer systems described here possess the desired properties for EIA: relatively high buffering capacity and low conductivity to minimize heat generation during electrophoresis.

(a) TMEDA/acetate buffer, pH 5.0, for use with carbamylated antibodies. Add 1.16 g of N,N,N',N'-tetramethyethylenediamine (TMEDA, molecular weight 116.21) to 800 ml of distilled water, add 100 ml of 1:1,000 Merthiolate, adjust the pH of the solution to 5.0 with 1 M acetic acid, and make to 1 liter.

(b) Tris-borate buffer, pH 8.6, for use with glutaraldehyde copolymerized sera. Add 27.7 g of 2-amino-2-hydroxymethyl-1,3-propanediol (Tris, Tromethamine, molecular weight 121.14), 7.6 g of boric acid (molecular weight 61.84), and 1.8 g of EDTA disodium salt dihydrate (molecular weight 372.21) to 800 ml of distilled water, add 100 ml of 1:1,000 Merthiolate, and make to 1 liter.

Diluent for copolymerizing sera: To 50 ml of 0.2 M sodium barbital, add 27.5 ml of 0.2 M HCl and 0.4 ml of 50% (wt/wt) glutaraldehyde, and dilute to 200 ml. Store at 2 to 8 C.

Carbamylation (4)

(a) 7 mg of the IgG portion of the antisera in 1 ml of 0.1 M NaCl (for preparation of antisera IgG, see antisera section).

(b) 7 ml of borate buffer, pH 8.0 (9.03 g of H_3BO_3, 2.13 g of NaCl, and 5.18 g of $Na_2B_4O_7 \cdot 10H_2O$; make to 1 liter).

(c) 2 ml of 1.0 M potassium isocyanate (KOCN). Prepare fresh each day of use.

The mixture of a and b is heated to 45 C and the reaction is started by addition of the isocyanate solution. Incubation is continued for 2 h and stopped by desalting on a column of Sephadex G-25 equilibrated with a 0.01 M sodium phosphate buffer, pH 6.0. Carbamylation is a mild procedure, and, when carried out to a point where the antibody is isoelectric in agarose at pH 5.0, the antibody retains about 80% of its titer. Such antibodies are quite stable and can be used for several months.

Agarose gel (1%): The same procedure is followed as in RID, but 1 g of agarose is used per 100 ml of the appropriate buffer (i.e., TMEDA/acetate for carbamylated antibody and Tris-borate for copolymerized sera).

Determination of appropriate antiserum dilution. Just as for RID, the antiserum concentration for EIA must be determined empirically. The gel plates hold 3.4 ml of warm (56 C) agarose. Appropriate initial dilutions of antisera are 1:10, 1:20, and 1:30.

1. Mark three 10-ml test tubes 1:10, 1:20, and 1:30. In the first test tube pipette 9 ml, in the second 2.5 ml, and in the third 3.0 ml of agarose solution, and place in a 56 C water bath.

2. To the first test tube, add 1 ml of warmed (56 C) antiserum and mix thoroughly.

3. Pipette 2.5 ml of the mixture in the first test tube into the second (1 to 20) test tube and mix thoroughly.

4. Pipette 1.5 ml from first test tube into the third test tube and mix thoroughly. Hold all test tubes in a 56 C water bath until ready to prepare the immunoplate.

5. With the three plates (marked 1:10, 1:20, and 1:30) on a level surface, and using warmed wide-orifice 5-ml pipettes, pipette 3.4 ml from each test tube into the corresponding plates, using the pipette tip to spread gel evenly. Avoid air bubbles.

6. Cover each plate and allow to stand for 20 to 30 min for gel to solidify. Plates may be stored in a humidity chamber at 2 to 8 C for several days or longer if wrapped in Saran.

7. When ready to use, replace the lid of the immunoplate with the template, and, using the #14 syringe needle punch, punch eight holes in the gel. Remove the agarose plugs with a Pasteur pipette and suction.

8. Dilute the reference serum or working standard 1:50 for IgG and 1:10 for IgA and IgM (100%).

9. When using the carbamylated-antibody method, fill wells 1, 2, and 3 with undiluted sample (100%) of the above dilutions, 1:2 dilution (50%), and 1:4 dilution (25%). Repeat in wells 6, 7, and 8. When testing patients, wells 4 and 5 will contain low and high internal standards diluted as in 8, and wells 6, 7, and 8 will contain patient sera diluted as in step 8. Use a micropipette capable of delivering 2 μliters accurately. The wells should be filled and electrophoresis should be started as rapidly as possible, consistent with accuracy, to prevent broadening of the rocket base by diffusion.

10. Place the plates in the electrophoresis chamber, making certain plates are aligned exactly parallel to the flow of the current and with

wells nearest the *anode*. Be sure wicks are making good contact, and turn on the current. The amount of current per plate must be predetermined in each laboratory for the equipment and conditions used. The highest current consistent with no alteration (drying or distortion) of the agarose bed should be used. With the ICL system using the plates described here and sponge wicks, a current of 4 mA/plate is used at 5 C or room temperature.

11. When using glutaraldehyde copolymerized sera (antigen) with unmodified antibody, first make the 25 and 50% dilutions and the undiluted (100%) serum with physiological saline; then make the 1:50 (IgG) or the 1:10 (IgM, IgA) dilutions with the glutaraldehyde diluent. After 30 min (timed), apply samples (2 μliters) as rapidly as possible and proceed as in step 10 but with holes nearest the *cathode*.

12. The best total time for electrophoresis should also be determined in each laboratory since this will vary with the system, current, antibody concentration, and amount of antigen applied. What is desired are rockets of approximately 6 mm (lowest concentration) to 20 mm (highest concentration) with well-developed, pointed tips which, when graphed on arithmetic graph paper (height versus percentage of reference serum), will give a straight line (Fig. 7).

Quantitation of patient sera (see chapter 98). When the correct antiserum concentration, current, and time of electrophoresis has been determined for each immunoglobulin, a standardized procedure has been established and should be adhered to scrupulously for testing of patient sera.

Three patients sera can be tested per plate. Add 2 μliters each of diluted low and high

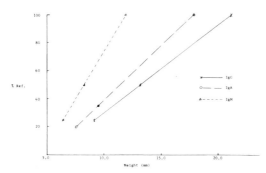

FIG. 7. *Standard reference curve for EIA. Rocket heights in mm are plotted versus percentage of reference serum on arithmetic graph paper. The best straight line should not be extended above or below points measured. Unknowns are converted to IU/ml or mg% from Table 1.*

internal standard to wells 1 and 8, respectively, add 2 μliters of each diluted patient serum in wells 2, 3, and 4, and add diluted reference serum or working standard to wells 5, 6, and 7. Follow the standardized procedure for current and time. Measure the rocket heights as described and plot the standard curve. Using the rocket height for each patient, find the percentage of reference serum and convert to mg/100 ml or IU/ml from Table 1.

If the rockets with patient sera are too small to be read accurately, the test should be repeated with lower dilution of the sera. If rockets are found without "points," the immunoglobulin concentration is too high and the test must be repeated using higher dilutions of the patient serum.

Sources of error.

1. Poor sample application, resulting in inaccurate volumes of sample, cutting of sample well, splattering of sample on agarose bed which produces secondary rockets.

2. Too long a period between application of samples and start of electrophoresis, producing short, broad-based rockets.

3. Too much current or not enough cooling during electrophoresis, causing drying or distortion of agarose bed.

4. Change of pH in buffer solution.

5. Poor contact between wicks and agarose gel, giving wavy precipitin patterns.

6. Immunoplates not aligned properly in electrophoresis chamber, giving skewed rockets.

7. Improper leveling when pouring plates, resulting in uneven bed thickness and inconsistent results.

8. Electrophoresis time too short, resulting in rockets without tips.

9. Inaccurate dilutions.

10. Uneven cooling between upper and lower surface of agarose bed, resulting in "tunneling" (i.e., more rapid movement of antigen near one surface than near the other).

11. Evaporation and drying of plates during storage.

LITERATURE CITED

1. Axelsen, N. H., J. Krøll, and B. Weeke (ed.). 1973. A manual of quantitative immunoelectrophoresis. Universitetsforlaget, Oslo.
2. Bergsma, D., R. A. Good, J. Finstad, and N. W. Paul (ed.). 1975. Birth defects. Original Article Series, vol. 11, no. 1, The National Foundation-March of Dimes. Sinauer Associates, Inc., Sunderland, Mass.
3. Berne, B. H. 1974. Differing methodology and equation used in quantitating immunoglobulins by radial immunodiffusion: a comparative evaluation of reported and commercial

techniques. Clin. Chem. 20:61–69.

4. Bjerrum, O. J., A. Ingild, H. Løwenstein, and B. Weeke. 1973. Carbamylated antibodies used for quantitation of human IgG: a routine method, p. 145–148. *In* N. H. Axelsen, J. Krøll, and B. Weeke (ed.), A manual of quantitative immunoelectrophoresis. Universitetsforlaget, Oslo.

5. Bjerrum, O. J., A. Ingild, H. Løwenstein, and B. Weeke. 1973. Quantitation of human IgG by rocket immunoelectrophoresis at pH 5 by use of carbamylated antibodies: a routine laboratory method. Clin. Chim. Acta 46:337–393.

6. Clark, H. G. M., and T. Freeman. 1966. A quantitative immunoelectrophoresis method (Laurell electrophoresis). Protides Biol. Fluids, Proc. Colloq. 14:503–509.

7. Fahey, J. L., and E. M. McKelvey. 1965. Quantitative determination of serum immunoglobulins in antibody-agar plates. J. Immunol. 94:84.

8. Heremans, J. P., and P. L. Masson. 1973. Specific analysis of immunoglobulins: techniques and clinical value. Clin. Chem. 19:294–300.

9. Hosty, R. A., M. Hollenbeck, and S. Shane. 1973. Intercomparison of results obtained with five commercial diffusion plates supplied for quantitation of immunoglobulins. Clin. Chem. 19:524–526.

10. Killingsworth, L. M., and J. Savory. 1971. Automated immunochemical procedures for measurement of immunoglobulins IgG, IgA, and IgM in human serum. Clin. Chem. 17:936–940.

11. Larson, C., B. Orenstein, and R. F. Ritchie. 1971. An automated method for quantitation of proteins in body fluids, p. 101–104. *In* Advances in automated analysis, Technicon International Congress, 1970, vol. 1. Thurman Associates, Miami.

12. Laurell, C. B. 1966. Quantitative estimation of proteins by electrophoresis in agarose gel containing antibodies. Anal. Biochem. 15:45–52.

13. Laurell, C. B. 1966. Quantitative estimation of proteins by electrophoresis in antibody-containing agarose gel. Protides Biol. Fluids, Proc. Colloq. 14:499–502.

14. Mancini, G., A. O. Carbonara, and J. F. Heremans. 1965. Immunochemical quantitation of antigens by single radial immunodiffusion. Immunochemistry 2:235.

15. Merrill, D., R. F. Hartley, and H. N. Claman. 1967. A simple, rapid method for quantitation of immunoglobulins in dilute biological fluids. J. Lab. Clin. Med. 69:151–159.

16. Palmer, D. F., and R. Woods. 1972. A procedural guide to the performance of the radial immunodiffusion test and the immunoelectrophoresis test for qualitation and quantitation of immunoglobulins. Immunology series, no. 3. Department of Health, Education and Welfare Publication no. (HSM) 72-8102, Center for Disease Control, Atlanta, Ga.

17. Ritchie, R. F. 1967. A simple, direct and sensitive technique for measurement of specific proteins in dilute solutions. J. Lab. Clin. Med. 70:512–517.

18. Ritzmann, S. E., and J. C. Daniels (ed.). 1975. Serum protein abnormalities: diagnostic and clinical aspects. Little, Brown and Co., Boston.

19. Ritzmann, S. E. (ed.). 1975. ICL scientific methodology. ICL Scientific, Fountain Valley, Calif.

20. Rowe, D., B. Grob, and S. G. Anderson. 1972. An international reference preparation of human immunoglobulins G, A and M—content of immunoglobulins by weight. Bull. WHO 46:67.

21. Steinbuch, M., and R. Audran. 1969. The isolation of IgG from mammalian sera with the aid of caprylic acid. Arch. Biochem. Biophys. 134:279–284.

22. Verbruggen, R. 1975. Quantitative immunoelectrophoretic methods: a literature survey. Clin. Chem. 21:5–43.

23. Weeke, B., and J. P. Thomsen. 1968. A puncher for agar gels. Scand. J. Clin. Lab. Invest. 22:165.

24. U. S. Department of Health, Education and Welfare. 1974. Center for Disease Control, proficiency testing: non-syphilis serology quantitative immunoglobulins, 1973. Public Health Service, Atlanta, Ga.

Chapter 3

Immunoelectrophoresis (Including Zone Electrophoresis)

SHAUL KOCHWA

INTRODUCTION

Principles of electrophoresis were defined in the early 19th century. In 1879, Helmholz suggested the existence of an electrical double layer at the interface of solvent and solid, but it was only in the 1930s that a group of Swedish physicists put the theory into practice and designed the first electrophoretic instruments. Theorell and Tiselius developed apparatus for preparative and analytical electrophoresis in liquid phase. But these instruments were costly, bulky, and difficult to operate, and they required large amounts of sample. The use of electrophoresis in clinical sciences advanced notably when the idea of using a porous support was introduced in the early 1940s (zone electrophoresis). The first supporting medium was paper, and within two decades numerous materials were used to separate practically any charged molecules. Today, the most widely used support matrices are cellulose acetate, starch, acrylamide, agar, and agarose.

Although electrophoresis can achieve separation of molecules that differ in charge, combination with other techniques results in an increased analytical power of this method. Thus, a combination of electrophoresis and the sieving effect of acrylamide gels of different pore size (disc electrophoresis) permits added separation of molecules on the basis of their molecular dimensions. A combination of electrophoresis and immunological reactions (immunoelectrophoresis) allows the identification of different components having similar electrophoretic mobility but dissimilar antigenic determinants. A vast literature covers all aspects of electrophoresis and immunoelectrophoresis, and references 1, 2, 3, and 5 are books recommended for basic reading.

PRINCIPLES OF ELECTROPHORESIS

Electrophoresis is in general any movement of a solid phase with respect to a liquid phase under the influence of an externally applied electrical field.

Electrophoretic mobility *(m)* of a particle or molecule is a physical constant under defined conditions. It is the distance in centimeters traveled by a particle in a unit of time (centimeters/second) per unit of field strength expressed as a voltage drop per cm $\left(\dfrac{V}{cm}\right)$. The dimensions are $m = \dfrac{cm^2}{V\ s}$.

For a particle to move in an electrical field, a certain resistance of the medium has to be overcome (frictional resistance). The frictional resistance in solution obeys Stocke's law, but in gels, in suspensions, or on solid matrix theoretical equations have not yet been developed. Therefore, in general, calculation of a relative electrophoretic mobility allows comparison of materials. Relative mobility is a distance traveled by a molecule or a particle in a unit of time under identical electrical field conditions. When a mixture of particles or molecules having different net charges and sizes is placed in a uniform electric field, the differing molecules move with different velocities, and, as a result, complete or partial separation occurs.

The major application of electrophoresis in clinics is to separate constituents of plasma and other body fluids, and, since the original work of Tiselius and Kabat in 1939, the designations of major components (peaks) observed in human serum have remained unchanged. Today, we discern albumin and α_1, α_2, β, and γ globulins, and we refer to any pathological changes as located in these positions.

The final position and resolution of constituents of a protein mixture after electrophoresis is dependent on the factors dicussed below.

Structure of proteins

Proteins are polymers of amino acids and may be composed of one or more polypeptide chains with or without carbohydrate or lipid attached to them. The building blocks of proteins are amino acids that all have the following basic structure:

$$\begin{array}{c} \quad\quad R_2 \quad O \\ \quad\quad | \quad\quad \| \\ R_1{-}C{-}C{-}OH \\ \quad\quad | \\ \quad\quad HN_2 \end{array}$$

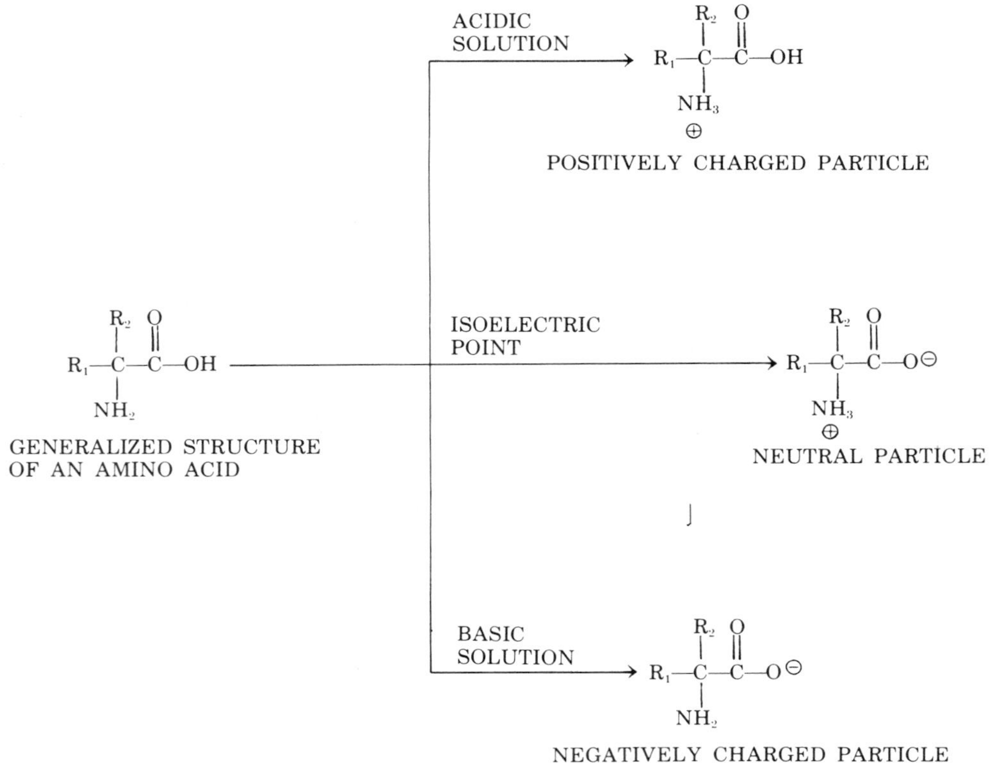

Fig. 1. *Effect of pH on amino acid structure.*

Formation of a peptide bond occurs between the carboxyl group of one amino acid and the amino group of another.

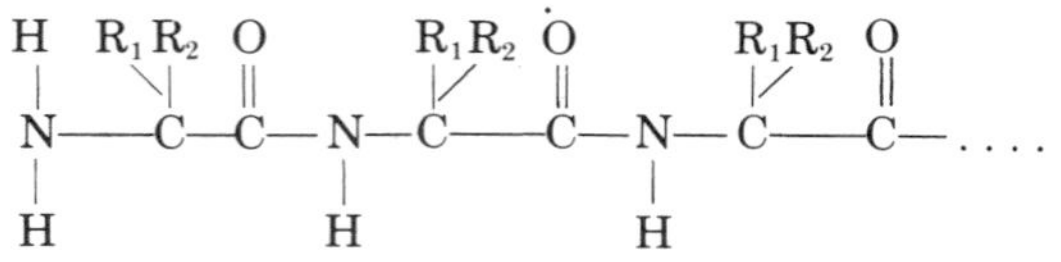

Polypeptide chains may have a length up to several hundred amino acids. Amino acids are amphoteric; i.e., depending on pH they are either positively or negatively charged (Fig. 1).

In a polypeptide chain where only one positive and one negative group are present, total electrical charge is actually determined by side chains (R) of the amino acids in the polypeptide backbone.

Several types of side chains exist: aliphatic apolar (glycine, alanine, valine, leucine, isoleucine, and methionine), heterocyclic and aromatic apolar (proline, threonine, tryptophan, and tyrosine), aliphatic polar (serine, phenylalanine, cysteine, asparagine, and glutamine), and ionizable side chains (aspartic acid, glutamic acid, histidine, lysine, arginine, and neuraminic acid of the carbohydrate moiety). The polar and apolar side chains are responsible primarily for folding and for the three-dimensional structure of the molecule, whereas the ionizable side chains confer on the molecule its electrical charge. Therefore, each protein molecule, depending on pH, behaves as an ampholyte and can exist in three states: positively charged (acidic solution), negatively charged (alkaline solution), and neutral (isoelectric point). At a given pH, the net charge of protein molecules and, therefore, the electrophoretic mobility depend on the content of amino acids with ionizable side chains. At its isoelectric point, the molecule has no electrophoretic mobility and will remain at the point of origin. Electrophoretic mobility thus depends on how far the pH of the buffer is from the pH of the protein's isoelectric point; the bigger this difference, the farther and faster the molecule will move in a constant electrical field. A mixture of proteins, as in serum or plasma, will separate at neutrality: some molecules will move to the positive pole; others will move to the negative;

and some will remain stationary. Proteins usually have minimal solubility at their isoelectric point and may precipitate out of solution. For these reasons, in routine electrophoresis of serum, the pH of the buffer is chosen so that all molecules will be negatively charged (alkaline buffer) and will all move to the positive pole. Under these conditions, the highest mobility will be of prealbumin and albumin and the lowest will be of gamma globulin.

Buffer

As explained in the preceding section, the pH of the buffer used in electrophoresis has to be such that all proteins have the same electrostatic sign.

The suitability of a buffer to be used in electrophoresis is determined by both its concentration and its ionic strength. Concentration is expressed as molarity (M), and the ionic strength (μ) is $\mu = \frac{1}{2}\Sigma Mc^2$, where c is the valence of each ion.

For serum proteins, barbital buffers (a mixture of diethyl barbituric acid and sodium barbital at pH 8.0 to 9.0) are commonly used. Their advantage over other systems such as borate buffers is that they are monovalent, they do not interact or denature proteins to any great extent, and, being large molecules, they migrate slowly and contribute relatively little to the generation of heat.

The main role of buffer is to maintain pH and conduct electricity. Current is carried by ions in solution, and, therefore, the larger the number of buffer ions (high ionic strength), the larger the portion of current that they will carry. But the concentration of buffer can influence the migration pattern of proteins. At high buffer concentrations, the mobility of protein molecules decreases; the sharpness of the protein bands increases, but the amount of heat generated also increases and may cause damage to both the supporting medium and the sample. Reduction in ionic strength will increase protein mobility, broaden the protein band zones, and decrease the amount of heat generated. At very low buffer concentrations, flocculation and partial denaturation of protein may occur. In general, an ionic strength of about 0.05 is used where the adverse result of low concentration of salts is minimal and the electrophoretic mobility and delineation of protein zones is satisfactory.

Electrical field

Ionic concentration of buffer and the nature of the supporting medium both introduce resistance to the flow of an electric current. Ohm's law governs this relationship, $V = RA$ (V = voltage, R = resistance, A = current). The amount of heat (H) generated by a current passing through a medium in a unit of time is $H = \frac{VA}{Q}$, where Q is the mechanical equivalent of heat 4.185×10^7 erg/cal.

Since the resistance of buffer is more or less constant, it follows that an increase in current will cause an increase in voltage and the amount of heat generated. But even at a constant voltage the current will increase during the electrophoretic run because, as heat is generated, solvent evaporates from the supporting medium, concentration of the buffer increases, and resistance to electrical conductance decreases so that more current flows through the system.

To keep generation of heat at a minimum, either a relatively low voltage must be applied or other means of heat dissipation must be used, such as placing the supporting medium on a cooled plate or putting the whole apparatus into a cold room. It is evident that in order to obtain reproducible results either voltage or current must be kept constant. Under constant voltage conditions, current will increase in time and electrophoretic mobility will also increase. Under constant current conditions, voltage will drop in time and electrophoretic mobility will remain almost constant. For all practical purposes, it is not important whether current or voltage is regulated for very short runs, as performed on acetate, cellulose, or agar. However, for runs that take 24 h or longer, a constant voltage is advisable. Such long runs have the disadvantage of broadening the separated bands as a result of diffusion. Determination of the best conditions for electrophoresis is dependent on interrelationships of buffer, electrical conditions, and the time period over which the separation is conducted.

Electroendosmosis and wick flow

Supports used in routine electrophoresis (paper, cellulose acetate, agar, or agarose) all display various degrees of a negative charge when impregnated with alkaline buffer. As a result of this charge, water becomes positively charged. But the bond is not a strong one, and, because the support cannot move, the water molecules move to the negative pole when current is applied. The magnitude of this movement depends on the nature of the support (agar the biggest, agarose the smallest), the nature of the buffer (ionic strength, pH), and the applied potential. As a result of the endosmotic flow, some proteins, although negatively charged, appear to move to the cathode (gamma globulin). This occurs when the velocity of the endosmotic flow is greater than the electrophoretic mobility of the molecule. The endosmotic flow may be counterbalanced by a hydrostatic pressure. If the cathodic buffer vessel is filled with buffer to a higher level than the anodic, the buffer will flow from cathode to anode even without an applied potential and, as a result, will counteract the endosmotic flow when current is applied. The electroendosmotic flow does not affect the electrophoretic mobility, and the separation of protein molecules is not disturbed. The relative mobilities of one protein to the other remain unchanged; only their position relative to point of origin is displaced toward the cathode. Endosmotic flow may be determined by use of an uncharged molecule, e.g., dextran; its position in relation to the origin will indicate the net electroendosmotic flow.

Another consideration related to the flow of the buffer is so-called wick flow. This flow is a result of the evaporation of water from the support because of heat generated by the electric current (see above, Electrical field). The support is connected by wicks with the two reservoirs of buffer and, because of capillary flow, water lost by evaporation is constantly replaced. This replacement is equal from both reservoirs and prevents an increase in the ionic strength of buffer in the support and a subsequent change in conditions of electrophoresis.

Nature the supporting media

It is beyond the scope of this chapter to review the characteristics and applications of supporting media for zone electrophoresis. Two types of such support are available, one where the molecules are separated mainly on the basis of their charge (paper, cellulose acetate, starch, Pevicon), and another where the pore size of the support decreases the electrophoretic mobility of proteins in accordance with their size (gels prepared from starch, agar, agarose, acrylamide, and other polymeric substances). For routine analytical electrophoresis of serum proteins, the most convenient support is cellulose acetate. Its advantages over paper and other support media are numerous. To name just a few: (i) adsorption of proteins is minimal, there is no trailing, and the background after staining is colorless, accentuating the sharpness of bands; (ii) the pore size of the matrix is uniform and the endosmotic flow is low; (iii) very small quantitites of sample are necessary; and (iv) the time of separation is short.

Proteins separated on cellulose acetate membranes can be stained with a variety of dyes, and to facilitate quantitation the membrane can be made transparent. During this clearing process, the porous structure of the membrane collapses, the fiber mesh closes, and a material very similar to cellophane is obtained.

Cellulose acetate membranes are obtained by treating cellulose with acetic anhydride. The resulting polymers are soluble in organic solvents and can be cast in any form, size, and thickness. The microporous membranes are brittle when dry and consist of a three-dimensional mesh containing about 80% dead air space. When saturated with buffer, they regain their strength and provide a conductor for current and an excellent support for separation of proteins. This polymer is insoluble in organic alcohols, benzene, toluene, etc., but will dissolve in glacial acetic acid, chloroform, acetone, etc. The thickness of the membrane used for electrophoresis is about 120 μm with a pore size of 0.4 μm (diameter).

Cellulose acetate membranes are available from several manufacturers, of which the most popular are

Sepraphore III ..	Gelman Instruments
Sartorius Membranes	Brinkman Instruments
Celotate	Millipore Corp.
Oxoid	Oxo Ltd.
Titan III	Helena Laboratories

Each of these manufacturers produces electrophoresis apparatus designed for their special membranes, and at least a dozen other manufacturers of electrophoresis apparatus use membranes made by others. For example, the Beckman microzone electrophoresis system uses cellulose acetate membranes manufactured by Millipore Corp.

Of other supporting media, agar and agarose are widely used in immunoelectrophoresis. They are solid at room temperature in low concentrations, are transparent, and permit rapid separation of proteins, and agarose has a very low endosmotic flow. For preparative purposes, starch, Pevikon, and acrylamide, and, for analytical purposes, starch gel and especially acrylamide gel, are in general use (see reference 5 for further information).

PRINCIPLES OF IMMUNOELECTROPHORESIS

Very few techniques have had as much of an impact on progress in biomedical sciences as the introduction of immunoelectrophoresis by

Grabar and Williams in 1953. This method combines principles of zone electrophoresis with antigen-antibody reactions in gels.

Immunoelectrophoresis is a two-step procedure: in the first step, the mixture of proteins is separated by zone electrophoresis; in the second step, groups of proteins separated by their electrophoretic mobility are analyzed with specific antisera to allow development of arcs of precipitation.

Electrophoresis

Practically any support medium used in zone electrophoresis can be adapted to further use for immunological analysis. However, the most widely used is agar gel. These gels dissolve easily in hot buffer solutions, they are solid at ambient temperatures, even at low agar concentrations they are elastic and homogeneous, their pore size is relatively large so that the diffusion can take place, and they are sufficiently transparent to allow observation of immunological reactions. Furthermore, electrophoresis in agar gel differs little from free electrophoresis in solution because, at the 1% agar commonly used, 99% of the gel consists of buffer. This allows a rapid separation of serum into albumin and α_1, α_2, β, and γ globulins, with minimal diffusion. Because of endosmotic flow, β globulins seem not to move and are found near the point of application.

Immunological reactions

After electrophoresis, immunological identification of separated components is performed in the same gel. For this purpose, a long narrow trough is cut in the agar gel parallel to the direction of electrophoretic separation at an appropriate distance from the application point. This trough is filled with antibody solution. As in all other types of immunological reaction in gels, antigens and antibodies diffuse toward each other. Because of differences in diffusion patterns (antibodies diffuse as a linear front from the trough, whereas antigens diffuse radially from electrophoretically separated foci), the precipitation lines appear as ellipsoid arcs. Because the mixture of antigens is applied into a well in the agar, after electrophoretic separation each antigen focus preserves the shape of the application well and then diffuses radially. As a result, the position of the equivalence zone, where precipitation is visible, will depend on the concentration of both antigen and antibody. When the concentration of antigen is too high, precipitation may occur in the antibody trough, and only the ends of the arc, where the concentration of antigen is lower, will be visible. When the concentration of antigen is very

low, no visible precipitation will be formed. The position of the precipitin arc in respect to the antibody trough can indicate the antigen concentration if the characteristics and potency of the antiserum used are known.

The procedure for immunoelectrophoresis is illustrated in Fig. 2. The three steps are (i) electrophoresis of human serum sample in agar or agarose, (ii) removal of gel to create trough and addition of antiserum, and (iii) development of precipitation arcs.

The minimal number of recognizable protein components in a mixture is represented by the number of arcs, and this depends on the presence of appropriate antibodies. There is very little probability that two proteins will simultaneously (i) have the same electrophoretic mobility, (ii) have the same molecular dimensions that govern diffusion, and (iii) be subject to identical respective antibody concentrations to produce overlapping equivalence zones with a single precipitin line. Any immunoelectrophoretic analysis is dependent primarily on having appropriate antibodies of correct concentration.

The shape of the precipitin arc reflects the electrophoretic homogeneity of the protein. For example, albumin is a very homogeneous protein and on immunoelectrophoresis forms a very narrow, heavy precipitin line. On the other hand, gamma globulin forms a precipitin line that extends from the γ to α_2 region. However, if a homogeneous, monoclonal gamma globulin protein is present, its precipitation

1. ELECTROPHORESIS OF SAMPLE IN AGAR

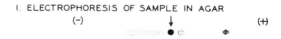

2. PREPARE TROUGH FOR ANTIBODY DIFFUSION

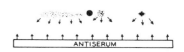

3. DEVELOPMENT OF PRECIPITATION LINES

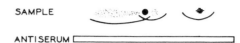

FIG. 2. *Immunoelectrophoresis procedure. Three major steps in serum analysis are illustrated. (1) Serum sample is added to small well in agar plate and electrophoresis is performed to separate the major serum components. (2) Trough is cut in agar and antiserum is added to fill trough. The human serum components (antigens) in the central agar and the antibodies in the trough diffuse through the agar toward each other. (3) Precipitation arcs become visible where antigen-antibody complexes indicate the presence of individual serum proteins (IgG, etc.).*

characteristics will be similar to those of albumin.

In immunoelectrophoretic analysis both specificity and source of antibody require consideration. Equine antibodies produce soluble complexes in the presence of either antigen or antibody excess, whereas most antibodies from other animals do this only with antigen excess. It is a good practice to test each new antibody batch in several dilutions with various concentrations of antigens to define optimal working concentrations of reactants.

In general, two types of antibodies are sought: monospecific, containing antibodies to one protein, one antigenic determinant, or one portion of a molecule (e.g., Fc portion of gamma globulins), or polyvalent, containing a mixture of antibodies to multiple antigens (e.g., anti-whole human serum, anti-immunoglobulin serum). When immunoelectrophoretic analysis is used to evaluate purification of an antigen, the antibodies used should be prepared against and react with all antigens in the initial mixture. This must be followed by antibodies prepared against partially purified fractions, always keeping in mind the fact that this method will detect only components against which antibody was formed.

ANALYTICAL ZONE ELECTROPHORESIS ON CELLULOSE ACETATE

The following description is limited to the use of the Microzone Electrophoresis System manufactured by Beckman Industries Inc., Fullerton, Calif. However, the procedure is valid in general for any other manufactured or self-made instrument. The following description follows recommendations of the manufacturers, with changes resulting from experience in my laboratory.

Equipment

Microzone electrophoresis cell, power supply, sample applicator, squeegee, electrophoresis membranes, microzone densitometer.

Reagents

Veronal buffer, pH 8.6, $\mu = 0.075$ (2.76 g of diethyl barbituric acid and 15.40 g of sodium diethyl barbiturate in 1 liter of water), can be obtained as B-2 buffer from Beckman in packages sufficient for 1 liter of $\mu = 0.075$ or for 1.5 liters of $\mu = 0.05$ solution. It dissolves in cold water in several hours or at about 80 C in 0.5 h with constant stirring. Use a volumetric flask for preparation. Store at 4 C but bring to room temperature before use.

Fixative dye solution consists of 0.2% Ponceau-S stain solution (wt/vol), 3% trichloroacetic acid (wt/vol), and 3% sulfosalicylic acid (wt/vol). This can be obtained from Beckman Instruments in concentrated form to be diluted in distilled water to 250 ml. Stored in a closed bottle, it can be reused many times, adding unused solution as required.

Rinse solution: 5% glacial acetic acid (wt/vol) in distilled water.

Alcohol dehydration solution: 95% ethyl alcohol.

Clearing solution: 75 ml of 95% ethyl alcohol mixed with 25 ml of glacial acetic acid. (Manufacturers suggestion: 30% reagent grade cyclohexanol in denatured alcohol.) Prepare fresh before use.

Parafilm is supplied in rolls by American Can Co., Neenah, Wis. Prepare sheets 4 × 7 inches (10 × 17.8 cm).

Procedure

Sample preparation. Any solution of proteins can be analyzed, but the optimal concentration to be tested will vary depending on the number of different proteins to be discerned and on their electrophoretic and staining characteristics. In general, mixtures of proteins should be between 3 and 8 g/100 ml, and single components can be visualized at about 0.5 g/100 ml. Therefore, it is necessary, especially when performing routine serum analysis, to determine first the protein concentration and, whenever total protein concentration is higher than 11 g/100 ml, to dilute the sample 1:2 in 0.9% NaCl solution. After concentration of solutions of proteins (e.g., body fluids, fractions obtained from separation procedures), they must be dialyzed to remove excess salt. Blood obtained from patients must be completely clotted before separated serum can be tested. Heparin may change the electrophoretic mobility of many proteins, especially lipoproteins.

Sample application.

1. Fill six plastic trays (supplied by Beckman with the Microzone electrophoresis kit) with 100 ml of the following solutions: 1, buffer; 2, fixative dye; 3 and 4, rinse (5% acetic acid); 5, dehydration (95% ethyl alcohol), and 6, clearing solution with an immersed $2^{3}/_{8} \times 6^{3}/_{16}$ inch (6 × 15.7 cm) clean glass plate.

2. To fill up the Microzone cells with buffer, remove the upper lid, the cover, and the bridge assembly, and pour enough buffer to each half of the cell so that the levels on either side are at the lower line (total about 230 ml). Tilt the cell forward for few seconds (electrode terminals facing the operator) until the buffer flows over the center divider. The buffer level on both sides should be equal and within the two buffer

lines engraved on the cell. When necessary, add more buffer and repeat the leveling step. Close the cell.

3. Cellulose acetate membrane is removed by forceps from the package. *Never during the whole operation touch the membrane with fingers, because this can produce irregular patterns.* The membrane is floated on the buffer in tray 1 and saturated with buffer from beneath. After the membrane is uniformly wet, it is submerged by agitating the tray sidewise. If during saturation dry spots are present (areas where the buffer did not penetrate because of trapped air), leave the membrane floating on the buffer for additional time to permit the trapped air to escape; otherwise, discard the membrane.

4. After saturation, remove the membrane quickly from the tray with forceps, grasping by one edge, and blot gently between two pieces of Whatman 3 MM paper or two paper towels. Do not blot dry, or white spots will appear and cause irregular patterns, but too little blotting will leave the membrane wet and result in smeared patterns. Do not leave the membrane on the blotter for a long time (10 to 20 s is sufficient); work fast.

5. Remove the bridge assembly from the electrophoresis cell, lift the membrane guides, take the blotted membrane, and place the reference hole end of the membrane on the movable membrane mount (the membrane has, in addition to two rows of eight holes, one additional hole that serves as a marker). Push the movable mount to the extreme right, to permit engagement of the second set of holes on the stationary mount. Release the movable mount, return the membrane guides to the horizontal position, and secure them with screws. The membrane is now under slight tension, and the sides are straight down. If the membrane is too loose or sags, the pattern will be irregular because the sample will not be evenly applied; on the other hand, too much tension may tear the membrane. Place the bridge assembly with the membrane into the cell with the reference hole of the membrane in the left lower corner (to indicate either sample no. 1 or no. 8). Check that both ends of the membrane are submerged in the buffer. Replace the cover and the upper lid, and permit the membrane to equilibrate for at least 2 min. Connect the socket from the power supply to the cell and make the proper connection to determine the position of the anode (+) and the direction of the electrophoretic migration. If the Beckman Duostat power supply is used, the red plug indicates that the anode will be to the right, and the black plug indicates that the anode will be to the left.

6. While the membrane is equilibrating, place on a 4 × 7 inch Parafilm sheet drops of specimens to undergo electrophoresis. A small pea-size drop covered with a small plastic or glass beaker to prevent excessive evaporation is required. It is good practice to put the Parafilm sheet over a paper on which the names of patients or numbers of samples are marked in the spots where the sample is to be applied. The protein concentration of the specimen is also required to determine the time of application.

7. The application of the sample to the membrane must be very rapid. The applicator supplied by Beckman Instruments has two buttons, a white one that releases the tip and a red one that retracts it. The tip has two wires that must be parallel when viewed from the top and slightly curved or flat when viewed from the side. Any imperfection in the tip will result in a defective pattern. Before application, release the tip, rinse with distilled water, and remove excess water by touching the tip to adsorbent tissue. Without breaking the surface of the sample drop on the Parafilm, pick up a specimen with the tip of the applicator. Blot the tip by touching adsorbent tissue, and repeat the step of sample pick-up. This double procedure will prevent any possible dilution of the sample by traces of rinse water that may be present on the applicator tip. Press the red button to retract the pen. Position the rider of the applicator in the last groove on the right of the cover of the cell; insert the strip selection pin on the front of the applicator into the hole opposite to the selected number. Under these conditions the application tip will be in the center of the membrane, and the electrophoretic separation can be performed in either direction. Depress the white button so that the tip will fall and touch the membrane. Simultaneously start a stop watch. Time of application depends on the concentration of proteins in the solution. For normal serum concentrations 3 to 5 s are sufficient (3 s for 8 to 9 g/100 ml, 4 s for 7 to 8 g/100 ml, and 5 s for 6 to 7 g/100 ml). For lower protein concentrations, up to 10 s can be used, and if necessary double application can be made. After the desired time has elapsed, press the red button, retract the pen, rinse the tip, and repeat the procedure of application, as above, for the next sample. A total of eight samples can be applied on one membrane. After all samples have been applied, replace the lid of the electrophoretic cells and turn on the power supply.

Electrophoresis and staining.

1. Use the constant voltage setting on the power supply at 250 V. Time the run for 18 min. During this period of time, the initial current of

4 to 6 mA will increase to 6 to 8 mA. The buffer can be reused up to eight times, provided that the direction of the current is reversed for each run. Before changing buffer, the cell must be thoroughly cleaned of salt deposits.

2. At the end of the run, turn off the power, disconnect the plugs, remove the upper lid and cover, lift the bridge with the membrane, blot the buffer-saturated ends of the membrane, lift both hinges, remove the membrane with a pair of forceps, and float it on the fixative dye solution in tray 2. After saturation, submerge by agitation and stain for at least 8 min. Shorter staining time will result in spuriously low albumin values, whereas longer staining time has little effect on the final result.

Transfer the membrane successively into trays 3 and 4 for 4 min each. The time of destaining is not critical and can be extended up to 2 h. After use, discard the solution from tray 3, replace it with fresh solution, and use this in the next run as tray 4. Move tray 4, previously used as a second destainer, to position 3. In this manner, the final destaining is always done in fresh solution. The destaining is followed by an alcohol rinse (tray 5) for exactly 1 min to dehydrate the membrane. Finally, the membrane is placed on the glass plate immersed in clearing solution (tray 6) for exactly 1 min. With a pair of forceps in each hand remove the plate with the membrane from the clearing solution, permit the fluid to drain at an angle for a few seconds, and draw the squeegee from top to bottom with one motion to remove excess clearing solution.

Clearing and alcohol rinsing solutions should be prepared daily and not used for longer than 6 h. The longer the clearing solution stands, the more stretched the membrane becomes, causing distortion of the pattern.

3. The glass plate with the membrane is placed into an incubator at 37 C for 25 min. An oven at 100 C can be used for a shorter time. There is no odor of clearing solution after adequate incubation of the clear film. After the glass plate has cooled to room temperature, the film is loosened at one corner with a scalpel, and an open membrane holder is slid under the membrane so that the pattern of separated fractions is in the center. Protruding membrane edges should be trimmed.

4. The holder is a transparent, firm, plastic envelope that fits into the densitometers and protects the fragile membrane. Scan each pattern in a Beckman Microzone densitometer at 520 mm. For calculation of results, align the densitometer tracings to the center of albumin fractions and, for each of a membrane's separate samples, use the same distances to demonstrate the α_1, α_2, β, and γ electrophoretic frac-

tion. This will allow localization of abnormalities. Count the integrator units for each specimen and calculate the relative (%) and absolute (g/100 ml) concentrations, for the latter using total protein concentration obtained by any method that is in use in the laboratory (Auto-Analyzer, Refractometry, VV adsorption, etc.).

PREPARATIVE ZONE ELECTROPHORESIS

Zone electrophoresis on starch is a general method for preparative separation of relatively large samples of proteins, especially of monoclonal immunoglobulins (Ig's). The following description is for an instrument manufactured by Buchler Instruments, Fort Lee, N.J., but any system consisting of two buffer vessels and a covered tray can be used.

Equipment

Migrating chamber (Buchler) or two separate buffer vessels with platinum electrodes, starch tray, power supply (500 V, 100 mA), large metal spoon, large metal spatula, Büchner fritted-glass funnels (coarse, about 30-ml volume), 250-ml filter flasks, source of vacuum.

Reagents

Potato starch: Purified powder (not hydrolyzed), obtainable from Fisher Scientific Co., Fair Lawn, N.J., can be used without any further purification. If the purity of the starch preparation is not known, wash the powder several times with distilled water, each time permitting the starch to settle. This removes small particles and electrolytes present in the preparation.

Pevikon C-870 can be obtained from Mercer Chemical Co., New York, N.Y. It should be washed several times with distilled water to reduce the amount of fine material.

Barbital buffer, pH 8.8 (stock solution), 41.2 g of sodium barbital, and 7.36 g of barbituric acid derivative in 2 liters of distilled water. Dissolve separately. Warm barbituric acid derivative in about 1,000 ml of distilled water in a water bath at ~80 C until it goes into solution. Dissolve sodium barbital in about 500 ml of distilled water at room temperature. Mix both solutions and fill up to 2 liters. For use, dilute one part of buffer with three parts of distilled water.

Indicator: Bromophenol blue can be obtained from any reagent supply company. Add about 1 mg of the dye to the sample as a marker for albumin. The progress of electrophoretic separation can be observed by noting the progress of the blue line of albumin.

Staining solution: 1% bromophenol blue in

HgCl₂-saturated 95% ethanol. Mercuric chloride must be in excess, and a few crystals will be present on the bottom of the flask. Store in a dark bottle.

Decolorizing solution: Methanol-acetic acid-distilled water, 45:10:45.

Procedure

Preparation of block. Prepare a slurry of about 500 g of potato starch or 850 g of Pevikon and 400 ml of diluted buffer. Add the buffer slowly, mixing with a metal spoon until a smooth, thick paste is formed. Pour the slurry into the tray in which, on each end, a 4-inch wick of Whatman 3 MM filter paper was placed so that about 1 inch is on the bottom of the tray. After the starch is poured, excess buffer is removed by placing paper towels on the ends of the trays on top of two filter-paper wicks until a firm, but damp, potato starch mass is left in the tray. Allow about 1 h for this procedure.

Make slits in the starch block with a metal spatula. These should be located about one-third of the distance between the cathode and the anode. About 1 ml of specimen can be applied per 1 cm of slit on a starch block 1.5 cm thick. The number of slits made depends on the number of samples to be separated. Leave a 2-cm distance from the edges of the starch. To prevent overlap, leave at least 2 cm between samples.

Selection of block thickness represents a compromise between size of sample to be fractionated and the degree of separation needed. Thicker blocks will accept larger samples but will also have a greater temperature gradient between center and surface, which will contribute to greater diffusion of each component and reduce the sharpness of electrophoretic resolution.

Sample application. Slowly apply the specimens, with added bromophenol blue, to allow good adsorption. For uniform application, a paste can be made of sample with a small amount of starch. For small volumes, Whatman 3 MM filter paper the size of the slit can be saturated with the sample and inserted into the slit. After any application, press with a metal spatula on the starch block next to the slit to close the gap and achieve electrical continuity.

Electrophoresis. Place the tray in the electrophoretic chamber, and immerse the filter-paper wicks in the buffer chambers filled with diluted buffer. The cathode is always nearer to the application slit (short part of the block). Use constant voltage, 10 to 12 V per cm of block. The current (mA) will depend on the width and the thickness of the starch block. The separation must be performed for 16 to 48 h at 4 C

(either in a cold room or on a cooling plate equipped with a circulation of alcohol at 0 to 2 C). The length of the electrophoresis time is determined by observation of the position of the blue line albumin and by the degree of separation required.

Identification of position for elution of protein fractions. Cut 5-mm wide strips of Whatman no. 1 filter paper, each the length of the starch block. Place these strips on the starch block in the direction of the electrophoretic separation. Separate the strips by 4 to 5 cm for a large sample, or use one per small sample. Mark the position of the origin on each strip. Press gently on the strip and permit it to absorb buffer with dissolved proteins from the block. Remove each strip and immerse in staining solution. Stain for about 5 min, rinse with distilled water, and destain in decolorizing solution. Locate the position of protein fractions in the starch block from the stained bands on the paper strips, and cut out starch block sections containing each desired protein.

Fractions obtained by block electrophoresis are valuable for further characterization of Ig components. Chemical typing of Ig's and their subtypes is possible with these fractions (4).

Elution of proteins. Transfer each starch fraction into a fritted-glass funnel and press with the flat top of a glass stopper. Any buffer or salt solution in which the protein is soluble can be added for elution; use a volume equal to about 60% of the volume of the starch fraction. Connect the funnel to vacuum and separate the eluant. Wash once with a small additional quantity of the same solvent. Under these conditions, about 95% of proteins will be separated from the starch. Centrifuge the eluant to remove starch particles, dialyze against distilled water, and lyophilize. If small samples for identification are needed, the starch can be centrifuged and washed with saline.

IMMUNOELECTROPHORESIS

Scheidigger's microimmunoelectrophoresis technique on microscope slides is suitable for clinical work. The following description is limited to the use of the immunoelectrophoretic equipment obtainable as a kit from Gelman Instrument Co., Ann Arbor, Mich. However, the procedures described are valid for any other immunoelectrophoretic set-up, including self-made instruments.

Equipment

The power supply and the electrophoretic chamber can be obtained commercially or adapted from available equipment. The requirement is that the two buffer containers will be $10^1/_2$ inches (26.7 cm) apart to accommodate $10^3/_4$-inch (27.3-cm) immuno-frames, and that the frames be confined during electrophoresis in a limited air space to reduce evaporation.

The equipment supplied in the Gelman immunoelectrophoresis kit consists of punch set, leveling table, plastic immuno-frames each holding six microscopic slides, metal frame holders each holding three frames, gel knife, suction needles, and polystyrene tanks for storage, incubation, staining, and rinsing of immuno-frames each accommodating one frame holder.

Reagents

Buffer: 5.778 g of tris(hydroxymethyl)aminomethane, 2.466 g of barbituric acid derivative, and 9.756 g of sodium barbital, dissolved in 1 liter of distilled water. This buffer, pH = 8.8, $\mu = 0.06$, is supplied by Gelman as High Resolution Buffer in packages sufficient for 1 liter of solution.

Merthiolate: Eli Lilly & Co., Indianapolis, Ind. Prepare a 1% solution in distilled water.

Agar and agarose powder: Several purified agar powder preparations are available for use without further purification (Noble agar, Difco Laboratories, Detroit, Mich.; Rein Agar, Behring Werke, Marburg Lahn, Germany). Agarose is available from Mann Research Laboratories, New York, N.Y., Bio-Rad Laboratories, Richmond, Calif., Pharmacia Fine Chemicals, Uppsala, Sweden, and others.

Other sources of agar, in powder or in fibers, should be purified to remove electrolytes. For this purpose, agar is washed in distilled water and then suspended in acetone. The powder is dried after the acetone is removed.

Agar or agarose gel: Disperse 10 g of purified agar or agarose powder in 1 liter of dilute high-resolution buffer (500 ml of high-resolution buffer + 500 ml of distilled water). This buffer has $\mu = 0.03$. Heat the suspension with constant stirring, either in a boiling-water bath or on a free flame without bringing the suspension to boiling, until a clear solution is obtained. The heating time is not critical when distilled water is used for dissolving the agar and after melting an equal volume of undiluted buffer warmed to 56 C is added. Add 10 ml of 1% Merthiolate, distribute in 10-ml portions in tubes, seal with Parafilm, and store refrigerated until use. When purified agar powder is not available, prepare a 4 to 6% agar gel by dissolving the agar at 100 C in distilled water. Pour the solution into a flat tray and, after solidification, cut out small 1-cm^3 cubes; wash in several changes of distilled water. Dry a

small volume of agar cubes to constant weight at 110 C. Dissolve the remaining agar gel cubes in enough distilled water to make a 2% solution. Add an equal volume of high-resolution buffer. This will produce 1% agar, $\mu = 0.03$.

Adhesive agar: Dissolve 0.1 g of agar and 0.05 ml of glycerol in 100 ml of distilled water in a boiling-water bath. Store 5-ml portions refrigerated until use.

Rinsing solution: Methyl alcohol-glacial acetic acid-distilled water, 45:10:45.

Staining solution: Dissolve 9 g of Amido Black 10 B (can be obtained from many laboratory supply companies) in 1,500 ml of rinsing solution. Filter before use.

Antisera: Polyvalent and monovalent antibodies can be obtained from many companies. To name just a few:

Behring Werke, Marburg Lahn, Germany
Cappel Laboratories, Downingtown, Pa.
Hyland Laboratories, Costa Mesa, Calif.
Kalestad Laboratories, Inc., Minneapolis, Minn.
Kent Laboratories, Vancouver, B.C., Canada
Meloy Laboratories, Springfield, Va.
Miles Laboratories, Elkart, Ind.

Some of the companies label their product with antibody content. However, each batch should be checked separately against appropriate antigen to determine suitability and concentration at which the antiserum should be used. Antibodies especially to light chains must be carefully selected. In many cases these antibodies are prepared against Bence Jones proteins and react poorly with the intact Ig molecule. The antibody content of these antisera, especially anti-λ, is often low and formation of a visible precipitin arc may be prevented by antigen excess.

Procedure

Preparation of slides. Clear glass microscope slides, 75 mm × 25 mm, are numbered by engraving with a diamond pencil on the top and the bottom of one side. Coat each slide with a thin layer of adhesive agar, using a wooden applicator stick or small paint brush for application. The adhesive agar, when dry, facilitates firm adherence of agar gel to the glass slide and prevents the sample from dissipating between the agar gel and glass surface.

Place coated glass slides in an immuno-frame (six per frame), and place the frame on the leveling table so that the slides will be horizontal. Melt agar or agarose and keep it above 60 C. A Temp-block from Lab Line Instruments, Melrose Park, Ill., can be used for individual test tubes. With a capillary pipette, apply a small quantity of agar around the edges of the slide so that the slide will be sealed to the frame to prevent seepage. Melted agar is then evenly distributed over the slides from a 10-ml pipette that was rinsed several times with hot agar solution. Use 12 to 13 ml of melted agar per half of a frame (three slides). The agar surface after solidification must be smooth and free from air bubbles and agar lumps, and the overall depth of agar on a slide must be uniform. Cover the leveling table and leave the frames to set for 15 to 20 min. Prepare a humidity chamber by placing several layers of Whatman 3 MM filter paper on the bottom of a polystyrene tank. Saturate the paper with water. Insert the immuno-frames into a frame holder, and transfer the holder into the tank until time for use.

Specimen application. Fill the chambers of the electrophoresis apparatus with high-resolution buffer, take out the immuno-frames, and, with a Gelman gel punch, cut the sample wells and the antibody trough in each slide. The arrangement most widely used for serum analyses is to apply two specimens (two unknown or one unknown and one known) to a slide and use one antibody trough between. The trough is 1 mm wide, and distance between the trough and the sample is 5 mm. The sample well is 1.5 mm in diameter and is placed in the center of the slide. This arrangement permits analysis of two specimens with six antisera on a single frame. The most commonly used combination of antibodies is anti-whole human serum, anti-IgG, anti-IgA, anti-IgM, anti-κ, and anti-λ. For special purposes, the gel cutter can provide several other patterns, such as two antibody troughs with one or three samples, different distances between antigen and antibody, and others.

After the sample well and the antibody trough have been punched on all six slides, the plug of each sample well is sucked out with a suction needle, and about 3 μliters of a sample (in case of serum, dilute 1:2 with saline) is applied with a microsyringe.

Immunoelectrophoresis. The immuno-frames are placed into the electrophoresis chamber that accommodates up to three frames and is connected with buffer reservoirs with Whatman 3 MM filter paper wicks that have been saturated with buffer (Gelman microporous wicks are supplied precut to size 1 × 2.5 inches). The chamber is covered, and the power supply is connected. Use 250 V constant voltage. The current at the beginning is about 6 mA per frame and increases during the 75-min run to about 8 to 9 mA per frame. Do not use more than 11 mA per frame. After the zone electrophoresis in agar or agarose is completed,

the immuno-frames are taken out from the chamber, the agar is removed from the prepunched antibody trough with the gel knife, and the trough is filled with about 0.08 ml of antibody. The immuno-frames are inserted into the frame holder and returned to the humidity chamber for incubation at room temperature. Precipitin arcs start to be visible after 6 to 8 h, and the reaction is completed after 24 h. At this time, with diffuse transmitted light, a picture can be taken for records. The immuno-frames in a slide holder are now transferred to a polystyrene tank filled with saline. Overnight, all proteins not precipitated by antibodies will diffuse from the agar. The saline is now replaced for 2 h with distilled water to allow removal of salt. After this washing, each half of an immuno-frame is covered by a strip of Whatman no. 1 filter paper, 3 cm × 29 cm, which has been moistened with water, and placed in incubator at 37 C for overnight drying.

The dry slides are moistened with tap water and the filter paper is removed. The slide surface is washed with tap water, returned to its frame holder, stained in a tank for 5 min, washed under tap water, and destained in three changes of rinsing solution. The stain can be reused many times; the rinsing solution can be decolorized by filtering through charcoal on filter paper and reused.

The destained slides can be photographed on a light box and analyzed by inspection. These slides can be preserved for 1 to 2 years.

ANALYSIS OF BODY FLUIDS

Body fluids (urine; cerebrospinal, synovial, seminal, and amniotic fluids; peritoneal and pleural exudates; milk and colostrum; lymph; and others) have all been studied by immunoelectrophoresis. Many serum proteins are present in varying quantities and, when concentrated, can be readily identified.

More information is often obtained when specimens are studied without concentration. For example, in unconcentrated normal urine only traces of albumin will be detected on immunoelectrophoresis, and any increase in other serum proteins, especially excessive excretion of light chains, will be easily discerned. Under certain conditions, however, concentration of urine is necessary. When myeloma patients that excrete Bence Jones protein are followed during chemotherapy, it is important to know, in addition to the total protein excretion, whether the ratio of albumin to Bence Jones protein changes. This can be determined after concentrated urine is analyzed by zone electrophoresis on cellulose acetate membranes.

In normal cerebrospinal fluid, only an albumin precipitin line is seen on immunoelectrophoresis; appearance of an IgG precipitin arc indicates increased Ig.

IDENTIFICATION OF PRECIPITIN LINES

Antigens in mixtures can be identified with monospecific antisera. When only multivalent antibodies are available, an individual precipitin line can be identified by electrophoresis of the sample in the center of the slide and between two parallel troughs. After electrophoresis, one trough is filled with multivalent antibody and the other, with purified marker antigen (6). With incubation for 24 h, the antigen from the trough diffuses in a linear front, and in absence of the antigen in the sample a straight line of precipitation will be formed at the equivalence zone between the troughs. However, if the sample subjected to electrophoresis contains a similar antigen, there will be at a certain point (depending on its electrophoretic mobility) a focus of this antigen. At this point, the total concentration of antigen will be higher than at other points on the line of precipitation, giving the appearance of an arc with two long "whiskers" parallel to the antibody well. By this method, antigen at very low concentration can be augmented and identified even in an otherwise negative specimen.

Precipitin lines parallel to the antibody trough may be artifacts under certain conditions. Such a line may appear when two antibody troughs contain antibodies of different specificity and one of these antibodies was rendered specific by absorption with a soluble antigen that will react with antibody in the second trough. Solid-phase adsorption of antisera will prevent this artifact.

EVALUATION OF PATTERNS

1. Zone electrophoresis on a cellulose acetate membrane will usually indicate an abnormal pattern of serum proteins. A narrow, deeply stained band anywhere from the α_2 to γ region reflects an increase in protein of restricted mobility. Very light stain in the γ region indicates hypogammaglobulinemia, whereas heavy diffuse staining of the region indicates hypergammaglobulinemia. Albumin is usually the fastest and heaviest stained region.

2. Immunoelectrophoresis is used to characterize abnormalities, but it is advisable for all samples because an abnormality not evident from zone electrophoresis may be found. This is especially true for small monoclonal Ig peaks which can be obscured by other proteins that

migrate similarly. In hypogammaglobulinemia, light chains may be found only by immunoelectrophoresis.

Six slides allow use of anti-whole human serum, anti-IgG, anti-IgA, anti-IgM, anti-κ, and anti-λ, so that most of the abnormalities in Ig's will be recognized in the first run. This arrangement of reagents identifies heavy chains (γ, α, μ) and light chains (κ, λ), and the position of the arc of the monoclonal protein in respect to the origin must be identical for appropriate slides.

In some cases of monoclonal (restricted mobility) Ig, two arcs of precipitation of different electrophoretic mobility are found on tests with appropriate anti-light-chain serum, whereas only one is present with anti-heavy-chain serum. Such a finding indicates the presence of free light chains in addition to intact molecules of Ig's.

3. In many instances (especially with IgA and IgM proteins), the reaction with anti-light-chain antibodies is negative. In most of these cases, the quaternary structure of the molecule obscures the light-chain antigenic determinants and does not permit light chains to react with antibody. In such cases, reduction (10 μliters of 2-mercaptoethanol per 1 ml of serum) without alkylation is sufficient to ·induce changes in these molecules that will allow a reaction to take place and light chains to be identified.

4. In certain diseases, IgM monoclonal protein is found in monomeric form (7S IgM). On immunoelectrophoresis, the appearance of the arc resembles IgG myeloma protein, rather than IgM, and no change in the shape of the arc is found after treatment with 2-mercaptoethanol.

5. Positive euglobulin test (insolubility of proteins in low ionic strength solutions) may pose a problem on zone and immunoelectrophoretic analysis. The low ionic strength concentration of buffer in the supporting medium may cause precipitation around the application well. As a result, distorted patterns can be produced and, especially for IgM, a precipitation line may not be formed. A partial remedy for this problem is to dilute serum 1:2 in 4% NaCl to increase the ionic strength of the sample and prevent local precipitation of euglobulin.

6. Cryoprecipitation is a relatively common (5 to 7%) feature of monoclonal proteins and, depending on the individual proteins, the transition temperature may vary. It is important to allow the agar gel to equilibrate at room temperature before application of the sample. When current is applied, the temperature of

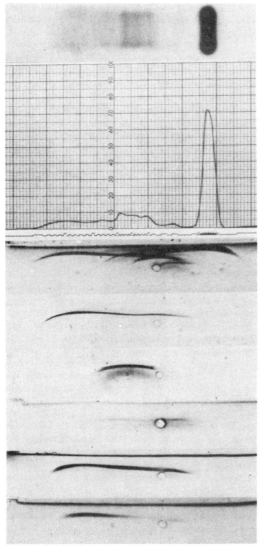

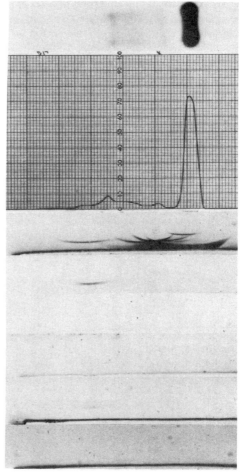

Fig. 4. *Hypogammaglobulinemic serum. Note weak reaction with anti-IgG and practical absence of IgA and IgM. See Fig. 3 for details.*

Fig. 3. *Normal human serum. Figures 3–10 show representative examples of electrophoretic and immunoelectrophoretic patterns of human serum and urine (anode to the right). The order of antibodies used in the trough of all immunoelectrophoretic patterns is, from the bottom, anti-lambda, anti-kappa, anti-IgM, anti-IgA, anti-IgG, and anti-whole human serum. In Fig. 3–6 and 8, the cellulose acetate picture is positioned on top to coincide with both its analytrol tracing (second from top) and immunoelectrophoretic patterns. Two antigens are seen in the paired immunoelectrophoretic pictures of Fig. 7, 9, and 10 where cellulose acetate pictures (top) and their analytrol tracing (just beneath) are positioned to the right. In Fig. 7 and 10 both electrophoretic and immunoelectrophoretic pictures are paired to show urine on top and serum immediately below. In Fig. 9, immuno-*

the gel rises so that normal patterns can be obtained.

7. Specimens of sera containing mixed cryoglobulins (in general, complexes of IgM and IgG with or without the C1q component of the complement) give a characteristic immunoelectropherogram. A small precipitin arc is found at the application well, and this has the same appearance with anti-IgG, anti-IgM, and anti-light-chain sera. Not all of IgG and IgM is in complex form, and individual antibodies will produce normal-appearing arcs in appropriate positions as well.

electrophoresis pairs show mercaptoethanol-treated serum above and untreated serum below.

INTERPRETATION OF RESULTS

No single method is adequate for the diagnosis of protein abnormalities. Correlation of results of zone electrophoresis, immunoelectrophoresis, and protein concentration represents a sound approach for the analysis of serum and body fluid proteins.

It is impossible in this short chapter to review the vast biochemical and clinical data that have accumulated in the past quarter century, but several guidelines for interpretation will be

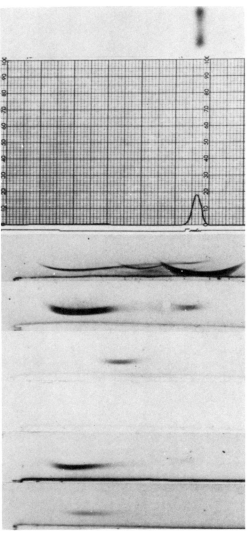

FIG. 6. *Urine, generalized proteinuria. Many more proteins are found on immunoelectrophoresis than on cellulose acetate electrophoresis. See Fig. 3 for details.*

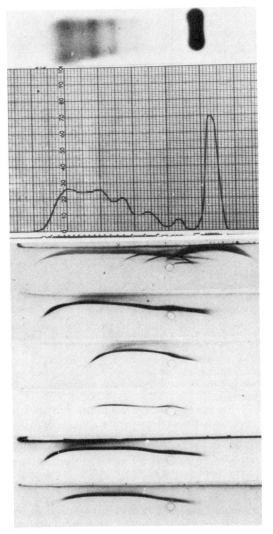

FIG. 5. *Hypergammaglobulinemic serum. Note diffuse increase in all Ig's of both light-chain types. See Fig. 3 for details.*

provided, especially those related to abnormalities of Ig's.

Inherited deficiencies in human proteins can be detected by immunoelectrophoresis if the antibody is present and the antigen is in a concentration sufficient to produce a precipitation arc. Genetically determined absence of albumin, haptoglobin, transferrin, low- and high-density lipoproteins, ceruloplasmin, IgA, all Ig's, and fibrinogen can be easily determined by immunoelectrophoresis with the use

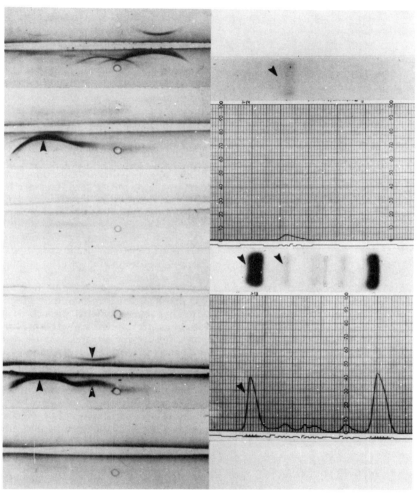

FIG. 7. *IgG, kappa myeloma with kappa Bence Jones proteinuria. Note both myeloma protein and light chains in serum (arrow) and Bence Jones protein of identical mobility in the urine (arrow). See Fig. 3 for details.*

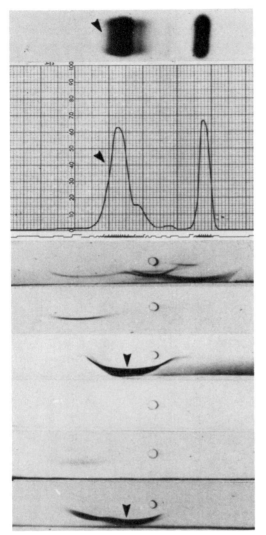

FIG. 8. *IgA lambda myeloma serum. Arrows indicate myeloma protein. See Fig. 3 for details.*

of specific antisera that are commercially available. Genetic variants of serum protein can be readily demonstrated by immunoelectrophoresis (e.g., bisalbuminemia, Gc, and haptoglobin polymorphism).

Clinical syndromes classified as plasma cell dyscrasias are all characterized by uncontrolled proliferation of potentially antibody-producing cell clones that produce large quantities of homogeneous intact Ig's, free light chains, or fragments of such molecules.

The following broad conclusions can be inferred from the appearance of homogeneous bands on zone electrophoresis and from restricted mobility of precipitin arcs on immunoelectrophoresis.

1. A homogeneous band with α_2 to γ mobility on zone electrophoresis and arc of restricted mobility with one of the specific Ig antisera (anti-IgG, -IgA, and -IgM) and a corresponding arc with the same mobility produced by anti-light-chain serum (κ or α) indicates presence of a monoclonal Ig molecule and may indicate multiple myeloma (IgG or IgA), macroglobulinemia (IgM), or benign monoclonal hypergammaglobulinemia. Differentiation between malignant disease (myeloma or macroglobulinemia) and benign monoclonal hypergammaglobulinemia must be made by clinical criteria, and the urine must be tested for corresponding light-chain excretion (Bence Jones proteinuria).

2. Two arcs of different electrophoretic mobility are revealed by immunoelectrophoresis and anti-κ or anti-λ sera. One arc has the mobility corresponding to the myeloma protein while the other, usually fainter, arc indicates in most cases presence of free light chains. On rare occasions, a double myeloma may be present and a check with anti-IgD and anti-IgE sera is required. The urine should be tested for Bence Jones protein.

3. A homogeneous band with α_2 to γ mobility on zone electrophoresis and an arc of restricted mobility seen only with anti-κ or -λ antiserum. Immunoelectrophoresis with anti-IgD, anti-IgE specific sera is required because a positive result indicates IgD or IgE gammopathy. If negative, however, several possibilities must be considered: (i) light-chain disease with renal insufficiency and accumulation of serum light chains (seen frequently); (ii) presence of light-chain tetramer (molecular weight ~90,000) that will not be filtered by glomeruli (rare); (iii) presence of an Ig of unknown heavy-chain characteristics. Molecular weight determination is needed to indicate such a rare possibility.

4. A homogeneous band with α_2 to γ mobility on zone electrophoresis, an arc of restricted mobility with anti-IgG, -IgA, or -IgM, but absence of a reaction with either anti-κ or anti-λ even after reduction with 2-mercaptoethanol. Probably heavy-chain disease, but requires confirmation by isolation and determination of molecular weight.

5. A homogeneous band with α_2 or γ mobility on zone electrophoresis but no reaction with standard test sera. This must be tested with anti-IgD and anti-IgE for the possibility of δ or ϵ heavy-chain disease. If negative, the nature of the abnormal band found on zone electrophoresis must be characterized further by physi-

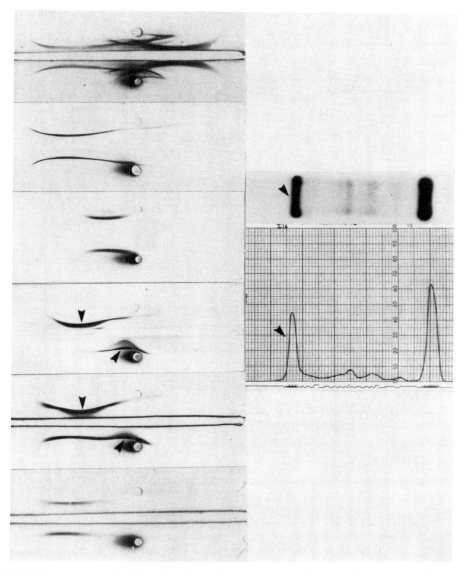

Fig. 9. *IgM kappa macroglobulinemia. Observe change in electrophoretic mobility when 19S macroglobulin is reduced to 7S subunits (arrows). The appearance of arc with 7S subunits resembles arcs of myeloma proteins. See Fig. 3 for details.*

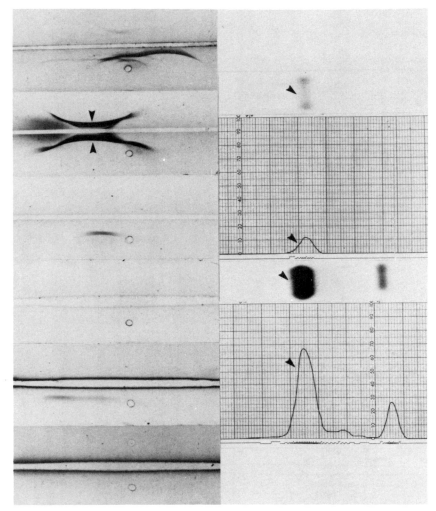

FIG. 10. *IgG heavy-chain disease. Observe complete lack of reaction with anti-kappa and anti-lambda sera, and identical mobility on immunoelectrophoresis developed with anti-IgG. See Fig. 3 for details.*

cochemical and immunochemical methods.

6. No abnormality on both zone electrophoresis and immunoelectrophoresis except hypogammaglobulinemia, but clinical myeloma has been diagnosed. Nonsecretory myeloma does occur (about 1% of cases).

Other gammopathies: Monoclonal Ig's are found in 0.1 to 0.3% of normal healthy persons over 21 years of age (studies performed on blood bank donors). This frequency increases with age to 3% for persons over 70 years and almost 20% for persons over 95 years of age. The relation of this to the incidence of myeloma and macroglobulinemia of 2 to 4 per 100,000 people is unclear, and considerations that they represent pre-myeloma states are controversial. In all such cases of benign monoclonal hypergammaglobulinemia, the concentration of the monoclonal protein is constant over the years and there is no reduction in other serum Ig's.

Monoclonal Ig's are also found in some malignant and nonmalignant diseases, and they are frequent in such lymphoreticular malignancies as lymphoma and leukemia. Therefore, each accidental finding of monoclonal gammopathy should be clinically evaluated. For clinical evaluation and diagnosis, consult references 7 and 8.

LITERATURE CITED

1. Bier, M. 1959. Electrophoresis, theory, methods and applications, vol. 1. Academic Press Inc.,

New York.

2. Bier, M. 1967. Electrophoresis, theory, methods and applications, vol. 2. Academic Press Inc., New York.

3. Grabar, P., and P. Burtin. 1964. Immunoelectrophoretic analysis. Elsevier, New York.

4. Kochwa, S., E. Makuku, and B. Frangione. 1975. Arch. Intern. Med. 135:37–39.

5. Maurer, M. R. 1971. Disc electrophoresis and related techniques of polyacrylamide gel electrophoresis. W. de Gruyter.

6. Osserman, E. S. 1960. A modified technique of immunoelectrophoresis facilitating the identification of specific precipitin arcs. J. Immunol. 84:93–97.

7. Waldenstrom, J. G. 1968. Monoclonal and polyclonal hypergammaglobulinemia: clinical and biological significance. Vanderbilt Univ. Press, Nashville.

8. Wintrobe, M. M., et al. 1976. Clinical hematology, 7th ed. Lea & Febiger, Philadelphia.

Chapter 4

Complement

HENRY GEWURZ AND LISBETH A. SUYEHIRA

INTRODUCTION

Overview

"Complement" refers to a group of interacting serum proteins, of which many are enzymes, originally detected by its ability to bring about cytolysis of antibody-sensitized bacteria and erythrocytes; its name derives from this ability to complement certain reactivities initiated by antibody. It is now clear that the complement system mediates many reactivities in addition to cytolysis which contribute to inflammation and host defense, and that the sequence can be initiated in multiple ways rather than by antibody only. Complement long was measured as the dilution of test fluid (usually serum) required to induce hemolysis under standardized conditions. As additional functions of complement have been recognized and the proteins which comprise the system were isolated and characterized, additional assays have become available; of the newer methods, radial immunodiffusion using monospecific antisera has been the most valuable and widely used. In this chapter we detail a methodology for hemolytic complement and complement protein concentrations evolved by others which we have found to be useful in the clinical evaluation of the complement system.

The primary complement pathway

Eleven complement proteins are involved in mediating the usual antibody-initiated hemolysis. These comprise the "primary complement pathway" and are termed complement (abbreviated C) "components" or "subcomponents." Certain of their reactivities are shown in Fig. 1. They are designated with numerals in order of their sequence of action with two exceptions: (a) C1 long after its discovery was found to be a macromolecule consisting of three proteins linked by calcium, and these are designated C1q, C1r, and C1s, respectively; and (b) the fourth component to be discovered emerged as the second to react in the hemolytic sequence, but its original designation as "C4" has been retained. The reaction sequence is shown in Fig. 1; activated components are designated by an overlying bar (e.g., $C\overline{1s}$), and cleavage products by letters in the lower case (e.g., C3b). The primary C pathway has been divided into recognition (C1q, C1r, C1s), activation (C4, C2, C3), and attack (C5, C6, C7, C8, C9) portions with respect to its function in cytolysis, and these interactions have recently been reviewed (17–19).

The alternative C pathway

The existence of an additional interacting group of proteins, alternative to C1, C4, and C2 but sharing the ability to activate the C system at the level of C3, has recently been appreciated. It involves at least four additional proteins which have been termed initiating factor (IF), factor D, factor B, and properdin, along with C3 and C3b, and has been designated the "properdin" or "alternative" C pathway. Certain properties of two properdin system factors are shown in Table 1, and this pathway has recently been reviewed (19). Other pathways to activation of the terminal C components have been shown; one involves interaction of C1 with properdin system factors and another involves a new enzyme termed "properdin convertase." Certain of these considerations and some of the multiple modes of initiating the C sequence at various entry points are shown in Fig. 1.

Inhibitors of C components

Several proteins which act as inhibitors of C components or split fragments already have been identified (Fig. 1). The first discovered and presently the most important in clinical assays is the C1-esterase inhibitor ($C\overline{1}$-INH), which as one of its many functions inhibits the ability of $C\overline{1s}$ to act upon C4 and C2; inborn deficiency or abnormality of this inhibitor has been associated with and apparently is responsible for hereditary angioedema (HAE) (2, 22). An inactivator of C3b, termed C3b-INA, has been defined, and its deficiency (to date reported in a single patient) has been associated with hypercatabolism and therefore depletion of C3 associated with deposition upon bystander cells (3). An inactivator of the C3a and C5a anaphylatoxins has been characterized, and activities inhibitory to C5, C6, C7 and the C567 trimolecular complex, respectively, have been reported, but have not yet been associated with clinical symptomatology.

Assays of C function

Each of the eleven proteins of the primary C pathway is required in order to obtain hemolysis in the standard assays for hemolytic C activity including those described below. However, multiple functions in addition to hemolysis not requiring the activity of all the C components result from the activation of individual or

Table 1. *Normal serum concentrations and properties of commonly assayed complement and properdin system proteins*

Protein	Normal serum concn (μg/ml)	Mol wt[a]	Relative electro- phoretic mobility[a]
C1q	110–220	400,000	γ_2
C4	200–800	206,000	B_1
C3	800–1,800	180,000	B_2
Factor B	175–275	93,000	B
Properdin	10–20	184,000	γ_2

[a] Cited in reference 19.

groups of C components. These include reactions of agglutination, adherence, opsonization for phagocytosis, generation of anaphylatoxins (which initiate the release of histamine from mast cells), and factors chemotactic for leukocytes (particularly neutrophils); these may involve the native proteins (C1q), large cleavage products (C4b, C3b, C5b), activation peptides (C3a, C5a), or multimolecular assembly units (C567) and are shown in Fig. 1. Each function mediated by C can in turn be adapted to an assay for the C components and activities involved, and indeed these may have real usefulness in the clinical evaluation of the C system in certain circumstances. However, since hemolysis of sensitized erythrocytes requires *all* the primary pathway factors, is suitably convenient and quantitative, and has been the most widely used, it remains the *functional* C assay of greatest value. Functional assays selective for the properdin pathway have not yet reached general clinical usefulness.

Assay for C proteins

Immunochemical assays for the C and properdin proteins in recent years have received a wider usage by far than have any of the hemo-

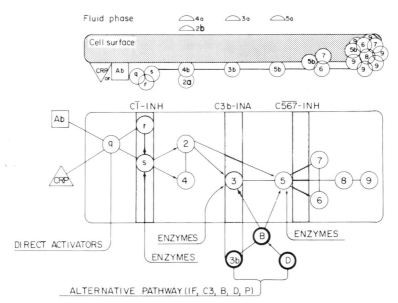

Fig. 1. *Diagrammatic representation of the primary C pathway (enclosed in rectangle), showing the alternative (properdin) pathway and additional modes of C activation. Enzymatic cleavages are represented by arrows, and inhibitory activities are shown by shading. The interactions of C components at the cell surface (stipple) and cleavage products released into the fluid phase are shown above. The activation peptides C3a and C5a have anaphylatoxin and neutrophil chemotactic activity; C4b and C3b each mediate attachment of B-lymphocytes and macrophages, immune adherence, and (as does C5b) opsonization for phagocytosis; C567 has neutrophil chemotactic activity; the C5-9 complex mediates cytolysis and bacterial growth inhibition.*

lytic assays. This seems due in part to their simplicity; accuracy; less rigid requirement for serum volume, collection and storage; concern with absolute rather than activity values; and easy adaptability into laboratory routines which generally involve similar immunochemical assays for other serum proteins. Of these, radial immunodiffusion assays for C3, C4, and perhaps C1q in the primary pathway, and for factor B and properdin in the alternative pathway, have been of the greatest clinical value. A technology directed to identification and quantification of cleaved or otherwise altered components also has been developed, but this remains of greater usefulness to the specialty laboratory.

CLINICAL INDICATIONS

Overview

The C system presently is evaluated in patients predominantly to detect individuals with depleted or deficient levels in order (a) to determine the presence, extent, and/or consequences of ongoing immune processes and, when found, to serve as an index of the therapeutic response; and (b) to detect individuals with inborn deficiencies of C components or inhibitors.

Acquired deficiencies

The acquired deficiencies are by far the most frequent (5, 25). C levels regularly are depressed in active systemic lupus erythematosus (SLE), acute post-streptococcal glomerulonephritis (AGN), and membranoproliferative chronic glomerulonephritis (MPGN), and thus serve as valuable diagnostic aids and therapeutic guides. The C depressions usually are associated with hypercatabolism, although prolonged intervals of decreased synthesis occur in AGN and MPGN. Serum C levels also are secondarily depressed in patients with acute serum sickness reactions to simple proteins (e.g., horse gamma globulin), viruses (e.g., hepatitis B), and protozoa (e.g., malaria). C is decreased in some but not all patients with (a) collagen diseases other than SLE (such as in 10% of patients with rheumatoid arthritis); (b) various forms of renal and hepatic disease; (c) subacute bacterial endocarditis; (d) endotoxemia; (e) septicemia; (f) hypergammaglobulinemia, such as that associated with multiple myeloma; (g) cryoglobulinemia; (h) rapidly rejecting allografts; and (i) hemolytic anemia. Depressed synovial (and in certain instances pleural or pericardial) fluid C levels have been useful in the differential diagnosis of rheumatoid arthritis.

Inborn deficiencies

Patients with inborn deficiencies of each of the primary C pathway proteins excepting C9 have now been detected (2, 4, 5, 28). Individuals lacking C1r, C1s, C4, C2, and C5 have presented with an unusually frequent incidence of SLE as well as renal and other collagen diseases, again emphasizing the value of C determinations in these conditions. Other patients with inborn errors of C (C3, C6, C8) have presented with repeated or unusual responses to certain infections. Plasma therapy for interval restoration of the deficient component has been therapeutic in at least two such individuals, indicating a value for C determinations in patients presenting in these ways as well. The association of C1-INH deficiency with HAE already has been cited.

The usefulness of the determination of the pattern of depletion of the individual C components, the so-called C component depletion profile, is discussed below.

ASSAYS OF HEMOLYTIC COMPLEMENT ACTIVITY

Overview

Numerous methods for the titration of hemolytic C activity have been presented. For the most part these quantify the dilution of serum required to lyse a given proportion of the indicator cells under standardized conditions, and utilize variations in buffers, reaction conditions and volumes, indicator cells, end points, and modes of quantitating hemolysis. These factors were studied extensively by Mayer and his colleagues (16, 20). Their methodology, worked out completely for guinea pigs and suitably adapted to human serum, has been the most widely used. The quantitative determination outlined below follows their procedure with only minor modifications. Hemolytic C activity also has been quantitated in part or completely by automated techniques (e.g., 32), or by assays based on the rate of hemolysis (13).

We also have found it valuable to screen samples by hemolytic radial diffusion the day they are received, and we present a methodology for this purpose. This may serve as a convenient qualitative method to identify samples with decreased C activity and/or to screen samples on which the more quantitative assay is to be performed. In the latter instance, a second specimen may be obtained with careful attention to collection and storage. This screening assay may also be useful in laboratories in which quantitative assays are not performed.

Quantitative assay of hemolytic C activity (based on the CH_{50} unit of Mayer)

Principle of the assay. This test depends upon the ability of the primary C pathway to induce hemolysis of erythrocytes sensitized with optimal amounts of anti-erythrocyte antibodies. The relationship between the amount of C present and the proportion of cells lysed follows a sigmoidal curve. This curve is steep in the central area, where the degree of lysis is sensitive to small changes in the amount of C present. Therefore, for precise titrations of hemolytic C, the dilution of serum which will lyse 50% of the indicator erythrocytes under defined conditions is determined, and is designated the 50% hemolytic unit of C, or the CH_{50}. This is an arbitrary unit, since its magnitude depends upon such factors as the erythrocyte concentration and fragility, the quantity and nature of the antibody used for sensitization, the ionic strength, Mg^{2+} and Ca^{2+} concentrations and pH of the reaction system, and the reaction time and temperature. Therefore, this assay must be carefully standardized in each laboratory with attention to these factors. References (16, 20, 24, 31) are valuable sources for this method.

Reagents and test samples. The reagents required are (a) gelatin-veronal-buffered saline supplemented with magnesium (GVB^+) and (b) sheep erythrocytes sensitized with rabbit antibody (ShEA); instructions for their preparation are detailed below. The assay can be performed using serum, plasma, or extravascular (synovial, pleural or pericardial, but not cerebrospinal) fluids. Special attention must be given to collection and storage of specimens. When serum is used, blood should be clotted for 15 to 30 min at room temperature and 30 to 60 min at 4 C, centrifuged at 4 C, and either assayed immediately or stored at −70 C. Inappropriate collection or storage can result in loss of C activity, particularly in certain pathological sera.

Procedure. The assay should be set up at 0 to 4 C with the tubes prechilled, in order to uniformly preserve C activity. Test and control (see below) samples should be removed from the freezer just prior to use and thawed quickly at 37 C. The following procedure is used to measure C activity in serum or plasma (see Table 2):

1. Prepare a row of five tubes (four 16 × 100 mm; one 17 × 150 mm) labeled A to E for each sample to be tested.

2. Add GVB^+ in the volumes indicated in Table 2 to tubes A to E.

3. Add 0.25 ml of test sample to tube E to give a dilution of 1:51. Mix thoroughly and add the volumes indicated in Table 2 to tubes A to D. Add 5.0 ml of GVB^+ to the volume remaining in tube E, which now serves as a control to measure the color contributed by the serum itself.

4. Include two "standard" sera with each assay, in order to monitor technical and reagent variations. Standard A (the reference standard) is used to establish an adjustment factor to correct for such variables as indicator cell reactivity and precise incubation times and temperatures. Standard B (the internal control) is used to monitor variations in standard A as well as the reproducibility of the test. Both standards should be handled identically to patient serum samples.

TABLE 2. *Sample protocol for titration of hemolytic C activity in human serum or plasma*[a]

Tube designation	ShEA 5 × 10^8/ml (ml)	GVB^+ (ml)	C source 1:51 (ml)	C dilution	OD	OD′	y	$\dfrac{y}{1-y}$	CH_{50}/ml
A	1.0	1.5	5.0	1:10	.642	.619	.89	8.1 ⎫	
B	1.0	4.0	2.5	1:20	.468	.455	.66	1.9 ⎪	
C	1.0	5.0	1.5	1:34	.220	.211	.30	.43 ⎬ 25	
D	1.0	5.5	1.0	1:51	.041	.034	.05	.05 ⎭	
E[b]	–	4.0	2.5	1:20	.010				
Cell control									
A	1.0	6.5	–	–	.002 ⎫ .003	–	–	–	–
B	1.0		–	–	.004 ⎭	–	–	–	–
Complete lysis									
A	1.0	H_2O − 6.5 ml	–	–	.690 ⎫ .697	–	–	–	–
B	1.0		–	–	.704 ⎭	–	–	–	–

[a] Adapted from reference 16.

[b] Tube E is used both to prepare the initial (1:51) C dilution and to serve as a serum blank; it is prepared by first adding 0.25 ml of undiluted serum to 12.5 ml of GVB^+. After the amounts indicated have been delivered to tubes A to D, an additional 5.0 ml of GVB^+ is added to tube E, enabling the contents to be used to correct for the original sample color.

5. Prepare cell control tubes to measure spontaneous lysis during the assay by adding 6.5 ml of GVB$^+$ to each of two appropriately labeled tubes. Experiments with cell controls showing >2% spontaneous hemolysis should be discarded.

6. Prepare complete-lysis tubes for use in the calculation of the percent lysis by adding 6.5 ml of water to each of two appropriately labeled tubes.

7. Add 1.0 ml of EA (5×10^8/ml) to tubes A to D as well as to the cell control and complete lysis tubes, bringing the final volume to 7.5 ml. Mix well.

8. Incubate for 1 h in a 37 C water bath, with occasional agitation.

9. Centrifuge to sediment the cells, usually 3,000 rpm for 5 min.

10. Transfer the supernatant fluids to separate tubes, and measure the amount of oxyhemoglobin released spectrophotometrically at 541 nm in optical density (OD) units.

Note: Extravascular fluids contain lower amounts of hemolytic C activity than does serum or plasma. Therefore, the CH$_{50}$ assay is performed with lower dilutions of these fluids in tubes A to D (usually 1:5, 1:10, 1:20, 1:40). This procedure is not suitable for assay of cerebrospinal fluid (see below).

Calculations.

1. Calculate the OD of the serum present in each test dilution based on the OD of tube E, which is equivalent to a 1:20 serum dilution, by the formula: OD of serum dilution = (20/reciprocal of serum dilution) $\times$ OD of tube E.

2. Subtract the sum of the OD of the averaged cell controls and the OD of the appropriate serum dilution from each test serum dilution; this represents the corrected OD, or OD'. Thus: OD' of sample = OD of sample − (OD of cell controls + OD of sample serum dilution).

3. Calculate the percent lysis (y) by the formula: y = OD' sample/OD complete lysis − OD of cell control.

4. Using 2×3 cycle log-log graph paper, plot the log of $y/(1 - y)$ on the x axis, and the log of the reciprocal of the C dilution on the y axis, using only y values between 20 and 80% for the greatest accuracy. Construct the best straight line for the points of each sample; if only one graphable point is obtained, the line may be constructed based on the slope of a sample run concurrently with only a minor loss of accuracy. The CH$_{50}$ is the reciprocal of the dilution at which point the line crosses the 50% lysis point, where $y/(1 - y) = 1.0$. The CH$_{50}$ may also be derived from the y values by use of factors

derived from the von Krogh equation (16), which serves as a mathematical description of the sigmoidal hemolytic C response curve, and/or with use of a programmable calculator.

5. Correct the CH$_{50}$ of each test sample by multiplying with the following factor: designated CH$_{50}$ of reference standard/CH$_{50}$ of reference standard in assay.

6. Normal levels in our laboratory are 20 to 40 CH$_{50}$/ml. The normal range should be established in each laboratory.

Limitations and advantages. As emphasized, this assay measures C in arbitrary activity rather than in absolute protein units, and thus is subject to fluctuations based on minor alterations of reaction conditions. It is insensitive to depletions of up to 50 to 80% of the normal levels of individual components and fails to detect depletion of most of the properdin system factors. It requires careful collection and handling of specimens, as well as utilization of cold storage equipment, and is relatively time-consuming. However, these disadvantages pertain to assays of virtually all C functions and, once established as a routine procedure, the hemolytic titration is a most valuable tool in the evaluation of the C system. It represents the assay of C function which best combines the features of sensitivity, precision, reproducibility, and convenience, and thus is the method of choice for this purpose. Since each of the primary C pathway components are required for hemolysis, by its use all of the inborn and most of the acquired C deficiencies can be detected.

Qualitative screening by hemolytic radial diffusion

Principle. The hemolytic activity of C also can be demonstrated by using sensitized erythrocytes incorporated into agarose-containing immunodiffusion plates. Fresh sera added to wells introduced into the agarose produce a circular zone of hemolysis as radial diffusion of C occurs. The diameter of the zone of lysis gives a qualitative measure of the amount of hemolytic C activity present in a way analogous to that seen in single radial immunodiffusion assays. This procedure is useful as a rapid, convenient screen for hemolytic C activity.

Procedure. The hemolytic screen plates are prepared to contain 0.3% agarose and 1×10^9 sensitized sheep erythrocytes in a total volume of 3.5 ml (see reagent section). Samples for assay should be collected and handled as described in the section "Quantitative assay of hemolytic C activity."

1. Introduce wells into the agarose using a

sharpened 13-gauge cannula. The wells should be approximately 8 mm from each other and 4 mm from the edge of the plate.

2. Use a Hamilton syringe to add 5 μl of an undiluted standard serum and of each test sample to the appropriate well, rinsing the syringe between samples.

3. After 15 min, invert and incubate the plate(s) in a moist chamber for 1 h at 37 C, and score as indicated below; incubation may be continued overnight at room temperature.

Interpretation. The assay serves to rapidly identify samples with decreased hemolytic activity. Lysis is scored as (a) *normal,* (b) *low,* or (c) *absent,* based on comparison with the activity of the standard serum. Occasionally sera that show deficient hemolytic activity in this screen will have normal activity in the quantitative CH_{50} assay; this discrepancy is probably due to interaction of the sera with the agarose. In addition, two unusual visually striking phenomena have been observed: (a) a "target" appearance, which is based upon the protection of a zone of cells near the well by "blocking" anti-erythrocyte antibodies (29), and (b) a linear zone of lysis between two adjacent wells which has been observed when certain acute-phase sera were used; the latter phenomenon reflects a fluid-phase activation of and bystander hemolysis by the C attack mechanism termed "reactive lysis" (30).

Usefulness of assay. This assay has been useful in (a) allowing rapid qualitative evaluation of C activity as a diagnostic aid; (b) screening samples in which additional C studies might be informative; and (c) serving as a qualitative assay for hemolytic C activity in laboratories where more elaborate techniques are not available.

ASSAYS FOR COMPLEMENT PROTEIN

Overview

With isolation and characterization of the components of both the primary and alternative C pathways, immunochemical techniques utilizing monospecific antisera have become the main assays for serum C in humans. Adaptation of the single radial immunodiffusion method has allowed quantification of C component levels on an absolute weight basis rather than by arbitrary units; a markedly increased ease of performance; a high degree of reproducibility; less rigid requirements for serum volume, collection, and storage; and easy adaptability into laboratory routines, permitting measurement of C levels in any laboratory. Current applications of electroimmunodiffusion

and automated nephelometric procedures are further making C measurements more convenient in large hospitals and specialty laboratories. The principles underlying these methods have been reviewed in an earlier chapter. Their adaptation to the assay of C3 and C4 and, to a lesser extent, C1q, C1-INH, properdin and factor B is briefly outlined here.

Assays by single radial immunodiffusion (see chapter 2)

Assay of C3 and C4 (12). The reagents needed for these assays include immunodiffusion plates prepared with appropriate amounts of monospecific antisera incorporated into the agarose, and reference standard and internal control sera. Formulae for preparation of the gels are listed in the REAGENTS section. A calibration curve must be constructed for each batch of plates. The C3 calibration curve is prepared by assaying in duplicate dilutions (1:3; 1:4; 1:6; 1:8; and 1:12) of the C3 standard on each of three separate plates. The C4 calibration curve is prepared by assaying in duplicate dilutions (1:1, i.e., undiluted; 1:2; 1:4, and 1:8) of the C4 standard. Once the calibration curves and the reproducibility of the assay are established, it is possible to utilize these as reference data and to assay only appropriate single dilutions of the reference standard in the daily assays. At least one such standard should appear on every plate. The procedure is as follows:

1. For the assay of C3, prepare a 1:6 dilution of the reference standard, internal control, and test samples by adding 0.1 ml of serum to 0.5 ml of ethylenediaminetetraacetic acid (EDTA)-veronal buffer. C4 is assayed undiluted.

2. Prepare wells in the C3 and C4 plates, respectively, using a sharpened 12-gauge cannula. The wells should be at least 8 mm apart and 4 mm from the edge of the plate to avoid distortion of the precipitin rings.

3. Using a Hamilton syringe, add 5 μl of the reference standard, internal control, and test samples to their respective wells. Rinse the syringes with distilled water between samples. Include the standard and control sera on each plate.

4. Allow 10 min at room temperature for diffusion, invert and place the plates in a humidity chamber, and continue incubation at room temperature for at least 24 h.

5. Score the plates over an illuminated viewbox by measuring the diameters of the precipitin rings to the nearest 0.1 mm with a calibrated ocular. Read the values in micrograms per milliliter from the calibration curve.

6. If the standard varies from the expected

diameter by 0.2 mm or less, correct the value of the patient samples using a factor derived from a ratio of the expected value of the reference standard as compared to the value achieved. Variations greater than 0.2 mm indicate unacceptable technical variability or reagent instability, and the assay should be repeated.

7. Until a universal reference standard is generally available for the assay of C proteins, a laboratory may determine the protein concentrations of its reference standard (a) by preparing or obtaining C components in an immunochemically pure form, or (b) by obtaining standardized sera from a laboratory in which this value already has been established. Once such a primary standard is obtained, the laboratory should establish a value for its own "secondary" standard by multiple assays comparing these two samples. This serum should be stored in small aliquots at -70 C, each of which should be used only once and discarded. Repeated freeze-thawing of standard or test samples may result in fluctuations of values that reflect changes in antigenic determinants due to alteration of the protein structure (see below).

8. Normal levels are cited in Table 2.

Assays of C1q, factor B, properdin, and C̄1-INH. C1q (11), factor B (15,26), and properdin (15) can be assayed in similar ways using commercially available reagents. References for the procedures are cited, as are normal levels (Table 2), and suggested formulae for preparation of suitable immunodiffusion plates are cited in the REAGENTS section. C̄1-INH may also be measured by immunodiffusion (22).

Pitfalls. The advantages of the radial immunodiffusion assay have been cited, and its limitations are considered in this section. It permits accurate detection of proteins only in amounts above 2.5 μg/ml and thus is much less sensitive than hemolytic titrations. Since it quantifies proteins on the basis of antigenicity, it may not detect functional variations and one obtains data only for the component(s) assayed rather than a survey of the function of the entire system. Intervals upwards of 24 h are usually required for the reactions to reach end points, and this prolonged diffusion time favors the appearance of falsely elevated values when cleaved C components are present. This also enhances the potential for interactions between the suspending medium and the test serum, favoring the possibility that such cleavage products might be formed.

An example is found in the assay of C3. Native C3 contains three antigenic determinants — A, B, and D. However, C3 in "aged" or "converted" serum may exist as at least two antigenically distinct forms: C3d (or α2D) with antigenic site D, and C3c (or β1A) with antigenic site A — the B antigen is "lost" when C3 is converted. These forms of C3 can be present in varying amounts depending upon the degree of conversion. Further, when a determinant is present on a smaller molecule, it diffuses at a faster rate and presents as a larger ring of precipitation. The commercially available antisera as usually prepared contain specificities for both C3 (β1C) and C3c (β1A). However, uncontrolled collection, handling, and/or storage may yield relatively larger amounts of β1A, which would then appear as a precipitation ring of larger diameter than if C3 had remained in its native unconverted state. This phenomenon thus can contribute to a variability in the radial immunodiffusion assay. Freeze-thawings, immune complexes, and multiple additional factors may lead to similar effects, which can also affect C components other than C3.

Additional assays of C protein

The electroimmunodiffusion assay of Laurell, based upon the principle of electrophoresis of antigen into antiserum-containing agarose, has been used for measurement of C proteins (3). By this method, the rocket-shaped peak heights are compared to those of a series of standards in order to quantitate the antigen in the test samples. This method offers the advantage of greater sensitivity and less total time required to obtain the results, minimizing the effects of diffusion as well as of conversion of C components which may occur during the radial immunodiffusion. It has been claimed to be the most generally applicable, reliable, precise, accurate, and reproducible means for measuring C proteins (3); the absence of more extensive current usage may relate to the decreased convenience involved in establishing and performing the assay.

An automated immunoprecipitation method has been introduced based on a continuous-flow system (21). Serum is reacted with monospecific antisera, currently commercially available for C3, C4, and C̄1-INH, and the amount of precipitation is measured nephelometrically. This method is extremely sensitive, uses relatively small amounts of reagents, and seems most valuable for the larger laboratory concerned with numerous assays of multiple proteins. The major current disadvantages to this assay seem to be cost of the system and availability of commercial antisera suitable for assay of additional C components.

A prominent feature of the interactions of the

C system is the limited proteolytic cleavage and/or alteration of structure of multiple C components which occurs upon activation of both the primary and the properdin pathway (18, 19). These alterations have been adapted into attempts to assay for altered C components as indicators of C activation in vivo, and such have been reported for C3 antigens (including C3c, C3d, and C3a), as well as for C1s, C4 factor B, and properdin (5, 15, 24–26). Similarly, the ability of sera from certain patients to induce alterations in the structure of given components during preincubations in vitro has been assayed, and indeed, the initiating factor (IF; C3NeF) of the properdin pathway was first detected by its ability to induce conversion and therefore loss of the B antigen of C3 during such incubations (26). However, these assays would seem still to be in the province of the specialty laboratory.

INTERPRETATIONS

Overview

C levels fluctuate in response to a variety of stimuli and disease processes. These alterations can be characterized by appropriate functional and immunochemical tests; those described herein serve for most purposes. Further analyses of individual component hemolytic activities (methodologies for which are cited in references 13 and 24) or protein levels, as well as assays of additional C-dependent functions, serve in further characterization of underlying conditions, but usually are in the province of the specialty laboratory.

The complement profile

The most frequently occurring alterations of C are elevations of levels, since most of the components respond as acute-phase reactants (27). However, the main clinical application of C assays presently is in the detection of individuals in whom C activity and/or proteins are decreased. This occurs predominantly in one of three ways: (i) increased utilization in vivo; (ii) decreased synthesis in vivo; and (iii) increased utilization or conversion (post-venipuncture) in vitro.

C levels most frequently are determined in order to detect processes in the first category, in evaluation of patients with known or suspected immune-mediated diseases. Immune (or inflammatory) reactions, which consume C efficiently in vitro, seem only rarely to result in decreased C levels in vivo, apparently because utilization must be intense in order to overcome the increased rate of C formation also associated with inflammation. The C-consuming insult which does decrease the serum C level frequently induces a characteristic alteration of the C components and the C-dependent activities to which they contribute. This can be represented as a "complement profile," and may help identify the nature of the insult and the disease with which it is associated. This usually involves depression of both total hemolytic C activity and of the levels of *multiple* C components, as occurs in SLE. We have found it useful to group assays for other parameters frequently altered during the immune-mediated diseases, e.g., C-reactive protein, antinuclear antibodies, and rheumatoid factor, along with the C assays usually performed for this purpose.

The second indication for C determinations clinically is in the detection of the *rare* patient with unexplained repeated or unusual responses to infections, in whom inability to form a given C component is the underlying basis. Decreased synthesis of a C component also occurs on an acquired and transitory basis, as in certain diseases associated with C consuming processes (e.g., AGN and MPGN). Patients in both categories frequently present with a distinctive C profile, in which total hemolytic C activity is *greatly* depressed or absent, while the protein level of only a single component is depleted. This diagnosis must be established with care, because C-consuming processes do occur with increased frequency in patients with inborn C deficiencies.

The depressions of C levels which occur post-venipuncture also tend to be associated with characteristic alterations of the C profile, which usually show decreased total hemolytic C activity with normal levels of all of the C components tested. These changes may derive from simple "aging" or improper handling of sera, but also occur in well-handled specimens when potent C-consuming activity is present, e.g., in HAE, cryoglobulinemia, certain immune complex diseases, or a recently-appreciated coagulation-associated C-consuming process (6). Obviously, improper handling will result in greater perturbations in such pathological sera.

The C profile in given diseases

C levels in diseases must be interpreted as aids to suggesting and confirming given diagnoses, and not definitive of themselves. There are enormous variations in the C component patterns during the course of a disease in a given patient, as well as in different patients presenting with a given disease. The various alterations consequent to venipuncture add additional cause for precaution. However, a brief *generalization* for interpreting results obtained by the methods suggested herein (involving total hemolytic C4 and C3 protein levels) may be presented (Table 3).

Determination of additional C component levels (by hemolytic and immunochemical methods) is valuable in individual instances and methodologies for these purposes have been presented (13). Thus, immunoassay for factor B and properdin can indicate the participation of the alternative C pathway (9, 15, 25, 26), e.g., among the hypocomplementemic renal diseases, factor B is usually decreased in MPGN and properdin is usually decreased in AGN. Similarly, selected C1q deficiency has been seen in a distinctive form of hypocomplementemic vasculitis (1) and also in agammaglobulinemia syndromes. More elaborate descriptions and interpretations of C levels and their utilization in disease have appeared in multiple recent articles (5, 7–9, 25, 28).

C levels have been useful in determining the presence of rheumatoid processes in closed spaces by the evaluation of synovial, pleural and pericardial fluids, in which case depressed levels (as compared to total protein or expected fluid/serum ratios) have been seen (23). An assay for C4 activity, performed with C4-deficient guinea pig serum, has been of use in detecting central nervous system SLE (10).

Additional C assays

Assays of additional C-mediated functions can lead to improved characterization of the status of the C system. An assay for the ability of serum to neutralize the ability of C$\overline{1}$ to hydrolyze synthetic amino acid ester substrates provides the definitive procedure for the diagnosis of HAE (14); we have found it convenient first to define C4 protein levels in patients suspected of having this disease, and if this is decreased, to perform a definitive assay for C1-INH such as that just cited. Other assays frequently performed in the immunology laboratory, such as measurements for B-cell rosettes using an intermediate involving complement components, as well as assays for C-dependent phagocytosis and bactericidal activities, can also be adjusted to serve for assays of C as well. In this respect, an assay for phagocytosis of yeast particles revealed an abnormality of the fifth component of C (C5) to be characteristic of, and probably responsible for, the susceptibility to infection in the severe form of Leiner's disease; this abnormality would not have been detected by C5 hemolytic or protein assays (17a). Immune adherence, chemotaxis and anaphylatoxin assays similarly may be of value in testing the status of the C system. Complement deposition in vivo can be recognized by using anti-C antibodies on frozen tissue specimens with conventional immunofluorescent methods, and anti-C reagents have been valuable in detecting the presence of C components on erythrocytes. Finally, immunoconglutinins, which are antibodies to C components C4 and C3, may serve to reflect the role of C in disease. It therefore is anticipated that with further investigations, an increasingly useful protocol for determining C profiles will be designed which will serve as well for the interpretation of immune-related diseases as the basic serum electrolyte profile has served for the interpretation of many metabolic diseases.

REAGENTS

Stock solutions (16, 20)

5× Veronal (1 liter). Dissolve 41.2 g of NaCl and 5.095 g of Na–5,5 diethyl barbiturate in 700 ml of distilled water. Adjust the pH to 7.35 ± 0.05 with 1 N HCl. Bring the volume to 1 liter with distilled water.

2.0 M MgCl$_2$. Prepare 100 ml of approximately 3 M MgCl$_2$. Measure the specific gravity and interpolate the concentration of MgCl$_2$ from the "Concentration Properties of Aqueous

TABLE 3. *A guide for interpreting C4 and C3 protein levels in patients with decreased total hemolytic C activity*[a]

C protein level	Normal C4	Decreased C4
Normal C3	Alterations in vitro[b] (e.g., improper handling) Coagulation-associated C consumption Inborn errors[c] (other than C4 or C3)	Immune complex disease Hypergammaglobulinemic states Cryoglobulinemia Hereditary angioedema[c] Inborn C4 deficiency[c]
Decreased C3	AGN MPGN Immune complex disease Inborn C3 deficiency[c]	Active SLE Serum sickness (e.g., in association with infections) Chronic active hepatitis Subacute bacterial endocarditis Immune complex disease

[a] With awareness of extreme variability.
[b] Most frequent.
[c] Extremely rare; consider especially when total hemolytic C activity is completely absent.

Solutions Conversion" tables in the *Handbook of Chemistry and Physics*. Adjust the concentration to 2.00 M by addition of the appropriate amount of distilled water.

0.3 M CaCl$_2$. Prepare 100 ml of approximately 0.5 M CaCl$_2$. Determine the concentration of CaCl$_2$ as in solution 3 above and adjust to 0.300 M CaCl$_2$ with distilled water.

Stock metals. Add equal volumes of 2.0 M MgCl$_2$ and 0.3 M CaCl$_2$.

0.1 M stock EDTA (500 ml). Dissolve 18.6 g of Na$_2$H$_2$–EDTA in 400 ml of distilled water, with constant mixing to aid dissolution. Adjust the pH to 7.65 ± 0.05 with freshly prepared 2 N NaOH. Bring to 500-ml volume with distilled water.

Glycine-saline buffer (500 ml). Dissolve 3.75 g of glycine, 4.25 g of NaCl, and 1.25 ml of 1.0 N NaOH in 450 ml of distilled water. Adjust the pH to 8.2 with 10% Na$_2$CO$_3$ and bring to 500-ml volume.

0.1 M sodium azide (1 liter). Dissolve 6.5 g of sodium azide in distilled water and bring to 1 liter.

Working solutions (16, 20)

GVB$^=$ (1 liter). Dissolve 1 g of gelatin in 600 ml of hot, distilled water. Cool to room temperature. Add to 200 ml of 5× veronal and bring to 1 liter with distilled water.

GVB$^+$ (1 liter). Add 0.5 ml of 2.0 M MgCl$_2$ to 1 liter of GVB$^=$.

GVB^{++} (1 liter). Add 1.0 ml of Stock Metals (see above) to 1 liter of GVB$^=$.

GGVB^{++} (1 liter). Mix 500 ml of 5% dextrose, 200 ml of 5× veronal, and 1.0 ml of Stock Metals in a volumetric flask. Bring to 1-liter volume with distilled water.

0.01 M EDTA (1 liter). Dilute 100 ml of 0.1 M stock EDTA to 1 liter with GVB$^=$.

EDTA-VB (1 liter). Mix 200 ml of 5× veronal and 100 ml of 0.1 M stock EDTA. Bring to 1 liter with distilled water.

Preparation of optimally sensitized erythrocytes (EA at 1×10^9/ml)

Preparation of sheep erythrocytes (E). Wash sheep erythrocytes (E) twice with 0.15 M NaCl and once with 0.01 M EDTA. Resuspend to a known volume (V$_1$) in 0.01 M EDTA. Lyse 0.5 ml of the cell suspension in 7.0 ml of distilled water, and adjust the cell concentration to 1×10^9/ml spectrophotometrically, using the following equations:

(a) (OD of V$_1$ at 541 nm/0.703) × V$_1$ = V$_2$, where V$_2$ is the volume of EA at 1×10^9/ml.

(b) V$_2$ − V$_1$ = milliliters of 0.01 M EDTA to add to cell suspension V$_1$ in order to obtain a final concentration of 1×10^9 EA/ml.

Sensitization of E. Mix equal volumes of E (1×10^9/ml) and hemolysin (antibody; see below) diluted in GVB$^+$. Incubate at 37 C for 30 min; mix frequently. Incubate at 0 C for 30 min, again mixing frequently. Centrifuge and wash once with GVB$^+$. Resuspend in GGVB$^+$ and readjust (spectrophotometrically as above) to 1×10^9 cells/ml. Add sodium azide to a final concentration of 0.001 M. EA usually remain stable at 0 C for 1 to 3 weeks.

Selection of optimal hemolysin concentration. To determine the dilution of hemolysin for preparation of optimal EA, test a series of dilutions of fresh human C absorbed 5× with E (10 min, 0 C, 5% [vol/vol]) against E sensitized with varying dilutions of hemolysin. A C dilution yielding 50 to 70% lysis (usually 1:25) should be included. Prepare hemolysin dilutions of 1:400, 1:800, 1:1,000, 1:1,200, and 1:1,600. Prepare EA by adding 15 ml of the respective dilutions to 15 ml E at a concentration of 1×10^9/ml. For each hemolysin dilution used, prepare a set of tubes A to E as in section on Quantitative assay of hemolytic C activity; prepare a separate cell control and complete lysis tube for each set of EA. Assay and determine *y* for each reaction tube also as in section on Quantitative assay of hemolytic C activity. On standard graph paper, plot the hemolysin dilution on the X axis and the percent lysis (*y*) on the Y axis for each C dilution used. A plateau should be apparent for each C dilution, and the hemolysin dilution to be used for subsequent C titrations is twice that concentration at which the plateau ends. This helps to neutralize natural antibody as a variable in this assay and renders the assay more dependent upon the C concentration selectively.

Immunodiffusion plates

Hemolytic screen plates.

1. Prepare a solution containing 2.0 g of agarose (l'Industrie Biologique Francaise), 5 ml of 0.1 M sodium azide, and 95 ml of GVB$^+$.

2. Heat with constant stirring to dissolve the agarose. Do not allow the agarose to boil or scorch. Cool to 50 to 60 C in a water bath.

3. Mix 3 ml of agarose, 1.5 ml of GVB$^+$, and 1.0 ml of EA (1×10^9/ml) in a 13 × 100 mm tube for each plate to be prepared and pour into a 3.5-ml empty immunodiffusion plate (Hyland). Quickly spread the mixture to the edges of the plate and allow solidification on a level surface.

4. Label, cover, and store the plates inverted in a moist bag at 4 C.

C3 plates.

1. Prepare a solution containing 1.7 g of Noble agar (Difco), 20 ml of 5× veronal, 10 ml of

0.1 M EDTA, 5 ml of 0.1 M sodium azide, and 65 ml of distilled water.

2. Heat with constant stirring to dissolve the agar. Do not let the agar scorch or boil. Cool to 60 C in a water bath set at that temperature.

3. Determine the amount of antiserum per plate that will produce diameters of 4.5 to 5.0 mm with a 1:6 dilution of the Reference Standard. Dilute the antiserum in EDTA-veronal buffer in order to deliver that amount in a volume of 0.5 ml.

4. For each plate, mix 3.0 ml of agar and 0.5 ml of diluted antiserum in a 13 × 100 mm test tube. Quickly pour into an empty immunodiffusion plate (Hyland), and spread the mixture to the edges of the plate. Allow the plate to solidify on a level surface.

5. Label the plates, cover, and store inverted in a moist bag at 4 C.

C4 plates.

1. Prepare a solution containing 1.4 g of SeaKem agarose (Marine Colloids), 10 ml of 0.1 M EDTA, 20 ml of 5× veronal, 5 ml of 0.1 M sodium azide, and 65 ml of distilled water.

2. Heat with constant stirring to dissolve the agarose. Do not let the agar scorch or boil. Cool to 60 C in a water bath.

3. Determine the amount of antiserum that will produce diameters of 4.5 to 5.0 mm with a 1:1 dilution of the Reference Standard; dilute the antiserum in EDTA-veronal buffer in order to deliver that amount in a volume of 0.5 ml.

4. Proceed as from step no. 4 above.

C1q plates.

1. Prepare a solution containing 1.0 g of SeaKem agarose (Marine Colloids), 5 ml of 0.1 M sodium azide, and 95 ml of glycine-saline buffer.

2. Proceed as from step no. 2 above.

Factor B plates.

1. Prepare a solution containing 1.4 g of SeaKem agarose (Marine Colloids), 10 ml of 0.1 M EDTA, 20 ml of 5× veronal, 5 ml of 0.1 M sodium azide, and 65 ml of distilled water.

2. Proceed as from step no. 2 above. Antiserum is commercially available from Behring Diagnostics.

Properdin plates.

1. Prepare a solution containing 1.0 g of SeaKem agarose (Marine Colloids), 10 ml of 0.1 M EDTA, 20 ml of 5× veronal, 5 ml of 0.1 M sodium azide, and 65 ml of distilled water.

2. Proceed as from step no. 2 above. Antiserum is commercially available from Atlantic Antibodies.

Internal control

A normal serum pool should be prepared from a single individual, and aliquoted and stored at −70 C in order to serve as the "internal control" sample during repeated testing over a prolonged period of time. In the calibration of this pool, fresh aliquots (each discarded after use) should repeatedly be assayed along with the reference standard in order to obtain an arithmetic mean ±2 standard deviations for the parameter in question. Results of each assay should be compared with this "known" value. If they fall outside 2 standard deviations, that entire assay should be discarded; if this experience is repeated, it should be taken as a signal to reevaluate all the reagents used in the assay, including both the reference standard and the internal control.

LITERATURE CITED

1. Agnello, V., S. Ruddy, R. J. Winchester, C. L. Christian, and H. G. Kunkel. 1975. Hereditary C2 deficiency in systemic lupus erythematosus and acquired complement abnormalities in an unusual SLE-related syndrome, p. 312–317. In D. Bergsma, R. A. Good, and N. W. Paul (ed.), Immunodeficiency in man and animals. Birth Defects Original Article Series, vol. 11, no. 1. The National Foundation March of Dimes.

2. Alper, C. A., and F. S. Rosen. 1971. Genetic aspects of the complement system. Adv. Immunol. 14:251.

3. Alper, C. A., and F. S. Rosen. 1975. Complement in laboratory medicine, p. 47–68. In G. N. Vyas, D. P. Stites, and G. Brecher (ed.), Laboratory diagnosis of immunologic disorders. Grune & Stratton. New York.

4. Day, N. K., and R. A. Good. 1975. Deficiencies of the complement system in man, p. 306–311. In D. Bergsma, R. A. Good, and N. W. Paul (ed.). Immunodeficiency in man and animals. Birth Defects Original Article Series, vol. 11, no. 1. The National Foundation March of Dimes.

5. Frank, M. M., and J. P. Atkinson. 1975. Complement in clinical medicine. Disease-a-month. Yearbook Publication, Chicago.

6. Gewurz, H., and N. Ertel. 1973. Non-immune activation of complement: two new phenomena, p. 340–349. In W. Braun and J. Ungar (ed.), "Non-specific" factors influencing host resistance. S. Karger, Basel.

7. Gewurz, H., R. J. Pickering, S. E. Mergenhagen, and R. A. Good. 1968. The complement profile in acute glomerulonephritis. Systemic lupus erythematosus and hypocomplementemic chronic glomerulonephritis: contrasts and experimental correlations. Int. Arch. Allergy Appl. Immunol. 34:557–570.

8. Gewurz, H., R. J. Pickering, P. S. Clark, A. R. Page, J. Finstad, and R. A. Good. 1968. The complement system in the prevention, media-

tion, and diagnosis of disease and its usefulness in the determination of immunopatho-
genic mechanisms, p. 396–417. *In* D. Bergsma
and R. A. Good (ed.), Immunologic deficiency
disease in man. Birth Defects Original Article
Series, vol. 4, no. 1.

9. Gewurz, H., R. J. Pickering, G. Naff, R. Snyderman, S. E. Mergenhagen, and R. A. Good.
1969. Decreased properdin activity in acute
glomerulonephritis. Int. Arch. Allergy Appl.
Immunol. **36**:592–598.

10. Hadler, N. M., R. A. Gerwin, M. M. Frank, J.
N. Whitaker, M. Baker, and J. L. Decker.
1973. The fourth component of complement in
the cerebrospinal fluid in systemic lupus erythematosus. Arthritis Rheum. **16**:507–521.

11. Hanauer, L. B., and C. L. Christian. 1967. Clinical studies of hemolytic complement and the
11s component. Am. J. Med. **42**:882–890.

12. Kohler, P. F., and H. J. Muller-Eberhard. 1967.
Immunochemical quantitation of the third,
fourth and fifth components of human complement: concentrations in the serum of healthy
adults. J. Immunol. **99**:1211–1216.

13. Lachmann, P. J., M. J. Hobart, and W. P. As-
ton. 1973. Complement. *In* D. M. Weir (ed.),
Handbook of experimental immunology, 2nd
ed. Blackwell Scientific Publications, Oxford,
England.

14. Levy, L., and I. H. Lepow. 1959. Assay and
properties of serum inhibitor of C'1-esterase.
Proc. Soc. Exp. Biol. Med. **101**:608–611.

15. McLean, R. H., and A. F. Michael. 1973. Properdin and C3 proactivator. Alternate pathway
components in human glomerulonephritis. J.
Clin. Invest. **52**:634–644.

16. Mayer, M. M. 1971. Complement and complement fixation, p. 133–240. *In* E. A. Kabat
(ed.), Experimental immunochemistry, 2nd
ed. Charles C Thomas, Publisher, Springfield, Ill.

17. Mayer, M. M. 1973. The complement system.
Sci. Am. **229**:54–66.

17a. Miller, M. E., and V. R. Nilsson. 1974. A major
role of the fifth component of complement (C5)
in the opsonization of yeast particles. Partial
dichotomy of function and immunochemical
measurement. Clin. Immunol. Immunopathol.
2:244–255.

18. Müller-Eberhard, H. J. 1972. The molecular
basis of the biologic activities of complement,
p. 75–104. *In* The Harvey lectures, 1970–71.
Academic Press Inc., New York.

19. Müller-Eberhard, H. J. 1975. Complement.
Ann. Rev. Biochem. **44**:697–724.

20. Rapp, H. J., and T. Borsos. 1970. Molecular
basis of complement action. Appleton-Century-Crofts, New York.

21. Ritchie, R. F., C. A. Alper, J. Graves, N. Pearson, and C. Larson. 1973. Automated quantitation of proteins in serum and other biologic
fluids. Am. J. Clin. Pathol. **59**:151–159.

22. Rosen, F. H., C. A. Alper, J. Pensley, M. R.
Klemperer, and V. H. Donaldson. 1971. Genetically determined heterogeneity of the C1-
esterase inhibitor in patients with hereditary
angioneurotic edema. J. Clin. Invest. **50**:2143–
2149.

23. Ruddy, S., and K. F. Austen. 1970. The complement system in rheumatoid synovitis. I. An
analysis of complement component activities
in rheumatoid synovial fluids. Arthritis
Rheum. **13**:713–723.

24. Ruddy, S., and K. F. Austen. 1975. Complement
and its components, p. 131–157. *In* A. S.
Cohen (ed.), Laboratory diagnostic procedures in the rheumatic diseases. Little,
Brown & Co., Boston.

25. Ruddy, S., I. Gigli, and K. F. Austen. 1972. The
complement system of man. N. Engl. J. Med.
287:489–494, 545–549, 592–596, 642–646.

26. Ruley, E. J., J. Forristal, N. C. Davis, C.
Andres, and C. D. West. 1973. Hypocomplementemia of membranoproliferative nephritis. Dependence of the nephritis factor reaction on properdin factor B. J. Clin. Invest.
52:896–904.

27. Schutte, M., R. DiCamelli, P. Murphy, M. Sa-
dove, and H. Gewurz. 1974. C3 proactivator
(C3PA) as an acute phase reactant. Clin. Exp.
Immunol. **18**:251–256.

28. Stroud, R. M. 1974. Genetic abnormalities of the
complement system of man associated with
disease. Transplant Proc. **6**:59–65.

29. Thompson, R. A., and D. S. Rowe. 1967. Immune haemolysis in agar: demonstration of
the protective action of antibodies. Immunology **13**:411–420.

30. Thompson, R. A., and D. S. Rowe. 1968. Reactive haemolysis — a distinctive form of red cell
lysis. Immunology **14**:745–762.

31. Townes, A. S., C. R. Stewart, Jr., and A. G.
Osler. 1963. Immunologic studies of systemic
lupus erythematosus. Bull. Johns Hopkins
Hosp. **112**:202–219.

32. Vargues, R. M., and W. Henley. 1974. Automation of immune hemolytic and complement
fixation reactions by AutoAnalyzer. Mt. Sinai
J. Med. **41**:1–59.

Section B

TESTS FOR CELLULAR COMPONENTS OF THE IMMUNOLOGICAL RESPONSE

Chapter 5

Introduction

ROSS E. ROCKLIN AND JOHN R. DAVID

This section deals with various techniques currently available for evaluating the cellular components of the immune responses in humans. The cell types which comprise the cellular hypersensitivity reaction include lymphocytes, macrophages, and granulocytes. These techniques are used to assess in vitro cellular function in patients who have certain types of recurrent infections (fungal, mycobacterial, and pyogenic), depressed cellular immunity (sarcoidosis and cancer), and autoimmune disease (glomerulonephritis and thyroiditis).

At present, however, the best in vivo screening procedure that the clinician can employ to evaluate cellular hypersensitivity is still the 24- to 48-h skin test (chapter 6). The development of one or more positive cutaneous responses to environmental antigens such as tuberculin purified protein derivative, monilia, streptokinase-streptodornase, or mumps, or being newly sensitized to a contact allergen such as dinitrochlorobenzene, usually indicates intact cellular immunity. A positive delayed skin test response results from lymphocyte-macrophage interaction as well as certain components of the inflammatory response. In vitro testing in such patients will not usually provide more information. However, polymorphonuclear leukocyte function is not evaluated by delayed hypersensitivity skin testing, and such tests would therefore not detect defects in this system. Failure to respond to a battery of environmental antigens or to be sensitized to a new antigen is referred to as "cutaneous anergy" and is associated with depressed cellular immunity and lowered resistance to infection. Since cutaneous anergy may result from abnormalities in the lymphocyte, the macrophage, or both, the in vitro tests are valuable in defining the level of the defect. The ensuing chapters in this section describe techniques for the qualitative and quantitative evaluation of lymphocyte, macrophage, and polymorphonuclear leukocyte functions. Basophil and eosinophil functions are covered in another section of this book, section G.

The tests which assess lymphocyte function measure surface markers and their ability to proliferate, produce mediators, and mount cytotoxic responses. The enumeration of lymphocyte subpopulations (T cells and B cells) utilizes the observation that unique receptors are present on each cell type. Immunofluorescence techniques are used to identify immunoglobulin receptors on B cells, and rosetting techniques are used for the identification of T cells and B cells (chapter 7). These observations can also be used to develop methods for purifying lymphocyte subpopulations so that the investigator can study each cell type separately (chapter 8).

Lymphocyte proliferative responses can be evaluated by using nonspecific mitogenic stimulants such as phytohemagglutinin, concanavalin A, or pokeweed mitogen, and by specific stimuli such as soluble antigens (chapter 9). The nonspecific activation of lymphocytes measures both T cell and B cell function, although the kinetics of these responses differ. In contrast, specific antigenic challenge appears to measure only T cell function. By using autologous as well as homologous serum in the cultures, one can also determine whether the patient's serum contains factors which may interfere with the proliferative response.

The elaboration of soluble mediators by lymphoctyes indicates that these cells are capable of producing factors which alter the function of a variety of cells involved in cellular immune reactions. Some examples include migration inhibitory factor (chapter 10), leukocyte inhibitory factor (chapter 11), chemotactic factor (chapter 12), lymphotoxin (chapter 13), interferon (chapter 14), and lymphocyte mitogenic factor (chapter 15). The production of these mediators by lymphocytes, as well as their unique biological assay systems, are described in the above chapters. Although the elaboration of these factors can be shown to correlate with in vivo delayed hypersensitivity in humans, they do not necessarily measure the function of a particular cell type (T or B cells).

The mixed lymphocyte culture and cytotoxicity tests, which measure responses to allogeneic antigens on the surface of target cells and are indicators of T cell function, are covered in another section (J).

Whenever possible, the clinician should use more than one in vitro test of lymphocyte function, since each assay may measure a distinct subpopulation of cells. Furthermore, present evidence indicates that lymphocytes are compartmentalized; that is, cells in the blood may be functionally different from those in lymph nodes or spleen. Therefore, sampling blood lymphocytes alone may not yield representative results. An evaluation should include a quantitation of the numbers of T and B cells, proliferative responses to mitogens and specific antigens, measurement of at least one lymphocyte mediator, and a cytotoxic response.

Assessment of macrophage and polymorphonuclear leukocyte function is performed by measuring the ability of these cells to ingest particles, to kill microorganisms, and to respond to certain stimuli by increased directed movement (chemotaxis), by identifying certain surface receptors, and by determining their response to lymphocyte mediators. These procedures are covered in chapters 12, 16, and 17. Chapter 18 is also included in this section to present a comprehensive evaluation of patients with certain viral diseases. This chapter utilizes several of the in vitro cellular assays described in other chapters and demonstrates how the investigator may apply these techniques to a particular problem.

Because of their complexity, these in vitro assays are not routinely carried out in most clinical laboratories and are restricted at present to research centers which specialize in basic and applied investigation. Moreover, because of the nature of these assays, that is, they are biological phenomena and subject to considerable variation, the results should be interpreted with caution. There is a fairly high incidence (10 to 20%) of false-negative values being obtained with these tests. Therefore, in an individual patient a negative result should be repeated once or twice to confirm abnormal cellular function. For this reason, these tests are more useful when applied to the study of groups or populations of patients with certain diseases rather than individual patients. Although they are not usually diagnostic, these tests are of value clinically for the purposes of identifying certain pathogenetic factors and monitoring the results of therapy and the clinical course of patients with depressed cellular function.

Chapter 6

Delayed Hypersensitivity Skin Testing

LYNN E. SPITLER

INTRODUCTION

Skin testing remains by far the most important means currently available for the clinical assessment of the status of cellular immune responses in patients, despite the recent development of newer in vitro techniques. If a red bump (a delayed hypersensitivity[1] reaction) develops at the site of injection of the test antigen, it means that the afferent, central, and efferent limbs of the immune response are intact and also that the patient's ability to mount a nonspecific inflammatory response is intact (16). Few other tests can provide so much information.

The first description of a delayed hypersensitivity reaction was probably that of Jenner, published in 1798, who described the reaction which followed injection of antigen into the arm of a patient who had recovered from cowpox.

Tuberculin reactivity, considered to be the classic example of a delayed hypersensitivity reaction, was recognized almost 100 years later when Koch reported that the injection of tubercle bacilli or an extract of tubercle bacilli into the skin of humans or guinea pigs with tuberculosis caused typical signs of inflammation consisting of rubor, tumor, dolor, and calor with microscopic lesions characteristic of the tuberculous inflammatory process. This has been termed the "Koch phenomenon."

Von Pirquet performed experiments using varying concentrations of tuberculin and recognized that there was a period of latency in the development of the reaction regardless of the concentration used (26).

In 1924–1925, Zinsser distinguished this from other forms of hypersensitivity and recognized that it could take place without antibody. He termed it bacterial allergy and referred to "delayed skin reactions" (27, 28).

[1] In this chapter, the term "delayed hypersensitivity" will be used to refer to the immune response which is characterized by a positive skin test, whereas "cellular immunity" will refer not only to the delayed hypersensitivity reaction but also to the constellation of in vitro parameters which have also come to be associated with this type of response.

Landsteiner and Chase firmly laid the groundwork for our current understanding of the delayed hypersensitivity reaction as a part of cellular immunity by showing that sensitivity to a simple chemical (picryl chloride) could be transferred by means of cells (17). Chase later confirmed this with the transfer of tuberculin reactivity (10), and Lawrence demonstrated that the same phenomenon applied to humans when he transferred reactivity to tuberculin (19) and subsequently to streptococcal antigen (20) using whole leukocytes derived from the peripheral blood.

CLINICAL INDICATIONS

Skin tests are useful in the following circumstances.

To assess whether there is diminished delayed hypersensitivity or anergy in selected patients

There are a number of circumstances in which assessment of the status of delayed hypersensitivity will aid in the diagnosis and/or treatment of a patient. In patients who have usually severe or recurrent infections, or who develop infections with unusual organisms, the question frequently arises as to whether there might be an underlying congenital or acquired defect in delayed hypersensitivity. Skin tests may also be used to assist in diagnosis and evaluation of the patient with a disease associated with a defect in delayed hypersensitivity, such as Hodgkin's disease or sarcoidosis (see full list below). Similarly, an assessment of delayed hypersensitivity may be helpful in determining the prognosis in patients with certain kinds of malignancy since diminished reactivity may be associated with a poorer prognosis.

Screening for anergy should also be performed in children with conditions known to be associated with defective delayed hypersensitivity. These include patients with hypoparathyroidism and cardiac disease, known to be associated with the Di George syndrome, those with telangiectasia, ataxia, and absent immunoglobulin A, known to be associated with ataxia telangiectasis, and those with thrombocytopenia and eczema, known to be associated with the Wiskott-Aldrich syndrome.

In all of the above examples, the standard procedure is to apply a panel of skin test antigens in an intermediate test strength; if the results with the intermediate strength are negative, a higher test strength of the antigen is applied. The antigens selected for this purpose are those to which the patients are commonly exposed, and therefore most normal subjects will respond to at least some of the antigens. Apparent lack of reactivity could occur in patients who actually have normal delayed hypersensitivity in the following circumstances:

1. Choice of antigens, application of the tests, or reading of the test may be inappropriate. This can be avoided by careful attention to technique as described below.

2. The patient might not have been exposed to the test antigens. This will rarely, if ever, be the case with adult subjects being tested with common antigens, such as candida, coccidioidin, mumps, purified protein derivative of tuberculin (PPD), streptokinase-streptodornase (SK-SD), and trichophyton, but it could occur in children. If this is a concern, it is possible to gain more information by sensitizing the patient to an agent known to cause delayed hypersensitivity, such as dinitrochlorobenzene (DNCB) or keyhole limpet hemocyanin (11), and subsequently testing for reactivity by applying a test dose of the same antigen. Another test which may be of value in this circumstance is the use of the phytohemagglutinin (PHA) skin test (3, 5, 18). This test seems especially useful for evaluation of immunodeficiency in infants and children, but it has been less useful for the evaluation of adults and is not an approved procedure.

3. The patient may have a condition in the skin which precludes demonstration of a positive response (atopic dermatitis may represent such a condition), or there may be a defect in the nonspecific inflammatory response. Perhaps the latter is the case in some patients with malignancy. One means of assessing whether the inflammatory response is intact is by the application of croton oil; however, since this substance is recognized to be a co-carcinogen, its use for this purpose cannot be recommended. Another agent which can be used to assess the nonspecific inflammatory response is sodium lauryl sulfate (W. L. Epstein, in preparation). Since this is not a co-carcinogen, and it produces positive results in over 90% of normal subjects, its use is recommended rather than croton oil, which is more commonly used for this

purpose. If there is a strong suspicion that the lack of skin test reactivity may be due to local conditions or lack of inflammatory response, it may be necessary to perform in vitro studies to gain additional information as to the status of the patient's cellular immune system.

4. A strong immediate reaction at the site of injection of the test antigen may result in a false-negative delayed reaction. This should be suspected if there is a strong immediate reaction and absent delayed reaction. Local or systemic administration of antihistamines may suppress the immediate reaction and permit visualization of the delayed reaction (6). Others have been unable to confirm this work (23).

To assess the results of immunotherapy

Skin tests remain the best means of assessing the results of attempts to increase the cellular immune response with agents such as transfer factor, levamisole, or BCG. It is important in this regard to be sure that the second-strength antigens are applied if testing with the intermediate strength produces a negative result. Administration of transfer factor usually causes conversion only of reactions to second-strength antigens and not to intermediate-strength antigens.

To follow the course of the disease process

There are a number of diseases in which disease activity and/or dissemination of disease is associated with loss of skin test reactivity to antigen of the infecting organism. Return of skin reactivity to the infecting organism is associated with recovery. Coccidioidomycosis is an example of such a disease. Patients with progressive or disseminated disease will frequently have a negative skin test to intermediate (1:100) and second (1:10) strength coccidioidin. During the course of therapy with amphotericin B, conversion of the skin test to positive is often the first sign heralding clinical improvement. In this regard, it is important always to apply the intermediate-strength test antigen before proceeding to the second-strength test, even if the second-strength test was previously negative, because a severe local reaction could occur to the second-strength antigen if the patient has regained reactivity. This phenomenon also has been observed in candidiasis.

TEST PROCEDURES

Skin testing is an important aspect in the evaluation of patients for possible defects in cellular immunity. The keys to success in the use of these tests to determine whether there is a defect in delayed hypersensitivity are as follows:

1. Use the complete battery of six skin test antigens.

2. Repeat the test in higher antigen concentration when the tests are negative with the intermediate strength.

3. Carefully observe and record the results in millimeters of erythema and induration at 24 and 48 h. This will aid future observers much more than a simple recording of positive or negative.

Skin tests

1. Question the patient as to whether he has ever had skin tests in the past and whether he has ever had a severe local reaction to such a test. Patients frequently have previously had skin tests for tuberculosis, and occasionally one will recall having had a severe local response. Also question the patient as to whether he has had tuberculosis or BCG vaccination. Inquire about places of residence for tests with histoplasmin, blastomycin, and coccidioidin.

2. Prepare syringes containing antigens. If there is not history of a severe local reaction and no history of tuberculosis or BCG vaccination, it is appropriate to administer the tests in the intermediate strength (see below, Reagents). If there is reason to suspect that the patient may be unusually sensitive to one or more of the antigens, this antigen should first be applied in a lower concentration (first test strength or a dilution thereof). An example of a panel of antigens commonly used to screen for anergy is the following: candida (dermatophyton O), 1:100; coccidioidin, 1:100; mumps; PPD, 5 tuberculin units (TU) (0.2 µg); SK-SD, 4 U/1 U of test dose; and trichophyton (dermatophyton), 1:30 (see below, Reagents).

Use a separate, sterile 1-ml tuberculin syringe with a 0.5-inch 27-gauge needle for each injection. Label each syringe with the name of the antigen it will contain. Draw a little over 0.1 ml of the antigen solution into the syringe and express air bubbles with tapping, so that needle is filled and 0.1 ml of solution remains in the syringe. Be sure that the needle is filled; it will hold almost 0.05 ml so that inadequate filling would result in injection of less than the appropriate test dose.

3. Examine the patient and choose an appropriate location for injection of the test antigen. Usually, the forearms are the most convenient place for such injections. Occasionally, the arms may be involved in the disease process (as in patients with mucocutaneous candidiasis, Wiskott-Aldrich syndrome, or atopic dermatitis), in which case it is necessary to choose some other area which is free from disease, such as the back.

Clean the selected area with a sterile alcohol swab and allow to dry. It is convenient always to inject the series of antigens in the same order (such as in alphabetical order) to avoid confusion in reading which test was at which site. Insert the tip of the needle, bevel up, just underneath the surface of the skin, and inject 0.1 ml of the antigen solution (intracutaneous injection). This should result in a bleb about 5 to 10 mm in diameter. If the injection is associated with a flat area with flat pseudopods radiating out, it indicates that there was air present in the needle. If no bleb is formed, it indicates that the injection was subcutaneous rather than intracutaneous and should be repeated at another site. Circle the site of the injection with a circle about 5 cm in diameter, using an indelible marking pencil. If the tests are not being done regularly in a standard order, also label each circle with the code for the test antigen (Fig. 1). Instruct the patient not to wash off the circles until the tests are completed.

4. Read and record results 24 h later. Measure the diameter of erythema and of induration in two directions, and record each in millimeters (e.g., erythema = 10×12 mm, induration = 8×9 mm). A form convenient for these records is illustrated in Fig. 2. If there is a very large reaction, the true extent of the reaction may sometimes be missed and only the central area of increased reactivity is observed; observe the entire area carefully in making readings. Occasionally, in black-skinned individuals it may not be possible to see the erythema, and it is necessary to rely solely on induration in making the readings.

5. Apply second-strength antigens if the 24-h readings are negative for intermediate-strength antigen. For the antigens listed in the panel, second test strengths are available for the following: candida 1:10, coccidioidin 1:10, PPD 250 TU (5.0 µg), and SK-SD 40/10. If the patient shows less than 5 mm of erythema and induration 24 h after the injection of the intermediate-strength antigen, the second strength may be applied. (Some physicians may wish to wait until the 48-h readings are obtained before applying the second-test strength. In my experience, applying the second strength when the intermediate test is negative at 24 h has not resulted in severe local reactions, and it has the advantage of saving 1 day in the evaluation, which may be especially important for patients

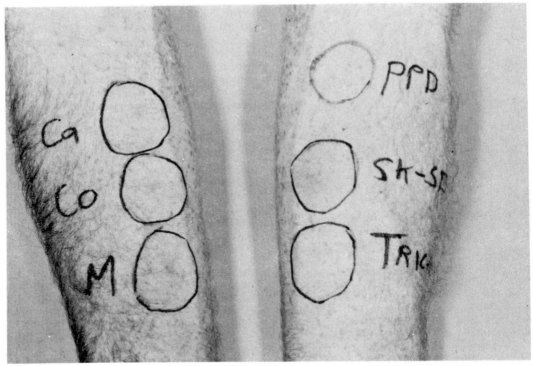

FIG. 1. *Application of skin tests.*

who are traveling considerable distances for the evaluation.)

Label and fill the syringes as described above. It is convenient to inject the second test strength of the antigen next to and about 4 cm from the intermediate-strength test to avoid confusion as to the location of the various test antigens. Circle and label the sites as above.

Dinitrochlorobenzene sensitization

Note: Food and Drug Administration (FDA) approval is required.

WEAR DISPOSABLE PROTECTIVE GLOVES DURING PROCEDURE. The sensitization and testing procedure described below is a slight modification of the method described by Epstein and Kligman (13) and may produce severe local reactions in immunologically normal subjects. Therefore, it should only be performed in selected subjects in whom immunological deficiency is strongly suspected, for example, in subjects who show no response to the panel of intermediate-strength skin tests antigens. For routine testing of patients who may have good immunological reactivity (such as patients with early stages of malignancy), use of a lower sensitizing dose of DNCB is recommended.

1. Dissolve DNCB in acetone in a concentra-

tion of 10 mg/ml (sensitizing solution). This may be kept in a refrigerator in a foil-wrapped or light-impenetrable bottle for a period up to 2 weeks, but must be freshly prepared every 2 weeks.

2. Cleanse the medial aspect of the upper arm with alcohol, and apply 0.2 ml of the sensitizing solution (a total of 2 mg of DNCB) within a metal ring 2 to 3 cm in diameter. Allow to dry with gentle blowing. Cover with a Band-Aid.

3. Instruct the patient to remove the Band-Aid 24 h later and to watch the area for a spontaneous flare reaction at about 10 to 14 days after the application. This would consist of erythema with or without induration and vesicle formation.

4. Fourteen days later, prepare test solutions of DNCB in acetone in the following concentrations: 500, 250, 150, and 50 μg/ml. Ask the patient whether or not a flare occurred, examine the sensitizing site, and record the response. If a strong flare occurred, use only the lower doses of the test solutions. Cleanse the forearm with alcohol, and apply 0.2 ml of the DNCB test solutions within the 2- to 3-cm ring at separate sites (test doses applied = 100, 50, 30, and 10 μg). Air-dry as above and cover with Band-Aids.

5. If possible, examine the test sites 2, 4, and 6

NAME: _____
Date: _____

ADDRESS: _____

PHONE: _____

HOSPITAL NUMBER: _____

REFERRED BY: _____

ADDRESS: _____

PHONE: _____

DIAGNOSIS: _____

	INTERMEDIATE TEST STRENGTH				SECOND TEST STRENGTH			
	24°		48°		24°		48°	
	ERY	IND	ERY	IND	ERY	IND	ERY	IND
CANDIDA 1:100			1:10					
COCCI 1:100			1:10					
MUMPS								
PPD INTERMED.			2nd					
SK - SD 4/1			40/10					
TRICHOPHYTIN 1:30								

REMARKS: _____

_____

_____

_____

_____

FIG. 2. *Form for recording results of skin tests.*

days after application of the test doses. Record results as follows: 0, no reaction; 1+, erythema only; 2+, erythema with induration; 3+, vesicles, erythema, and induration; 4+, bullae and/or ulceration.

If it is not possible to examine the test sites on 3 separate days, examine the site on the *4th* day after application of the test solutions. (*Note:* This is different in timing than examining the usual intradermal delayed sensitivity skin tests, which are read at 24 and 48 h after application.)

6. If results of the 2-week reading are negative, repeat the application and reading of the test doses 2 weeks later (1 month after sensitizing dose).

Nonspecific inflammatory response: sodium lauryl sulfate

WEAR DISPOSABLE PROTECTIVE GLOVES DURING PROCEDURE.

1. Make up a stock solution of sodium lauryl sulfate in saline in a concentration of 100 mg/ml. Store in a refrigerator.

2. For use, prepare a 1:10 dilution of the stock solution (10 mg/ml).

3. Prepare a 2.0-cm square of nonwoven cotton cloth (Webril, Curity) and saturate it with 0.5 ml of the 10-mg/ml sodium lauryl sulfate solution.

4. Cleanse the skin of the forearm with alcohol, and press the saturated gauze firmly to the skin.

5. Apply overlapping strips of impermeable plastic tape (3M Blenderm). Further buttress

the patch with overlapping strips of Micropore or Dermiclear tape (Johnson & Johnson Co.) followed by wrapping with Webril. In hot weather, take the further precaution of spraying the skin around the patch with Aeroplast Spray-on Bandage (Parke-Davis & Co.) before sealing with 3M Blenderm. Complete occlusion is imperative.

6. Remove the dressing 48 h later. Record results as positive if erythema and induration are present and negative if there is no reaction.

REAGENTS

The first six antigens, listed here with their trade names, strengths (intermediate followed by second), and source, represent a standard panel which may be used for assessing anergy:

1. Candida, Dermatophyton O; 1:100, 1:10; Hollister-Stier Laboratories, Spokane, Wash.

2. Cocci (25), Coccidioidin; 1:100, 1:10; Cutter Laboratories, Berkeley, Calif.

3. Mumps (2, 12); Eli Lilly & Co., Indianapolis, Ind. At the present time, the mumps skin test antigen is no longer available from Eli Lilly & Co. We find that over 90% of normal adult subjects react to staphylococcus antigen (a 1:5 dilution of Staphage lysate; Delmont Laboratories, Inc., Swarthmore, Pa.), and we have substituted this antigen in the panel.

4. PPD (15), PPD stabilized solution; 50 TU/ml (test dose = 5 TU); Parke-Davis & Co., Detroit, Mich. PPD, PPD stabilized solution; 2,500 U/ml (test dose = 250 TU); Panray Division, Ormont Drug and Chemical Co., Inc., Englewood, N.J.

5. SK-SD, Varidase; 40 U/10 U per ml (test dose = 4 U/1 U), 400 U/100 U per ml (test dose = 40 U/10 U); Lederle Laboratories, Div. American Cyanamid Co., Pearl River, N.Y. This preparation is marketed as a product for fibrinolytic activity. FDA approval may be required for use for the purpose of skin testing.

6. Trichophyton, Dermatophyton; 1:30; Hollister-Stier Laboratories.

For further evaluation of possible anergy, the following tests may also be helpful. (*Note:* Some of these preparations are approved and marketed as vaccines rather than as skin test antigens. FDA approval may be required for their use for the purpose of skin testing.

Aspergillus (Aspergillus mixed antigen), Allermed, San Diego, Calif.

Candida antigen, 1:1,000, Allermed.

DNCB (1-chloro-2,4-dinitrobenzene), 10 mg/ml

(sensitizing dose = 2 mg), 500 μg/ml (test dose = 100 μg), 250 μg/ml (test dose = 50 μg), 150 μg/ml (test dose = 30 μg), 50 μg/ml (test dose = 10 μg), K & K Laboratories, Inc., Plainview, N.Y.

Mixed respiratory vaccine (MRV): *Staphylococcus aureus, Streptococcus, Diplococcus pneumoniae, Neisseria catarrhalis, Klebsiella pneumoniae,* and *Haemophilus influenzae,* 1:10, Hollister-Stier Laboratories

Monilia antigen, 1:500, Hollister-Stier Laboratories

PHA (phytohemagglutinin), 10 μg/ml (test dose = 1 μg), 50 μg/ml (test dose = 5 μg), Burroughs-Wellcome Co., Tuckahoe, N.Y.

Sodium lauryl sulfate, 10 mg/ml

Staphyloccal toxoid, 100 U/ml, 1,000 U/ml, 10,000 U/ml, Lederle Laboratories

Sources for other antigens which may prove useful in selected patients are as follows:

Diphtheria, Diphtheria Toxin Test Kit, Massachusetts Institute of Public Health, Jamaica Plains, Boston, Mass.

Histoplasmin, Parke-Davis & Co., Detroit, Mich.

Lymphogranuloma venereum, Lederle Laboratories

Staphylococcus, Staphage lysate (21), Delmont Laboratories, Inc., Swarthmore. Pa.

Tetanus toxoid (14), Wyeth Biological Laboratories, Marietta, Pa.

Trichinella extract, Lederle Laboratories

Tularemia (7), Chief, Immunobiologics Activity, Biologic Reagents Section, Center for Disease Control, Atlanta, Ga.

The use of some of the above antigens for diagnostic purposes has recently been reviewed (8, 24). We know of no commercial source for the following skin tests: actinomycosis, atypical mycobacteria including PPD-F, PPD-G, and PPD-B (Battey), aspergillosis, blastomycin, brucellosis, cat scratch fever, cryptococcosis, dharmendra, echinococcus, leishmaniasis, lepromin, sporotrichosis, or toxoplasmosis.

NOTES ON THE ANTIGENS

Candida

There are two preparations of candida antigen available from Hollister-Stier Laboratories. One, called monilia antigen, is prepared by grinding the organism. This antigen is generally used for testing for immediate sensitivity. The other is the preparation called Dermatophyton O, which is prepared from a culture filtrate of the organism in a manner analogous to the preparation of PPD. It is the preparation most

commonly used for delayed hypersensitivity testing. This preparation should not be confused with Dermatophyton, which is also produced by Hollister-Stier and contains trichophyton antigens.

Streptokinase-streptodornase

The SK-SD is a preparation used in patients for its fibrinolytic activity. However, the preparation contains the streptococcal antigens, and, when appropriately diluted, the fibrinolytic activity is insignificant and the antigens are ideal for skin testing. For the intermediate-strength tests, the preparation is diluted so that it contains 40 U of SK and 10 U of SD per ml. Thus, the injected dose in 0.1 ml will be 4 U of SK and 1 U of SD. For the second-strength test, the solution contains 400 U of SK and 100 U of SD/ml. It is the procedure in many laboratories to allow the solution to remain in a refrigerator for 2 days before use to allow the fibrinolytic activity to diminish. The antigenic activity remains, however, and appears to be stable for several months.

Purified protein derivative

In the past, PPD was regularly supplied in the form of tablets to be dissolved in a diluent before use. It has now been recognized that, once these tablets are redissolved, the PPD will adhere to the glass of the bottle, and the solution will undergo a progressive loss of potency. Accordingly, it is necessary that these solutions be freshly prepared for use. Alternately, a preparation is now available to which Tween-80 has been added. This solution, termed "PPD stabilized solution," is stable for prolonged periods.

Coccidioidin

Coccidioidin is included in the standard test panel because the author of this chapter works in the West, where it is a useful antigen. Accordingly, all results were analyzed with this included. Since reactivity to the intermediate strength of this antigen is fairly low (19%), the analysis of results using the panel would probably only be slightly changed if coccidioidin were not included in the panel.

Dinitrochlorobenzene

It should be noted that the time of maximal response to DNCB is usually not 48 h as it is for the intradermal skin tests, but rather is 4 days after application of the test dose; thus, a positive response might be missed if the test site is examined only at 48 h (W. L. Epstein, personal communication). Moreover, in examining the time course of sensitization, Epstein noted that some normal subjects did not show conversion of reactivity until 3 or 4 weeks after application of the sensitizing dose. Thus, although it is convenient and standard practice to test patients 2 weeks after the sensitizing dose, it is recommended that, if this test is negative, the test be repeated 2 weeks later to test for a later conversion.

Since application of the 2-mg sensitizing dose may result in a severe local reaction in subjects whose delayed hypersensitivity is not generally or seriously impaired, it may be desirable to use a lower sensitizing dose in these subjects or first to do the challenge test. The percentage of normal subjects showing a positive response to a test dose of 250 μg 1 month after sensitization with various doses of DNCB are as follows (13), with sensitizing dose followed by percentage: 25 μg (5%), 100 μg (16%), 250 μg (62%), 0.5 mg (62%), 2.5 mg (91%), 25 mg (89%), 50 mg (87%).

The antigens described (except DNCB) all appear to be relatively stable in solution and can be kept in a refrigerator for periods up to 1 year. To prevent contamination, a solution containing phenol as a preservative is usually used for preparing the dilution, recognizing that phenol itself may occasionally cause delayed hypersensitivity reactions.

COMPLICATIONS OF TESTING

Occasional patients who are very sensitive will have severe local reactions at the test site. These include pain, erythema, and induration, and there may be blister formation and necrosis. Scar formation and/or hyperpigmentation may result. There may be associated epitroclear or axillary adenopathy which is usually tender. Systemic effects, including fever and tachycardia, may occur rarely. The occurrence of severe local reactions is reduced by using the intermediate test strength antigens first (or lower strengths if the patient has a history suggesting that he may react strongly). This is followed by the second-strength test only if the intermediate test is negative. Severe local reactions may be well controlled by the local injection of steroids, such as a dilute solution of Kenalog (inject intracutaneously 0.2 to 0.5 ml of a solution containing 0.25 mg/ml). Systemic administration of a short course of steroids will also be effective but is rarely, if ever, necessary.

INTERPRETATION

What constitutes a positive response?

For the purposes described in this chapter, i.e., to determine whether or not the patient has delayed hypersensitivity to the test antigen, *a positive response is considered to consist of 5 mm or more of induration at the test site 48 h after injection of the test antigen.* It should be noted that such a reaction may not always represent a delayed hypersensitivity reaction (it could be the remnants of a previous arthus or other type of reaction); however, the only reliable way to distinguish these possibilities is through biopsy of the test site, which is not practical on a routine basis.

The package insert for the mumps skin test antigen indicates that a positive reaction is considered to be 15 mm of erythema. This is because previous studies showed that subjects with this reactivity were immune to the development of mumps, whereas those with negative reactions were susceptible. Since the purpose for which we are now using the skin test is usually not to determine susceptibility to disease but rather to determine the presence or absence of a delayed hypersensitivity reaction, it seems reasonable to accept 5 mm of induration as a positive response for this antigen, as it is for the other antigens.

What constitutes a diminished delayed hypersensitivity response or anergy?

For individual *adult* patients, diminished delayed hypersensitivity may be considered to exist if:

1. The patient shows positive responses (5 mm of induration) to fewer than two of the panel of six skin test antigens described above. The defect is more profound if the patient also shows lack of reactivity to second-strength antigens.

2. There is diminished strength of reactivity, i.e., if the *total* sum of millimeters of induration resulting from all six test antigens at 48 h after testing is less than 10.

3. The patient does not become sensitized after administration of DNCB.

Details regarding the above conclusions are as follows. Skin test reactivity was determined in 100 *adult* subjects including normal subjects and patients hospitalized for diseases not known to be associated with diminished delayed hypersensitivity.

Percentage of responses to individual antigens (Table 1). Mumps represents the best single antigen for evaluation for anergy, with SK-SD the next best. It is commonly believed that candida and trichophyton antigens represent good test antigens for the evaluation of anergy; however, this was not the case in this study. The candida antigen used in testing the control subjects reported herein was Dermato-

TABLE 1. *Skin test reactivity to intermediate- and second-strength test antigens in 100 control subjects*

Antigen	Intermediate strength (%)[a]	Second strength (%)[b]
Candida	39	92
Coccidioidin	19	45
Mumps	78	—
PPD	26	83
SK-SD	55	93
Trichophyton ...	28	—

[a] Numbers represent percentage of subjects showing 5 mm of induration at the test site 48 h after injection of the test antigen.

[b] Numbers represent percentage of subjects showing positive response to the intermediate-strength or, if negative, to the second-strength test antigen.

phyton O. This was selected originally because it is the antigen which has been most widely used for this purpose and also because the preparation was analogous to the preparation of PPD. Indeed, this preparation was useful for assessing delayed hypersensitivity, but it was found that only 39% of normal subjects responded to the intermediate-strength test dose. If subjects who did not show reactivity to the intermediate-strength test were then tested with the second test strength (1:10), over 90% were shown to respond (see below). Charles Kirkpatrick, however, reports that 27 of 32, or 84%, of normal subjects responded to the 1:100 dilution of Dermatophyton O (personal communication).

Other candida preparations have been tested. There has been no study in which the various preparations were compared. Palmer and Reed (22) used a 1:500 dilution of the Hollister-Stier preparation of monilia and reported that 63% of 752 hospitalized patients showed a positive response of 5 mm of induration. Antonino Catanzaro reports that about 75% of normal subjects show a positive response to a 1:1,000 dilution of the candida antigen prepared by Allermed (personal communication).

This variation may, in part, represent differences in reactivity in populations in different parts of the country, but more likely reflects differences in the antigens used. These results stress the importance of appropriate testing of a control group of subjects in the same location with the same lot of antigen when comparing response rates in various groups rather than relying on literature references for controls. Percentage responses to individual antigens are useful only when comparing groups of patients, not for evaluating individual subjects, since an individual may well lack prior exposure to individual antigens. For evaluating individuals for diminished delayed hypersensitivity, evaluation of responses to a panel of antigens (described below) is necessary.

Evaluation of the number of responses to the panel of six test antigens (Fig. 3). Occurrence of 5 mm of induration at 48 h is considered a positive response, and the number of positive responses to the panel of six antigens is counted. As indicated in Fig. 3, more than 90% of the normal population will show a response to two or more antigens. Accordingly, the delayed sensitivity response is considered to be diminished if the individual responds to fewer than two antigens.

Evaluation of the strength of skin test reactivity (Fig. 4). The mean of the recordings of the two diameter readings of millimeters of induration at the test site 48 h after injection of the test antigen is determined for each antigen. These means are summed. As shown in Fig. 4, over 90% of the normal population will show reactions totaling 10 mm of induration or more. Accordingly, a sum of less than 10 indicates diminished reactivity.

DNCB reaction. Occurrence of a spontaneous flare at the site of application of the sensitizing dose of DNCB indicates a positive response. There is a wide variation in the incidence of spontaneous flare in normal subjects. Epstein has found that this occurs in 20% of subjects (personal communication), whereas Catalona et al. reported it to be present in 97% of normal subjects (9). A positive response to the test dose of DNCB is considered to be a reaction of 2+ or more. That is, there must be induration and/or vesicle formation. Erythema alone does not constitute a positive response. A

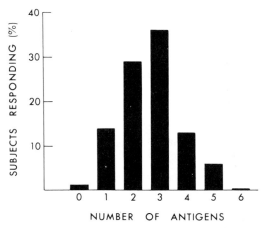

FIG. 3. *Skin test reactivity in 76 normal subjects.*

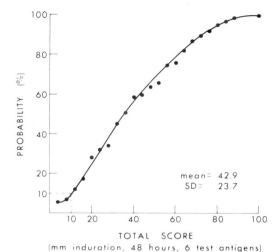

FIG. 4. *Evaluation of strength of skin test reactivity in 76 normal subjects.*

positive response to the 100-μg test dose of DNCB will occur in 90 to 100% of normal subjects.

Recently, methods have been described for performance of the DNCB test in a quantitative fashion (4, 9). Although these approaches certainly are appealing, they are not really practical for the routine testing of patients. The method of Catalona et al. requires that the subjects be examined daily for 16 days, whereas the method of Bleumink uses reagents and methods uncommon in the United States. Use of a series of test doses of DNCB as described herein is recommended to provide quantitative information regarding the patient's reactivity.

PHA response. The test produces a reaction similar in timing and appearance to that produced by other skin test antigens. On biopsy, the cellular infiltrate is also characteristic of a delayed hypersensitivity reaction (3). A positive response (5 mm of induration) to the 1-μg test dose of PHA is shown by 92 to 100% of normal infants, children, and adults (18). In children with immunodeficiency diseases, there is a fairly good correlation between diminished PHA response and other parameters of cellular immunity; however, there are notable exceptions in which reactivity or lack of reactivity did not correlate with other parameters (3, 5, 16). In adult subjects with disorders associated with anergy (e.g., sarcoidosis, Hodgkin's disease, etc.), there is a poor or no correlation between anergy and lack of PHA response (3, 5).

Results in children. There are few studies of the incidence of positive delayed hypersensitivity responses in children of various ages. It has

been shown that newborns may respond to DNCB by 2 to 3 weeks of age (5). Skin reactivity to candida is low before 7 to 8 months.

What causes diminished delayed sensitivity or anergy?

The conditions associated with diminished delayed hypersensitivity or anergy can be summarized as follows:

Hodgkin's disease
Sarcoidosis
Congenital immunodeficiency disease
    Severe combined immunodeficiency disease
    DiGeorge syndrome
    Nezelof's syndrome
    Ataxia telangiectasia
    Wiskott-Aldrich syndrome
    Mucocutaneous candidiasis
    Immunodeficiency with short-limbed dwarfism
    Immunodeficiency with cartilage-hair hypoplasia
Immunosuppressive therapy
Steroid therapy
Uremia
Radiation therapy
Acute leukemia
Advanced age
Infections
    Viral
        Mumps
        Infectious mononucleosis
        Rubella
        Influenza
        Measles
        Varicella
    Bacterial
        Tuberculosis
        Leprosy
        Products of gram-negative bacilli
    Fungal
        Coccidioidomycosis
        Aspergillosis
        Cryptococcosis
Viral vaccination
    Measles
    Polio
    Yellow fever
    Rubella
    Mumps
    Smallpox
Leukocytosis
Hypothyroidism
Vitamin C (ascorbic acid) deficiency
Malignancy (other than those listed above)
Iron deficiency
Liver disease
    Primary biliary cirrhosis

Active chronic hepatitis
Laennec's cirrhosis
Intestinal lymphangiectasia
Hypnosis
Immobilization
Immunodeficiency with thymoma
Immunological amnesia
Protein calorie malnutrition
Conditions in which delayed hypersensitivity is intact or reports conflict
Graves disease
Chronic lymphocytic leukemia
Rheumatoid arthritis
Systemic lupus erythematosis
Chronic marijuana use

Hodgkin's disease is by far the most outstanding cause of anergy in adults. In general, the occurrence of diminished reactivity is correlated with the stage of disease activity, but it may occur early in the course of disease. The degree of anergy may be profound in these patients, and this is one group where one may not observe any reactivity to either the intermediate- or second-strength antigens. By contrast, in sarcoidosis, anergy occurs in less than one-third of the patients. Accordingly, observation of positive skin test responses in a patient suspected of having sarcoidosis in no way eliminates this disease as a diagnosis.

ACKNOWLEDGMENTS

I am the recipient of National Institutes of Health Research Career Development Award AI 43012. This work was supported by Public Health Service grants AI 10686, NS 12133, and MS 777-B-2.

LITERATURE CITED

1. Aisenberg, A. C. 1966. Manifestations of immunologic unresponsiveness in Hodgkin's disease. Cancer Res. 26:1152–1160.

2. Angle, R. M. 1961. The use of mumps skin test antigen. J. Am. Med. Assoc. 177:126–127.

3. Blaese, R. M., P. Weiden, J. J. Oppenheim, and T. A. Waldmann. 1973. Phytohemagglutinin as a skin test for the evaluation of cellular immune competence in man. J. Lab. Clin. Med. 81:538–548.

4. Bleumink, E., J. P. Nater, S., Koops, and T. H. The. 1974. A standard method for DNCB sensitization testing in patients with neoplasms. Cancer 33:911–915.

5. Bonforte, R. J., M. Topilsky, L. E. Siltzbach, and P. R. Glade. 1972. Phytohemagglutinin skin test: a possible in vivo measure of cell-mediated immunity. J. Pediat. 81:775–780.

6. Brostoff, J., and I. M. Roitt. 1969. Cell-mediated (delayed) hypersensitivity in patients with summer hay-fever. Lancet 2:1269–1272.

7. Buchanan, T. M., G. F. Brooks, and P. S. Brachman. 1971. The tularemia skin test. Ann. Intern. Med. 74:336–343.

8. Buechner, H. A., J. H. Seabury, C. C. Campbell, L. K. Georg, L. Kaufman, and W. Kaplan. 1973. The current status of serologic, immunologic and skin tests in the diagnosis of pulmonary mycoses. Chest 63:259–270.

9. Catalona, W. J., P. T. Taylor, and P. B. Chretien. 1972. Quantitative dinitrochlorobenzene contact sensitization in a normal population. Clin. Exp. Immunol. 12:325–333.

10. Chase, M. W. 1945. The cellular transfer of cutaneous hypersensitivity to tuberculin. Proc. Soc. Exp. Biol. Med. 59:134–135.

11. Curtis, J. E., E. M. Hersh, J. E. Harris, C. McBride, and E. J. Freireich. 1970. The human primary immune response to keyhole limpet haemocyanin: interrelationships of delayed hypersensitivity, antibody response and in vitro blast transformation. Clin. Exp. Immunol. 6:473–491.

12. Enders, J. F., S. Cohen, and L. W. Kane. 1945. Immunity in mumps. II. The development of complement-fixing antibody and dermal hypersensitivity in human beings following mumps. J. Exp. Med. 81:119–135.

13. Epstein, W. L., and A. M. Kligman. 1958. The interference phenomenon in allergic contact dermatitis. J. Invest. Dermatol. 31:103–108.

14. Facktor, M. A., R. A. Bernstein, and P. Fireman. 1973. Hypersensitivity to tetanus toxoid. J. Allergy Clin. Immunol. 52:1–12.

15. Holden, M., M. R. Dubin, and P. H. Diamond. 1971. Frequency, of negative intermediate-strength tuberculin sensitivity in patients with active tuberculosis. N. Engl. J. Med. 285:1506–1509.

16. Johnson, M. W., H. I. Maibach, S. E. Salmon. 1971. Skin reactivity in patients with cancer. Impaired delayed hypersensitivity or faulty inflammatory response? N. Engl. J. Med. 284:1255–1257.

17. Landsteiner, K., and M. W. Chase. 1942. Experiments on transfer of cutaneous sensitivity to simple compounds. Proc. Soc. Exp. Biol. Med. 49:688–690.

18. Lawlor, G. J., Jr., E. R. Stiehm, M. S. Kaplan, D. P. S. Sengar, and P. I. Terasaki. 1973. Phytohemagglutinin (PHA) skin test in the diagnosis of cellular immunodeficiency. J. Allergy Clin. Immunol. 52:31–37.

19. Lawrence, H. S. 1949. The cellular transfer of cutaneous hypersensitivity to tuberculin in man. Proc. Soc. Exp. Biol. Med. 71:516–522.

20. Lawrence, H. S. 1952. The cellular transfer in humans of delayed cutaneous reactivity to hemolytic streptococci. J. Immunol. 68:159–178.

21. Mudd, S., J. H. Taubler, and A. G. Baker. 1970. Delayed-type hypersensitivity to *Staphylococcus aureus* in human subjects. RES, J. Reticuloendothel. Soc. 8:493–498.

22. Palmer, D. L., and W. P. Reed. 1974. Delayed hypersensitivity skin testing. I. Response rates in a hospitalized population. J. Infect. Dis. 130:132–137.

23. Rocklin, R. E., H. Pence, H. Kaplan, and R. Evans. 1974. Cell-mediated immune response

of ragweed-sensitive patients to ragweed antigen E. J. Clin. Invest. **53:**735–744.

24. Salvin, S. B. 1963. Immunologic aspects of the mycosis. Prog. Allergy **7:**213–331.

25. Smith, C. E., E. G. Whiting, E. E. Baker, H. G. Rosenberger, R. R. Beard, and M. T. Saito. 1948. The use of coccidioidin. Am. Rev. Tuberc. **57:**330–360.

26. Von Pirquet, C. F. 1909/10. Quantitative experiments with the cutaneous tuberculin reaction. J. Pharmacol. Exp. Ther. **1:**151–174.

27. Zinsser, H. 1924. Bacterial allergy and tissue reactions. Proc. Soc. Exp. Biol. Med. **22:**35–39.

28. Zinsser, H., and J. H. Mueller. 1925. On the nature of bacterial allergies. J. Exp. Med. **41:**159–177.

Chapter 7

Methods for Enumerating Lymphocyte Populations

R. J. WINCHESTER AND G. ROSS

INTRODUCTION

Despite the seeming morphological uniformity of lymphocytes, the methods described in this chapter make possible the division of these cells into several subpopulations on the basis of differing surface structures that serve as population markers. The typical B lymphocyte (1, 15, 18) has readily detectable membrane immunoglobulin (mIg) and receptors for complement and the Fc region of IgG. B lymphocytes account for 1 to 15% of all peripheral blood lymphocytes. These markers are absent from typical T cells. T lymphocytes are recognized by formation of rosettes with sheep erythrocytes (E rosettes), a property not shared by B lymphocytes. Such T cells comprise approximately 75 to 85% of peripheral blood lymphocytes. This broad division of peripheral blood lymphocytes into typical T and B cells thus accounts for all but perhaps 5 to 15% of peripheral blood lymphocytes.

There is some difference of opinion about the nature and characteristics of the cell populations comprising this remainder, with evidence for heterogeneous populations that cannot be classified as either B or T cells. For example, a number of findings demonstrate a lymphoid cell population characterized by readily demonstrable Fc receptors and an absence of mIg, but with the property of forming E rosettes. Also, the K lymphocytes that have been defined in functional terms as the effector cells for antibody-dependent cell-mediated cytolysis are found among these cells. K cells express both complement and Fc receptors but lack IgG. Another example of a minor cell population is the lymphoid cell without any detectable markers; these are usually termed "null cells." It is clear, however, that the significance of a null cell population is dependent both on the number of markers assayed and on the sensitivity of the methods used. The section on Interpretation contains additional comments on these special populations.

There are two broad kinds of problems that recur in the methods used in this chapter and in the interpretation of their results. The first is how to measure unambiguously the presence of a particular marker without technical interference, and the second is the proper inference concerning lymphocyte type that is to be made from the finding of a given marker. The latter problem relates in particular to the minor cell populations. In general, there has been considerable progress in the delineation of solutions to these problems.

The choice of methods used to determine surface markers at the present time represents, to some degree, a compromise between technically demanding investigative procedures and the practical requirements of a clinically oriented laboratory. This is particularly true for B cell evaluation. For example, there are two entirely distinct complement receptors that usually, but not always, are found together. In the case of mIg determination, with some techniques, immune complexes are formed that nonspecifically stain all cells with Fc receptors, giving falsely elevated levels. In both examples, specialized reagents are required to make the exact determinations. The basic methods described in detail here represent the most simplified methods that retain the necessary specificity for determining the population markers and that avoid the major technical pitfalls.

In most situations, it is desirable to know the percentage of lymphocytes with mIg, Fc receptors, and complement receptors, and the percentage forming E rosettes. Methods for each of these determinations are described. Each of these determinations is relatively specialized, and they vary in their difficulty and demand for special equipment; however, all can be accomplished with commercially available starting reagents and equipment. Three methods involve rosette formation as the indicator system, and two methods utilize fluorescence microscopy (Table 1). Since many features are common to all of these assays, much of the section on Test Procedures has been organized to avoid repetition where possible.

CLINICAL INDICATIONS

An assessment of lymphocyte populations by these methods enumerates and to a degree characterizes the different lymphocytes that

TABLE 1. *Lymphoid cell population markers and methods used for their demonstration*

Marker	Cell population	Method described
mIg	B	Antibody tagged with fluorochrome
Fc receptor	B, plus	Immune complex tagged with fluorochrome
		Rosette formation with IgG antibody-coated erythrocytes
Complement receptors	B, plus	Rosette formation with erythrocyte coated with particular complement components
E rosette	T, plus	Spontaneous rosettes with sheep erythrocytes

comprise the central units of the immune system (12). There are several clinical areas in which information of this type is useful. The first is an analysis of an increased number of, or of morphologically abnormal, peripheral blood lymphocytes with the objective of determining whether a malignant proliferation is present. A related aspect that is receiving increased attention is the analysis of bone marrow aspirates or lymphocytes obtained from lymph node biopsies to supplement the classic histopathological methods.

B lymphocytes give rise to a spectrum of lymphoproliferative malignancies that vary in character from acute lymphatic leukemia, chronic lymphatic leukemia, and Waldenstrom's macroglobulinemia, to multiple myeloma (4, 20). The cells of each of these malignancies can be thought of as analogous to a step in the differentiation of the B lymphocytes from primitive cell to mature plasma cell. A smaller number of acute and chronic leukemias apparently arise from T cells. Some chronic lymphocytic leukemias have unusual combinations of surface markers that suggest an origin from the minor cell populations. The clinically diverse group of lymphomas and reticulum cell sarcomas are also being analyzed in this manner to determine their T or B cell character, and what differentiation step they represent. It is hoped that an improved understanding of their natural history and susceptibility to therapy can be made from such findings. Repetition of the studies during courses of therapy can permit a more precise determination of the degree of therapeutic response.

A second area of clinical application is in the study of a patient with a suspected primary deficiency of the immune system (4, 5, 8, 20). Attention is usually directed to it because of recurrent or unusual infections. A variety of differentiation failures and functional defects are included in this group. The assessment of lymphocyte markers and of the accessory cells of the immune system such as monocytes, coupled with the appropriate test of lymphocyte function, should permit an accurate definition of the nature of the cellular defect and a prediction of the most probable complications facing the patient. They will form the basis of an approach to correct or compensate for the deficiency.

The third principal area is broad and includes a wide variety of acute and chronic diseases associated with evidence of some alteration in the immune system. In some diseases such as infectious mononucleosis, the objective of the study is to characterize the cellular response to a known organism. In other infections such as leprosy, the objective is to characterize the elements of an ineffective immune response. In diseases of unknown etiology such as rheumatoid arthritis, systemic lupus erythematosus, and sarcoidosis, the studies are primarily made with a view towards uncovering features of the abnormal immune response that might lead to a better understanding of the nature of these diseases. In general, these have not led to major insights in this respect, but a number of abnormalities have been found that remain to be fully interpreted. These include changes in B and T cell ratios, increases both in Fc (+) mIg (−) cells and in null cells, and an appreciation of the quantity and reactivity to autoreactive antilymphocyte antibodies (24). Studies of synovial and other fluids such as pleural effusions occurring during rheumatoid arthritis have revealed considerable changes in the composition of the lymphocyte populations compared with peripheral blood.

TEST PROCEDURES

The five different methods fall into two categories: those using rosette assays and those using fluorescence analysis. The common features of each category of assay will be presented first followed by sections dealing with particular techniques and preparation of the specific reagents.

Cell preparation

The Ficoll-Hypaque method described in chapter 9 is used to obtain mononuclear cells. Particular care should be directed to obtaining yields of 70% or greater in order to assure representative results. Viability should approach 100%. The procedures need not be carried out under sterile conditions although the reagents must be kept free from bacterial or fungal contamination.

Monocyte labeling. The lymphocyte preparations obtained from Ficoll-Hypaque are not depleted of monocytes. Thus monocytes comprise approximately one-third of the cells isolated from normal individuals by this method. As will be discussed later, the monocytes, if not properly identified as such, can simulate B cells in several of the assays and lead to serious errors of interpretation. The best approach to the solution of this problem is to label the monocytes by latex ingestion. Labeling monocytes by latex ingestion is, therefore, essential for accurate determinations of lymphocyte receptors. The labeling procedure has the advantage of permitting cold-reactive antilymphocyte antibodies to be eluted as described below. This is a useful feature if many samples to be analyzed come from patients with autoimmune diseases.

Adjust the mononuclear cell preparation to about 10^6 cells/ml in Hanks balanced salt solution (HBSS). Add 1 drop (0.020 ml) of a 5% suspension of latex particles per $2 \pm 0.5 \times 10^7$ cells and incubate at 37 C for 45 min with occasional suspension. Wash three times with 30 to 40 ml of HBSS or phosphate-buffered saline-glucose (PBS-G) under the same conditions described in chapter 9. Monitor a drop of the suspended pellet to determine whether there are fewer than 1 free latex particle per 5 to 10 cells; if not, an additional wash is necessary. If monocytes are abundant, clumps of monocytes can form, incorporate other cells, and interfere with the analysis; they usually can be broken up by Vortex mixing. Re-isolation with prior monocyte depletion is rarely necessary. Some points on the discrimination between lymphocytes and monocytes are included in the section on fluoresence analysis.

Latex reagent. Latex particles 1.1 μm in diameter are obtained from Dow Diagnostics as a 10% suspension. They are washed five times in PBS by centrifugation at $15,000 \times g$ for 10 min and are stored as a 5% suspension in PBS at 4 C. The particles are resuspended before use.

Antilymphocyte antibodies. Antilymphocyte antibodies and other substances found in certain pathological states can cause serious interference with the assays (24). If their presence is suspected, such as in patients with systemic lupus erythematosus or Sjogren's syndrome, this effect can usually be minimized by carrying out the latex incubation procedure or an equivalent incubation at 37 C in the absence of autologous serum and washing with buffers

warmed to 37 C. In certain uncommon circumstances described below, overnight incubation in a medium such as RPMI 1640 supplemented with 10% fetal calf or normal human serum may be necessary to allow shedding of absorbed antibody.

Assays involving rosette formation

E rosette assay (spontaneous sheep erythrocyte rosettes). Delicate rosettes between T lymphocytes and sheep erythrocytes are formed during incubation at 4 C (1, 3, 4, 12, 15). There are a number of methodological variations in use. The procedure outlined below gives a high level of E rosette-forming cells.

In a 12×75 mm plastic, capped test tube, place 0.1 ml of 0.5% sheep erythrocyte suspension and 5×10^5 mononuclear cells in 0.1 ml of BSS. Add 0.020 ml of sheep erythrocyte-absorbed heat-inactivated human serum. Centrifuge slowly ($50 \times g$) for 5 min, and place tubes in a refrigerator (4 C) overnight without disrupting the pelleted cells. Just before examining a sample, remove it from the cold and add 1 drop of 0.2% trypan blue freshly diluted in physiological saline. Very gently resuspend the cells by tipping the tube so it is nearly horizontal and slowly twisting it about its long axis. In 1 or 2 min, the air-fluid interface will suspend essentially all of the pellet. A drop of the suspension is transferred to a hemocytometer chamber by means of capillary action in a Pasteur pipette without a bulb. Tapping, shaking, or in any way roughly suspending the rosettes will disrupt a variable number and should be avoided. After the cells have been allowed to sediment for 1 or 2 min, 200 lymphocytes are promptly counted under a $40\times$ to $95\times$ objective with the use of phase or conventional optics. A lymphocyte is scored as rosette-forming if three or more erythrocytes adhere. Cells taking up trypan blue and monocytes are excluded from the count. A thin-based hemocytometer chamber such as that used for platelet counting allows use of phase optics and thus affords superior cell identification and exclusion of monocytes. The use of a chamber is essential to avoid disruption of the rosettes by cover slip pressure.

Fc receptor assay (rosette method; 10). Easily disruptable rosettes are formed between IgG-coated ox erythrocytes and lymphocytes or monocytes bearing Fc receptors according to the method of Coombs et al. (13). The general resuspension and counting procedures are performed as described in the E rosette assay.

In a 12×75 mm plastic, capped test tube, place 0.1 ml of sensitized ox cell reagent and 2.0 $\times 10^5$ lymphocytes in 0.1 ml of HBSS. Mix and incubate at 37 C for 15 min. Centrifuge very gently, approximately $25 \times g$, for 5 min, incubate for 2 h or more at 4 C, and proceed to resuspend and enumerate rosettes as described above. The proper setting of the centrifuge may require optimization in each laboratory. The objective is to use sufficient force to pellet all cells yet not produce a button that is difficult to resuspend.

Assay for complement receptor lymphocytes (6). Human lymphocytes contain two different types of complement receptors: the immune adherence receptor and the C3d receptor. Most complement receptor lymphocytes in normal blood have both types of complement receptors, but some normal lymphocytes may have only one or the other of these two types of complement receptors. Some normal lymphoid cells have only one type of receptor. The two different complement receptors are antigenically distinct, have different complement specificities, and are located on separate molecules in the lymphocyte membrane (6, 16–18, 21). Complement receptor lymphocytes are detected by rosette formation with sheep erythrocytes coated with antibody and complement (EAC). EAC14 (EAC containing only the first two reacting components of complement, C1 and C4) form rosettes only with cells bearing immune adherence receptors, whereas EAC3d (EAC containing primarily only C3d) form rosettes only with cells bearing C3d receptors. Procedures for detection of each complement receptor are given below.

To perform the assay, add 5×10^5 mononuclear cells in 0.2 ml of HBSS to a 10×75 mm plastic test tube, add 0.2 ml of EAC (0.5%, of the appropriate specificity) and cap the tubes. Place them on a slow rotator (20 to 40 rpm) in the horizontal position for 30 min at 37 C to mix the cells and keep them in suspension. Then examine a drop of the suspension for the number of rosette-forming lymphocytes as outlined in the E rosette procedure. In the case of EAC rosettes, a slide and a cover slip sealed with nail polish may be used in place of the chamber.

Reagents for rosette procedures

Sheep erythrocytes. Before use, the sheep blood cells from 10 ml of sheep blood in Alsever's solution should be washed four times with 50 ml of ice-cold saline (10 min, $1,000 \times g$, 4 C). The sheep leukocyte layer ("buffy coat") on top of the erythrocyte pellet should be aspirated from the erythrocyte pellet (along with some of the erythrocytes) and discarded after the first centrifugation of the sheep blood. After

the last wash, the sheep erythrocytes should be resuspended at a concentration of 5%, vol/vol (i.e., 1 ml of packed sheep erythrocytes in 20 ml), in 0.01 GVBE (see below) and warmed to 37 C. For small volumes, the concentration of the sheep erythrocytes should be checked spectrophotometrically. For this purpose, a 0.5-ml sample of the 5% sheep erythrocyte suspension is lysed by addition of 14.5 ml of water (1:30 dilution). The optical density at 541 nm (OD_{541}) of this lysed sample should be 0.350 if the sheep erythrocytes are correctly suspended at 5% (vol/vol). If the OD_{541} is more than 0.350, for example, 0.700, then the sheep erythrocytes must be diluted 1:2. If the OD_{541} is less than 0.350, then the sheep erythrocytes must be pelleted and resuspended in a smaller volume.

In the case of erythrocytes for E rosettes, some laboratories report that optimal results are obtained if the blood in Alsever's solution is stored for 5 to 7 days after shedding before it is used. Blood stored more than 5 to 6 weeks is no longer suitable. The dilution to 0.5% for E rosettes need not be as accurate as for preparation of EAC; 0.1 ml of packed cells diluted to 20 ml in HBSS will suffice.

Heat-inactivated human serum. Fresh human AB serum is heated at 56 C for 30 min. Next, washed sheep erythrocytes are pelleted into each of three tubes. After aspirating as much of the sheep erythrocyte supernatant fluid as possible, 10 volumes of serum are added to the first tube and suspended by use of a Vortex mixer. After incubation at 37 C for 15 min, followed by centrifugation to pack the sheep erythrocytes, the once-absorbed serum is transferred by aspiration to the second tube of packed sheep erythrocytes and the process is repeated. After the third absorption, the heat-inactivated and absorbed serum is dispensed in 0.5-ml volumes and frozen at -70 C until used.

HBSS is available as prepackaged powders that are reconstituted with distilled water according to instructions (Difco, Grand Island Biological Co., Microbiological Associates).

Buffers and medium.

Veronal buffer stock solution:

1. Dissolve 4.6 g of barbituric acid in 600 ml of boiling water.

2. Dissolve 2.0 g of sodium barbital and 83.8 g of NaCl in 1 liter of cold water.

3. Mix the dissolved barbituric acid with the cold solution and add enough water to give a total volume of 2 liters. A 1:5 dilution of the stock solution with water should have a pH of 7.2 to 7.4 and a conductivity approximately equal to that of normal saline.

Ca^{2+}-Mg^{2+} stock solution: Dissolve 0.44 g of

$CaCl_2 \cdot 2H_2O$ and 2.03 g of $MgCl_2 \cdot 6H_2O$ in 100 ml of water.

Gelatin, 2%:

1. Dissolve 40 g of gelatin powder in 2 liters of boiling water (stir slowly until dissolved).

2. Cool to room temperature and add additional water to bring the volume up to 2 liters.

3. Dispense into autoclavable bottles, 50 ml per bottle.

4. Autoclave.

5. Store at 4 C.

EDTA, 0.2 M, pH 7.2:

1. Dissolve 37.23 g of disodium ethylenediaminetetraacetate (EDTA) and 38.02 g of tetrasodium EDTA in 1 liter of boiling water.

2. Cool to room temperature and bring up to 1 liter with water.

3. Check that the pH is 7.2 to 7.4

Gelatin-veronal buffer (GVB):

1. Melt 50 ml of 2% gelatin at 37 C.

2. Pour 200 ml of veronal buffer stock solution into a 1-liter graduated cylinder.

3. Add the 50 ml of melted gelatin and 5 ml of the Ca^{2+}-Mg^{2+} stock solution.

4. Bring up to 1 liter with water.

5. Check that the pH is 7.2 to 7.4 and that the conductivity is approximately equal to that of normal saline.

0.01 M EDTA-GVB (0.01 GBVE):

1. Prepare 1 liter of GVB but omit the 5 ml of Ca^{2+}-Mg^{2+} solution.

2. Add 50 ml of the 0.2 M EDTA, pH 7.2, to a 1-liter graduated cylinder and bring the volume up to 1 liter with the Ca^{2+}-Mg^{2+}-free GVB.

0.04 M EDTA-GVB (0.04 GVBE):

1. Prepare 1 liter of Ca^{2+}-Mg^{2+}-free GVB.

2. Add 200 ml of 0.2 M EDTA, pH 7.2, to a 1-liter graduated cylinder and bring the volume up to 1 liter with the Ca^{2+}-Mg^{2+}-free GVB.

Anti-sheep erythrocyte antibodies (EA). The IgM fraction of rabbit anti-sheep erythrocyte serum can be purchased from Cordis Laboratories, Miami, Fla. This antibody has been titrated by the manufacturer and is supplied with information concerning the optimal dilution necessary for formation of EA.

C1. C1 is prepared from fresh human serum by low-ionic-strength precipitation. Ice-cold serum is adjusted to pH 7.0 with 1 N HCl and then diluted 1:3 with ice-cold distilled water. After 30 min of stirring at 0 to 4 C, the precipitate is pelleted by centrifugation at $1,000 \times g$ for 30 min at 4 C. The supernatant fluid is decanted and discarded. The precipitate is washed by careful resuspension in five times the original serum volume of ice-cold veronal buffer stock solution diluted 1:15 with water, followed by recentrifugation at $1,000 \times g$ for 30

min at 4 C. The washed precipitate is partially dissolved by stirring for 15 min at 0 to 4 C after resuspension in one-fourth the original serum volume of ice-cold veronal buffer stock solution diluted 1:2.5 with water and containing onetenth part of Ca^{2+}-Mg^{2+} stock solution. The suspension, containing dissolved C1, is then diluted 1:2 with water, dispensed in 0.5-ml volumes, and frozen at -70 C until use. C1 should be thawed rapidly in a 37 C water bath and then kept on ice until added to the EA.

C5-deficient mouse serum. Many different strains of mice are genetically deficient in C5. A complete list of C5 (MuB1 antigen)-deficient and normal strains of mice is given in reference 7. Some examples of strains that are C5 deficient are AKR, A/HeJ, DBA/2J, NZB/B1, and A/J. Commercially available mouse serum should not be used. Mice should be bled directly into a glass tube in an ice bath. Mice can be easily bled from the tail without killing them. Mice are restrained in a box with a small hole at one end through which the tail is drawn and held in one hand over the glass tube. With the other hand, a razor blade or scalpel blade is drawn perpendicularly across the bottom of the tail at a point about one-third of the length down the tail from the base. The cut should not be more than one-third of the way through the tail. After 20 drops of blood have been allowed to drip into the tube, the bleeding is stopped by holding a piece of tissue tightly over the cut. Before bleeding the mice, it is necessary to warm them in an incubator at 45 C for 15 to 20 min to dilate the blood vessels in their tail. After allowing the pooled blood from several mice to clot for 3 to 4 h on ice, the serum is separated by centrifugation and absorbed three times with 0.1 volume of packed sheep erythrocytes. The absorptions with the sheep erythrocytes are performed similarly as with the heat-inactivated serum (see above) except that each absorption is incubated in an ice bath (0 to 2 C) for 10 min, rather than at 37 C for 15 min. After absorption, the serum is dispensed in 4-ml volumes and stored at -70 C until used.

EDTA-inactivated C5-deficient mouse serum. Just before use, fresh or thawed mouse serum is mixed with an equal volume of 0.04 GVBE and incubated at 37 C for 10 min.

Preparation of EA ($EA_{\gamma M}$). EA are prepared by sensitizing sheep erythrocytes with the IgM antibody fraction of rabbit anti-sheep erythrocyte serum.

The IgM anti-sheep erythrocyte antibody should then be diluted (information concerning the appropriate dilution is supplied by the manufacturer) in 0.01 GVBE and warmed to 37 C.

Equal volumes of sheep erythrocytes and anti-sheep erythrocyte antibody are then mixed together, incubated with occasional gentle agitation at 37 C for 30 min, and then transferred to an ice bath for 30 min. The EA are ready to use after one wash with ice-cold 0.01 GVBE and two washes with ice cold GVB.

Preparation of EAC14. EAC14 are prepared by sequential addition of C1 and C4 (heat-inactivated serum) to EA. A 10-ml amount of EA, suspended at 2.5% (vol/vol) in GVB (OD_{541} of a 0.5-ml sample lysed with 14.5 ml of water = 0.175) and warmed to 37 C, is mixed with 0.5 ml of C1. After 15 min of incubation at 37 C, the EAC1 are washed two times with 37 C GVB in a room temperature centrifuge. The C1 contained on the EAC1 is labile and comes off the EAC1 even more rapidly when the EAC1 are cooled below 37 C. It is therefore important to wash the EAC1 with 37 C GVB and as rapidly as possible, so that the C1 does not come off the EAC1 before the C4 is added. After resuspending the EAC1 at 2.5% (vol/vol) in 37 C GVB, heat-inactivated serum is added as a C4 source (see below), and the cells are incubated for 15 min at 37 C. Immediately at the end of this incubation period, the cell suspension is diluted with 4 to 5 volumes of ice-cold GVB and centrifuged. If incubation with the serum is prolonged beyond 15 min, inactivation by the serum C4 inactivator becomes appreciable. After two washes with ice-cold GVB, the EAC14 are suspended at 0.5%, vol/vol (OD_{415} of a 0.5-ml sample lysed with 14.5 ml of water = 0.300), in HBSS and stored at 0 to 4 C for up to 5 days until used.

There is a characteristic optimal amount of heat-inactivated serum that is required. This sharp optimum varies with individual sera and thus must be determined with each new batch of serum. If too much serum is added to the EAC1, the amount of bound C4 that is generated on the EAC14 will be diminished as a result of the action of the serum C4 inactivator. The amount of C4 fixed with increasing amounts of heated serum is determined by measuring EAC14 rosette formation with human erythrocytes (immune adherence). That amount of heat-inactivated serum found to produce a maximal number of EAC14 rosettes with human erythrocytes (usually 0.12 to 0.16 ml/10⁹ EAC1) is then used in all future EAC14 preparations that utilize that particular serum.

Preparation of EAC3d. EAC3d are prepared by addition of C5-deficient mouse serum to EA. C4 and C3b, which are also fixed onto the EAC from the mouse serum, are subsequently cleaved away by the enzyme-like inactivators contained in the mouse serum, so that C3d is the only component bound to the EAC that reacts with complement receptors. It is, however, absolutely necessary to check the EAC3d after they are prepared to ascertain that all of the C4 and C3b have been cleaved. Since inactivation of C4 and C3b is usually incomplete, it is necessary to treat the EAC3d with EDTA-inactivated mouse serum (which permits C4 and C3b inactivation and prevents additional C4 and C3b fixation).

A 10-ml amount of EA, suspended at 1%, vol/vol (OD_{415} of a 0.5-ml sample lysed with 14.5 ml of water = 0.600), in 37 C GVB, is mixed with 10 ml of C5-deficient mouse serum diluted 1:2.5 in GVB. After 30 min of incubation at 37 C, the EAC3d are washed two times in 37 C 0.04 GVBE and incubated in 40 ml of 0.04 GVBE for 30 min at 37 C. Next, the EAC3d are washed two times in 37 C 0.04 GVBE, suspended in 2 ml of 37 C 0.04 GVBE, and mixed with 8 ml of EDTA-inactivated C5-deficient mouse serum. After 30 min of incubation at 37 C, the EAC3d are washed once with ice-cold 0.04 GVBE and twice with ice-cold GVB, and then are resuspended at 0.5% (vol/vol) in HBSS.

Control procedure for EAC. Human E rosette formation with EAC, the immune adherence phenomenon, is assayed in the same way as lymphocyte rosette formation except that the human erythrocytes, suspended at 3×10^6/ml, are used instead of the lymphocytes. A single drop of blood obtained by pricking a finger is sufficient for more than 20 ml of human erythrocytes diluted to 3×10^6/ml. Before use, the human erythrocytes should be washed three times in normal saline. Using a four-button counter, count 200 to 300 human erythrocytes in random fields in four different categories: unrosetted (zero or one attached EAC) and rosetted with two, three, or four attached EAC. Human E rosettes with more than four attached EAC are rare. From the number of each of the three types of rosettes, the total number of EAC bound in rosettes (of two or more attached EAC per rosette) is determined. From the total number, the average number of EAC bound to 100 human erythrocytes is calculated by dividing the total number of EAC bound by the number of human erythrocytes counted and multiplying by 100.

Testing EAC for specificity and potency. EAC14 prepared as described above will react specifically with immune adherence receptors. However, the amount of C4 fixed onto the EAC14 may vary with different sera, and it is therefore essential to determine the optimal amount with each serum. Also, the amount of

EAC14-human E rosettes obtained will vary with the human erythrocyte donor. It is desirable that the reference erythrocytes come from the same O-positive individual available each week and that the erythrocytes form strong rosettes in the range of 50 to 100 EAC14 bound in rosettes to 100 human erythrocytes. It is absolutely essential to test the EAC3d for human E rosettes, using the same human erythrocytes, to assure that they are specific for C3d receptors. The EAC3d should produce 10% or less of the number of EAC bound per 100 human erythrocytes as the EAC14. Testing EAC3d for potency is more specialized, and potency may have to be inferred from the range of normal values. The best way to test the EAC3d for potency is by rosette formation with cells from an established lymphoblastoid line. The cell line termed "Raji" is well suited since it forms almost no EAC14 rosettes and nearly 100% EAC3d rosettes.

Ox cell EA reagent. Fresh ox blood is shed into ACD solution and remains usable for 2 weeks when stored at 4 C. Every 2 to 3 days, wash a portion of the cells four times with PBS and adjust to a 0.5% suspension. Incubate the cell suspension with an equal volume of a sub-agglutinating dilution of rabbit anti-ox erythrocyte serum for 2 h at 22 C. Wash the sensitized cells twice with PBS and resuspend to 0.5% in 10% fetal calf serum. HBSS should be added if the lymphocyte-EA mixture is incubated for more than 2 h. The adequacy of ox cell sensitization by the rabbit antibody should be verified by a hemagglutination assay using microtiter plates and an anti-rabbit IgG antiserum, e.g., sheep anti-rabbit. The cells are used at 0.5% suspension.

The rabbit anti-ox erythrocyte serum is readily obtained by an initial course of four weekly injections of 0.2 ml of packed washed ox cells. The subagglutinating zone of the antiserum is also determined by hemagglutination with the use of the 0.5% suspension of ox cells and serial dilutions of the rabbit antiserum. Certain oxen vary in the amount of neuraminic acid that is present on the erythrocytes; if low, the cells are readily agglutinated and not satisfactory (13).

Fluorescence microscopy analysis for membrane immunoglobulin or Fc receptor

The number of cells with mIg and the number with receptors for Fc regions of IgG are both determined by nearly identical staining procedures, but with different reagents. The procedure for staining is given first, followed by sections on the reagents.

Staining procedure. Mononuclear cell preparations previously incubated with latex and washed as described above are given a final wash with PBS-BSA (PBS containing 2% bovine serum albumin and 0.02% sodium azide) and are resuspended at a concentration of 2×10^7 to 2.5×10^7/ml in PBS-BSA. The staining is usually done at room temperature although, as noted below, for special purposes 4 C is sometimes used. A 0.025-ml amount of cell suspension is placed in a 10×75 mm plasic test tube and the appropriate reagent is added. For mIg this is usually 0.025 ml of an antiserum conjugate. For determination of the Fc receptor, the reagent is 0.025 ml of a preparation of aggregated IgG labeled with fluorochrome or sequentially added antibody and antigen labeled with fluorochrome to form an immune complex system. The cells are then mixed with the added reagent. This can be done by quickly and forcibly rubbing the test tube tip over the top of a wire test tube rack. After a 30-min incubation, 2 ml of PBS-BSA is added and the cells are centrifuged. After centrifugation, the wash is poured out with a continuous motion, the tube top is blotted while inverted, and the pellet is resuspended as described above before the next portion of wash solution is added. The cells are washed three times. After each centrifugation, any residual foam is aspirated off. The remainder of the final wash is not poured off until immediately before making the slide; then the top of the tube is briefly pressed against a towel to dry it and the pellet is resuspended with several forcible strokes across a test tube rack. A Pasteur pipette is quickly put in the tube, and a column of 0.5 to 1.0 cm of cell suspension is removed by capillary action and expressed on the slide by thumb pressure. The importance of these maneuvers is to achieve a cell density of 15 to 25 per oil immersion field. After 15 to 20 s, a cover glass is placed on the drop and pressed firmly down with the eraser of a pencil. The edges are sealed with a high-quality, quick-drying clear nail polish. The slides are examined with a high-resolution oil or water immersion objective of at least $45\times$. Phase optics alternating with the incident fluorescent illumination of a Ploem-type device are used to identify the cell type and perform the fluorescence analysis. A total of 200 to 500 cells are counted depending on the percentage of positive cells encountered. Cells with homogeneous cytoplasmic staining due to early cell death are not counted. They are readily recognized by the absence of the circumferential ring of fluorescence and greater fluorescence intensity in the cell center.

Discrimination of lymphocytes from monocytes is essential and requires some practice. The majority of monocytes will have ingested latex particles, and these are seen to be clearly within the cytoplasm. However, other cells shown to be monocytes by specialized criteria fail to ingest latex. These may be recognized by an irregular profile of the cell membrane, granular cytoplasm, and an indistinct nuclear membrane. Occasionally, one or two latex particles can be found adhering to the surface membrane of a typical lymphocyte. These are not excluded from the lymphocyte population.

Reagents for determining Fc receptors (9, 23). The principle involved is the formation of fresh immune complexes with an antiserum that is conjugated to a fluorochrome. These immune complexes bind to the Fc receptor, and cells are identified by their positive fluorescence. Nearly any antigen-antibody system could in principle be used, and the following system is given as an example. The antigen is rabbit IgG purchased as fraction II (FII) and made up in PBS-BSA at 10 mg/ml. The antibody is sheep anti-rabbit IgG conjugated to either fluorescein or tetramethyl rhodamine. It may be prepared as outlined below or obtained commercially. The optimal ratio of antigen will vary according to the strength of the antiserum and is found empirically. Dilutions of the antigen are made at 0.01, 0.05, 0.10, and 0.20 mg/ml in PBS-BSA. To each separate tube containing cells, 0.025 ml of the antibody conjugate is added followed by 0.025 ml of the antigen solution. The procedure of incubation, washing, slide preparation and examination described above is carried out. The optimal amount of antigen is selected by determining which concentration gives the highest percentage of staining cells. This standardization curve should show a distinct maximum zone with higher and lower concentration of antigen giving lower values. Preference is given to a concentration that produces a fine granular pattern of staining. In some instances, additional concentrations of antigen will have to be explored if there is doubt that the maximum has been reached. Since the high dilutions of antigen are not stable, they should be prepared freshly each day from the stock solution. The antiserum ratio standardization procedure should be repeated with any change in antiserum. A known standard cell preparation should be run each week. Although normal peripheral blood cells can be used, the use of a lymphocyte preparation from a patient with chronic lymphatic leukemia or a B cell line such as DAUDI will greatly simplify the standardization and control of the proce-

dure. It should be emphasized that use of a F(ab')$_2$ fragment of antibody to form immune complexes is not suitable.

Reagents for determining mIg. Among several factors influencing the choice of methods, the primary ones are as follows:

1. IgD and IgM comprise the dominant mIg classes on peripheral blood B cells. IgA and IgG account for a minority of less than one-tenth of the mIg-positive cells (19, 22, 23). IgM and IgD occur together on the majority of mIg-positive cells.

2. The presence of the Fc receptor for IgG introduces stong constraints on the methods since any immune complexes formed with minute residual amounts of serum Ig will confer positive staining due to formation and uptake of immune complexes (23). In addition, aggregates present in the antiserum preparation will be nonspecifically taken up and similarly produce false-positive staining (4).

Two different approaches to avoid these problems will be presented, the first using standard reagents and the second involving specially prepared antibody fragments.

Procedure I

Whole IgG fraction of antisera specific for human IgM and IgD conjugated to a fluorochrome are used as a mixture. Anti-whole Ig reagents or mixtures with specificity for IgG or light chains will all give significantly high false-positive staining and should not be used. It must be emphasized that no soluble absorptions should have been used in preparing the IgM or IgD specific reagents since when they are mixed, further absorption will occur. Each day, prior to staining, the sera should be centrifuged at $20,000 \times g$ for 30 min to remove larger aggregates. Two important controls should be carried out once on each new batch of serum:

1. The plateau test determines the relative strength of the conjugated antiserum for surface staining. To a series of tubes containing mononuclear cells with latex-labeled monocytes, add 0.1, 0.05, 0.025, and then 0.025 ml of twofold serially diluted conjugated antiserum up to a dilution of 1:16. Separate tests should be made for the IgM and the IgD antisera. The cells are stained and processed as described above. The numbers of lymphocytes positive in fluorescence are plotted versus the dilutions. The plateau percentage reflects the maximal number of positive cells bearing the Ig. As the amount of antiserum is reduced, only cells with the greatest abundance of mIg are stained, resulting in lower percentages. The amount of

serum used in routine staining should be sufficient to place the reaction on the plateau by a factor of two.

2. In the monocyte staining test, the presence of Fc receptors on monocytes serves as a built-in control for nonspecific staining due to complexes or aggregates (9). Careful search for stained monocytes should be made, particularly at the higher concentrations used in the plateau test, and reagents should be returned to the manufacturer as not suitable for surface staining if they fail this test. It should be emphasized that complete specificity of fluorescent reagents, established by other standard immunological criteria such as intracellular staining, does not assure that a reagent is suitable for lymphocyte surface staining. These reagents are available from a number of companies.

Procedure II

In this procedure the Fc regions of the anti-Ig antibodies are removed by pepsin digestion, and then they are conjugated with fluorochrome (23). This treatment minimizes the uptake of any immune complexes formed during staining and removes the requirement for ultracentrifugation prior to each staining. Antibodies to all Ig classes can be used for surface staining. The drawback is that at present $F(ab')_2$ reagents are not widely available from commercial sources. Cappell Laboratories (Downington, Pa.) has recently announced their production. A procedure for preparing them is given below. The $F(ab')_2$ reagents are also tested for potency and specificity as described under Procedure I. Some monocytes will retain IgG on their Fc receptors, and this is stained by $F(ab')_2$ anti-IgG reagents, but not by the other class-specific reagents. We employ a screening mixture composed of a pool of separately conjugated and absorbed $F(ab')_2$ reagents specific for IgG, IgA, IgM, and IgD, respectively. Alternatively, a screening mixture with specificity for kappa and lambda determinants can be used. Immunization and absorption procedures cannot be dealt with in this section. In general, absorptions should be performed with the use of insolubilized myeloma proteins of documented high purity prepared according to methods such as those clearly outlined in the Pharmacia product literature. The definition of reagent specificity after absorption is greatly aided by the availability of lymphocytes from patients with chronic lymphatic leukemia. The method of $F(ab')_2$ fragment preparation and conjugation, while containing a number of steps, is basically a series of chromatographic preparations that

are readily standardized and do not require fraction collector pumps or monitors.

Preparation of $F(ab')_2$ reagents for immunofluorescence. A 30- to 50-ml amount of strong antiserum is mixed with an equal volume of saturated ammonium sulfate, and the precipitate is harvested by centrifugation. This is dissolved in and dialyzed against 0.05 M $NaCl_2$-0.01 M phosphate buffer, pH 7.5, and passed over a diethylaminoethyl (DEAE)-cellulose column equilibrated with the same buffer. The rabbit IgG fraction is digested with pepsin, yielding $F(ab')_2$ fragments. The protein content is measured and the solution is dialyzed against 0.1 M sodium acetate buffer, pH 4.1. Then 2 mg of pepsin per 100 mg of IgG is added, and the mixture is incubated at 37 C for 18 h. The mixture is neutralized by adding Trizma base (1.0 M) and is dialyzed against 0.01 M sodium phosphate buffer, pH 7.5. The mixture is passed over a DEAE-cellulose column (Whatman DE 52) equilibrated with the same buffer, and the "fall through" peak is retained. If gel filtration techniques with fraction collectors are available, it is preferable to omit the last DEAE-cellulose chromatography and apply the neutralized digest to a G-150 Sephadex column equilibrated with 0.05 M phosphate buffer, pH 7.3, and 0.5 M NaCl. Gel filtration will eliminate any undigested 150,000-molecular-weight material as well as Fab fragments, along with the other smaller fragments removed on DEAE-cellulose chromatography. The $F(ab')_2$ fragments will elute in a large peak following the void volume. At this point or at any other point in the procedure, the sample volume can be reduced by adding ammonium sulfate to half saturation and dialyzing the precipitate against the appropriate buffer, in this case 0.15 M NaCl.

The optical density is measured at 280 nm and divided by 1.35 to obtain the protein concentration. A known volume of the rabbit $F(ab')_2$ preparation containing about 100 mg is adjusted to a concentration between 5 and 10 mg/ml. A 0.1-ml amount 1.0 M sodium bicarbonate-sodium carbonate (pH 9.5) buffer is added per ml of protein solution, and the mixture is put in a small beaker with a small magnetic stirring bar gently turning. A 1.0 mg/ml suspension of tetramethyl rhodamine isothiocyanate in 0.15 M saline is prepared by first weighing out 5 to 10 mg of the fluorochrome in a plastic test tube, adding saline, and finely suspending the reagent by ultrasound. In a Branson ultrasound machine the microtip unit is used to deliver 60 to 70 W/cm^2 for three 30-s intervals (23). A volume of the fluorochrome suspension sufficient to give 0.035 mg of fluorochrome/1.0 mg of protein is added dropwise. The mixture is stirred in a 4 C room overnight after being covered with Parafilm.

Unconjugated fluorochrome is removed by passing the mixture over a 25 × 3 cm column of G-50 Sephadex equilibrated with 0.01 M phosphate buffer, pH 7.5. The first colored peak is then applied to a 15 × 1 cm column of DE-52 cellulose equilibrated with 0.1 M phosphate buffer, pH 7.5. The "fall through" is reserved but usually contains hypoconjugated F(ab′)$_2$ fragments and gives weak staining. The major peak is obtained by eluting with 0.01 M phosphate buffer, pH 7.5, which has been rendered 0.125 M in NaCl. The yield should be greater than 50% and with some sera can be above 90% (2). Conjugate still remaining on the column is usually hyperconjugated and can nonspecifically adhere to cells by charge-charge interactions; a 0.15 M NaCl elution can be attempted if significant material remains on the column, but nonspecific staining should be evaluated. The conjugate is made 2% in bovine serum albumin and dialyzed against PBS containing azide.

The conjugation step requires additional comment (2, 14). Tetramethyl rhodamine is chosen as a superior fluorochrome for surface Ig demonstration for a variety of technical reasons; however, the conjugation is sometimes more difficult to perform satisfactorily than with fluorescein. Lot-to-lot variations result in appreciably different solubility properties, shelf life, and ultimate conjugation efficiency of tetramethyl rhodamine isothiocyanate. Also, the fluorochrome is hygroscopic, and water uptake diminishes solubilization. It is recommended to test new lots of fluorochrome on dialyzed human or rabbit FII IgG and determine whether they give a suitable yield of properly conjugated IgG, to avoid wasting antibody preparations. The technical service divisions of the manufacturer can be of assistance in solving problems that arise. We have had satisfactory results with fluorochromes obtained from Baltimore Biological Laboratories. Procedures for rendering the antisera specific for an Ig class and verifying this procedure cannot be gone into in detail. The central points are to use myeloma proteins of documented purity to remove known unwanted specificities. The resulting reagent must have its specificity assayed by direct fluorescence with the use of cells from chronic lymphatic leukemia, lymphoid cell lines, or erythrocytes coated with defined immunoglobulins. DE-52 is a convenient form of DEAE-cellulose manufactured by Whatman that requires only

washing with the phosphate buffer before use. Stock solutions of 1.0 M sodium chloride and 0.5 M sodium phosphate buffer are both maintained, and dilute solutions are prepared on the day of use by accurate dilutions.

INTERPRETATION

In addition to the basic problem of determining the clinical significance of cell markers in relation to the indication of the test, the clinical immunologist must be aware of several technical considerations that can alter the basic interpretation of the test result. Two important concerns must be (i) the adequacy of monocyte identification and (ii) the potential of interference from antilymphocyte antibodies.

Since the monocyte shares several markers with the B lymphocyte, it is possible that in pathological situations where monocytes are significantly increased they could be erroneously counted as B lymphocytes. Elevated levels of monocytes are more likely to occur in malignancies, in chronic infections, especially in immunodeficiency states, and in disorders such as rheumatoid arthritis. Since the monocyte is an accessory cell to the immune system, the percentage and calculated absolute number of monocytes can be a useful datum.

The second problem, that of autologously reacting antilymphocyte antibodies, merits particular comment. These antibodies, by adhering to the surface of the lymphocyte, can confer positive surface staining to an otherwise Ig-negative cell (24). The presence of these antibodies can usually be recognized when the sum of surface staining plus E rosettes exceeds 100%. These antilymphocyte antibodies may occur in a number of diseases such as infectious mononucleosis, chronic infections, rheumatoid arthritis, Sjögren's syndrome, and lupus erythematosus. The fact that in most instances they are primarily of the IgM class also contributes to their being confused with mIg. Since the bulk of the antibodies show diminished activity at 37 C incubation, washing at 37 C serves to elute considerable amounts of the antibodies. Occasionally, overnight incubation of the cells in medium at 37 C prior to analysis is necessary to allow shedding of more avid antilymphocyte antibodies. This should be performed if the sum of E rosettes plus surface staining is greater than 100% after three washes. The sensitivity of the mIg method to this type of interference can, however, be turned to good advantage, for by performing the staining reaction for surface Ig at 4 C on samples of cells incubated in patient serum or normal serum, the finding of an elevated proportion of positive cells in the former situation indicates the presence of anti-lymphocyte antibodies. The sensitivity of this method is equal to lymphocytotoxic assays. The antilymphocyte antibodies show inhibition of a number of the lymphocyte function assays such as the mixed lymphocyte culture reaction or mitogen stimulation. The antilymphocyte antibodies can inhibit E rosette assays under circumstances of short 4 C incubation periods such as 1 h but have not been found to cause inhibition when the E rosette incubation is carried out overnight (24).

The range of normal adult values has not definitely been determined, and the following values should be used only as general guidelines (1, 10, 12, 13, 16, 23). The figures are presented as percentages of lymphocytes bearing the marker, rather than in terms of absolute number of lymphocytes with the marker: mIg, 1 to 15%; Fc receptor, 5 to 20%; EAC1–4 rosettes and EAC3d rosettes, each 5 to 20%, although the percentages for each variety of complement rosette were not usually the same in any given patient. In an average individual the percentage of cells with mIg is in the range of 9% while complement rosettes are in the range of 12 to 15, whereas the number of lymphocytes with Fc receptors is one and one-half to two times the level of mIg. The level of E rosettes is 85%.

From the percentages of lymphocytes found with each of the markers, certain inferences can be made concerning the lymphocyte populations comprising the sample. The number of lymphocytes with mIg are, by generally agreed definition, B cells. However, at certain stages of B cell development, mIg is not detectable, and thus the true percentage of B cells is slightly higher.

In certain literature the percentage of cells staining with anti-Ig reagents was sometimes considerably higher. To a varying extent this reflected staining of monocytes or lymphocytes bearing only Fc receptors by immune complexes or aggregates. This was particularly a problem with membrane IgG staining. It is now clear that IgD and IgM constitute the major membrane immunoglobulins. Most peripheral blood B cells have both IgM and IgD although roughly one-quarter of the cells have only either one or the other class detectable. IgA- and IgG-bearing cells together account for under 2% of peripheral blood lymphocytes in the average normal person (23).

Cells with Fc receptors are found in at least two lymphocyte populations: the typical B cell and a second cell type that lacks mIg but has to a considerable degree the property of forming E rosettes as mentioned in the Introduction (10, 23).

The complement receptor-bearing lymphocytes are also heterogeneous and include in addition to the B cells an mIg-negative population that is not well understood at present. The relationship between the two complement receptors is complicated. The immune adherence receptor is specific for C4 or the C3c region of C3b. The C3d receptor is specific for the C3d region of C3b and is unreactive with C4. C3b is bound preferentially to immune adherence receptors when both types of complement receptors are present on a single cell. However, C3b can also be bound to C3d receptors by way of its C3d region, and some cells that contain only C3d receptors can bind immune complexes containing only C3b. These two receptors are usually expressed together on most B cells but are capable of independent expression. This independent expression is most apparent in varieties of lymphoproliferative disease as discussed subsequently (16).

Recently, several laboratories have described differentiation alloantigens expressed on B lymphocytes but not on the vast majority of T lymphocytes. Pregnancy sera and heterosera have been used in fluorescent-antibody or cytotoxicity assays to demonstrate these antigens. These antigens are expressed in the absence of surface Ig and have been used as a marker of a B cell precursor (11). These HL-B antigens are also expressed on monocytes and polymorphonuclear leukocyte precursors.

The principal technical factors responsible for diminished levels of E rosette-forming cells relate to mechanical or thermal disruption after formation, and failure to adequately exclude monocytes. As discussed above, antilymphocyte antibodies can also cause interference. Monocytes and classic B cells have not been demonstrated to form E rosettes, with the rare exception of chronic lymphatic leukemias that have a Forssman type of antibody specificity in their mIg. Although what might be termed the "classic" T lymphocyte has as its only marker the property of forming E rosettes, the E rosettes are also formed with some lymphocytes bearing Fc or complement receptors (23). The nature of this population of cells is a matter of current discussion. In many patients with rheumatoid arthritis, and notably in certain immune deficiency states such as X-linked hypogammaglobulinemia, this latter population of E rosette-forming cells is considerably increased.

Null cells are difficult to enumerate in normal peripheral blood using the techniques described here. In pathological states such as the joint fluids of patients with rheumatoid arthritis, null cells are readily identified, comprising up to one-quarter of all the lymphocytes (24). These null cells lack mIg, Fc receptors, and complement receptors, and fail to form E rosettes. The vast majority of these null cells lack the B cell alloantigen system and thus are possibly more related to T cells.

The most readily recognized abnormalities are those due to an abnormal proliferation of lymphoid cells in diseases such as, for example, chronic lymphatic leukemia. Here the leukemic lymphocyte is usually of the classic B variety with mIg and receptors for Fc region and complement (4, 20, 21). The proportion of cells staining for IgD to IgM and a single light-chain class is a characteristic for each leukemia and provides evidence that they are "monoclonal" in origin. Very rare but well-documented examples of chronic leukemia with IgG on the membrane have been reported. Typically the proportion of cells with C3d receptor is increased while the relative proportion of cells with immune adherence receptors is greatly diminished. In some few cases, only the C3d receptor is detectable (16, 17). Occasional leukemic patients have proliferating cells with other surface markers such as isolated E rosette formation or E rosette formation plus complement or Fc receptors (21). These uncommon chronic leukemias probably represent, respectively, malignant transformation of a T cell and a cell from a minor population not readily classified as a T or B cell, such as the K cell. The acute lymphoblastic leukemias are more difficult to classify. The pathological cells from about one-fourth of the patient population lack B cell receptors and will form E rosettes, and thus may be T cell derived. However, the leukemic cells from the other patients do not form E rosettes and also lack mIg and Fc and complement receptors. There is evidence that they are in the B cell lineage by virtue of the detection of B cell alloantigens (11). In some patients with Waldenströms macroglobulinemia, elevated percentages of B lymphocytes are found in peripheral blood (20). In contrast to the situation in chronic lymphatic leukemia, these patients have lymphoid cells with immune adherence receptors that lack C3d receptors. There are also a number of other malignant proliferations with distinctive surface markers such as Sezary cells, hairy cells, etc., that cannot be described in detail here. Insufficient experience has been obtained in the analysis of moderate increases in the lymphocyte count, and it is possible that states

of benign monoclonal lymphocytosis analogous to benign Ig bands will be found. For this reason, the diagnosis of leukemia with its implications of malignancy should not be based solely on these immunological analyses. Autoreactive antilymphocyte antibodies are encountered in certain cases of leukemia and lymphoma. These can markedly interfere with interpretation. They are usually cold reactive and of the IgM class.

The analysis of situations where the competency of the immune system is being evaluated is less advanced. The better-studied frank immune deficiency syndromes serve to illustrate the variety of findings that can be encountered (4, 5, 8, 20). At one extreme of the spectrum is X-linked infantile hypogammaglobulinemia of Bruton where no mIg-bearing cells are found. The percentage of E rosette-forming cells can be 95% or higher. A variable and often increased number of lymphoid cells with Fc receptors and complement receptors are present. At the opposite extreme is the thymic hypoplasia syndrome of Di George. Here, the percentage of E rosette-forming cells is much decreased, and reciprocally two-thirds or more of the lymphocytes have mIg consisting of primarily IgM and IgD as determined by F(ab')$_2$ reagents. IgG- and IgA-bearing cells were increased to levels of 5 to 10%. In other forms of immunodeficiency, typical B cells with mIg are also present at increased levels, yet they fail to differentiate into plasma cells.

The wide variation in percentages and numbers of peripheral blood B cells in ostensibly normal individuals makes a delineation of a mild derangement of the immune system difficult to define in terms of changes in populations of lymphocytes. For example, a number of healthy young adults have been identified with true B cells in the range of 1%. Similarly, in normal infants, although the percentage of B cells is considerably elevated at birth, the variation in composition of peripheral blood lymphocytes with maturation is not fully defined.

LITERATURE CITED

1. Aiuti, F., J.-C. Cerottini, R. R. A. Coombs, M. Cooper, H. B. Dickler, et al. 1974. Identification, enumeration, and isolation of B and T lymphocytes from human peripheral blood. Scand. J. Immunol. 3:521–532.
2. Amante, L., A. Ancona, and L. Forni. 1972. The conjugation of immunoglobulins with tetra methyl rhodamine isothio cyanate. A comparison between the amorphous and the crystalline fluorochrome. J. Immunol. Methods 1:289–301.
3. Bach, J.-F. 1973. Evaluation of T cells and

thymic serum factors in man using the rosette technique. Transplant. Rev. 16:196–217.

4. Bentwich, Z., and H. G. Kunkel. 1973. Specific properties of human B and T lymphocytes and alterations in disease. Transplant. Rev. 16:29–50.

5. Bergsma, D., R. A Good, and J. Finstad (ed.). 1975. Immunodeficiency in man and animals. Sinauer Associates, Inc., Sunderland, Mass.

6. Bianco, C., R. Patrick, and V. Nussenzweig. 1970. A population of lymphocytes bearing a membrane receptor for antigen-antibody-complement complexes. J. Exp. Med. 132:702–720.

7. Cinader, B., S. Dubiski, and A. C. Wardlaw. 1964. Distribution, inheritance and properties of an antigen, MUB1, and its relation to hemolytic complement. J. Exp. Med. 120:897–924.

8. Cooper, M. D., R. G. Keightley, L.-Y. F. Wu, and A. R. Lawton III. 1973. Developmental defects of T and B cell lines in humans. Transplant. Rev. 16:51–84.

9. Dickler, H. B., and H. G. Kunkel. 1972. Interaction of aggregated gamma globulin with B lymphocytes. J. Exp. Med. 136:191–196.

10. Froland, S. S., and J. B. Natvig. 1973. Identification of three different human lymphocyte populations by surface markers. Transplant. Rev. 16:114–162.

11. Fu, S. M., R. J. Winchester, and H. G. Kunkel. 1975. The occurrence of the HL-B alloantigens on the cells of unclassified acute lymphoblastic leukemias. J. Exp. Med. 142:1334–1338.

12. Greaves, M. F., J. T. T. Owen, and M. C. Raff. 1973. T and B lymphocytes; origins, properties and roles in immune responses. American Elsevier, New York.

13. Haegart, D. G., T. Hallberg, and R. R. A. Coombs. 1974. B and T lymphocyte subpopulations in human peripheral blood. Int. Arch. Allergy 46: 525–538.

14. Hijmans, W., and M. Schaeffer. 1975. Fifth International Conference on Immunofluorescence and related staining techniques. The New York Academy of Sciences. Vol. 254.

15. Jondal, M., H. Wigzell, and F. Aiuti. 1973. Human lymphocyte subpopulations: classification according to surface markers and/or functional characteristics. Transplant. Rev. 16:163–195.

16. Ross, G. D., and M. J. Polley. 1975. Specificity of human lymphocyte complement receptors. J. Exp. Med. 141:1163–1180.

17. Ross, G. D., M. J. Polley, E. M. Rabellino, and H. M. Grey. 1973. Two Different Complement Receptors on Human Lymphocytes. J. Exp. Med. 138:798–811.

18. Ross, G. D., E. M. Rabellino, M. J. Polley, and H. M. Grey. 1973. Combined studies of complement receptor and surface immunoglobulin bearing cells and sheep erythrocyte rosette-forming cells in normal and leukemic human lymphocytes. J. Clin. Invest. 52:377–385.

19. Rowe, D., K. Hug, L. Forni, and B. Pernis. 1973. Immunoglobulin D as a lymphocyte receptor. J. Exp. Med. 138:965–972.

20. Seligman, M., J.-L. Preud'Homme, and J.-C. Brouet. 1973. B and T cell markers in human proliferative blood diseases and primary immunodeficiencies, with special reference to membrane bound immunoglobulins. Transplant. Rev. 16:85–113.

21. Shevach, E. M., E. S. Jaffe, and I. Green. 1973. Receptors for complement and immunoglobulin on human and animal lymphoid cells. Transplant. Rev. 16:3–28.

22. Warner, N. L. 1974. Membrane immunoglobulins and antigen receptors on B and T lymphocytes. Adv. Immunol. 19:67–216.

23. Winchester, R. J., S. M. Fu, T. Hoffman, and H. G. Kunkel. 1975. IgG on lymphocyte surfaces; technical problems and the significance of a third cell population. J. Immunol. 114:1210–1212.

24. Winchester, R. J., J. B. Winfield, F. Siegal, P. Wernet, Z. Bentwich, and H. G. Kunkel. 1974. Analyses of lymphocytes from patients with rheumatoid arthritis and systemic lupus erythematosus J. Clin. Invest. 54:1082–1092.

Chapter 8

Methods for the Separation of Unique Human Lymphocyte Subpopulations

LEONARD CHESS AND STUART F. SCHLOSSMAN

INTRODUCTION

The cellular basis of the immune response involves the complex interactions between thymus-derived (T) lymphocytes and bone marrow-derived (B) lymphocytes, and indeed subpopulations of both. Since these heterogeneous subclasses of lymphocytes are in general morphologically indistinguishable and are found together in all peripheral lymphoid tissues, their study has been facilitated by methods allowing for their separation. In recent years, a variety of techniques have been developed for the isolation of T and B lymphocytes. Many of these methods are based on physical-chemical properties of the lymphocyte subpopulations, which include the property of surface adherence, capacity to bind to sheep cells directly or to antibody and complement-coated sheep cells, size, density, and surface charge (3, 4, 6, 11). Although most of these approaches have been extremely useful in providing enriched populations of cells, significant overlap often occurs between the populations isolated. Furthermore, in some procedures quantitative recovery of both depleted and enriched populations is often difficult to achieve.

Recently, a number of specific cellular immunoabasorbents have been developed which, when used in conjunction with other techniques, allow for both specific depletion as well as quantitative recovery of individual lymphocyte subsets (1, 7, 9, 10).

In the present chapter we describe, in detail, the specific column immunoabsorbent chromatography and rosetting techniques used in our laboratory. The former technique permits the isolation of highly purified populations of surface immunoglobulin (Ig) negative cells (predominantly T cells) and surface Ig positive populations (predominantly B cells). The rosetting techniques allow for the subsequent fractionation of these populations. The principle underlying the affinity column techniques is simply that B cells, by virtue of their surface Ig, will bind to columns to which anti(Fab)$_2$ is covalently linked. Non-Ig cells pass through these columns without binding. Moreover, the Ig positive cells can be quantitatively recovered from the columns by competitive inhibition with free Ig or, under special circumstances, by enzyme digestion of the insoluble immunoabasorbent. Following separation of the human lymphocytes into Ig negative and Ig positive populations of cells, the rosette depletion techniques are used for further subfractionation of these populations. Rosette techniques are dependent on the observations that T cells alone form spontaneous rosettes with sheep erythrocytes, whereas B cells and to a certain extent monocytes form rosettes only when the sheep cells are coated with antibody or antibody and complement (EAC rosettes). The sheep cell-coated lymphocytes are of higher density than the nonrosetted lymphocytes and can be subsequently fractionated by sedimentation through Ficoll-Hypaque, with the nonrosetting cells isolated at the interface. Both techniques, i.e., column immunoabsorbent fractionation and rosetting techniques, allow for the isolation of three distinct surface membrane subpopulations of human lymphocytes. Perhaps of greater importance, the functional properties of these isolated populations have been documented and indicate that they are unique subpopulations (1, 2, 5, 8).

MATERIALS

Solutions, chemicals, and reagents

Human gamma globulin (Miles-Pentex, Kankakee, Ill.)

Crystallized pepsin (Miles-Pentex)

Sodium acetate, 0.1 M, pH 4.5 (Fisher Scientific)

Sodium sulfate (Fisher Scientific)

Phosphate-buffered saline (PBS), pH 7.4

Complete Freund's adjuvant (Difco Laboratories, Detroit, Mich.)

Cyanogen bromide (Eastman Kodak Co., Rochester, N.Y.)

Glycine buffer, 0.1 M, pH 2.5

Phosphate buffer, 2 M, pH.8.0

Sepharose 4-B (Pharmacia Fine Chemicals)
Sephadex G-200 (Pharmacia Fine Chemicals)
Medium 199 (Grand Island Biological Co.,
  Grand Island, N.Y.)
Penicillin-streptomycin solution (Grand Island
  Biological Co.)
Ethylenediaminetetraacetate (EDTA) (2.5 mM)
Fetal calf serum (Microbiological Associates,
  Inc., Bethesda, Md.)
Hanks balanced salt solution, HBSS (Microbio-
  logical Associates)
Ficoll (Pharmacia, Uppsala, Sweden)
Hypaque (Sigma Chemical Co.)
Sheep erythrocytes (Microbiological Associ-
  ates)
EAC cells (Cordis Laboratories, Miami, Fla.)

Special equipment

Light microscope
Fluorescence microscope
Refrigerated centrifuge
Disposable syringes
Plastic stopcocks
Polyethylene sintered disks (Bell Art Products,
  Benawalk, N.J.)
Glass columns (1 × 40 cm)
Spectrophotometer
pH meter

Animals

Rabbits and animal care facilities

TEST PROCEDURES

Cellular immunoabsorbent chromatography

Preparation of rabbit anti(Fab)$_2$ sera.

1. To obtain human (Fab)$_2$ fragments, dissolve 500 mg of human gamma globulin in 0.1
M sodium acetate buffer (pH 4.5) containing 5
mg of pepsin, and incubate the mixture at 37 C
for 20 h. Adjust the digested gamma globulin
solution to pH 8.0, and add 50 ml of Na$_2$SO$_4$ (25
g/100 ml) dropwise.

2. Dissolve the white precipitate [containing
(Fab)$_2$] in water. Then dialyze it against 0.1 M
sodium acetate followed by PBS, and bring it to
a concentration of 5 mg/ml in PBS.

3. To prepare rabbit anti(Fab)$_2$, emulsify 1
mg of (Fab)$_2$ in complete Freund's adjuvant and
inject it intramuscularly weekly for 3 weeks.
One week after the last immunization, the rabbits are bled and sera are collected.

Purification of rabbit anti(Fab)$_2$ sera.

1. Activate 30 ml of Sepharose 4-B with cyanogen bromide (20 ml of 50 mg/ml solution) for 12

min, maintaining the pH at 11.0 with 1 N
NaOH.

2. Wash the activated Sepharose in borate-
buffered saline (pH 8.3), and add 200 mg of
human gamma globulin for 18 h at 4 C.

3. Wash the conjugated Sepharose exhaustively with PBS, and pack it in a glass column.

4. Pass 100 ml of rabbit anti(Fab)$_2$ sera
through 10 ml of packed human gamma globulin conjugated Sepharose.

5. Then elute the retained anti(Fab)$_2$ antibody from the column with 0.1 M glycine-HCl
buffer (pH 2.5) and collect it in 2 M phosphate
buffer (pH 8.0).

6. Dialyze the purified antibody against PBS,
concentrate it to approximately 10 mg/ml, and
store it at −70 C.

Preparation of Sephadex G-200 anti(Fab)$_2$ immunoabsorbent columns.

1. Activate 60 ml of Sephadex G-200, sieved to
achieve uniform bead size (88 to 120 μm), with
100 mg of cyanogen bromide, maintaining the
pH at 10.2 with 1 N NaOH, for 10 min. Proper
activation should result in a 20 to 30% loss in
volume.

2. Wash the activated Sephadex G-200 with
borate-buffered saline (pH 8.3), and add 20 mg
of purified anti(Fab)$_2$ for 4 h at room temperature without mechanical stirring.

3. Wash the resulting Sephadex G-200
anti(Fab)$_2$ conjugate with PBS over a sintered-
glass funnel without suction. Mix every 15 min
with a glass rod.

4. Fit disposable syringes (12 ml) with polyethylene disks, and pack them with 8 to 10 ml of
the anti(Fab)$_2$ conjugated Sephadex.

5. Wash columns with medium 199 containing 5% fetal calf serum, 2.5 mM EDTA,
and 1% penicillin-streptomycin. At this point,
the columns are ready for cell fractionation.

Cell preparation and fractionation.

1. The mononuclear cells from whole peripheral blood or from other peripheral lymphoid
tissues should be isolated and purified by Ficoll-Hypaque centrifugation, to remove erythrocytes, granulocytes, and debris. The cells are
then washed three times in medium 199 containing 5% fetal calf serum and made monocyte
deficient by use of the iron carbonyl technique
(10). One should avoid using nylon wool columns for depletion of monocytes since these
columns will also selectively deplete B cells.
The resulting highly purified lymphocyte population, which should contain greater than 98%
lymphocytes, is then brought to a concentration

of 10×10^6 to 20×10^6 per ml in medium containing 5% fetal calf serum and 2.5 mM EDTA (starting medium) before application to Sephadex anti-human Fab columns.

2. A 5- to 10-ml amount of the lymphocyte suspension is applied to each 8-ml column at room temperature, and eluates are collected by stepwise elution with 15-ml amounts of starting medium at a flow rate of approximately 0.3 to 0.5 ml per min. Elution with starting medium is continued until the effluent is virtually cell-free.

3. The retained cells are eluted by competitive inhibition with the use of two 15-ml portions of medium containing 10 mg of human gamma globulin per ml. During the elution of bound cells, the column can be gently mixed by simply drawing the column material up and down in a Pasteur pipette.

4. The recovered cell populations are then washed three to four times in medium 199 containing fetal calf serum before analysis of surface characteristics or before other investigations are carried out in cell culture. All cells passing directly through the column are surface Ig negative, whereas more than 98% of the cells eluted with human Ig stain with fluorescein-conjugated anti(Fab)$_2$ reagents. Greater than 90% of all cells applied to the immunoabsorbent columns are routinely recovered.

Comments.

1. Sephadex G-200 serves as an excellent filter for lymphocytes since cells are not nonspecifically retained. This property allows for "total" cell recovery.

2. The anti(Fab)$_2$ must be purified and tested for antibody activity prior to conjugation to Sephadex G-200. Use of anti(Fab)$_2$ serum without purification of the antibody is not advised.

3. Once prepared, anti(Fab)$_2$ conjugated Sephadex can be stored in sodium azide at 4 C for as long as 3 months without loss of activity.

4. The Ig negative fraction isolated from anti(Fab)$_2$ immunoabsorbent columns is composed predominantly of T cells but is heterogeneous in that there exists an Ig negative, E rosette negative subset (null cell) within this population (see below).

5. The Ig positive fraction is routinely more than 98% B cells by surface markers and functional properties.

6. Residual monocytes, not removed by the iron carbonyl technique, are found distributed in both the Ig negative and Ig positive populations and can be removed by nylon wool for special studies.

Rosetting techniques for further fractionation of human lymphocyte subpopulations

Isolation of the E rosette negative, Ig negative subset from the non-Ig-bearing population.

1. Sheep erythrocytes (E cells) are washed three times in HBSS and made up to a final concentration of 5% cells in HBSS.

2. Non-Ig-bearing lymphocytes isolated from the immunoabsorbent column above are washed three times in HBSS and brought to a concentration of 15×10^6 cells per ml.

3. Equal volumes of the washed non-Ig lymphocytes are mixed with the 5% suspension of E cells, spun for 5 min at $250 \times g$, and placed at room temperature for 1 to 2 h.

4. The E rosetted cells are then gently resuspended, layered over Ficoll-Hypaque, and spun at $400 \times g$ for 40 min at 20 C. The interface containing the nonrosetted cells is then aspirated and washed three times in medium 199 with 5% fetal calf serum. The recovered lymphocyte population is surface Ig negative and E rosette negative, and represents a population of null cells.

Isolation of the E rosette positive (T cell) subset from the non-Ig population

1. Sheep erythrocytes coated with antibody and complement (EAC cells) are washed three times in HBSS and brought to a 5% concentration.

2. Equal volumes of EAC cells and HBSS-washed non-Ig-bearing lymphocytes are gently mixed, incubated for 0.5 h at 37 C, and centrifuged at $250 \times g$ for 5 min.

3. The EAC rosettes are then gently resuspended, layered over Ficoll-Hypaque, and spun at $400 \times g$ at 37 C for 40 min. The non-EAC rosetting lymphocytes recovered from the interface are washed three times in medium 199 with 5% fetal calf serum. This population of cells is E rosette positive and surface Ig negative and represents a highly purified T cell population.

Comments.

1. Fresh E and EAC cells (<1 week old) are required for optimal separation to be achieved.

2. The temperature requirements outlined above are crucial for adequate cell separation.

3. With both the E and the EAC depletion techniques, one routinely has a 20 to 40% cell loss. This makes use of these techniques for the separation of whole lymphocytes into T and B cell populations subject to the criticism that

unique subpopulations may be lost.

4. Utilizing rosette depletion techniques alone, one requires two depletions before highly purified populations are obtained.

With all cell separation techniques it is extremely important to characterize each isolated population not only by surface marker criteria but also by functional studies.

LITERATURE CITED

1. Chess, L., R. P. MacDermott, and S. F. Schlossman. 1974. Immunologic function of isolated human lymphocyte subpopulations. I. Quantitative isolation of human T and B cells and response to mitogens. J. Immunol. 113:1113–1221.

2. Chess, L., R. P. MacDermott, P. M. Sondel, and S. F. Schlossman. 1974. Isolation and characterization of cells involved in human cellular hypersensitivity. Prog. Immunol. 3:125.

3. Eisen, S. A., H. J. Wedner, and C. W. Parker. 1972. Isolation of pure human peripheral blood T-lymphocytes using nylon wool columns. Immunol. Commun. 1:571–577.

4. Geha, R. S., F. S. Rosen, and E. Merler. 1973. Identification and characterization of subpopulations of lymphocytes in human peripheral blood after fractionation on discontinuous gradients of albumin. J. Clin. Invest. 52:1726–1734.

5. Rocklin, R. E., R. P. MacDermott, L. Chess, S. F. Schlossman, and J. R. David. 1974. Studies on mediator production by highly purified human T and B lymphocytes. J. Exp. Med. 140:1303–1316.

6. Mendes, N. F., M. Tolnai, N. Silveira, R. Gilbertsen, and R. Metzgar. 1973. Technical aspects of the rosette tests used to detect human complement receptor (B) and sheep erythrocyte-binding (T) lymphocytes. J. Immunol. 111:860–867.

7. Schloosman, S. F., and L. Hudson. 1973. Specific purification of lymphocyte populations on a digestible immunoabsorbant. J. Immunol. 110:313–315.

8. Sondel, P. M., L. Chess, R. P. MacDermott, and S. F. Schlossman. 1975. Immunologic function of isolated human lymphocyte subpopulations. III. Specific allogeneic lympholysis mediated by human T cells alone. J. Immunol. 114:982–987.

9. Wigzell, H. 1971. Cellular immunosorbents. Prog. Immunol. 1:1105–1114.

10. Wofsy, L., J. Kimura, and P. Truffa-bachi. 1971. Cell separation on affinity columns: the preparation of pure populations of anti-hapten specific lymphocytes. J. Immunol. 107:725–729.

11. Zeiller, K., G. Pascher, and K. Hannig. 1972. Preparative electrophoretic separation of antibody forming cells. Prep. Biochem. 2:21–37.

Chapter 9

Lymphocyte Transformation

JOOST J. OPPENHEIM AND BILHA SCHECTER

INTRODUCTION

Cell-mediated immunity (CMI) can be evaluated by a considerable number of methods. Skin tests for delayed hypersensitivity reactions provide a relatively easy, reproducible, and informative means of assessing immunological competence (see chapter 00). However, skin tests assay predominantly the effector limb of CMI (9). They are contraindicated in sensitized subjects and, since skin tests also result in the administration of immunogenic doses of antigens, they alter the immunological status of the subject. A variety of in vitro assays of CMI have been developed during the past decade which avoid these pitfalls. These have all been developed since the discovery by Nowell in 1960 (53) that phytohemagglutinin (PHA), a lectin extracted from kidney beans, transforms small lymphocytes into proliferating lymphoblasts in tissue culture. Since then, such mitogen-induced, as well as antigen-induced, lymphocyte transformation has become a widely used experimental tool of great utility for biochemists, cell biologists, geneticists, immunologists, and virologists, as well as clinicians.

There are a variety of in vitro tests for evaluating CMI. Assays of lymphocyte transformation provide the simplest, most reproducible, rapid semiquantitative, and widely used in vitro correlate of CMI (12, 13, 33, 51, 54). Although in vitro assays of mediator production can correlate more closely with skin tests (60), they are in general more difficult to perform. Dissociation of cutaneous delayed hypersensitivity, in vitro mediator production, and lymphocyte transformation have also been observed (17, 61, 62, 65). Sometimes only lymphocyte transformation detects defects in CMI, because some antigenic components induce only lymphocyte transformation whereas others induce only mediator production (67). At times, only lymphoproliferative reactions, but not other assays of CMI, detect defective immune function (7). Lymphocyte transformation can be defective, even in the absence of lymphopenia (46), and therefore provides a sensitive indicator of defective lymphocyte function.

In this review, we will critically evaluate various methods for assessing lymphocyte transformation and provide references only to recent and some classical papers. For additional information, there are older relevant reviews (16, 55) and books (10, 27). We will describe in detail two practical, mechanized micromethods used by us to assess lymphocyte transformation. They involve assaying protein synthesis by transforming lymphocytes, which has the advantage of rapidity, or assaying deoxyribonucleic acid (DNA) synthesis, which provides greater sensitivity. These methods enable lymphocyte transformation to be used both as a routine clinical test and as a widely applicable investigative tool for experimental studies.

The lymphocyte transformation test has an enormous range of applications as follows:

1. Clinically, assays of lymphocyte transformation provide an appropriate and practical means of assessing and monitoring both genetic and acquired immunological deficiency states (40). In addition to providing a sensitive indicator of depressed lymphocyte function, the effects of various immunoenhancing and immunosuppressive therapies can be sequentially monitored by assays of lymphocyte transformation. For example, a variety of treatments of congenitally immunodeficient subjects such as bone marrow (40) and thymic grafts (40), as well as treatment with transfer factor (42) and thymic hormone (64), have been monitored by their beneficial effect on deficient in vitro lymphocyte transformation. The suggestion that both the degree of impairment of lymphocyte reactivity in cancer patients and the improvement in the in vitro lymphocyte reactions following resections or chemotherapy can be used as prognostic indicators is also worthy of further exploration (73).

2. Only by comparing the in vitro lymphoproliferative reactions of cells cultured in the patient's own versus a pool of normal homologous serum or plasma can it be established whether a lymphocyte defect is intrinsically cellular or due to extrinsic toxic (20, 46, 52) or inhibitory factors present in patients' sera. A

variety of specific (3, 4, 29, 32, 36, 74, 75) as well as nonspecific factors (50) that interfere with normal lymphocyte function of a patient can be detected only by comparing sera in this fashion.

3. Assays of lymphocyte transformation have great potential clinical applicability as a diagnostic tool for detecting previous exposure to various pathogens. For example, in malaria (76), hepatitis (77), *Mycoplasma pneumoniae* infections (7), periodontal disease (34, 44), and certain viral infections (68), previous exposure can be detected only by in vitro lymphoproliferative reactions in response to the relevant antigen because many of the subjects no longer have detectable serum antibodies. Similarly, since the relevant antigens that are etiological agents in various autoimmune conditions specifically stimulate lymphocytes only from patients with these conditions (1, 6, 19), this lymphocyte reaction provides a powerful diagnostic tool for detection of autoimmune conditions. Furthermore, antigens responsible for allergies can also stimulate specific in vitro lymphoproliferative reactions because immediate allergic as well as contact and drug reactions frequently occur in response to thymus-dependent antigens. Therefore, lymphocyte transformation also can be used as a diagnostic aid in allergic conditions (4, 22, 24, 48, 62).

4. It is becoming apparent that accurate and relevant histocompatibility typing of candidates and donors for transplants can be achieved only by using mixed leukocyte reactions (MLR). This is based on the observation that in vitro transformation responses result from mixing leukocytes from unrelated but not from identical subjects (5). Although this provides a more cumbersome approach than histocompatibility locus A (HL-A) typing, one can use banks of frozen stored typed cells (14) for MLR typing. Graft survival correlates best in MLR rather than HL-A identical subjects. In fact, so-called anti-HL-B from pregnancy sera are becoming available which react with the relevant non-HL-A cell surface antigens that are responsible for the MLR. These antibodies can be detected best by their inhibitory effects on the MLR. It is hoped that these antisera will make these types of crucial typing studies practicable (75). An additional utility of this approach is that the genetic susceptibility to various illnesses of individuals may eventually become predictable on the basis of their HL-A or MLR type (28).

5. There are several additional experimental applications for lymphocyte transformation that warrant brief mention. The functional capacity of subpopulations of thymus-derived (T) and bone marrow-derived (B) lymphocytes can be determined, thus permitting more exact localization of a patient's immunological defects (18, 31, 37). The assay can be used to detect hyperactivity of the subpopulation of T suppressor cells, as indicated by the observations that T cells from patients with variable immunodeficiency when added to cultures of normal lymphocytes suppress their in vitro production of immunoglobulin (72). Finally, the same procedures used for assaying lymphocyte transformation can be used to generate culture supernatant fluids containing mediators of cellular immunity, as will be discussed in subsequent chapters.

TEST PROCEDURES

General problems

Tissue culture techniques require careful, patient workers and a few months of practice before optimal results are obtained. Instruments such as laminar flow hoods, although they diminish the incidence of contamination, cannot substitute for good sterile techniques. As with most well-established techniques, variations abound, and laboratories modify the assay to fulfill their own requirements. When the technique is first established, it is crucial to determine the kinetics, cell density, culture medium, volume, source of plasma, type of culture vessels, and other conditions that produce optimal results. Even under optimal experimental conditions, there is considerable variability in the lymphoproliferative response of normal individuals, and the degree of reactivity of the same individual varies considerably upon repeated testing. Some of this is due to unavoidable variations in tissue culture techniques, and some is due to the effects of uncontrollable environmental influences on a donor's lymphocyte reactivity. It is, therefore, crucial to control for technical variability by always testing age- and preferably sex-matched normal controls at the same time as experimental subjects (15, 21). It is also essential to use some potent stimulants as positive controls in each experiment and to use multiple doses of a stimulant since only the reaction to suboptimal doses may be abnormal (21, 54, 78).

Preparation of cell suspensions

Human peripheral blood (20 to 500 ml) for all types of lymphocyte cultures can be obtained by venipuncture and heparinized (10 to 50 units of heparin/ml) or defibrinated (15). When other lymphoid organs such as tonsils, thymuses, or spleens are used, lymphocyte suspensions are prepared as described elsewhere (23). The red blood cells in whole blood are sedimented at $1 \times g$ at 37 C for 1 to 2 h in tubes which are slanted at a 15° angle to increase surface area. The occasional blood samples from males and defibrinated samples that do not sediment will do so 30 to 60 min after the addition of 1:4 (vol/vol) sterile 6% dextran in isotonic saline (molecular weight 2×10^5 to 3×10^5). The leukocyte-rich plasma can be aspirated, and the cell and plasma concentrations of the cell suspensions can be adjusted by the addition of appropriate amounts of medium. Alternatively, the cells can be washed free from plasma and resuspended in the proper volume of serum-containing medium. Such leukocyte suspensions are usually cultured at a concentration of 10^6 to 2×10^6/ml in a volume of 1 to 3 ml in vials or tubes. Leukocyte counts are performed by standard hematological techniques either manually or with a Coulter counter.

The disadvantage inherent in culturing unfractionated leukocytes is that on rare occasions, when less than 30% of them are lymphocytes, the excessive numbers of neutrophils even in macrocultures interfere with optimal reactions (49). This leads to the impression of impaired lymphocyte function in patients with lymphopenia or marked granulocytosis. This problem is avoided by eliminating the neutrophils and culturing the mononuclear cell fraction obtained from Ficoll-Hypaque gradients. In contrast to unfractionated leukocytes, the mononuclear cells from relatively lymphopenic subjects, if not intrinsically defective, will react normally. In the case of microcultures, it is essential to eliminate neutrophils to obtain optimal results.

Mononuclear cells can be obtained by centrifuging either whole blood or leukocytes in plasma or saline on Ficoll-Hypaque (2.4:1) gradients as described by Boyum (11). Alternatively, one can use a premixed commercial preparation, such as Lymphoprep. One can add 9 ml of a 1:3 dilution of whole blood or leukocyte-rich plasma in isotonic saline to 3 ml of the prepared Ficoll-Hypaque in a relatively narrow (diameter 15 to 16 mm) sterile tube. We have achieved optimal separation by adding 9 ml of leukocytes containing no more than 10^8 cells resuspended in isotonic saline to the 3 ml of Ficoll-Hypaque. With the tube held at a slant, the leukocytes are gently layered with a pipette on top of the Ficoll-Hypaque. The tubes are then centrifuged at room temperature for 40 min at $400 \times g$ in a centrifuge (PR$_2$ International) with the brake off so it does not decelerate too

rapidly. Mononuclear lymphocytes and monocytes are recovered at the Ficoll-Hypaque plasma interface and thoroughly washed, whereas red blood cells and neutrophils pass through the Ficoll-Hypaque and are eliminated. Some laboratories use the Technicon Lymphocyte Separator in which the majority of cells that have phagocytized iron filings are removed by attraction to a magnet. However, this method puts some constraint on the volumes of cell suspensions that can be processed and provides no advantage over other methods of purifying lymphocytes.

Alternatively, one can eliminate the neutrophils by filtering the leukocytes on sterile glass bead or nylon columns which provide a large surface on which adherent phagocytic cells are retained. However, this removes most of the adherent monocytes, and the resultant fraction of nonadherent lymphocytes does not manifest optimal lymphoproliferative reactions to antigenic stimulants unless monocytes or macrophages are readded (8). Although this technique is too laborious for routine studies, it does provide the possibility of assessing the functional capacity of macrophages to restore the response of normally reactive lymphocytes in vitro (8, 71). For example, it has been observed that, when lymphocyte transformation is inhibited by poliovirus, the macrophages rather than the lymphocytes are defective (29).

Recently, several feasible and reasonably reproducible techniques that fractionate human lymphocytes into either 95% pure thymus-dependent (T) cells or bone marrow-derived (B) cells have been developed (see chapter 8). Populations of lymphocytes rich in T cells can be obtained by eluting the least adherent fraction of cells from nylon columns (25). In our hands, the best means for obtaining B cells is to selectively deplete them of T cells by rosetting them twice with sheep red blood cells and differentially centrifuging them on Ficoll-Hypaque to recover the nonrosetted B cell fraction from the gradient (47). Alternatively, a fluorescent cell sorter which uses laser beams to separate lymphocyte subpopulations that fluoresce with specific antisera can be obtained for about $75,000 (18). These methods enable one to evaluate the in vitro lymphoproliferative response to these two major subpopulations of lymphocytes in clinical conditions.

Culturing lymphocytes

Macrocultures. We have previously reviewed the methodology for performing "macrocultures" (55). This includes cultures performed in a great variety of individual tubes, vials, or bottles ranging in volume from 0.5 to 500 ml (66). The crucial principle to keep in mind when performing such cultures is that the density of cells that settle on the bottom of the culture vessel determines whether the lymphocytes will grow. As a rule, 10^6 to 2×10^6 leukocytes or mononuclear cells/cm^2 will be optimal. Lymphocytes at lower densities will not grow as well, if at all, and at higher densities they will inhibit one another. The depth of medium can range from 0.5 to 3 cm, which indicates that the cell concentration can be varied over a much wider range than the cell density.

The mononuclear or leukocyte cell suspensions are prepared in medium containing 15 to 20% autologous or pooled homologous plasma or serum. Pooled homologous plasma or serum is almost as effective as autochthonous plasma provided it is less than 1 month old. To replace autochthonous plasma, the cells should be "gently" centrifuged at $300 \times g$ for 10 min, washed three times with serum-free medium, and evenly resuspended by repeated aspirations in the desired plasma-containing medium. Although it is commonly used, it is not necessary to use AB plasma since blood group substances are not lymphocyte stimulants. However, use of heterologous sera such as fetal calf sera should be avoided because they do stimulate a limited degree of lymphocyte proliferation and therefore raise the background response of "control" cultures. Although nutritionally sufficient, plasma concentrations of less than 10% favor an increased incidence of "nonspecific" reactions to antigens by unsensitized lymphocytes. In the absence of serum or plasma, only reactions to the more potent mitogens can be elicited, but antigen-induced lymphoproliferative reactions fail to occur (41). In contrast, at concentrations >40% plasma the maximal lymphoproliferative responses to both mitogens and antigens become progressively lower, and detection of reactivity to weaker stimulants may be lost. This may be due to the presence of nonspecific immunosuppressive factors such as α-macroglobulins or competitive binding of mitogens to other plasma constituents (50).

Adequate nutritional support is provided by media ranging in complexity from Eagle's minimal essential medium (MEM) to enriched Roswell Park Memorial Institute 1640 (RPMI-1640) supplemented with 2 mM glutamine, 50 units of penicillin, and 50 μg of streptomycin per ml. In donors who are allergic to penicillin, one should use gentamicin (5 μg of reagent/ml of medium). Contamination with fungus or molds can be countered by the addition of 10 μg of 5-fluorocytosine/ml. Although antibiotics minimize contamination, strict sterile techniques must still be used. If the medium is to be reutilized over longer intervals, it must be resupplemented with freshly thawed 2 mM glutamine once a month. In macrocultures, optimal DNA synthesis by mitogen-stimulated lymphocytes usually occurs after 2 to 3 days and to antigens after 5 to 7 days of incubation. The methods for assaying either DNA or protein synthesis in macrocultures are as described below in the sections on microassays.

Microassay of DNA synthesis. For clinical laboratory studies, we currently advocate the use of microculture techniques because they are more economical in use of tissue culture materials and patients' blood, and they require less space and labor than macrocultures (30, 47, 60). The only disadvantage of microcultures is that they are significantly less sensitive in the presence of polymorphonuclear leukocytes. Therefore, they require the time-consuming step of fractionation of leukocytes to obtain mononuclear cells.

For microculture assays plastic plates that are specified for tissue culture purposes are used. They contain 96 flat-bottomed wells which hold a volume of 0.2 ml with 10^5 to 2×10^5 mononuclear cells. Operationally, it is simplest to add the desired cell number in a 0.1-ml volume of medium, as previously described, to the appropriate number of wells, followed by 0.1-ml volumes of medium containing twice the desired final concentration of stimulant. Either 1-ml sterile disposable pipettes or automatic pipettes such as those made by Eppendorf with disposable sterile plastic tips can be used to dispense the cells and stimulants. They are then covered with sterile plastic lids and incubated.

Water-jacketed incubators usually provide more stable temperature regulation than those in which the atmosphere is circulated with fans, but both types are adequate. Incubation of cells in a humidified atmosphere at 5 to 10% CO_2 and air is necessary for optimal reactivity of microcultures. The presence of CO_2 maintains the bicarbonate-buffered media at the proper pH of 7.2. When macrocultures are incubated in the absence of CO_2, the cells can be grown in tightly capped vials or tubes. Microtiter plates can be closed with sealing tape. In both cases, the cells can generate sufficient CO_2 when adequately stimulated. However, weak stimulants do not induce sufficient metabolic activity by the cells to support growth under these conditions. The use of N-2-hydroxyethylpiperazine-N'-2-ethanesulfonic acid (HEPES) buffer only partially alleviates this problem.

It takes from 2 to 4 days of incubation to

detect optimal DNA synthesis in response to mitogens, whereas optimal lymphocyte reactions to antigenic stimulants take from 4.5 to 7 days (Fig. 1). In fact, the response to suboptimal doses of potent mitogens also peaks after 4 days, indicating a direct relationship between the size of the reactive cell population and the rate of DNA synthesis.

The great utility and widespread use of lymphocyte assays has been made possible by the development of quantitative assays of incorporation of radioisotope precursors, which has liberated the technique from the vagaries of laborious morphological evaluation. The uptake of either tritiated thymidine ([^{3}H]TdR, 0.5 μCi/well, specific activity 2 Ci/mmol) or [^{14}C]-

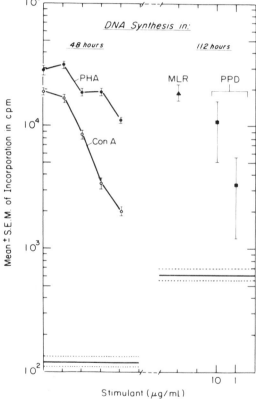

FIG. 1. *Mean ± SE of the mean incorporation of ^{3}H-TdR by triplicate microcultures of 2 × 10^5 normal human peripheral blood mononuclear cells/well. Mitogen-stimulated cultures were incubated with serial twofold dilutions of either phytohemagglutinin (1 μg/ml) or concanavalin A (8 μg/ml) for 48 h. Cultures were stimulated with antigens including a bidirectional mixed leukocyte reaction and 10 and 1 μg of purified protein derivative. The mean counts per minute of [^{3}H]Tdr incorporated by unstimulated cultures is shown by the solid horizontal lines.*

thymidine (0.05 μCi/well, specific activity 50 mCi/mmol) is most commonly used to determine DNA synthesis by cells in S phase. Investigators who wish to avoid the problem of reutilization of isotope use [^{125}I]5-iododeoxyuridine, 200 Ci/mmol (New England Nuclear Corp., Boston, Mass.), which also has the advantage that ^{125}I can be measured in a gamma rather than beta scintillation counter (59). To ensure that the radiolabeled precursor is present in excess, it is very important to add a radiolabeled precursor with low specific activity (38). One can usually demonstrate significant incorporation by adding radiolabeled precursors from 4 to 16 h prior to processing. The shorter 4-h exposure to radioisotope is preferable, but, for the sake of convenience, overnight labeling is often used. Cultures are either immediately harvested or stored as described in the next section. It must be emphasized that incorporation of [^{3}H]TdR is only an estimate of proliferation since cells synthesizing DNA in S phase do not necessarily go on to divide.

Microassay of protein synthesis. A microculture as well as a macroculture technique has been developed which accurately assesses lymphocyte transformation by determining radioactive leucine incorporation into proteins of responding mononuclear leukocytes. The major advantage of this technique is its speed, low incidence of contamination, and lack of requirement for serum. Only 6 to 48 h of incubation are needed to assess lymphocyte competence by this method. It requires the use of leucine-free media to avoid dilution of the radiolabeled leucine precursor in these studies. The absence of leucine does not affect lymphocyte transformation (2). The medium is supplemented with antibiotics, as previously discussed, and the labile essential amino acid glutamine (2 mM). The medium can also be enriched by addition of 1 ml of a nonessential amino acid concentrate (100 ×) per 100 ml of medium. Alternatively, leucine-free RPMI-1640 can be used. Under these conditions, 90% of the lymphocytes remain viable for 48 h of incubation (2). After 48 h, in the absence of serum, the viability of lymphocyte cultures decreases drastically.

Portions of 0.1 ml of the cell suspension are added to microtiter tissue culture plates with 96 V-shaped wells by use of automatic pipettes with sterilized disposable plastic tips. The stimulants are added to the appropriate wells in 10-μliter volumes of medium or phosphate-buffered saline (PBS) at 10 times the desired final concentration. The cells and stimulants are then mixed by placing the plates on a microshaker for 15 s. The plates are incubated in a humidified mixture of 5 to 10% CO² in air at 37 C for 6 to 48 h.

Two to three hours before harvesting the cultures, 1 to 2 µCi of [³H]leucine (specific activity 1 to 2 Ci/mmol) or 0.25 µCi of [¹⁴C]leucine (350 mCi/mmol) is added to each well in a volume of 0.01 ml of PBS with a repeating dispenser Hamilton syringe. The plates are reshaken and reincubated. The culture is stopped by the addition of 0.02 ml of 50% trichloroacetic acid to each well at room temperature. The plates can either be processed immediately or stored at 4 C for up to 1 week.

It has been observed that the incorporation of radiolabeled leucine by both unstimulated and stimulated cultures increases proportionately over a wide concentration range of 2×10^5 to 10^6 mononuclear cells/0.1 ml. Therefore, the stimulation ratio of counts per minute of radiolabeled leucine in experimental stimulated to control unstimulated cultures (E/C) remains stable over this range of cell concentrations. Since the amount of blood that can be used for such studies is usually limiting, only 2.5×10^5 cells/0.1 ml are incubated for 24 h to assay the response to potent mitogens. If necessary, as few as 10^4 cells can be used to obtain significant reactions to potent mitogens, albeit with lower E/C ratios (2).

The degree of background protein synthesis in control cultures decreases slowly over a 48-h period of incubation. In contrast, mitogen-stimulated cultures already show increases in protein synthesis by 4 to 6 h of incubation. This continues to increase for 24 h and plateaus by 48 h. When lower doses of mitogens are used, one obtains optimal sensitivity of the assay and reproducibility of ±10% standard deviation (SD) of the mean counts per minute of replicate cultures by 24 h. However, in the case of weaker antigenic stimulants and the MLR, higher cell concentrations of $10^6/0.1$ ml and a longer incubation period of 48 h are needed to obtain a significant difference in E/C (Fig. 2). We therefore recommend that the more rapid microassay of protein synthesis be used for assaying efficacy of response to mitogens to diagnose immunodeficiency states (Table 1). The assay of DNA synthesis, although slower, is more sensitive and requires fewer cells, and we therefore recommend it be used for detection of prior antigenic sensitization and for the unidirectional MLR.

Processing of lymphocyte cultures

One of the great advantages of microculture assays is that they can be rapidly processed

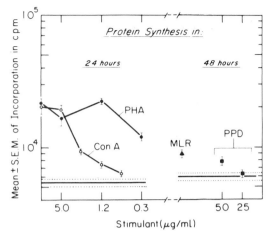

FIG. 2. *Mean ± SE of the mean of [¹⁴C]leucine incorporation by triplicate microcultures of 2.5 × 10⁵ normal human peripheral blood mononuclear cells/ well. Their dose responses to some mitogens and antigens are shown. The mean counts per minute of [¹⁴C]leucine incorporated by unstimulated cultures is shown by the solid horizontal lines.*

with automated harvesting machines (30) which aspirate and wash cells onto glass-fiber filters. This method results in more reproducible data and saves time and effort in comparison with other approaches. In measuring incorporation into DNA, the filters can be washed many times sequentially with isotonic saline, 5% trichloroacetic acid, and absolute methanol. However, repeated washing of the filters with only isotonic saline or water gives similar results. Apparently, the filters retain predominantly macromolecules with incorporated radioisotope, since the cells are broken up on the filter and unincorporated isotope is washed out. In the case of the assay for protein synthesis, the incorporation into acid-precipitable material (i.e., proteins) is measured. In this case, the filters usually are washed with 5% trichloroacetic acid and methanol. The filters are then dried overnight at room temperature or for 30 min under infrared lamps, punched out, and dropped into scintillation vials which contain scintillation fluid; they are then cooled and counted in a beta scintillation counter at the appropriate settings to determine the counts per minute. Although more expensive than homemade mixtures, versatile commercially prepared scintillation fluids are available for counting dried or dissolved samples (Liquifluor), or for samples containing some residual water.

Alternatively, one can use a less expensive or

TABLE 1. *T cell mitogen-induced lymphocyte transformation in immune deficiency determined with the microassay for protein synthesis*

Diagnosis	Mitogen		
	Phytohemagglutinin	WBA[a]	Concanavalin A
Normal	1.09 ± 0.74[b] (20)	1.08 ± 0.86 (12)	1.05 ± 0.62 (18)
Hodgkin's disease	0.17 (1)	0 (1)	0.07 (1)
Chronic lymphatic leukemia	0.33 (1)	0.40 (1)	0.47 (1)
Acute lymphatic leukemia	0.19 (1)	0.16 (1)	0.50 (1)
Acute lymphoma	0.05 (1)	0.07 (1)	0 (1)
Ataxia telangiectasia	0.21 ± 0.05 (3)	0.056 ± 0.06 (2)	0.15 ± 0.20 (5)
Down's syndrome	1.01 ± 0.72 (9)	1.00 ± 1.00 (4)	1.12 ± 0.82 (7)

[a] Wax bean agglutinin obtained from N. Sharon, Weizmann Institute of Science.

[b] Mean $\pm$ 2 SD of ratio of counts per minute of radiolabeled leucine incorporated by mitogen-stimulated mononuclear cell cultures from paired normal subjects or a normal subject and patient tested at the same time. Since the stimulation ratios E/C of a given individual can vary markedly over a period of time, one means by which this variable can be minimized is by analyzing the responses of paired subjects' lymphocytes tested at the same time. The ratio of response of paired normal subjects is close to 1, whereas patients whose reactivity falls *below* the 95% confidence limits of the response (mean $\pm$ 2 SD) were significantly hyporeactive. This approach permits comparison of the response of single patients as well as groups of patients with normal subjects. However, it is preferable because it is statistically less demanding to demonstrate abnormalities in a group of subjects by use of a Student's *t* test (45).

[c] Number of pairs tested. Data obtained from a collaborative study with Stanley Levine of Kaplan Hospital, Rehovot, Israel.

nonautomated filtering device composed of a single filtering unit or of 10 coupled filtering units. For processing the microtiter plates, if one does not have a filter unit, one can use a technique in which the entire plate is centrifuged and washed four times by use of special plate holders which fit into an International centrifuge head (#276). The acid-precipitable material is then dissolved in 1 N NaOH and transferred with an automatic pipette into scintillation vials (63). A scintillation fluid is used that is miscible with water-containing samples.

In the case of macrocultures, if a modified multiple automated sample harvester (MASH) or filter units are not available, one can remove the excessive unincorporated radiolabeled precursor by the laborious procedure of sequentially centrifuging (500 $\times$ g for 10 min) and washing the cells at least four times. Usually the cells are washed once with isotonic saline, twice with 5% trichloroacetic acid to obtain only that fraction of [^{3}H]TdR which has been incorporated by the macromolecular ($>$5,000 molecular weight) constituents of the cells, and finally with absolute methanol to dehydrate the pellet. Alternatively, one can wash the cells with isotonic saline only, since only up to 15% of the intracellular thymidine is in the precursor pool, and this is taken up in proportionately greater amounts by stimulated than unstimulated cells. Then the cell pellet is dissolved in 0.2 ml of Hyamine or NCS solubilizer at 60 C for 15 min, added to scintillation vials, and counted as

above. Beware of the fact that NCS dissolves plastic!

There are some ardent advocates of the technique of culturing whole blood directly diluted 1:10 to 1:40 with medium. This obviously provides the simplest and most economic approach. Although in our hands this method was lacking in sensitivity (55), convincing data have been published which show marked mitogen- and antigen-stimulated proliferative reactions by such whole blood cultures (58, 59). Since the responses in these cultures peak later, there is the disadvantage that it takes 4 days to obtain mitogen-induced and 7 days for antigen-induced reactions. There is the additional disadvantage that these cultures have to be decolorized with acetic acid and/or hydrogen peroxide as well as repeatedly centrifuged and washed to be harvested. There is one report, however, in which as little as 7 μliters of whole blood diluted in medium has been used in microcultures (39). If this is confirmed as being a sensitive and reproducible approach, it promises to become the most applicable means of assaying lymphocyte transformation.

Morphological evaluation

After an appropriate period of 3 to 7 days of incubation, cell suspensions in macrocultures or a pool of a number of microcultures can be pelleted by gentle centrifugation at 200 $\times$ g for 10 min, gently smeared on glass slides, fixed with methanol, and stained with Jenner Giemsa or Wright stain. The proportions of transformed lymphoblasts can then be differentiated from typical small lymphocytes on the basis of increased size (12 to 30 μm in diameter) and an increase in cytoplasmic basophilia and vacuolization. The enlarged nucleus becomes euchromatic, develops readily apparent nucleoli, and can be arrested at various stages of mitosis by colchicine (16). However, such an analysis is easier said than done for the following reasons:

1. There is a significant proportion of intermediate size lymphoblasts which are difficult to classify. Either they appear early in the response or when they appear later in the response they actually represent the progressively smaller progeny of precursor lymphoblasts that have undergone repeated divisions. (70). This can be overcome to some extent by adding [^{3}H]TdR (1 μCi/ml or 0.5 μCi/well) to the cultures for the final 4 to 16 h of incubation and preparing radioautographs (35). Most lymphocytes undergoing DNA synthesis will be labeled by this procedure. However, radioautography also has its limitations since only a proportion of the lymphoblasts will be labeled because some of the transformed lymphocytes will not be synthesizing DNA at the time of exposure to [^{3}H]TdR.

2. The proportion of monocytes, as a result of their enhanced survival, becomes relatively increased, and they can look like transformed lymphocytes. The addition of a 1:10,000 dilution of 1.3-μm (diameter) polystyrene particles which are phagocytized only by monocytic lymphocytes differentiates them from nonphagocytic lymphocytes.

Despite these problems, morphological analyses still provide the only way to determine the proportion of the lymphocyte population that is reacting to a stimulant. Occasionally, stained smears can be used to detect bacterial contamination, although streaking the culture supernatant fluids on blood agar provides an easier means of detecting this problem.

Nonspecific and specific lymphocyte stimulants

The battery of stimulants that can be used to evaluate lymphocyte reactivity forms two groups. Those grouped into "nonspecific" mitogens transform from 60 to 90% of lymphocytes from all normal adults, as well as newborns, independent of immunization. The other group of stimulants are classified as antigens because they stimulate lymphocytes only from sensitized donors. Antigens initially activate only a small clone of the previously sensitized lymphocyte population to transform, but after repeated divisions, during the 5 to 7 days of incubation, 5 to 35% of the lymphocytes appear to be transformed. Therefore, antigen-induced lymphoproliferation represents a secondary response in vitro and fails to stimulate unsensitized adults and the majority of cultures of newborn cord blood lymphocytes. Stimulants can be further characterized by whether they are thymus dependent and stimulate purified T but not B cells or, conversely, are thymus independent and stimulate purified B but not T cells. It must be emphasized that, in the usual heterogeneous mixtures of T and B lymphocytes, the so-called T cell stimulants activate both lymphocyte populations, presumably because they stimulate T cells to make factors that in turn enhance the reactions of B cells (26). Readily available T cell mitogens that are commonly used include PHA (1 to 5 μg/ml) and concanavalin A (ConA, 1 to 10/μg/ml). Pokeweed mitogen (1:20 dilution) stimulates both T and B cells. In humans pokeweed is a thymus-dependent stimulant which can stimulate B cells only in the presence of some T cells (26). In contrast, B cell mitogens will activate only B cells, even in mixtures of B and T lymphocytes (38). Unfortunately, the best known B cell mitogens, such as thymus-independent lipopolysaccharide endotoxins (LPS) and anti-immunoglobulin antibodies are too limited in potency to permit evaluation of B lymphoproliferative reactivity in humans (57). In the case of humans, LPS stimulates only B cells of sensitized subjects and does so only in presence of some T cells; it, therefore, behaves like a T-dependent B cell antigen (37, 56).

In assessing immunocompetence of lymphocytes, it is very important to test the lymphocyte reactivity to suboptimal doses of a mitogen, such as PHA. This can be achieved by determining the dose response to five twofold dilutions of PHA, which will at times detect obvious hyporeactivity of lymphocytes in subjects that have normal reactions to the optimal doses of potent stimulants. For example, in a number of immunodeficiency states (21, 45, 78), including Wiskott-Aldrich syndrome (54), the proliferative response to optimal doses of PHA will be normal, whereas subnormal reactivity can be detected only in response to suboptimal doses of PHA (Table 2).

Antigens that are also commonly used to evaluate the efficacy of human lymphocyte transformation are all thymus dependent and activate T as well as B cell proliferation. They include purified protein derivative (PPD, at 20 μg/ml), streptolysin O (1:20 final dilution), *Candida albicans* (1:100 final dilution of glyc-

TABLE 2. *Detection of impaired lymphoproliferative response in Wiskott-Aldrich syndrome to suboptimal doses of PHA*

Concn of PHA (μg/ml)	Normal subjects	Patients
None	$2,250 \pm 120^a$	$7,500 \pm 2,500$
8	$45,000 \pm 18,000$	$51,000 \pm 15,000$
2	$74,000 \pm 16,000$	$53,000 \pm 20,000$
1	$92,000 \pm 20,000$	$38,000 \pm 13,000$
0.5	$88,000 \pm 8,000$	$23,000 \pm 14,000$
0.25	$49,000 \pm 10,000$	$13,000 \pm 8,000$

[a] Mean ± SE of the mean counts per minute of tritiated thymidine incorporated by duplicate macrocultures from five controls and patients (54).

erol saline extract), and tetanus toxoid (2 LFU/ml or 6 μg/ml, from L. Levine, Massachusetts Department of Health, Boston). Some investigators have proposed that a cocktail consisting of a pool of antigens be used to evaluate in vitro lymphocyte reactivity (43). All the stimulants can be dissolved in sterile water, PBS, or medium. The activity of these stimulants is usually best preserved by storing them in portions at 4 C, except that streptolysin O can only be kept frozen and thawed once, which avoids subjecting it to denaturation by repeated freezing and thawing.

In the case of the bidirectional MLR, equal numbers of leukocytes or lymphocytes from two unrelated individuals are mixed and serve as stimulants that induce an in vitro response to one another (Fig. 1 and 2). To be able to determine the response of one subject's cells, one must perform a "unidirectional" MLR. This can be achieved by preparing viable but nonproliferating leukocytes as stimulants. Such viable stimulator cells can be obtained either by irradiating leukocytes with 1,000 to 4,000 R or by incubating them for 25 min at 37 C with mitomycin C (25 μg/ml, which must then be thoroughly washed off), both of which will block proliferative responses by the cells. Since they will not block protein synthesis, attempts to obtain unidirectional MLRs with assays of protein synthesis have been unsuccessful (2).

REAGENTS

Stimulants

PHA (phytohemagglutinin; Burroughs-Wellcome Co., Tuckahoe, N.Y.) is dissolved in PBS and kept frozen at −20 C at a concentration of 1 mg/ml. Higher dilutions used for routine work will be stable at 4 C for up to 1 month.

ConA (concanavalin A; Miles-Yeda Ltd.,

Rehovot, Israel) can be handled in the same manner as PHA.

Pokeweed mitogen (Grand Island Biological Co., Grand Island, N.Y.) is diluted with medium and frozen at −20 C in small portions prior to use.

LPS (lipopolysaccharide endotoxin) is prepared from *Salmonella typhosa* 0901 (Difco Laboratories, Detroit, Mich.). LPS solution is prepared by dissolving it at 10 mg/ml in PBS and heating it in boiling water for 1 h. This stock solution is then kept at 4 C and diluted for use at 50 μg/ml.

PPD (purified protein derivative; Connaught Laboratories, Toronto, Ontario, Canada) can be stored at 4 C and diluted for use.

Streptolysin O (Difco Laboratories) is unstable; it must be kept at −20 C in small portions and thawed only once.

Candida albicans (Hollister-Stier, Spokane, Wash.) is used at 1:100 final dilution of glycerol saline extract and can be stored at 4 C.

Assay reagents

Media. Can be kept indefinitely at 4 C.

Eagle's minimal essential medium (MEM)—Grand Island Biological Co.

Roswell Park Memorial Institute 1640 (RPMI-1640)—Grand Island Biological Co.

Eagle's medium without leucine—Microbiological Associates, Inc., Bethesda, Md.

Nonessential amino acids (100×)—Grand Island Biological Co.

HEPES buffer—Calbiochem, Gaithersburg, Md.

Phosphate-buffered saline (PBS)—0.15 M sodium chloride, 0.01 M sodium phosphate, pH 7.2.

L-Glutamine—Nutritional Biochemicals Corp., Cleveland, Ohio. Concentration in medium, 0.59 μg/ml. It must be kept at −20 C.

Antibiotics and fungicides.

Penicillin and streptomycin—Microbiological Associates, Inc. Store at −20 C.

Gentamicin (effective concentration 5 μg/ml)—Schering Corp., Port Reading, N.Y.

5-Fluorocytosine—Hoffman-La Roche, Inc., Nutley, N.J.

Reagents for cell preparation.

Heparin, preservative free, approximately 150 units/mg—Mann Research Laboratories, New York, N.Y., or Connaught Laboratories.

Dextran, type 200c—Sigma Chemical Co., St. Louis, Mo. Dissolve in sterile distilled water at a concentration of 6% (6 g/100 ml).

Ficoll, molecular weight 400,000—Sigma Chemical Co. (9% in distilled water).

Hypaque—Winthrop Laboratories, New York, N.Y. (33.9% dissolved in water by heating to 56 C for 30 min).

Lymphoprep—Nyegard and Co., Oslo, Norway.

Radioactive materials. [^{14}C]thymidine (50 mCi/mmol), [^{3}H]thymidine (2 Ci/mmol), [^{14}C]-leucine (350 mCi/mmol) and [^{3}H]leucine (1 Ci/mmol) were obtained from Schwarz/Mann, Rockville, Md., or the Radio Chemical Centre, Amersham, England.

[^{125}I]5-iododeoxyuridine (200 Ci/mmol) was from New England Nuclear Corp., Boston, Mass.

Solubilizers.

Hyamine—Packard Instrument Co., Inc., Downers Grove, Ill.

NCS solubilizer—Amersham, England. Cannot be used in plastic tubes.

Scintillation liquids. For counting dried samples on membrane or glass-fiber filters: 2,5-Diphenyloxazole (PPO), 4 g, and dimethyl-1,4-bis-(5-phenyloxazolyl)benzene (dimethyl-POPOP), 100 mg (Packard Instrument Co., Inc.) dissolved in 1 liter of toluene.

Liquifluor (New England Nuclear Corp.) diluted in toluene as directed.

For counting samples dissolved in aqueous solutions:

Mixture of toluene with PPO and POPOP (1 liter) as described above + Triton X-100 (550 ml) + water (150 ml).

Hydromix (Yorktown Research, New York, N.Y.).

Instruments and other facilities

Liquid scintillation spectrometer, model 3320 automatic counter—Packard Instrument Co., Inc.

Coulter counter—Coulter Electronics, Inc., Hialeah, Fla.

PR-2 International centrifuge—Damon, IEC Div. model, Needham, Mass.

Technicon lymphocyte separator—Technicon Instruments Corp., Tarrytown, N.Y.

Automated harvesting machine, Mash II, Microbiological Associates, Inc.

Multiple membrane filter—Yeda Scientific Instruments, Rehovot, Israel.

Automatic pipettes and sterile disposable tips —Eppendorf, Hamburg, West Germany, or Oxford Laboratories, Oxford, Calif.

Micromedic System model 25000 automatic pipette—Micromedic System Inc., Philadelphia, Pa.

Microshaker—Cooke Microtiter System, Alexandria, Va.

Hamilton Syringe—Hamilton Co., Whittier, Calif.

V-shaped microtiter plates—Cooke Microtiter System

Flat-bottom microtiter plates, Microtest II tissue culture plates and lids—Falcon Plastics, Oxnard, Calif.

Sealing tape—Cooke Microtiter System.

Glass-fiber filters (934AH), Reeve Angel and Co., Clifton, N.J.

Nylon wool—DuPont de Nemours & Co. Textile Fibers, Portsmouth, Va.

Superbrite glass beads (#100–500 s) Minnesota Mining & Manufacturing Co., Minneapolis, Minn.

INTERPRETATION

Experimental points should be performed at least in duplicate and preferably in triplicate or quadruplicate. The arithmetic mean and standard error of the mean of the counts per minute of the samples should be determined. Some laboratories correct the "raw" counts per minute for both degree of quenching and efficiency of their counter and express their results in disintegrations per minute (dpm). When, as usually is the case, the degree of quenching of samples within a given experiment is similar and machine efficiency is constant, this additional step does not really affect the interpretation of the data and can be omitted. The counts per minute of replicate samples, except in the case of very weak stimulants and unstimulated cultures, should vary by less than 20% from the mean. Variations in excess of 20% in replicate stimulated cultures are indicative of technical problems. It is not valid to eliminate replicate samples that vary too much from the mean unless they completely failed to incorporate or incorporated too much radioisotope. This is often due to bacterial contamination, cell death for unknown causes associated with evidence of alkalinity of medium (purple phenophthalein indicator), or omission of the [^{3}H]TdR pulse.

The large changes in magnitude of [^{3}H]TdR incorporation by cultured lymphocytes with increasing duration of incubation are based on their exponential growth rate. Therefore, small differences in growth rate become magnified with time and result in a non-normal distribution of data. For a proper statistical assessment, data of this type must be normalized. This can be achieved by logarithmic conversion of the counts per minute, which can then be analyzed by Student's t test, analysis of variance, or other statistical methods. The data can then be reconverted to counts per minute and the geometric mean ± confidence limits can be expressed. Although the same approach can be used to analyze the radiolabeled leucine uptake, analysis of arithmetic means is probably adequate since the duration of culture is shorter and the exponential changes therefore are not as great.

Frequently, only the ratios of experimental to control (E/C) cultures are shown. Although this normalizes the data to some extent, it is based on the assumption that the degree of reactivity of control and experimental cultures will be affected by variables in the same way and will remain proportional. Unfortunately, this is sometimes not the case. There may be uncontrollable prior in vivo excitation of immunological reactivity that elevates the response in "control" cultures and interferes with the reactivity to other stimuli, as in Wiskott-Aldrich patients (Table 2). Stimulants present in vivo may be transferred into the cultures and may be responsible for the progressive increases in proliferation in unstimulated cultures that occur with longer periods of incubation. Alternatively, lymphoproliferative reactions in control cultures may be induced by media components, cell products, or too vigorous handling which may damage and stimulate some cells. Factors that stimulate control cultures appear to lower the E/C, although the actual degree of experimental response may remain stable. Therefore, although it is more cumbersome, the control as well as experimental results always ought to be indicated to permit proper evaluation of the data.

The thymidine incorporation by unstimulated cultures is usually low because only stimulated lymphocytes go on to synthesize DNA. This low background is responsible for the sensitivity of this assay, and it has been estimated that the repeated divisions of an initial clone with fewer than 10 stimulated cells in a population of 10^6 lymphocytes theoretically can result in significant increases (E/C) in thymidine uptake. Provided background counts per minute of thymidine incorporation are at reasonably low levels and the variation between replicates is $< 20\%$, reproducible threefold or greater differences between E and C are indicative of significant lymphocyte proliferation. Smaller differences than that must be consistently reproduced many times to be indicative of a biologically meaningful reaction.

Since protein synthesis, in contrast to DNA synthesis, is an ongoing process in the resting lymphocyte, there is considerable uptake of radiolabeled leucine by unstimulated cultures (Fig. 2). However, "small" increases in protein synthesis by stimulated cultures can be quite significant since the variation between replicate cultures is much smaller ($\pm 10\%$) than in the case of [^{3}H]TdR uptake ($\pm 20\%$). The only valid criterion for determining significant stimulation of protein synthesis depends on comparison with the corresponding unstimulated controls (E/C), and ratios of 1.5 or greater are usually significant. Repeated tests of the response of a normal individual's lymphocytes will result in considerable variation in the incorporation of radiolabeled leucine, but his E/C will fluctuate much less and remain in the normal range (45; Table 1).

To establish whether an individual's lymphocytes are functioning within the normal range, one should compare his response with that of concomitantly tested normally reactive controls. In addition, this reactivity must be assessed relative to the 95 or 99% confidence limits of the reactivity of a large number of age-matched normal subjects, previously tested by the laboratory (Table 1). Whether a group of patients have normally transforming lymphocytes can be determined by comparing them with a concomitantly tested group of normal subjects by use of Student's t test.

CONCLUSIONS

The time has come to establish assays for lymphocyte transformation as a routine diagnostic tool in the clinical laboratory. As indicated in the Introduction, the assay provides a very useful means of assessing immunological competence in genetic and acquired immunodeficiency states and a sensitive tool for detecting immunological reactions to pathogens, allergens, and self-antigens. Tissue culture techniques have been developed which permit economical, reproducible and rapid, partially mechanized microassays to be performed. Consequently, results can be obtained in 1 to 2 days which enable the physician to determine the functional immunological capacity of a patient's cell-mediated immunological reactions.

ACKNOWLEDGMENTS

We are very grateful for the constructive criticisms of the manuscript by Ronald Levy and Larry Steinman.

LITERATURE CITED

1. Abramsky, O., A. Aharonov, C. Webb, and S. Fuchs. 1975. Cellular immune response to ace-

tylcholine receptor rich fraction in patients with myasthenia gravis. Clin. Exp. Immunol. **19**:11–16.

2. Adkinson, N. F., Jr., S. A. Rosenberg, and W. D. Terry. 1974. Early detection of lymphocyte stimulation and mixed lymphocyte interactions in man with a semimicro protein assay. J. Immunol. **112**:1426–1434.

3. Ahmed, A., D. M. Strong, K. W. Sell, G. B. Thurman, R. C. Knudsen, R. Wistar, Jr., and W. R. Grace. 1974. Demonstration of a blocking factor in the plasma and spinal fluid of patients with subacute sclerosing panencephalitis. I. Partial characterization. J. Exp. Med. **139**:902–924.

4. Anderson, J. A., S. R. Lane, W. A. Howard, S. Leikin, and J. J. Oppenheim. 1974. The effect of a "blocking" plasma factor induced by hyposensitization on alternaria induced lymphocyte transformation. Cell. Immunol. **10**:442–449.

5. Bain, B., M. Vas, and L. Lowenstein. 1964. The development of large immature mononuclear cells in mixed leucocyte cultures. Blood **23**:108–111.

6. Behan, P. O., J. B. Lamarche, R. G. Feldman, and W. A. Sheramata. 1970. Lymphocyte transformation in the Guillain-Barre Syndrome. Lancet **1**:421.

7. Biberfeld, G., P. Biberfeld, and G. Stermer. 1974. Cell mediated immune response following mycoplasma pneumoniae infection in man. I. Lymphocyte stimulation. Clin. Exp. Immunol. **17**:29–41.

8. Blaese, R. M., J. J. Oppenheim, R. C. Seeger, and T. A. Waldmann. 1972. Lymphocyte macrophage interaction in antigen-induced *in vitro* lymphocyte transformation in patients with the Wiskott Aldrich syndrome and other diseases with anergy. Cell. Immunol. **4**:228–242.

9. Blaese, R. M., P. Weiden, J. J. Oppenheim, and T. A. Waldmann. 1973. Phytohemagglutinin as a skin test for the evaluation of cellular immune competence in man. J. Lab. Clin. Med. **81**:538–549.

10. Bloom, B. R., and P. Glade (ed.). 1971. *In vitro* methods in cell-mediated immunity. Academic Press Inc., New York.

11. Boyum, A. 1966. Ficoll Hypaque method for separating mononuclear cells and granulocytes from human blood. Scand. J. Clin. Lab. Invest. Suppl., p. 77.

12. Catalona, W. J., J. L. Tarpley, C. Potvin, and P. B. Chretien. 1975. Correlations among cutaneous reactivity to DNCB, PHA induced lymphocyte blastogenesis and peripheral blood E rosettes. Clin. Exp. Immunol. **19**:327–333.

13. Catanzaro, A., L. E. Spitler, and K. M. Moser. 1975. Cellular immune response in coccidioidomycosis. Cell. Immunol. **15**:360–371.

14. Chess, L., G. N. Bock, and M. R. Mardiney, Jr. 1972. Restoration of the reactivity of frozen stored human lymphocytes in the mixed lymphocyte reaction and in response to specific antigens. Transplantation **14**:728–733.

15. Delespesse, G., J. Duchateau, P. A. Bastenie, J. P. Lauvaux, H. Collet, and A. Govaerts. 1974. Cell mediated immunity in diabetes mellitus. Clin. Exp. Immunol. **18**:461–467.

16. Douglas, S. D. 1971. Human lymphocyte growth *in vitro*: morphological, biochemical and immunological significance. Int. Rev. Exp. Pathol. **10**:41–114.

17. Eife, R. F., G. Eife, C. S. August, W. L. Kuhre, and K. Staehr-Johansen. 1974. Lymphotoxin production and blast cell transformation by cord blood lymphocytes: dissociated lymphocyte function in newborn infants. Cell. Immunol. **14**:435–442.

18. Epstein, L. B., H. W. Kreth, and L. A. Herzenberg. 1974. Fluorescence activated cell sorting of human T and B lymphocytes. II. Identification of the cell type responsible for interferon production and cell proliferation in response to mitogens. Cell. Immunol. **12**:407–421.

19. Esiri, M. M., I. C. M. MacLennan, and B. L. Hazleman. 1973. Lymphocyte sensitivity to skeletal muscle in patients with polymyositis and other disorders. Clin. Exp. Immunol. **14**:25–35.

20. Espanol, T., E. B. Todd, and J. F. Soothill. 1974. The effect of anaesthesia on the lymphocyte response to phytohemagglutinin. Clin. Exp. Immunol. **18**:73–79.

21. Foad, B. S. I., L. E. Adams, Y. Yamauchi, and A. Litwin. 1974. Phytomitogen responses of peripheral blood lymphocytes in young and older subjects. Clin. Exp. Immunol. **17**:657–664.

22. Gatien, J. G., E. Merler, and H. R. Colten. 1975. Allergy to ragweed antigen E: effect of specific immunotherapy on the reactivity of human T lymphocytes *in vitro*. Clin. Immunol. Immunopathol. **4**:32–37.

23. Geha, R. S., and E. Merler. 1974. Response of human thymus derived (B) lymphocytes to mitogenic stimulation *in vitro*. Eur. J. Immunol. **4**:193–199.

24. Glass, D., L. Roffe, R. N. Maini, D. G. Wraith, and G. Nuki. 1975. Adverse reactions to An[124] ACTH therapy associated with specific cellular immunity. Clin. Exp. Immunol. **20**:55–63.

25. Greaves, M. F., and G. Brown. 1974. Purification of human T and B lymphocytes. J. Immunol. **112**:420–423.

26. Greaves, M., G. Janossy, and M. Doenhoff. 1974. Selective triggering of human T and B lymphocytes *in vitro* by polyclonal mitogens. J. Exp. Med. **140**:1–18.

27. Greaves, M. F., J. J. T. Owen, and M. C. Raff. 1973. T and B lymphocytes, origins, properties and roles in immune responses. American Elsevier Publishing Co., Inc., New York.

28. Greenberg, L. J., E. D. Gray, and E. J. Yunis. 1975. Association of HL-A5 and immune responsiveness *in vitro* to streptococcal antigens. J. Exp. Med. **141**:935–943.

29. Handin, R. I., W. P. Piessens, and W. C. Moloney. 1973. Stimulation of nonimmunized lymphocytes by platelet antibody complexes in

idiopathic thrombocytopenic purpura. N. Engl. J. Med. **289**:714–718.

30. Hartzman, R. J., M. L. Bach, F. H. Bach, G. Thurman, and K. W. Sell. 1972. Precipitation of radioactively labeled samples: a semi-automatic multiple sample processor. Cell. Immunol. **4**:182–187.

31. Hedfors, E. 1974. Activation of peripheral T cells of sarcoidosis patients and healthy controls. Clin. Exp. Immunol. **18**:379–390.

32. Heilman, D. H., and W. McFarland. 1966. Inhibition of tuberculin induced mitogenesis in cultures of lymphocytes from tuberculous donors. Int. Arch. Allergy **30**:58–60.

33. Horsmanheimo, M. 1974. Correlation of tuberculin induced lymphocyte transformation with skin test reactivity and with clinical manifestations of sarcoidosis. Cell. Immunol. **10**:329–337.

34. Horton, J. E., S. Leikin, and J. J. Oppenheim. 1972. Human lymphoproliferative reactions to saliva and dental plaque deposits: an *in vitro* correlation with periodontal disease. J. Periodontol. **43**:522–527.

35. Hsu, T. C. 1969. Mammalian Chromosome Newsletter **10**:104–108.

36. Ivanyi, L., S. J. Challacombe, and T. Lehner. 1973. The specificity of serum factors in lymphocyte transformation in periodontal disease. Clin. Exp. Immunol. **14**:491–500.

37. Ivanyi, L., and T. Lehner. 1975. Stimulation of human lymphocytes by B cell mitogens. Clin. Exp. Immunol. **18**:347–356.

38. Janossy, G., M. F. Greaves, M. J. Doenhoff, and J. Snajar. 1973. Lymphocyte activation. V. Quantitation of the proliferative response to mitogens using defined T and B cell populations. Clin. Exp. Immunol. **14**:581–596.

39. Kaplan, J. M., and A. F. Razzano. 1973. A miniature phytohemagglutinin assay using disposable microtiter plates. Immunol. Commun. **2**:507–519.

40. Kazimiera, J., Gajl-Peczalska, B. H. Park, W. D. Biggar, and R. A. Good. 1973. B and T lymphocytes in primary immunodeficiency in man. J. Clin. Invest. **52**:919–918.

41. Kirchner, H., and J. J. Oppenheim. 1972. Stimulation of chicken lymphocytes in a serum-free medium. Cell. Immunol. **3**:695–699.

42. Lawrence, H. S. 1974. Transfer factor in cellular immunity. Harvey Lect. **68**:239–350.

43. Leguit, P., A. Meinesz, L. Huismans, and V. P. Eijsvoogel. 1973. The use of an antigen cocktail in the lymphocyte transformation test. Clin. Exp. Immunol. **14**:149–152.

44. Lehner, T., M. A. Wilton, S. J. Challacombe, and L. Ivanyi. 1974. Sequential cell mediated immune responses in experimental gingivitis in man. Clin. Exp. Immunol. **16**:481–492.

45. Levy, R., and H. S. Kaplan. 1974. Impaired lymphocyte function in untreated Hodgkin's disease. N. Engl. J. Med. **290**:181–186.

46. Lopez, C., R. L. Simmons, J. L. Touraine, B. M. Park, D. F. Fiszkiss, J. S. Najarian, and R. A. Good. 1975. Discrepancy between PHA responsiveness and quantitative estimates of T cell numbers during chronic renal failure and immunosuppression after transplantation. Clin. Immunol. Immunopathol. **4**:135–142.

47. Mackler, B. F., L. Altman, D. L. Rosenstreich, and J. J. Oppenheim. 1974. Activation of human B lymphocytes: induction of lymphokine production by EAC and blastogenesis by soluble mitogens. Nature (London) **249**:834–837.

48. Miller, A. E. and W. R. Levis. 1973. Lymphocyte transformation during dinitrochlorobenzene contact sensitization. J. Clin. Invest. **52**:1925–1930.

49. Moore, D. L., B. Heyworth, and J. Brown. 1974. PHA induced lymphocyte transformation in malarious, malnourished and control Gambian children. Clin. Exp. Immunol. **17**:647–656.

50. Murgita, R. A., and T. B. Tomasi, Jr. 1975. Suppression of the immune response by α fetoprotein. II. Effect on MLR and mitogenic reactions. J. Exp. Med. **141**:440–452.

51. Myrvang, B., T. Godal, D. S. Ridley, S. S. Froland, and Y. K. Song. 1973. Immune responsiveness to mycobacterium leprae and other mycobacterial antigens throughout the clinical and histopathological spectrum of leprosy. Clin. Exp. Immunol. **14**:541–553.

52. Nelson, D. S., and J. M. Penrose. 1975. Effect of hemodialysis and transplantation on inhibition of lymphocyte transformation by sera from uremic patients. Clin. Immunol. Immunopathol. **4**:143–146.

53. Nowell, P. C. 1960. Phytohemagglutinin: an initiator of mitosis in cultures of normal human leucocytes. Cancer Res. **20**:462–466.

54. Oppenheim, J. J., R. M. Blaese, and T. A. Waldmann. 1970. Impaired lymphocyte transformation and delayed hypersensitivity in Wiskott Aldrich syndrome. J. Immunol. **104**:835–844.

55. Oppenheim, J. J., S. Dougherty, S. C. Chan, and J. Baker. 1975. Utilization of lymphocyte transformation to assess clinical disorders, p. 87–109. *In* G. N. Vyas (ed.), Laboratory diagnosis of immunological disorders. Grune and Stratton, New York.

56. Oppenheim, J. J., and S. Perry. 1965. Effects of endotoxins on cultured leukocytes. Proc. Soc. Exp. Biol. Med. **118**:1014–1019.

57. Oppenheim, J. J., G. N. Rogentine, and W. D. Terry. 1969. The transformation of human lymphocytes by monkey antisera to human immunoglobulins. Immunology **16**:123–138.

58. Pauly, J. L., J. E. Sokal, and T. Han. 1973. Whole blood culture technique for functional studies of lymphocyte reactivity to mitogens, antigens and homologous lymphocytes. J. Lab. Clin. Med. **82**:500–512.

59. Pellegrino, M. A., S. Ferrone, A. Pellegrino, and R. A. Reisfeld. 1973. A rapid microtechnique for *in vitro* stimulation of human lymphocytes by phytohemagglutinin. Clin. Immunol. Immunopathol. **2**:67–73.

60. Penhale, W. J., A. Farmer, A. C. Maccuish, and W. J. Irvine. 1974. A rapid micromethod for the phytohemagglutinin induced human lymphocyte transformation test. Clin. Exp. Immunol. **18:**155–167.

61. Rocklin, R. E., O. L. Meyers, and J. R. David. 1970. An *in vitro* assay for cellular hypersensitivity in man. J. Immunol. **104:**95–102.

62. Rocklin, R. E., H. Pence, H. Kaplan, and R. Evans. 1974. Cell-mediated immune responses of ragweed-sensitive patients to antigen. *In vitro* lymphocyte transformation and mediator production. J. Clin. Invest. **53:**735–744.

63. Rosenberg, S. A., R. Levy, B. Schechter, S. Ficker, and W. D. Terry. 1972. A rapid microassay of cellular immunity in the guinea pig and mouse. Transplantation **13:**541–545.

64. Rotter, V., and N. Trainin. 1975. Increased mitogenic reactivity of normal spleen cells to T lectins induced by thymus humoral factor (THF). Cell. Immunol. **16:**413–421.

65. Ruhl, H., W. Vogt, G. Bochert, S. Schmidt, H. Schaou, and R. Moelle. 1974. Lymphocyte transformation and production of a human mononuclear leucocyte chemotactic factor in patients with Hodgkin's disease. Clin. Exp. Immunol. **17:**407–415.

66. Sengar, D. P. S., and P. I. Terasaki. 1971. A semi micro mixed leucocyte culture test. Transplantation **11:**260–268.

67. Seravalli, E., and A. Taranta. 1974. Lymphocyte transformation and macrophage migration inhibition by electro focused and gel filtered fractions of group A streptococcal filtrate. Cell. Immunol. **14:**366–375.

68. Smith, K. A., L. Chess, and M. R. Mardiney. 1973. The relationship between rubella hemagglutination inhibition antibody (HIA) and rubella induced *in vitro* lymphocyte tritiated thymidine incorporation. Cell. Immunol. **8:**321–327.

69. Soontiens, F. J. C. J., and J. Van der Veen. 1973. Evidence for a macrophage mediated effect of polio virus on the lymphocyte response to phytohemagglutinin. J. Immunol. **111:**1411–1419.

70. Steward, C. D., S. J. Cramer, and P. G. Steward. 1975. The response of human peripheral blood lymphocytes to phytohemagglutinin: determination of cell numbers. Cell. Immunol. **16:**237–250.

71. Twomey, J. J., and O. Sharkey. 1972. An adaptation of the mixed leukocyte culture test for use in evaluating lymphocyte and macrophage function. J. Immunol. **108:**984–990.

72. Waldmann, T. A., S. Broder, M. Durm, B. Meade, R. Krakauer, M. Blackman, and C. Goldman. 1975. T cell suppression of Pokeweed mitogen induced immunoglobulin production. *In* J. J. Oppenheim and D. Rosenstreich (ed.), Role of mitogens in immunobiology, Academic Press Inc., New York, in press.

73. Watkins, S. M. 1973. The effects of surgery on lymphocyte transformation in patients with cancer. Clin. Exp. Immunol. **14:**69–76.

74. Wernet, P., and H. G. Kunkel. 1973. Antibodies to a specific surface antigen of T cells in human sera inhibiting mixed leukocyte culture reactions. J. Exp. Med. **138:**1021–1026.

75. Winchester, R. J., S. M. Fu, P. Wernet, H. G. Kunkel, B. Dupont, and C. Jersild. 1975. Recognition by pregnancy sera of non-HLA alloantigens selectively expressed on B lymphocytes. J. Exp. Med. **141:**924–929.

76. Wyler, D. J., and J. J. Oppenheim. 1974. Lymphocyte transformation in human plasmodium falciparum malaria. J. Immunol. **113:**449.

77. Yeung Laiwah, A. A. C., A. K. R. Chandhuri, and J. R. Anderson. 1973. Lymphocyte transformation and leucocyte migration inhibition by Australia antigen. Clin. Exp. Immunol. **15:**27–34.

78. Ziegler, J. B., P. Hansen, and R. Penny. 1975. Intrinsic lymphocyte defect in Hodgkin's disease: analysis of the phytohemagglutinin dose response. Clin. Immunol. Immunopathol. **3:**451–460.

Chapter 10

Production and Assay of Human Migration Inhibitory Factor

ROSS E. ROCKLIN

INTRODUCTION

Sensitized lymphocytes, when activated in vitro by a specific antigen, produce a soluble factor termed migration inhibitory factor (MIF) which retards the migration of macrophages or monocytes from capillary tubes (2, 4, 6, 7). The MIF system of migration inhibition utilizing macrophages or monocytes as indicator cells has been shown to be distinct from the system of migration inhibition which uses polymorphonuclear (PMN) leukocytes as indicator cells (9). The inhibition of migration of PMN leukocytes is mediated by a separate factor termed leukocyte inhibitory factor, which is covered in chapter 6. Human MIF has the properties of a protein with a molecular weight of 23,000 (13). The production of antigen-induced MIF in vitro correlates with the in vivo state of cellular hypersensitivity of the lymphocyte donor (12, 14). Lymphocytes from normal subjects who manifest cutaneous delayed hypersensitivity to various antigens produce MIF in vitro to the same antigens, whereas lymphocytes from normal subjects who lack delayed hypersensitivity to these antigens fail to elaborate MIF when challenged in vitro. There are several recent reviews covering the MIF test (1, 3, 5) and its application to clinical disease (10).

There are currently two methods available for the assay of human MIF. The direct assay (one-step procedure) involves the use of sensitized human lymphocytes mixed with guinea pig macrophages or human monocytes in capillary tubes. Specific antigen is added to the system, MIF is made locally by the lymphocytes, and the MIF then acts upon the macrophages or monocytes within the 24-h assay period to inhibit their migration. In the indirect system (two-step procedure), sensitized lymphocytes are first cultured separately with antigen to produce MIF over a 1- to 2-day period. The culture fluid (cell-free supernatant) is then assayed for MIF activity on nonimmune guinea pig macrophages or human monocytes in capillary tubes. The main advantage of the direct MIF system is the short time required to perform the test (24 h) and the fact that it is technically less complicated than the indirect method. The main disadvantage with this method is that a negative result, that is, no MIF activity detectable in the system, is difficult to interpret. A negative result may reflect depressed lymphocyte production (no mediator production) or a failure of the indicator cell (macrophage or monocyte) to respond to MIF. The main advantage of the indirect method is that it permits a dissection of the lymphocyte-macrophage interaction by testing each component separately. By culturing lymphocytes first to produce MIF, one can then proceed to test for mediator production using heterologous or autologous indicator cells. The direct method should be used as a screening procedure. If a positive result is obtained, then one may assume that this particular function is normal. If a negative result is obtained, then the indirect method should be used so that each component can be tested separately.

The following sections deal primarily with the indirect MIF test, but a brief description of the direct assay is also included. A description of lymphocyte isolation and culture techniques is given as well as the procedure for the assay for MIF activity with the use of guinea pig macrophages and human monocytes in capillary tubes as indicator cells. The reason for using guinea pig macrophages as a routine procedure instead of using human monocytes relates to the difficulty in obtaining the latter cell population in sufficient quantities.

CLINICAL INDICATIONS

The indications for the use of the migration inhibition test fall into two main categories: evaluation of lymphocyte function in general and detection of sensitized lymphocytes to tissue antigens or drugs. In the former, the production of MIF in response to environmental antigens such as purified protein derivative (PPD), monilia, or streptokinase-streptodornase gives one an estimation of lymphocyte function as it relates to the expression of cellular hypersensitivity in the skin. In regard to the latter situation, since in vivo skin testing to tissue antigens or drugs is not recommended because of the possibility of clinical reactions or sensitization of the patient, there is a great advantage in using an in vitro test which does not alter the immunological response of the patient.

TEST PROCEDURES

Sterile technique is used throughout the procedures described here.

Production of migration inhibitory factor-containing supernatant fluids by human lymphocytes

1. Draw 50 to 100 ml of venous blood into plastic syringes containing 1 ml of sodium heparin and 5 ml of dextran per 50-ml syringe. Invert the syringes several times to mix the blood, dextran, and heparin solutions, and place them in an upright position in a ring stand for approximately 1 h at 37 C.

2. After the incubation period or when approximately 50% of the red cells have sedimented in the syringe, use an 18-gauge needle to express the leukocyte-rich plasma from the syringe into a 50-ml conical centrifuge tube.

3. Centrifuge the leukocyte-rich plasma from each 50 ml of blood at room temperature at $180 \times g$ for 10 min. Then suction off the plasma using a Pasteur pipette.

4. Resuspend the leukocytes from each 50 ml of blood in 8 ml of warm tissue culture (TC) medium 199 containing 30 mM N-2-hydroxyethylpiperazine-N'-2-ethanesulfonic acid (HEPES) buffer.

5. Slowly layer 4 ml of the cell suspension over 3 ml of a Ficoll-Hypaque solution which is contained in a 12-ml conical centrifuge tube. Care should be taken not to disturb the interface; that is, the cell suspension should be pipetted over the Ficoll very gently.

6. Centrifuge the tubes containing the cell suspension and Ficoll at $400 \times g$ for 35 min at room temperature. Then carefully remove mononuclear cells which are present at the medium-Ficoll interface, using a Pasteur pipette.

7. Wash the mononuclear cells in 10 ml of TC medium 199 for 10 min at $180 \times g$ at room temperature.

8. On the final wash, resuspend the cells to 10 ml and perform a white count. A total white count is recorded, and a small sample of cells is placed on a slide, air-dried, and stained with Wright's stain. A differential cell count is then performed.

9. The final volume of the cell suspension should be adjusted to 5×10^6 lymphocytes/ml

in TC medium 199 containing 10% AB+ serum.

10. The lymphocyte suspension is then divided into 2-ml portions and placed in 12×125 mm screw-top tubes.

11. The experiment is set up with one tube containing cells without any antigen and other tubes containing cells plus each antigen being tested for MIF production (for example: PPD, 10 μg/ml; monilia, 0.01 ml of stock solution/ml of cell suspension; and streptokinase-streptodornase, 50 units/ml of cell suspension). If more than one antigen is being tested for MIF production, then a separate set of tubes should also be set up. These tubes, termed antigen controls, consist of one tube containing tissue culture medium alone (without cells) and others containing medium plus each antigen (without cells) at the same concentration used above.

12. The cultures are then placed in a 37 C incubator containing a 5% CO_2-95% air atmosphere.

13. After incubation for 48 h, the cells are centrifuged at $180 \times g$ for 10 min at room temperature, and the supernatant fluids are carefully removed with a Pasteur pipette. Prior to assay, 0.1 ml of normal guinea pig serum is added to each 2 ml of supernatant fluid. These supernatant fluids are then used to fill chambers containing the indicator cells.

Migration inhibitory factor assay with guinea pig peritoneal exudate cells as indicator cells

1. To obtain a peritoneal exudate, inject 30 ml of light mineral oil intraperitoneally into male albino guinea pigs (approximately 400 to 500 g) about 72 h prior to the time when the cells are needed. It is helpful to remove food from the animals the night before this procedure since this reduces vomiting and simplifies the process of injecting into the peritoneum without hitting the intestine. The animals have been anesthetized with ether, and their abdomens have been shaved and wiped thoroughly with 70% alcohol. The 30 ml of oil is injected at the midline, through the linear alba, to minimize bleeding.

2. The animals' food should be removed the night before the cells are to be harvested. Sacrifice the animals under ether by cardiac puncture and exsanguination. (The blood from normal animals is collected with the use of aseptic technique, allowing the blood to clot, and the serum collected that day is pooled with serum from other animals and is used in future experiments.) The abdomen is swabbed with alcohol, and a 6- to 7-cm skin incision, down to

the peritoneum, is made starting at the xyphoid process. Using a 30-ml syringe containing a three-way stopcock or repeater unit, inject a total of 150 ml of cold Hanks balanced salt solution (BSS) intraperitoneally. The abdomen is gently agitated to mix the oil with the wash solution. Carefully introduce a trocar and sheath. Remove the trocar and replace it in the sheath with a canula which is attached to polyethylene tubing. The other end of the tubing should already be in a sterile separatory funnel.

3. The oil and Hanks wash solution should begin to drain by gravity. Because the oil emerges first, the flow begins slowly, and as the Hanks BSS emerges the flow will speed up. When all of the wash has drained into the separatory funnel, recap it, shake it, and allow it to sit briefly so that the oil separates from the Hanks BSS. Then drain the wash containing the cells into 250-ml flat-bottomed centrifuge bottles, leaving the oil behind. Cover the bottles with sterile gauze, and centrifuge them for 15 min at 5 C and $450 \times g$. Aspirate the supernatant fluid, removing any remaining oil first, by vacuum, and gently swirl the cells from the bottom of the bottles with fresh Hanks BSS. Transfer the cells into 12-ml centrifuge tubes and wash them twice more, with Hanks BSS, centrifuging for 5 min at 5 C and $250 \times g$. After the final wash, the cell suspension to be used in the capillaries is made up to 10% by volume (for example, 0.1 ml of cell-packed volume is made up to 1.0 ml), in TC medium 199 containing 15% normal guinea pig serum and 100 units of penicillin and 100 μg of streptomycin/ml. Each 1 ml of cell suspension will make 12 to 15 filled capillaries or a maximum of 6 to 7 chambers (2 capillaries per chamber).

4. To prepare cell suspension in capillary tubes, melt two beakers of paraffin wax and cool until soft (until the beaker feels just warm to the touch). Set up a sterile towel in a hood with a basin or dry sterile 2×2 gauze, an ear bayonet from the instrument kit (see below, Reagents and Supplies), and a sterile petri dish of capillary tubes. Also set out a test tube rack which will hold the tube containing the cell suspension and other tubes for the placement of the capillaries, once filled. Mix the cell suspension well before drawing into the capillaries. Using the ear bayonet, pick up a capillary tube and allow it to fill with the cell suspension to approximately 5 mm from the top; put the instrument down (keeping it sterile) and take the capillary from the tube by hand. Dry it with the sterile gauze (keeping the capillary level so that the cell suspension does not drain out), and plug the other end with warm wax. The wax plug should

be about 2 to 3 mm long. As the capillaries are sealed with wax, they are dropped into a tube which contains cotton at the bottom. Keep at room temperature until the capillaries are ready to spin. Centrifuge the capillaries at $250 \times g$ at room temperature for 5 min. Then place the capillary tubes in a petri dish and keep on ice.

5. The capillaries are then placed in chambers, and medium from the lymphocyte cultures is added in the following way. The trays of chambers are prepared in advance to the point where the bottom cover slips are in place and sealed with wax. As they are to be used, invert the chambers in small groups and, using a syringe containing silicone grease, place two spots of silicone grease inside where the capillaries are to be attached. Wipe each capillary with a 2×2 gauze square moistened with 70% alcohol and then with a dry gauze. Rest the end of the capillary containing the cells on a sterile petri dish and cut with an ampoule file (the file is sterilized by wiping several times with gauze wet with alcohol and then with a sterile dry gauze). The capillary is cut with the ampoule file by making a ridge in the capillary at a point 0.5 mm below the cell-fluid interface on the cell side. The capillary is rotated 180° so that the ridge is at the bottom. Applying upward pressure while holding the tip of the capillary down with the file will break the capillary. With the thumb forceps, pick up the portion containing the cells and place it in the chamber on one of the spots of silicone. Tap it down with the forceps to be sure that it is lying flat on the bottom of the cover slip.

6. After two capillaries are in place in the chamber, inspect to be sure that no silicone grease is near the open end of the capillary where the cells will be migrating out. Then place the second cover slip on top of the chamber, seal with melted wax, and fill the chamber with the test supernatant fluids. Each chamber will contain approximately 0.8 ml of fluid, and therefore each test supernatant fluid can fill two chambers. The filling holes are sealed with wax, and the chamber is placed on a tray fitted with glass rods approximately 4 cm apart, so that the chamber is suspended in air and does not touch the bottom of the tray. This is important because the wax becomes sticky at 37 C, and the bottom cover slip may become loose if it is stuck to the tray. Care should be taken to fill the chamber without leaving any air bubbles since, during the 24-h incubation period, any air in the chamber will form larger bubbles and disturb the migration when the chambers are moved. Also, in filling the chambers with medium, use a glass disposable sy-

ringe and # 25-gauge needle so that the fluid can be introduced smoothly without too much pressure. Do not point the needle at the open end of a capillary, as this may wash some cells out and cause variability in migration. After the chambers are filled and assembled on the trays, inspect them before they are placed in a 37 C incubator for 18 to 24 h.

7. After the cells have been allowed to migrate onto the glass cover slip for 18 to 24 h, measure the area of migration. The chambers are placed on a microscope, and the area of migration is projected onto a piece of paper through a projecting prism. The area is then drawn and measured with a planimeter. Since the planimeter measures large areas with greater accuracy than small ones, it is advisable that the microscope be placed at such a distance that the control area of migration is projected with about 7 to 8 cm at its widest diameter. The percent migration inhibition is calculated from the following formula:

$$\% \text{ inhibition} = 1.0 - \frac{\text{test area}}{\text{control area}} \times 100$$

where test area is the area of migration of cells in the presence of supernatant fluid with antigen and control area is the area of migration of cells in the control supernatant fluid.

8. The mean migration of four capillaries containing cells from one animal is calculated and used in the formula. One can determine whether the mean migration in the presence of the control supernatant fluids is statistically different from that in the presence of the test supernatant fluid by performing a Student t test for paired means. In general, greater than 20% inhibition of migration is considered to be a positive MIF response, although in some instances 15% inhibition may be significant. If control media are used, calculate whether any nonspecific inhibition due to the test antigens occurs. Toxicity due to antigen alone should be subtracted from the inhibition obtained from the test supernatant fluids.

Migration inhibitory factor assay with human monocytes in capillary tubes as indicator cells

1. Mononuclear cells from 100 ml of blood are obtained by use of the Ficoll-Hypaque centrifugation technique described above (Production of migration inhibitory factor-containing supernatant fluids by human lymphocytes). After one washing procedure, the cells are resuspended in 5.0 ml of TC medium 199 containing 20% fetal calf serum.

2. The 5.0-ml cell suspension of mononuclear cells is pipetted into a plastic petri dish (15×60 mm) and allowed to sit for 1 h at 37 C in an incubator containing a 5% CO_2-95% air mixture.

3. The nonadherent cells, which contain approximately 80 to 90% lymphocytes, are poured off and can then be used to make MIF for subsequent experiments. Greater than 95% of the cells which adhere to the bottom of the petri dish are monocytes. To remove these cells, add 5.0 ml of Hanks BSS without calcium or magnesium containing 10^{-4} M ethylenediaminetetraacetate. Allow the monocytes to incubate for 10 min in this solution at room temperature; then, using a rubber policeman, gently scrape the bottom of the petri dish to remove these cells.

4. The monocytes thus obtained are washed in TC medium 199 and resuspended in this medium containing 10% horse serum to a volume of approximately 0.4 to 0.5 ml. This volume of cell suspension will make up approximately 25 to 30 capillaries. The capillaries are prepared as above except that 20-μliter microcapillaries are used instead of the 50-μliter capillaries used for the guinea pig cells. These capillaries are then placed in chambers and filled with medium as above. The area of migration is drawn at 18 h, and the percent migration inhibition is calculated by use of the formula given in the preceding section.

Direct migration inhibitory factor assay

The method described here was modified from the work of Rajapakse and Glynn (8). Human mononuclear cells and guinea pig peritoneal exudate cells are obtained as described above. Human mononuclear cells are mixed with guinea pig peritoneal exudate cells in a ratio of 1:3 (human to guinea pig) so that a total of 40×10^6 cells/ml are placed in capillaries. The cells are suspended in TC medium 199 (100 units of penicillin and 100 μg of streptomycin/ml) containing 15% normal guinea pig serum. This amount of cells (40×10^6) will suffice to make 15 to 20 capillaries. The capillaries are placed in chambers as above and filled with medium alone or medium plus each test antigen (same concentrations as above). Antigen controls utilize medium alone and medium plus antigen placed in chambers with capillaries containing macrophages *without* human mononuclear cells. The migration is drawn at 18 to 24 h, and the inhibition is calculated as above (area with antigen/area without antigen).

REAGENTS AND SUPPLIES

Tissue culture medium: TC medium 199 in Hanks BSS

HEPES buffer (1 M)

Agammaglobulinemic horse serum

Ficoll-Hypaque solution: 10 parts 37.5% Hypaque (sodium diatrizoate) to 24 parts 9% Ficoll

Dextran: Macrodex, 6% (wt/vol) in saline

Heparin sodium injection USP, 1,000 units/cc

Antigens (dialyze for 24 h against 200 volumes of 0.15 N saline prior to use):

Tuberculin PPD without preservative

Streptokinase-streptodornase (Varidase) at 100,000 units of streptokinase and 25,000 units of streptodornase

Candida albicans (Dermatophytin "O" undiluted)

Sterile light mineral oil, Marcol 52, Humble Oil Co.

Male Hartley guinea pigs (400 to 500 g)

Instrument kit (collecting cells) containing two hemostats, one #4 knife handle, one #20 knife blade, and one large toothed forcep

Duke cannulated trocars (Sklar #215-25)

Polyethylene tubing from I.V. Saftisets

Separatory funnel, 250 ml (sterilized with a test tube over the draining tip)

Wide-mouthed, flat-bottomed centrifuge bottles (250 ml volume)

Hanks BSS

Penicillin (5,000 units) and streptomycin (5,000 μg) solution

Instrument kit (preparing capillary tubes and chambers) containing one ear forcep (bayonet, Sklar #3350-65), one thumb forcep, two cover slip forceps, one hemostat

Glass or stainless steel beakers (50 ml) containing sterile paraffin wax (melting point 56.5 C)

Capillary tubes: 1.2 to 1.4 mm inner diameter, 50-μliter; 0.6 to 0.8 mm inner diameter, 20-μliter

Cover slips (#1, ½, 22 mm round)

Stainless steel trays, 9 × 12 inches, each containing 20 chambers

Mackaness-type lucite chambers (Berton Plastics, Hackensack, N.J.)

Silicone stopcock grease

Microscope with projection prism and 3.5 objective

Compensating polar planimeter (Kueffel & Esser)

Fetal calf serum

INTERPRETATION

The human MIF test measures the production of a soluble lymphocyte mediator in response to specific antigen which is responsible for inhibiting the random migration of either guinea pig macrophages or human monocytes. The in vitro production of MIF in normal subjects correlates with the in vivo state of cellular hypersensitivity of the lymphocyte donor. Recent evidence indicates that MIF production is not solely the function of human T cell subpopulations (11). Human B cell subpopulations also elaborate MIF in response to specific antigen which is similar in size to the T cell mediator. Furthermore, B cells make more of this material. Therefore, the MIF test may be used to assess cellular hypersensitivity per se but cannot be used to measure the in vitro response of a particular cell type (T versus B). If MIF production is absent in patients with cutaneous anergy, this presumably indicates a defect in both T and B cell function. It is not clear at present exactly how the B cell functions in delayed hypersensitivity or what is the role of B cell MIF.

Although the detection of MIF in response to certain tissue antigens may indicate sensitization related to the pathogenesis of a disease, it in no way proves a causal relationship. One does not know how the sensitization occurred, whether as a primary event or secondary to tissue damage. The test may be used to follow the effects of treatment in patients as well as to determine their responses during the course of their illness. There is a 10 to 20% incidence of false-negative results with this assay, but it is rare to find false-positive results. Therefore, it is recommended that one carry out population studies in a particular disease rather than rely heavily on the results of individual patients. In addition, negative results should be repeated in an individual patient to confirm abnormal lymphocyte function.

LITERATURE CITED

1. Bloom, B. R. 1971. In vitro approaches to the mechanism of cell-mediated immune reactions Adv. Immunol. **13**:101–208.
2. Bloom, B. R., and B. Bennett. 1966. Mechanism of a reaction in vitro associated with delayed-type hypersensitivity. Science **153**:80–82.
3. Bloom, B. R., and P. Glade (ed.). 1971. In vitro methods in cell-mediated immunity. Academic Press Inc., New York.
4. David, J. R., S. Al-Askari, H. S. Lawrence, and L. Thomas. 1964. Delayed hypersensitivity in vitro. I. The specificity of cell migration by antigen. J. Immunol. **93**:264–273.
5. David, J. R., and R. A. David. 1972. Cellular hypersensitivity and immunity: inhibition of macrophage migration and lymphocyte mediators. Prog. Allergy **16**:300–449.

6. George, M., and J. H. Vaughan. 1964. In vitro cell migration as a model for delayed hypersensitivity. Proc. Soc. Exp. Biol. Med. **111**:514–521.

7. Krejci, J., J. Pekarek, J. Johanovsky, and J. Svefcar. 1969. Demonstration of the inflammatory activity of the supernatant of hypersensitive lymph node cells incubated with a high degree of antigen. Immunology **16**:677–684.

8. Rajapakse, D. A., and L. E. Glynn. 1970. Macrophage migration inhibition test using guinea pig macrophages and human lymphocytes. Nature (London) **226**:857–858.

9. Rocklin, R. E. 1974. Products of activated lymphocytes: leukocyte inhibitory factor (LIF) distinct from migration inhibitory factor (MIF). J. Immunol. **112**: 1461–1466.

10. Rocklin, R. E. 1974. Clinical application of in vitro lymphocyte tests. Prog. Clin. Immunol. **2:** 21–67.

11. Rocklin, R. E., R. P. MacDermott, L. Chess, S. F. Schlossman, and J. R. David. 1974. Studies on mediator production by highly purified human T and B lymphocytes. J. Exp. Med **140:** 1303–1316.

12. Rocklin, R. E., O. L. Meyers, and J. R. David. 1970. An in vitro assay for cellular hypersensitivity in man. J. Immunol. **104**:95–102.

13. Rocklin, R. E., H. G. Remold, and J. R. David. 1972. Characterization of human migration inhibitory factor (MIF) from antigen-stimulated lymphocytes. Cell. Immunol. **5**:436–445.

14. Thor, D. E., R. E. Jureiz, S. R. Veach, E. Miller, and S. Dray. 1968. Cell migration inhibition factor released by antigen from human peripheral lymphocytes. Nature (London) **219**:755–757.

Chapter 11

Leukocyte Migration Inhibitory Factor

JENS E. CLAUSEN

INTRODUCTION

During the past decade, antigen-induced migration inhibition of human peripheral blood leukocytes has been used extensively as an in vitro parameter of cell-mediated immunity in humans. The migration inhibition of leukocytes has many similarities to the migration inhibition of macrophages. However, two distinct migration inhibitory factors (MIF) seem to be responsible for the two inhibition reactions: a *granulocyte-MIF* which does not inhibit either monocytes or macrophages, and a *macrophage-MIF* which also inhibits monocytes, but not granulocytes (12).

The antigen-sensitive cell in the leukocyte migration inhibition reaction is the lymphocyte, whereas the polymorph is merely an indicator cell which migrates. Even if human monocytes are inhibited by supernatant fluids from stimulated lymphocyte cultures, the monocyte is without importance in the antigen-induced migration inhibition of nonseparated peripheral blood leukocytes (2).

Preformed cytophilic antibodies may be present on the polymorphs. This, however, cannot explain the antigen-induced migration inhibition of nonseparated leukocytes, since purified polymorphs from sensitized subjects migrate uninhibited by antigen (2). Correspondingly, even after preincubation with plasma from a sensitized subject, nonimmune leukocytes migrate uninhibited by the appropriate antigen (8).

In 1967, Søborg and Bendixen (1, 13) adapted the capillary tube technique for human peripheral blood leukocytes. Since then, this technique, with or without minor modifications, has been used in a great number of studies within clinical immunology. Nevertheless, several groups have reported their inability to use the capillary tube technique in humans, especially in demonstrating tuberculin hypersensitivity. This may in part be caused by the escape phenomenon (i.e., no migration inhibition in the later culture period although a migration inhibition does occur during the first few hours of culture). Similar difficulties led me to develop an agarose migration technique (3). The agarose technique has been used both in a direct test (3) and in an indirect two-stage assay in which cell-free supernatant fluids from stimulated lymphocyte cultures are assayed for migration inhibitory activity on normal nonseparated leukocytes or purified polymorphs (4, 5).

TEST PROCEDURES

Preparation of tissue culture media

Liquid medium. HEPES-buffered tissue culture (TC) medium is prepared from 100 ml of 10-fold concentrated TC medium 199, 6.2 g of N-2-hydroxyethyl piperazine-N'-2-ethanesulfonic acid (HEPES), 500,000 IU of penicillin, 500 mg of streptomycin, and distilled water added to 1,000 ml. The pH of the medium is adjusted to 7.40 with 5 N NaOH. The medium is sterilized by filtration through membrane filters, 0.22-μm pore size (Millipore Corp., Bedford, Mass.).

Agarose medium. A 2% agarose solution in distilled water is prepared every 2 weeks and stored at 5 C. Fresh agarose culture medium is prepared every day. The 2% agarose gel is heated in boiling water. After dissolution, the agarose is cooled to 47 C in a water bath. For preparing 100 ml of agarose culture medium, 50 ml of 2% agarose solution is added to a mixture (prewarmed to 47 C) of 31 ml of sterile distilled water, 9 ml of 10-fold concentrated TC medium 199, 10 ml of horse serum, 200 μliters of penicillin-streptomycin in sterilized water (containing 6,600 IU of penicillin and 6.6 mg of streptomycin), and 540 μliters of 10% sodium bicarbonate. The reagents are measured by use of disposable plastic syringes.

Thus, the final agarose medium contains 1% agarose, single-strength TC medium 199, 10% horse serum, 66 IU of penicillin/ml, and 66 μg of streptomycin/ml.

The 47 C agarose culture medium is sucked into a prewarmed 25-ml burette, and 5-ml volumes are transferred to 48 × 8.5 mm disposable plastic petri dishes (Millipore Corp.). After the gel medium has solidified, the dishes are incubated at 37 C in a humidified atmosphere of 2% CO_2 in air. When leukocyte cultures are to be made, six to eight wells are punched in the gel with a 2.5-mm (external diameter) gel puncher (Dansk Laboratorieudstyr, Copenhagen, Denmark).

The bicarbonate/CO_2 buffer, which results in a pH between 7.20 and 7.40, can be replaced by HEPES, 0.62 g per 100 ml of agarose medium (9).

Preparation of nonseparated leukocytes

Venous blood (8 ml/tube) is collected in 115 × 13 mm polystyrene tubes each containing 250 IU of heparin and 2 ml of 5% dextran 250 in saline (0.9%) solution.

After sedimentation for 0.75 to 1 h at 37 C, the leukocyte-rich plasma is removed with a disposable polystyrene pipette.

The leukocyte count (cells per microliter) of the leukocyte-rich plasma is determined. The volume of medium for resuspending the cells after the washing procedure (see below) is calculated from the total leukocyte number of the leukocyte-rich plasma (i.e., leukocyte count × 10^3 × milliliters of plasma).

Leukocytes for use in direct migration tests. The leukocyte-rich plasma is distributed into 80 × 16 mm polyethylene tubes and centrifuged at 220 × g for 5 min at room temperature. The supernatant plasma is tipped off, and the cells are resuspended in Hanks balanced salt solution and transferred into one of the tubes.

The resuspended cells are centrifuged at 220 × g for 5 min, and the wash with Hanks balanced salt solution is repeated two more times.

After the third wash, the cells are resuspended in HEPES-buffered TC medium 199 (or TC medium 199) containing 10% horse serum to give a leukocyte concentration of 2.4 × 10^8/ml (for the agarose migration test) or 1.5 × 10^8/ml (for the capillary tube migration test).

Leukocytes for assaying migration inhibitory activity of cell-free culture supernatant fluids. The leukocyte-rich plasma is divided into a number of 80 × 16 mm polyethylene tubes corresponding to the number of cell-free culture supernatant fluids which are to be tested for MIF activity.

The cells are washed three times in Hanks balanced salt solution. After the last centrifugation, the salt solution is tipped off, and the cells are resuspended in the different culture supernatant fluids to give a leukocyte concentration of 2.1 × 10^8/ml.

The migration inhibitory activity of culture supernatant fluids can also be tested on purified polymorphs (4).

Preparation of purified mononuclear leukocytes for first-stage cultures of the indirect migration inhibitory factor assay

Venous blood with 250 IU of heparin per 10 ml of blood is diluted with an equal volume of Hanks balanced salt solution. Then 7 ml of the diluted blood is carefully layered upon 3 ml of Isopaque-Ficoll solution in 110 × 17 mm polystyrene tubes.

After centrifugation at 400 × g for 40 min at room temperature, the mononuclear leukocytes (lymphocytes plus monocytes) in the interface between the plasma and the Isopaque-Ficoll solution are pipetted off with a Pasteur pipette, washed three times in Hanks balanced salt solution, and resuspended in HEPES-buffered TC medium 199 containing 20% horse serum (with or without antigen) to give a cell concentration of 2 × 10^6/ml.

Leukocyte migration capillary tube test

Amounts of 50 μliters of the suspension of nonseparated leukocytes (1.5 × 10^8 cells/ml; see above, Leukocytes for use in direct migration tests) are drawn into glass capillary tubes (see below, Reagents). The capillaries are closed by melting the empty end in a gas flame.

After cooling, the capillaries are placed in 80 × 16 mm polyethylene tubes and centrifuged at 900 × g for 10 min at room temperature. A 3- to 5-mm length of the cell pellet is desirable.

The capillary tubes are cut 1 mm below the cell-fluid interface and are immediately placed in culture chambers (see below, Reagents) containing about 0.5 ml of TC medium 199 with 10% horse serum. The closed tip of the capillary tube is fixed on the bottom at the periphery of the chamber by a dab of silicone grease (Dow Corning Corp., Midland, Mich.).

Antigen is added to some of the chambers.

The chambers are carefully filled up with TC medium 199 containing 10% horse serum and sealed with cover slips (20 × 20 mm) applied to the previously siliconized rim of the chamber. Care should be taken to avoid any air bubbles within the culture chambers.

After incubation for 20 h at 37 C, the migration areas are studied under a projection microscope and measured by planimetry. The migration inhibition is expressed as a migration index which indicates the ratio between the average area of four to six antigen-containing cultures and that of the same number of control cultures.

Under some circumstances, it is advisable to measure the migration areas after 4 h as well as after 20 h, since the antigen-induced migration inhibition may be more pronounced during the early culture period (7).

Microcapillary tube technique. The microcapillary tube technique devised by Maini et al. (10, 11) differs especially in two points from the original capillary tube technique described above. First, the leukocyte suspension is drawn into 10-μliter capillaries obtained by halving 20-μliter microcapillaries (Hemocaps, Drummond Scientific Co., Broomall, Pa.). Second, the cells are cultured in 0.5-ml chambers of a sterile disposable polystyrene tray containing 12 chambers (Sterilin Ltd., Hill Rise, Richmond, England).

Leukocyte migration agarose test

Part of the suspension of nonseparated leukocytes (2.4 × 10⁸ cells/ml; see above, Leukocytes for use in direct migration tests) is mixed with antigen-containing medium in the proportion 9:1, and an equal part is mixed with medium without antigen (e.g., 90 μliters of the leukocyte suspension is mixed with 10 μliters of purified protein derivative [PPD] of tuberculin [1 mg of PPD/ml] in phosphate buffer, and, as a control, 90 μliters is mixed with 10 μliters of the phosphate buffer without PPD).

The highest concentration of antigen which does not inhibit leukocytes from nonsensitized subjects is often used as the routine concentration. However, more information is obtained if the migration inhibition is measured also at various lower antigen concentrations.

After incubation for 30 min at 37 C, 7-μliter portions from each of the cell suspensions are placed in wells in agarose medium by means of micropipettes. The same number of control and stimulated cultures is made on each agarose plate.

The agarose cultures are incubated at 37 C in a humidified atmosphere of 2% CO_2 in air (see below, Reagents). During the following hours, the cells will migrate out in the capillary cleft beneath the gel.

After 20 h of culture, the migration areas around the wells are studied under a projection microscope and measured by planimetry. The bottom of the well is not included in the migration area.

Since the migration inhibition is more pronounced early in the culture period, it can be useful to measure the migration areas after 4 h as well as after 20 h (6).

The migration inhibition is expressed as a migration index which indicates the ratio between the average area of six to eight antigen-stimulated cultures and that of the same number of control cultures.

Indirect two-stage migration inhibitory factor agarose assay

First stage: preparation of culture supernatant fluids. The suspensions of purified mononuclear leukocytes with or without antigen (prepared as described above) can be treated in two different ways:

Cells cultured in the presence of antigen. The cell suspensions are divided into three or four 500-μliter portions and cultured for 24 h at 37 C in 38 × 12.5 mm polypropylene tubes. At the end of the culture period, the supernatant fluids within each group are pooled and centrifuged at 2,000 × g for 15 min.

Antigen is added to the control supernatant fluid to reconstitute it to the concentration present in the supernatant fluid from the antigen-containing cultures.

Cells preincubated with antigen for 2.5 h and then cultured in antigen-free medium. After incubation of the control as well as the antigen-containing cell suspension for 2.5 h at 37 C, the cells are sedimented by centrifugation at 220 × g for 5 min, washed three times in HEPES-buffered TC medium 199, and resuspended in HEPES-buffered TC medium 199 with 20% horse serum to a final cell concentration of 2 × 10⁶/ml. Both cell suspensions are divided into three or four 500-μliter portions and cultured for 2 days. At the end of the culture period, the supernatant fluids within each group are pooled and centrifuged at 2,000 × g for 15 min.

Second stage: migration inhibition of indicator leukocytes by supernatant fluids. The migration inhibitory effect of culture supernatant fluids containing antigen has to be tested on leukocytes from donors without immunity to the specific antigen. In contrast, supernatant fluids containing no antigen can be tested on leukocytes without regard to the specific immune state of the cell donor.

Nonseparated leukocytes or purified polymorphs are resuspended in the supernatant fluids from control and activated cultures (see above, Leukocytes for assaying migration inhibitory activity of cell-free culture supernatant fluids).

After incubation for 1.5 h at 37 C, six to eight 7-μliter portions from each of the cell suspensions are placed in wells in agarose medium.

The migration inhibitory effect of a supernatant fluid from an antigen-stimulated culture is expressed as a migration index which indicates the ratio between the average migration area of indicator cells resuspended in supernatant fluid from antigen-stimulated cultures and that of cells resuspended in supernatant fluid from corresponding control cultures.

REAGENTS

Sodium bicarbonate: TC bicarbonate solution 10% (Difco Laboratories, Detroit, Mich.)

HEPES (Sigma Chemical Co., St. Louis, Mo.)

Agarose (Litex, Glostrup, Denmark)

Horse serum (Statens Seruminstitut, Copenhagen, Denmark)

Penicillin-streptomycin: TC penicillin-streptomycin, desiccated (Difco Laboratories)

TC medium 199 (Difco Laboratories)

Tenfold concentrated TC medium 199: TC medium 199, $10\times$ (Difco Laboratories)

Heparin: Heparin Leo, 5,000 IU per ml (Leo, Copenhagen, Denmark)

Dextran 250, molecular weight 250,000 (Pharmacia, Uppsala, Sweden)

Isopaque-Ficoll solution: 10% Isopaque (Nyegaard and Co., Oslo, Norway) and 6.4% Ficoll (Pharmacia) in distilled water

Other supplies

Test tubes (Nunc, Roskilde, Denmark) used are 115×13 mm and 110×17 mm polystyrene (Nunclon) tubes, 80×16 mm polyethylene tubes, and 38×12.5 mm polypropylene tubes.

Syringes are disposable B-D plastic syringes (Plastipak), 1, 5, 10, and 20 ml.

Needles are disposable 18- and 19-gauge B-D needles.

Pipettes include Carlsberg micropipettes (Dansk Laboratorieudstyr, Copenhagen, Denmark), 7, 10, 15, 20, 90, 135, and 180 μliters; Pasteur pipettes; and disposable polystyrene pipettes (Nunc).

Glass capillary tubes are 200 mm long with 1.4-mm external and 1.1-mm internal diameter (Nordisk Glasteknik, Copenhagen, Denmark). The capillaries are siliconized and sterilized by dry heat (180 C for 3 h).

Culture chambers are made by glass rings (6-mm height with 18-mm external and 15-mm internal diameter) mounted on a 3-mm glass plate by means of Araldite. The culture chambers are siliconized and sterilized by dry heat.

Incubator: 37 C, 2% CO_2 in humidified air. If an incubator with gas supply is not available, the agarose culture dishes can be placed on well-moist filter papers on a thick glass plate under the upper part of an exsiccator (26-cm opening diameter) which closes airtight to the glass plate. This homemade incubator is placed at 37 C and gassed (5 liters/min) for 10 min with 2% CO_2 in humidified air. Continuous gassing is unnecessary.

COMMENTS

In a great number of investigations, antigen-induced inhibition of human leukocyte migration has been strongly correlated with delayed skin hypersensitivity, but a quantitative correlation has only rarely been demonstrated. This is not surprising, but is an obvious consequence of the differences between the in vitro and the in vivo reaction with regard both to complexity and to time course. In the in vitro situation, antigen-sensitive lymphocytes as well as migrating polymorphs are present in great numbers when the antigen is added, and the migration inhibition will depend mainly on the MIF production during the first few hours. In contrast, only few leukocytes are present locally in the skin when the antigen is injected. Therefore, the cutaneous inflammatory reaction will be delayed, depending on the influx of blood leukocytes.

In human investigations, it is of great importance that the in vitro tests, as opposed to the skin test, do not induce or increase immunity to transplantation antigens or autoantigens. Furthermore, antigen preparations may be contaminated by infectious agents, making them unusable for in vivo experiments.

When uniform procedures of the macrocapillary, as well as the microcapillary, and the agarose technique have been used, several groups have obtained reproducible results. In my hands, the agarose technique has been much more sensitive than the original capillary tube technique in demonstrating direct tuberculin (PPD)-induced migration inhibition of leukocytes from Mantoux-positive subjects and in demonstrating migration inhibitory activity of cell-free culture supernatant fluids (7). However, the microcapillary tube technique is probably more sensitive than the original capillary tube technique (11). Furthermore, like the agarose technique, the microcapillary technique offers the considerable advantage of allowing a large number of replicates on small amounts of blood (i.e., about 20 cultures per 10 ml of blood).

An advantage of the agarose technique is that the cell cultures can be fixed and the gel can be removed, leaving the cells in situ for microscopic studies.

A disadvantage of the direct test is that the result will depend not only on the response of the antigen-sensitive lymphocytes, but also on the MIF sensitivity of the migrating polymorphs. Although the MIF sensitivity of polymorphs may be of importance in vivo, it is desirable to separate this characteristic of the polymorph from the lymphocyte function. Such a separation is obtained by the two-stage assay in which the migrating polymorphs are from normal donors.

Migration inhibitory activity of culture supernatant fluids can be demonstrated by the agarose technique with the use of only 50 to 100 μliters of nondialyzed, unconcentrated supernatant fluid. Therefore, this technique is most valuable when only a limited number of cells (i.e., blood) are available for the first-stage cultures.

LITERATURE CITED

1. Bendixen, G., and M. Søborg. 1969. A leucocyte migration technique for in vitro detection of cellular (delayed type) hypersensitivity in man. Dan. Med. Bull. 16:1–6.

2. Clausen, J. E. 1970. Polymorphonuclear leucocytes in the specific antigen-induced inhibition of the in vitro migration of human peripheral leucocytes. Acta Med. Scand. 188:59–64.

3. Clausen, J. E. 1971. Tuberculin-induced migration inhibition of human peripheral leucocytes in agarose medium. Acta Allergol. 26: 56–80.

4. Clausen, J. E. 1972. Migration inhibitory effect of cell-free supernatants from mixed human lymphocyte cultures. J. Immunol. 108:453–459.

5. Clausen, J. E. 1973. Migration inhibitory effect of cell-free supernatants from tuberculin-stimulated cultures of human mononuclear leukocytes demonstrated by two-step MIF agarose assay. J. Immunol. 110:546–551.

6. Clausen, J. E. 1973. Tuberculin-induced migration inhibition of human peripheral blood leukocytes after 2, 4, and 20 hours in agarose culture. Acta Allergol. 28:28–41.

7. Clausen, J. E. 1973. Comparison between capillary tube and agarose migration technique in the study of human peripheral blood leukocytes. Acta Allergol. 28:145–158.

8. Clausen, J. E. 1973. Leukocyte migration agarose test: inability to transfer tuberculin hypersensitivity by incubating nonsensitive leukocytes with plasma from persons with tuberculin-sensitive leukocytes. Acta Allergol. 28:172–179.

9. Clausen, J. E. 1973. Leukocyte migration agarose technique: some technical details. Acta Allergol. 28:351–364.

10. Federlin, K., R. N. Maini, A. S. Russell, and D. C. Dumonde. 1971. A micro-method for peripheral leucocyte migration in tuberculin sensitivity. J. Clin. Pathol. 24:533–536.

11. Maini, R. N., L. M. Roffe, I. T. Magrath, and D. C. Dumonde. 1973. Standardization of the leucocyte migration test. Int. Arch. Allergy 45:308–321.

12. Rocklin, R. E. 1974. Products of activated lymphocytes: leukocyte inhibitory factor (LIF) distinct from migration inhibitory factor (MIF). J. Immunol. 112:1461–1466.

13. Søborg, M., and G. Bendixen. 1967. Human lymphocyte migration as a parameter of hypersensitivity. Acta Med. Scand. 181:247–256.

Chapter 12

Chemotaxis

PETER A. WARD

INTRODUCTION

Chemotaxis of white blood cells (leukotaxis) is the unidirectional migratory response of cells to an increasing chemical gradient of attractant. That leukocytes have the ability to respond to chemotactic stimuli has been demonstrated for neutrophils, basophils, eosinophils, monocytes, and, also, lymphocytes. Attractant factors derive from several sources, the chief being the complement proteins of plasma, although antigen-activated lymphocytes and other cell types may also serve as a source for the production or release of chemotactic factors. In general, enzymatic cleavage of the third (C3) and the fifth (C5) components of complement results in the release of chemotactic peptides or, in the case of C5, the additional mechanism involving assemblage of a macromolecular complex, C567. Bacteria may also serve as a source of chemotactic factor production, either by the production of small chemotactic peptides or through the action of elaborated proteases which cleave C3 or C5 into chemotactic fragments.

The earlier in vitro methods for assessing leukotaxis were cumbersome and nonquantitative, largely relying on visualization with time-lapse photography of the migrational tracks of leukocytes. Approximately one decade ago, the micropore filter technique was introduced by Boyden, utilizing a membrane that allows the diffusion of soluble materials and, at the same time, permits leukocytes to migrate toward the diffusing substance. Details will be discussed below. The methods for assessing in vivo leukocyte chemotaxis in humans are not well established. The Rebuck skin window consists of a superficially abraded area (induced by a sharp scalpel), the surface of which is covered with a glass slide that is removed several hours later, air-dried, and stained for leukocyte content (see chapter 82). Mediators responsible for the inflammatory response in the Rebuck skin window are not presently known. Furthermore, because the cellular response in the skin window cannot be readily and reproducibly quantitated, this technique cannot be considered a reliably quantitative assay for leukocyte function. However, it does have some useful clinical application where interpretation of results does not depend on quantitation of cellular accumulations. In sum, there is no good in vivo assay in humans for leukotactic functions. Useful review articles have been published (2, 5, 6).

GENERAL INDICATIONS

Leukotactic assays are performed to determine the extent to which leukocytes can respond to chemotactic stimuli. Leukotactic disorders are found most commonly in patients who present histories of chronic, recurrent bacterial infections. Leukotactic disorders may be due to internal abnormalities in leukocytes, or they may be caused by defects in the plasma substrate system (complement) that accounts for generation of leukotactic factors. Cellular defects may be acquired or familial, examples being diabetes mellitus and the Chediak-Higashi syndrome, respectively (see references 5 and 6 for a review of clinical disorders). Chemotactic testing most frequently involves functional assessment of blood neutrophils, since these are readily obtainable. Blood monocytes, which are isolated in adequate amounts only with considerable difficulty, can also be studied (4). In addition, it is possible to test serum for the generation of leukotactic factors or for the presence of leukotactic inhibitors. Advantages of these techniques include the ready availability of test materials by venipuncture and the in vitro nature of the assay. The major disadvantage is the requirement for experienced laboratory personnel and the somewhat time-consuming nature of the assay. Aside from the in vitro assay for chemotaxis, there is no other (in vivo) definitive and unequivocal method for measuring chemotaxis. Chemotaxis of basophils or eosinophils is not feasible for the clinical laboratory, inasmuch as the isolation of adequate numbers of these cells is technically difficult.

TEST PROCEDURES

Two different quantitative techniques for chemotactic assessment are available, the first employing a radioassay and the second involving visual counting of cells. The former technique is not feasible for the clinical laboratory because it requires radiolabeling of patient leukocytes (with ^{51}Cr) and subsequently measuring radioactivity in a scintillation counter (1). The second technique, that of visual counting, is the method commonly used in clinical testing (2, 5, 6). The following technical aspects of chemotaxis are important.

Leukocytes

Neutrophil testing is most commonly employed. The cells are obtained by sedimentation of red cells in anticoagulated blood (5 units of heparin/ml) in an inverted syringe into which the blood has been drawn. Dextran-induced sedimentation of red cells can also be used to reduce the time required (to 30 min from 1 to 2 h) for obtaining a leukocyte-rich suspension. For the dextran technique, 1 volume of 6% dextran in saline is added to 1 volume of blood; sedimentation is carried out in a 50-ml plastic centrifuge tube. (Leukocytes will adhere to glass surfaces.) The yield of neutrophils will vary with the leukocyte count of the donor and with conditions of sedimentation, but 15 ml of blood should suffice. (In pediatric cases 5 to 8 ml may be used). Once the suspension of neutrophils is obtained, the cells are gently pelleted by centrifugation (approximately 900 rpm for 10 min, or 500 $\times$ g) and then resuspended in medium 199 at a concentration of 2.5×10^6 neutrophils/ml. Serum is added to the cell suspension at a concentration of 10% (i.e., 1:10 dilution of serum). The protocol given in Table 1 describes a typical chemotactic assay.
For monocyte chemotaxis, special fractionation of blood is required with a Ficoll-Hypaque gradient, as described by Snyderman et al. (4).

Chemotactic factors

To test chemotactic responsiveness of leukocytes, chemotactic factors are obviously essential. For most assays, two different chemotactic factor preparations can be used. The first is a culture supernatant fluid obtained by overnight growth of *Escherichia coli* in medium 199. Bacteria are removed by centrifugation, and the pH is adjusted to neutrality with 1 M NaOH. This batch of bacterial chemotactic factor can be frozen in small portions for storage. Dilutions of the factor 1:5 in medium 199 should provide a potent chemotactic factor. The second factor, the C5 fragment, is generated in fresh human serum by the addition of zymosan, 10 mg/ml of serum, and incubation at 37 C for 1 h. This preparation has potent chemotactic activity at a 1:20 dilution in medium 199.

Chemotactic chambers

All leukotactic assays employ chambers that have two compartments separated by a micropore filter. Chambers commonly used consist of a steel housing with rubber gaskets, between which the filter is held. The upper compartment contains the cell suspension, and the lower compartment contains the culture medium (medium 199) with or without the chemotactic factor. The lower compartment is filled with 1.0 ml of fluid that is injected with a tuberculin syringe and needle (26 gauge) by perforating the rubber gasket of the chamber. When the lower compartment is filled, the chamber is placed on the countertop, and the cell suspension (1.0 ml containing 2.5×10^6 neutrophils) is added by use of a plastic pipette. If plastic chambers are used, the lower compartment contains a larger volume (approximately 2.4 ml) and can be filled by pipetting the diluted chemotactic factor preparation. Most plastic chambers have upper compartments that contain smaller volumes (approximately 0.4 ml). When these chambers are used, the same relative concentration of leukocytes (2.5×10^6 ml) is employed.

Incubation

Chambers are incubated in air at 37 C for 3 h.

Staining of filters

After the appropriate period of incubation, chambers are disassembled. The filters are dipped in propanol (absolute), which allows fixation, then stained for 15 min in hemotoxylin (Harris), dipped in distilled water for washing, and moved into 70%, 95%, and absolute propanol (1-propanol; 3 to 5 min each), followed by clearing in xylene. To facilitate processing of filters, special brass cassettes are available (see below). This permits the simultaneous staining of 25 to 50 filters. The filters are then placed on conventional glass slides with Permount as the mounting medium. It is convenient to invert the filters at the time of mounting them on glass, that is, to have the original lower surface of the filter facing upward. This facilitates the visualization of cells that have moved completely across the filter. Glass cover slips are then applied.

Assessment of cell migration

The original upper and lower surfaces of the filters can be readily distinguished. The upper surface will contain mononuclear cells (lymphocytes and monocytes) that have not responded chemotactically under the conditions described above. The original lower surface (distal to the starting monolayer of leukocytes) will contain only migrated neutrophils. By light microscopy and under high (dry)-power magnification (ca. $\times 240$), the number of migrated leukocytes is counted. Five fields in high power are selected at random. The total number of migrated leukocytes in response to a chemotactic stimulus will usually be approximately 250, whereas the negative control (culture medium alone) will be around 30.

Typical protocol and results

A typical protocol with typical results is given in Table 1.

Assessment of monocyte chemotaxis

Monocytes respond chemotactically most effectively to the C5 fragment and to a product of antigen-stimulated lymphoid cells (6). In clinical medicine two different aspects of monocyte chemotaxis are usually studied: the monocytes themselves and the chemotactic factors produced from lymphoid cells, particularly in patients with suspected underlying immunological dysfunction (deficiency states). If monocyte function is to be studied, the cells must be fractionated from blood by the Ficoll-Hypaque method (see reference 4). In this case, plastic chambers are employed to keep to a minimum the numbers of cells required (0.3 ml of cells in 10% serum, 2.5×10^6/ml). Factors employed are the C5 fragment generated in zymosan-activated serum (described above) or the culture fluid (diluted 1:5) from antigen-stimulated lymphoid cells. Chapter 10 of this *Manual* contains details concerning preparation of this lymphocyte product. A detailed description of

the monocyte chemotactic factor assay involving human cells was presented by Snyderman et al. (3).

REAGENTS

Chemotaxis chambers

Chemotaxis chambers are available from Schleicher & Schuell Co., Keene, N.H., or Bellco Glass Co., Vineland, N.J. (These companies also supply rubber gaskets and glass cover slips used in chamber assembly.) Plastic chambers can be obtained from AHLCO Scientific, Inc., Granby, Conn. 06035.

Micropore filters

Filters used are of 5 μm porosity and are made of mixed esters of cellulose; they are coded as SMWP 02500 (Millipore Corp., Bedford, Mass.). Other types of filters are made from polycarbonate and can be obtained from Nucleopore Corp., Pleasanton, Calif.

Culture medium

Medium 199 can be obtained from any tissue culture supplier. This should be buffered with tris(hydroxymethyl)aminomethane-chloride, 0.05 M, pH 7.4. (A stock solution of 0.5 M with pH adjusted is usually convenient to keep at 5 C for use.) Alternatively, *N*-2-hydroxyethyl piperazine-*N'*-2-ethanesulfonic acid buffer (0.01 M) may be used.

Chemotactic factors

Overnight culture fluid from *E. coli* or any other bacterial species that replicates rapidly in medium 199 at 37 C is used. Bacteria are removed by centrifugation. The factor is diluted 1:5 for use. The C5 fragment from complement can be generated in fresh human serum by incubation with 10 mg of zymosan/ml of serum, at 37 C for 1 h. Zymosan can be purchased from Sigma Chemical Co., St. Louis, Mo.. Schwarz/Mann Biochemicals, New York, N.Y., or Nutritional Biochemicals Corp., La Jolla, Calif.

INTERPRETATION

The protocol listed in Table 1 describes a routine assay. The protocol listed in Table 2 shows examples of these screening assays in which three different kinds of defects were found. The following defects can be detected: cellular hyporesponsiveness, the presence of an inhibitor, and defective generation of complement-derived chemotactic activity.

The three different results (A, B, C) in Table 2 are diagnosed as follows:

TABLE 1. *Typical protocol with typical results*

Upper compartment (1.0-ml vol)		Lower compartment (1.0 ml)	Chemotactic count
Cells (2.5×10^6, 1 ml)	Serum (10%)		
Normal[a]	Normal	Blank	20
Normal	Normal	Bacterial factor (1:5)	250
Normal	Normal	Zymosan-activated normal serum[b]	300
Normal	Normal	Normal serum	40

[a] Donor source.

[b] A 1-mg amount of zymosan in 0.1 ml of serum, incubated at 37 C for 1 h followed by dilution to 1.0 ml.

TABLE 2. *Protocols showing examples of screening assays with three different kinds of defects[a]*

Upper compartment		Lower compart- ment	Chemotactic counts		
Cells	Serum		Expt A	Expt B	Expt C
N	N	—	20	20	20
N	N	bf	200	200	200
N	P	bf	50	200	200
N	N	Z·Sn	250	250	250
N	N	Z·Sp	250	250	60
P	P	—	10	10	10
P	P	bf	20	20	200
P	N	bf	200	20	200

[a] Abbreviations: bf = bacterial factor 1:5 to 1:15; Z·Sn = zymosan-activated normal serum; Z·Sp = zymosan-activated patient serum; N = normal volunteer; P = patient volunteer.

A = Presence of chemotactic inhibitor in patient volunteer serum.

B = Chemotactically defective patient volunteer cells.

C = Defective generation of chemotactic activity in patient volunteer serum.

It will require more elaborate studies to determine the nature of any inhibitor found in serum (that is, whether the inhibitor is cell-directed or chemotactic factor-directed).

ACKNOWLEDGMENTS

This work was supported by Public Health Service grants AI 09651, AI 11526, and AI 12225 from the National Institute of Allergy and Infectious Diseases.

LITERATURE CITED

1. Gallin, J. I., R. A. Clark, and H. R. Kimball. 1973. Granulocyte chemotaxis: an improved in vitro assay employing chromium-51 labelled granulocytes. J. Immunol. 110:233–240.
2. Keller, H. U., and E. Sorkin. 1968. Chemotaxis of leukocytes. Experientia 24:641–752.
3. Snyderman, R., L. C. Altman, A. Frankel, and R. M. Blaese. 1973. Defective mononuclear leukocyte chemotaxis: a previously unrecognized immune dysfunction. Studies in a patient with chronic mucocutaneous candidiases. Ann. Intern. Med. 78:509–513.
4. Snyderman, R., H. S. Shin, and M. H. Hausman. 1971. A chemotactic factor for mononuclear leukocytes. Proc. Soc. Exp. Biol. Med. 138:387–390.
5. Stossel, T. P. 1974. Phagocytosis. N. Engl. J. Med. 250:717–723, 774–780, 833–839.
6. Ward, P. A. 1974. Leukotaxis and leukotactic disorders. Am. J. Pathol. 77:520–538.

Chapter 13

In Vitro Detection of Human Lymphotoxin

JOHN E. LEWIS, DARYL S. FAIR, ANNE-MARIE PRIEUR, ROBERT L. LUNDAK, AND GALE A. GRANGER

INTRODUCTION

Host cellular immunity is a complex reaction both in vivo and in vitro. These reactions, mediated by host lymphocytes and macrophages, have been associated with tissue destruction, typified by the reactions seen in delayed hypersensitivity, allograft rejection, tumor immunity, and certain autoimmune disease states. Although the relationships of these various reactions to one another are not yet known, it is clear that they all share certain fundamental steps at the cell and molecular level in vitro (11, 13, 15). The first step is recognition of the foreign antigen or cell, presumably mediated by receptors on the immune lymphocyte surface (13, 15). The second step, termed "activation" and triggered by the recognition phase, produces dramatic changes in lymphocyte biosynthesis, energy metabolism, and cellular morphology, resulting in the formation of the effector cell (15, 24). The third step is the cytolytic phase, in which the "activated" aggressor cell by a yet unknown mechanism causes either cytolysis or growth inhibition of cells and tissues in vitro (13, 15). Recent studies have revealed that the "activated" lymphoid cell can release a complex family of soluble molecules which may be important effectors in causing the various manifestations of cell-mediated immunity in vitro and in vivo (6, 22, 28).

Our studies have dealt with a family of lymphocyte effector molecules (LEM) with cytotoxic or cytostatic activity in vitro, termed lymphotoxin (LT), proliferation inhibition factor (PIF), and colony inhibition factor (CIF; 7, 10, 16). Collectively, we shall refer to these activities as the inhibitory LEM. These materials are released by "activated" lymphocytes from humans and other animal species in vitro (6, 22). The agents which trigger their release can be grouped into several categories: (i) *specific stimulation* occurs when lymphoid cells from preimmunized donors are cultured with the specific soluble or particulate antigen (induction and secretion of LEM is highly specific

for the particular antigen in these situations); (ii) *nonspecific stimulation* occurs when lymphoid cells from nonimmunized donors are co-cultured with any one of a family of substances termed mitogens, i.e., phytohemagglutinin (PHA) or concanavalin A (ConA), which induce cellular activation; (iii) *allogeneic stimulation* occurs in mixed lymphocyte cultures, when lymphoid cells are obtained from genetically dissimilar, nonimmunized individuals; and (iv) *continuous human lymphoid cell lines* have been shown to release LEM spontaneously (6). Production of LEM requires induction of lymphocyte activation, cellular metabolism, and biosynthesis (22). Studies by a number of investigators indicate that, once released, the inhibitory family of LEM is nonspecific. There is, however, a wide spectrum of sensitivity of cells to these substances in vitro (17, 32).

Interaction of human LT with a cell(s) in culture is a complex reaction and can manifest itself in several different ways. The first occurs at high LT concentrations, or with a sensitive cell, and results in cytolysis. At intermediate LT levels, or with a more resistant target cell, the interaction can irreversibly block cell division without cytolysis. At lower levels, or with very resistant target cells, there is only a transitory and reversible inhibition of cell division (6, 17, 32). The step(s) involved in LT-target cell interaction in vitro appears to be initially a rapid binding to trypsin-sensitive cell surface receptors. This binding is irreversible, and the material is consumed in the reaction (14). The subsequent steps result in either cytotoxicity or cytostasis. Numerous studies suggest that the cytolytic event probably involves a direct effect on the cell membrane by a mechanism not yet understood (14, 30, 31). ·

Recent studies show that the induction and release of this family of molecules appear to be under very stringent regulatory controls in vitro (1). These studies may hold the key to how a nonspecific "soluble" molecule(s) could be employed by the lymphoid cell to cause both specific and nonspecific cytolysis or cytostasis.

Figure 1 is a schematic representation of our interpretation of how the lymphoid cell could employ this family of molecules as short-range mediators.

There are a number of different in vitro tests available for measuring the presence of inhibitory LEM in the supernatant fluid from activated lymphoid cells. Isotope uptake, isotope release, and direct cell count are methods employed by various investigators to measure direct LT-induced cytotoxicity of cells in vitro. Isotope uptake requires the addition of radioactive precursors to the culture medium to determine the number of viable cells remaining in the cultures. Isotope release monitors cell destruction by the release of isotopes from prelabeled target cells. The final methods involve the enumeration of cells directly, either by observation under a microscope in the presence of vital stains or by passage through a mechanical particle counter. Variations of the above methods utilize LT assays which include inhibitors of cellular biosynthesis and metabolism. These agents either accentuate the degree of cytolysis or accelerate the rate of destruction and shorten the incubation period. There are methods for measuring the inhibition of cell division, the event observed when either low levels of LT are present or the target cells employed are resistant. These techniques assess the capacity of treated cells to divide by measuring their ability to form colonies when plated at low density or their ability to synthesize deoxyribonucleic acid (DNA). Our own experience indicates that the most crucial aspects of testing for the presence of LEM are as follows: (i) the requirement that lymphocytes be activated, (ii) the differential effects of the concentration of LEM on target cells, and (iii) a sensitive indicator target cell.

The LT activities found in a cell-free supernatant fluid from activated human lymphoid cells were previously identified as a single component (8). Recent evidence, however, indicates that these activities are associated with a family of molecules. There are at least four proteins that have LT-like functions identified in the supernatant fluids of stimulated lymphocytes. It appears, moreover, that each member has LT, PIF, and CIF *activities* (17). Preliminary evidence indicates that certain of these molecules may be related to or derived from one another. The major component has a molecular weight of 80,000 and accounts for at least 50 to 80% of the activity in a given supernatant fluid. General physical properties of the LT(s) released by activated human lymphocytes in vitro are as follows:

Molecular species: protein

Molecular weight: 90,000, 65,000, and 10,000 (four separate molecules)

Effect of heating: inactivated in 15 min at 85 C

Stability: resists nuclease, freezing and thawing; trypsin sensitive

Electrophoretic mobility: alpha globulin and albumin

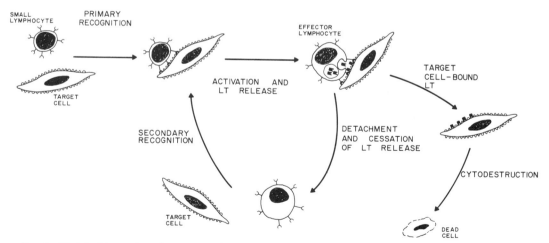

FIG. 1. *Model of how a lymphocyte may induce destruction of cells in vitro, employing lymphocyte effector molecules. The immune lymphocyte first recognized the "target" cell by specific receptors on its surface. This induces activation of the lymphocyte, and it secretes LT or LT-like materials onto the target cell surface. The lymphoid cell may then detach itself from the target cell, stop LT secretion, and move away to destroy another cell. The LT-coated target cell will die or be growth-inhibited.*

CLINICAL INDICATIONS

Little is known regarding the in vivo relevance of LEM. As "short-range" mediators, they may only exist in vivo free in the space between the activated lymphocyte and the target cell. This is supported by the observation that human lymphocytes require continual membrane stimulation to maintain LT secretion and that once the stimulating agent is removed from the membrane receptor secretion stops (1). LT secretion is regulated by agents which modulate the levels of intracellular cyclic nucleotides. Those agents which raise intracellular cyclic adenosine monophosphate suppress the release of LT from stimulated lymphocytes in vitro (23). Immunosuppressive agents have also been shown to diminish LT release (32).

Clinically, the role of LT in certain disorders may be of great importance. LT may be present in fluids, bathing accumulations of interacting lymphoid cells and affected tissue(s). It is possible that it may be found free in various fluids obtainable from an in vivo reaction site(s) associated with cell-mediated immune phenomena. In certain systemic reactions, these materials may be present in the blood vascular system.

In vitro methods have been reported that can determine whether lymphocytes collected from an in situ reaction center are releasing LT. In brief, these techniques involve removing biopsies or tissue slices from the reaction area, placing them in culture for an interval of time, and measuring the presence of LT in the supernatant fluid from the culture. LT-releasing cells have been described in rat allografts (9) and in the joint tissues of patients with rheumatoid arthritis. The use of fluorescent antibodies would allow studies to be performed on fixed sections, much as one now detects the presence of immunoglobulins in situ. The collection of lymphocytes from peripheral blood would be an alternative to tissue biopsy. Lymphoid cells can be collected, purified, and mixed in culture with the antigen in question, and the release of LT can then be assessed in the culture supernatant fluids.

It is important to establish the in vivo relevance or role of the effector molecules in cell-mediated immune reactions. There are certain obvious sequelae which could be examined. For example, the various manifestations of immunodeficiency diseases(s) as they relate to both B and T cell dysfunction. Studies have related certain cell-mediated deficiency diseases to low levels of LEM release (25). These situations represent hyporesponsive patients. LEM assays may be valuable indicators for assessing syndromes in which an immunological reaction is suspected, such as the putative autoimmune diseases. Chronic infections with bacteria or fungi indicate, rather than a general immune dysfunction, a very specific deficiency with regard to particular antigens. Studies would be interesting and relevant in clinical situations where there is pathological tissue destruction occurring in allograft rejection, delayed hypersensitivity, and tumor immunity.

The capacity to measure the state of a patient's cell-mediated immune system in vitro has distinct clinical advantages. Whereas a battery of sophisticated methods are available for assessing the patient's humoral response, DNA synthesis is the only method currently available for monitoring cellular events. The wide spectrum of LEM may provide important probes with which to begin to dissect and understand the nature of the cellular immune system. Of the various tests, LT and interferon are the only ones which allow a semiquantitative evaluation of the amount of material present in a given supernatant fluid. These assays have the advantage of giving not just a qualitative answer but also a relative level and the ability to compare this level with normal individuals.

There are certain disadvantages and criticisms that must be considered when employing in vitro testing methods. The first is the test system itself. Certain physical parameters must be carefully and critically controlled to insure a valid test. These will be mentioned in detail later, but they are briefly outlined here: (i) temperature is important because a 3 C drop from 37 to 34 C inhibits more than 50% of human LT-induced target L cell destruction in the standard assay system; (ii) certain sera optimize the degree of LT-induced destruction; (iii) the use of biosynthetic inhibitors, such as mitomycin C, makes target cells more susceptible and enhances the degree of destruction; (iv) a sensitive target indicator cell must be used; and (v) the reproducibility and stability of the test must be considered. Variability in the test system may occur even when all the above parameters are controlled. Some ways to minimize variability include the use of an internal control or standard sample of supernatant fluid containing LT. Although the actual end point titer may vary, the ratio of the test titer to the standard titer stays constant. Another method is to accumulate experimental samples and test them all in a single assay. Controls should include supernatant fluids from nonstimulated lymphocytes and, when feasible, cells from a healthy subject and/or a patient recovering from the same disease.

TEST PROCEDURES AND CULTURE METHODS

The culture methods and in vitro test procedures described in this chapter have been designed primarily for clinicians employing human cells. They are, however, generally applicable to other animal species, as previously described for basic research (22).

Lymphocyte culturing

In humans, lymphocytes derived from peripheral blood, tonsils, adenoids, lymph node, or spleen are capable of secreting LT. The most readily obtainable source of lymphocytes is peripheral blood. Tonsils and adenoids are lymphoid tissues that also give exceptionally high yields of very pure and responsive lymphocytes.

Peripheral blood lymphocyte preparation.
1. Obtain 20 ml of heparinized blood (100 U/ml) by venipuncture.
2. Dilute 15 ml of blood with 15 ml of phosphate-buffered saline (PBS) and layer it carefully over 17 ml of Ficoll-Hypaque (density, 1.077 g/cc) in a 50-ml centrifuge tube.
3. Centrifuge the gradients at 400 × g at room temperature for 40 min.
4. Remove lymphocytes at the blood-Hypaque interphase with a Pasteur pipette.
5. Wash the lymphocytes three times by centrifugation (300 × g for 10 min) and resuspend them in PBS. The cell concentration is adjusted to the final density needed.
6. After thoroughly resuspending the cells, take 10 μliters of the suspension and mix in a serological test tube containing 500 μliters of Eosin-Y (0.2% in PBS) and 490 μliters of PBS with 1% serum added.
7. Using a hemacytometer, count the cells immediately. Viable cells are unstained; dead lymphocytes stain pink.

The viability and purity of the lymphocyte preparations are an important parameter to consider, since granulocytes are known to release substances which can mimic mediators. Lymphocyte preparations having less than 70% viability should not be used.

Solid tissue collection. The method described below can be used for tonsils, adenoids, lymph node, and spleen. Tonsils and adenoids will be cited as an example. Ideally, tissues should be collected in a medium containing high concentrations of antibiotics and processed

the same day as surgery. Refrigeration and same-day processing give 80 to 90% lymphocyte viability. Cell suspensions can be stored overnight at 4 or 37 C, after preparation, if kept in media. Pathology laboratories are requested to refrigerate tonsils and adenoids immediately and to avoid formalin contamination when examining tissues. The medium used for tissue collection is Eagle's minimal essential medium (MEM) supplemented with nonessential amino acids, 4 mM glutamine, 1 mM sodium pyruvate, 200 U of penicillin/ml, 200 μg of streptomycin/ml, 5 μg of amphotericin B/ml, and 62 μg of amikacin/ml. (The antibiotic concentration in the medium is twice normal to minimize bacterial and fungal contamination [2×-AM].)

Solid tissue preparation (tonsils and adenoids). (See Fig. 2.) Use sterile techniques and tissue culture methodology when preparing tissues. When possible, work in a laminar airflow hood to avoid microbial contamination.
1. Wash the tissues at least twice with 2×-AM before removal from the collecting jars.
2. Scalpel-mince the tissues in a sterile petri dish while they are bathed in 2×-AM. Mince until there are no large pieces of tissue remaining.
3. Pour the petri dish contents into a sterile fine-mesh household strainer suspended over a sterile petri dish, and gently homogenize the tissues with a chemistry pestle. Rinse the strainer frequently with 2×-AM.
4. Aseptically pipette the cell suspension into a 50-ml centrifuge tube, and centrifuge at 80 × g for 30 s to remove tissue debris.
5. Carefully aspirate the supernatant fluid into another 50-ml centrifuge tube, and centrifuge at 300 × g for 5 min.
6. Aspirate and discard the supernatant fluid.
7. Resuspend the cell pellet in 5 to 10 ml of 2×-AM.
8. After thoroughly resuspending the cells, take 10 μliters of the suspension and mix thoroughly in a serological test tube containing 500 μliters of Eosin-Y and 490 μliters of PBS. Count viable cells.

The mean yields of lymphocytes obtainable from a single tonsil and adenoid are 2.5×10^9 and 1.4×10^9, respectively. Lymphocyte suspensions from spleen homogenates require Ficoll-Hypaque separation because of the heterogeneous cell population.

Lymphocyte culture media. Lymphocyte culture media can be purchased from a number of vendors or prepared de novo (see below, Reagents).

Culture vessels. Lymphocyte culturing can

successfully be achieved in a variety of culture vessels. Glass and plastic ware are most commonly employed. If plastic ware is used, it is advisable to use tissue culture grade. Glassware should be thoroughly washed and sterilized.

Lymphocyte supernatant preparation (Fig. 2). Lymphocytes release more lymphokines if cultured under optimal conditions. Lymphocyte culture density varies with the volume of culture medium and the stimulating agent employed.

1. Suspensions of lymphocytes are cultured at a density of 10^6 to 4×10^6 cells/ml. For example, a cell density of 4×10^6 cells/ml is used with a 32-oz glass or plastic flasks containing 200 ml of medium, whereas 10^6 cells/ml is sufficient for a 1-ml tube culture.

2. Add the stimulating agent to the cell culture. This step is critical. An optimal concentration of the agent chosen is required for maximal LT secretion. For example, a cell concentration of 4×10^6 cells/ml in 200 ml of culture medium can be adequately stimulated with 20 μg of PHA-P/ml (see Reagents).

3. Serum (5 to 10%) is added to provide an enriched medium. Cells are maintained for 4 to 5 days in a 5% CO_2–95% air environment. Although LT can be detected within hours in a strongly stimulated culture, maximal levels are reached in 4 to 5 days.

Stimulating agents. There is a broad range of agents that activate or transform lymphocytes. One of the most commonly used strong mitogens is PHA. This plant extract converts normally quiescent small lymphocytes to a biosynthetically active and morphologically enlarged blast cell. Figure 3 depicts the kinetics of LT production as it relates to biosynthetic events with PHA, ConA, and a tissue allogeneic mix as the activating agents.

Kinetics of lymphocyte culturing and lymphokine production. Figure 4 depicts the relationship of LT release to ribonucleic acid, deoxyribonucleic acid, and protein synthesis after stimulation with a strong mitogen (PHA-P). LT concentrations plateau on day 5. Optimally, lymphocytes in culture remain viable for 10 days. Supernatant fluids can be harvested on the 5th day (cells are resuspended in fresh medium, plus the activating agent at reduced levels) and again on the 10th day, allowing for a doubling of the volume collected from a single preparation.

Supernatant harvesting

Lymphokines are not released unless lymphocytes have been adequately stimulated. Some visual signs will indicate whether a culture is healthy and whether the cells have been activated. Lymphocytes in culture at the end of 5 days at 37 C show aggregation, and the container, if agitated, shows turbidity and a drop in pH. Microbial contamination can be determined by observing the clear fluid before agitation; if the fluid above the clumped, settled cells is turbid, fungal or bacterial contamination

LYMPHOID TISSUE	PERIPHERAL BLOOD	STOCK CULTURES
Mince and homogenize		Mouse fibroblast L-929 cells (alpha subline)
Lymphocytes	Ficoll-Hypaque gradients	
Lymphocytes cultured at 10^6 to 4×10^6 cells/ml + activating agent		Trypsinize and adjust cell density to 10^5 cells/ml
		Add mitomycin C (0.5 μg/ml)
		Establish 1.0-ml cultures in screw-capped tubes
Collect supernatant fluid		
Dilutions of supernatant fluids prepared for quantitative assay		After 24 h, examine L cells for confluent, healthy cultures
	Add LT-containing dilutions to L cell monolayers; incubate at 37 C for 16 to 24 h	Discard supernatant fluid
	Wash and trypsinize, and determine the number of viable cells	
	Units of LT in the original medium equals the reciprocal of the LD_{50} dilution or that which kills 50% of the target cells	

FIG. 2. *Schematic outline of general steps involved in inducing, collecting, and testing for LT in human lymphocyte cultures.*

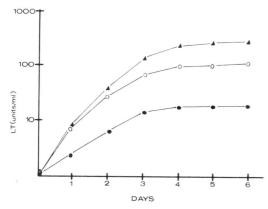

Fig. 3. *Kinetics of LT production by human lymphocytes in vitro after stimulation with PHA (▲), Con A (○), and allogeneic lymphocytes (●).*

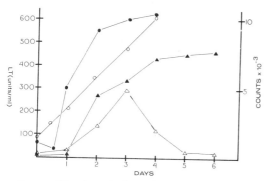

Fig. 4. *Kinetics of ribonucleic acid (●), protein (○), and deoxyribonucleic acid (△) synthesis and LT secretion (▲) in PHA-P-activated cultures of human lymphocytes in vitro.*

might be suspected. Supernatant fluids are collected by centrifugation or filtering. Collect them in sterile bottles and immediately freeze them. If cells are to be recultured with fresh media, collect the LT-rich supernatant fluid by centrifugation ($300 \times g$ for 10 min), and resuspend the pellet in fresh medium.

Target cells

Cell lines. The choice of a target indicator cell is important. It has been shown that different target cell lines (32) and sublines (21) exhibit different sensitivities to cytotoxic supernatant fluids. A particular subline (alpha) of L-929 mouse fibroblast (L cells) is an extremely sensitive indicator of in vitro cytolytic activity (see below, Reagents, for additional information on this cell line).

Maintenance of stock cultures. The procedure given below outlines a laboratory protocol

for maintaining culture lines in vessels with a surface area of 75 cm^2 (16-oz prescription bottle or T75 tissue culture flask). Various-sized containers can be employed for culture; however, volumes and cell numbers should be correspondingly adjusted.

1. Alpha-L cells are maintained as monolayers in 16-oz prescription bottles. Cultures are grown in MEM supplemented with penicillin, streptomycin, and 3 to 5% fetal or newborn calf serum, and are incubated at 37 C in a 5% CO_2-95% air atmosphere.

2. Healthy cells are passed just prior to or at the time of monolayer confluency as determined by examination with a microscope. Discard the used medium, and wash the cells with 30 ml of sterile PBS to remove proteins and divalent cations.

3. Discard the PBS and add 1.0 ml of 0.05% trypsin-10^{-4} M ethylenediaminetetraacetic acid solution in PBS. Gently distribute the enzyme over the entire monolayer by tilting the bottle. Incubate at 37 C for 1 to 2 min.

4. Add 5 to 6 ml of medium, and dislodge the cells from the glass by vigorous shaking.

5. Determine the cell density by use of a hemacytometer or particle counter.

6. Cells are passed biweekly by seeding a new bottle(s) with 4×10^5 cells in 17 ml of fresh medium. These cells may be used in the LT assay (see below).

Storage of cell lines.

1. Cells are kept frozen to minimize loss of viability.

2. Ampoules containing 5×10^6 cells/ml are suspended in fresh medium containing 10% dimethylsulfoxide (DMSO), sealed, and frozen by setting on dry ice. Decrease the temperature at a rate of 1° C/min until frozen.

3. Ampoules are then stored frozen in the liquid phase of a nitrogen container.

Lymphotoxin assay (Fig. 2)

1. Set up assay tubes 24 h prior to performing the cytotoxicity test.

2. Alpha-L fibroblast cells are harvested by trypsinization, and the concentration is adjusted to 10^5 cells/ml by the addition of fresh medium (see above, Maintenance of stock cultures).

3. Add mitomycin C to a final concentration of 0.5 μg/ml.

4. Mix and pipette 1 ml of the cell suspension into screw-capped tubes.

5. Mark all tubes to identify the location of cell attachment once the monolayer of L cells has been established.

6. Incubate the tubes at a 5° slant (commercial racks are available; see below, Reagents) for 24 h at 37 C in the absence of light in a 5% CO_2-95% air atmosphere (mitomycin C is light sensitive).

Addition of test supernatant fluids.

1. Target cell monolayers *must be* examined with a microscope to insure that only confluent, healthy cultures are used.

2. Test supernatant fluids can be used undiluted if a qualitative answer is desired. For quantitatively determining the amount of LT activity, dilute the supernatant fluids, using threefold serial dilutions in MEM.

3. Discard cell medium and replace with 1.0 ml of the appropriate dilution of the LT-containing material to be tested. Control cultures receive fresh MEM, MEM containing the stimulating agent, or media from unstimulated lymphocyte cultures. Each dilution should be run in duplicate or triplicate cultures.

4. Incubate cultures at 37 C for 24 h in a 5% CO_2-95% air atmosphere in the 5° slant racks. All tubes are realigned to insure that the cell monolayers are covered with medium.

Counting target cells.

1. Visually examine the tubes for cell destruction by using a regular or tissue culture microscope for qualitative estimate of LT activity (Fig. 5).

2. Discard the medium from each tube and add 4.5 ml of PBS to wash off dead cells.

3. Decant and realign the tubes in the 5° slant rack. Add 0.5 ml of a 0.005% trypsin solution. Be sure that the trypsin solution "wets" the monolayer. Incubate for 1 to 3 min at 37 C. Longer incubation can result in cellular aggregation.

4. Add 4.5 ml of filtered formalin-treated PBS (0.1% formalin) and vortex each tube. Examine a random number to determine whether detachment has been achieved.

5. The intact cells are counted on a model F Coulter counter or in a hemacytometer.

6. Data are plotted by the percentage of cell destruction versus the LT dilution.

7. A unit of LT activity is defined as the quantity of LT which results in a 50% reduction in mitomycin C-treated alpha L-929 target cells. The titer or units of LT in a supernatant fluid is expressed as the reciprocal of the dilution effecting the 50% reduction in cells (29).

Other testing methods

Although we have described one assay method for LT, investigators have employed other techniques which include either micromethods or the use of radioisotopes. Outlines below are some common procedures.

In vitro microassay for LT (19).

1. Small amounts of supernatant fluids can be analyzed by use of microtiter plates.

2. To each well, add 0.2 ml of alpha L-929 cells (1,000 to 5,000 cells/ml). The cells should be thoroughly suspended in a conditioned medium obtained from a 24-h stock culture. Clarify the cells by centrifugation at $300 \times g$ for 5 min, and adjust the pH to 6.7 with 7% sterile acetic acid.

3. Seal the microplate with a gas-impervious, pressure-sensitive film, and incubate overnight at 37 C.

4. After incubation, remove the seal, decant the medium, and add 0.2 ml of fresh medium containing the various dilutions of test and control supernatant fluids. Be sure healthy monolayers are present in the well, as verified by visual inspection.

5. The microplates are again sealed with the gas-impervious film and incubated for 24 h at 37 C.

6. Killing of target cells is monitored by decanting LT-containing medium and counting the remaining cells.

Advantages of the microassay over the tube assay are that it requires smaller amounts of cytotoxic supernatant fluids and that no CO_2 incubator is required. Disadvantages of this system include variability in target cell densities from well to well and the requirement for gentle washing of target cells with PBS to avoid dislodging cells from the sides of the well.

Release of ^{51}Cr from target cells.

1. Mouse L-929 target cells (27) or mouse DBA/2 mastocytoma cells (12) are established in culture for 24 h at 37 C in a 5% CO_2-95% air atmosphere in the presence of 1 to 2 μCi of ^{51}Cr/ml.

2. After incubation, the cells are washed thoroughly to remove free ^{51}Cr, and the cytotoxic supernatant fluids in the appropriate dilutions are added. Control cultures include: supernatant fluids from nonstimulated lymphocyte cultures (nonspecific release control), fresh MEM medium (nonspecific release control), and water to measure the maximal release of radioactivity from target cells.

3. Incubate for 16 to 24 h; then carefully remove the media from the cultures and save. Both the media and the cells are counted for the presence of ^{51}Cr.

An advantage of the ^{51}Cr release assay is that

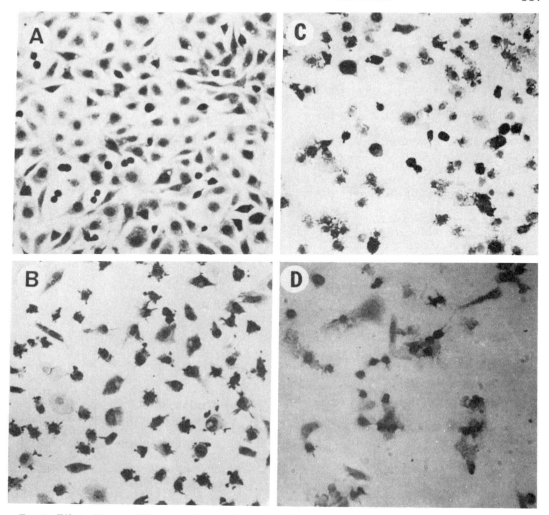

FIG. 5. *Effect of human LT on monolayer cultures of C$_3$H mouse alpha L cells in vitro (A) before addition of LT, (B) after 6 h of exposure to LT, (C) after 10 h of exposure to LT, and (D) after 16 h in LT. L cell cover slip cultures were exposed to LT-containing medium, removed, and stained with May-Grunewald-Giemsa. ×100.*

it is a sensitive method for measuring cellular lysis. Disadvantages include the number of manipulations required to monitor the radioactivity in both cellular supernatant fluids and intact cells, and the high background values of spontaneous release.

Other radioisotopic assays. Recently, a technique has been described (18) for measuring cytolytic activity by using microculture plates and the multiple automated sample harvester (MASH). The degree of cytolysis is measured by the ability of the remaining viable cells to incorporate [^{3}H]methyl-thymidine ([^{3}H]TdR). The major advantage of this microassay is that large numbers of assays can be handled easily

and that the sensitivity of [^{3}H]TdR makes the task of counting viable cells simpler.

Target cells can be tested for viability after exposure to cytotoxic supernatant fluids by the ^{86}Rb uptake method (4). After the ^{86}Rb has been taken up and free label has been washed away, the intracellular label is released by lysis with 0.02% saponin and then counted.

The use of metabolic inhibitors in tissue culture interferes with the biosynthetic mechanisms of target cells. The advantages of using, for example, mitomycin C and actinomycin D, is that target cells show an increased susceptibility to LT destruction and a decrease in the time required for observing cytolysis.

REAGENTS

Preparation in the laboratory

Lymphocyte culture medium. For 100 ml of finished medium:

Minimal essential medium	90.0 ml
20,000 of U penicillin/20,000 μg of streptomycin (100×)	1.0 ml
Glutamine, 200 mM (100×)	1.0 ml
Nonessential amino acids (100×) ..	1.0 ml
Sodium pyruvate, 100 mM	1.0 ml
Mercaptoethanol, 5 mM	1.0 ml
Serum ....e........	5.0 ml

Target cell culture medium. For 100 ml of finished medium:

Minimal essential medium	95.0 ml
Glutamine, 200 mM (100×)	1.0 ml
20,000 U of penicillin/20,000 μg of streptomycin (100×)	1.0 ml
Serum	3.0 ml

Phosphate-buffered saline. For 1 liter of solution:

NaCl	8.18 g
$NaH_2PO_4 \cdot 12H_2O$	3.58 g
Distilled water	981 ml
pH to 6.9 with 5 M NaOH	

Trypsin solution, 0.05%. For 100 ml of finished solution:

Trypsin (1:250)	50 mg
Ethylenediaminetetracetic acid ...	29 mg
PBS	100 ml

Ficoll-Hypaque. Combine 47.6 g of Ficoll and 625 ml of distilled water. Stir until dissolved. Add 100 ml of Hypaque. Check density (1.077 g/cc).

Commercial sources

Suppliers' names are abbreviated as follows: Bellco—Bellco Glass, Inc., Vineland, N.J.; Corning—Corning Glass Works, Corning, N.Y.; GIBCO—Grand Island Biological Co., Grand Island, N.Y.; MBA—Microbiological Associates, Inc., Bethesda, Md.; Schwartz-Mann—Schwartz-Mann Co., Orangeburg, N.Y.; Scientific Products—Scientific Products, Irvine, Calif.; Sigma—Sigma Chemical Co., St. Louis, Mo.; Wellcome—Wellcome Reagents Order Department, Burroughs-Wellcome Co., Greenville, N.C.; Winthrop—Winthrop Laboratories, Menlo Park, Calif.

Catalog numbers are given in parentheses after the suppliers' names.

Reagents.

Minimal essential medium: GIBCO (157), MBA (12-127)

Glutamine: GIBCO (M12-20403), MBA (17-605F)

Penicillin/streptomycin: GIBCO (507), MBA (17-603F)

Newborn calf serum: GIBCO (601), MBA (14-416)

Fetal calf serum: GIBCO (629), MBA (14-414)

Nonessential amino acids: GIBCO (114), MBA (13-114)

Sodium pyruvate: GIBCO (136), MBA (13-115)

Trypsin (1:250): GIBCO (505), MBA (17-162)

2-Mercaptoethanol: Schwartz-Mann (901542)

Phytohemagglutinin
  PHA-P: Wellcome (MR68)
  PHA-W: Wellcome (MR10)

Concanavalin A, grade IV: Sigma (C2010)

Ficoll: Sigma (F-4375)

Hypaque M-75: Winthrop (H351)

Equipment.

Tissue culture plastic ware
  Large culture flask (75 cm²): Corning (25110)
  Small culture flask (25 cm²): Corning (25100)
  Assay culture tubes (16 × 125 mm): Corning (25200)

Tissue culture glassware
  Large culture flask (60 cm²): Bellco (1932-18060)
  Small culture flask (30 cm²): Bellco (1932-18030)
  Tube rack: Bellco (1917-00016)
  Assay tubes (16 × 125 mm): Scientific (T 1350-4)

Special materials. Mouse L-929 fibroblast (alpha strain) and lymphotoxin standards are available from G. A. Granger, Department of Molecular Biology and Biochemistry, University of California, Irvine.

LITERATURE CITED

1. Daynes, R. A., and G. A. Granger. 1974. The regulation of lymphotoxin release from stimulated human lymphocyte cultures: the requirement for continual mitogen stimulation. Cell. Immunol. **12**:252–262.

2. Eife, R. F., and C. S. August. 1973. Detection of lymphotoxin produced in mixed lymphocyte cultures (MLC): variation in target cell sensitivity. Cell. Immunol. **9**:163–168.

3. Eife, R. F., G. Eife, C. S. August, W. L. Kuhre, and K. Staehr-Johansen. 1974. LT production in blast cell transformation by cord blood lymphocytes—dissociated function in newborn infants. Cell. Immunol. **14**:435–442.

4. Eifel, P. J., S. M. Walker, and Z. J. Lucas. 1975. Standardization of a sensitive and rapid assay for lymphotoxin. Cell. Immunol. **15**:208–221.

5. Gottoff, S. P., S. Lolekha, and S. Dray. 1971. The in vitro macrophage aggregation, p. 327–331. In B. R. Bloom and P. R. Glade (ed.), In vitro methods in cell-mediated immunity. Academic Press Inc., New York.

6. Granger, G. A. 1972. Lymphokines—the media-

tors of cellular immunity. Ser. Haematol. **4:**8–40.

7. Granger, G. A., and W. P. Kolb. 1968. Lymphocyte in vitro cytotoxicity: mechanisms of immune and non-immune small lymphocyte mediated target L-cell destruction. J. Immunol. **101:**111–120.

8. Granger, G. A., E. C. Laserna, W. P. Kolb, and F. Chapman. 1973. Human lymphotoxin purification and some properties. Proc. Natl. Acad. Sci. U.S.A. **70:**27–30.

9. Granger, G. A., and T. C. Moore. 1974. Accumulation of lymphotoxin secreting lymphoid cells in rat heart allografts. Surgery **76:**542–545.

10. Green, J. A., S. R. Cooperband, J. H. Rutstein, and S. Kilbrick. 1970. Inhibition of target cell proliferation by supernatants from cultures of human peripheral lymphocytes. J. Immunol. **105:**48.

11. Hellstrom, K. E., and I. Hellstrom. 1969. Cellular immunity against tumor antigens. Adv. Cancer Res. **12:**167–223.

12. Henney, C. S. 1971. Quantitation of the cell-mediated immune response. I. The number of cytolytically active mouse lymphoid cells induced by immunization with allogeneic mastocytoma cells. J. Immunol. **107:**1558–1566.

13. Henney, C. S. 1973. On the mechanism of T-cell mediated cytolysis. Transplant. Rev. **17:**36–71.

14. Hessinger, D. A., R. A. Daynes, and G. A. Granger. 1973. The binding of human lymphotoxin to target cell membranes and its relationship to cell-mediated cytodestruction. Proc. Natl. Acad. Sci. U.S.A. **11:**3082–3086.

15. Holm, G. 1969. Cytotoxic effects of lymphoid cells in vitro. Adv. Immunol. **11:**117–193.

16. Holzman, R. S., A. S. Lebowitz, F. T. Valentine, and H. S. Lawerence. 1973. Preparation and properties of cloning inhibitory factor. I. Inhibition of HeLa cell cloning by stimulated lymphocytes and their culture supernatants. Cell. Immunol. **8:**249–258.

17. Jeffes, E. W. B., III, and G. A. Granger. 1975. Relationship of cloning inhibition factor, lymphotoxin factor and proliferation inhibition factor release in vitro by mitogen activated human lymphocytes. J. Immunol. **114:**64–69.

18. Knudsen, R. C., A. A. Ahmed, and K. W. Sells. 1974. An in vitro microassay for lymphotoxin using microculture plates and the multiple automated sample harvester. J. Immunol. Methods **5:**55–63.

19. Kramer, J. J., and G. A. Granger. 1972. An improved in vitro assay for lymphotoxin. Cell.

Immunol. **3:**144–149.

20. Kramer, J. J., and G. A. Granger. 1975. Relationship of lymphotoxin secretion and DNA synthesis in the human mixed lymphocyte reaction in vitro. Cell. Immunol. **17:**192–201.

21. Kramer, S. L., and G. A. Granger. 1975. The role of lymphotoxin in target cell destruction by mitogen-activated human lymphocytes. I. Correlation of target cell sensitivity to lymphotoxin and the intact lymphocyte. Cell. Immunol. **15:**57–68.

22. Lawrence, H. S., and M. Landy (ed.). 1969. Mediators of cellular immunity. Academic Press Inc., New York.

23. Lies, R. B., and J. B. Peter. 1973. Cyclic AMP inhibition of cytotoxin ("lymphotoxin") elaboration by stimulated lymphocytes. Cell. Immunol. **8:**332–335.

24. Ling, N. R. 1968. Lymphocyte stimulation. John Wiley & Sons, Inc., New York.

25. Oppenheim, J. J., R. M. Blaese, J. E. Horton, D. E. Thor, and G. A. Granger. 1973. Production of macrophage migration, inhibition factor and LT by leukocyte from normal and Wiskott-Aldrich syndrome patients. Cell. Immunol. **8:**62–70.

26. Peter, J. B. 1971. Cytotoxin(s) produced by human lymphocytes: inhibition by anti-inflammatory steroids and anti-malarial drugs. Cell. Immunol. **2:**199–202.

27. Peter, J. B., J. A. Stratton, K. E. Stempel, D. Yu, and C. Cardin. 1973. Characteristics of a cytotoxin ("lymphotoxin") produced by stimulation of human lymphoid tissue. J. Immunol. **111:**770–782.

28. Ruddle, N. H. 1972. Approaches to the quantitative analysis of delayed hypersensitivity. Curr. Top. Microbiol. Immunol. **57:**75–110.

29. Spofford, B. T., R. A. Daynes, and G. A. Granger. 1974. Cell-mediated immunity in vitro: a highly sensitive assay for human lymphotoxin. J. Immunol. **112:**2111–2116.

30. Walker, S., and Z. Lucas. 1972. Cytotoxic activity of lymphocytes: assay for cytotoxicity by ribidium exchange of isotopic equilibrium. J. Immunol. **109:**1223–1232.

31. Walker, S. M., and Z. J. Lucas. 1972. Cytotoxic activity of lymphocytes: studies on mechanisms of lymphotoxin-mediated cytotoxicity. J. Immunol. **109:**1233–1244.

32. Williams, T. W., and G. A. Granger. 1973. Lymphocyte in vitro cytotoxicity: mechanism of human lymphotoxin-induced target cell destruction. Cell. Immunol. **6:**171–185.

Chapter 14

Assay of Human Immune Interferon from Lymphocyte-Macrophage Cultures by a Virus Plaque Reduction Method

LOIS B. EPSTEIN

INTRODUCTION

The interferons are antiviral glycoproteins, active against a wide range of viruses and produced by animal cells in response to viruses as well as to other stimuli. Many live and inactivated viruses and viral antigens have been shown to stimulate interferon production, as have polynucleotides, synthetic polymers, bacterial products and antigens, and plant-derived mitogens. Interferons are considered to be generally species or order specific, as, with a few exceptions, they afford the best protection to animal cells of the homologous species, or order. Interferons are produced in vivo and in vitro by many and diverse types of cells (11, 12). Interferons do not have a direct effect on viruses. Rather, they act by conferring on cells resistance to virus infection.

Various methods for the assay of interferons have been developed, and several authors have described and evaluated them in detail (1, 10, 12, 13, 22, 23). Grossberg et al. (13) summarized the methods employed as (i) reduction in the number or size of viral plaques; (ii) reduction in yield of virions, viral ribonucleic acid, viral hemagglutinin, or viral associated enzyme; (iii) inhibition of generalized viral cytopathic effects in a monolayer culture of cells determined visually or by the incorporation of a vital dye; (iv) reduction in quantitative hemadsorption; and (v) maintenance of cellular metabolic activity unimpaired by viral growth, especially as indicated by pH change.

The method chosen for use in my laboratory is a virus plaque reduction method, modified from that originally described by Merigan et al. (18, 19). This type of method was chosen because it was the one most frequently employed by research scientists in the field of interferon (13) and because the results are easy to quantitate. The assay is based on the ability of interferon-containing fluids to confer protection against viral plaque formation in confluent monolayers of fibroblasts. Because of the general species-specific nature of human interferon, fibroblasts of human origin, obtained from neonatal foreskins, are used as the indicator cells. Foreskins were chosen as the source of fibroblasts because they are readily available from newborn nurseries and the fibroblasts prepared from them are very sensitive to the effects of interferon. Bovine vesicular stomatitis virus is used as the challenge virus, as it produces distinct plaques in the foreskin fibroblast monolayers and it is very sensitive to the effects of interferon. The number of manipulations in the assay is kept to a minimum as the assay is run from start to finish in the same group of petri dishes. Another good feature of the assay is that the viability of the indicator cells at the termination of the assay can be assessed readily by their uptake of a supervital stain. In this way nonspecific cellular-destructive effects of the complex fluids which contain interferons can be ruled out.

The term "interferons" has been used in the plural because there is evidence that there may be more than one substance which fits the criteria for acceptance of a viral inhibitor as an interferon (17). The principal evidence for this is twofold. Some of the physical properties of the interferons (i.e., stability to heat and low pH) vary depending on the nature of the inducer and the cell of origin (21). In addition, antigenically distinct species of human interferon have been shown to exist (14).

Recently, two broad categories of human interferon have been designated on the basis of physical properties and type of stimulus (21). One, designated as type I or "classical interferon," is produced in vitro by buffy coat leukocytes or by nonlymphoid cells in response to viruses and is stable to low pH (pH 2) and heat (1 h at 56 C). The other, designated as type II or "immune interferon," is produced in vitro by lymphocytes as a mediator of cellular immunity in response to mitogens or specific antigens and is acid and heat labile. The remainder of this chapter will be concerned only with immune interferon, although the same techniques could be applied for the assay of classical interferon as well.

It should be noted at the outset, however, that the assay of interferon is not as yet a routine clinical laboratory test. The assay can be performed only in a laboratory that has tissue culture facilities and personnel trained in sterile and tissue culture techniques and in the handling and propagation of viruses. Both the clinician and the clinical immunologist should be aware, however, that such a research tool as the assay of interferon is available in specialized laboratories and that new and important information about the immunological status of patients with a wide variety of disease states can be obtained by its use, as well as basic information concerning the role of interferon in the immune response.

CLINICAL INDICATIONS

The three types of situations for which my laboratory uses this test and the rationale for doing so are as follows:

1. *To study the in vitro production of immune interferon by highly purified populations of human T or B lymphocytes as a measure of the effector competence of these cells.* The test is performed on normal donors or patients in which it is desired to evaluate or follow the effect of a given disease state, course of the disease, or therapy on this parameter of the cellular immune response. Both human T and B lymphocytes can produce interferon in vitro in response to the mitogens phytohemagglutinin (PHA-P) and pokeweed (PWM; 8). However, T cell interferon is detectable earlier, after 3 days of culture, whereas B cell production of interferon is delayed 5 to 7 days. Thus, the measurement of interferon after 3 days of in vitro mitogenic stimulation of lymphocytes has become a new tool with which T lymphocyte effector competence can be assessed. Similarly, B cell effector function can be evaluated by using 5- to 7-day cultures of purified B cells. To date, studies indicate that certain patients with selective immunoglobulin A (IgA) deficiency have a defect in the ability of their T lymphocytes to produce interferon in vitro (3), and patients with chronic lymphocytic leukemia (CLL) have a defect in both T and B cell interferon production (5).

2. *To study the ability of human macrophages from normal donors or patients to augment in vitro lymphocyte interferon production as a measure of the functional integrity of the macrophages.* Macrophages present in vitro in mitogen-stimulated cultures augment lymphocyte production of interferon (2, 6) and many other mediators of cellular immunity (2). It is thus possible to test the efficacy of macrophages in autochthonous macrophage-lymphocyte cultures from either normal subjects or patients or in allogeneic cultures in which normal macrophages are combined with a patient's lymphocytes or a patient's macrophages are combined with normal lymphocytes. For example, the defect in T lymphocyte interferon production exhibited by the cells from patients with CLL is not corrected by normal macrophages (5), but the macrophages from these patients are competent in augmenting interferon production by normal lymphocytes.

3. *To study the interaction of lymphocytes and macrophages from normal donors or patients and the in vitro effect of drugs on this interaction and on interferon production.* Several agents which increase intracellular cyclic adenosine monophosphate content or mimic the action of the endogenous nucleotide inhibit the production of interferon by human lymphocytes (4). One of these agents, cholera toxin, prevents PHA-induced interferon production by an action on the ability of lymphocytes to produce the interferon, rather than on the ability of macrophages to augment production by the lymphocytes. Thus, this system could be used to test established drugs or screen new ones for their effects on this in vitro model of the cellular immune response.

In our in vitro system in which the competence of lymphocytes and/or macrophages is evaluated by their ability, respectively, to produce or augment interferon, mitogens are usually used to induce the interferon. Various antigens could be used as well, however, as previously sensitized human lymphocytes will produce, and macrophages will augment, interferon produced in response to bacterial (7) and viral antigens (9, 20). It should be noted, however, that, whereas mitogen-stimulated T lymphocyte interferon levels peak after 3 days in culture, bacterial or viral antigen-stimulated interferon levels peak after 7 to 8 days.

In the system to be described, combined macrophage-lymphocyte cultures are prepared and are stimulated with mitogen or antigen, the cell pellet is studied for the incorporation of ³H-thymidine into deoxyribonucleic acid (DNA), and the supernatant fluids are assayed for interferon. Thus, the system allows for the monitoring of the proliferative capability of the mitogen- or antigen-stimulated lymphocytes as well as the mediator response. Our system requires two donations of blood 1 week apart, the first for the preparation of macrophage cultures and the second for the isolation of lymphocytes by their passage through a nylon fiber column. Despite the disadvantage of the double donation requirement, we prefer the use of lymphocyte-macrophage cultures to lymphocyte-monocyte cultures which can be prepared from Ficoll gradient-isolated cells from a single donation of blood for the following reasons:

1. The nylon fiber column-separated human T cell preparations used in the lymphocyte-macrophage system are more pure than lymphocyte preparations obtained from Ficoll gradients. The proportion of B cells in the former as determined by fluorescence microscopy (8) is 6.5% (range, 4 to 9.5%) and, in the latter, after absorption of monocytes, 18.0% (range, 15 to 21%).

2. Monocytes appear to elaborate an antagonist to interferon, which inhibits the antiviral expression of the mediator in low dilutions of the culture supernatant fluids. Well-differentiated macrophages do not elaborate this antagonist (2).

3. Interferon is never observed in control lymphocyte-macrophage cultures from which mitogen or antigen has been omitted, whereas it is often found in unstimulated lymphocyte-monocyte cultures if sufficient dilutions of the culture supernatant fluids are made.

4. If a viral antigen preparation is used as the interferon-inducing agent, the lymphocyte-macrophage culture system reflects the prior immunological history of the donor, whereas the lymphocyte-monocyte culture system does not (15). Varicella-zoster antigen-stimulated interferon production by lymphocytes in lymphocyte-monocyte cultures occurred whether or not the donor had had previous exposure to the virus, whereas with the lymphocyte-macrophage system interferon was produced only on an immune specific basis.

TEST PROCEDURES

There are two aspects to this test. The first is the macrophage-lymphocyte tissue culture system used to generate the immune interferon, and the second is the assay of immune interferon itself. Because there are numerous descriptions of the macrophage-lymphocyte tissue culture system in the literature (2, 5, 6), it will be described only briefly below, whereas the interferon assay will be described in much greater detail.

Macrophage-lymphocyte tissue culture system

Preparation of macrophage monolayers (5, 6). Using sterile technique throughout, withdraw venous blood into one or more 50-ml plastic syringes which contain 750 units of aqueous, preservative-free sodium heparin. The blood of a normal donor is always run in parallel whenever a patient's blood is being studied. Separate leukocyte-rich plasma by gravity sedimentation at 37 C in sterile siliconized or plastic tubes

for 1.5 to 2 h. Wash cells twice with an equal volume of McCoy's medium and resuspend them in McCoy's medium supplemented with 30% pooled human AB sera (McCoy's-30 AB). Count the cells and prepare a Giemsa-stained cytocentrifuge smear (Shandon-Elliott Cytocentrifuge, London, England) for a differential count. Adjust the cell concentration to 1.5×10^6 monocytes per ml, and add 0.75 ml of the cell suspension to Leighton tubes (16×85 mm) which contain glass cover slips. Permit the cells to adhere for 2 h at 37 C and decant the nonadherent cells; wash the adherent cells gently three times with 1 ml of warm McCoy's medium, and reincubate them with 1 ml of McCoy's-30 AB. Repeat the washing procedure at midweek. After 1 week, the macrophage cultures contain 2×10^4 to 5×10^4 macrophages, are 99 to 100% pure, and are ready for combination with lymphocytes. From 100 ml of blood, 15 to 20 macrophage cultures can be obtained.

Preparation of purified lymphocytes (5). Using sterile technique throughout, obtain a second sample of blood (50 to 100 ml) 1 week after the initial donation of blood. Using nonsiliconized glassware, isolate leukocyte-rich plasma as described above, wash once with McCoy's medium, and resuspend in 40 ml of McCoy's-30 AB with 0.2 ml of aqueous sodium heparin. Apply the cell suspension via a separatory funnel at a flow rate of 10 to 15 drops per min to a 37 C water-jacketed glass column which has been packed to a length of 12.7 cm with 1.75 g of nylon fiber (Fenwal Co., Morton Grove, Ill.) and prewashed with 30 ml of McCoy's-30 AB. After the cell suspension has been applied to the column, add 40 ml of McCoy's-30 AB via a second separatory funnel to elute additional lymphocytes. Count and do a differential count on the cell effluent, and adjust the lymphocyte concentration to 10^6 per ml in fresh McCoy's-30 AB. Such eluates are usually 99% pure lymphocytes, of which > 93% are T cells. From 100 ml of blood, 50×10^6 to 100×10^6 lymphocytes are obtained in this manner. Lyse erythrocytes accompanying the T lymphocytes by exposure to NH_4Cl (9).

With the exception of one set of studies, my laboratory has concentrated on aspects of interferon production by T lymphocytes. The one exception (8) was at a time when we had access to a fluorescence-activated cell sorter (FACS) which provides highly enriched populations of B cells as well as highly purified T cells. Because of the scarcity of the FACS machines as well as the expense, the reader is referred to chapter 8 in this *Manual* for details on other techniques for isolating purified preparations of human B lymphocytes.

Preparation of combined macrophage-lymphocyte cultures (3, 5, 8).

Decant the medium from Leighton tube cultures of macrophages and replace it with 1 ml of the lymphocyte suspension. Prepare control cultures of macrophages alone with fresh McCoy's-30 AB and cultures of lymphocytes alone in Leighton tubes. Add mitogens or antigens over a wide dose range at the initiation of culture, and maintain cultures at 37 C in a CO_2 incubator. The dose schedule we employ is as follows: PHA-P (Difco), 8, 17, 33, or 50 $\mu g/ml$ (3, 5, 8); PWM (Grand Island Biological Co., Santa Clara, Calif.), 24, 45, or 84 $\mu g/ml$ (3, 5, 8); PPD, 2nd strength, 3.3 $\mu g/ml$ (7); and vaccinia antigen, 2×10^4 to 4×10^4 plaque-forming units (PFU)/ml (9).

Harvesting the cultures (9).

To allow for detection of maximal proliferative response as well as maximal interferon response, harvest cultures which contain T lymphocytes, macrophages, and mitogen at 3 days and those which contain antigen at 5 to 10 days. Harvest cultures which contain B lymphocytes, macrophages, and mitogen at 5 to 10 days as well. The time course relationship for antigenic stimulation of B cell interferon is not yet known. To harvest the cultures, add 1 μCi of [^3H]thymidine (specific activity, 2.1 Ci/mmol; New England Nuclear Corp., Boston, Mass.) 1 h prior to termination of the cultures. Incubate at 37 C. Using sterile technique, collect the culture supernatant fluids after their passage through a multiport filtration apparatus (Hoefer Scientific Instruments, San Francisco, Calif.) and refrigerate at 4 C for subsequent interferon assay. To determine the amount of incorporation of [^3H]thymidine into DNA, collect the cell pellets on glass filter-paper circles and wash twice with cold phosphate-buffered saline (pH 7.4), cold 5% trichloroacetic acid, and cold absolute methanol. Transfer the circles to counting vials containing 1 ml of Nuclear-Chicago Solubilizer; after 1 h add 10 ml of toluene base 2,5-diphenyloxazole-1,4-bis-(5-phenyloxazolyl)benzene scintillation fluid and count.

Interferon assay

Preparation of human foreskin fibroblast monolayer stocks.

Distribute to newborn nurseries sterile glass vials containing 5 ml of minimal essential medium (MEM) supplemented with 10% fetal calf serum (FCS), 100 units of penicillin/ml, 100 μg of streptomycin/ml, and 100 μg of mystatin/ml (MEM-FCS-PSM) for use by the obstetrical and nursing staff to collect foreskin samples obtained at circumcision. Keep foreskin samples at 5 C prior to use as the source of fibroblast monolayers. Also, prior to use check sterility of each foreskin sample by culturing a few drops of the media from each vial in thioglycolate broth at 37 C for 24 to 48 h. Discard any contaminated vials. Using sterile technique throughout, combine 10 to 15 foreskins, mince with scissors, and wash three times with Dulbecco's phosphate-buffered saline deficient in Ca and Mg ions (PDS) to remove serum and blood. Transfer the tissue chunks to a 500-ml trypsinization flask which contains a magnet and is mounted on a magnetic stirrer. Trypsinize the samples with 50 ml of 0.25% trypsin solution at 37 C for 20 min, and decant the cell suspension to 40-ml centrifuge tubes kept on ice which contain 2 ml of FCS. Repeat the trypsinization procedure on the original tissue samples with fresh 0.25% trypsin three additional times. Centrifuge the pooled cell suspensions at 1,000 rpm for 10 min, decant the supernatant fluid, and resuspend the cell pellet in MEM-FCS-PSM. To make the primary monolayer, add 10^7 cells in 15 ml of MEM-FCS-PSM to a 100×20 mm plastic culture dish and maintain at 37 C in a CO_2 incubator. Replace with fresh MEM-FCS-PSM every 5 days, and periodically monitor the monolayer with an inverted microscope until confluence is observed, after about 10 to 14 days.

To pass the primary monolayer to a 32-oz prescription bottle (Owens Glass Co., Toledo, Ohio), decant the media from the monolayer, add 10 ml of 0.25% trypsin solution in PDS at 37 C, and incubate at 37 C for 15 min. Transfer the cell suspension to centrifuge tubes which contain 2 ml of FCS, centrifuge at 1,000 rpm for 10 min, aspirate the supernatant fluid, resuspend the cells in MEM-FCS-PSM, count the cells, adjust the cell concentration, and transfer 2×10^6 cells in 50 ml to a 32-oz prescription bottle. Periodically monitor the monolayer with an inverted microscope. Once confluence occurs (after about 1 week), the cells from the one 32-oz bottle can be trypsinized in the same fashion and used to seed six other 32-oz prescription bottles, each with 2×10^6 cells in 50 ml of MEM-FCS-PSM.

Thus, this procedure involves the preparation of a primary fibroblast monolayer, its passage to a 32-oz prescription bottle, and its passage at confluence to six other bottles. Once the monolayers in the six prescription bottles are confluent, they can be trypsinized and used for one of three purposes: (i) to seed the 60×15 mm plastic culture dishes used for the interferon assay, (ii) for continued propagation of the foreskin line either by direct passage or by freezing down cells for future use, for future assays, or (iii) for the preparation of an internal laboratory interferon standard. Allow at least 4 to 5 weeks from the time that foreskin samples are received to the time that sufficient fibroblast stocks are available to start an assay. Also, once the stocks are sufficient, the line is passed only 10 additional times over a 10-week period, as these lines occasionally lose their sensitivity to virus or interferon. Consequently, after the 5th or 6th passage of one line, we routinely start a primary monolayer on another, and we always have additional stocks of fibroblasts at low passage number frozen in liquid nitrogen for emergency use.

Preparation of NDV-induced foreskin fibroblast interferon as an internal laboratory interferon standard. Decant the media from one 32-oz prescription bottle containing a confluent foreskin fibroblast monolayer. Wash with 20 ml of serum-free MEM, decant, and add 5 ml of MEM which contains 10^7 to 5×10^7 PFU of Newcastle disease virus (NDV; Herts, California, or Victoria strain); incubate at 37 C for 1 h to allow for virus attachment. Add 15 ml of MEM-PSM and maintain the culture at 37 C in a CO_2 incubator for 48 h. Decant the interferon-containing supernatant media, and acidify with 4 N HCl at 4 C for 5 days to destroy residual virus. Neutralize to pH 7.0 with 4 N NaOH, and freeze at -70 C in small portions. Use this interferon sample as an internal laboratory standard with every assay as a measure of the relative sensitivity to interferon of the fibroblasts being used. If the internal laboratory standard is calibrated against the international interferon standard (available from the Reference Reagents Branch, National Institute of Allergy and Infectious Diseases, Bethesda, Md.), it will be possible to compare directly the results obtained in one laboratory with those obtained in others.

Propagation of VSV for use as the challenge virus in the interferon assay. Prepare in 32-oz prescription bottles confluent monolayers of chick embryo fibroblasts by standard procedures (16) in medium 199 supplemented with 5% FCS (199-FCS). $TCID_{50}$ is defined as the highest dilution of virus-containing solution that will produce infection in 50% of susceptible cultures. Decant media from each bottle and add 10^4 $TCID_{50}$ of bovine vesicular stomatitis virus (VSV), Indiana strain, to each bottle in 5 ml of 199-FCS for 30 min at room temperature to allow for virus adsorption. Add an additional 15 ml of 199-FCS, and incubate at 37 C for 24 h or until cytopathic effect is noted in more than 75% of each culture. Collect the supernatant fluids and spin in a Sorvall centrifuge at 10,000 $\times$ g for 10 min at 4 C to sediment coarse cellular debris. Remove and pool supernatant fluids,

and freeze at -70 C in small portions. To determine which dilution of VSV will be suitable for use in the interferon assay, run dilutions of virus in MEM from 10^{-1} to 10^{-8} on confluent monolayers of foreskin fibroblasts in 60×15 mm plastic culture dishes, just as the virus challenge is performed in the interferon assay described below. That dilution of VSV which, in a 0.5-ml volume, results in 60 to 100 viral plaques per 60×15 mm culture dish will be used as the virus dilution for subsequent interferon assays on a given fibroblast line. Each time a new fibroblast line is established, i.e., about every 10 weeks (assuming that an interferon assay is run every week), a virus titration must be run, to establish the sensitivity of a given line to the virus.

The interferon assay itself—exposure of monolayers to interferon-containing fluids. Once fibroblast and viral stocks and internal laboratory interferon standard are prepared, the interferon assay can proceed. Using the trypsinization procedure described above for 32-oz prescription bottles, remove the confluent foreskin fibroblast monolayers from six prescription bottles, wash cells, resuspend in fresh MEM-FCS-PSM, and seed the desired number of 60×15 mm plastic culture dishes with 2×10^5 fibroblasts in 5 ml of media for use in the interferon assay. In addition, seed six 32-oz prescription bottles with 2×10^6 cells in 20 ml for use in an assay the following week.

It is feasible for one individual to run 120 plates per week (40 culture dishes on each of three trays) for an interferon assay. This allows for the proper virus controls, determination of interferon titer of from 20 to 30 samples (depending on whether three or four dilutions are made), and determination of the internal interferon standard. We routinely run two assays per week, each by a separate individual, and hence the monolayers from six 32-oz prescription bottles are sufficient to seed 240 60×15 mm plates and six fresh 32-oz bottles. The seeding is usually performed on Wednesday of each week, as, at the concentrations indicated, the 60×15 mm plates will become confluent by the following Monday or Tuesday, and the bottles will become confluent within 1 week, by the following Wednesday. If it is desired to use the plates or bottles at a somewhat later date, they can be "held" at or near confluence by reducing the FCS in the media from 10% to 2%.

With sterile technique used throughout, samples to be tested for interferon are diluted in serial half log dilutions of MEM-PSM. For example, to make 1:3, 1:10, and 1:30 dilutions, add 1.82 ml of the solution to be tested to 4 ml of MEM-PSM; then add 1.82 ml of the 1:3 to 4 ml of

MEM-PSM to make the 1:10 dilution; and then add 1.82 ml of the 1:10 to 4 ml of MEM-PSM to make a 1:30 dilution. Remove 1.82 ml from the 1:30 dilution, and each dilution will have a 4-ml volume to be applied to the confluent monolayers of fibroblasts. Vortex each tube after a given dilution is made. For dilutions of 1:10, 1:30, and 1:100, start with 0.58 ml of sample and 5.25 ml of MEM-PSM; remove 1.82 ml of the 1:10 and add to 4 ml of MEM-PSM to make the 1:30, etc. For 1:30, 1:100, and 1:300 dilutions, start with 0.19 ml of sample and 5.63 ml of MEM-PSM; remove 1.82 ml of the 1:30 and add to 4 ml of MEM-PSM to make the 1:100, etc. For 1:100, 1;300, and 1:1,000 dilutions start with 0.06 ml of sample and 5.75 ml of MEM-PSM; remove 1.82 ml of the 1:100 and add to 4 ml of MEM-PSM to make the 1:300, etc. Always remove 1.82 ml from the final dilution so that the volume of samples applied to the monolayers is always 4 ml.

Check that all the monolayers in the 60 × 15 mm culture dishes are confluent prior to use in the assay. Label each plate with the number of sample and dilution of sample to be employed. On every tray of 40 plates, allow 3 plates for virus controls, with no interferon sample. For every 120 plates, allow 3 to 4 plates for dilutions of the internal laboratory interferon standard and 3 to 4 plates if the international interferon standard is run. Decant MEM-FCS-PSM from confluent monolayers, and replace with 4 ml of serial half log dilutions of the interferon samples to be assayed for antiviral activity, i.e., lymphocyte-macrophage culture supernatant fluids. Use 4 ml of MEM-PSM for virus control monolayers. Maintain culture dishes at 37 C in a 5% CO_2 atmosphere for 18 to 24 h. This interferon assay can also be used to detect interferon in human serum or other body fluids, such as the fluid contained in virus-caused vesicles.

The interferon assay itself — virus challenge. Remove the serial dilutions of samples to be tested from the monolayers and wash all plates gently with 4 ml of MEM-PSM. Return plates to the incubator while making virus dilutions. Make serial log dilutions of VSV virus stock on ice with cold MEM-PSM to achieve that dilution of VSV in 0.5 ml which had been determined on previous titration to give 60 to 100 plaques per 60 × 15 mm culture dish. Be certain that virus dilutions are kept at 5 C and that they are thoroughly mixed. Gently aspirate the MEM-PSM from the plates, add 0.5 ml of VSV to each with an automatic syringe, and incubate them at 37 C for 45 min in a 5% CO_2 environment to allow for adsorption of virus. During this period of time, prepare the solution to be used as an agar overlay by combining 250

ml of 2 × agar, 1.9% (Difco) which had been previously autoclaved and then maintained at 45 C, and 250 ml of 2 × MEM-FCS-PSM also maintained at 45 C. Gently aspirate excess virus off plates with a Pasteur pipette and discard virus solution in Wescodyne (West Chemical Products, New York, N.Y.). With a 5-ml automatic syringe, add 4 ml of agar overlay, aiming the stream of warm agar toward the side of the culture dish, so as not to disturb the monolayer, and let the agar solidify for 10 to 15 min. Return to a CO_2 incubator at 37 C for 48 h.

The interferon assay itself — neutral red staining of plates. Using an automatic syringe, stain plates with 2 ml of 0.025% neutral red solution in phosphate-buffered saline for 2 h at 37 C. Aspirate off stain and incubate for an additional 2.5 to 3 h; then count virus plaques, which will appear as clear areas on each plate. Thus, a typical weekly time schedule would be as follows: expose monolayers to supernatant fluids on Monday, do virus challenge on Tuesday, stain and read on Thursday, and pass cells for next assay on Wednesday.

Characterization of an antiviral substance as an interferon. If greater than 50% virus plaque reduction is observed for a given culture situation, then further tests must be performed to determine whether the antiviral effect is caused by an interferon. To qualify as an interferon, the antiviral effect must be destroyed by the action of trypsin (thus indicating it is a protein). Also, unlike a virus, it should be nonsedimentable when exposed to 100,000 × g for 2 h in an ultracentrifuge, it should have a broad antiviral spectrum, and it should exert general species specificity. Its response to low pH and heat should be well documented so that it can be classified as a particular type of interferon, i.e., immune or classical. The techniques for characterization of an antiviral substance as an interferon have been recently reiterated in detail (21).

REAGENTS

All media used for the preparation of lymphocyte-macrophage cultures or for the interferon assay may be obtained from Grand Island Biological Co., Santa Clara, Calif. MEM (Earle's base) is purchased as 10 × and diluted out with sterile distilled water. To each 100 ml of 1 × MEM is added 3 ml of 7.5% $NaHCO_3$, 10,000 units of penicillin, 10,000 μg of streptomycin, and 10,000 units of mystatin.

To prepare 250 ml of 2 × MEM for use in agar overlay after virus challenge in the interferon assay, combine 50 ml of 10 × MEM, 5 ml of penicillin and streptomycin solution, 5 ml of mystatin, 15 ml of $NaHCO_3$, and 50 ml of FCS, and make up to 250 ml with distilled water. Combine this with 250 ml of 1.9% agar solution.

Trypsin is obtained from Nutritional Biochemicals Corp., Cleveland, Ohio.

Neutral red is obtained from the same company. Add 1 g of neutral red and 9 g of NaCl to 1 liter of distilled water. Autoclave for 20 min. Store at 5 C. At the time of use, use 1 part of this stock solution with 3 parts of sterile phosphate-buffered saline. For 120 plates use 65 ml of neutral red stock and 195 ml of phosphate-buffered saline.

All other sources for reagents have been listed in the text.

appear to decline significantly if stored at 5 C for as little as 7 days or up to several months. No significant differences were found between mean titers obtained by two different laboratory personnel assaying the same samples.

The variability inherent in the lymphocyte-macrophage interferon-producing system has also been assessed. When supernatant fluids from several (five to nine) replicate cultures are analyzed at the same time, the interferon titers fall within the range of the mean ±32%. The variability is, of course, the result of the intra-interferon assay variability already mentioned and the actual differences among individual

INTERPRETATION

Calculations

Interferon titer is defined as the dilution of sample which in a 4-ml volume results in 50% reduction in viral plaques. The formula for calculation of the interferon titer is as follows:

Interferon titer

$$= \frac{(\text{1/2 control number} - \text{the plaque number of low neighbor}) \times (\text{difference in the dilution})}{(\text{difference in plaque number})}$$

$$+ \text{ low dilution}$$

A typical calculation is as follows:

Plaque no. at dilution:				Control plates	Mean control	1/2 control
1:30	1:100	1:300	1:1,000	58	58	29
				56		
0	3	30	56	60		

It is apparent that the titer lies somewhere between the 1:100 and 1:300 dilution, and, using the numbers above, the value is computed as 293.

$$\text{Interferon titer} = \frac{(29 - 3) \times (300 - 100)}{(30 - 3)} + 100 = 293$$

Reproducibility of the assay and interferon-producing system

The reproducibility of the interferon assay system discussed above has been analyzed in several ways. When several assays of a single immune interferon preparation are carried out simultaneously using replicate fibroblast plates and the same virus preparation, the interferon titers fall within a range of the mean ±21% (mean ± 2 standard deviations). On the other hand, when a single sample of an interferon standard is assayed repeatedly on different days over a period of 4 months, the values obtained are within the range of the mean ± 49% (2 standard deviations). In addition, titers of interferon in replicate or pooled lymphocyte-macrophage supernatant fluids do not

cultures which occur as they are prepared.

Normal range

The range of interferon titers observed in the supernatant fluid of PHA-stimulated T lymphocyte-macrophage cultures from normal donors is very broad. For example, in a study of 10 normal donors (3), the range of interferon titers was 50 to 212 when the final PHA concentration in culture was 8 μg/ml, 40 to 308 at 17 μg/ml, 69 to 364 at 33 μg/ml, and 49 to 371 at 50 μg/ml. For PWM-stimulated cultures from the same donors, the range of interferon titers was 20 to 221 when the final PWM concentration was 24 μg/ml, 47 to 320 at 45 μg/ml, and 24 to 316 at 84 μg/ml. However, in patients in whom a defect in mitogen-stimulated T lymphocyte interferon was reported, i.e., three with selective IgA deficiency (3) and five with CLL (5), there was no detectable interferon production (titer <10). Thus, to date the defects described in patients have been gross ones.

Perhaps by doing serial studies on patients it will be possible to detect less severe or transient defects in lymphocyte interferon production. The performance of such studies in the future will be facilitated by the use of micromethods for the culture system and for the interferon assay which are currently being developed.

ACKNOWLEDGMENTS

The work described is supported by Public Health Service grants CA 14508 and AI 12481.

I thank Della Goldblatt and Miriam Seelig for technical assistance and Carol Stadum and Dorothy Metcalf for typing the manuscript.

LITERATURE CITED

1. Baron, S. 1969. Interferon: production, assay, and characterization, p. 399–410. In K. Habel and N. P. Salzman (ed.), Fundamental techniques in virology. Academic Press Inc., New York.
2. Epstein, L. B. 1976. The ability of macrophages to augment in vitro mitogen and antigen stimulated production of interferon and other mediators of cellular immunity by lymphocytes, p. 201–234. In D. Nelson (ed.), Immunobiology of the macrophage. Academic Press Inc., New York.
3. Epstein, L. B., and A. J. Ammann. 1974. Evaluation of T lymphocyte effector function in immunodeficiency diseases: abnormality in mitogen stimulated interferon in patients with selective IgA deficiency. J. Immunol. 112:617–626.
4. Epstein, L. B., and H. R. Bourne. 1976. Interferon production by mitogen-stimulated lymphocytes: cyclic AMP mediated inhibition by cholera toxin. In D. L. Rosenstreich and J. J. Oppenheim (ed.), Mitogens in immunobiology. Academic Press Inc., New York.
5. Epstein, L. B., and M. J. Cline. 1974. Chronic lymphocytic leukemia: studies on mitogen stimulated lymphocyte interferon as a new technique for assessing T lymphocyte effector function. Clin. Exp. Immunol. 16:553–563.
6. Epstein, L. B., M. J. Cline, and T. C. Merigan. 1971. The interaction of human macrophages and lymphocytes in the PHA stimulated production of interferon. J. Clin. Invest. 50:744–753.
7. Epstein, L. B., M. J. Cline, and T. C. Merigan. 1971. PPD-stimulated interferon: in vitro macrophage-lymphocyte interaction in the production of a mediator of cellular immunity. Cell. Immunol. 2:602–613.
8. Epstein, L. B., H. W. Kreth, and L. A. Herzenberg. 1974. Fluorescence-activated cell sorting of human T and B lymphocytes. II. Identification of the cell type responsible for interferon production and cell proliferation in response to mitogens. Cell. Immunol. 12:407–421.
9. Epstein, L. B., D. A. Stevens, and T. C. Merigan. 1972. Selective increase in lymphocyte interferon response to vaccinia antigen after revaccination. Proc. Natl. Acad. Sci. U.S.A. 69:2632–2636.
10. Finter, N. B. 1966. Interferon assays and standards, p. 87–118. In N. B. Finter (ed.), Interferons. North Holland Publishing Co., Amsterdam.
11. Finter, N. B. (ed.). 1973. Interferon and interferon inducers, North Holland Research Monographs Frontiers of Biology, vol. 2. American Elsevier Publishing Co., New York.
12. Grossberg, S. E. 1972. The interferons and their inducers: molecular and therapeutic considerations. N. Engl. J. Med. 287:13–19, 79–85, 122–128.
13. Grossberg, S. E., P. Jameson, and J. J. Sedmak. 1974. Interferon bioassay methods and the development of standard procedures: a critique and analysis of current observations, p. 26–34. In C. Waymouth (ed.), The production and use of interferon for the treatment and prevention of human virus infections, Proceedings of a Tissue Culture Association Workshop. Tissue Culture Association, Rockville, Md.
14. Havell, E. A., B. Berman, C. A. Ogburn, K. Berg, K. Paucker, and J. Vilcek. 1975. Two antigenically distinct species of human interferon. Proc. Natl. Acad. Sci. U.S.A. 72:2185–2187.
15. Jordan, G. W., and T. C. Merigan. 1974. Cell-mediated immunity to Varicella-zoster virus: in vitro lymphocyte responses. J. Infect. Dis. 130:495–501.
16. Lennette, E. H., and N. J. Schmidt (ed.). 1969. Diagnostic procedures for viral and rickettsial diseases, p. 113. American Public Health Association, Inc., New York.
17. Lockart, R. Z., Jr. 1973. Criteria for acceptance of a viral inhibitor as an interferon and a general description of the biological properties of known interferons, p. 11–27. In N. B. Finter (ed.), Interferon and interferon inducers, North Holland Research Monographs Frontiers of Biology, vol. 2. American Elsevier Publishing Co., New York.
18. Merigan, T. C. 1971. A plaque inhibition assay for human interferon employing human neonate skin fibroblast monolayers and bovine vesicular stomatitis virus, p. 489–499. In B. R. Bloom and P. R. Glade (ed.), In vitro methods in cell mediated immunity. Academic Press Inc., New York.
19. Merigan, T. C., D. F. Gregory, and J. K. Petralli. 1966. Physical properties of human interferon prepared in vitro and in vivo. Virology 29:515–522.
20. Rasmussen, L. E., G. W. Jordan, D. A. Stevens, and T. C. Merigan. 1974. Lymphocyte interferon production and transformation after

Herpes simplex infections in humans. J. Immunol. 112:728–736.

21. Valle, M. J., G. W. Jordan, S. Haahr, and T. C. Merigan. 1975. Characteristics of immune interferon produced by human lymphocyte cultures compared to other human interferons. J. Immunol. 115:230–233.

22. Vilcek, J. 1969. Interferon. Springer-Verlag, New York.

23. Wagner, R. R., A. H. Levy, and T. J. Smith. 1968. Techniques for the study of interferons in animal virus-cell systems, p. 2–52. *In* K. Maramorosch and H. Koprowski (ed.), Methods in virology, vol. 4. Academic Press Inc., New York.

Chapter 15

Detection and Measurement of Lymphocyte Mitogenic Factor

R. A. WOLSTENCROFT, R. N. MAINI, AND D. C. DUMONDE

INTRODUCTION

The proposition that sensitized lymphocytes generate special mediators of cellular immunity was based upon the discovery of dialyzable leukocyte transfer factor in humans (44) and the demonstration of macrophage migration inhibition factor in guinea pigs (10, 16). A variety of soluble nonantibody materials, with a wide range of biological activities, have now been extracted from the supernatant fluids of lymphoid cells cultured with or without deliberate stimulation, and from lymphoid cell populations themselves, in attempts to delineate the molecular nature of substances which might have such mediator function (17, 46). Included among the biological activities are those which have the property of stimulating fresh lymphocytes (9, 66, 67) and which would therefore appear to amplify and perhaps coordinate the recruitment and activation of lymphocytes in the local environment of a cellular immune response (18). The existence of such physiological mediators would imply that, in clinical circumstances, abnormality in their production or action might represent a significant attribute of a disease entity (20). Accordingly, the purpose of this chapter is threefold: (i) to present a simplified classification of lymphocyte-stimulating "factors" which are being considered in terms of their contribution to cellular immune function in humans; (ii) to describe the production and measurement of one such factor, whose activity we have termed "lymphocyte mitogenic factor" (LMF); and (iii) to consider the potential significance of attempting to measure the activity of LMF in the assessment of immunological disease.

Categories of lymphocyte-stimulating "factors"

Table 1 illustrates how a whole variety of names may be assigned to extracts of leukocytes, lymphoid cells, or lymphoid tissues, or to soluble products of lymphoid cells or leukocytes, which have the common general property of stimulating some aspects of lymphocyte behavior or function in a variety of environmental circumstances. Much of the evidence for the separate identity of these lymphocyte-stimulating factors derives from animal experiments, and, with the notable exception of dialyzable transfer factor, work on the characterization of lymphocyte-stimulating factors of human origin is in its infancy. Table 1 thus throws into perspective our current state of ignorance concerning the classification of human lymphocyte-stimulating "mediators" and emphasizes the need to establish rigorous biological criteria whereby these may be delineated in humans.

Applying the above classification, Table 2 reveals how knowledge is beginning to accumulate concerning the different attributes of lymphocyte function which appear to be modulated by different categories of lymphocyte-stimulating factors. Particular confusion reigns at the present time concerning the use of the terms "mitogenic," "blastogenic," "transforming," "recruiting," "potentiating," "augmenting," "replacing," "reconstituting," "helper," and "enhancing." (The Oxford English Dictionary provides the interested worker with a rich source of material as a basis for semantic arguments, which will not be discussed here.) However, it is likely that, whenever lymphoid cells are activated in vivo or in vitro, a variety of metabolically active substances are generated whose biological effects on other neighboring lymphoid cells will depend upon the existing patterns of cellular activation and cellular traffic in that microenvironment. In biological and clinical terms it will be necessary to define more closely the test systems in vitro which permit the identification of these different activities in order to determine eventually: (i) whether some of them are due to the same molecular entity; (ii) the extent to which they are represented in humans; (iii) whether there is sufficient evidence to implicate some of the "factors" in the normal physiology of the immune system; and (iv) the extent to which abnormalities in their production or action can be faithfully associated with defined disease states in humans.

The "mediator" concept

Critical appraisal that any of the categories of lymphocyte-stimulating factors act as molec-

TABLE 1. *Suggested nomenclature of principal nonantibody lymphocyte-stimulating factors derived by extraction or culture of leukocytes, lymphoid cells, or lymphoid tissue*[a]

Generic term(s) in frequent use	Circumstances in which production usually described	Usual implication of nomenclature
(Mitogenic) lymphokine(s)	(a) Lymphocyte activation in vitro with sufficient soluble antigen, allogeneic cells, or phytomitogen (b) Lymphoblast cell line culture supernatant fluid	Soluble factor increases deoxyribonucleic acid (DNA) synthesis nonspecifically by allogeneic or autologous lymphocytes without supplementation by inducing or unrelated antigen
Lymphocyte-"recruiting" or "transforming" factor(s)	Lymphocyte stimulation with soluble antigen in low concentration or in "pulse" culture or with insolubilized antigen	In the presence of additional specific (inducing) antigen, the soluble factor induces DNA synthesis or blast cell development in otherwise unresponsive cell cultures
"Potentiating" or "augmenting" factors	(a) Antigen- or phytomitogen-stimulated lymphocyte cultures (b) Supernatant fluids of adherent cell cultures (c) Extraction of polymorphs, macrophages, or leukocytes	Soluble factor or extract increases DNA synthesis by lymphocytes responding to the presence of antigen or phytomitogen
T cell-replacing or "helper" factor(s)	(a) Antigen-specific T-lymphocyte stimulation (b) Mitogen-stimulated T-lymphocyte cultures	In the presence of specific antigen, the soluble factor "restores" antibody or immunoglobulin production by T cell-depleted lymphocyte populations in vitro or in vivo
"Immune" ribonucleic acid	Preparation from lymph nodes or spleen of specifically immunized donors	Ribonucleic acid extract confers upon "naive" lymphocytes a "donor" pattern of responsiveness to specific antigen
(Dialyzable) transfer factor	(a) Extraction of peripheral (human) leukocytes or lymphoid tissue from hypersensitive donor (b) Short-term "pulse" culture of hypersensitive lymphocytes with specific antigen	Injection of extract into healthy-unresponsive or immunodeficient subject confers specific cell-mediated immunity responsiveness, implying conversion of lymphocyte reactivity
Thymus factors	Extraction of polypeptide fractions from (bovine) thymus or human sera	Polypeptide "hormones" accelerate T cell maturation in vivo and in cell culture

[a] For principal references, see Table 2.

ular mediators of lymphocyte function in experimental animals and humans requires the classical approach of endocrine and neurotransmitter physiology that established criteria (15) which potential mediators should satisfy. These "Dale" criteria are essentially: (i) the "substance" (e.g., lymphocyte-stimulating factor) must be identified by biological or pharmacological tests which measure its amount or activity; (ii) the substance must be recoverable in an appropriate time course, from cell cultures or body fluids, during application of the stimulus whose effects it is supposed to mediate (i.e., lymphocyte activation); (iii) the substance must induce similar effects as the stimulus, preferably in both qualitative and quantitative terms; (iv) physiological mechanisms must exist for destruction or elimination of the potential mediator substance; (v) antagonism or potentiation of the release, action, or destruction of the

substance must appropriately modify the effects of the stimulus (e.g., antigenic "challenge" in vivo and in vitro); and (vi) antagonists or potentiators of the stimulus process itself (e.g., cellular immune response in vivo or in vitro) must appropriately modify the release, action, or destruction of the proposed mediator (lymphocyte-stimulating factor).

When the different categories of lymphocyte-stimulating "factors" (Table 1) are viewed in this light, it is apparent that no single category currently fulfills all the classical criteria for acceptance as a physiological mediator of lymphocyte function. Elsewhere (11, 52), we have discussed the definition and measurement of lymphokines, which despite their heterogeneity would seem to be susceptible to the "classical" approach, particularly in animal systems. In culturing human lymphocytes with antigen or phytomitogen and observing the production of a soluble "factor" with lymphocyte-stimulating activity in a particular test system, it is at present an article of faith that one is studying an important component of immunological homeostasis in humans (20).

Use of the term "lymphocyte mitogenic factor"

In this introduction we have considered it important to point out how slender is current evidence for the separate physiological identity of any of the proposed lymphocyte-stimulating substances which have been obtained from leukocytes or lymphoid cells. We shall therefore use the term (and its abbreviation, "LMF") in both a generic and operational sense to describe the following circumstances:

(i) where antigen- or phytomitogen-activated lymphocyte-rich cell populations generate culture supernatant fluids which stimulate cellular incorporation of radiolabeled thymidine when they are added (in unfractionated or fractionated form) to fresh ("test") cultures of allogeneic, autologous, or even xenogeneic lymphocytes, under conditions where no other stimulant is present in the test cultures; and

(ii) where the lymphocyte-stimulating effects of these supernatant fluids or their derivatives are greater than that obtained by adding corresponding amounts of antigen or phytomitogen to control supernatant fluids from operationally unactivated lymphocytes.

In some circumstances, the lymphocyte-stimulating effects of these supernatant fluids are greater than the sum of separate effects of corresponding amounts of (i) antigen or phytomitogen remaining in supernatant fluids or their derivatives, together with (ii) effects of a similar quantity of culture supernatant fluid from operationally unactivated lymphocytes. In many reports, this information is not presented, but we would draw attention to the desirability of obtaining such data.

In the generic sense this approach allows for the demonstration of lymphokines, recruiting factors, potentiating factors, etc., in the culture products whose activities indicate the presence of a "mitogenic" agent. In the operational sense the term LMF implies a product or products of lymphocyte activation, and, if it is an antigen that is being used to activate the primary lymphocyte cultures, there is clinical interest in whether the activity of LMF runs parallel with

TABLE 2. Biological activities of principal categories of lymphocyte-stimulating factors as delineated in Table 1 [a]

Category or specification of lymphocyte-stimulating "factor(s)"	Stimulation of DNA synthesis in vitro			Functional stimulation of cultured lymphocytes			Stimulation of lymphocyte function in vivo		
	Mitogenic	Specific antigen-dependent	Augmenting	T cell rosettes	Cytotoxicity	a AB/Ig synthesis b MIF production	Cell-mediated immunity reaction	Antibody/immunoglobulin production	Lymphoid histology
Lymphokine	+ (21, 52)	− (68)	− (32)	NK	+ (13, 24)	a (59)	+ (42)	+ (43, 37)	+ (38, 39)
Lymphocyte-"recruiting" or "transforming" factor(s)	− (63)	+ (63)	−	NK	NK	a (?28)	NK	NK	NK
"Potentiating" or "augmenting" factor(s)	− (4)	− (35, 36)	+ (34, 41)	NK	NK	a (?28)	NK	NK	NK
T cell-replacing or "helper" factor(s) for B cell function	− (3, 28)	+ (1)	− (1)	NK	NK	a (1, 3, 25, 64)	NK	+ (53)	NK
"Immune" ribonucleic acid	NK	NK	NK	NK	NK	a, b (7, 55, 61)	+ (31, 51)	+ (8)	NK
"Transfer" factors	−	+ (?2)	+ (29, 30)	+ (62)	+ (PC)[b]	b (48, 56)	+ (44, 45)	− (45)	+ (45)
"Thymus" factors	−	−	+ (14)	+ (5)	NK	NK	+ (65)	+ (23)	+ (23)

[a] Numbers in parentheses are references. NK, Not known; +, positive effect; −, no effect in test system, or not applicable.

[b] L. E. Spitler, personal communication.

other parameters of sensitization in the cell donor. At the investigational level one can seek to determine whether the LMF activity is independent of the retention of inducing antigen in the culture supernatant fluids, whether separate (and recombined) lymphocyte subpopulations selectively generate LMF activity, and whether simple biochemical fractionation of LMF-rich supernatant fluids reveals that several categories of lymphocyte-stimulating agents (e.g.,mitogenic lymphokine, potentiating or recruiting factors) are present in and separable within the original supernatant fluids.

With these real qualifications we describe a convenient method for the production of LMF-rich supernatant fluids, by antigen-activated human blood lymphocytes, which was developed (49, 50) following the demonstration of LMF in the guinea pig (19, 67) and which provides sufficient material for simple clinical and biological investigation.

PREPARATION AND DETECTION OF LYMPHOCYTE MITOGENIC FACTOR IN HUMAN LYMPHOCYTE CULTURE

Materials and equipment

Blood collection. Blood taking set (Baxter Division Travenol Laboratories Ltd., Thetford, U.K.). Sterile collecting bottle. Lignocaine 1% and syringe fitted with a 27-gauge needle. Preservative-free sodium heparin (Evans Medical Ltd., Liverpool, U.K.) freshly constituted from powder at 10,000 units/ml in Eagle's minimal essential medium (MEM).

Column and water bath for lymphocyte separation (see Fig. 1). A glass column 50 cm long and 3 cm in diameter, with a 4.5-cm nozzle of 0.5-cm diameter. A water jacket for the column with a thermostatically controlled heating coil. Ballotini glass beads, no. 11 size, 176 to 249 μm in diameter (Jencons Scientific Ltd., Hemel Hempstead, U.K.); the beads are soaked for 18 h in 5% HCl, washed well with tap water, rinsed with deionized water, and dried in a hot-air oven. Silicone rubber tubing attached to column nozzle with a screw clip to control drip rate. Glass wool (Scientific Supplies Co. Ltd., London, England.)

Culture media. Waymouth's MB 752/1 medium supplied in powder form or Eagle's MEM supplied as a 10× concentrate (Flow Laboratories Ltd., Irvine, U.K.) are constituted with distilled water, and sodium bicarbonate is added to a final concentration of 2.0 g/liter (pH 7.2). L-Glutamine is also added according to the supplier's instructions. Benzyl penicillin and streptomycin sulfate (Glaxo Laboratories Ltd.,

Greenford, U.K.) at final concentrations of 200 units/ml and 100 μg/ml, respectively, are added to the culture media before use.

Other solutions. Dextraven 150:6% dextran (average molecular weight, 150,000) in saline (Fisons Pharmaceuticals Ltd., Loughborough, U.K.). Hanks balanced salt solution (Oxoid, London, England). Eosin Y (G. T. Gurr Ltd., London, England): 8 mg/ml in phosphate-buffered saline.

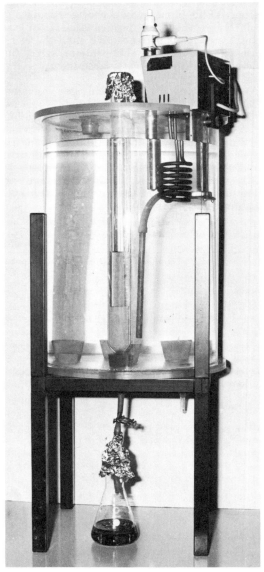

FIG. 1. *Lymphocyte separation column containing Ballotini beads and immersed in constant-temperature cylindrical water bath at 37 C.*

Antigens. PPD: acetone-dried or neutralized and freeze-dried purified protein derivative of tuberculin (Ministry of Agriculture, Fisheries and Food, Weybridge, U.K.). Mixed grass pollen antigen (Beecham's Research Laboratories, Brockham Park, U.K.). Other stimulants, viz., reagent-grade or purified phytohemagglutinin (PHA; Wellcome Reagents Ltd., Beckenham, U.K.) and concanavalin A (Con A; Miles Laboratories Ltd., Slough, U.K.) have also been used for the production of LMF and/or for the assessment of the test system.

General apparatus. Conical and round-bottomed glass centrifuge tubes (50 ml) siliconized before use with Repelcote (Hopkins and Williams, Romford, U.K.). Conical flasks. Cylinders. Culture vessels: 16 × 125 mm rimless test tubes or Bijoux bottles. Aluminum test tube caps. Sterilizing filters (0.2 μm) and filter holders (Millipore [U.K.] Ltd., London). Hemocytometer. Aluminum foil. Disposable Pasteur pipettes. Graduated pipettes of different sizes: 0.1 ml to 10 ml. Refrigerated centrifuge. Incubator fitted with 5% CO_2 in air apparatus. Microscope.

Measurement of tritiated (^{3}H) thymidine uptake by lymphocytes. [^{3}H]thymidine, 5 Ci/mmol (Radiochemical Centre, Amersham, U.K.), diluted to 20 μCi/ml in Eagle's MEM. Hyamine hydroxide (Packard Instruments Ltd., Caversham, Berks., U.K.); 5% trichloroacetic acid in water. Phosphate-buffered saline (pH 7.4). Methanol. Toluene phosphor scintillation fluid (Fisons Scientific Apparatus Ltd., Loughborough, U.K.).

Sterilization/washing. Glassware and other apparatus are washed in tissue culture detergent, rinsed well in tap water and then with deionized water, and sterilized by dry heat or autoclaving. Solutions are sterilized by membrane filtration or autoclaving.

Preparation of glass columns for lymphocyte separation

The column is plugged with enough glass wool to fill the neck and base and then filled with 50 ml of Ballotini glass beads. The top of the column is covered with an aluminum foil cap, and the nozzle is inserted through a hole in a silicone-rubber bung which fits into the base of the water jacket. A piece of silicone-rubber tubing, with a screw-clip attached, is fitted onto the nozzle, and the complete outlet is wrapped in aluminum foil. After sterilizing in a dry-air oven for 1 h, the column is allowed to cool and then is placed in the water jacket which is filled with water and heated to a constant temperature of 37 C. The silicone tube is unwrapped

and placed into a sterile collecting vessel with a foil cover. Hanks solution, prewarmed to 37 C, is poured into the column to completely wet the glass beads and glass wool. The column is then allowed to flow, by use of the screw-clip adjuster, and a sufficient volume of Hanks solution (i.e., 200 to 500 ml) is used to wash the column until the effluent attains a pH of 7.4. (To minimize disruption of the glass bead bed, all solutions applied to the column should be loaded down the side of the glass column.) The flow is then stopped, leaving a small column of Hanks solution above the beads, and the column is maintained at 37 C until the leukocyte mixture is prepared.

Collection of blood and separation of lymphocytes

A 0.5-ml amount of 1% lignocaine is injected intradermally, superficial to the median antecubital vein in the elbow, and the vene-section cannula of the blood taking set is inserted into the vein, the other end of the taking set having previously been punctured into the collection bottle containing 0.2 ml of heparin. A 100-ml sample of venous blood is collected, the bottle being gently swirled during the procedure to maintain even heparinization. It is convenient to collect a further volume of blood into a non-heparinized vessel for the serum required in culture.

To 100 ml of the blood, 30 ml of Ringer's solution and 30 ml of 6% dextran are added, and the blood is poured into five 50-ml round-bottomed glass tubes, care being taken to avoid formation of air bubbles at the fluid/air interface. If bubbles form, these are removed with a Pasteur pipette. The tubes are placed upright in a rack at 37 C for about 1 h to allow sedimentation of erythrocytes. The upper leukocyte-rich layer is collected with a Pasteur pipette (care being exercised to avoid contamination with erythrocytes) and poured into the glass column. After incubation for 10 min (to re-equilibrate the temperature), the screw-clip is loosened and the eluate is collected aseptically at the rate of 2 ml/min. Complete elution is effected by washing the column with 100 ml of Hanks solution at the same flow rate. The combined lymphocyte-rich eluates are divided into 50-ml conical tubes and centrifuged at 500 × g for 15 min at 20 C. The fluid is aspirated by a Pasteur pipette attached to a vacuum pump. The cells in the pellet at the bottom of the tube are washed in Waymouth's medium containing 15% autologous serum and resuspended in 5 ml of 15% serum-Waymouth medium for cell counting and assessment of cell viability by nuclear exclusion of Eosin Y. The separation procedure yields about 10^8 viable lymphocytes per 100 ml of blood. Mononuclear cells comprise 95 to 100% of the total white cells, and a two- to eightfold excess of erythrocytes is usual.

Production of lymphocyte mitogenic factor-containing supernatant fluids

Lymphocytes are cultured at 6×10^6 to 10×10^6 viable cells/ml in 3-ml amounts in tubes or Bijoux bottles containing 15% autologous serum-Waymouth's medium together with an appropriate concentration of antigen or mitogen at a concentration known to produce optimal deoxyribonucleic acid synthesis. For example, PPD (Weybridge) was used at a concentration of 10 to 50 μg/ml and mixed grass pollen, at 150 μg/ml. Similar amounts of the same cell suspension are also cultured *without* any additions for "control" supernatant fluids. After culture at 37 C for 3 days, the supernatant fluids are "harvested" by centrifugation at $1,000 \times g$ for 20 min. The "control" supernatant fluids are then "reconstituted" with antigen to give the same final concentration present in the stimulated cultures. The supernatant fluids are sterilized by membrane filtration and stored at −20 C. Supernatant fluids from lymphocytes cultured in the presence of antigen are termed "preincubated" ("P") in contrast to the "reconstituted" (R) control supernatant fluids prepared from the same population of lymphocytes cultured in the absence of antigens.

Detection of lymphocyte mitogenic factor activity in culture supernatant fluids

For this purpose, allogeneic or autologous peripheral blood lymphocytes are separated from fresh blood by means of the previously described techniques, on a suitable occasion after preparation of the culture supernatant fluids. The separated lymphocytes are washed and suspended at 1.5×10^6 cells/ml in 15% fresh autologous serum-Waymouth's medium and distributed in 2-ml portions in the requisite number of culture vessels (usually 16×125 mm rimless test tubes with loose aluminum caps). Undiluted P and R supernatant fluids as well as dilutions are added in 1-ml volumes to the cells, giving final culture volumes of 3 ml, a cell concentration of 10^6/ml, and final dilutions of P and R supernatant fluids of 1:3, 1:6, and 1:12. Each dilution of P and R is tested in triplicate. Other control treatments should include (i) serum-Waymouth's medium alone and (ii) antigen or mitogen at concentrations equivalent to that present in the supernatant fluids.

The cultures are incubated at 37 C in 5% CO_2

in air, and 18 h before termination, 2 μCi of [³H]thymidine is added to each culture (contained in 0.1 ml of Waymouth's medium). At 144 h, the culture test tubes are centrifuged at $500 \times g$ for 5 min at 4 C and the supernatant fluid is poured off. By use of a Whirlimixer, the cell pellet is dispersed and washed in 3 ml of ice-cold phosphate-buffered saline (pH 7.4). After recentrifugation at $1,500 \times g$, the cells are washed twice with 3 ml of ice-cold 5% trichloroacetic acid. The precipitate is dried by washing with 3 ml of ice-cold methanol and is solubilized in 0.5 ml of Hyamine hydroxide in an agitating water bath at 56 C for 30 min. The solubilized material is flushed into counting vials with 15 ml of toluene phosphor and counted in a liquid scintillation counter. Total incorporation of [³H]thymidine is expressed as quench-corrected disintegrations per minute per culture, and the value for each single treatment is the mean of the replicate determinations.

Table 3 cites data from our experiments (49, 50) which show the detection of LMF activity in tests where P−R has a positive value. No clinical significance has yet been attached to circumstances where P−R has a negative value; there are a variety of possibilities, but these await investigation.

Operational notes

1. In comparing LMF production by groups of subjects selected merely to show a given form of hypersensitivity (e.g., Mantoux-positive versus Mantoux-negative or atopic versus nonatopic), the prevalence of LMF positivity has been expressed by the proportion of subjects that exhibit P−R values greater than zero. Where P−R differences are small, it may be argued that replicate variation in thymidine incorporation within the test should be examined, and that LMF should only be cited as "positive" if the P value (as mean disintegrations per minute ± the standard deviation) is statistically greater than the corresponding R value. This reasoning acquires greater force where isolated investigations are undertaken of LMF production by an individual subject.

2. The value of an "R-type" supernatant fluid as control allows a correction to be made for any nonspecific (i.e., non-antigen-induced) activity (stimulatory or suppressive) which would influence the results. For this reason LMF activity is recorded as P−R (in disintegrations per minute per culture) rather than as P−C values (where C represents basal uptake of test lymphocytes).

3. Both autologous and allogeneic lymphocyte populations can be used to test for LMF

TABLE 3. *Data illustrating detection of LMF activity in human lymphocyte culture supernatant fluids (see 49, 50)*

Features of clinical hypersensitivity	LMF production		[³H]thymidine uptake[a] by test cells in presence of supernatant fluids		LMF activity[b]
	Antigen dose	Superna-tant dilu-tion	R	P	
Type IV (tuber-culin PPD) Mantoux-posi-tive (1:10³)[c] Mantoux-neg-ative	PPD, 30 µg/ ml	1:3 1:3	17,685 8,500	28,269 8,433	10,584 (present) −67 (absent)
Type I (grass pollen) Allergen-posi-tive (14 mm)[c] Allergen-neg-ative	Pollen, 150 µg/ ml	1:3 1:3	3,034 4,135	10,376 3,174	7,342 (present) −961 (absent)

[a] [³H]thymidine uptake by test cells (autologous lymphocytes) expressed as Δdisintegrations per minute per culture (mean of triplicates). R = reconstituted; P = preincubated.
[b] LMF activity recorded as Δdisintegrations per minute (P − R) and expressed as "present" or "absent."
[c] Skin reactivity: type IV response to 1:1,000 tuberculin or type I response (14-mm erythema) to 25,000 Noon units of grass pollen allergen.

activity, although in Table 3 we illustrate data obtained with autologous test cells.

4. The fact that LMF activity can be generated in type I as well as in type IV hypersensitivity suggests that more than one type of mechanism may be involved in LMF production (49, 50, 58).

5. Little is known of the dose-response characteristics of human LMF; we stress the desirability of testing for LMF at more than one supernatant dilution.

6. In animal experiments, dialysis of supernatant fluids frequently results in removal of substances which interfere with the expression of LMF activity (68); similar comparisons are needed with human supernatant fluids.

7. The inclusion of specific or nonspecific antigens in the test system allows for detection of augmenting or potentiating effects of LMF. By testing the LMF preparation together with added antigens, the antigen dependence and specificity of augmentation can be determined (see also Table 1).

MEASUREMENT OF LYMPHOCYTE MITOGENIC FACTOR ACTIVITY IN LYMPHOCYTE CULTURE FLUIDS

The foregoing description indicates that subjects can be classified as LMF "producers" or nonproducers (in respect of stimulation by a given antigen) but fails to indicate how the relative activities of two or more LMF prepara-

tions may be quantitated. A second problem arises from the selection of clinically hypersensitive (i.e., "allergic") subjects in available studies, for the "normal" range of LMF production to any one antigen is at present unknown. For example, 90% of Mantoux-positive subjects and 90% of subjects with type I (pollen) sensitivity appear to be LMF producers, whereas 90% of subjects without Mantoux reactivity or pollen sensitivity are LMF nonproducers to the corresponding antigens. These studies (49, 50) were done on deliberately selected "positive" and "negative" reactors, and methods have not yet been applied by which LMF production could be followed through clinically defined stages in the manifestations of allergic disease. Recent advances in the measurement of mitogenic lymphokine activity in the guinea pig have led to the development of quantitative measurements which are now briefly described with the implication that they might be applicable to the study of human LMF.

Measurement of LMF activity by reference to a working standard

Figure 2a illustrates the problem of comparing two preparations of mitogenic lymphokine with widely different activities. The dose-response curves AA and BB depict the thymidine-incorporation values obtained by testing P-type supernatant fluids only. In this example, the relative potency of the two preparations is

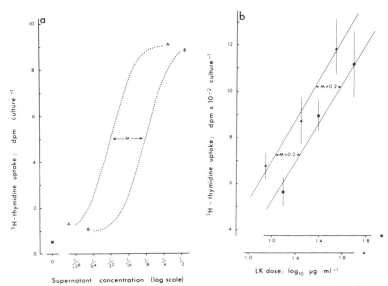

FIG. 2. *Representation of dose-response curves for two LMF-containing ("P-type") supernatant fluids (A and B). Response data ([³H]thymidine uptake, in arbitrary units, by test lymphocytes) plotted against logarithmically spaced supernatant concentrations. The relative potency of the two preparations is measured from the horizontal distance between equipotent doses (i.e., antilog M; on the graph, 32 ÷ 8 = 4). (b) Parallel line assay of guinea pig mitogenic lymphokine. Response of test lymphocytes to three concentrations of "unknown" preparation (▲) and "standard" (●) recorded as disintegrations per minute ([³H]thymidine uptake)/culture (mean of quadruplicate cultures ± SD). Regression lines for the two preparations are drawn by eye and, for clarity, the log-dose scales for the unknown (▲) and standard (●) are displaced by 0.2 log unit. Potency ratio = antilog M, in this experiment = 1.05, with 95% fiducial limits (calculated from Fieller's theorem) of 0.85 to 1.31. Analysis of variance (26) showed assay data to be statistically valid.*

given by the horizontal distance (as an antilog) between the two curves measured at equal response points lying on linear and parallel parts of the log dose-response curves. The figure shows a fourfold difference between the activities of these two preparations and represents the sort of results that might be anticipated in clinically different situations. In principle, a desirable objective would be to prepare a sufficient quantity of active LMF to serve as a working standard with designated "units" of activity, to include the standard in each LMF test, and to express the LMF activity of unknown preparations according to their potency relative to the "standard" preparation.

In practice, however, studies are needed to determine whether unfractionated human lymphocyte culture supernatant fluids will fulfill the necessary criteria of linearity and parallelism of dose-response relationships to permit the application of this quantitative approach. Figure 2b shows an example of data which do fulfill these criteria where an "unknown" guinea pig lymphokine preparation was assayed against a standard preparation. In this assay the three doses of each lymphokine (i.e., a 3 + 3 assay)

are equally spaced on a logarithmic scale, and equal numbers of replicates (actually four) are used at individual dose levels. Usually the potency ratio is determined by calculation, and the "best" (i.e., least squares) estimate is obtained by simple trigonometry using a pooled regression value for the two preparations (see 26). The calculated potency ratio of the unknown preparation illustrated in Fig. 2b was 1.05, and the 95% fiducial limits of this estimate, calculated by Fieller's theorem (see 26), were 0.85 and 1.31. Repeated assay of the same lymphokine preparation gave the following potency ratio values and confidence limits: 1.34 (1.13 to 1.63), 0.91 (0.73 to 1.14), and 0.71 (0.62 to 0.81). Chi-square analysis of these estimates confirmed their homogeneity and indicated the reproducibility of the assay method (11).

The successful application of quantitative bioassay to the measurement of LMF activity in guinea pigs suggests its applicability to humans. With human LMF, assay format and data handling techniques will naturally be determined by the precision and dose-response characteristics of the results obtained. With this qualification, experience of measuring lymphokines in animal systems generates confidence in the view that quantitative approaches to the measurement of any human lymphokine activity will eventually be fruitful.

BIOLOGICAL AND CLINICAL SIGNIFICANCE OF LYMPHOCYTE MITOGENIC FACTOR PRODUCTION

Although the LMF activity of lymphocyte activation products was delineated shortly after the discovery of their migration-inhibitory (MIF) activity, until recently the study of LMF as a lymphocyte "mediator" in either animal or human systems has been a relatively minor pursuit. However, five sets of observations may be viewed as contributing to a recent growth of interest in LMF: (i) evidence that LMF is produced by the peripheral blood leukocytes of bursectomized but not thymectomized chickens (54); (ii) evidence that LMF is preferentially produced by T cell-enriched lymphocyte populations in humans (27, 57); (iii) demonstrations (see Table 2) that LMF-containing lymphocyte supernatant fluids induce accelerated antibody production by cultured rabbit or human lymphocytes and accelerated cytodifferentiation of antibody-forming cells in guinea pig lymph nodes; (iv) demonstration that, in allergic states of both immediate and delayed hypersensitivity, LMF is produced by antigen-stimulated human lymphocytes (49, 50, 57, 58); and (v) evidence that quantitative bioassays of LMF have been established in the guinea pig whereby LMF activity can be measured in "units" by reference to a material lymphokine standard (11). Accordingly, there is now much interest in defining the nature of LMF as a lymphocyte-mediator system in animals and humans, and in assessing the potential significance of LMF production in physiological and pathological states.

Occurrence and principal properties of lymphocyte mitogenic factor in humans

The production of LMF by antigen-stimulated human lymphocytes can now be regarded as a normal attribute of healthy subjects exhibiting delayed hypersensitivity, lymphocyte transformation, and MIF production to soluble antigens such as tuberculin PPD, candida somatic protein, streptokinase-streptodornase, and tetanus toxoid. Furthermore, where investigated, LMF production by antigen-stimulated human lymphocytes runs parallel with lymphocyte transformation responses in clinical states of both immediate and delayed hypersensitivity. What little information exists concerning

the production of, or response to, lymphocyte-stimulating factors in disease syndromes, suggests that LMF may be a useful parameter of lymphocyte function (Table 4). Chromatographic separation studies of antigen-stimulated human LMF indicate that its activity is nondialyzable, with a molecular weight smaller than that of serum albumin, possibly in the range of 20,000 to 30,000 (57). Like MIF, human LMF production is inhibited by puromycin, and its activity is destroyed by proteolysis (27). Again, like MIF, LMF can be generated by phytomitogen-stimulated human lymphocytes, suggesting that a mitogenic lymphokine may be largely responsible for its activity (47). However, several lines of evidence indicate that, as in the guinea pig, LMF in humans is "different" from MIF: (i) both B cell- and T cell-enriched subpopulations produce MIF, but only T cell-rich subpopulations produce LMF (57); (ii) lymphocyte transformation and LMF production run parallel but dissociate from MIF production in clinical states of immediate hypersensitivity and severe infection (12, 50).

At present, it seems that LMF production in humans, in the sense implied by use of the term "mitogenic lymphokine," may be a preferential

TABLE 4. *Lymphocyte-stimulating factors: abnormality in production or response in disease states*

Disease entity	Mediator production or response to preformed mediators
Mantoux-positive sarcoidosis	Depressed production of "lymphocyte-transforming" factor (33)
Disseminated candidiasis with positive DH or MIF	Depressed production of "lymphocyte mitogenic" factor (PC)[a]
Anergic coccidioidomycosis and candidiasis; some Wiskott-Aldrich; some sarcoidosis	Diminished response to injections of dialyzable transfer factor (40, 45)
Atopic sensitization to pollen	Excessive production of "lymphocyte-mitogenic" factor(s) (50, 58)
Allergic cutaneous leishmaniasis	Some patients produce a "lymphocyte mitogenic" factor (12)
Rheumatoid disease	(i) Synovial fluid contains "lymphocyte mitogenic" and "helper" factors (60, 69) (ii) Serum of some older patients has raised thymosin levels (6)

[a] H. Valdimarsson, personal communication.

property of a subpopulation of lymphocytes that possesses certain of the accepted characteristics of T cells. There is clearly a great need for further clinical study, in survey and in depth, to define more closely the circumstances of LMF production by human lymphocytes in health and disease.

Lymphocyte mitogenic factor activity viewed as a lymphocyte function test

In the general sense, LMF may be viewed as mediating antigen-induced lymphocyte transformations, as being physiologically produced by a small proportion of specifically antigen-sensitive T cells in a lymphocyte population, and normally as acting on a larger subpopulation of lymphocytes, which may include cells otherwise classified as of both T and B varieties. The existence of LMF activity as a physiological entity presumably illustrates how lymphocyte subpopulations, which differ in origin and life cycle, do not necessarily function in isolation, but interact in the positive sense. The demonstration that human peripheral blood lymphocytes are capable of generating and responding to LMF would therefore imply the integrity of such a cooperating pathway. If more precise modes of action could be ascribed to the substances mediating LMF activity (e.g., cell cooperation mechanisms in antibody production; amplification of T cell protective mechanisms), then the measurement of LMF activity and response to LMF could be viewed as an important component of lymphocyte function tests. There is great need for the development of techniques to test the ability of human lymphocytes to initiate antibody responses in lymphoid cells of human origin (22). The possibility arises that among lymphocyte-stimulating factors detected by the LMF test there resides a special mediator of T cell-B cell cooperation whose functional assessment may prove to be of great interest in the whole range of immunological disease.

The detection of human LMF activity is a technically simple procedure, although much further work needs to be done concerning the optimal conditions of antigen concentration and timing, and the development of precise methods for measurement for LMF activity. As with any other lymphocyte function test in clinical use, variations in the sequestration of lymphocytes in diseased tissues may well distort the picture in peripheral blood. However, with that single qualification, and against the growing background of knowledge of lymphocyte-stimulating factors in general, the time would seem to be ripe for the wider introduction of an LMF test into the clinical laboratory.

Technical improvements and future trends

Recent technical innovations in the study of lymphocyte activities may help the development of work on human LMF. These could be (i) the use of miniaturized techniques of blood and lymphocyte culture in tests of LMF activity; (ii) the development of "standard" preparations of human (or animal) LMF against which to assay the potency of preparations in units of mitogenic activity; (iii) the standardization of antigens used in the induction of transformation responses and in LMF production; (iv) the use of standard cell lines of human origin as "targets" for the lymphocyte-stimulating activities of LMF-rich supernatant fluids; (v) the possible use of murine thymocytes as test cells; (vi) the incorporation of a simple separation technique (e.g., differential membrane filtration) to remove, from lymphocyte supernatant fluids, low- or high-molecular-weight substances which might interfere with [^{3}H]thymidine incorporation in test cultures; and (vii) the regular use of a simple lymphocyte separation technique to concentrate a subpopulation found to be largely responsible for generating LMF activity.

Future trends in the study of LMF are likely to emerge in parallel with the study of lymphocyte mediators in general. Examples of these would be (i) the precise measurement of mediator activity against defined clinical criteria; (ii) the development of biological standards of LMF as diagnostic reagents to assist quantitation of lymphocyte function; (iii) the recognition and classification of abnormalities in LMF production or responsiveness; and (iv) the development of agonists and antagonists of LMF activity or production in therapeutic attempts to control defined aspects of the immune response in humans.

ACKNOWLEDGMENTS

We thank the Medical Research Council, the Wellcome Trust, the Arthritis and Rheumatism Council, and the Multiple Sclerosis Society for continued support.

LITERATURE CITED

1. Armeding, D., and D. H. Katz. 1974. Activation of T and B lymphocytes *in vitro*. II. Biological and biochemical properties of an allogeneic effect factor (AEF) active in triggering specific B lymphocytes. J. Exp. Med. 140:19–35.
2. Ascher, M. S., W. J. Schneider, F. T. Valentine, and H. S. Lawrence. 1974. *In vitro* properties of leukocyte dialysates containing transfer factor. Proc. Natl. Acad. Sci. U.S.A. 71:1178–1182.
3. Askonas, B. A., A. Schimpl, and E. Wecker.

1974. The differentiation function of T-cell replacing factor in nu/nu spleen cell cultures. Eur. J. Immunol. 4:164–169.

4. Bach, F. H., B. J. Alter, S. Solliday, D. C. Zoschke, and M. Janis. 1970. Lymphocyte reactivity *in vitro*. II. Soluble reconstituting factor permitting response of purified lymphocytes. Cell Immunol. 1:219–227.

5. Bach, J. F., M. Dardenne, A. L. Goldstein, A. Guha, and A. White. 1971. Appearance of T cell markers in bone-marrow rosette-forming cells after incubation with thymosin, a thymic hormone. Proc. Natl. Acad. Sci. 68:2734–2738.

6. Bach, J.-F., F. Reyes, C. Judet, and M. Dardenne. 1975. Significance of IgG-binding cells in rheumatoid arthritis: their possible relation to thymic function. *In* D. C. Dumonde (ed.), Infection and immunology in the rheumatic diseases. Blackwell, London.

7. Bell, C., and S. Dray. 1971. Conversion of non-immune rabbit spleen cells from an immunised rabbit to produce IgM and IgG of foreign heavy-chain allotype. J. Immunol. 107:83–95.

8. Bell, C., and S. Dray. 1973. RNA conversion of lymphoid cells to synthesise allogeneic immunoglobulins *in vivo*. Cell. Immunol. 6: 375–393.

9. Bloom, B. R. 1971. *In vitro* approaches to the mechanism of cell-mediated immune reactions. Adv. Immunol. 13:101–208.

10. Bloom, B. R., and B. Bennett. 1966. Mechanism of a reaction *in vitro* associated with delayed type hypersensitivity. Science 153:80–82.

11. Bray, M. A., D. C. Dumonde, J. M. Hanson, J. Morley, J. V. Smart, and R. A. Wolstencroft. 1976. Heterogeneity of guinea pig lymphokines revealed by parallel bioassay. Clin. Exp. Immunol. 23:333–346.

12. Bray, R. S., A. D. M. Bryceson, R. N. Maini, E. J. Bowers, P. H. Holmes, and D. C. Dumonde. 1975. *In vitro* correlates of delayed hypersensitivity in human leishmaniasis. Clin. Exp. Immunol., in press.

13. Butterworth, A. E. 1973. Non-specific cytotoxic effects of antigen-transformed lymphocytes. Kinetics, cell-requirements and the role of recruitment. Cell. Immunol. 7:357–369.

14. Cohen, G. H., and A. L. Goldstein. 1975. Mixed lymphocyte reaction bioassay for thymosin. *In* D. van Bekkum (ed.), Biological activity of thymic hormones. Kooker Scientific Publications, Rotterdam.

15. Dale, H. H. 1933. Progress in autopharmacology. Bull. Johns Hopkins Hosp. 53:297–310.

16. David, J. R. 1966. Delayed hypersensitivity *in vitro* and its mediation by cell-free substances formed by lymphoid cell-antigen interaction. Proc. Natl. Acad. Sci. U.S.A. 56:72–77.

17. David, J. R., and R. R. David. 1972. Cellular hypersensitivity and immunity. Inhibition of macrophage migration and the lymphocyte mediators. Prog. Allergy 16:300–449.

18. Dumonde, D. C. 1970. 'Lymphokines': molecular mediators of cellular immune responses in animals and man. Proc. R. Soc. Med. 63:899–902.

19. Dumonde, D. C., W. T. Howson, and R. A. Wolstencroft. 1968. The role of macrophages and lymphocytes in reactions of delayed hypersensitivity, p. 263–278. *In* P. A. Miescher and P. Grabar (ed.), Immunopathology, 5th International Symposium: mechanisms of inflammation induced by immune reactions. Schwabe, Basel.

20. Dumonde, D. C., and R. N. Maini. 1971. The clinical significance of mediators of cellular immunity. Clin. Allergy 1:123–139.

21. Dumonde, D. C., R. A. Wolstencroft, G. S. Panayi, M. Matthew, J. Morley, and W. T. Howson. 1969. Lymphokines: non-antibody mediators of cellular immunity generated by lymphocyte activation. Nature (London) 224:38–42.

22. Editorial. 1975. Lymphocyte subpopulations in chronic inflammatory diseases. Br. Med. J. 2:1–2.

23. Edwards, D. C. 1975. The influence of thymus extracts on immune systems. Behring Inst. Mitt. 57:3–10.

24. Falk, R. E., J. A. Falk, E. Möller, and G. Möller. 1970. Lymphocyte-activating factors released *in vitro* by sensitised and non-sensitised human lymphocytes. Cell. Immunol. 1:150–161.

25. Feldmann, M., and A. Basten. 1972. Cell interactions in the immune response *in vitro*. IV. Comparison of the effects of antigen-specific and allogeneic thymus derived cell factors. J. Exp. Med. 136:722–736.

26. Finney, D. J. 1964. Statistical method in biological assay, 2nd ed. Griffin, London.

27. Geha, R. S., and E. Merler. 1974. Human lymphocyte mitogenic factor: synthesis by sensitised thymus-derived lymphocytes, dependence of expression on the presence of antigen. Cell. Immunol. 10:86–104.

28. Geha, R. S., E. Schneeberger, F. S. Rosen, and E. Merler. 1973. Interaction of human thymus-derived and non-thymus-derived lymphocytes *in vitro*. Induction of proliferation and antibody synthesis in B-lymphocytes by a soluble factor released from antigen-stimulated T lymphocytes. J. Exp. Med. 138:1230–1247.

29. Hamblin, A. S. 1975. The effect of transfer factor on cultured lymphocytes. Behring Inst. Mitt. 57:25–31.

30. Hamblin, A. S., R. N. Maini, and D. C. Dumonde. 1975. Human transfer factor *in vitro*. I. Augmentation of lymphocyte transformation to tuberculin PPD. Clin. Exp. Immunol. 23:290–302.

31. Han, T., J. L. Pauly, and A. Mittleman. 1975. Adoptive transfer of cell-mediated immunity to tuberculin using RNA from tuberculin-sensitive subjects. Immunology 28:127–132.

32. Havemann, K., and S. Burger. 1971. *In vitro* studies on the release of mitogenic factor by sensitised human lymphocytes. Eur. J. Immunol. 1:285–290.

33. Horsmanheimo, M. 1974. Lymphocyte transforming factor in sarcoidosis. Cell. Immunol. 10:338–343.

34. Janis, M., and F. H. Bach. 1970. Potentiation of *in vitro* lymphocyte reactivity. Nature (London) 225:238–239.

35. Janis, M., and F. H. Bach. 1971. Blastogenic factor production by PHA-stimulated leucocytes, p. 335–344. *In* O. R. McIntyre (ed.), Proceedings of the fourth annual leucocyte culture conference. Appleton-Century-Crofts, New York.

36. Kasakura, S. 1970. Heterogeneity of blastogenic factors produced *in vitro* by antigenically stimulated and unstimulated leukocytes. J. Immunol. 105:1162–1167.

37. Kelly, R. H., V. S. Harvey, T. E. Sadler, and D. C. Dumonde. 1975. Accelerated cytodifferentiation of antibody-secreting cells in guinea pig lymph nodes stimulated by sheep erythrocytes and lymphokines. Clin. Exp. Immunol. 21:141–154.

38. Kelly, R. H., and R. A. Wolstencroft. 1974. Germinal centre proliferation in response to mitogenic lymphokines. Clin. Exp. Immunol. 18:321–336.

39. Kelly, R. H., R. A. Wolstencroft, D. C. Dumonde, and B. M. Balfour. 1972. Role of lymphocyte activation products (LAP) in cell-mediated immunity. II. Effects of lymphocyte activation products on lymph node architecture and evidence for peripheral release of LAP following antigenic stimulation. Clin. Exp. Immunol. 10:49–65.

40. Kirkpatrick, C. H., and D. Rifkind (ed.). 1974. Workshop on basic properties and clinical applications of transfer factor, Tucson, Arizona. Cell. Immunol. 10:165–168.

41. Kirkpatrick, C. H., D. P. Stites, T. K. Smith, and R. A. Johnson. 1971. A factor which enhances DNA synthesis in cultures of stimulated lymphocytes, p. 219–225. *In* O. R. McIntyre (ed.), Proceedings of the fourth annual leucocyte culture conference. Appleton-Century-Crofts, New York.

42. Krejci, J., J. Pekarek, J. Svejcar, and J. Johanovsky. 1973. The effect of lymphokines on the development of delayed hypersensitivity to an unrelated antigen. Immunology 25:875–879.

43. Krejci, J., J. Pekarek, J. Svejcar, and J. Johanovsky. 1973. Role of mediators of cellular hypersensitivity in the stimulation of the antibody formation to unrelated antigen. Cell. Immunol. 7:322–327.

44. Lawrence, H. S. 1960. Some biological and immunological properties of transfer factor. Ciba Found. symposium on cellular aspects of immunity, p. 243–271.

45. Lawrence, H. S. 1974. Transfer factor in cellular immunity. Harvey Lect. Ser. 68:239–350.

46. Lawrence, H. S., and M. Landy (ed.). 1969. Mediators of cellular immunity. Academic Press Inc., New York.

47. Mackler, B. F., R. A. Wolstencroft, and D. C. Dumonde. 1972. Concanavalin A as an inducer of human lymphocyte mitogenic factor. Nature (London) New Biol. 239:139–142.

48. Maddison, S. E., M. D. Hicklin, B. P. Conway, and I. G. Kagan. 1972. Transfer factor: delayed hypersensitivity to *Schistosoma mansoni* and tuberculin in *Macaca mulatta*. Science 178:757–759.

49. Maini, R. N., A. D. M. Bryceson, R. A. Wolstencroft, and D. C. Dumonde. 1969. Lymphocyte mitogenic factor in man. Nature (London) 224:43–44.

50. Maini, R. N., D. C. Dumonde, J. A. Faux, F. E. Hargreave, and J. Pepys. 1971. The production of lymphocyte mitogenic factor and migration-inhibition factor by antigen-stimulated lymphocytes of subjects with grass pollen allergy. Clin. Exp. Immunol. 9:449–465.

51. Mannick, J. A., and R. H. Egdahl. 1962. Transformation of non-immune lymph node cells to state of transplantation immunity by RNA. Ann. Surg. 156:356–365.

52. Morley, J., R. A. Wolstencroft, and D. C. Dumonde. 1973. The measurement of lymphokines. *In* D. M. Weir (ed.), Handbook of experimental immunology, 2nd ed. Blackwell, Oxford.

53. Munro, A. J., and M. J. Taussig 1975. Two genes in the major histocompatibility complex control immune response. Nature (London) 256:103–106.

54. Oates, C. M., J. F. Bissenden, R. N. Maini, L. N. Payne, and D. C. Dumonde. 1972. Thymus and bursa dependence of lymphocyte mitogenic factor in the chicken. Nature (London) New Biol. 239:137–139.

55. Paque, R. E., and S. Dray. 1972. Monkey to human transfer of delayed hypersensitivity *in vitro* with RNA extracts. Cell. Immunol. 5:30–41.

56. Paque, R. E., P. J. Kniskern, S. Dray, and P. Baram. 1969. *In vitro* studies with 'transfer factor.' Transfer of the cell migration inhibition correlate of delayed hypersensitivity in humans with cell lysates from humans sensitised to histoplasmin coccidioidin or PPD. J. Immunol. 103:1014–1021.

57. Rocklin, R. E., R. P. MacDermott, L. Chess, S. F. Schlossman, and J. R. David. 1974. Studies on mediator production by highly purified human T and B lymphocytes. J. Exp. Med. 140:1303–1316.

58. Rocklin, R. E., H. Pence, H. Kaplan, and R. Evans. 1974. Cell-mediated immune response of ragweed-sensitive patients to ragweed antigen E. *In vitro* lymphocyte transformation and elaboration of lymphocyte mediators. J. Clin. Invest. 53:735–744.

59. Rosenthal, M., P. Stastny, and M. Ziff. 1973. Stimulation of γ-globulin synthesis and specific antibody production by a factor released by activated lymphocytes. J. Immunol. 111: 1119–1127.

60. Stastny, P., M. Rosenthal, M. Andreis, and M. Ziff. 1975. Lymphokines in the rheumatoid

joint. Arthritis Rheum. 18:237–243.

61. Thor, D. E., and S. Dray. 1968. The cell migration-inhibition correlate of delayed hypersensitivity: conversion of human non-sensitive lymph node cells to sensitive cells with an RNA extract. J. Immunol. 101:469–480.

62. Valdimarsson, H. 1975. The influence of dialysable leucocyte extracts on immune systems. Behring Inst. Mitt. 57:11–16.

63. Valentine, F. T., and H. S. Lawrence. 1969. Lymphocyte stimulation: transfer of cellular hypersensitivity to antigen in vitro. Science 165:1014–1016.

64. Waldmann, H., and A. Munro. 1974. T-cell dependent mediator in the immune response. II. Physical and biological properties. Immunology 27:53–64.

65. Wara, D. W., A. L. Goldstein, N. E. Doyle, and A. J. Amann. 1975. Thymosin activity in patients with cellular immunodeficiency. N. Engl. J. Med. 292:70–74.

66. Wolstencroft, R. A. 1971. Lymphocyte mitogenic factor in relation to mediators of cellular immunity, p. 130–153. In J.-P. Revillard (ed.), Cell-mediated immunity: in vitro correlates. Karger, Basel.

67. Wolstencroft, R. A., and D. C. Dumonde. 1970. In vitro studies of cell-mediated immunity. I. Induction of lymphocyte transformation by a soluble mitogenic factor derived from interaction of sensitised guinea-pig lymphoid cells with specific antigen. Immunology 18:599–610.

68. Wolstencroft, R. A., M. Matthew, C. M. Oates, R. N. Maini, and D. C. Dumonde. 1971. Lymphocyte mitogenic factor in cell-mediated immunity, p. 28–37. In D. C. Dumonde (ed.), The role of lymphocytes and macrophages in the immunological response. Springer, Berlin.

69. Ziff, M. 1974. Autoimmune processes in rheumatoid arthritis, p. 37–46. In L. Brent and E. J. Holborow (ed.), Progress in immunology II, vol. 5. American Elsevier, New York.

Chapter 16

Macrophage Activation and Function

MARY C. TERRITO, DAVID W. GOLDE, AND MARTIN J. CLINE

INTRODUCTION

Mononuclear phagocytes (M Φ, monocytes and macrophages) have numerous functions: (i) they are scavengers clearing the body of dead or damaged cells, inorganic crystals, and organic debris; (ii) they are an important defense system against certain classes of microorganisms, particularly facultative and obligate intracellular parasites; (iii) they are involved in antigen presentation to certain lymphocyte subpopulations in the afferent limb of the immune response and in the interaction with lymphoid cells in the expression of cell-mediated immune reactions; (iv) finally, they are thought to be involved in the in vivo regulation of granulopoiesis. This last function is probably mediated via the production of colony-stimulating activity, which is also a requirement for granulocyte proliferation and differentiation in vitro.

To accomplish these functions, M Φ have certain well-developed characteristics: highly developed phagocytic and pinocytic activity; ability to adhere to a charged surface (related to phagocytic ability); motility with ability to respond to certain chemotactic stimuli; membrane receptors for the Fc portion of certain classes of immunoglobulin G molecules and for certain complement components; and a well-developed arsenal of lysosomal (granule) acid hydrolases, oxygenases, and cationic proteins (6).

Many of these characteristics appear to be enhanced or exaggerated in humans or animals responding to intracellular microorganisms or with well-developed cell-mediated immune reactions. M Φ in such circumstances are said to be "activated," and compared with nonactivated cells, show a higher rate of cell metabolism as demonstrated by glucose oxidation, more rapid adherence to and spreading on glass, a richer content of lysosomal enzymes, and more effective killing of microorganisms (19). Activation is thought to be mediated by the soluble products of certain lymphoid cells.

Despite this multiplicity of M Φ functions and the numerous experimental systems used in measurement of these functions, no codified system for measuring M Φ performance has yet been widely accepted in clinical practice. This lack of a uniform system of measurement is reflected in the paucity of documented diseases of monocytes or of abnormalities of M Φ function. This situation stands in contrast to the well-documented abnormalities of granulocyte function (15). Given these limitations, we have selected procedures for cell isolation and measurement of M Φ function that we have found useful and that we believe are relevant to studying human disease. In addition, the reader may wish to consult general reviews (6, 20) and original articles describing specific aspects of M Φ function, composition and metabolism, or activation. In each subsection, alternative modes of testing function are enumerated.

MONOCYTE ISOLATION

Principle

Monocytes may be conveniently isolated from other peripheral blood leukocytes by sequential buoyant density centrifugation in Ficoll-Hypaque gradients and adherence to glass or plastic. Monocyte density is similar to that of other blood mononuclear leukocytes but is considerably less than that of polymorphonuclear leukocytes (4). In separating monocytes from lymphocytes of similar density, advantage is taken of the greater adherent properties of the mononuclear phagocyte.

Reagents

Ficoll-Hypaque solution (475 ml): dissolve 29.5 g of Ficoll in 375 ml of doubly distilled warm water, add 100.5 ml of 50% Hypaque (Winthrop Laboratories, New York, N.Y.), mix well, and sterilize by filtration through a 0.4-μm filter (Millipore Corp., Bedford, Mass.).

Heparin, preservative-free or containing benzyl alcohol (no phenol), 5 units per ml of blood.

Sterile phosphate-buffered saline (PBS).

Sterile fetal calf serum (FCS).

McCoy's 5A tissue culture medium.

Procedure (4)

Heparinized venous blood is diluted with an equal volume of PBS, and 15-ml volumes are carefully layered over 3 ml of Ficoll-Hypaque solution in 16 × 150 mm sterile plastic tubes. The diluted blood is added carefully so as to avoid turbulence, which will disturb the interface.

The tubes are centrifuged at 520 × g in a refrigerated centrifuge cooled to 18 to 20 C for 40 min. For the International PRJ centrifuge, the #269 head is used and is spun at 1,450 rpm. When the tubes are removed from the centrifuge, a distinct band can be seen between the plasma and Ficoll-Hypaque layers as shown in Fig. 1. Aspirate and discard the top layer containing the diluted plasma. Then harvest cell band A with a sterile Pasteur pipette, using a circular motion and without taking up more than half of the Ficoll-Hypaque layer. Combine the A band from two tubes in a new 16 × 150 mm tube, add 10 ml of PBS, mix, and centrifuge at 180 × g for 10 min. Then resuspend the cells in 2 ml of Hanks balanced salt solution (HBSS) containing 15% FCS and wash them two times in the same HBSS-FCS, using centrifugations of 150 × g for 8 min. The cell pellet is free from platelets and erythrocytes, and it contains from 60 to 85% lymphocytes and 15 to 40% monocytes with less than 0.5% contamination by granulocytes. The B band (Fig. 1) contains mostly mature granulocytes.

The mixture of lymphocytes and monocytes is resuspended in McCoy's medium with 20% FCS or human AB serum to a concentration of 10^6 to 2×10^6 per ml. The mixed cell suspension may be used for studying phagocytosis, microbial killing, or chemotaxis. If pure monocytes are desired, this suspension is added to glass Leighton (L) tubes or petri dishes. The volume of suspension added depends on the differential cell count; a volume yielding 10^6 monocytes per L tube is often used. The tubes are gassed with 5% CO_2 in air and tightly stoppered with white rubber tissue culture stoppers, or they are loosely capped and placed in an incubator at 37 C with 7.5% CO_2 for 3 h or overnight to allow the monocytes to adhere to the glass cover slip. The tubes or petri dishes are then washed twice with HBSS-FCS at 37 C. Monocyte purity then varies between 70 and 99%. If additional purity is required, the cells may be cultivated for 1 to 2 days, and the tubes are washed twice more with complete medium. The additional washing procedures will reduce the total yield of monocytes but will increase the purity to 96 to 100%. The purity of the monocyte preparation may be

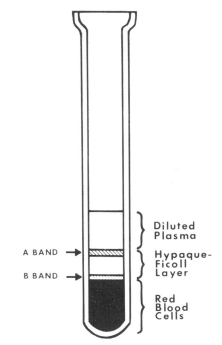

FIG. 1. *Hypaque-Ficoll gradient of peripheral blood showing approximate levels of cellular bands. The mononuclear leukocytes are found in the A band.*

gauged by a number of procedures, but we prefer the histochemical stain for α-naphthyl butyrase, which is found in monocytes but not in granulocytes or lymphocytes (1). Adherent monocytes can be removed from the monolayers with a rubber policeman or with 0.25% trypsin.

MONOCYTE CULTURE

Monocyte-derived macrophages can be prepared from human blood by continued cultivation of the purified monocyte populations (12). The Leighton tube cultures should be re-fed with McCoy's 5A medium with 20% human AB serum approximately every 5 days. Fetal calf serum produces less satisfactory results. The Leighton tubes should be gassed with 5% CO_2 prior to incubation, and a loose-fitting cap is applied to allow for adequate gas exchange. The tubes should be positioned in racks so that the tissue culture medium evenly covers the glass cover slip. After 5 days in culture, the monocytes will begin to transform into macrophages and subsequently will spread out on the glass and become multinucleated. After 5 to 10 days of culture, the macrophage populations are almost 100% pure.

PULMONARY MACROPHAGE ISOLATION AND CULTURE

Pulmonary macrophages can be obtained from human subjects by bronchopulmonary lavage (9). Under local anesthesia and fluoroscopic control, a #16 to #19F Metras catheter is passed transnasally into a lower lobe bronchus. The balloon is then inflated with approximately 5 ml of air, and the tube patency is checked by injecting 100 ml of air with a glass syringe. The procedure may be done with the patient in the sitting position. Segmental lavage is then performed by infusing 100 to 300 ml of physiological saline solution and withdrawing with a 100-ml syringe after each 100 ml of saline is injected. The retrieved material is a clear to opalescent, foamy fluid. This material is then diluted with equal volumes of HBSS with 20% FCS.

The lavage effluent-culture medium mixture is then transferred to 50-ml plastic or siliconized glass centrifuge tubes and centrifuged at 150 × g for 10 min. The cell pellets are washed twice by centrifugation and suspended in McCoy's 5A with 20% FCS or 20% AB human serum. They may be cultured on plastic or glass in a CO_2 incubator (7). Macrophages from human bone marrow can be cultured in a similar manner with the use of diffusion chambers (11).

PHAGOCYTOSIS

Principle

A variety of methods of determining particle uptake by leukocytes exist. All involve mechanisms for differentiating intracellular from extracellular particles. Some require cell suspensions for the procedure, whereas others are performed with surface-adherent cells. Quantitation of phagocytosis by the visual counting of intracellular particles is a simple method. It has the advantage of being applicable to mixed leukocyte suspensions as well as to isolated monocyte or macrophage preparations. Occasionally, with the visual method difficulties arise in differentiating particles that are simply adherent to the cell from those that have been completely engulfed. Therefore, procedures in which labeled particles are used have also been described (24).

Reagents

Sabouraud-2% dextrose broth.
Human AB serum (or other source of opsonins).
HBSS with 10% FCS (HBSS-FCS).
Giemsa stain.
Candida albicans or *C. pseudotropicalis*.

Procedure (modified from reference 16)

Tests should be run in duplicate with sterile techniques used throughout.

1. M Φ suspensions are prepared by use of the A band from Ficoll-Hypaque separation as described in preceding sections. (Mixed leukocyte suspensions can also be used.) The working solution is made up to 10^6 M Φ/ml in HBSS-FCS.

2. *Candida* cells are cultured overnight at 37 C in broth, washed twice in saline, and resuspended at 10^6 yeast/ml in HBSS-FCS. (A variety of other particles can be used, including *Cryptococcus* [8], polyvinyl toluene [2], BCG, or *Listeria* [21].)

3. Into 12 × 75 mm plastic capped tubes are placed 0.3 ml of yeast suspension, 0.1 ml of M Φ suspension, and 0.1 ml of AB serum. The tubes are incubated at 37 C on a rocker panel or mixing wheel for 30 min.

4. After incubation, cytocentrifuge preparations are made, fixed in methanol, stained with Giemsa, and then examined microscopically. The number of *Candida* cells ingested by 200 consecutive M Φ is determined and expressed as the mean number of yeast/M Φ (the "phagocytic index").

Alternative methods

Alternative methods include radioisotopic measurement of bacteria ingested (24), bacterial colony counting (23), and albumin-paraffin oil emulsion ingestion (18).

MICROBIAL KILLING

Principle

The microbicidal capacity of leukocytes is generally measured by use of modifications of the method of Maaløe and of Hirsch and Strauss (14), in which the leukocytes are allowed to ingest a given number of organisms. Once inside the leukocyte, the microbe is exposed to the cidal element of the cell. The leukocytes are later lysed, and the intracellular organisms are assayed by colony-counting methods to determine the number of viable organisms remaining.

Pitfalls and errors

Since neutrophils and eosinophils are also active phagocytes, this assay cannot be used for mixed leukocyte preparations.

Nonphagocytized organisms will remain viable and increase the final number of viable organisms remaining at any time. Various modifications have been used to differentiate defects in the engulfment phase from the killing phase. These involve an elimination or separation of the extracellular organisms and include differential centrifugation, antibiotics, and enzymes (23), or decreasing the microbe-to-phagocyte ratio.

Many organisms tend to clump together and give falsely low readings on colony counting.

Reagents

Trypticase soy broth (TSB) and agar (TSA).
Human AB or autologous serum.
HBSS with 20% heat-inactivated FCS (HBSS-FCS).
Saline.

Procedure (23)

All tests are run in duplicate with sterile technique used throughout.

1. M Φ suspensions are prepared from the A band of Ficoll-Hypaque separation as described in preceding sections and resuspended at 10^7 M Φ/ml of HBSS-FCS.

2. Bacterial suspensions are prepared as follows. *Staphylococcus aureus* is cultured for 16 h at 37 C in TSB. Other organisms such as *Escherichia coli*, *Listeria monocytogenes*, *Salmonella typhimurium* (23), or *Candida* (17) can also be used with minor modifications. The culture is centrifuged at 4,000 × *g* for 10 min at 4 C, washed twice in saline, and adjusted to a concentration of 10^8 bacteria/ml by measuring turbidity spectrophotometrically at 620 nm. (The turbidity at which 10^8 bacteria/ml are in the suspension needs to be determined previously by plating and counting the number of colonies formed after 48 h of incubation at 37 C by use of various optical densities of bacterial suspension.) The 10^8 suspension is diluted with HBSS-FCS to obtain a final working concentration of 10^7 bacteria/ml.

3. Autologous or normal AB serum can be used as a source of opsonin.

4. Into 12 × 75 mm plastic tubes are placed 0.3 ml of HBSS-FCS, 0.1 ml of bacterial suspension, 0.5 ml of M Φ suspension, and 0.1 ml of serum. Control tubes containing the same concentrations of HBSS, bacteria, and serum, but without M Φ (to determine bacterial viability), as well as tubes containing HBSS, serum, and M Φ (to insure sterility) are run simultaneously. The tubes are incubated at 37 C on a mixer.

5. At 0, 2, and 4 h, a 0.1-ml sample is removed from each tube, placed in 0.9 ml of isotonic saline, and sonically treated for 15 s at a level of 40% with the low probe setting of a Bronwill

sonic oscillator. (Alternatively, 0.1 ml of the leukocytes can be lysed in 9.9 ml of distilled sterile water and mixed on a Vortex mixer to disperse the bacteria.)

6. Serial 10-fold dilutions of the sonically treated suspension are made and spread on TSA.

7. The culture plates are incubated at 37 C for 48 h, and the colonies formed are counted to determine the number of viable bacteria. Results can then be expressed as the percent killed at *x* hours.

Alternative methods

Alternative methods include the measurement of viable intracellular organisms by their ability to incorporate [³H]thymidine (5) and by their Giemsa staining characteristics (16). Both of these methods can be used in mixed leukocyte preparations.

CHEMOTAXIS

Principle

A basic biological property of M Φ is their ability to undergo directional migration in response to specific (chemotactic) stimuli. Chemotaxis in these cells is measured by modifications of a method initially described by Boyden (3). The leukocytes are placed in the upper compartment of a chamber, separated from the lower compartment by a filter of suitable pore size through which the cells can migrate actively but not drop passively. When solutions of chemotactically active substances are placed in the lower compartment of the chamber, the leukocytes will actively migrate through the pores and adhere to the lower surface of the filter.

Pitfalls and errors

Although all the cells that migrate through are presumed to adhere to the lower surface of the filter, there have been some studies with neutrophils in which the cells dropped off the filter and would cause a falsely low count. This has not been described yet for M Φ but should be considered a possibility.

There is occasionally a tendency for clumping of the leukocytes on the lower surface of the filter, making it difficult to get a representative cell count. Techniques described for neutrophil chemotaxis using chromium-51-labeled cells and counting the filters in a gamma counter (10) may be helpful in eliminating the counting difficulties for M Φ.

Reagents and equipment

Gey's balanced salt solution, pH 7.0 (GBSS).
AB serum.
Giemsa stain.
Xylene.
Human serum albumin (HSA).
Rabbit anti-HSA (heated 30 min at 56 C).
Boyden chemotaxis chambers (Ahlco Machine Co., New Briton, Conn.).
Membrane filters (Nuclepore; Wallabs Inc., San Rafael, Calif.). Diameter, 13 mm. Pore size, 5 μm (for monocytes) and 8 μm (for macrophages).

Procedure for monocytes (22)

All tests are run in duplicate or triplicate.

1. Monocytes are isolated as in preceding sections and resuspended to 10^6 monocytes/ml in GBSS.

2. Chemotactic factor: A number of substances chemotactic for monocytes have been described. The cleavage product of the fifth component of complement (C5a) is useful as a standard assay. This can be produced from serum by a variety of methods of which antigen-antibody complex stimulation is an example (25). To make the antigen-antibody complex, 100 μg of HSA in 0.1 ml of GBSS is mixed with 1 mg of antibody nitrogen/ml. Normal serum is incubated with this complex for 10 min at 37 C to activate complement and produce the chemotactic complement factors. This is followed by heating at 56 C for 30 min to inactivate serum chemotactic inhibitors, and the mixture is then diluted to a 20% concentration with GBSS and used as the chemotactic solution.

3. Boyden Chambers are prepared and filled as follows. The 5-μm membrane filter is inserted into the chamber with microforceps. The dull side of the Nuclepore should be up and the shiny side down. The upper compartment is then screwed into place.

The chemotactic solution is introduced into the lower compartment by use of a Pasteur pipette. The chambers should be tipped slightly while adding this solution to avoid getting air trapped beneath the filter. In control chambers, plain GBSS without a chemotactic agent is added to the lower compartment.

The cell suspension is then *immediately* added to the upper compartment.

4. The chambers are then incubated in a humidified atmosphere at 37 C for 90 min.

5. After incubation, the solutions are decanted from the upper and lower compartments. The filters are removed, rinsed in saline, and fixed in methanol (3 min). The filters are then stained with Giemsa (30 min) and cleared in xylene (3 min). They are subsequently *inverted* and mounted on glass slides so that the lower surface of the filter (the surface to which the cells have migrated) is now on top.

6. The monocytes that have migrated through the filter are counted by use of a microgrid in 10 vertical and 10 horizontal oil-powered fields. This is then multiplied by the factor for the microgrid to obtain the number of cells per high-power field.

Procedure for macrophages

The procedure for macrophages is similar to that for peripheral blood monocytes with the following modifications (13, 25):

Step 1. Prepare macrophages as described in preceding sections. Resuspend in GBSS with 2% human serum albumin at a concentration of 10^6 macrophages/ml.

Step 2. A 20% solution of *untreated* serum in GBSS is used as the chemotactic agent.

Step 3. An 8-μm pore size filter is used.

Step 4. The chambers are incubated for 3 to 5 h.

LITERATURE CITED

1. Ansley, H., and L. Ornstein. 1970. Enzyme histochemistry and differential white cell counts on the technicon hemalog$_{TM}$ D. Adv. Automated Anal. 1:5–15.

2. Axline, S. G., and E. P. Reaven. 1974. Inhibition of phagocytosis and plasma membrane mobility of the cultivated macrophage by cytochalasin B. J. Cell Biol. 62:647–659.

3. Boyden, S. 1962. The chemotactic effect of mixtures of antibody and antigen on polymorphonuclear leukocytes. J. Exp. Med. 115:453–466.

4. Boyum, A. 1968. Isolation of mononuclear cells and granulocytes from human blood. Scand. J. Clin. Lab. Invest. 21:77–83 (Suppl. 97).

5. Cline, M. J. 1973. A new white cell test which measures individual phagocyte function in a mixed leukocyte population. I. A neutrophil defect in acute myelocytic leukemia. J. Lab. Clin. Med. 81:311–316.

6. Cline, M. J. 1975. The white cell. Harvard University Press, Cambridge.

7. Cohen, A. B., and M. J. Cline. 1971. The human alveolar macrophage: isolation, cultivation in vitro, and functional characteristics. J. Clin. Invest. 50:1390–1398.

8. Diamond, R. D., R. K. Root, and J. E. Bennett. 1972. Factors influencing killing of *Cryptococcus neoformans* by human leukocytes in vitro. J. Infect. Dis. 125:367–376.

9. Finley, T. N., and A. J. Ladman, 1972. Low yield of pulmonary surfactant in cigarette smokers. N. Engl. J. Med. 286:223–227.

10. Gallin, J. I., R. A. Clark, and H. R. Kimball. 1973. Granulocyte chemotaxis: an improved in vitro assay employing ^{51}Cr-labeled granulocytes. J. Immunol. **110**:233–240.

11. Golde, D. W., and M. J. Cline. 1973. Growth of human bone marrow in liquid culture. Blood **41**:45–57.

12. Hanifin, J., and M. J. Cline. 1970. Human monocytes and macrophages. Interaction with antigen and lymphocytes. J. Cell Biol. **46**:97–105.

13. Hausman, M. S., R. Snyderman, and S. E. Mergenhagen. 1972. Humoral mediators of chemotaxis of mononuclear leukocytes. J. Infect. Dis. **125**:595–602.

14. Hirsch, J. G., and B. Strauss. 1964. Studies on heat-labile opsonin in rabbit serum. J. Immunol. **92**:145–154.

15. Klebanoff, S. J. 1971. Intraleukocytic microbicidal defects. Annu. Rev. Med. **22**:39–62.

16. Lehrer, R. I. 1970. Measurement of candidacidal activity of specific leukocyte types in mixed cell populations. I. Normal, myeloperoxidase-deficient, and chronic granulomatous disease neutrophils. Infect. Immun. **2**:42–47.

17. Lehrer, R. I., and M. J. Cline. 1969. Interaction of *Candida albicans* with human leukocytes and serum. J. Bacteriol. **98**:996–1004.

18. Mason, R. J., T. P. Stossel, and M. Vaughan. 1973. Quantitative studies of phagocytosis by alveolar macrophages. Biochim. Biophys. Acta **304**:864–870.

19. Nathan, C. F., M. L. Karnovsky, and J. R. David. 1971. Alterations of macrophage functions by mediators from lymphocytes. J. Exp. Med. **133**:1356–1376.

20. Nelson, D. S. (ed.). 1976. Immunobiology of the macrophage. Academic Press, Inc. New York.

21. Ratzan, K. R., D. M. Musher, G. T. Keusch, and L. Weinstein. 1972. Correlation of increased metabolic activity, resistance to infection, enhanced phagocytosis, and inhibition of bacterial growth by macrophages from *Listeria*- and BCG-infected mice. Infect. Immun. **5**:499–504.

22. Snyderman, R., L. C. Altman, M. S. Hausman, and S. E. Mergenhagen. 1972. Human mononuclear leukocyte chemotaxis: a quantitative assay for humoral and cellular chemotactic factors. J. Immunol. **108**:857–860.

23. Steigbigel, R. T., L. H. Lambert, Jr., and J. S. Remington. 1974. Phagocytic and bactericidal properties of normal human monocytes. J. Clin. Invest. **53**:131–142.

24. Thomas, W. R., P. G. Holt, and D. Keast. 1974. Phagocytosis and processing of bacteria by peritoneal macrophages. RES, J. Reticuloendothel. Soc. **15**:16–21.

25. Wilkinson, P. C., J. F. Borel, V. J. Stecher-Levin, and E. Sorkin. 1969. Macrophage and neutrophil specific chemotactic factors in serum. Nature (London) **222**:244–247.

Chapter 17

Phagocytosis

THOMAS P. STOSSEL AND MARILYN TAYLOR

INTRODUCTION

Neutrophil hypofunction is a cause of recurrent pyogenic infection. To combat pyogenic infection, neutrophils must respond to chemotactic factors by locomoting toward the source of inflammation, must ingest microorganisms, and must kill them. Many microbes resist ingestion because they are not recognized by neutrophils. Serum interacts with most of these microorganisms and deposits opsonins on them which render them palatable to the neutrophils. During ingestion, granules in the neutrophil cytoplasm fuse with the membrane of the vacuole forming around the microbe and discharge their contents into the vacuole. Some of this material ends up in the medium surrounding the neutrophil. Since the granules disappear during this process, it is called degranulation. The granule contents include hydrolytic enzymes, bactericidal proteins, and myeloperoxidase. Myeloperoxidase, in combination with hydrogen peroxide and other oxygen metabolites such as superoxide anions, is extremely active in killing ingested microorganisms (9).

Since susceptibility to infection is as much determined by the exposure to the pathogen as by the status of the host, the clinical presentation of patients with neutrophil abnormalities may vary enormously, and the laboratory assessment is an essential feature in diagnosis. The approach to chemotactic functions of neutrophils is covered in chapter 5 of this *Manual*. This chapter will focus on assessment of ingestion, degranulation, and neutrophil oxygen metabolism.

Many of the tests commonly used for evaluating neutrophil function have been devised or successfully applied in the setting of clear-cut, usually genetic disorders where certain neutrophil functions were grossly impaired. Some of these tests are not necessarily applicable to more subtle types of neutrophil dysfunction. The degranulation and oxygen metabolism rates are determined by the magnitude of membrane stimulation, usually the ingestion rate. Therefore, it is important that the measurements of degranulation or oxygen metabolism

be correlated with equally precise determinations of the ingestion rate. Finally, the tests to be presented are bioassays which are quite complex and which are subject to a large amount of variability. The laboratory performing the tests must be prepared to do adequate numbers of control determinations for comparison with patients' samples and must be conservative in interpreting the results.

EVALUATION OF INGESTION

The ingestion process may be analyzed qualitatively, semiquantitatively, or quantitatively. The first of these approaches is usually achieved by morphological means. A semiquantitative impression of ingestion can be obtained by microscopic examination of the phagocytic process, but the error factor is large. The methods which involve inactivation of a population of bacteria by phagocytes can also be considered semiquantitative because of the complexity of systems utilized. True quantitation of ingestion is attained with chemically or radiochemically measurable substrates for phagocytosis. The factors that are important for accurate determination of true phagocytic rates have been discussed elsewhere (5, 10). Rate in this context refers to initial rates of particle uptake as opposed to phagocytic capacity. The latter is measured when the incubation period is sufficiently long and the particle concentration high enough to allow the cells to surfeit themselves. If the particle concentration is low, it may not be known whether rate or capacity is being determined. Detailed time course studies under such conditions are preferable to single time determinations but are still not as reliable as measurement of initial rates. It is preferable to measure the accumulation of particles within cells rather than the disappearance of particles from the extracellular medium. In the former case, uningested particles are usually removed, and therefore it is possible to use saturating quantities of particles. Initial rates of ingestion can then be determined by use of short incubation periods since the base line is zero. When the disappearance of extracellular particles is measured, long incubation periods are required if large particle concentrations are used, since it is difficult to measure small changes in large quantities. This approach is acceptable if the differences in ingestion among various experimental conditions are great. Subtle alterations may go undetected. Certain kinetic data must be obtained for a given test system. These should include: proportionality of ingestion rate with cell concentration, proportionality of the ingestion rate with particle concentration at low particle to cell ratios, and independence of ingestion rate with respect to particle concentration at high particle to cell ratios. This latter point is especially important because the ability to demonstrate independence from particle concentration implies that nonspecific adherence of particles to cells is not being confused with true engulfment. Also relevant to this issue is the ability to demonstrate complete inhibition of ingestion by incubating cells and particles together at zero degrees or with high concentrations of metabolic inhibitors.

When the rate of ingestion of particles requiring opsonization is under investigation, a complex interaction comes into consideration. The opsonic activity of serum is first exerted upon the particle, altering it in such a way that its entry into the cell is facilitated. If all reagents, i.e., cells, opsonin source, and test particles, are incubated simultaneously, the measured rate of ingestion will in actuality be a combination of two rates, opsonization and ingestion. Different variables introduced into such a system may influence one process and not the other. Therefore, it is best to design experiments in such a way, e.g., by preincubating the particles with the opsonin source, that the rates may be separated.

EVALUATION OF DEGRANULATION

Degranulation may be assessed by measuring the rate of appearance of granule-associated enzymes in phagocytic vacuoles, in the extracellular medium, or both. The first may be determined in a semiquantitative manner by histochemical techniques with light or electron microscopy used to visualize the results. Quantitative assessment of intravacuolar degranulation is possible by means of techniques in which phagocytic vacuoles are isolated in pure form and the quantity of granule-associated enzyme in them is compared with the amount of ingested material also in the phagosomes (11). Extracellular degranulation is quantified by measuring granule-associated enzymes appearing in the extracellular medium (12). Although

it has not been proven that the extracellular secretion of granule contents is absolutely correlated with intravacuolar degranulation, this approach is the simplest.

EVALUATION OF NEUTROPHIL OXYGEN METABOLISM

In recent years, attention has been directed at metabolic perturbations thought to be associated with phagocytic microbicidal activity, particularly those having to do with the generation of hydrogen peroxide. This interest has been stimulated by recognition of the antimicrobial activity of hydrogen peroxide and its potentiation by myeloperoxidase, and by discovery of a syndrome, chronic granulomatous disease, in which phagocytes of patients with recurrent infections fail to produce hydrogen peroxide and other oxygen metabolites (3). In addition to its significance for phagocytic functions related to inactivation of ingested microbes, activation of oxygen metabolism is a useful indirect marker for the ingestion process per se. Precise quantitative methods for direct measurement of hydrogen peroxide and superoxide under conditions of phagocytosis are currently available (7), but related processes including hexose monophosphate shunt activity, nitroblue tetrazolium (NBT) reduction (1), and iodination (6) can be quantified effectively.

SPECIFIC TESTS

Assay for the rate of ingestion by blood phagocytes (neutrophils, bands, and monocytes) and simultaneous assay of the rate of ingestion and of nitroblue tetrazolium reduction

Principle. Phagocytic cells isolated from human blood are fed *Escherichia coli* lipopolysaccharide-coated paraffin oil droplets containing oil red O. The phagocytes ingest these particles only if the particles are first treated with fresh human serum which opsonizes them by depositing C3 on the particle surfaces in a form that makes them palatable. The rate of ingestion of the opsonized particles by the cells is constant for 5 min. After cells and particles have been incubated for 5 min, the uningested oil particles, because of their low density, are efficiently separated from the cells containing ingested particles by centrifugation: the cells sediment and the unengulfed particles float. Oil red O is extracted from the washed cell pellets with dioxane and spectrophotometrically measured. This system measures true ingestion rates as discussed above in the Introduction (8).

During ingestion, superoxide anions are formed. When NBT, a yellow redox compound, is present in the extracellular medium, it is swept into the phagocytic vacuole with the ingested particle, and there it is reduced by the superoxide anions. The reduction product of NBT, a purple insoluble formazan, can be extracted with the dioxane solution used to extract the oil red O. The optical density (OD) of the formazan is determined at a different wavelength from that of oil red O.

Preparation of phagocytes. Blood is collected in ACD anticoagulant, 2 ml per 8 ml of blood. The large amount of anticoagulant prevents platelet clumping which fosters leukocyte agglutination. One duplicate assay can easily be performed with 8 ml of blood although, if available, 16 ml is preferable. Then 6% dextran 75 in isotonic saline (McGaw Laboratories, Glendale, Calif.) is taken into the syringe (0.5 volume per volume of blood), the syringe is stood on its hub, and the erythrocytes settle at room temperature (45 to 60 min is usually required). After settling, the supernatant plasma is expressed through a bent venipuncture needle into 50-ml plastic conical centrifuge tubes (15 ml per tube). A sample is taken for differential count (the morphology is well preserved at this point). Ice-cold 0.87% ammonium chloride is added (35 ml), and the tubes are inverted once and immediately centrifuged (80 × g for 10 min). The ammonium chloride solution lyses erythrocytes remaining. The lysis is relatively inefficient, but it is gentle and has less damaging effects on the leukocytes than hypotonic lysis. The cell buttons are suspended in ice-cold isotonic saline, pooled, and washed once with isotonic saline (centrifuge at 800 × g for 10 min). If a delay in performing the assay is anticipated, the cells can be kept for several hours in cold saline or plasma—this is better than buffered media with divalent cations which allow for clumping. The final cell buttons are suspended in any buffered isotonic medium with divalent cations (Krebs-Ringer phosphate, Hanks balanced salt solution, etc.) such that the leukocyte count is about 20,000 to 60,000/mm³. With experience the count can be approximated by judging the turbidity of the suspension. A sample is taken for cell count at this time.

Preparation of paraffin oil plus oil red O. Approximately 2 g of oil red O (Allied Chemical, Morristown, N.J.) is added to 50 ml of *heavy* paraffin oil (mineral oil; Fisher Scientific Co., Fair Lawn, N.J.) in a large porcelain mortar and ground with a pestle. The saturated suspension is centrifuged in plastic tubes (top speed in a Sorvall or International clinical centrifuge) to remove undissolved dye (which can be reutilized). The dye-containing paraffin oil is stable and can be stored indefinitely at room temperature. Since the amount of dye in the oil varies, a factor is computed which converts OD to milligrams of paraffin oil to permit normalization and comparison of results. A 10-μliter amount of oil red O-paraffin oil is added to 10 ml of dioxane, and the OD at 525 nm is determined. The following formula gives the conversion factor, the units of which are mg/OD:

$$0.89/OD$$

where 0.89 is the density of the paraffin oil and OD is the actual reading.

Preparation of particles. To prepare the droplets, dissolve 40 mg of *E. coli* lipopolysaccharide O26:B6 (Boivin preparation; Difco catalogue no. 3920-25) in 3 ml of balanced salt solution in a 10- to 15-ml glass or thick-walled plastic test tube, and disperse the lipopolysaccharide by brief sonic treatment (any model Sonifier will do). Layer 1 ml of the paraffin oil-oil red O over the aqueous lipopolysaccharide suspension, and sonically treat the mixture. The Sonifier probe should be just below the oil-aqueous interface; the length of sonic treatment is about 90 s, just until the tube becomes hot to handle. The output can be low; the sonic treatment details are unimportant except that it is better to err on the side of treating too long. The final preparation should look like a strawberry milkshake. The particle suspension can be used immediately (after cooling) or frozen. Brief sonic treatment after thawing is advisable.

Opsonization. The particles are opsonized, usually just before the ingestion step, by adding an equal volume of fresh human serum and incubating the mixture at 37 C for 25 to 30 min. Maximal C3 deposition has occurred by that time; if the particles are allowed to sit longer in serum, proteolytic activity slowly removes the opsonically active C3. Therefore, the opsonized particles must be kept cold, frozen, or washed (see below) until use. Opsonized particles can be frozen and thawed and are still palatable to the phagocytes.

Ingestion. To assay ingestion, add 0.2 volume of opsonized particle suspension (prewarmed to 37 C) to 0.8 volume of cell suspension (also prewarmed). The reaction can be started by adding either particles to cells or cells to particles. The reaction can be run in siliconized glass 15-ml conical centrifuge tubes in a system with a total volume of 1 ml (in which case 0.2 ml of particles is added to 0.8 ml of cell suspension). After 5 min, during which the tubes are occasionally tapped to keep the actors in suspension, add 6 ml of ice-cold isotonic saline containing 1 mM N-ethylmaleimide (126 mg/liter), which poisons the cells and stops ingestion. Centrifuge the tubes at $250 \times g$ (1,000 rpm for 10 min in a centrifuge with 19-cm radius). Dislodge the rim of uningested particles at the top by shaking the tube vertically; discard the supernatant fluid, but do not drain the pellets completely. The small amount of residual supernatant fluid is used to suspend the cell pellet by tapping the bottom of the tube. Add more N-ethylmaleimide-saline, and repeat the washing. After the second wash, discard the supernatant fluid, invert the tubes to drain the pellets, and, finally, wipe the sides of the tubes with tissue. To disrupt the cell pellets and make the oil red O soluble, add 1 or more ml of dioxane with tapping or vortexing of the tubes. Centrifuge the extracts at $500 \times g$ for 15 min to remove debris, and read the OD of the extracts in a colorimeter or spectrophotometer at a wavelength of 525 nm against a dioxane blank.

Combined assay of NBT reduction and ingestion. NBT (nitroblue tetrazolium; Sigma Chemical Co., St. Louis, Mo.) is "dissolved" in balanced salt solution at a concentration of 2 mg/ml. In fact, the solubility of this material is variable and only about 0.6 mg ends up dissolved in 1 ml. The solution-suspension therefore must be carefully filtered, either through an apparatus with 0.8-μm pores (Millipore Corp.) or through Whatman no. 1 filter paper. If sterile equipment is used, the former technique has the advantage that the filtrate can be considered sterile and stored in lots for longer periods of time than unsterile solution, since the balanced salt solution promotes microbial growth. It is important that microbial contamination be minimized, since bacteria will enhance NBT reduction by the cells.

Incubations are set up as follows:

	Tube 1	Tube 2
Opsonized particles	0.2 ml	0.2 ml
Cell suspension	0.4 ml	0.4 ml
Balanced salt solution	0.4 ml	—
NBT in balanced salt solution	None	0.4 ml

The reaction is started by adding the cells to the other premixed, prewarmed reagents. Tube 1 gives the ingestion rate, and tube 2 gives the NBT reduction rate. The rest of the assay is done as described above except that the NBT-formazan must be extracted with dioxane by heating the tube in a boiling-water bath for 15 to 30 min. The optical density of NBT-formazan is read at 580 nm and converted to micrograms of formazan by multiplying the OD by 14.14.

Calculation of results.

$$\frac{OD_{525} \times \text{conversion factor}}{\text{time of} \atop \text{incubation} \times \text{phagocytic cells in} \atop \text{total system} \times 10^7} = \text{initial ingestion rate}$$

where the phagocytic cells in the total system include polymorphonuclear leukocytes, bands, and monocytes, and the initial ingestion rate is expressed in milligrams of paraffin oil per 10^7 phagocytes per minute.

To determine NBT reduction, the OD of tube 1 at 580 nm must be substracted from that of tube 2, since oil red O absorbs somewhat at 580 nm. Thus

$$\frac{OD_{580} \text{ of tube } 2 - OD_{580} \text{ of tube } 1 \times 14.14}{\text{time of incubation} \times \text{phagocytic cells} \times 10^7}$$
$$= \text{initial NBT reduction rate}$$

where the initial NBT reduction rate is expressed in micrograms of formazan per 10^7 phagocytes per minute.

Comments. Depending on the question being asked, one may wish to compare different sera against a set of control cells, to compare the same serum against different cells, or to test a patient's serum and cells together as a screening procedure.

If assay of serum opsonic activity is in question, the number of samples can be markedly increased by obtaining 30 to 50 ml of blood from a consenting individual with neutrophilia secondary to acute infection. Since the ingestion rate per cell may be increased in infected patients, several control sera (or pooled control serum) should be tested against the test sera, and then the results are compared for that day's determination. External comparisons can be made in that setting by keeping lots of frozen (-70 C) control or pooled control sera and including a sample in each run.

As discussed above, there is marked variation in test results because of the many factors that contribute to the final value. Figure 1 shows a frequency distribution for ingestion rates of 57 control determinations. In our laboratory we do not consider an initial ingestion rate abnormal that is greater than 0.05 mg of paraffin oil ingested per 10^7 phagocytes/min.

Patients with chronic granulomatous disease have ratios of NBT reduction/ingestion that are less than 1.5. In some families, the inheritance of this disease is X-linked, and mothers of patients have a population of cells which do not reduce NBT in accordance with the Lyon hypothesis. These "carriers" have ratios that range from 1.5 to 3, which does overlap with the

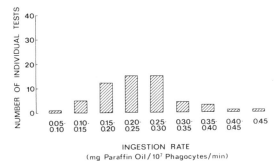

FIG. 1. *Frequency distribution of initial ingestion rates by normal blood phagocytes of lipopolysaccharide-coated paraffin oil droplets opsonized with the phagocyte donors' serum.*

lower limit of normal (2.5). The ratios vary enormously and are high in acute inflammatory states. We do not attempt to interpret the meaning of high reduction/ingestion ratios in our laboratory. Absent NBT reduction has also been found for neutrophils of rare patients lacking neutrophil glucose-6-phosphate dehydrogenase (9). These patients behave clinically in a similar way to patients with chronic granulomatous disease.

Assay of degranulation by measurement of extracellular release of β-glucuronidase activity

Preparation of phagocytes and particles. Peripheral blood phagocytes are prepared as described above. Particles are also prepared and opsonized as described except that fluorochemical liquid, FC 80 (Minnesota Mining & Mfg. Co., St. Paul, Minn.), is substituted for the paraffin oil containing oil red O. This heavy liquid results in an emulsion of heavy particles which sediment easily during centrifugation. The effect of these particles on degranulation can be compared with the ingestion rate of paraffin oil particles assayed as described above.

Incubation. About 10^7 leukocytes are incubated in small plastic test tubes (Falcon Plastics Co.) in 0.8 ml of balanced salt solution for 5 min in a shaking water bath at 37 C. Opsonized lipopolysaccharide-coated fluorochemical liquid particles, prewarmed at the same time, are added (0.2 ml) to the cell suspensions (zero time). At 15 and 30 min, the tubes are cooled on ice and then centrifuged in a refrigerated centrifuge at $250 \times g$ for 10 min. The supernatant fluid contains the extracellular medium to be assayed for enzyme activity. A 0.5-ml amount of this fluid is aspirated and kept on ice until

assayed later the same day or else frozen at -20 C until assay at a later date. The enzyme is stable in the frozen state for months. Controls to be included in each run are 0.2 ml of balanced salt solution added at zero time in place of opsonized particles and 0.2 ml of particles which have not been opsonized. Each incubation condition should be run at least in duplicate.

Assay of enzyme activity. A substrate mixture is prepared by dissolving 31.5 mg of p-nitrophenyl-β-glucuronide (Sigma Chemical Co.) and 100 μliters of Triton-X 100 (Packard Instrument Co., Downers Grove, Ill.) in 100 ml of 0.05 M sodium acetate-acetic acid buffer, pH 5. The substrate mixture can be kept frozen at -20 C and thawed before each use. Enzyme assay incubations consist of 0.9 ml of substrate mix to which 0.1 ml of sample is added. The mixtures are incubated for 18 h (overnight) at 37 C. The reaction is terminated by addition of 2 ml of 0.1 N NaOH. The OD of the solution is determined spectrophotometrically at 410 nm.

Calculation of results. For the system described:

$$(OD_{410} \times 20)/(1.84 \times 18)$$

gives the number of nanomoles generated per hour at each time of sampling by 10^7 leukocytes.

As mentioned previously, the results of degranulation assays are best expressed as a function of the initial ingestion rate assayed as described above. Then the results can be expressed as degranulation (nanomoles of p-nitrophenyl-β-glucuronide released at a given time per milligram of paraffin oil ingested per minute).

EVALUATION OF NEUTROPHIL BACTERICIDAL ACTIVITY

The basis of bactericidal tests is the rapid killing of the test organisms once placed in the cytoplasm of the phagocyte or the removal of the bacteria from the extracellular medium. The method of Maaløe (4) with various modifications (2) has been extensively employed.

The bactericidal assay measures the end point of several processes including opsonization, ingestion, and the metabolic alterations prerequisite for bacterial killing. The limitations of this approach include those mentioned above having to do with separation of ingestion from nonspecific adherence. Because of the diverse number of processes involved, the interpretation of the final killing "rate" is somewhat difficult. Moreover, the test requires prolonged incubation times since the disappearance of viability is determined under nonsaturating conditions. For this reason, agglutination of phagocytes and of bacteria on phagocytes or membranes can occur. A clump of bacteria will produce a single colony, thus leading to an underestimation of the number of viable organisms actually present. The test is most useful when the anticipated experimental conditions will yield a result that is much different from that of the controls. A description of the technique is included because of its widespread use. It is a tricky, laborious test which should only be performed by those familiar with bacteriological methodology and the pitfalls of interpreting the test.

Reagents

1. Bacteria grown overnight in Trypticase soy broth (or other, depending on the organism), centrifuged, washed, and adjusted in salt solution to an appropriate concentration by turbidimetry at 650 nm.
2. Bovine albumin, 100 mg/liter in distilled water.
3. Nutrient agar.

Organisms may be harvested at any phase of the growth cycle. If taken at the early lag phase, populations usually remain stable in phagocytic systems for a period of 1 to 2 h. In contrast, lag-phase organisms will begin multiplying within 1 h and, unless the period of phagocytosis is short, will alter the initial multiplicity of bacteria/phagocyte. It is usually simpler to harvest from liquid media since the bacteria can be collected by centrifugation, are not in large clumps, and may be easily washed. Solutions used to wash and resuspend viable organisms are similar to those employed for phagocytes. Certain bacteria are rapidly killed in saline or balanced salt solution. This bactericidal action can be reversed by the addition of as little as 0.01% bovine serum albumin.

The quantitation of viable populations may be performed by a number of methods. The most rigorous is colony counting after preparing pour plates or streaking a measured sample on the surface of quadrant plates. If the same cultural conditions are employed from day to day, it is easier to assay the optical density of the washed suspension at 650 nm and construct a standard curve of OD versus viable units. When late lag-phase organisms are employed, there may be many nonviable bacteria which influence the nephelometric method but go undetected by plate counts. Under these conditions it is best to do a total particle count with a Petroff-Hausser counting chamber.

Procedure

Phagocytes suspended in balanced salt solution are dispensed to sterile siliconized 15×150 mm tubes. Serum and bacteria are then added to appropriate concentrations, and the tubes are sealed and mixed. The total volume of each tube is 2.0 ml and contains 20×10^6 to 30×10^6 phagocytes/ml, 10^6 to 30×10^6 bacteria/ml, and concentrations of serum ranging from 1 to 50% depending on the nature of the experiment. It is usually best to employ not more than three bacteria/phagocyte and to use lag-phase organisms which do not multiply readily. The tubes are then incubated at 37 C either in a reciprocating water bath or end over end in a warm room. At varying periods of time from 0 to 3 or more h, samples are removed to measure (i) the total viable bacterial population, (ii) the extracellular population, and (ii) the cell-associated organisms.

The total count is obtained by diluting 0.01 to 0.2 ml of the suspension in the dilute albumin solution and homogenizing to disrupt the leukocytes. Homogenization can be performed with a high-speed Teflon pestle in a tight-fitting tube. Serial 10-fold dilutions are then prepared and plated either on the surface of nutrient agar or by pour plate techniques. This procedure liberates most organisms and is an index of both intracellular and extracellular viable bacteria.

Simultaneously, a 1.0-ml sample is taken to evaluate extracellular and cell-associated microorganisms. This sample is diluted 1:5 with cold salt solution and centrifuged for 3 to 4 min at $45 \times g$. This deposits the leukocytes, leaving a clear supernatant fluid, a sample of which is plated for the extracellular population. The pellet is then resuspended in buffer, homogenized, and plated to obtain cell-associated bacteria. The number of viable organisms per milliliter in the original suspension is then calculated, and each of the three bacterial counts per sample is plotted semilogarithmically.

Appropriate controls must be conducted to rule out: (i) an extracellular bactericidal effect of the medium, which can be accomplished by incubating bacteria and leukocytes in a stationary system in which contact is minimal, and (ii) major trapping of particles with leukocytes during low-speed centrifugation, which becomes apparent if the difference between total and cell-associated counts at time zero is less than 1 log unit. Under these conditions the "rate" of phagocytosis can be followed for long periods of time, and the influence of components of the medium as well as cell-oriented factors can be evaluated in detail.

ACKNOWLEDGMENTS

This work was supported by Public Health Service grant HL-17742. T.P.S. is an Established Investigator of the American Heart Association.

LITERATURE CITED

1.. Baehner, R. L., and D. G. Nathan. 1968. Quantitative nitroblue tetrazolium test in chronic granulomatous disease. N. Engl. J. Med. **278:**971–976.

2. Cohn, Z. A., and S. I. Morse. 1959. Interactions between rabbit polymorphonuclear leucocytes and staphylococci. J. Exp. Med. **110:**419–443.

3. Johnston, R. B., Jr., and R. L. Baehner. 1971. Chronic granulomatous disease: correlation between pathogenesis and clinical findings. Pediatrics **48:**730–739.

4. Maaløe, O. 1946. On the relation between alexin and opsonin. Ejnar Munksgaard, Copenhagen.

5. Michell, R. H., S. J. Pancake, J. Noseworthy, and M. L. Karnovsky. 1969. Measurement of rates of phagocytosis: the use of cellular monolayers. J. Cell Biol. **40:**216–224.

6. Pincus, S. H., and S. J. Klebanoff. 1971. Quantitative leukocyte iodination. N. Engl. J. Med. **284:**744–750.

7. Root, R. K., J. Metcalf, N. Oshino, and B. Chance. 1975. H_2O_2 release from human granulocytes during phagocytosis. I. Documentation, quantitation, and some regulating factors. J. Clin. Invest. **55:**945–955.

8. Stossel, T. P. 1973. Evaluation of opsonic and leukocyte function with a spectrophotometric test in patients with infection and with phagocytic disorders. Blood **42:**121–130.

9. Stossel, T. P. 1974. Phagocytosis. N. Engl. J. Med. **290:**717–723, 774–780, 833–839.

10. Stossel, T. P. 1975. Phagocytosis: recognition and ingestion. Semin. Hematol. **12:**83–116.

11. Stossel, T. P., R. K. Root, and M. Vaughan. 1972. Phagocytosis in chronic granulomatous disease and the Chediak-Higashi syndrome. N. Engl. J. Med. **286:**120–123.

12. Zurier, R. B., S. Hoffstein, and G. Weissmann. 1973. Cytochalasin B: effect on lysosomal enzyme release from human leukocytes. Proc. Natl. Acad. Sci. U.S.A. **70:**844–848.

Chapter 18

Assays of Cell-Mediated Immunity to Viruses

JOSEPH A. BELLANTI, STEPHEN M. PETERS, AND MAREK ROLA-PLESZCZYNSKI

INTRODUCTION

Cell-mediated immunity (CMI) to viruses is now a well-established parameter of host resistance (3). In recent years, tests for the measurement of CMI to specific viruses have become available in many laboratories throughout the world and are providing useful tools for the study of disease susceptibility in humans (4). Most of these assays represent research methods which are at present in an active stage of development in different laboratories. Because of their clinical importance, however, there is every reason to suspect that they will soon become available in most clinical laboratories as licensure and certification of clinical immunology laboratories become a reality.

CLINICAL INDICATIONS

Tests of CMI to viruses should be performed in clinical states in which there is susceptibility to viral infection related to immune deficiency (primary or secondary) or in which congenital, recurrent, latent, or chronic viral infection is suspected. These indications are shown in Table 1 together with their clinical presentation and pathogenetic mechanism(s).

Those patients with primary immune deficiencies, particularly those with depressed T cell function, e.g., DiGeorge syndrome, are unusually predisposed to certain viral infections such as the herpes group. Similarly, patients who have deficient immune function secondary to certain physiological states (e.g., pregnancy) or secondary to disease (e.g., malignancy) or treatment (e.g., steroids, cytotoxic chemicals) also fall prey to recurrent viral infection as a consequence of T cell function. Therefore, any patients who manifest such recurrent viral infection should not only have their general immune status evaluated but should also be tested for specific viral CMI.

Another group which is usually susceptible to viral infection is the fetus and the newborn. This susceptibility derives from a variety of immune deficiencies characteristic of this period, but in particular those of the T cell system. For example, congenital rubella syndrome has been associated not only with deficient lymphoproliferative responses to phytohemagglutinin (PHA) but also with deficiency in specific CMI to rubella virus. Other viruses which are prevalent in this age group include infection with cytomegalovirus and herpes simplex virus types 1 and 2.

In the older age group, recurrent or latent viral infection is not unusual in the general population who otherwise have normal immune function. Recent studies of patients with herpes labialis or herpes genitalis have demonstrated subtle defects of specific CMI to herpesvirus type 1 and type 2, respectively. In any patient with recurrent herpes zoster, a diligent search for underlying lymphoma should be undertaken since this infection may be the heralding sign of this malignancy in which anergy is often seen. In patients with herpes zoster, more subtle defects of specific CMI to varicella-zoster virus may be detected as these patients are studied.

Finally, one of the most recent findings in certain chronic demyelinating central nervous system diseases such as subacute sclerosing panencephalitis and multiple sclerosis has been that of depressed or inhibited CMI responses which appear to be related to the presence of "blocking factors" in both the plasma and cerebrospinal fluid (36). Although the activity of lymphocytes from these patients appears to have normal immune T cell function, their responses appear to be extirpated by the presence of these "blocking factors."

ASSAYS OF CELL-MEDIATED IMMUNITY

At present, there are basically three types of in vitro approach to the study of CMI to viruses: (i) lymphocyte activation, (ii) macrophage inhibition factor (MIF) assay, and (iii) lymphocytotoxicity. Since most of these tests have only recently become available, it is difficult to describe categorically their advantages or pitfalls. Tests of lymphocyte activation are easily performed and measure the "afferent" lymphoproliferative limit of immunity. They suffer from day to day variations owing to fluctuations

155

TABLE 1. *Clinical indications for performing tests of cell-mediated immunity to viruses*

Clinical entity	Clinical presentation	Pathogenetic mechanism(s)
Immune deficiency		
Primary or secondary (pregnancy, steroids, cytotoxic drugs)	Recurrent or severe viral infection (e.g., herpes, vaccinia)	Depressed T cell function
Congenital infection		
Rubella	Congenital rubella syndrome	Depressed virus-specific cell-mediated immunity
Cytomegalovirus (CMV)	Congenital CMV	
Herpes simplex (types 1 and 2)	Neonatal herpes infection	
Recurrent infections		
Herpes simplex (types 1 and 2)	Herpes labialis	Depressed virus-specific cell-mediated immunity
Varicella-zoster (lymphoma)	Herpes genitalis	
	Herpes zoster	
Chronic viral infections		
Subacute sclerosing panencephalitis	Chronic demyelinating central nervous system diseases	Genetic susceptibility; "blocking" factors
Multiple sclerosis		

within a given individual or intercurrent infections which may depress specific responses. Other pitfalls include nonspecific responses due to impurities of the test antigen (e.g., tissue culture contaminants) and the difficulty in maintaining cell viability in long-term cell cultures, particularly in microassay systems. The advantages of the MIF assay are its great sensitivity and its measurement of the efferent limb. It suffers from technical difficulties in performance of the assay and also in nonspecificity due to qualitative differences in antigen preparations. The lymphocytotoxicity assay also measures the "efferent" limb. The great advantages of this assay are its specificity and its ability to be controlled adequately. The lack of available target cells may limit the test, but the recent description of cryopreserved acutely infected target cell lines may alleviate this problem (39). Another theoretical pitfall of the lymphocytotoxicity procedure recently described by Doherty et al. (6) and Zinkernagel and Doherty (46) is a requirement of syngeneic lymphocytes and target cells for maximal sensitivity in animal systems. However, this has not appeared to be a limitation for the lymphocytotoxicity assay in humans.

LYMPHOCYTE ACTIVATION

Antigen-induced lymphocyte transformation has been reported for a wide variety of viruses which are summarized in Table 2. The principle underlying the test procedure is that, upon exposure of specifically sensitized lymphocytes to viral antigen, the cells undergo a series of morphological, biochemical, and biological changes. The increase in deoxyribonucleic acid (DNA) synthesis is usually measured by the incorporation of tritiated thymidine into the

newly synthesized DNA. Both T and B lymphocytes are involved in the lymphoproliferative response to antigen, although T cells appear to play a more important role. The presence of adherent cells, e.g., macrophages, has been shown to be essential for maximal stimulation in this assay, although further work is required.

Materials and reagents

Medium. Medium for leukocyte cultures and for dilution of all reagents consists of RPMI 1640 medium with glutamine (Grand Island Biological Co., Grand Island, N.Y.) supplemented with heat-inactivated fetal calf serum (in varying concentrations ranging from 10 to 50%), 100 units of penicillin/ml, and 100 μg of streptomycin/ml.

Preparation of leukocytes. A variety of methods currently available for the purification of lymphocytes for use in the in vitro assays of CMI are described in chapter 8. The most widely used technique is the Hypaque-Ficoll method. Briefly, whole blood is obtained by venipuncture under aseptic conditions into heparinized syringes (20 units/ml of blood). Purified suspensions of lymphocytes are obtained from the Hypaque-Ficoll gradient after centrifugation at $400 \times g$ for 40 min. This method yields approximately 2×10^6 mononuclear cells/ml of peripheral blood with a purity averaging 90% lymphocytes and 10% monocytes.

Test antigens. Test antigens vary according to the viral antigen employed, as shown in Table 2. The viral antigens can be prepared in the laboratory or can be purchased from several commercial vendors including the following:

Rubella (complement-fixing antigen)—Microbiological Associates, Inc., Bethesda, Md.; Flow Laboratories, Rockville, Md.

TABLE 2. *Lymphocyte activation assays used for measurement of specific cell-mediated immunity to viruses in the human*

Virus	Source of test antigen	Status of antigen[a]	Reference
Togaviruses			
Sindbis[b]	Suckling mouse brain	L	Griffin and Johnson (13)
Venezuelan equine encephalitis[b]	Mouse spleen cells	I	Adler and Rabinowitz (1), Rabinowitz and Proctor (22)
Dengue[c]	Monkey kidney tissue (LLC-MK2)	I	Halstead et al. (14)
Rubella	Baby hamster kidney (BHK-21)		Smith et al. (34)
Herpesviruses			
Cytomegalovirus	Human embryonic lung (WI-38)	L	Thurman et al. (41)
Epstein-Barr virus	Human lymphoid cell line ("AV")	I	Gerber and Lucas (9)
Herpes simplex type 1	Primary rabbit kidney (PRK)	I	Rosenberg et al. (26, 27)
Herpes simplex type 2	Hamster embryo fibroblasts (HEF)	I	Rapp and Duff (24)
Varicella	Human embryonic lung	I	Russell et al. (29)
Paramyxoviruses			
Subacute sclerosing panencephalitis (SSPE)	SSPE-infected HeLa cells	L	Thurman et al. (41)
Rubeola	Monkey kidney cells (Vero)	I	Graziano et al. (11)
Mumps	Chicken embryo	I	Smith et al. (33)
Orthomyxovirus			
Influenza	PR-8-infected mouse lung tissue	L	Hellman et al. (15)
Rhabdovirus			
Rabies	Baby hamster kidney (BHK-S13)	I	Wiktor et al. (44)
Hepatitis virus			
Hepatitis B	Hepatitis B-antigen rich serum	L	Pettigrew et al. (21)
Poxvirus			
Vaccinia	Primary rabbit kidney (PRK)	I	Rosenberg et al. (25, 27)

[a] L = live; I = inactivated.
[b] In mice.
[c] In monkeys.

Rubeola (complement-fixing antigen)—Microbiological Associates, Inc.

Mumps (complement-fixing antigen)—Microbiological Associates, Inc.

Mumps (skin test antigen)—Eli Lilly & Co. Indianapolis, Ind.

A number of recent studies have indicated that the use of whole cells or cell membrane-associated antigens may be preferable or even essential for the measurement of lymphoproliferative responses to viruses. This may allow the detection of CMI which could not be measured with the use of non-cell-associated antigens. A control antigen consisting of tissue cultures derived from uninfected parent lines should also be included for the measurement of background activity.

For every viral antigen tested a dose reponse curve should be established in which different dilutions of test antigen are employed at different incubation periods, e.g., 3 to 7 days, in order to obtain optimal concentrations of antigens and incubation times for use in the test system.

Radionuclides. Tritium-labeled thymidine (^{3}[H]thymidine, 18 to 20 Ci/mmol) can be ob-

tained from New England Nuclear Corp., Boston, Mass., or Amersham-Searle Corp., Arlington Heights, Ill.

Test procedure

The details of the test procedure are described in chapter 9. Although both macro- and microassays are available, most laboratories utilize microassay procedures because of their simplicity, reproducibility, and economy.

The following is a brief description of the microassay procedure used in our laboratory. To each of 12 wells of a microtest tissue culture plate (Falcon Plastics) is added 0.1 ml of leukocyte suspension containing 10^6 cells/ml; an additional 0.1 ml of test antigen, control antigen, or medium is then added to each of 3 additional wells. A 0.1-ml amount of a 0.1% solution of PHA is added to an additional 3 wells as a positive control of nonspecific lymphoproliferation. All plates are covered with sterile plastic lids and incubated at 37 C for 72 h in a 5% CO_2 atmosphere.

After incubation, 1 μCi of [^{3}H]thymidine is added to each culture for the final hours of incubation. The cells are washed and collected in a multiple automated sample harvester (MASH II, Microbiological Associates Inc.) designed to harvest, wash, and separate the cells from supernatant fluid. After harvesting, the aspirated cell suspensions are collected on individual disks, transferred to vials containing scintillation fluid, and counted in a liquid scintillation spectrometer.

The results are expressed either as the mean counts per minute of triplicate cultures or as the ratio (stimulation ratio) of counts per minute of [³H]thymidine incorporated in the presence of test antigen divided by the counts per minute of [³H]thymidine incorporated in the presence of medium or control antigen as follows:

$$\text{stimulation index} = \frac{\text{counts/min in test antigen}}{\text{counts/min in control antigen}}$$

Stimulation indices vary with different viral antigens. However, indices from 2-fold to 30-fold have been considered normal.

MIGRATION INHIBITION FACTOR ASSAY

The inhibition of macrophage migration in vitro has been shown to be a useful correlate of delayed-type hypersensitivity to a wide variety of antigens, but has had limited application to the study of CMI to viruses. Some of the presently described assays are shown in Table 3. The principle underlying the procedure is that specifically sensitized lymphocytes upon exposure to viral antigen release a soluble factor which inhibits the migration of macrophages (MIF) or leukocytes (LIF). A variety of techniques are available for the specific assays and are described in chapters 10 and 11. These include the indirect MIF assay and the agarose plate method. The following is a brief description of the LIF assay described by Ütermohlen and Zabriskie (42).

Materials and reagents

Medium. Medium for the leukocyte cultures and dilution of all reagents consists of Eagle's-Earle's balanced salt solution (BSS) supplemented with 20% fetal calf serum (Flow Laboratories).

Preparation of leukocytes. Under aseptic conditions, whole venous blood is collected by venipuncture into heparinized syringes (20 units/ml) and mixed with a solution of 2% Knox gelatin in 0.15 M NaCl. After sedimentation at 37 C at a 45° slant for 15 min and upright for 5 min, the leukocyte-rich plasma is removed and centrifuged at $700 \times g$ for 10 min. The pellet is then treated with 0.85% NH₄Cl for 5 to 10 min to lyse residual erythrocytes. The leukocytes are then washed three times in saline and concentrated in Eagle's-Earle's BSS to 20×10^7 leukocytes per ml.

Test antigens. Test antigens vary but essentially consist of tissue culture-derived viral antigens which can be either prepared in the laboratory or purchased commercially (Table 3). In the case of measles, rubella, and parainfluenza I, the test antigens are further purified by freeze-thawing the virus-infected cells, followed by sonic treatment and mild centrifugation to remove large cellular debris. The supernatant fluids containing the viral antigen are used as the test antigen. None of the antigens contains preservatives. Control antigens consist of uninfected parental cell lines treated in an identical fashion.

Test procedures

Samples of leukocyte suspensions are loaded into 20-μliter capillaries. The bottom of the capillary is sealed with clay, and the capillar-

TABLE 3. *Assays for migration inhibition factor in the assessment of cell-mediated immunity to viruses in the human*

Virus	Source of test antigen	Reference
Togavirus		
Rubella	BHK-21	Ütermohlen and Zabriskie (42)
Herpes virus		
Herpes simplex type 1	Monkey kidney tissue	Wilton et al. (45)
Paramyxoviruses		
Measles	African green monkey kidney	Ütermohlen and Zabriskie (42)
Parainfluenza type 1	Embryonated chicken egg	Ütermohlen and Zabriskie (42)
Orthomyxovirus		
Influenza	Embryonated chicken egg	Waldman et al. (43)
Hepatitis virus		
Hepatitis B	Hepatitis-antigen positive serum	Gerber et al. (10)

ies are then centrifuged at $300 \times g$ for 10 min. The capillaries are cut at the medium-cell interface, and the pieces containing the cell pellets are placed in planchettes (York Scientific, Ogdensburg, N.Y.) to which appropriate concentrations of test antigen or control antigen (e.g., 1:10 or 1:100) are added. The planchettes are covered with glass cover slips, sealed with stopcock grease or paraffin, and incubated at 37 C for 18 h. The resultant fans are projected onto tracing paper, cut out, and weighed; the area is directly proportional to the weight.

The migration inhibition index (MII) is calculated as follows:

$$MII = 100 - \left[\frac{\text{leukocyte migration in antigen-stimulated supernatant}}{\text{leukocyte migration in control-stimulated supernatant}} \times 100 \right]$$

Migration inhibition indices greater than 15% are considered indicative of significant CMI.

LYMPHOCYTOTOXICITY

Among the several techniques available for the study of specific CMI to viruses is the assay of in vitro lymphocyte-mediated cytotoxicity employing the release of ^{51}Cr from virus-infected cell lines. These assays have been derived from techniques originally described in tumor and transplantation immunology. Lymphocytotoxicity assays have now been developed for a number of viral agents, some representatives of which are shown in Table 4. The principle underlying this procedure is that, following the interaction of specifically sensitized lymphocytes with viral antigens on the surface of acutely or persistently infected tissue culture lines, a sequence of events leads to the lysis of infected target cells which can be measured either by morphological techniques or through the release of radiolabled cytoplasmic constituents from these cells. The morphological changes which are seen in tests of viral lymphocytotoxicity to measles virus are shown in Fig. 1.

TABLE 4. *Characteristics of viruses and cell culture lines used in lymphocytotoxicity assays of cell-mediated immunity to viruses in the human*

Virus	Cell culture line	Infection[a]	Reference
Togaviruses			
Sindbis[b]	Mouse embryo fibroblasts	A	McFarland (19)
Rubella	Baby hamster kidney (BHK-21)	P	Steele et al. (37)
Herpesviruses			
Cytomegalovirus	Human lung fibroblasts (WI-38)	A	Thong et al. (39)
Herpes simplex type 1	Human prostatic adenoma (MA-160)	P	Thong et al. (40), Steele et al. (38)
	Human amniotic cells	A	Russell et al. (30)
	Vero cells	A	Ramshaw (23)
Epstein-Barr virus	Lymphoblastoid 8392	P	Royston et al. (28)
Paramyxoviruses			
Subacute sclerosing panencephalitis	Human prostatic adenoma (MA-160)	P	Steele et al. (36)
Rubeola	Human lung fibroblasts (WI-38)	P	Steele et al. (36), Labowskie et al. (17)
Mumps	Conjunctival epithelia	P	Speel et al. (35)
	Vero cells	A	Andersson et al. (2)
Orthomyxovirus			
Influenza	Baby hamster kidney (BHK-21)	A	Greenberg et al. (12)
Arenavirus[b]			
Lymphocytic choriomeningitis (LCM)	L cells infected with LCM	A	Cole et al. (5)
	L cells infected with LCM	A	Doherty et al. (6), Zinkernagel and Doherty (46)
Murine leukemia[b]			
Moloney	MSV-induced tumors	A	Lamon et al. (18)
C-type	BALB/c fibroblasts	P	Hirsch et al. (16)
Poxvirus[b]			
Ectromelia	Ectromelia-infected fibroblasts	P	Gardner et al. (7, 8)

[a] A = acute; P = persistent.
[b] In mice.

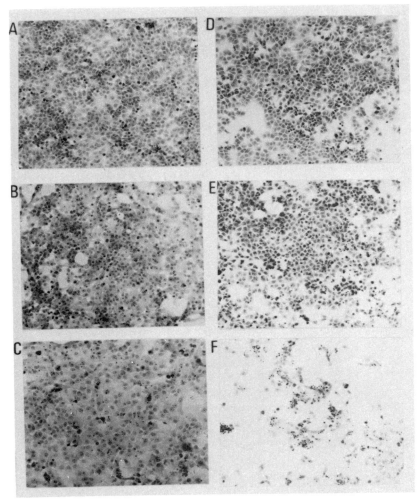

FIG. 1. *Measurement of lymphocytotoxicity by cytopathic effects (hematoxylin and eosin, ×118). Cultures of parent uninfected HeLa cell lines are shown in A, B, and C, and K11 sublines persistently infected with measles virus are shown in D, E, and F. Control uninfected and infected cultures without lymphocytes are shown in panels A and D, respectively. Addition of lymphocytes from a measles-seronegative individual to target cells reveals no destruction of the uninfected (B) or the infected K11-S subline (E). Addition of lymphocytes from an individual seropositive for measles shows no destruction of the uninfected subline (C), but significant destruction of the infected K11-S subline (F) with adsorption of lymphocytes adherent to remnants of target cells. From Labowskie et al. (17).*

The lymphocytotoxicity assay depends upon several technical points of importance. These include (i) selection of an optimal cell line which exhibits minimal background release in the absence of effector cells and maximal release in their presence, (ii) the physiological state of the target cell, e.g., acute or persistent (chronic) infection which can influence the concentration of virus-specific antigens or non-virion antigens on the surface of the infected target cell and in turn can influence the lym-phocyte-target cell interaction, (iii) optimal ratios of effector to target cells (most assays require at least a ratio of 50:1 or 100:1), and (iv) optimal incubation time for assay, e.g., 12 to 24 h.

Among the mechanisms suggested to explain the cytotoxic action of lymphocytes in vitro are (i) direct cell-mediated cytotoxicity by sensitized T lymphocytes (20), (ii) antibody-dependent lymphocyte-mediated (non-T cell, or killer [K] cell) cytotoxicity (32), and (iii) lymphokine-induced cytotoxicity (e.g., lymphotoxin). Also included within the matrix of cellular immunity has been the description of activated macrophages in target cell destructiion. Although a number of techniques have been described which are based on any or all of these various mechanisms, the present discussion will be restricted to that of direct T cell-mediated lymphocytotoxicity. In the various lymphocytotoxicity assays which have been described in our laboratory, T cells have been shown to be the active effector cell. In others, non-T cells have been shown to be the active cells in mediating lysis, and in still others antibody-dependent lymphocytotoxicity appears to be operative.

Recently, an additional facet of cellular immunity to viruses has been the modulation of lymphocytotoxicity by humoral ("blocking") factors which appear to interfere with the expressions of lymphocytes on target cells. These "blocking factors" are similar to those described in cancer patients and have been detected in both the serum and cerebrospinal fluid of patients with certain forms of chronic demyelinating diseases such as subacute sclerosing panencephalitis and multiple sclerosis. These "blocking factors" may represent either free viral antigen or antigen-antibody complexes.

Materials and reagents

Medium. The culture medium used in all cytotoxicity assays in our laboratory is RPMI 1640 medium supplemented with glutamine, 10% fetal calf serum, 100 units of pencillin/ml, and 100 μg of streptomycin/ml. Some laboratories use Eagle's minimal essential medium with equally good results.

Preparation of leukocytes. Peripheral venous blood is collected by venipuncture and transferred to heparinized 16 × 125 mm glass test tubes (Microbiological Associates, Inc.). Purified suspensions of mononuclear cells are prepared by the Hypaque-Ficoll gradient method as described above. After separation from the gradient, the leukocytes are washed three times in medium and adjusted to a final concentration of 5 × 10^6/ml.

Target cells. Several cell culture lines which are either acutely or persistently infected with viruses have been used in tests of lymphocytotoxicity to viruses. These have either been prepared in our laboratory or obtained from Microbiological Associates, Inc. A list of several of the available culture lines which have been used in lymphocytotoxicity is shown in Table 4.

1. *Preparation of acutely infected target cell*

lines. The method for the preparation and monitoring of acutely infected target cells for use in the lymphocytotoxicity assay is schematically represented in Fig. 2. Monolayer cultures are infected at a low multiplicity of infection (1:1) and kept in culture anywhere from 1 to 24 h at 37 C, depending upon the test virus to be employed. After an appropriate length of incubation, the cells are enzymatically dispersed and cryopreserved with dimethyl sulfoxide as a cryoprotective agent. The cells are then slowly frozen at rate of 1 C per min and stored in a vapor phase of liquid nitrogen until ready for testing; control uninfected cell cultures are similarly processed.

On the day of a typical experiment, the cells are rapidly thawed in a 37 C water bath and resuspended in a 10-fold volume of medium.

2. *Preparation of persistently infected target cell lines.* Persistently infected target cell lines are developed after acute infection of a susceptible cell line and recovery of the surviving cells. These cells are then passaged and form the basis of a continuing persistently infected cell line. Control uninfected cells are similarly processed after enzymatic dispersion and utilized in fashion identical to that described for the acutely infected cell lines.

3. *Monitoring of the target cell lines.* Monitoring of the cell lines can be performed by tests of infectivity, in the case of acutely infected cell lines, or by indirect immunofluorescence, electron microscopy, or hemadsorption, in the case of the persistently infected cell lines (Fig. 2). Preparations suitable for tests of lymphocytotoxicity should include target cells exhibiting evidence of cell surface antigens in greater than 90% of the cells.

Radionuclides. A variety of radionuclides have been employed for labeling the target cells, including ^{51}Cr, [^{3}H]thymidine ^{86}Rb, and ^{67}Ga. The most commonly used radioisotope for cytotoxicity assays is ^{51}Cr (Na$_2$ ^{51}CrO$_4$), and this can be obtained from Amersham/Searle, Arlington Heights, Ill.

Test procedure

A variety of techniques have been described for the lymphocytotoxicity assay which are generally applicable in all virus systems that have been studied. Although both macro- and microassays are available, most investigators employ the microassay procedures (37).

Radiolabeling the target cells. The infected and control target cells are radiolabeled by incubating a 5-ml sample of cell suspension containing 2 × 10^6/ml with 100 μCi of sodium ^{51}Cr chromate at 37 C for 1 h. The cells are then washed three times in 10-fold volumes of cold medium and resuspended to a final concentration of 5×10^4 cells per ml in RPMI medium.

Lymphocytotoxicity assay. For each experiment performed on lymphocytes from a single individual, a series of 12 wells is inoculated with the following constituents as shown in Fig. 3. Into each of the first 6 wells (1–6), 0.1 ml of infected target cells is pipetted (Biopipette, Schwarz/Mann); similarly, 0.1 ml of control target cells is pipetted into the last 6 wells (7–12). Subsequently, 0.1 ml of the lymphocyte suspension containing 5×10^6 cells/ml is pipetted into wells 1–3 and wells 7–9 (Fig. 3). Finally, 0.1 ml of medium is pipetted into the remaining wells (4–6 and 10–12). The microtest plates are

then covered with Falcon lids and are incubated in a moisture-laden atmosphere at 37 C containing 5% CO_2 for various lengths of time. The optimal incubation periods, the rates of spontaneous release of ^{51}Cr, and the optimal lymphocyte-to-target cell ratios should be determined for each virus system employed, as illustrated in Fig. 4. In addition, two types of incubation procedures have been employed: in the first the test plates are placed on a rocker platform when an automated harvesting procedure is utilized, and in the second method the plates are maintained in a stationary position to allow settling of the cells when a manual method of harvesting is employed.

Harvesting. After incubation of the test

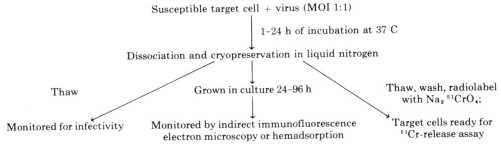

FIG. 2. *Preparation and monitoring of target cells acutely infected with viruses for use in the* ^{51}Cr-release *lymphocytotoxicity assay.*

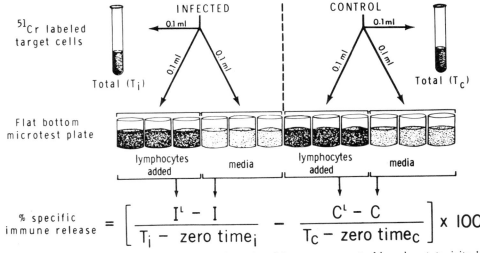

FIG. 3. *Schematic representation of the method employed for measurement of lymphocytotoxicity by* ^{51}Cr *release and method for calculation. With uninfected and persistently infected BHK-21 cultures, the spontaneous release of* ^{51}Cr *from infected target cells(I) and control cells (C) was subtracted from that released from the interaction of lymphocytes with either infected target cells (I^L) or control cells (C^C). The release at zero time was subtracted from the total amount of radioactivity in the infected (T_i) and control (T_c) target cells to determine the total amount of* ^{51}Cr *that was available for release during incubation periods. The specific immune release was calculated by subtracting the percentage of* ^{51}Cr *release in the control target cells from that released from the infected cells. From Steele et al. (37).*

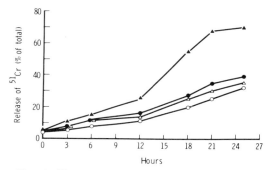

FIG. 4. *Time course study of the release of* ^{51}Cr *in the lymphocytotoxicity assay for viruses. The spontaneous release of* ^{51}Cr *from infected* ($\triangle$) *and control* (O) *target cells is shown together with the lymphocyte-mediated release of* ^{51}Cr *from infected* ($\blacktriangle$) *and control* ($\bullet$) *target cells over a 24-h period.*

plates, the harvesting of the cellular constituents from the microtest plates can be accomplished by either of two methods. In the original description of the test, a multiple automated sample harvester (MASH) was employed, and this method is suitable when persistently infected cell lines are employed (37). However, because of the high spontaneous release, owing to physical rupture of cells, particularly when acutely infected target cells are employed, this manner of collection is not satisfactory in some systems. Therefore, we have modified the original method to a manual method of harvesting in the latter situation.

The method of harvesting with the MASH is as follows. The contents of 12 wells in a row are aspirated through the inner channels of 12 double lumen tubes. The cells are then simultaneously aspirated, washed, and retained on a glass-fiber filter paper (Glass Fiber Filter, 934, A. Reeves-Angel, Clifton, N.J.). The combined supernatant fluid and washing fluid containing the released ^{51}Cr are collected in 16×125 mm gamma counting tubes for direct counting in a gamma spectrometer.

For the manual method of collection, the harvesting is performed by withdrawing 0.1 ml of the supernatant fluids from each well by use of a Biopipette. This is performed by gentle aspiration without resuspending the cells which have settled to the bottom. This sample is transferred into a 16×125 mm gamma counting tube for counting in the spectrometer. In the final calculation the values for released ^{51}Cr are expressed as total counts per minute per 0.2 ml by doubling the initial values which were obtained.

Calculation of specific CMI: specific immune release. In calculating the results, spontaneous release of ^{51}Cr from infected target cells (I) or control cells (C) is subtracted from that released from the interaction of lymphocytes with either infected target cells (I^L) or control cells (C^L), respectively. The release at zero time is then subtracted from the total amount of radioactivity in infected (T_i) and control (T_c) target cells to determine the total amount of ^{51}Cr that is available for release during the incubation periods. Some investigators use a freeze-thaw value for this figure instead of total amount of radioactivity. This is obtained by repetitively freeze-thawing the target cells three times and measuring the released ^{51}Cr in the supernatant fluids. The specific immune release is then calculated by subtracting the percent ^{51}Cr release in the control target cells from that released from the infected cells according to the formula shown in Fig. 3.

Testing for "blocking factors." In certain specialized tests it may be necessary to measure the presence of "blocking factors" either in the serum or cerebrospinal fluid of patients (36). Such factors may block or enhance specific lymphocytotoxicity. In performing these tests 0.05 ml of heat-inactivated autologous serum or cerebrospinal fluid is added to each of the 12 wells and the assay is performed as described above. An appropriate correction ($\times 2.5$) must be used for the additional dilution when calculating specific immune release.

ACKNOWLEDGMENT

These studies were supported by the U.S. Army Medical Research and Development Command (DA-49-193-MD-2633).

LITERATURE CITED

1. Adler, W. H., and S. G. Rabinowitz. 1973. Host defenses during primary Venezuelan equine encephalomyelitis virus infection in mice. II. In vitro methods for the measurement and qualitation of the immune response. J. Immunol. **110:**1354–1362.
2. Andersson, T., V. Stejskal, and B. Harfast, 1975. An in-vitro method for study of human lymphocyte cytotoxicity against mumps-virus-infected target cells. J. Immunol. **114:**237–243.
3. Bellanti, J. A. 1971. Immunology, p. 269–291. W. B. Saunders Co., Philadelphia.
4. Bloom, B. R., and B. Rager-Zisman. 1975. Cell-mediated immunity in viral infections, p. 113–136. *In* A. L. Notkins (ed.), Viral immunology and immunopathology. Academic Press Inc., New York.
5. Cole, G. A., R. A. Prendergast, and C. S. Henney. 1973. In vitro correlates of LCM virus-induced immune responses, p. 61–71. *In* F. Lehmann-Grube (ed.), Lymphocytic choriomeningitis virus and other arenaviruses. Springer-Verlag, Berlin.

6. Doherty, P. C., R. M. Zinkernagel, and I. A. Ramshaw. 1974. Specificity and development of cytotoxic thymus derived lymphocytes in lymphocytic choriomeningitis. J. Immunol. **112**:1548–1552.

7. Gardner, I., N. A. Bowern, and R. V. Blanden. 1974. Cell-mediated cytotoxicity against etromelia virus-infected target cells. I. Specificity and kinetics. Eur. J. Immunol. **4**:63–67.

8. Gardner, I., N. A. Bowern, and R. V. Blanden. 1974. Cell-mediated cytotoxicity against etromelia virus-infected target cells. II. Identification of effector cells and analysis of mechanisms. Eur. J. Immunol. **4**:68–72.

9. Gerber, P., and S. J. Lucas. 1972. In vitro stimulation of human lymphocytes by Epstein-Barr virus. Cell Immunol. 5:318–324.

10. Gerber, M. J., S. B. V. Vittal, and B. F. Clowdus. 1972. Hepatitis virus B and chronic alcoholic liver disease. Lancet **2**:1034–1035.

11. Graziano, K. D., J. C. Ruckdeschel, and M. R. Mardiney, Jr. 1975. Cell-associated immunity to measles (rubeola). The demonstration of invitro lymphocyte tritiated thymidine incorporation in response to measles complement-fixation antigen. Cell. Immunol. **15**:347–359.

12. Greenberg, S. B., B. S. Criswell, and R. B. Couch. 1975. Lymphocyte-mediated cytotoxicity against influenza virus infected cells: an in vitro method. J. Immunol. **15**:601–603.

13. Griffin, D. E., and R. T. Johnson. 1973. Cellular immune response to viral infection: in-vitro studies of lymphocytes from mice infected with Sindbis virus. Cell. Immunol. **9**:426–434.

14. Halstead, S. B., J. S. Chow, and N. J. Marchette. 1973. Immunological enhancement of dengue virus replication. Nature (London) New Biol. **243**:24–25.

15. Hellman, A., A. K. Fowler, H. G. Steinman, and P. M. Buzzerd. 1972. Studies of the blastogenic responses of murine lymphocyte. III. Specific viral transformation. Proc. Soc. Exp. Biol. Med. **141**:106–109.

16. Hirsch, M. E., A. P. Kelly, M. R. Proffitt, and P. H. Black. 1975. Cell-mediated immunity to antigens associated with endogenous murine C-type leukemia viruses. Science **187**:959–961.

17. Labowskie, R. J., R. Edelman, R. Rustigian, and J. A. Bellanti. 1974. Studies of cell-mediated immunity to measles virus by in-vitro lymphocyte-mediated cytotoxicity. J. Infect. Dis. **129**:233–239.

18. Lamon, E. W., H. Wigzell, E. Klein, B. Andersson, and H. M. Skurzak. 1973. The lymphocyte response to primary moloney sarcoma virus tumors in BALB/c mice. J. Exp. Med. **137**:1472–1493.

19. McFarland, H. F. 1974. In vitro studies of cell-mediated immunity in an acute viral infection. J. Immunol. **113**:173–180.

20. Perlmann, P., and G. Holm. 1969. Cytotoxic effects in vitro. Adv. Immunol. **11**:117–193.

21. Pettigrew, N. M., R. I. Russell, R. B. Goudie, and A. K. R. Chaudhuri. 1972. Evidence for a role of hepatitis virus B in chronic alcoholic liver disease. Lancet **2**:724.

22. Rabinowitz, S. G., and R. A. Proctor. 1974. In vitro study of antiviral activity of immune spleen cells in experimental Venezuelan equine encephalomyelitis infections in mice. J. Immunol. **112**:1070–1077.

23. Ramshaw, I. 1975. Lysis of herpesvirus-infected target cells by immune spleen cells. Infect. Immun. **11**:767–769.

24. Rapp, F., and R. Duff. 1972. In vitro cell transformation by herpesvirus. Fed. Proc. **31**:1660–1668.

25. Rosenberg, G. L., P. A. Farber, and A. L. Notkins. 1972. In vitro stimulation of sensitized lymphocytes by herpes simplex virus and vaccinia virus. Proc. Natl. Acad. Sci. U.S.A. **69**:756–760.

26. Rosenberg, G. L., and A. L. Notkins. 1974. Induction of cellular immunity to herpes simplex virus: relationship to the humoral immune response. J. Immunol. **112**:1019–1025.

27. Rosenberg, G. L., C. Wohlenberg, A. J. Nahmias, and A. L. Notkins. 1972. Differentiation of type 1 and type 2 herpes simplex virus by in vitro stimulation of immune lymphocytes. J. Immunol. **109**:413–414.

28. Royston, I., J. L. Sullivan, P. O. Periman, and E. Perlin. 1975. Cell-mediated immunity to Epstein-Barr-virus-transformed lymphoblastoid cells in acute infectious mononucleosis. N. Engl. J. Med. **293**:1159–1163.

29. Russell, A. S., R. A. Maini, M. Bailey, and D. C. Dumonde. 1972. Cell-mediated immunity to varicella-zoster antigen in acute herpes zoster (shingles). Cell. Immunol. **14**:181–185.

30. Russell, A. S., J. S. Percy, and T. Kovithavongs. 1975. Cell-mediated immunity to herpes simplex in humans: lymphocyte cytotoxicity measured by ^{51}Cr-release from infected cells. Infect. Immun. **11**:355–359.

31. Rustigian, R., S. H. Winston, J. A. Bellanti, and L. A. Clark. 1975. Neutralizing antibody and lymphocyte-mediated, colony-forming inhibition responses to measles infection in Cercopithecus aethiops monkeys. J. Infect. Dis. **132**:511–519.

32. Shore, S. L., A. J. Nahmias, S. E. Starr, P. A. Wood, and D. E. McFarlin. 1974. Detection of cell-dependent cytotoxic antibody to cells infected with herpes simplex virus. Nature (London) **251**:350–352.

33. Smith, K. A., L. Chess, and M. R. Mardiney, Jr. 1972. The characteristics of lymphocyte tritiated thymidine incorporation in response to mumps virus. Cell. Immunol. **5**:597–604.

34. Smith, K. A., L. Chess, and M. R. Mardiney, Jr. 1973. The relationship between rubella hemagglutination-inhibition antibody (HIA) and rubella-induced in-vitro lymphocyte tritiated thymidine incorporation. Cell. Immunol. **8**:321–327.

35. Speel, L. F., J. E. Osborn, and D. L. Walker. 1968. An immuno-cytopathogenic interaction between sensitized leukocytes and epithelial cells carrying a persistent noncytotocidal myxovirus infection. J. Immunol. **101**:409–417.

36. Steele, R. W. D. A. Fuccillo, S. A. Hensen, M. M. Vincent, and J. A. Bellanti. 1976. Cellular immunity in sclerosing panencephalitis. J. Pediat. **88**:56–62.

37. Steele, R. W., S. A. Hensen, M. M. Vincent, D. A. Fuccillo, and J. A. Bellanti. 1973. A ^{51}Cr microassay technique for cell-mediated immunity to viruses. J. Immunol. **110**:1502–1510.

38. Steele, R. W., M. M. Vincent, S. A. Hensen, D. A. Fuccillo, I. A. Chapa, and L. Canales. 1975. Cellular immune responses to herpes simplex virus type 1 in recurrent herpes labialis: in vitro blastogenesis and cytotoxicity to infected cell lines. J. Infect. Dis. **131**:528–534.

39. Thong, Y. H., S. A. Hensen, M. M. Vincent, D. A. Fuccillo, W. A. Stiles, and J. A. Bellanti. 1975. Use of cryopreserved virus-infected target cells in a lymphocytotoxicity ^{51}Cr release microassay for cell-mediated immunity to cytomegalovirus. Infect. Immun. **13**:643–645.

40. Thong, Y. H., M. M. Vincent, S. A. Hensen, D. A. Fuccillo, M. Rola-Pleszczynski, and J. A. Bellanti. 1975. Depressed specific cell-mediated immunity to herpes simplex virus type 1 in patients with recurrent herpes labialis. Infect. Immun. **12**:78–80.

41. Thurman, G. B., A. Ahmed, D. M. Strong, R. C. Knudsen, W. R. Grace, and K. W. Sell. 1973. Lymphocyte activation in subacute sclerosing panencephalitis virus and cytomegalovirus infections. In vitro stimulation in response to viral-infected cell lines. J. Exp. Med. **138**:839–846.

42. Ütermohlen, V., and J. B. Zabriskie. 1973. A suppression of cellular immunity in patients with multiple sclerosis. J. Exp. Med. **138**:1591–1596.

43. Waldman, R. H., C. S. Spencer, and J. E. Johnson. 1972. Respiratory and systemic cellular and humoral immune responses to influenza virus vaccine administered parenterally or by nose drops. Cell. Immunol. **3**:294–300.

44. Wiktor, T. J., I. Kamo, and H. Koprowski. 1974. In vitro stimulation of rabbit lymphocytes after immunization with live and inactivated rabies vaccines. J. Immunol. **112**:2013–2019.

45. Wilton, J. M. A., L. Ivanyi, and T. Lehner. 1972. Cell-mediated immunity in herpes virus hominis infections. Br. Med. J. **1**:723–726.

46. Zinkernagel, R. M., and P. C. Doherty. 1975. H-2 compatibility requirement for T-cell mediated lysis of target cells infected with lymphocytic choriomeningitis virus: different cytotoxic T-cell specificities are associated with structures coded for in H-2K or H-2D. J. Exp. Med. **141**:427–436.

Chapter 19

Principles of Radioimmunoassay

THOMAS J. GILL III

INTRODUCTION

The basic principles of radioimmunoassay have been reviewed in detail (1–3, 5), and a compendium of radioimmunoassay techniques has been published (4). Radioimmunoassay and competitive protein binding are essentially the same procedure, except that the former uses a specific antibody and the latter uses a specific binding protein which is not an antibody but usually a serum transport protein. The underlying principle of both procedures is to establish a stoichiometric relationship between the binding protein and the antigen, to select the most appropriate conditions as the standard, and then to perturb this equilibrium by adding the unknown sample. The extent to which the unknown competes for the binding protein is compared with a standard curve, and the concentration of the material being measured is read from the curve. The basic chemical reactions involved in this technique, given in terms of radioimmunoassay, are illustrated in Fig. 1. The establishment of a standard curve and its use in determining the amount of antigen in an unknown sample are shown in Fig. 2.

The derivations of the equations governing the radioimmunoassay method are given below:

1. The general case:

S = macromolecular binding site (antibody combining site)
L = ligand site (antigenic site)
K_a = association constant

$$S + L \rightleftharpoons SL$$

$$K_a = \frac{[SL]}{[S][L]}$$

$$[S] K_a = \frac{[SL]}{[L]} = \frac{\text{bound ligand } (B)}{\text{free ligand } (F)}$$

The concentration of free macromolecular binding sites is calculated according to:

[free sites] = [total sites] − [bound sites]

$$[S] \leq [S_t] - [SL]$$

2. If immunoglobulin G is used, there are 2 combining sites/molecule, and

$2[Ab_i]$ = $[Ab_o]$ = total concentration of antibody combining sites

where $[Ab_i]$ is the initial molar concentration of antibody used in the system. Hence

$$[Ab] = [Ab_o] - [AbAg]$$

and

$$([Ab_o] - [AbAg]) K_a = \frac{[AbAg]}{[Ag]}$$

$$([Ab_o] - B) K_a = \frac{B}{F}$$

where B = bound antigen and F = free antigen.

SENSITIVITY

The antibody concentration to be used in the radioimmunoassay should be selected such that measurements will be carried out between 10 and 90% antibody saturation, and the association constant (K_a) determines the lowest antibody concentration that can be used. As a rule of thumb, the antibody concentration should be approximately equal to $1/K_a$, at which point the bound to free (B/F) ratio is approximately 1. For maximal sensitivity, the lowest antibody concentration that will bind a measurable fraction of antigen should be used.

ANTIBODY REQUIREMENTS

The binding constant of the antibody is usually the most important factor in determining the success of radioimmunoassay: note that there is a direct relationship to the B/F ratio in the bindng equation. The selectivity of the antibody is also important, since the specificity for the antigen under question must be considerably greater than that for any interfering antigens. The antibodies should have the highest possible affinity (10^8 to 10^{11} L/M) for the native antigen. A major source of error in the development of a radioimmunoassay is the use of an inadequately characterized antibody, i.e., one whose specificity, affinity, and cross-reactivity have not been unequivocally established. The techniques for immunization to obtain such an antibody preparation are empirical, but they involve the use of relatively small amounts of

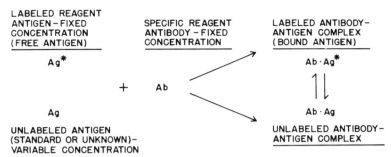

FIG. 1. *Basic chemical reaction in a radioimmunoassay procedure. The equilibrium between the antibody (Ab) and the radioactive antigen (Ag*) of the assay system and the antibody and the nonradioactive antigen (Ag) of the test system is dependent upon the amount of antigen added in the test system (standard solution or unknown sample).*

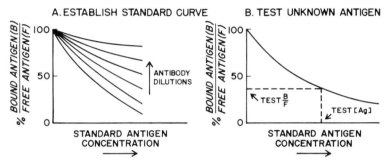

FIG. 2. *(A) A standard curve is constructed by taking a fixed amount of antibody and of radioactive antigen and adding a known concentration of standard antigen solution. This procedure is carried out at various antibody dilutions, and the antibody dilution that gives a moderate slope is chosen as the standard. (B) The antigen in the unknown is determined by adding a test sample to the standard (Ab + Ag*) mixture. The bound to free ratio (B/F) is measured, and the unknown antigen concentration is read from the standard curve.*

antigen and harvesting the antibody later in the course of immunization. Generally, the use of complete Freund's adjuvant is recommended for the immunization procedure. Since individual antisera vary widely in their binding constants and in their heterogeneity, each antiserum should be investigated individually and sera should not be pooled.

ANTIGEN REQUIREMENTS

The antigen used for immunization and for establishing the standard curve should be as pure as possible. Some of the problems that may arise in raising antisera are cross-reactivities with degradation products of the antigen or with a contaminant in the antigen preparation used for immunization. The radioactive labeling procedure should not alter the antigen to any detectable extent. For example, ^{125}I is a very common label for proteins, and the mildest oxidizing conditions for the shortest periods of time should be used to attach it to the protein. The higher the specific activity of the antigen, the greater the risk of damage, especially with proteins. Hence, there should be, on the average, less than 1 molecule of iodine per molecule of protein. The dilemma here is the choice between the very high specific activity that may be needed to detect antigens which are in very low concentrations under physiological conditions and the danger of degradation due to radioactive decay. This question must be addressed and settled in the context of each radioimmunoassay. The choice should be made in terms of the binding constant of the antibody and the minimal amount of radioactive antigen needed to establish the proper assay.

Although it is desirable to have the antigen always as pure as possible, the labeled antigen used in the assay system can be somewhat less pure provided that the antigen retains its capacity to bind to the antibody. The unlabeled antigen used as the immunogen should be as pure as possible, so that it will elicit highly specific antibody, and the unlabeled antigen used as a standard must be as pure as possible in order to be identical to the unknown antigen to be measured. Thus, any compromise that is necessary can be made with the labeled antigen used in the assay system, since both the standard and the unknown will be judged under the same assay conditions.

SEPARATION OF BOUND AND FREE ANTIGEN

The crux of the radioimmunoassay technique is the separation of bound and free antigen. Since one is dealing with an equilibrium situation that can shift, the separation must take place very rapidly and almost simultaneously in all samples being compared. Thus, the dissociation rate of the antibody-antigen complex is more critical than the association rate in determining the techniques of separation of bound and free antigen. The ideal situation is that in which the bound and free antigen are separated rapidly and simultaneously in all tubes in order to prevent a shift in equilibrium. In trying to approach this ideal, it is critical that experimental conditions be identical for the unknown and reference samples. This implies simultaneous handling of many tubes and a mechanism for keeping the temperature constant, since the equilibrium of the antibody-antigen reaction is a direct function of temperature. Many methods have been used: adsorption of the antigen on a solid phase, chromatography, electrophoresis, and precipitation of the antibody-antigen complex by salting out or by an antiglobulin reagent. Probably the most common technique is the adsorption of the free antigen onto a solid phase, and charcoal alone or coated with dextran or with serum albumin to prevent nonspecific adsorption is the most generally used adsorbent.

EVALUATION OF THE TECHNIQUE

After a radioimmunoassay has been developed, several points should be established to show that it is giving the appropriate answers:

1. The native antigen and the antigen used as a reference standard react identically with the antibody.

2. Other substances in physiological fluids must not interfere nonspecifically or by cross-reactivity with the antigen being measured. If they do, a prior fractionation step must be done to remove them.

3. The unknown antigen concentrations measured must be of the same magnitude as those which are physiologically active.

4. The measured antigen concentration must be independent of plasma dilution. The dilution profile of a standard sample of the antigen and a measured sample of the unknown should be superimposable.

5. The amount of antigen measured should vary systematically under different physiological conditions, and the physiological changes with changes in antigen concentration should be as expected.

LITERATURE CITED

1. Berson, S. A., and R. Yalow (ed.). 1973. Methods in investigative and diagnostic endocrinology, p. 84–135. North Holland Publishing Co., Amsterdam.

2. Haber, E., and K. Poulsen. 1974. The application of antibody to the measurement of substances of physiological and pharmacological interest, p. 249–275. *In* M. Sela (ed.), The antigens, II. Academic Press Inc., New York.

3. Hunter, W. M. 1973. Radioimmunoassay, p. 1–36. *In* D. M. Weir (ed.), Handbook of experimental immunology. Blackwell Scientific Publications, London.

4. Jaffe, B. M., and H. R. Behrman (ed.). 1974. Methods of hormone radioimmunoassay. Academic Press Inc., New York.

5. Odell, W. D., and W. A. Daugherty (ed.). 1971. Principles of competitive protein-binding assays. Lippincott Co., Philadelphia.

Chapter 20

Measurement of Insulin in Human Body Fluids

M. J. LEVITT AND K. W. SCHMITT

INTRODUCTION

Insulin is a polypeptide hormone synthesized in the β cells of the Islets of Langerhans in the pancreas. At one time, it was thought that the activity of this hormone could be attributed to a single chemical species, but it is now known that several molecules possess insulin-like biological or immunological properties (8, 34, 41, 45). It is generally agreed that the insulin monomer is the physiologically most important form of the hormone in normal individuals. Measurements of this "insulin" are complicated by the fact that other "insulins" are also found in body tissues (30, 35, 42, 54). A macromolecule is present in the pancreas that is antigenically similar to the insulin monomer (52). This "big, big insulin," with a molecular weight of approximately 100,000, may be an inactive intermediate in the biosynthesis of the insulin monomer. It is not understood how the macromolecular intermediate, or some other precursor, is converted into a smaller single chain polypeptide precursor of the insulin monomer. This "big insulin" or "proinsulin" precursor has a molecular weight of approximately 9,000 and is held in a folded configuration by three intrachain disulfide bonds (8, 39). Proinsulin has approximately 15% of the activity of the monomer. It is normally released from the β cell in an amount less than one-third the amount of insulin monomer released, but the proportion of proinsulin released is elevated in certain pathological conditions (8, 25).

Most of the proinsulin normally undergoes proteolysis within the Golgi apparatus or the secretory granules of the β cell. Proteolysis occurs at two specific sites, resulting in the splitting out of a peptide from the interior of the peptide chain. The insulin monomer formed by this reaction has a molecular weight of approximately 6,000 and consists of two dissimilar peptide chains. The A and B chains are held together by two of the three disulfide bonds that were intrachain linkages in the proinsulin precursor. Both the insulin monomer and the "connecting peptide" ("C peptide") are normally released together from the β cell (24, 29).

All of the precursor forms of the insulin mon-omer can be present in the circulation, in addition to partially metabolized or chemically altered monomers (18, 25). Furthermore, insulin monomer may be converted in the circulation to dimers or tetramers with biological and antigenic properties that may differ from those of the monomer (24, 25). The many forms of insulin or insulin-like material that may be present in a biological specimen mean that no single type of assay will be completely satisfactory for the measurement of insulin. Bioassays for insulin will detect only active forms of the hormone in proportion to their activities, not to their amounts. Immunological assays will detect molecules closely related structurally to insulin, whether or not they are active biologically.

Bioassays of insulin are often based on the ability of the hormone to increase the rate at which fatty or amino acids or glucose enter tissues (7, 34, 47). The insulin-like activity (ILA) measured in these assays probably includes active principles other than insulin (30, 34). This suspicion results from the observation that circulating ILA remains long after extirpation of the pancreas (18, 25). Further doubt about the specificities of insulin bioassays is based on the fact that insulin antibodies suppress far less than half of the original ILA (39, 41). It may yet be shown that the nonsuppressible ILA is due to some unknown form of insulin, but present evidence suggests that it is due to active principles other than insulin.

Radioimmunoassays have replaced bioassays as the preferred method for measuring tissue levels of insulin. Radioimmunoassays are far more sensitive, are simpler to perform, and correlate better with the clinical manifestations of patients (25, 30, 39). The immunoreactive insulin (IRI) measured in a radioimmunoassay will depend primarily upon the nature of the antibodies used in the test (25, 26). The immunogen used in preparing the antisera must be highly purified in order to obtain specificity in the radioimmunoassay. Even when the same immunogen is used, the antisera produced may react to different extents with different forms of insulin. It is to be expected that different radioimmunoassays for insulin monomer also detect, to varying degrees, proinsulin, insulin metabolites, and other antigenically related compounds (8, 9, 25).

Another source of analytical variation between different insulin radioimmunoassays is the possible presence of insulin antibodies in the specimen being tested (11, 18, 21, 40). It is not certain whether human insulin is antigenic in the human, but some patients may have altered forms of the hormone that are antigenic (17, 18, 34, 39). Antibodies must always be expected in patients receiving exogenous insulin because the hormone is derived from other species, and it may have been made more antigenically active by processing (18, 24, 25, 40). The presence of antibodies in a specimen can result in false assay results, but the direction and extent of the errors will depend upon the parameters of the radioimmunoassay (39). The use of a specimen control which does not receive added antiserum can sometimes reveal whether significant amounts of endogenous insulin antibodies are present in a sample (26).

Radioimmunoassays for insulin have been developed in which several different methods are used to separate antibody-bound insulin from unbound insulin (10, 26, 30, 43). Electrophoretic separations are elegant but not well suited to the processing of multiple specimens (10). In some radioimmunoassays, unbound insulin is removed by adsorption onto particulate matter such as charcoal, resin, cellulose, or talc (11, 26, 32, 39). If exposure to the adsorbent is not well controlled, falsely elevated results may be obtained because of "stripping" of previously bound insulin from the antiserum (11, 40). The presence of insulin antibodies in the specimen will cause falsely lowered results in this type of assay, since the fraction of insulin bound will be artifactually raised (39). A greater latitude in experimental details during the separation of bound from unbound insulin is possible in double-antibody radioimmunoassays. In this technique, insulin in the specimen and added trace-labeled insulin are first bound to insulin antibodies from another species, such as the rabbit; later addition of an antiserum directed against rabbit gamma globulins will cause precipitation of the first antibody along with the bound insulin (4, 9, 10). Unfortunately, insulin which is not chemically bound to the first antibody may co-precipitate, leading to falsely low results. The presence of endogenous antibodies to insulin can result in falsely elevated results in this type of assay since labeled insulin may bind to the human antibodies which are not precipitated by the second antibody (39). Greater ease in separating antibody-bound insulin from unbound insulin is afforded in solid-phase radioimmunoassays. In these tests, centrifugation is sufficient to sediment the insulin which is bound to antibodies which are either polymerized or chemically attached to inert particles. In those cases where the antibodies are chemically fixed to particles, the adhering unbound insulin may be washed off.

Additional analytical variations in radioimmunoassays for insulin occur as a result of the type of specimen tested. Higher levels of insulin can be found in the serum than in the heparinized plasma of the same individuals when double-antibody radioimmunoassays are performed (36). In some radioimmunoassays, the presence of heparin can cause the apparent plasma levels to exceed the levels measured in the serum of the same patients (2). In other radioimmunoassays heparin has no effect on the measured insulin value (19). The presence of other chemicals can also affect the measured insulin values in different direction and degrees, depending upon the particular radioimmunoassay conditions (53).

When radioimmunoassays are used to measure the amount of circulating foreign insulin administered to a patient, different results are likely to be obtained with different assay systems. This results from differences in cross-reactivity of the foreign insulins with different antiserum preparations used in the assays.

Fortunately, useful information can be gained from properly conducted radioimmunoassays performed in one laboratory using a constant set of reagents and a single type of specimen. The presence of interfering substances in a specimen can be detected by determining parallelism in the radioimmunoassay. Upon fourfold or higher dilution, the sample should behave antigenically the same as the purified standard; nonparallel behavior indicates the presence of interfering substances (32).

Radioimmunoassays for insulin are used in hospital laboratories for the measurement of circulating insulin levels in patients. No survey method for measuring insulin is available or necessary. The assay for insulin described here is a solid-phase radioimmunoassay in which insulin antibodies are chemically attached to Sephadex particles. All of the reagents necessary to perform the assay are provided in a test kit. This assay has been thoroughly tested and has been designated as a Selected Method of Clinical Chemistry (48, 49).

Measurements of circulating insulin antibodies or of proinsulin are beyond the ability of most laboratories to perform (11, 40, 43). These assays are available at major medical institutions and commerical testing laboratories.

CLINICAL INDICATIONS

The only universally recognized clinical application for insulin measurements is to distinguish insulomas from other causes of hypoglycemia. Measurements of circulating insulin levels have contributed to an understanding of the pathophysiology of diabetes mellitus but have not been of diagnostic value. The most sensitive, and the only generally accepted, test for the diagnosis of diabetes mellitus is an oral glucose tolerance test with analyses of true glucose blood levels. The results of this test can be compared to a criterion proposed for confirming a diagnosis of diabetes mellitus and staging the disease (15, 16, 20, 28, 31, 37, 51).

Insulin measurements are essential in patients with unexplained spontaneous hypoglycemia for the diagnosis of insulomas, small insulin-producing tumors of islet cell tissue that develop in pancreatic and ectopic sites. At one time, it was thought that insulomas could be diagnosed by the presence of Whipple's triad of symptoms: hypoglycemic symptomatology, hypoglycemia documented by a venous or capillary blood glucose concentration below 40 mg/100 ml, and relief of hypoglycemic symptoms by the ingestion of carbohydrates (1, 33). It is now realized that Whipple's triad of symptoms can occur in other conditions, including severe liver disease, hereditary enzyme defects, pituitary-adrenal disease, factitious administration of insulin or oral hypoglycemic agents, ethanol ingestion, and nonpancreatic neoplasms — sarcomas, fibromas, hepatomas, etc. (1).

If a patient is observed during an apparent episode of hypoglycemia, a blood sample should be drawn and the glucose level should be estimated by means of a dip-stick test. An indication of hypoglycemia can then be documented by a test that measures true glucose, and the serum insulin level can be measured (12). Since most patients with a history suggestive of hypoglycemia are not observed during such an episode, it is often necessary to employ insulin suppression or stimulation tests. Insulin suppression and stimulation tests are capable of producing life-threatening hypoglycemia and thus should be performed only when appropriate corrective therapy is readily available.

Insulin suppression tests are preferable to stimulation tests since the latter place the patient at a greater risk and may be of limited diagnostic value (33). Insulin stimulation tests on patients with surgically proven insulomas have been found to give false-negative results with the following frequencies: tolbutamide, 20%; glucagon, 30%; and L-leucine, 50% (33).

Suppression of insulin secretion can be achieved simply by fasting a patient. If a patient does not exhibit hypoglycemia after three fasts of 12- to 24-h durations, there is only about a 10% chance that the patient has an insuloma (1, 33). A patient with suspected insuloma who does not exhibit hypoglycemia under the above conditions may be stressed more severely with a fast extending to 72 h and including periods of moderate exercise. To confirm the presence of an insuloma, circulating levels of glucose and insulin should be determined at 6- or 12-h intervals and particularly whenever hypoglycemic symptoms occur (1, 33).

Other insulin suppression tests exist but are not as well established. In one test, ethanol is infused after a 36-h fast to produce hypoglycemia, and an inappropriately elevated insulin level is considered a positive result (1). Another test involves the administration of fish insulin to produce hypoglycemia. In this case, circulating insulin levels must be measured with an antiserum that does not recognize fish insulin (12).

TEST PROCEDURES

The Phadebas Insulin Test (Pharmacia Laboratories, Inc., Piscataway, N.J.) is supplied as a 100-test kit suitable for the duplicate measurement of the hormone in approximately 40 specimens. Included in the kit is a lyophilized standard consisting of porcine insulin of known activity which behaves antigenically identically to human insulin. The insulin antibody is chemically bound to Sephadex (a cross-linked dextran polymer) and is supplied in a lyophilized form. Trace insulin consists of approximately 3 μCi of lyophilized [^{125}I]insulin. Buffer salts are also provided as a dry powder.

To perform the assay, a portion of the sample is mixed with trace [^{125}I]insulin and the immunosorbent consisting of the Sephadex-anti-insulin complex. After overnight incubation, the immunosorbent is sedimented by centrifugation and the supernatant fluid is discarded. The immunosorbent is washed to remove physically adsorbed [^{125}I]insulin; then the radioactivity bound to the immunosorbent is determined. The amount of insulin present in the sample is determined by comparison of the bound radioactivity with the radioactivity bound in tubes containing known amounts of standard insulin.

Precautions

If glassware is used, it must be thoroughly siliconized to prevent errors due to the binding of insulin. It is simpler, and equally satisfactory, to use plastic pipette tips and assay tubes. (Tubes designed for this assay can be purchased from Pharmacia Laboratories, Inc.)

Water used in the assay should be of the greatest purity available; distilled water that is further purified is desirable. The immunosorbent particles must be kept suspended during addition to the assay tubes and during the incubation period. During addition, the immunosorbent suspension should be stirred magnetically at a rate such that a vortex appears at the surface only. As the suspension is depleted, the stirring rate should be reduced to maintain a small vortex since the particles can be fractured by excessive stirring. During the incubation period, the assay tubes should be agitated in a horizontal shaker at high speed, on a rocking platform, or on a rotator.

Errors can be introduced after the incubation period by dissociation of insulin from the immunosorbent. Washing and centrifugation of the immunosorbent should be performed in a reproducible manner and without undue delays. Centrifugation at a constant temperature helps to improve reproducibility. It is essential that the centrifugal force applied be sufficient to pack the immunosorbent particles into a pellet at the bottoms of the assay tubes.

Specimens

Either serum or heparinized plasma samples can be used in the assay. Specimens should be free from hemolysis since constituents of red blood cells can degrade insulin (5, 6). Specimens should be stored frozen until the day of the assay but not refrozen. If desired, specimens can be stored at 4 C for up to 2 weeks in case additional testing is required. Specimens containing particulate matter should be centrifuged at 5,000 rpm for 5 min, and the clear supernatant fluid used for the assay.

Preparation of buffer

Use 150 ml of ultrapure water in portions to transfer quantitatively the buffer salts from the vial and stopper into a 200-ml volumetric flask. Swirl the flask to dissolve the buffer salts; then add water to the mark. (Foam that obscures the mark may be removed and discarded.) Cap the flask and mix by inversion 10 times.

Preparation of stock standard

Add 4.0 ml of ultrapure water to the lyophilized insulin standard. Cap the vial and swirl it gently to dissolve all the protein. Mix by inversion 10 times.

Preparation of working standard

Label tubes A to H and prepare dilutions of the stock standard according to the protocol in Table 1. Use a fresh 0.5-ml pipette for each dilution. Mix each dilution thoroughly by shaking before preparing the next dilution.

Preparation of assay tubes

Label up to 100 tubes in duplicate A to H for standards and the remainder for samples and controls. Label two additional tubes TA. Pipette 0.1 ml of each working standard solution into the correspondingly labeled tubes. Similarly, pipette 0.1 ml of each sample or control into appropriately labeled tubes. When there is insufficient sample, as little as 0.025 ml can be used and the additional volume to 0.1 ml can be made up by the addition of buffer.

Preparation of labeled insulin

Add 10.0 ml of buffer to the vial of [^{125}I]insulin, cap the vial, and mix by inversion 10 times.

Preparation of immunosorbent

Add 100 ml of buffer in portions to transfer quantitatively the contents of the Sephadex-anti-insulin vial into a 150-ml beaker. Add a Teflon-coated stirring bar and place the beaker on a magnetic stirrer. Increase the speed of mixing until a vortex begins to be generated in the suspension.

Addition of labeled insulin and immunosorbent

A volume of 0.1 ml of labeled insulin solution and 1.0 ml of immunosorbent suspension can be added to each assay tube by separate pipettings. It is easier and more accurate, however, to add them concurrently by means of an automatic diluter (Model 25000 Automatic Pipette; Micromedic Systems, Inc., Philadelphia, Pa.). Set the diluter to sample 0.1 ml of labeled insulin and deliver this with 1.0 ml of immunosorbent suspension. Add this combination to each assay tube and to the tubes labeled TA.

TABLE 1. *Protocol for preparing working standard solutions*

Tube	Buffer (ml)	Add (ml)	Insulin (μU/ml)
A	0.0	0.5 of stock standard	320
B	0.5	0.5 of stock standard	160
C	0.5	0.5 of B	80
D	0.5	0.5 of C	40
E	0.5	0.5 of D	20
F	0.5	0.5 of E	10
G	0.5	0.5 of F	5
H	0.5	0.0	0

Incubation

Cap each tube tightly, set aside the tubes marked TA, and place the remaining tubes in a shaker or on a rocker. Allow the tubes to incubate at room temperature for 18 h with constant agitation.

Separation of antibody-bound insulin

Centrifuge each assay tube at 2,000 × g for 2 min at 15 C to drain all the liquid to the bottom of the tube. Remove the cap; then centrifuge the tube at 2,000 × g 10 min at 15 C to collect the immunosorbent as a pellet at the bottom of the tube. Withdraw the supernatant fluid down to 5 mm from the bottom by means of an aspirator connected to a waste bottle. A collar should be placed on the aspirator nozzle to adjust the depth of insertion so that the pellet is not disturbed. (A nozzle for this purpose is available upon request from the manufacturer of the assay kit.)

Washing of the immunosorbent

Squirt 2.0 ml of 0.9% saline into each assay tube to resuspend the immunosorbent particles. This addition can be done rapidly while the tubes remain in the centrifuge carriers by means of a spring-loaded syringe (Cornwall syringe; Becton-Dickinson & Co., Rutherford, N.J.). Again centrifuge the tubes at 2,000 × g for 10 min at 15 C, and remove the supernatant fluids down to 5 mm from the bottoms of the tubes. Repeat the washing, centrifugation, and aspiration a third time.

Measurement of radioactivity

Place each assay tube and the TA tubes in a gamma counter with the appropriate settings for the detection of ^{125}I radiation. Also place six empty tubes at random in the counting sequence to determine the radiation background level. Measure the radioactivity in each tube for 4 min.

Calculation

Average the radioactivity in the empty tubes to obtain the background count. Average the radioactivity in each pair of replicate assay tubes; then subtract the background count to obtain the average corrected count for each standard, control, and sample. Determine the corrected total activity by subtracting the background count from the average of the counts for the TA tubes. Calculate the percentage of bound counts in each standard as follows:

% bound, standard =
$$\frac{\text{corrected count for standard}}{\text{corrected total activity count}} \times 100$$

On a 3-cycle semilog graph paper, plot the percentage bound for the standards on the linear ordinate and the concentrations of insulin on the log abscissa. Calculate the percentage of bound counts in each sample as follows:

% bound, sample =
$$\frac{\text{corrected count for sample}}{\text{corrected total activity count}} \times 100$$

To find the insulin value in each sample, determine where the percent bound for the sample intersects the standard curve; then read off the insulin concentration corresponding to that point. If less then 0.1 ml of sample is used in the assay, the insulin value determined from the standard curve must be multiplied by a correction factor as indicated:

true insulin value = insulin value from curve
$$\times \frac{0.1 \text{ ml}}{\text{ml of sample used}}$$

Controls

In a properly performed assay the standard curve will approximate a straight line (Fig. 1). Significant deviations from linearity signify that the assay is invalid. The quality of the labeled insulin will decrease with time, and this may be monitored by calculating the efficiency of each assay as follows:

efficiency =
$$\frac{\text{corrected count for zero tube (H standard)}}{\text{corrected total activity count}} \times 100$$

Efficiency typically approximates 30% with a fresh kit, and good results may be obtained as long as it remains above approximately 15%.

Quality control specimens to be included in each assay can be purchased in lyophilized form

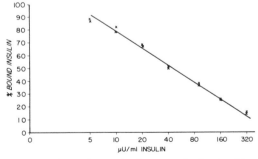

Fig. 1. *Typical standard curve obtained with a Phadebas Insulin Test Kit by an experienced operator. Individual values for replicate determinations of each standard are shown. Large deviation from linearity below approximately 10 µU/ml is clearly evident. A smaller deviation from linearity occurs above approximately 200 µU/ml.*

from many suppliers. It is equally satisfactory to prepare the needed quality control pools containing insulin equivalent to approximately 25, 50, and 75% bound insulin. These pools may be made easily by adding insulin standard left over from the assays to samples of outdated human plasma. These pools are stable for at least 3 months if stored at −40 C.

Assay parameters

The insulin values of quality control pools can be determined with a reproducibility of 5% within a single assay and of 10% between assays when performed by an experienced operator.

The standard curve deviates from linearity at values above approximately 80% and below approximately 20% bound, which results in uncertainty for insulin values below approximately 10 μU/ml and above approximately 200 μU/ml. Specimens containing more than 320 μU of insulin per ml can be assayed after up to fourfold dilution with buffer.

REAGENTS

A wide selection of insulin radioimmunoassay test kits are available commercially from the following sources:

Amersham/Searle Corp., Arlington Heights, Ill. 60005

Bio-RIA, Montreal, P.Q., Canada H3M 3A2

Calbiochem, San Diego, Calif. 92112

Corning Biological Products, Medfield, Mass. 02052

Curtis Nuclear Corp., Los Angeles, Calif. 90058

ICN Pharmaceuticals, Portland, Ore. 97208

Medvak, Columbia, Md. 21045

Pharmacia Laboratories, Piscataway, N.J. 08854

Schwarz/Mann, Orangeburg, N.Y. 10962

Kits will probably be preferred by most laboratories performing relatively few insulin assays; they should be used with sufficient control samples to detect when the manufacturer alters the composition or quality of the reagents. Purchase of reagents from different manufacturers may be more attractive economically to laboratories performing extensive insulin testing. It is necessary, however, to invest considerable time and effort to establish a suitable set of assay conditions with a given set of reagents. Where the necessary facilities and technical personnel are available, it may be most economical to prepare the insulin antiserum and labeled trace instead of purchasing them.

INTERPRETATION

Radioimmunoassays for insulin, intended to measure the monomeric form of the hormone, may also measure contributions from other forms, including proinsulin, dimers, and metabolic products. The degree of interference in the assay by other forms of insulin will depend primarily on the nature of the antiserum used, but other analytical parameters can also influence the specificities of the assays (9, 32, 39, 43). Interpretations of the results of insulin radioimmunoassays should be made with awareness of the interferences caused by anticoagulants, hemolysis, and drugs administered to the patient (53).

Differences between the results of insulin radioimmunoassays are not large when normal individuals are tested. Most laboratories find circulating insulin levels of approximately 5 to 30 μU/ml in nondiabetic individuals of normal weight after an overnight fast (3, 22). Different insulin radioimmunoassays are more likely to produce different results when elevated levels are measured in individuals who have pathological processes or who have received exogenous insulin. Elevated levels of insulin detected in double-antibody and similar radioimmunoassays should be interpreted with awareness that they may be due to the presence of insulin antibodies resulting from factitious administration of insulin (42).

The role of insulin in the etiology of diabetes mellitus is well documented, and insulin measurements are not required to diagnose this disease. A diagnosis of chemical diabetes mellitus can be made solely on the basis of true glucose levels in blood during an oral glucose tolerance test. Various criteria have been proposed for assessing the results of this test and to establish the stage of the disease (15, 16, 20, 28, 31, 37, 46, 50, 51).

When circulating insulin levels are obtained in an oral glucose tolerance test, different responses are seen in normal and diabetic individuals (Fig. 2). In normal individuals, circulating insulin levels rise four- to eightfold to a peak in 30 to 60 min and return to normal in 4 h. Untreated patients with juvenile or overt diabetes mellitus generally do not have detectable levels of circulating insulin; less often, they may demonstrate an ability to secrete insulin, but they have an essentially flat response to the glucose load. Patients with chemical diabetes mellitus have a response that differs from normal in that peak insulin levels are reached later, the peak value can be greater than normal, and the total amount of insulin secreted in response to the glucose load is greater. Obese

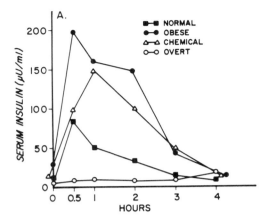

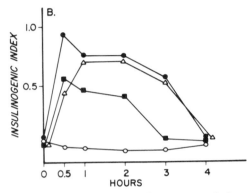

FIG. 2. *(A) Insulin values during an oral glucose tolerance test in various individuals:* ○, *individual with juvenile or overt diabetes mellitus;* ■, *normal individuals;* △, *individual with chemical diabetes mellitus;* ●, *obese individual without diabetes mellitus. (B) Insulinogenic Index values during an oral glucose tolerance test in the same individuals.*

individuals without diabetes mellitus secrete greater than normal amounts of glucose during the oral glucose tolerance test yet do not become hypoglycemic (13, 27, 38).

The circulating insulin and glucose levels in each sample obtained during an oral glucose tolerance test can be compared by calculating various indices (27). One of the most popular of these is calculated as follows:

insulinogenic index =
$$\frac{\text{plasma insulin value (in } \mu\text{U/ml)}}{\text{plasma glucose value (in mg/100 ml)}}$$

The insulinogenic index emphasizes the lack of insulin relative to glucose that is characteristic of juvenile or overt diabetes mellitus (Fig. 2). The index also demonstrates the hypersecretion of insulin during the oral glucose tolerance test

seen in nondiabetic obese individuals. A similar hypersecretion is seen in the third trimester of pregnancy, acromegaly, and Cushing's syndrome (38). The insulin hypersecretion in these conditions is necessary to compensate for anti-insulin factors; otherwise, a diabetic glucose tolerance curve would be exhibited.

The preferable method of diagnosing an insuloma is with a fasting insulin suppression test (1). An insulin stimulation test can also be used. Either type of test should be conducted only when therapy is readily available to counteract any severe hypoglycemia that may be produced in the patient.

The results of a fasting insulin suppression test can be used to calculate two ratios that compare the glucose level to the insulin response in each sample obtained during the test. The preferred glucose-insulin ratio is calculated as follows:

glucose-insulin ratio =
$$\frac{\text{plasma glucose value (in mg/100 ml}}{\text{serum insulin value (in } \mu\text{U/ml}}$$

Values of this ratio greater than 5.0 are considered normal, and values less than 2.5 are diagnostic for insulomas (Fig. 3). The diagnostic value of this ratio is improved in the presence of hypoglycemia: fasting venous or capillary plasma true glucose level below 40 mg/100 ml (23). The amended insulin-glucose ratio provides greater sensitivity but is probably too sensitive if the plasma glucose level is below 35 mg/100 ml. This ratio is calculated as follows:

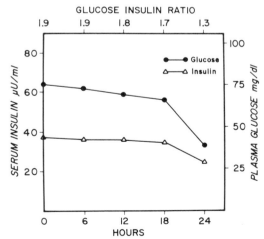

FIG. 3. *Typical glucose-insulin ratio in a patient with an insuloma during a 24-h fasting insulin suppression test.*

amended insulin-glucose ratio =
$$\frac{\text{serum insulin value (in } \mu\text{U/ml)} \times 100}{\text{plasma glucose value (in mg/100 ml)} - 30}$$

A value of less than 50 in this ratio is considered normal. Most patients with insulomas have values close to 200, although any value above 50 is considered diagnostic (44).

The tolbutamide stimulation test is not recommended because of the risk it presents to the patient and because 20% of patients with insulomas (especially children) fail to respond to the stimulus (33). Tolbutamide, which causes the release of insulin from the pancreas, is administered intravenously in a 1-g dose within 30 s to a patient fasted overnight. Blood samples are drawn for glucose and insulin measurements at 0, 2, 5, 15, 30, 45, 60, 90, 120, 150, and 180 min (note: the test may have to be stopped if severe hypoglycemia occurs). In patients with insulomas, a normal or excessive fall in blood glucose occurs within 30 min and is sustained for at least 150 min (14). Serum insulin levels in these patients rise to over 150 μU/ml within 5 min and return slowly to fasting levels. Patients with hepatic cirrhosis, acromegaly, Cushing's disease, and obesity may have excessive insulin rises, but the fall in blood glucose is lower and slower than in patients with insulomas (33).

A much safer insulin stimulation test involves the intravenous administration to a patient fasted overnight of 1 mg of glucagon, which causes an acute release of insulin from the pancreas and also stimulates hepatic glycogenolysis (33). Blood samples for insulin and glucose measurements are obtained at 0, 2, 5, 15, 30, 45, 90, and 120 min (14). Patients with insulomas exhibit serum insulin values greater than 180 μU/ml in 5 to 10 min and may have subnormal blood glucose values. Normal insulin values with a blunted glucose response are indicative of hepatic or endocrine organ dysfunction as the cause of hypoglycemia. In 30% of patients with insulomas, this test will not give a diagnostic pattern (33).

Another stimulation test involves the administration of L-leucine, which causes a release of insulin from the pancreas. The compound is given orally at a dose of 200 mg/kg of body weight in tomato juice (14). A fall in blood glucose of 40% or greater is considered diagnostic for insulomas in adults not pretreated with oral sulfonylurea compounds (33). This stimulation test has limited reliability since false-positive results can be obtained in children without insulomas, and up to 50% false-negative results can be obtained in patients with insulomas (33).

A diagnosis of insuloma should alert the physician to the possibility of the presence of other endocrine adenomas (41). This association of insulomas with other endocrine adenomas is referred to as the multiple endocrine adenomatosis syndrome (MEA type I).

LITERATURE CITED

1. Alsever, R. N., and M. R. Stjerholm. 1973. Current concepts in diagnosis of insulinoma. Rocky Mount. Med. J. 22:209–212.
2. Aynsley-Green, A., and K. G. M. M. Alberti. 1972. Serum-insulin or plasma-insulin? Lancet 1:318.
3. Berson, S. A., and R. S. Yalow. 1960. Immunoassay of endogenous plasma insulin in man. J. Clin. Invest. 39:1157–1175.
4. Blanks, M. C., and G. C. Gerritsen. 1974. An ultra-micro immunoassay for insulin. Proc. Soc. Exp. Biol. Med. 146:448–452.
5. Brodal, B. P. 1971. The influence of haemolysis on the radioimmunoassay of insulin. Scand. J. Clin. Lab. Invest. 28:287–290.
6. Cantrell, J. W., J. M. Hochholzer, and C. S. Frings. 1972. Effect of hemolysis on the apparent concentration of insulin in plasma. Clin. Chem. 18:1423–1425.
7. Christopher, A. B., and R. Aiman. 1974. Studies on rat diaphragm insulin bioassay method. Indian J. Med. Res. 62:1499–1510.
8. Clark, J. L., A. H. Rubenstein, P. E. Oyer, J. J. Mackenzie, S. Cho, and D. F. Steiner. 1970. Proinsulin and insulin biosynthesis, p. 339–348. In S. Falkmer, B. Hellman, and I.-B. Taljedal (ed.), The structure and metabolism of the pancreatic islets. Pergamon Press, New York.
9. Cotes, P. M., M. V. Musset, I. Berryman, R. Ekins, S. Glover, N. Hales, W. M. Hunter, C. Lowy, R. W. J. Neville, E. Samols, and P. M. Woodward. 1969. Collaborative study of estimates by radioimmunoassay of insulin concentrations in plasma samples examined in groups of five or six laboratories. J. Endocrinol. 45:557–569.
10. Daughaday, W. H., and L. S. Jacobs. 1971. Methods of separating antibody-bound from free antigen, p. 303–316. In W. D. Odell and W. H. Daughaday (ed.), Principles of competitive protein-binding assays. J. B. Lippincott Co., Philadelphia.
11. Dixon, K. 1974. Measurement of antibodies to insulin in serum. Clin. Chem. 20:1275–1281.
12. Editorial. 1974. Diagnosis of insulinoma. Lancet 2:385–386.
13. El-Khodary, A. Z., M. F. Ball, I. M. Oweiss, and J. J. Canary. 1972. Insulin secretion and body composition in obesity. Metabolism 21:641–655.
14. Ensinck, J. W., and R. H. Williams. 1974. Disorders causing hypoglycemia, p. 627–659. In R. H. Williams (ed.), Textbook of endocrinology, 5th ed. W. B. Saunders Co., Philadelphia.
15. European Association for the Study of Diabetes.

1970. A brief account of the European diabetes epidemiology study group recommendations and research. Diabetologia 6:453–454.

16. Fajans, S. S. 1971. Symposium on diabetes mellitus. Med. Clin. North Am. 55:793–805.

17. Faulk, W. P., J. P. Girard, and H. D. Welscher. 1974. Cell-mediated immunity to insulin and its polypeptide chains in man, p. 89–98. In P. A. Bastenie and W. Gepts (ed.), Immunity and autoimmunity in diabetes mellitus. Excerpta Medica, Amsterdam.

18. Federlin, K. 1971. Immunopathology of insulin. Monogr. Endocrinol., vol. 6.

19. Feldman, J. M., and B. A. Chapman. 1973. Radioimmunoassay of insulin in serum and plasma. Clin. Chem. 19:1250–1254.

20. Fitzgerald, M. O., and H. Keen. 1964. Diagnostic classification of diabetes. Br. Med. J. 1:1568.

21. Flier, J. S., C. R. Kahn, J. Roth, and R. S. Bar. 1975. Antibodies that impair insulin receptor binding in an unusual diabetic syndrome with severe insulin resistance. Science 190:63–65.

22. Grodsky, G. M., and P. H. Forsham. 1960. An immunochemical assay of total extractable insulin in man. J. Clin. Invest. 39:1070–1079.

23. Grunt, J. A., J. A. Pallotta, and J. S. Soeldner. 1970. Blood sugar, serum insulin and free fatty acid interrelationships during intravenous tolbutamide testing in normal young adults and in patients with insulinoma. Diabetes 19:122–126.

24. Hodgkin, D. C. 1974. Varieties of insulin. J. Endocrinol. 63:3P–14P.

25. Horowitz, D. L., and A. H. Rubenstein. 1974. Heterogeneity of circulating insulin and proinsulin in man. Israel J. Med. Sci. 10:1201–1211.

26. Kagan, A. 1975. Radioimmunoassay of insulin. Semin. Nucl. Med. 5:183–188.

27. Kipnis, D. M. 1970. Insulin secretion in normal and diabetic individuals. Adv. Intern. Med. 16:103–134.

28. Klimt, C. R., C. L. Meinert, C. L. Miller, and H. C. Knowles. 1967. A study of the relationship of therapy to vascular and other complications of diabetes, p. 261–269. In Tolbutamide after ten years, Brook Lodge Symposium, August 1967. Excerpta Medica, Amsterdam.

29. Lacy, P. E. 1975. Endocrine secretory mechanisms. Am. J. Pathol. 79:170–187.

30. Luyckx, A., and P. Lefebvre. 1970. Insulin, p. 143–162. In H. Van Cauwenberge and P. Franchimont (ed.), Assay of protein and polypeptide hormones. Pergamon Press, Oxford.

31. McDonald, G. W., J. P. Hoet, and W. J. H. Butterfield. 1965. Diabetes mellitus: report of a WHO expert committee. W.H.O. Tech. Rep. Ser. 310.

32. Malvano, R., T. Quesada, E. Rolleri, C. Gandolfi, and G. C. Zucchelli. 1974. Effects of methodological variables on insulin radioiuumnoassay. Clin. Chim. Acta 51:127–139.

33. Marks, V. 1971. Progress report, diagnosis of

insulinoma. Gut 12:835–843.

34. Marks, V., and E. Samols. 1968. Glucose homeostasis, p. 111–138. In V. H. T. James (ed.), Recent advances in endocrinology, 8th ed. J. & A. Churchill, London.

35. Nunes-Correa, J., C. Lowy, and P. H. Sonksen. 1974. Presumed insulinoma secreting a high-molecular-weight insulin analogue. Lancet 1:837–841.

36. Orosz, L., R. Michael, and M. Ziegler. 1971. Serum-insulin or plasma-insulin? Lancet 2:1149–1150.

37. O'Sullivan, J. B., and C. M. Mahan. 1968. Prospective study of 352 young patients with chemical diabetes. N. Engl. J. Med. 278:1038–1040.

38. Porte, D., and J. Bagdade. 1970. Human insulin secretion: an integrated approach. Annu. Rev. Med. 21:219–240.

39. Prout, T. 1974. Radioisotopic measurements of insulin, p. 267–279. In B. Rothfeld (ed.), Nuclear medicine in vitro. J. B. Lippincott, Philadelphia.

40. Rao, K. J., W. P. Faulk, J. H. Karam, G. M. Grodsky, and P. H. Forsham. 1975. Evidence in support of the concept of immune complex disease in insulin-treated diabetics, p. 255–263. In P. A. Bastenie and W. Gepts (ed.), Immunity and autoimmunity in diabetes mellitus. Excerpta Medica, Amsterdam.

41. Sawin, C. T. 1969. Endocrine physiology; the hormones, p. 202–243. Little, Brown and Co., Boston.

42. Schein, P. S., R. A. DeLellis, C. R. Kahn, P. Gorder, and A. R. Kraft. 1973. Islet cell tumors: current concepts and management. Ann. Intern. Med. 79:239–257.

43. Starr, J. I., and A. H. Rubenstein. 1974. Insulin, proinsulin, and c-peptide, p. 289–315. In B. M. Jaffe and H. R. Behrman (ed.), Methods of hormone radioimmunoassay. Academic Press Inc., New York.

44. Turner, R. C., N. W. Oakley, and J. P. N. Nabarru. 1971. Control of basal insulin secretion with special reference to the diagnosis of insulinomas. Br. Med. J. 2:132–135.

45. Unger, R. H. 1974. The pancreas as a regulator of metabolism, p. 179–204. In S. M. McCann (ed.), Endocrine physiology, Butterworths, London.

46. Valleron, A. J., E. Eschwege, L. Papoz, and G. E. Rosselin. 1975. Agreement and discrepancy in the evaluation of normal and diabetic oral glucose tolerance test. Diabetes 24:585–593.

47. Van Cauwenberge, H., P. Lefebvre, and P. Franchimont. 1970. Biological methods, p. 7–11. In H. Van Cauwenberge and P. Franchimont (ed.), Assay of protein and polypeptide hormones. Pergamon Press, Oxford.

48. Velasco, C. A., H. S. Cole, and R. A. Camerini-Davalos. 1974. Radioimmunoassay of insulin, with use of an immunosorbent. Clin. Chem. 20:700–702.

49. Velasco, C. A., W. Oppermann, and R. A. Camerini-Davalos. 1973. Critical variables in

the radioimmunological technique for measuring immunoreactive insulin with use of immunosorbents. Clin. Chem. **19**:201–204.

50. West, K. M. 1975. Substantial difference in the diagnostic criteria used by diabetes experts. Diabetes **24**:641–644.

51. Wilkerson, H. L. C. 1964. Diagnosis, oral glucose tolerance tests, p. 31–34. *In* Diabetes mellitus, diagnosis and treatment. American Diabetes Association, New York.

52. Yalow, R. S., and S. A. Berson. 1973. Big, big insulin. Metabolism **22**:703–713.

53. Young, D. S., L. C. Pestaner, and V. Gibberman. 1975. Effects of drugs on clinical laboratory tests. Clin. Chem. **21**:320D–321D.

54. Zacharewicz, F. A. 1974. The clinical significance of growth hormone and insulin assay, p. 18–32. *In* W. T. Newton and R. M. Donati (ed.), Radioassay in clinical medicine. Charles C Thomas, Springfield.

Chapter 21

Radioimmunoassay of Gastrin

JAMES E. McGUIGAN

INTRODUCTION

The gastrointestinal hormone gastrin, the most potent substance known to stimulate acid secretion, plays an important role in the control of acid secretion both in humans and in experimental animals. In 1964, Gregory and Tracy (4) purified two gastrins from porcine gastrin antral mucosa and subsequently from the gastric antral mucosa of man. These gastrins proved to be linear polypeptides, each containing 17 amino acids (heptadecapeptides). In one form of gastrin the tyrosine residue in position 12 was sulfated (gastrin II), and in the other form of gastrin the tyrosine was not sulfated (gastrin I). In all animal species thus far studied, both forms of gastrin heptadecapeptide exist in serum and in antral mucosa.

Prior to the advent of radioimmunoassay of gastrin, estimation of the gastrin activity was performed by bioassay. Bioasay methods proved insufficiently specific and insufficiently sensitive for satisfactory measurement of circulating gastrin levels. Radioimmunoassay of gastrin (6, 13, 14, 19, 20, 26) has provided a sensitive and specific method for measurement of serum gastrin concentrations in normal humans and in a variety of disease states and has also provided the capacity to measure gastrin content of extracts of tissues, including antral mucosa and tumor tissue rich in gastrin (e.g., in the gastrinoma of the Zollinger-Ellison [31] syndrome). As is the case for other radioimmunoassay techniques, radioimmunoassay of gastrin demands (i) the production of specific antibodies to gastrin, (ii) preparation of a radiolabeled form of the peptide (in this instance [125I]-gastrin), (iii) the availability of a pure peptide for purposes of radioiodination and for use as calibration standards, and (iv) a method of separation of antibody-bound and antibody-free radiolabeled peptide.

CLINICAL INDICATIONS

The primary clinical indication for measurement of serum gastrin concentration is the detection of increased serum gastrin levels in patients with the Zollinger-Ellison syndrome. It has been demonstrated conclusively that the Zollinger-Ellison syndrome, which is characterized by high rates of gastric acid secretion, severe peptic ulcer disease of the upper gastrointestinal tract, and non-beta islet cell tumors of the pancreas, is due to excessive release of gastrin from these tumors (gastrinomas, which are rich in gastrin content; 5, 14). Radioimmunoassay of gastrin provides a method for gastrin measurement which is much more sensitive and specific than previously utilized bioassay methods.

It must be recognized that there are other causes of increased fasting serum gastrin levels in addition to the Zollinger-Ellison syndrome. These include patients with pernicious anemia, as well as those with other forms of chronic atrophic gastritis with gastric atrophy, including patients with carcinoma of the stomach with decreased or absent gastric acid secretion (15, 16). The mechanism proposed for increased serum gastrin levels in patients with pernicious anemia and other forms of markedly reduced gastric acid secretion is that of the absence of gastric acid secretion, which normally serves to inhibit release of gastrin into the circulation. When the pH in the stomach is reduced to 3, gastrin release is reduced, and, when the pH is reduced to 1.5, release of gastrin into the circulation is eliminated. In addition, it has been shown that there are increased numbers of gastrin-containing cells in the gastric mucosa of patients with pernicious anemia. These patients with reduced acid secretion should be readily differentiated from the patients with the Zollinger-Ellison syndrome both on clinical grounds and by measurement of gastric acid secretory rates. Patients with renal failure may also have increased gastrin levels: this is believed due to disease-associated reductions in the effectiveness of the kidney in metabolizing gastrin. Under normal conditions, approximately 40% of gastrin is degraded by the renal cortex. Increased serum gastrin levels have also been described in both patients and experimental animals after massive resection of the small intestine (22, 25). Increases in serum gastrin levels have also been observed in the postoperative retained antrum syndrome (12). Modest increases in fasting serum gastrin levels have been noted in some patients with hyper-calcemic hyperparathyroidism; many such in-stances may represent patients with the multi-ple endocrine adenoma syndrome who harbor not yet detected Zollinger-Ellison tumors.

TEST PROCEDURES

Production of antibodies to gastrin

Two principal methods have been used for the production of antibodies to gastrin. The first method, which is recommended and is used in my laboratory, consists of the produc-tion of antibodies in rabbits which are repeat-edly immunized with human gastrin I cova-lently conjugated to bovine serum albumin (13). In this method 6 mg of human gastrin I hexa-decapeptide (residues 2 through 17) is dissolved in 0.4 ml of N,N-dimethylformamide to which 0.6 ml of 0.05 M potassium phosphate, pH 7.4, is added. Then bovine serum albumin, 12 mg in 0.4 ml of the same phosphate buffer, is added to the peptide solution. This is followed by addition of 50 mg of 1-ethyl-3-(3-dimethyl-aminopropyl) carbodiimide, 50 mg in 0.2 ml. The reaction mixture is gently stirred by means of a mag-netic mixer at room temperature for 20 to 24 h. The resultant slightly opalescent suspension-solution is then dialyzed for 48 h at 4 C against 2 liters of phosphate-buffered saline (0.15 M NaCl-0.01 M potassium phosphate, pH 7.4). With this technique, on the average from 8 to 12 human gastrin I molecules are conjugated to each bovine serum albumin molecule. For im-munization the resultant conjugate (5 mg/ml) is emulsified with an equal volume of complete Freund's adjuvant, and New Zealand white rabbits are immunized with 0.2 ml per footpad. Repeat immunization is performed 1 and 6 months after initial immunization and subse-quently at 2- to 4-month intervals. Antibodies satisfactory for radioimmunoassay are consist-ently obtained in blood procured 10 to 12 days after the third and subsequent immunizations. The second and alternative method of produc-tion of antibodies to gastrin was described by Yalow and Berson (26), in which they utilized partially purified porcine gastrin, without con-jugation to carrier protein, for immunization of guinea pigs. Partially purified procine gastrin was dissolved in 1 ml of 0.1 M glycine, pH 9.5, and titrated to pH 7.4 by addition of 0.25 M phosphate, pH 7.4. The resultant preparation was emulsified with complete Freund's adju-vant and administered to guinea pigs subcuta-neously. Immunizations were repeated at monthly intervals, and animals were bled 8 to 12 days later. With this technique, approxi-mately 40% of immunized guinea pigs develop circulating antibodies suitable for radioimmu-noassay of gastrin.

Radioiodination of gastrin

Because of the presence of a tyrosine residue in the gastrin molecule, human gastrin I can be readily radioiodinated (13) by application of the chloramine T method of Hunter and Greenwood (8). With this technique, 2 μg of human gastrin I in 50 μliters of 0.5 M potassium phosphate, pH 7.4, is placed in a 75 $\times$ 10 mm disposable glass tube. To this is added mCi of ^{125}INa. Then chloramine T (10 μliters containing 17.5 μg) is added with gentle mixing for 30 s. To this is then added 125 μg of sodium metabisulfite in 100 μliters of the same phosphate buffer. The resultant solution is applied to a Sephadex G-10 column (25 $\times$ 1.5 cm) and eluted in 2.0-ml frac-tions with 0.1 M potassium phosphate buffer, pH 7.4. Radiolabeled gastrin appears in the void volume (at approximately 16 ml). The ^{125}I which is not bound to the peptide is further retarded on the column and appears as a second major peak. With this method, radiolabeled gastrin may be prepared with an average spe-cific activity approximating 250 mCi/μmol. As an alternative to Sephadex G-10 filtration, Ya-low and Berson (26) have utilized starch gel electrophoresis for purification of [^{125}I]gastrin following radioiodination. More recently, Stadil and Rehfeld (21) described a method for radioiodination of gastrin which possesses the advantage of a more consistent preparation of monoiodinated gastrin. In this technique, ra-dioiodination is performed in 0.05 M potassium phosphate, pH 7.4. A 200-μCi amount of ^{125}INa is added to 4 μg of human gastrin I to which is added 5 μg of chloramine T in 10 μliters. After 30 s of incubation and mixing, 5 μg of sodium metabisulfite is added in 25 μliters. The result-ant mixture is applied to a column (0.9 $\times$ 15 cm) containing aminoethyl cellulose (AE 41, What-man) which has been charged appropriately and then equilibrated with 0.05 M ammonium bi-carbonate. The column is eluted by use of a linear gradient progressing from 0.05 M ammo-nium bicarbonate (300 ml) to 0.4 M ammonium bicarbonate (300 ml). With this technique, ^{125}I appears as a sharp peak, which is subsequently followed by fractions which may be demon-strated to contain monoiodinted human gastrin I.

Separation of antibody-bound from -free [^{125}I]-gastrin

A variety of techniques have been utilized for the separation of antibody-bound from antibody-free radiolabeled gastrin. The most rapid and convenient technique is that of utilization of an anion-binding resin (26), which tightly binds the strongly negatively charged [^{125}I]gastrin but does not bind antibody-bound [^{125}I]gastrin; Amberlite IRP-58M (Rohm and Haas) is an effective anion-binding resin for use in separation of antibody-bound from antibody-free [^{125}I]gastrin. An equally satisfactory alternative to resin separation of antibody-free from antibody-bound gastrin is that of double antibody precipitation, with the use of goat anti-rabbit gamma globulin, added in antibody excess (13). Other techniques which have been used, but which have been proven less satisfactory in my laboratory, include separation by use of charcoal binding (6) or ethanol precipitation (10).

Multiple molecular forms of gastrin

It has been well-established that gastrin in serum or plasma exists in a variety of molecular forms. These include heptadecapeptide gastrins (gastrins I and II) and larger forms of gastrin, which have been designated as big gastrin, G-34 (27, 28), and big, big gastrin (29, 30). Big gastrin is a linear polypeptide containing 34 amino acids, the carboxyl-terminal 17 of which are identical to heptadecapeptide gastrin. Big, big gastrin (molecular weight approximately 21,000) also appears to contain heptadecapeptide gastrin as part of its structure. It is probable that both big gastrin and big, big gastrin exist in the serum in both sulfated and nonsulfated forms (gastrins I and II). There also appear to be smaller molecular fragments of gastrin in the circulation (3, 17). Acceptable antibodies currently in use for radioimmunoassay of gastrin recognize and detect heptadecapeptide gatrin, big gastrin (G-34), and big, big gastrin in both their nonsulfated (gastrin I) and sulfated (gastrin II) forms. Serum gastrin concentrations may be expressed as picograms per milliliter relative to human gastrin I used as the reference standard; this is the more widely used designation. An alternative expression is that of femtomoles of gastrin per milliliter (1 fmol = 10^{-15} mol; in respect to heptadecapeptide gastrin, fmol/ml × 2.1 = pg/ml.)

The method for radioimmunoassay of gastrin to be described, and that used in my laboratory, utilizes antibodies to gastrin prepared in rabbits by immunization with human gastrin I conjugated to bovine serum albumin, radioiodination using Sephadex G-10 column separation or monoiodination, as described by Stadil and Rehfeld (21), separation of antibody-free from antibody-bound gastrin by use of Amberlite IRP-58M, and expression of serum gastrin con-

centrations as picograms per milliliter of serum relative to human gastrin I heptadecapeptide as standard.

Incubation contents and conditions

Incubations are performed in triplicate in 75 × 10 mm disposable glass test tubes. The calibration curve is established from which gastrin concentrations in unknown serum samples may be determined. All reagents are prepared in 0.02 M barbital buffer, pH 8.4, containing bovine serum albumin, 2.5 mg/ml. (It is necessary that all solutions be protein-containing to elim-

TABLE 1. *Example of constituents and volumes of reagents for gastrin radioimmunoassay calibration curve and serum gastrin determination*

Tube no.	BSA-Barb. buffer[a] (ml)	Human gastrin I, pg/ml (0.1 ml)	Serum unknowns[b] (ml)	Anti-serum to gastrin (ml)	^{125}I-labeled human gastrin I[c] (ml)
1	1.9	—	—	—	0.1
2	1.9	—	—	—	0.1
3	1.9	—	—	—	0.1
4	1.8	—	—	0.1	0.1
5	1.8	—	—	0.1	0.1
6	1.8	—	—	0.1	0.1
7	1.7	2,000	—	0.1	0.1
8	1.7	2,000	—	0.1	0.1
9	1.7	2,000	—	0.1	0.1
10	1.7	1,000	—	0.1	0.1
11	1.7	1,000	—	0.1	0.1
12	1.7	1,000	—	0.1	0.1
13	1.7	500	—	0.1	0.1
14	1.7	500	—	0.1	0.1
15	1.7	500	—	0.1	0.1
16	1.7	250	—	0.1	0.1
17	1.7	250	—	0.1	0.1
18	1.7	250	—	0.1	0.1
19	1.7	125	—	0.1	0.1
20	1.7	125	—	0.1	0.1
21	1.7	125	—	0.1	0.1
22	1.7	62.5	—	0.1	0.1
23	1.7	62.5	—	0.1	0.1
24	1.7	62.5	—	0.1	0.1
25	1.7	31.2	—	0.1	0.1
26	1.7	31.2	—	0.1	0.1
27	1.7	31.2	—	0.1	0.1
28	1.7	16.1	—	0.1	0.1
29	1.7	16.1	—	0.1	0.1
30	1.7	16.1	—	0.1	0.1
31	1.7	—	0.1 ⎫	0.1	0.1
32	1.7	—	0.1 ⎬ A	0.1	0.1
33	1.7	—	0.1 ⎭	0.1	0.1
34	1.7	—	0.1 ⎫	0.1	0.1
35	1.7	—	0.1 ⎬ B	0.1	0.1
36	1.7	—	0.1 ⎭	0.1	0.1

[a] Bovine serum albumin-barbital buffer.
[b] A and B represent two example unknown serum samples.
[c] 2,000 to 3,000 counts/min.

inate nonspecific peptide adsorption to glass, which for gastrin is not great. Alternatives to bovine serum albumin which have been used include ovalbumin, 2.5 mg/ml, or 2% normal animal or human serum.) Table 1 provides the constituents and volumes of reagents used in the preparation of a radioimmunoassay calibration curve and, in addition, the inclusion of two unknown sera, A and B. The total volume for each incubation tube is 2.0 ml. The initial three replicates contain 1.9 ml of bovine serum albumin-barbital buffer (BSA-Barb.) and 0.1 ml of ^{125}I-labeled human gastrin I (2,000 to 3,000 counts/min). These tubes constitute a determination of nonspecific binding, which should not exceed 10%. Each of the next three tubes contains 1.8 ml of BSA-Barb., 0.1 ml of [^{125}I]-gastrin, and, in addition, 0.1 ml of diluted antibodies to gastrin. Antibody dilutions, which may range from final dilutions of 1:20,000 to 1:2,000,000, are selected which yield [^{125}I]gastrin bound to free ratios in the range from 0.7 to 1.0. The value for these tubes yields the ratio of antibody-bound to antibody-free [^{125}I]-gastrin in the absence of additional unlabeled peptide (B_0). Subsequent tubes contain 1.7 ml of BSA-Barb., antibodies to gastrin, and radiolabeled gastrin as above, and, in addition 0.1 ml of human gastrin I standard or 0.1 ml of serum in which the gastrin content is to be measured. Gastrin standards are prepared in serial dilutions from 2,000 pg/ml to 16 pg/ml (Table 1). Incubation tubes are then sealed with Parafilm, mixed briefly with a Vortex mixer, and incubated for 2 to 4 days at 4 C. After the period of incubation, Amberlite IRP-58M (100 mg/ml) is suspended in 0.02 M barbital buffer, pH 8.4, and allowed to stand with continuous magnetic stirring at room temperature for at least 1 h. Immediately before addition of the resin, 0.1 ml of normal human serum is added to each of the 30 tubes in the calibration curve; 0.2 ml of the resin suspension is then transferred to each incubation tube. (Inasmuch as prolonged contact of resin with the incubation mixture can remove some bound gastrin from the gastrin antibody, no more than 48 tubes should be processed at one time. The remaining tubes should be kept at 4 C until processed with the resin.) As soon as the resin suspension is added, the tubes are agitated for 3 to 4 s with a Vortex mixer and then centrifuged for 5 min at 2,000 rpm at 4 C. Supernatant solutions are then transferred to a second 75 × 10 mm disposable test tube by means of Pasteur pipettes, and all tubes are sealed with Parafilm. Antibody-bound gastrin remains in the supernatant fluid, and antibody-free [^{125}I]gastrin is bound by the resin. Each tube is then counted in sequence (2 to 4 min) in an automatic gamma spectrometer.

It is strongly recommended that blood gastrin measuremnts be performed on serum rather than on plasma when the technique described here is used. This is necessary because excess heparin leads to increased nonspecific binding, probably by competing with gastrin for binding sites on the resin.

Calculations

Table 2 represents an example of counts per minute obtained and proportions of antibody-bound to antibody-free [^{125}I]gastrin for use in establishment of a calibration curve; it also includes data for two serum unknowns (A and B). Figure 1 is the graphic display of the calibration curve utilizing constituents and volumes of reagents indicated in Table 1 and antibody-bound to -free ^{125}I-labeled human gastrin I ratios and calculations from Table 2. The standard curve is prepared by plotting bound over free ratios of [^{125}I]gastrin I on the ordinate against picograms of gastrin per milliliter on the horizontal axis. Before this is done, bound over free ratios are corrected by subtracting the nonspecific binding blank (mean of supernatant counts from the first three tubes) from all subsequent supernatant tubes. The resultant calibration curve exhibits progressive decreases in bound over free ratios for [^{125}I]gastrin with increasing content of nonradiolabeled gastrin in the incubation tubes. Bound over free ratios may be expressed as the means of raw data of obtained bound over free ratios or, alternatively, as is shown in Table 1, may be corrected to ratios relative to B_0 (tubes 4, 5, 6) − 1.0. (I favor the latter procedure.) Precision of the assay may be assessed by determination of the standard error of the mean and coefficients of variations of unknown samples and for the calibration curve standards. Data obtained may then be plotted as a calibration diagram as in Fig. 1. This calibration curve may then be used to determine gastrin concentration in unknown serum samples. In general, the most precise portion of the calibraon curve is in its mid-portion. (Coefficients of variation in the mid-portion of the curve should not exceed 5%.)

Fasting serum samples A and B were included (Tables 1 and 2, Fig. 1) as examples for serum gastrin measurements. The gastrin concentration of serum sample A was determined to 64 pg/ml (based on B/F = 0.610, as applied to the calibration curve shown in Fig. 1); this value falls within the normal range. The serum

TABLE 2. *Example of counts per minute obtained, proportions of antibody-bound to -free [^{125}I]gastrin for calibration curve, and serum gastrin radioimmunoassay[a]*

Sample no.	Counts/ min free	Counts/ min bound	B/F	B/F-Corr.[b] (mean)	SEM[c]
1	2,640	39	0.015		
2	2,649	36	0.036	0	—
3	2,642	19	0.007		
4	1,111	1,236	1.086		
5	1,053	1,286	1.191	1.0	0.031
6	1,116	1,283	1.121		
7	2,455	208	0.072		
8	2,366	240	0.088	0.076	0.006
9	2,346	258	0.096		
10	2,152	350	0.148		
11	2,203	391	0.163	0.140	0.005
12	2,257	406	0.166		
13	1,976	513	0.244		
14	2,025	508	0.235	0.212	0.002
15	1,990	511	0.241		
16	1,859	702	0.361		
17	1,814	733	0.387	0.318	0.014
18	1,701	597	0.333		
19	1,580	931	0.588		
20	1,495	861	0.555	0.504	0.008
21	1,544	910	0.569		
22	1,369	985	0.697		
23	1,454	1,033	0.689	0.661	0.002
24	1,483	1,056	0.691		
25	1,356	1,094	0.784		
26	1,244	1,108	0.865	0.741	0.024
27	1,280	1,099	0.868		
28	1,245	1,187	0.928		
29	1,188	1,179	0.966	0.877	0.042
30	1,155	1,286	1.086		
31	1,380	1,001	0.702		
32	1,427	984	0.668	0.610	0.011
33	1,450	1,026	0.686	(A)	
34	2,275	328	0.131		
35	2,298	315	0.124	0.110	0.003
36	2,260	301	0.119	(B)	

[a] Tube numbers apply to those indicated in Table 1.

[b] Corrected bound/free [^{125}I]gastrin (B/F-Corr.) obtained by subtracting nonspecific binding (mean counts/minute of supernatants from initial three replicates) from each supernatant counts/minute, which is then divided by counts/minute in resin precipitates, with correction to B_o (tubes 4, 5, 6) = 1.0.

[c] Standard error of the mean.

gastrin level for serum sample B (B/F = 0.110) was 1,350 pg/ml, which represents an elevated serum gastrin concentration.

Controls for asessment of the precision and accuracy of test results may include utilization of human gastrin I standards (Medical Research Council of England) and serum samples

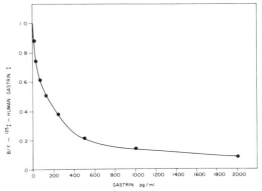

FIG. 1. *Calibration diagram indicating antibody-bound to antibody-free ^{125}I-labeled human gastrin I ratios (B/F) with inclusion of progressively increasing amounts of unlabeled human gastrin I in the incubation mixture. Gastrin contents of unknown serum samples are derived from application of B/F for each sample to the standard curve.*

of known gastrin concentration from previous authenticated asays.

Alternate methods and calculations

The techniques described above may also be performed similarly with antibodies to porcine gastrin (26). In addition, porcine gastrin (or gastrin from other mammalian species) may be used for radiolabeling and for calibration standards. In general, in the measurement of human serum gastrin, use of human gastrin I for radiolabeling and standards is preferable, since it does not require correction for potential differences in immunological reactivity of gastrin antibodies for gastrin from different mammalian species.

The double-antibody techniue, using goat anti-rabbit gamma globulin, may be used for separation of antibody-bound from antibody-free ^{125}I-labeled human gastrin I with incubation reactions performed at pH 8.4 (as above) or with phosphate-buffered saline, pH 7.4. The second antibody is added 2 days after initial incubation, and precipitates are obtained 20 to 24 h later by centrifugation at 2,000 rpm for 20 min at 4 C. Antibody-bound ^{125}I-labeled human gastrin I is contained in the precipitate, and antibody-free ^{125}I-labeled human gastrin I is in the supernatant fluid. This method possesses the advantages that the precipitates are stable and all incubation mixtures may be processed simultaneously.

The method for calculation of the proportion of [^{125}I]gastrin which is described above calculates individual B/F values using B_o corrected to 1.0 (Table 2, Fig. 1). A variety of other calculations and graphic methos have been used. These include calculation of the percentage of total [^{125}I]gastrin which is antibody-bound with B_0 adjusted to 100%, use of B/F ratios without corrections of B_0 to 1.0, and even use of F/B ratios. All may be used satisfactorily. The calibration curve may be depicted graphically in a linear-linear form as in Fig. 1 or alternatively in a semi-log form (26), in which the vertical axis is B/F and the horizontal axis is the log of the gastrin concentration (pg/ml). The latter method yields a sigmoid calibration curve, with a long linear mid-portion of the curve, which is the area of maximal assay precision.

REAGENTS

Human gastrin I (residues 1 to 17) and human gastrin I hexadecapeptide (residues 2 to 17) can be purchased from Imperial Chemical Industries, Ltd., Chesire, England. Standards for synthetic human gastrin I heptadecapeptide are available from the Medical Reserch Council of England. 1-Ethyl-3-(3-dimethyl-aminopropyl) carbodiimide can be purchased from Ott Chemical Co., bovine serum albumin, from Sigma Chemical Co., and ^{125}INa, from a variety of sources of radioisotopes including New England Nuclear Corp., Cambridge Nuclear Co., and Amersham/Searle. Other standard reagent-grade chemicals can be obtained from such companies as Fisher Chemical Co. (At the present time, E. R. Squibb & Sons makes available a radioimmunoassay kit which incorporates most of the procedure described in this protocol.)

Preparation and storage of reagents

Barbital buffer is prepared from barbituric acid and sodium barbital and kept in stock solution (1.0 M, pH 8.4) at 4 C. Dilutions of antibodies to gastrin are kept at a dilution 100-fold less than that used in the radioimmunoassay procedure, with storage in 0.02 M barbital, pH 8.4, containing 2.5 mg of bovine serum albumin/ml. Stock solutions for calibration curve materials are kept in the same protein-buffer solution in a concentration of 20,000 pg/ml. Gastrin, both in serum and in protein-containing solutions, is stable when maintained at -20 to -70 C for periods from many months to several years.

INTERPRETATION

Fasting serum gastrin levels

Normal fasting serum gastrin concentrations range from 20 to 160 pg/ml. Mean serum gastrin levels in fasting sera vary somewhat in different laboratories but average from 50 to 75 pg/ml in most laboratories. Fasting serum concentrations in patients with the Zollinger-Ellison syndrome are elevated when compared with those of normal human subjects and range from 175 to 350,000 pg/ml, with most patients with Zollinger-Ellison tumors having serum gastrin levels which are in excess of 800 pg/ml. Serum gastrin concentrations from 150 to 300 pg/ml may be viewed as indeterminate in respect to the Zollinger-Ellison syndrome and should be repeated. Fasting serum gastrin concentrations in patients with duodenal ulcer disease do not differ from those of normal subjects (24). Patients with gastric ulcer (24) may have slightly higher serum gastrin concentrations (mean, 160 pg/ml); however, this is probably related to decreases in gastric acid secretion. Fasting serum gastrin has been reported to be increased in the retained antrum syndrome (12). It must be stressed that gastric acid secretion should also be measured in all patients in whom the Zollinger-Ellison syndrome is suspected and in whom serum gastrin measurements are being determined for this consideration.

Provocative tests for the Zollinger-Ellison syndrome

Inasmuch as the measurement of serum gastrin concentrations has its principal application to the patient who may have the Zollinger-Ellison syndrome and since therapy may often be dictated by conclusions relative to the serum gastrin concentration, several provocative tests, in addition to measurement of the fasting serum gastrin level, have been evolved to assist in identifying patients with Zollinger-Ellison tumors. One such test is the calcium infusion test (1, 23). In this test the patient receives intravenous calcium (calcium gluconate) by constant intravenous infusion for a 3-h period (5 mg of Ca/kg·h). Serum gastrin levels are measured before institution of the infusion and at 30-min intervals for 4 h after the initiation of the infusion. Most patients with Zollinger-Ellison tumors will increase their serum gastrin level by greater than 500 pg/ml, whereas most normal subjects and patients with common peptic ulcer will increase their serum gastrin levels by less than 500 pg/ml. A second provocative test is that of secretin infusion. Intravenous secretin administration in normal individuals either slightly decreases fasting serum gastrin levels (7) or has no effect. In contrast, in patients with Zollinger-Ellison tumors, intravenous secretin infusion usually produces a paradoxical increase in serum gastrin concentration (2, 9, 11, 18). In this test secretin (GIH), 2 to 3 units/kg, is administered by intravenous injection over a 1-min period. Serum samples are obtained before intravenous administration of secretin and at 5-min intervals for 30 min after intravenous secretin injection. Normal individuals usually have decreases in their serum gastrin levels, whereas patients with the Zollinger-Ellison syndrome usually have increases in serum gastrin concentration. The major physiological stimulation to gastrin release is that of feeding, particularly the protein content of the meal. In response to the administration of a protein-containing meal (100 g of protein), serum gastrin concentrations in normal individuals as well as in patients with common peptic ulcer usually increase by 50 to 200%. Patients with Zollinger-Ellison tumors usually increase their serum gastrin concentrations in response to feeding by smaller increments or not at all.

ACKNOWLEDGMENTS

This work was supported by Public Health Service research grants AM13711 and CA15332 from the National Institutes of Health and by research grant DT-17 from the American Cancer Society.

LITERATURE CITED

1. Basso, N., and E. Passaro, Jr. 1970. Calcium-stimulated gastric secretion in Zollinger-Ellison syndrome. Arch. Surg. 101:399–402.
2. Bradley, E. L., II, J. T. Galambos, C. R. Lobley, and Y. K. Chan. 1973. Secretin-gastrin relationshps in Zollinger-Ellison syndrome. Surgery 73:550–556.
3. Dockray, G. J., and J. H. Walsh. 1975. Amino terminal gastrin fragment in serum of Zollinger-Ellison syndrome patients. Gastroenterology 68:222–230.
4. Gregory, R. A., and H. J. Tracy. 1964. The constitution and properties of two gastrins extracted from hog antral mucosa. I. The isolation of two gastrins from hog antral mucosa. Gut 5:103–107.
5. Gregory, R. A., H. J. Tracy, K. L. Agarwal, and M. I. Grossman. 1969. Amino acid composition of two gastrins isolated from Zollinger-Ellison tumor tissue. Gut 10:603–608.
6. Hansky, J., and M. D. Cain. 1969. Radioimmunoassay of gastrin in human serum. Lancet 2:1388–1390.
7. Hansky, J., C. Soveny, and M. G. Korman. 1971. Effect of secretin on serum gastrin as measured by radioimmunoassay. Gastroenterology 61:62–68.
8. Hunter, W. M., and F. C. Greenwood. 1962. Preparation of iodine-131 labeled human growth hormone of high specific activity. Nature (London) 194:495–496.
9. Isenberg, J. I., J. H. Walsh, E. Passaro, Jr., E. W. Moore, and M. I. Grossman. 1972. Unusual effect of secretin on serum gastrin, serum calium, and gastric acid secretion in a patient with suspected Zollinger-Ellison syndrome. Gastroenterology 62:626–631.
10. Jeffcoate, S. L. 1969. Radioimmunoassay of gastrin: specificity of gastrin antisera. Scand. J. Gastroenterol. 4:457–461.
11. Kolts, B. E., C. A. Herbst, and J. E. McGuigan. 1974. Calcium and secretin-stimulated gastrin release in the Zollinger-Ellison syndrome. Ann Intern. Med. 81:758–762.
12. Korman, M. G., D. F. Scott, J. Hansky, and H. Wilson. 1972. Hypergastrinemia due to an excluded gastric antrum: a proposed method for differentiation from the Zollinger-Ellison syndrome. Aust. N.Z. J. Med. 3:266–271.
13. McGuigan, J. E. 1968. Immunochemical studies with synthetic human gastrin. Gastroenterology 54:1005–1011.
14. McGuigan, J. E., and W. L. Trudeau. 1968. Immunochemical measurement of elevated levels of gastrin in the serum of patients with pancreatic tumors of the Zollinger-Ellison variety. N. Engl. J. Med. 278:1308–1313.
15. McGuigan, J. E., and W. L. Trudeau. 1970. Serum gastrin concentrations in pernicious anemia. N. Engl. J. Med. 282:358–361.
16. McGuigan, J. E., and W. L. Trudeau. 1973. Serum and tissue gastrin concentrations in patients with carcinoma of the stomach. Gastroenterology 64:22–25.
17. Rehfeld, J. F., and F. Stadil. 1973. Gel filtration studies on immunoreactive gastrin in serum from Zollinger-Ellison patients. Gut 14:369–373.
18. Schrumpf, E., H. Petersen, A. Berstad, J. Myren, and B. Rosenlund. 1973. The effect of secretin on plasma gastrin in the Zollinger-Ellison syndrome. Scand. J. Gastroenterol. 8:145–150.
19. Schrumpf, E., and T. Sand. 1972. Radioimmunoassay of gastrin with activated charcoal. Scand. J. Gastroenterol. 7:683–687.
20. Stadil, F., and J. F. Rehfeld. 1971. Radioimmunoassay of gastrin in human serum. Scand. J. Gastroenterol. Suppl. 9:61–65.
21. Stadil, F., and J. F. Rehfeld. 1972. Preparation of ^{125}I-labeled synthetic human gastrin I for radioimmunoanalysis. Scand. J. Clin. Lab. Invest. 30:361–368.
22. Straus, E., C. D. Gerson, and R. S. Yalow. 1974. Hypersecretion of gastrin associated with the short bowel syndrome. Gastroenterology 66:175–180.
23. Trudeau, W. L., and J. E. McGuigan. 1969. Effects of calcium on serum gastrin levels in the Zollinger-Ellison syndrome. N. Engl. J. Med. 281:862–866.
24. Trudeau, W. L., and J. E. McGuigan. 1971. Relations between serum gastrin levels and rates of gastric hydrochloric acid secretion. N. Engl. J. Med. 284:408–412.
25. Wickbom, G., J. H. Landor, F. L. Bushkin, and

J. E. McGuigan. 1975. Changes in gastric acid output and serum gastrin levels following massive small intestinal resection. Gastroenterology, in press.

26. Yalow, R. S., and S. A. Berson. 1970. Radioimmunoassa of gastrin. Gastroenterology 58:1–14.

27. Yalow, R. S., and S. A. Berson. 1970. Size and charge distinctions between endogenous human plasma gastrin in peripheral blood and heptadecapeptide gastrin. Gastroenterology 58:609–615.

28. Yalow, R. S., and S. A. Berson. 1971. Further studies on the nature of immunoreactive gastrin in human plasma. Gastroenterology 60:203–214.

29. Yalow, R. S., and S. A. Berson. 1972. And now "big, big" gastrin. Biochem. Biophys. Res. Commun. 48:391–395.

30. Yalow, R. S., and N. Wu. 1973. Additional studies on the nature of big, big gastrin. Gastroenterology 65:19–27.

31. Zollinger, R. M., and E. H. Ellison. 1955. Primary peptic ulcerations of the jejunum associated with islet cell tumors of the pancreas. Ann. Surg. 142:709–728.

Chapter 22

The Renin-Angiotensin System

EDGAR HABER AND KNUD POULSEN

INTRODUCTION

Renin is a proteolytic enzyme secreted by the juxtaglomerular cells of the kidney in response to changes in renal artery blood pressure, renal tubular sodium concentration, and the stimulation of the renal sympathetic nerves. This enzyme, which has not as yet been fully purified or characterized, reacts with a protein substrate, angiotensinogen (present in high concentration in plasma), to release a decapeptide fragment, angiotensin I (11).

The enzyme cleaves the substrate between leu^{10} and leu^{11} as shown in Fig. 1. Angiotensin I, which is inactive as a hormone, is further cleaved between phe^8 and his^9 to yield angiotensin II. This proteolytic cleavage occurs principally in the pulmonary circulation, and it is mediated by converting enzyme. Angiotensin II is a potent pressor hormone that causes systemic and pulmonary vasoconstriction, and it also acts as a major stimulus to the secretion of aldosterone by the adrenal gland. It has recently been found that a derivative of angiotensin II, the heptapeptide resulting from the cleavage between asp^1 and arg^2, may be more potent than angiotensin II in stimulating aldosterone secretion. It has tentatively been named angiotensin III (8).

Since renal renin has not yet been fully purified, a direct assay for this enzyme cannot be devised. Preliminary efforts at renin purification suggest that such a direct assay may soon be available (5, 7, 14). Indeed, a radioimmunoassay has been described for mouse submaxillary gland renin (6), which has now been fully purified. Renin is presently assayed by measuring its activity as an enzyme in determining the rate of generation of its product, angiotensin I. Angiotensin I has been measured by bioassay (10). The tedium and insensitivity of this approach have led to its replacement by an immunoassay for angiotensin I, which is presently the most common method of renin assay.

The results of renin assays may be expressed as either renin activity or renin concentration. The latter implies the rate of production of angiotensin I under a given set of conditions. The major variables in *renin activity* assays are renin itself and substrate concentration.

Both affect the rate of angiotensin I production. If renin is held constant, an increase in angiotensinogen concentration will increase angiotensin I generation. However, the relationship between substrate concentration and the rate of angiotensin I production is not a linear function (13). Results of renin activity assays are expressed as nanograms of angiotensin I produced per volume of sample per unit of time.

Performing *renin concentration* determinations in the presence of a constant high substrate concentration and comparing the rate of generation of angiotensin I under these defined conditions to a standard renin sample circumvent the variables in substrate concentration. The results are generally expressed in renin units (Goldblatt units). An alternative method is to add portions of standard renin to a plasma sample containing an unknown amount of substrate. The renin originally present in the sample may be computed from the amounts of angiotensin I released with and without the added renin (2, 13).

Renin activity is the parameter more commonly determined in clinical laboratories. This value is not only more easily obtained but it also correlates well with the concentrations of angiotensin II (the physiologically active hormone) in plasma (10). Renin activity values are of a diagnostic value in the various disease states to which this determination has been applied.

RENIN ACTIVITY ASSAY

Principle

A plasma sample is incubated at 37 C for a given period of time. Renin contained in the plasma reacts with intrinsic angiotensinogen to release angiotensin I. The released peptide must be protected from degradation by peptidases that are also present in the plasma. At the end of the incubation, the concentration of the peptide is measured by radioimmunoassay. Specific antibody and labeled angiotensin are added to a sample of the incubation mixture containing generated angiotensin I. After a further incubation period, the antibody-bound labeled angiotensin is separated from the un-

190

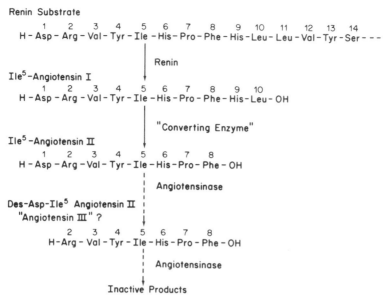

FIG. 1. *Biochemistry of the renin-angiotensin system. Ile⁵-angiotensin contains isoleucine in the 5 position and is the form of peptide that occurs in humans. The existence of des-Asp¹-angiotensin II as an intermediate in the pathway has not been definitely established. Modified from Oparil and Haber (8).*

bound labeled angiotensin, and the concentration of each is determined. The ratio of bound to free labeled angiotensin may be related to the concentration of unlabeled angiotensin present by reference to a standard curve.

Antiserum

A variety of means may be used to raise antisera to angiotensin I. We have found that an antigen produced by the coupling of the peptide to bovine immunoglobulin by a water-soluble carbodiimide when injected intradermally into rabbits frequently results in adequate antibodies (13). Antisera may also be purchased from several suppliers. Whether an antiserum is raised in one's own laboratory or purchased elsewhere, its suitability for radioimmunoassay should be determined. The criteria for selection are discussed in the section on Pitfalls.

Standards

There is considerable variability in the immunoreactivity of angiotensin I preparations that are available from commercial suppliers. A standard preparation is available from the Medical Research Council, Division of Biological Standards, Holly Hill, London, England, and it should be used for calibration of the commercial preparation that is used as the laboratory standard.

Labeled peptide

Labeled angiotensin I may also be purchased from several suppliers. A high specific activity is not essential in this assay. The material, however, should contain only monoiodinated angiotensin I, since the diiodinated product has diminished immunoreactivity, and radioactive decay may result in labeled products that are nonimmunoreactive and interfere with the assay. If desired, iodination may be done in the laboratory (3, 15).

TEST PROCEDURES

Two assay procedures will be discussed. The first uses a conventional approach which has been used widely for 7 to 8 years. The second procedure is a newer method which offers certain advantages and with which both of us have now had considerable experience.

I. Assay using peptidase inhibitors (3)

Blood is collected in chilled tubes containing ethylenediaminetetraacetate (EDTA; 1.29 mg/ml, final concentration). Vacutainer tubes from Becton, Dickinson (lavender top) containing EDTA are suitable. Blood should be conveyed to the laboratory on ice, and cells are sedimented in a refrigerated centrifuge.

Principle of the assay. Renin contained within a buffered plasma sample acts on intrinsic angiotensinogen at 37 C to produce angiotensin I, which is protected from further enzymatic degradation by EDTA, 8-hydroxyquinoline, and 2,3-dimercapto-1-propanol (BAL). The angiotensin I concentration in a sample of the incubation mixture is determined by radioimmunoassay. This value is corrected by subtracting the concentration of angiotensin I measured by radioimmunoassay in another sample of the same plasma that has been kept on ice. Thus, only the concentration of angiotensin I generated as a result of the 37 C incubation is reported as nanograms per milliliter per hour of incubation. In the radioimmunoassay, angiotensin I from the plasma sample, labeled angiotensin I, and specific antiserum are allowed to come to equilibrium in 18 h at 4 C. The sample is then exposed to charcoal in the presence of dextran, which selectively adsorbs the free ^{125}I-labeled angiotensin; antibody-bound ^{125}I-labeled angiotensin remains in the supernatant fluid. The concentration of antibody-bound ^{125}I-labeled angiotensin is inversely related to the amount of angiotensin generated in the plasma incubation.

Preparation of reagents.

Tris-acetate buffer, 0.1 M, pH 7.4

Dissolve 12.1 g of tris(hydroxymethyl)aminomethane (Tris) base in deionized water up to 1,000 ml. Add Merthiolate, 10 mg/100 ml (0.01%). Adjust to pH 7.4 with approximately 4.9 mg of glacial acetic acid. Use a pH meter. Store under refrigeration.

Tris-acetate buffer with lysozyme

Used for dilution of ^{125}I-labeled angiotensin and antibody. Prepare daily as needed: 1 mg of lysozyme/ml of Tris-acetate buffer.

Tris-hydrochloride buffer, 4 M, for pH control of plasma at pH 7.4

Dissolve 36.3 g of Tris base in 70 ml of water. Adjust to pH 7.2 with 6 N HCl (final volume, 75 ml). The pH should always be measured in a dilution 1:10 with distilled water.

Charcoal suspension

Prepare separately:

sodium barbital, 14.714 g, and sodium acetate, 9.714 g, in 500 ml of water + Merthiolate (1 mg/10 ml of solution). HCl, 0.1 N (5 ml of HCl in 600 ml of water).

NaCl (8.5 g/1,000 ml of water + 100 mg of Merthiolate or 17 g/2,000 ml of water + 200 mg of Merthiolate).

Withdraw 200 ml from 2,000 ml of NaCl solution. To 1,800 ml of NaCl solution, add 100 ml of sodium barbital-sodium acetate buffer and 100 ml of 0.1 N HCl. This is charcoal buffer.

Concentrated charcoal solution A is prepared by adding 2.5 g of Dextran 80 and 25 g of Norit A neutral (Fisher) to 1,000 ml of charcoal buffer. This is the stock solution. Store overnight.

Working solution B (for use in assay) is prepared by using a dilution 1:3 of the stock solution and charcoal buffer.

8-Hydroxyquinoline solution

Dissolve 1.3 g of 8-hydroxyquinoline sulfate (mol wt, 388) in distilled water to give 10 ml of solution; store in the dark. This is a 0.340 M solution.

^{125}I-labeled angiotensin I

Each assay requires 5,000 counts/min. Actual dilution depends on counter efficiency.

Preparation of incubation.

1. Centrifuge blood samples collected in chilled lavender-top tubes for 15 to 20 min at 2,500 rpm to obtain plasma; plasma should be kept frozen prior to use.

2. Prepare a duplicate set of tubes for each plasma sample.

3. Add 10 μliters of 8-hydroxyquinoline and 2.5 μliters of BAL solution in one tube.

4. Add 1 ml of cold plasma and 100 μliters of Tris-hydrochloride buffer, pH 7.2; shake well to insure proper mixing.

5. Transfer half the amount to a duplicate tube.

6. Stopper each tube; incubate one tube for 3 h at 37 C and refrigerate one at 4 C. These tubes can be frozen until ready for use; thawing should be done at 4 C.

Preparation of standard curve and sample assaying.

1. Number tubes 1 to 18 for the standard curve and 19 to 22 for the pool sample.

2. For each plasma sample (1 ml), prepare six plastic tubes, numbering them consecutively; these are three duplicated sets, one for nonincubated sample and the other two for incubated samples.

3. To each tube, add 500 μliters of ^{125}I-angiotensin diluted in Tris-lysozyme buffer; required counts, 5,000 counts/min per 500 μliters.

4. To tubes numbered 1 to 18, add angiotensin standard as follows:

Tube no.	Amt of A₁ (cold)
1,2	Control ⎫ no A₁ added
3,4	Trace ⎬
5,6	5 μliters
7,8	10 μliters
9,10	20 μliters
11,12	30 μliters
13,14	50 μliters
15,16	70 μliters
17,18	100 μliters

5. To tubes 19 to 22, add 50 and 25 μliters of plasma in duplicate.

6. For each plasma sample numbered tube, add cold plasma as follows:

Tube no.	Amt of plasma
23,24 (0 time)	50 μliters
25,26 (3-h incubation)	50 μliters
27,28 (3-h incubation)	25 μliters

followed by other samples.

7. Starting with tube 3, pipette in 500 μliters of antibody diluted 1:15,000 with Tris-lysozyme buffer.

8. Incubate all tubes for 18 to 20 h at 4 C.

Charcoal separation of bound from free ^{125}I-labeled angiotensin.

1. Add 1 ml of charcoal working solution B to each tube; it is important that all tubes be exposed to charcoal for approximately the same length of time, so a rapid, semiautomatic pipetting technique is desirable.

2. After 5 min, centrifuge at about 2,500 rpm at 4 C for 20 min.

3. Decant each clear supernatant fluid into a similarly numbered plastic tube.

4. Count supernatant fluid for 1 min in a gamma well counter; this represents antibody-bound counts (B); free ^{125}I-labeled angiotensin counts (F), in the charcoal, are determined by subtracting this value from the total counts added to the assay tube.

The supernatant counts are taken as the fraction of label that is antibody bound. Free counts are computed by subtracting this quantity from the total counts added. At each point, the ratio of free to bound counts is plotted against the amount of standard angiotensin I added. An almost linear plot results with many antisera. The amounts of angiotensin in the 50- and 10-μliter 37 C samples and the 50-μliter 0 C samples are read from the plot. The amount of angiotensin I per milliliter of plasma is then computed for 37 and 1 C. Subtracting these two values yields the amount of angiotensin generated in 3 h. The 50- and 10-μliter samples should give results that closely approximate each other if both fall within the range of the assay. Both samples are desirable since samples containing large amounts of angiotensin I may fall off scale with the 50-μliter sample, and samples containing very small amounts of angiotensin I may not be accurately assessed with the 10-μliter sample. Final results are expressed as nanograms per milliliter per hour. An alternative method to the reciprocal plot particularly suitable for use with a computer is the logit log method (16). Normal values are given in Table 1.

II. Antibody capture method (15)

Principle. This method has been developed to simplify the assay so that the entire procedure can be performed in a single tube with

TABLE 1. *Normal renin values^a (peptidase inhibitor assay)*

Na intake (mEq/day)	Posture	Renin activity (ng per ml per h)
110	Supine	1.91 ± 0.88
110	Upright	6.9 ± 4.7
10	Supine	3.14 ± 0.5
10	Upright	9.6 ± 3.9
After 80 mg of furosemide	–	9.8 ± 6.9

^{a} Subjects were young, white normal individuals, mostly males. Renin activity values tend to be lower in older people and in blacks.

microliter quantities of plasma without the need for adding the peptidase inhibitors. The principle, which was first described for angiotensin II (12) but recently detailed for angiotensin I (15), uses a high concentration of angiotensin I antibody during the plasma incubation at 37 C. All the angiotensin I generated is then captured by the antibody and thereby protected against degradation by peptidases. After incubation at 37 C, the generated angiotensin is quantified in the same tube by adding labeled angiotensin I. The amount and affinity of the antibody required are identical to that of other assays.

Detailed operating procedure. To determine renin activity in human plasma, 75 μliters of EDTA plasma (3 mM) is added to a tube (Fig. 2) at 0 C. A 10-μliter mixture consisting of 30% of 3 M Tris-hydrochloride, pH 7.2, and 70% of an appropriate dilution of angiotensin I specific antiserum is added. As a routine, if enough plasma is available, six such tubes are prepared for each plasma sample. Two tubes are kept at 0 C, and two tubes are incubated for 0.5 h and two for 3 h after which they are placed again at 0 C. To each tube is then added 1,000 μliters of 5,000 counts of ^{125}I-labeled angiotensin I (25 to 100 μCi/μg or higher specific activity) in a 0.08 M barbiturate buffer, pH 8.5. The cooling and dilution stop the enzymatic reactions and provoke the complex between antibody and angiotensin I to dissociate (13). By the addition of labeled angiotensin I, the mixture at this step is fully analogous to the radioimmunoassay step of the prior procedure. The tubes are kept at 4 C for 18 h to allow the new equilibrium to be established. Free and bound angiotensin are separated with 150 μliters of charcoal (63 mg of charcoal Norit A and 2 mg of Dextran 70 [Pharmacia] per ml of barbiturate buffer). The charcoal is retained on the inside of a plastic cap (Fig. 2), and all samples in a series, including the standards, are mixed simultaneously with the charcoal by inverting the rack of the tubes repeatedly for 30 s followed immediately by

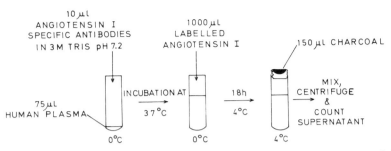

FIG. 2. *Principle of the antibody capture method. The antibody traps angiotensin I formed during incubation at 37 C. By dilution in the same tube with labeled angiotensin added in the cold, the mixture becomes that generally used for quantification of angiotensin by radioimmunoassay.*

centrifugation. The supernatant fluid is immediately decanted, and radioactivity is counted. A standard curve is made by adding standard angiotensin I (standardized against the Medical Research Council standard as indicated previously) in amounts from 0.1 to 2 ng contained in 10-μliter portions of 0.1 M Tris-hydrochloride, pH 7.5, containing 0.5% bovine serum albumin to a series of tubes containing 75 μliters of normal plasma and 10 μliters of the antibody-buffer mixture. The standards are kept at 0 C, tracer is added to them, and they are handled simultaneously with the unknown plasma samples. The counts determined in the supernatant fluid (bound fraction) are plotted against the added unlabeled angiotensin I (10). The amounts of angiotensin I in the unknown plasma samples are determined from the standard curve. The results are expressed as nanograms of angiotensin I generated per milliliter of plasma per hour of incubation. If significant, the unincubated plasma sample (zero time) is subtracted. To measure very high and very low renin values, the incubation time and not the amount of plasma is varied, as this results in the simplest assay procedure. The appropriate concentrations of antibody are determined initially by increasing the antibody concentration until maximal angiotensin I values are achieved or until the assay gives the same result with plasma samples with and without addition of BAL and 8-hydroxyquinoline. Rabbit renin, which may be present in the antiserum, does not influence the assay since it does not cleave human substrate.

INTERPRETATION

It is important to consider that renin activity may vary by as much as a factor of 10 in the normal individual. Posture and sodium intake are the major determinants, though diurnal variations have been described. Diuretics and antihypertensive medications have major ef-

fects on renin activity as do estrogens. Consequently, it is good practice to establish normal values in relation to posture, sodium intake, and time of day. Often, in clinical situations the sodium intake is not known. A 24-h urinary sodium excretion may substitute adequately. Nomograms have been constructed relating sodium excretion to renin activity. In adapting these, it is important to determine that the same method for renin activity measurement has been used, since different methods may result in very different rates of angiotensin I generation.

PITFALLS

Antisera

Most antisera raised to angiotensin I do not cross-react appreciably with angiotensin II. In any event, this is not a significant problem in the assay since the peptidase inhibitors used in the first assay method or the antibody capture of angiotensin I used in the second assay method prevent the conversion of angiotensin I to II by plasma converting enzyme. Antisera must, however, be selected for absence of cross-reactivity with plasma components. Such cross-reactivity leads to apparent high base-line or zero-time angiotensin I levels (as measured in the sample kept on ice) and consequent insensitivity of the assay. In normal plasma appropriately collected and kept on ice prior to assay, base-line values should not exceed 0.1 to 0.2 ng/ml. The dilution at which the antiserum is used is of little importance as long as the antibody that it contains is of adequate affinity. The amount of antiserum used is adjusted so that 50% of the added labeled angiotensin I is bound to antibody in the radioimmunoassay. The addition of 1 ng of standard angiotensin I should then result in a reduction of the bound tracer to at least 25%. When these conditions are satisfied, adequate antibody binding of angiotensin

I occurs at the higher concentrations used initially in the capture method.

Standards

When standard solutions are prepared in the microgram or nanogram concentration range, a protein carrier such as serum albumin or lysozyme must always be added to prevent adsorption to glass. Occasionally these proteins are contaminated with peptidases that rapidly degrade the standard. Bacterial growth may also cause degradation of the standard. This may be prevented by Merthiolate (0.1%) or sodium azide. It is good practice to store standard solutions at −20 C at a relatively high concentrations (20 to 400 ng/ml) in small portions so that each is thawed only once and then diluted or used directly to make the standard for that day's assay.

Buffers

The 3 M Tris-hydrochloride buffer varies in pH markedly with temperature and dilution. It should be adjusted at 37 C at a 1:10 dilution to a pH of 7.2, which results in a final pH of 7.5. When added to plasma, all buffers contain 0.01% Merthiolate to prevent bacterial growth.

Labeled angiotensin I

Labeled preparations containing significant amounts of free iodine are recognized by the fact that less than 95% of the radioactivity binds to charcoal in the absence of antibody. Appropriate immunoreactivity may be assessed by showing that more than 90% of the tracer can be bound by antibody at high antiserum concentrations. Each new lot of labeled peptide should be checked by these criteria as well as for sensitivity in a standard curve.

pH

Various pH levels have been recommended for the renin assay, ranging from 5.5 to 7.5. Two to three times as much angiotensin I is generated at pH 5.5 as at 7.4. The reasons for recommending pH 7.4 are as follows:

1. The assay, with an appropriate antiserum, is sufficiently sensitive to quantify even low renin values without the additional angiotensin generation afforded at low pH.

2. A low pH may introduce artifactually elevated apparent renin activity values because of nonrenin acid proteases which can release angiotensin I from angiotensinogen (9) or the acid activation of prorenin (4).

3. K_m for renin increases at a lower pH. This changes the influence that the substrate has on generation rate in a renin activity assay (1).

Inhibitors

The antibody capture method obviates the need for peptidase inhibitors. If other methods are used, the choice of the pH during the incubation dictates the inhibitors. BAL and 8-hydroxyquinoline are most effective at neutral pH. Diisopropylfluorophosphate is ineffective at neutral pH, but more effective at acidic pH. A more recently employed inhibitor, phenylmethylsulfonyl fluoride, appears to be effective over a wide pH range.

Storage

Plasma samples are probably stable over long periods of time when stored at −20 C. Recent reports, however, suggest that some samples may undergo activation of prorenin when stored up to 1 year in a freezer. Improper handling of a specimen after collection, such as exposure to room temperature, may result in considerable angiotensin I generation prior to incubation. The result may be a very high zero-time value.

Charcoal

Exposure of individual samples to charcoal for excessive periods of time may result in dissociation of the antigen-antibody complex, particularly with low affinity antibodies. Exposure for 5 min prior to centrifugation together with equal exposure of all tubes obviates these problems.

ASSAY FOR ANGIOTENSINOGEN ANGIOTENSIN I AND ANGIOTENSIN II CONCENTRATION

When large amounts of exogenous renin are added to a plasma sample, nearly all the angiotensinogen may be cleaved to angiotensin I. The molar concentration of angiotensin I then reflects the concentration of angiotensinogen. Assay for angiotensin I is performed as described previously.

Angiotensinogen concentration is known to rise in pregnancy, as the result of estrogen administration, and after nephrectomy. It is depressed in liver disease.

Circulating angiotensin I

Little work has been done in determining the concentration of circulating angiotensin I since it is difficult to inhibit fully the action of renin after blood collection. This measurement is of investigature interest only (10).

Circulating angiotensin II

A number of assays have been described for circulating angiotensin II. Great variability is apparent in the reported normal values (10). All present methods require some form of separation of the peptide from other plasma constituents, subjecting it to variable losses (10). Although losses may be controlled by use of a double isotope technique, another problem is that most angiotensin II antisera cross-react with metabolic products of the peptide. It is possible to measure the circulating concentrations of angiotensin II in plasma if angiotensin II is purified from plasma and separated from its metabolites, but the assay is cumbersome and difficult. It is apparent that a satisfactory assay for angiotensin II is not yet available for clinical use.

ACKNOWLEDGMENT

This work was supported by a Hypertension-SCOR Grant from the National Heart and Lung Institute, #14150, and by the Danish Medical Research Council.

LITERATURE CITED

1. Favre, L., and M. Vallotton. 1973. Kinetics of the reaction of human renin with natural substrates and tetradecapeptide substrate. Biochim. Biophys. Acta 327:471–480.
2. Haas, E., and H. Goldblatt. 1972. Indirect assay of plasma-renin. Lancet 1:1330–1332.
3. Haber, E., T. Koerner, L. B. Page, B. Kliman, and A. Pernode. 1969. Application of a radioimmunoassay for angiotensin I to the physiologic measurements of plasma renin activity in normal human subjects. J. Clin. Endocrinol. Metab. 29:1349–1355.
4. Leckie, B. J., and A. McConnell. 1975. A renin inhibitor from rabbit kidney. Conversion of a large inactive renin to a smaller active enzyme. Circ. Res. 36:513–519.
5. Lucas, C. P., W. K. Waldhausl, E. L. Cohen, F. G. Berlinger, W. J. McDonald, and R. S. Sider. 1975. A plasma inhibitor of the renin-antirenin reaction and the in vitro generation of angiotensin I. Metabolism 24:127–135.
6. Michelakis, A. M., H. Yoshida, J. Menzie, K. Murakami, and T. Inagami. 1974. A radioimmunoassay for the direct measurement of renin in mice and its application to submaxillary gland and kidney studies. Endocrinology 94:1101–1105.
7. Murakami, K., and T. Inagami. 1975. Isolation of pure and stable renin from hog kidney. Biochem. Biophys. Res. Commun. 62:757–763.
8. Oparil, S., and E. Haber. 1974. The renin-angiotensin system. N. Engl. J. Med. 291:389–401 and 446–457.
9. Oparil, S., T. J. Koerner, and E. Haber. 1974. Effects of pH and enzyme inhibitors on apparent generation of angiotensin I in human plasma. J. Clin. Endocrinol. Metab. 39:965–968.
10. Page, I. H., and F. M. Bumpus (ed.). 1974. Angiotensin. Springer-Verlag Berlin, Heidelberg.
11. Page, I. H., and J. W. McCubbin (ed.). 1968. Renal hypertension. Year Book Medical Publishers, Inc., Chicago.
12. Poulsen, K. 1971. Simplified method for radioimmunoassay of enzyme systems. Application on the human renin-angiotensin system. J. Lab Clin. Med. 78:309–315.
13. Poulsen, K. 1973. Kinetics of the renin system. The basis for determination of the different components of the system. Scand. J. Clin. Lab. Invest. 31(Suppl. 132):1–86.
14. Poulsen, K., J. Burton, and E. Haber. 1975. Purification of hog renin by affinity chromatography using the synthetic competitive inhibitor [D-Leu⁶]octapeptide. Biochim. Biophys. Acta 400:258–262.
15. Poulsen, K., and J. Jørgensen. 1974. An easy radioimmunological microassay of renin activity, concentration and substrate in human plasma and tissues based on angiotensin I trapping by antibody. J. Clin. Endocrinol. Metab. 39:816–825.
16. Rodbard, D., W. Bridson, and P. L. Rayford. 1969. Rapid calculation of radioimmunoassay results. J. Lab. Clin. Med. 74:770–781.

Chapter 23

Radioimmunoassay of Human Growth Hormone

RICHARD C. DIMOND

INTRODUCTION

The radioimmunoassay of human growth hormone (hGH) requires purified hGH as the antigen. It must be emphasized that the assay measures a substance in the unknown sample that is only immunochemically indistinguishable from the purified growth hormone standard; the method does not require or imply that the substance measured be structurally identical or biologically equipotent to the reference standard.

The assay has been applied, primarily, to the measurement of endogenous hormone in the peripheral circulation. The purpose of this chapter is to present specific details concerning the radioimmunoassay of hGH in plasma or serum. General methodological considerations, materials, preparation and purification of labeled hormone, a standard laboratory procedure for performing the actual determination itself, and the clinical application of the assay are discussed.

GENERAL CONSIDERATIONS

Antiserum

The hallmark of the method is that it allows measurement of low concentrations of a specific substance. These two features — sensitivity and specificity — are determined primarily by the antiserum. Both guinea pigs and rabbits have been immunized successfully for the production of hGH antisera (2). Although immunization techniques vary (2, 20), hGH appears to be highly antigenic in both species, and such methodological difference may not be critical. In general, animals are immunized with microgram quantities (e.g., 250 μg or less) of purified hGH in complete Freund's adjuvant at 1- to 4-week intervals, and satisfactory antisera may be obtained after four immunizing doses. Since antisera contain heterogeneous populations of antibody, they must be selected empirically on the basis of sensitivity and specificity.

Sensitivity is determined by the affinity of the antibody for hormone, and this is reflected in the slope of the standard curve such that small amounts of unlabeled hGH cause sub-stantial inhibition of binding to labeled hGH. If the concentration of high-affinity antibody is excessive, all hormone present will be bound, and competitive inhibition of binding will not be observed; accordingly, dilute antiserum is used. Thus, the dilution or titer of an antiserum is an expression of the quantity of high-affinity antibody present and not an expression of affinity per se. Theoretically, optimal sensitivity occurs when conditions provide 33% binding of labeled hormone in the absence of unlabeled hormone (2).

Specificity of the antiserum implies negligible cross-reation of hGH antibody with structurally related compounds. Thus, pituitary (10, 28) and plasma (10) growth hormones of nonprimate origin cross-react minimally with most hGH antisera, whereas simian growth hormone cross-reacts substantially (10, 28). However, hGH is structurally quite similar to human prolactin (hPRL) and human placental lactogen (hPL), and high circulating concentrations of hPRL (e.g., post-partum or certain pituitary tumors) and hPL (e.g., pregnancy or trophoblastic and certain nontrophoblastic neoplasms) may cross-react in a given hGH assay. To demonstrate that the substance measured behaves like hGH immunochemically, one must show that it is not distinguishable from the purified reference standard upon serial dilution.

Purified human growth hormone

hGH is a single-chain polypeptide with a molecular weight of ~21,500 (monomeric hGH). Various techniques, or modifications thereof, are available for its preparation and purification, including those of Li (17), Raben (21), Wilhelmi (19), and Roos (24). Higher yields and less structural alteration may occur with fresh or fresh-frozen rather than acetone-dried pituitaries (15, 17).

Labeled hormone

The development of a technique for preparing radiolabeled hormone of high specific activity was of major importance to radioimmunoassay methodology in general and to the hGH assay in particular. In 1962, Utiger, Parker, and Daughaday (28) reported the first radioimmunoassay of hGH, but nonspecific effects of unextracted plasma limited its widespread application. At about the same time, Greenwood, Hunter, and Glover (14) provided a method for labeling hGH to high specific activity with [131]I. Using this labeling technique, Glick et al. (10) developed a radioimmunoasay sensitive enough to measure hGH levels in small volumes of unextracted plasma from normal individuals.

Although hGH can be radiolabeled with several isotopes, ^{131}I and ^{125}I have been used most commonly. [125]I is preferred because of its availability in high isotopic abundance, its longer half-life, and the greater efficiency of equipment for counting it. The most popular method of radioiodination is that of Greenwood, Hunter, and Glover (14), though other methods are available (e.g., electrolytic, lactoperoxidase). [125]I is oxidized with chloramine T to an unknown reactive state and is substituted, primarily, onto tyrosyl residues of the hormone (histidyl- and sulfhydryl-containing residues as well); sodium metabisulfite is then added to reduce unreacted oxidized [125]I. Over-iodination and excessive exposure to chloramine T may result in substantial physicochemical alteration of the hormone, instability, and loss of immunoreactivity (2, 25); furthermore, the process of ^{125}I substitution is not uniform (25). Thus, it has been suggested that iodination be limited theoretically to not exceed an average of 1 mol of ^{125}I/mol of hGH (2, 25). At the conclusion of iodination, carrier protein (e.g., albumin) is added to prevent adsorption of ^{125}I]hGH to glass or plastic, to bind excess ^{125}I, and to "soak up" any free radicals formed from the radiolysis of water.

The ^{125}I]hGH may be purified by various methods (e.g., starch gel electrophoresis), but gel chromatography (22) has been employed most widely. With this technique, multiple radioactive species will be observed: free ^{125}I, monomeric ^{125}I]hGH with an apparent molecular weight of ~20,000, and several other minor components eluting earlier (and therefore with higher apparent molecular weights) than monomeric ^{125}I]hGH. The latter components may represent ^{125}I-labeled carrier protein or ^{125}I adsorbed to carrier protein, altered forms of hGH induced by the iodination procedure (so-called "damaged products"), or iodination of minor hGH components intrinsic to the unlabeled preparation. I use Sephadex G-100 (Pharmacia Fine Chemicals, Inc.) to separate monomeric ^{125}I]hGH from free ^{125}I and these other radioactive species.

The sensitivity of the assay will be influenced by the concentration of ^{125}I]hGH added. Although sensitivity is determined primarily by the antibody, competitive inhibition of binding at low concentrations of unlabeled hormone will be obscured by high concentrations of labeled hormone. Thus, low concentrations of ^{125}I]hGH are used. Unlabeled hormone, antibody, and ^{125}I]hGH can be incubated together initially, or the addition of ^{125}I]hGH can be delayed so that unlabeled hormone is allowed to "pre-incubate" with antibody. The latter method may be associated with improved sensitivity or a shortened assay time (2, 20).

Unknown samples

Endogenous hGH, unlike thyroid and steroid hormones, does not circulate bound to protein (1). Either plasma or serum samples are satisfactory for assay; under the conditions employed, I have found no systematic differences between hGH measurements in paired plasma and serum samples, and either may be stored frozen for years without loss of immunoreactivity.

Nonspecific influences

The immunochemical reactions involved are subject to the same general influences of the reaction medium, such as pH, ionic strength, and temperature, as are all chemical reactions. Most assays are performed in a pH range of 7.4 to 8.6. The ionic strength is particularly important: the assay buffer, solutions of standard hormone, and the unknown samples should have a similar salt content. Although the binding of antigen to antibody may be favored at low temperatures, the optimal temperature for a given assay is determined empirically: 4 C, room temperature, and 37 C have all been used. In addition, the concentrations of protein and other constituents in the unknown samples affect the assay. Plasma or serum may nonspecifically inhibit the binding of labeled hormone to antibody. Thus, one must demonstrate that a standard curve run in hormone-free plasma or serum is indistinguishable from one run in the assay buffer alone; otherwise, hormone-free plasma or serum must be added to the standard curve in the same volume as the unknown to be assayed. In my experience, this nonspecific effect is obviated by assaying plasma or serum samples at a 1:20 or greater dilution. Finally, labeled hormone may be unstable in the presence of only slightly diluted plasma or serum (so-called "incubation damage"). This effect is minimized by assaying plasma or serum at a 1:20 or greater dilution.

Separation techniques

Although paper-strip chromatoelectrophoresis was used originally to separate free and antibody-bound hormone, it has been largely replaced by a variety of test tube methods (2, 20). Of the latter, those employed commonly in the hGH assay include immunoprecipitation of soluble hormone-antibody complexes (i.e., second antibody), solid-phase adsorption of free hormone (e.g., charcoal, talc), and solid-phase adsorption of antibody (e.g., antibody-coated plastic tubes), but no single method has been entirely satisfactory. Since they are all influenced by nonspecific factors such as those that affect the reaction between free hormone and its antibody, optimal conditions of the separation procedure must be determined empirically.

In my laboratory, the double antibody technique of Skom and Talmage (27) as applied to the hGH assay by Schalch and Parker (26) is used. The method employs anti-gamma globulin serum (second antibody) that is homologous to the gamma globulin of the first antibody. Thus, if the hGH antiserum is prepared in a guinea pig, the second antibody (precipitating antibody) is prepared by immunizing an animal (e.g., goat or sheep) with guinea pig gamma globulin. Since low concentrations of first antibody are used in the assay, the bulk of the precipitate is increased by adding homologous gamma globulin or normal serum (e.g., normal guinea pig serum) to the reaction mixture.

MATERIALS

Buffers

The assay buffer (acetate-barbital, pH 7.4-0.35% [wt/vol] albumin) is prepared as follows: 9.7 g of sodium acetate and 14.7 g of sodium barbital are made up to 500 ml with distilled water; 100 ml of the acetate-barbital solution (stored at 4 C) is added to 1,800 ml of 0.85% (wt/vol) sodium chloride; the final pH is adjusted to 7.4 with 0.1 N HCl, and the volume is brought to 2,000 ml with water. On the day before any assay, sufficient buffer (stored at 4 C) is made 0.35% (wt/vol) in human albumin (Albumisol, Merck and Co., Inc.).

The iodination reaction is buffered with 0.25 M sodium phosphte, pH 7.4 (stored at -18 C).

Purified unlabeled hGH to be used for iodination is diluted 0.05 M sodium phosphate, pH 7.4 (stored at 4 C).

Antiserum and unlabeled hormone

The hGH antiserum and the purified unlabeled hGH that I have used were generously supplied by the National Institute of Arthritis, Metabolism, and Digestive Diseases (NIAMDD), Bethesda, Md., and the National Pituitary Agency. (These materials are made available by the NIAMDD for research purposes only.) Although analogous reagents are available commercially, I have no personal experience with such reagents (e.g., Calbiochem, La Jolla, Calif.: antiserum and hGH; Antibodies Inc., Davis, Calif.: antiserum).

The antiserum that I have used is a guinea pig anti-hGH serum (GP 2-5-19, Yalow and Berson) that was obtained after immunization with purified hGH (Raben). The antiserum is distributed at a 1:2,000 dilution in normal saline containing 1:5,000 Merthiolate and 1:100 normal guinea pig serum. The 1:2,000 antiserum is stored at -18 C in multiple 0.5-ml portions. I have not observed a decrease in sensitivity associated with storage or repeated freezing and thawing. However, it is noteworthy that Glick (9) has reported preferential loss of high-affinity hGH antibody in an antiserum stored at -20 C for 9 years.

Purified unlabeled hGH (Wilhelmi) that is to be iodinated is diluted in 0.05 M sodium phosphate, pH 7.4, to a final concentration of 250 μg/ml. Individual 20-μliter portions, each containing 5 μg of hGH, are put in iodination vials that have tapered conical bottoms, and are stored at -18 C. Purified unlabeled hGH that is to be used as the reference standard is diluted in the assay buffer to a final concentration of 2.5 ng/ml; individual 3-ml samples are made in separate vials and are stored at -18 C. Thus, multiple samples of purified unlabeled hGH are made in order to avoid potential structural alterations induced by repeated freezing and thawing. It is known that hGH may undergo deamidation while frozen; however, immunoreactivity does not appear to be affected by this process (1).

Iodination

Chloramine T and sodium metabisulfite (Matheson, Coleman, and Bell, Norwood, Ohio) are prepared fresh, 2 mg/ml and 1.2 mg/ml, respectively, in 0.05 M sodium phosphate, pH 7.4, immediately prior to use.

Sodium iodide-125 (Amersham/Searle Corp.) that is carrier-free and without added reducing agent is available in high concentrations specifically for iodination. Freshly prepared reagent in dilute sodium hydroxide, pH 8 to 11, is available every 2 weeks.

Phosphotungstic acid (PTA), 1% (vol/vol) in 0.5 N HCl, is used as a protein precipitant in assessing the efficiency of iodination.

I have no personal experience with commercially available [^{125}I]hGH (e.g., New England Nuclear Corp.).

Sephadex column

A 1.5 × 90 cm column of Sephadex G-100 (bead size, 40 to 120 μm) is prepared and equilibrated at 4 C in 0.01 M sodium phosphate (pH 7.4)-0.15 M sodium chloride-0.02% (wt/vol) sodium azide (phosphosaline-azide buffer) according to standard techniques (22). After calibration with globular reference proteins of known molecular weight (Pharmacia Fine Chemicals, Inc.) and a substance to mark the salt peak (e.g., ^{125}I), the column is equilibrated in phosphosaline-azide buffer containing 0.1% (wt/vol) albumin (human albumin; Miles Laboratories, Inc.). Labeled hormone is eluted from the gel column with the latter buffer. Both phosphosaline buffers are stored at 4 C. With care (22), the same gel column can be reused continually for years.

Separation

Undiluted normal guinea pig serum (NGPS; Miles Laboratories, Inc.) is stable during prolonged storage (1 year) at −18 C and may be repeatedly thawed and frozen.

Undiluted goat anti-guinea pig gamma globulin serum (Antibodies Inc.) is stable during prolonged storage (2 years) at −18 C and may be repeatedly thawed and frozen.

PREPARATION AND PURIFICATION OF ^{125}I-LABELED hGH

The original chloramine T method (14) for the preparation of high specific activity radioiodinated hGH has been modified over the years by many investigators. The method I employ is similar to that of Berson and Yalow (2). The iodination is limited theoretically not to exceed an average of 1 mol of ^{125}I/mol of hGH (2, 25). Since 5 μg or ~0.25 nmol of hGH is routinely iodinated, the amount of ^{125}I is limited not to exceed 500 μCi or ~0.25 nmol (the specific activity of carrier-free ^{125}I is ~17 mCi/μg). Therefore, the theoretical average specific activity of the product will not exceed ~100 μCi of ^{125}I/μg of hGH.

Small volumes of concentrated reagents are used. The reaction is performed under a hood, with usual precautions for the handling of radioisotopes. A 10-μliter glass syringe (Hamilton Co.) is used for pipetting ^{125}I; other reagents are pipetted with disposable plastic micropipette tips. All reagents are added to the conical vial containing the freshly thawed sample of unlabeled hGH to be iodinated. The reagents are added in rapid (~30 s) sequential order as

follows: to 20 μliters containing 5 μg of hGH (~0.25 nmol) in 0.05 M sodium phosphate, pH 7.4, add (i) 40 μliters of 0.25 M sodium phosphate, pH 7.4, (ii) ~400 to 500 μCi of ^{125}I (~0.2 to 0.25 nmol; I add ~ 4 μliters of a solution containing ~ 100 Ci of ^{125}I/μliter), (iii) 25 μliters of chloramine T (50 μg, ~175 nmol) in 0.05 M sodium phosphate, pH 7.4, and (iv) 100 μliters of soium metabisulfite (120 μg ~630 nmol) in 0.05 M sodium phosphate, pH 7.4. Then add (v) 100 μliters of phosphosaline-azide buffer containing 4% (wt/vol) albumin to prevent adsorption of labeled hormone to glass.

To estimate rapidly the efficiency of iodination (incorporation of ^{125}I into protein), place a minute sample of the iodination mixture in 1 ml of column eluant, and add 2 ml of PTA solution, which immediately precipitates the protein. After centrifugation, ^{125}I incorporation into protein is estimated by measuring radioactivity in the supernatant fluid and precipitate and calculating the percent protein-bound radioactivity. This estimate is in good agreement with the analogous calculation made from the Sephadex G-100 elution chromatogram. Routinely, 50 to 75% of the ^{125}I added is incorported into protein. Thus, based upon a theoretical specific activity of ~100 μCi of ^{125}I/μg of hGH, actual specific activities achieved are ~50 to 75 μCi of ^{125}I/μg of hGH. [^{125}I]hGH is then purified by gel chromatography at 4 C on a 1.5 × 85 cm column of Sephadex G-100 operated at a flow rate of 5 ml/h with the use of standard techniques (22). Fractions (1 ml) are collected in 15 × 125 mm glass tubes by use of an automatic fraction collector (LKB Instruments, Inc.) and are counted manually in a well-type gamma spectrometer. Finally, an elution chromatogram is plotted expressing radioactivity as a function of elution volume (Fig. 1).

Since gel chromatography separates compounds sequentially in order of decreasing molecular size, large molecules elute from the gel before small molecules. For globular proteins (such as hGH), a linear relationship exists between the partition coefficient (K_{av}) and log molecular weight (22). Having calibrated the column earlier, one knows the expected elution positions of hGH (mol wt ~21,500) and ^{125}I, respectively. The latter is indicated as such in Fig. 1. Monomeric [^{125}I]hGH in Fig. 1 refers to the highly immunoreactive component of ^{125}I-labeled protein which elutes with an apparent molecular weight of ~20,000 (K_{av} ~0.4), and therefore almost indistinguishably from purified unlabeled monomeric hGH. The three other components of ^{125}I-labeled protein present are apparently larger than monomeric [^{125}I]hGH (Fig. 1). Although these components may bind

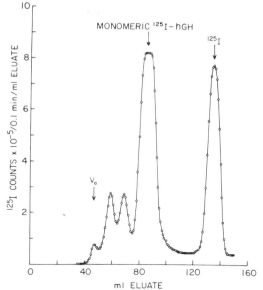

FIG. 1. *Purification of radioiodinated human growth hormone (hGH) by gel chromatography on Sephadex G-100. V_o indicates the void volume of the column. ^{125}I indicates the elution position of iodide-125. Monomeric [^{125}I]hGH indicates the immunoreactive component eluting with an apparent molecular weight of ~20,000.*

to antibody to varying degrees, their chemical nature is not known, and they are not used. To avoid potential structural alterations induced by repeated freezing and thawing, several fractions of monomeric [^{125}I]hGH (hereafter referred to as [^{125}I]hGH) are pooled, divided into small portions, and stored at 4 C. Immunoreactivity of fresh [^{125}I]hGH should be assessed before use in an assay, and a standard curve (or an abbreviated standard curve) is an appropriate test system. Alternatively, since this may take several days, one can quickly (1 day) assess binding of [^{125}I]hGH to a marked excess of antibody (in the absence of unlabeled hormone) as an index of immunoreactivity. In addition, we have found that the K_{av} of [^{125}I]hGH (labeled to appropriate specific activity) correlates highly with its immunoreactivity; thus, if the elution profile of the [^{125}I]hGH is as expected, we use it without further testing.

Since the sensitivity of the assay is partially determined by the concentration of [^{125}I]hGH added, the amount of [^{125}I]hGH used depends, in part, upon the sensitivity desired or needed; I routinely add 50 pg of [^{125}I]hGH/assay tube. In my experience, the [^{125}I]hGH has been stable and satisfactory for use in the assay for 4 to 6 weeks without further repurification. If accu-

mulation of free ^{125}I is excessive (>10 to 15%), it can be removed with an appropriate anion exchange resin.

RADIOIMMUNOASSAY PROCEDURE

Serum hGH is measured by a homologous radioimmunoassay employing a 1-ml incubation volume and a double antibody separation technique. The general procedure is as follows: (i) unlabeled hormone and antibody are allowed to react for 24 h at 37 C; (ii) [^{125}I]hGH and NGPS are added, and the reaction mixture is incubated for another 24 h at 37 C; (iii) after adding the second antibody, the tubes are placed at 4 C for the final 20 to 24 h.

Six determinations are made of [^{125}I]hGH binding to antibody in the absence of unlabeled hormone (B_0, "O" point, or "tracer" binding). The rest of the standard curve and four quality control sera are assayed in triplicate; unknown sera are assayed in duplicate. The mean coefficients of variation for intra- and inter-assay variability over the entire range of the standard curve are both less than 10%. Under the conditions employed, the antiserum (final dilution 1:2,000,000) routinely binds 40 to 50% of the [^{125}I]hGH (50 pg) in the absence of unlabeled hormone (B_0). The sensitivity of our assay is defined statistically by rejecting binding measurements of unlabeled hormone that fall within 3 standard deviations of the mean B_0. Under these conditions, the assay routinely detects 25 pg of hGH standard per assay tube or 0.5 ng of hGH per ml of serum diluted 1:20 (Fig. 2).

Tubes 1 to 3 receive no anti-hGH antibody ("non-immune" tubes) and generate a correction factor used in the calculation of binding to correct for free [^{125}I]hGH counts that are nonspecifically precipitated, trapped, or incompletely decanted during the separation procedure (~5% of the total counts added "precipitate" in tubes 1 to 3; % binding = 100 × bound counts/total counts; % binding corrected = 100 × bound counts corrected/total counts corrected). In my experience and in many radioimmunoassays employing a double antibody separation technique, it has not been necessary to set up individual "non-immune" tubes for each unknown sample. Such may not be the case for other assay systems, particularly those that are separated by adsorption of free hormone to solid-phase material (e.g., charcoal). Tubes 4 to 9 receive no unlabeled hGH (B_0 tubes). Tubes 10 to 33 receive varying amounts of unlabeled hGH standard: 10, 20, 40, 60, 80, 100, 140, and 200 μliters of hGH (2.5 ng/ml) are added; thus, these tubes contain 25, 50, 100, 150, 200, 250, 350, and 500 pg of hGH, respectively. Tubes 34

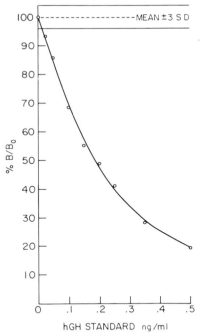

FIG. 2. *Radioimmunoassay standard curve of human growth hormone (hGH). B_0 represents the binding of $[^{125}I]hGH$ to antibody in the absence of unlabeled hGH and is assigned the value of 100%; B represents the binding of $[^{125}I]hGH$ in the presence of unlabeled hGH and is expressed as a fraction of B_0 (%B/B_0). The horizontal broken and solid lines at the top of the figure indicate the mean ±3 standard deviations for six determinations of B_0.*

to 45 (quality control tubes) receive 50 μliters of known sera containing ~0.8, 2.0, 5.0, and 8.0 ng hGH/ml, respectively (or ~40, 100, 250, and 400 pg of hGH/50-μliter sample). The remaining tubes receive not more than 50 μliters of serum from the unknown samples. Thus, our standard curve covers a 20-fold range for measuring 0.5 to 10 ng of hGH/ml of serum diluted 1:20; if an unknown sample is believed or found to contain >10 ng of hGH/ml, the sample is diluted in assay buffer and assayed at multiple dilutions.

With 12 × 75 mm glass tubes and an automatic pipette (Micromedic Systems, Inc.), tubes 1 to 3 receive 900 μliters of assay buffer, tubes 4 to 9 receive 800 μliters of assay buffer, and the remaining tubes receive sufficient assay buffer to bring their volumes to 800 μliters. Solutions of antiserum, $[^{125}I]hGH$ + NGPS, and second antibody are added by means of glass syringes with repeating dispensers (Hamilton Co.). The antiserum is used at a final dilution of 1:2,000,000 and is added as follows. An interme-

diate dilution of antiserum is made to 1:200,000/ml of assay buffer, and 100 μliters is added to all tubes except no. 1 to 3. After incubation for 24 h at 37 C, all tubes receive 100 μliters of a solution containing 500 pg of $[^{125}I]hGH$ + 50 μliters of undiluted NGPS/ml of assay buffer. After incubation for another 24 h at 37 C, all tubes receive 50 μliters of undiluted second antibody and are placed at 4 C for 20 to 24 h. The assay tubes are then centrifuged at ~1,200 × g for ~15 min at 4 C; the precipitate and supernatant fractions are separated by decantation, and both fractions are counted in a well-type automatic gamma spectrometer (one may also count only the bound or the free fraction).

A variety of methods are available for calculating the assay data, and the reader is referred to recent reviews for complete discussions of data analysis (20, 23). Our data are analyzed by use of a computerized calculator as follows: (i) the standard curve expresses percentage binding (corrected) as a function of hormone concentration, and is normalized by setting B_0 = 100%, and by expressing binding in the presence of unlabeled hormone, B, as a fraction of B_0 (% B/B_0); later, the standard curve is plotted arithmetically to facilitate comparison with previous and subsequent standard curves; (ii) a log-logit transformation of the standard curve data is performed (23), and the rest of the assay is calculated; (iii) hormone concentration (ng/ml) in unknown samples is determined by computer extrapolation from the standard curve and multiplication by the appropriate dilution factor for the sample.

CLINICAL APPLICATION

Regulation of growth hormone secretion

Clinical application of the hGH assay is based upon an understanding of those factors that regulate pituitary secretion of hGH (8, 18). Recent evidence suggests that specific substances within the hypothalamus both stimulate (growth hormone releasing factor, GHRF) and inhibit (somatotropin release inhibiting factor, SRIF) hGH secretion (18); although the chemical nature of GHRF has not yet been identified, SRIF has been purified and synthesized (3). This dual hypothalamic regulatory system is under the further influence of higher brain centers. In addition, it appears that dopamine, serotonin, and norepinephrine, which are present within the hypothalamus in high concentration, may act as neurotransmitters and mediate the effects of many hGH stimuli: L-dopa, 5-hydroxytryptophan, alpha-adrenergic agents, and beta-adrenergic blockade may stimulate or facilitate hGH release, and alpha-adrenergic blockade and beta-adrenergic agents may inhibit hGH secretion (18). Thus, acute hGH secretion has been associated with deep sleep (18) and a variety of both physical and psychological stresses, including general anesthesia and major surgery, administration of bacterial endotoxin, electroconvulsive therapy, blood sampling, and anxiety (8, 18). Physiological regulation of hGH secretion is subject to a wide variety of biochemical influences as well. Of these, the effects of alterations in carbohydrate and protein metabolism are well known: acute hypoglycemia, a falling blood sugar without hypoglycemia, exercise, interference with intracellular glucose utilization, protein ingestion, arginine administration, prolonged starvation, and protein depletion all stimulate relese of hGH, whereas hyperglycemia usually suppresses hGH secretion (8, 18).

A variety of other factors interact with this neuroendocrine regulatory system. Marked elevaion of hGH levels occurs in the neonate and, to a lesser degree, during infancy, compared with later childhood and adulthood (8). Ambulatory women have higher hGH levels than men, and estrogen treatment enhances hGH responsiveness to provocative stimuli in men and prepubertal children (8, 18). In contrast, emotional deprivation, obesity, hypo- and hyperthyroidism, Cushing's syndrome, chronic glucocorticoid therapy, and administration of medroxyprogesterone acetate are associated with blunted hGH responsiveness to provocative stimuli (8). Finally, hGH elevation itself may exert negative feedback inhibition of further hGH secretion (18).

Evaluation of growth hormone secretion

Assessment of hGH secretion is desirable as part of an evaluation of three clinical problems: namely, short stature possibly due to isolated hGH hyposecretion, hGH deficiency in association with other anterior pituitary deficits, and hypersecretion of hGH by a pituitary tumor resulting in gigantism (in children) or acromegaly (in adults). To evaluate such states of hGH hypo- or hypersecretion, one attempts to provoke or inhibit normal hGH secretion, respectively. In view of the effects of feeding, exercise, and stress mentioned previously, hGH stimulation and suppression tests in hospitalized patients are performed at bed rest after a 10- to 12-h fast (basal conditions), and serial blood samples are obtained after administration of the test agent; outpatient testing procedures should include at least a 1-h rest period.

Commonly employed hGH stimulation tests include insulin-induced hypoglycemia, administration of arginine, and L-dopa administration (4). In our laboratory, normal basal and stimulated hGH levels are <3 and >10 ng/ml, respectively. Peak hGH levels between 5 and 10 ng/ml are probably normal, whereas peak hGH levels <5 ng/ml represent inadequate stimulation. Since normal individuals may show variable hGH responses either to repeat testing or to multiple stimuli, an inadequate hGH response to a single test must be interpreted cautiously (8). Furthermore, other factors associated with blunted hGH responsiveness must not be overlooked. Whereas an adequate response implies a functionally normal hypothalamic-pituitary hGH axis, an inadequate response does not, by itself, differentiate between primary hypothalamic and primary pituitary disease. Recent evidence suggests that monotropic hGH deficiency may be due to hyposecretion of GHRF rather than to pituitary hGH deficiency per se (18).

Under basal conditions, hGH levels in normal individuals are usually suppressed to <1 ng/ml during the first 3 h after 100 g of oral glucose; by contrast, patients with gigantism or acromegaly have elevated mean basal hGH levels that rarely suppress to <5 ng/ml (7, 11). Since patterns of hGH secretion in individual patients may be highly variable under basal conditions and following glucose administrtion (5), multiple basal samples are indicated, and repeat suppression tests should be obtained if the diagnosis is in doubt. Although a "paradoxical" rise in hGH may follow glucose loading in acromegaly, similar responses have been reported in normal neonates and in patients with other conditions including hypothalamic tumors, acute intermittent porphyria, renal failure, and breast carcinoma (8, 18).

Heterogeneity of circulating human growth hormone

In the past several years, much attention has been focused on the heterogeneity of peptide hormones in general, and of hGH in particular (29). Recent studies suggest that at least four forms of immunoreactive hGH, with apparent molecular weights of ~20,000, ~40,000, ~80,000, and >150,000, are secreted into the peripheral circulation by the normal pituitary and by certain pituitary tumors (R. C. Dimond and S. W. Rosen, Clin. Res. 23:235A, 1975). Such studies raise the possibility that the immunoassay of hGH may measure bioltgcally inactive components and thereby contribute to the poor correlation between elevated hGH levels and clinical manifestations in certain disorders such as Laron dwarfism (16) and acromegaly. However, monomeric hGH is the major immunoreactive component of both pituitary and circulating hGH (29). Since the larger forms of hGH are immunochemically similar to monomeric hGH (6, 12), their quantitation by radioimmunoassy appears valid. Although these larger components of immunoreactive hGH may be biologically less active than monomeric hGH (13), they are not present in sufficient quantity to account for such clinical and laboratory discrepancies (12). Thus, even though the nature and significance of these larger forms of hGH are obscure, their measurement does not diminish the clinical utility of the hGH radioimmunoassay.

ACKNOWLEDGMENTS

I am grateful to Yvonne Lukes for technical assistance, to Alice Franklin for secretarial assistance, and to Saul W. Rosen for critical review of the manuscript.

LITERATURE CITED

1. Berson, S. A., and R. S. Yalow. 1966. State of human growth hormone in plasma and changes in stored solutions of pituitary growth hormone. J. Biol. Chem. 241:5745–5749.

2. Berson, S. A., and R. S. Yalow. 1973. p. 84–125, 302–308. In S. A. Berson and R. S. Yalow (ed.), Methods in investigative and diagnostic endocrinology, vol. 2A. North-Holland Publishing Co., Amsterdam.

3. Brazeau, P., W. Vale, R. Burgus, N. Ling, M. Butcher, J. Rivier, and R. Guillemin. 1973. Hypothalamic polypeptide that inhibits the secretion of immunoreavive pituitary growth hormone. Science 179:77–79.

4. Daughaday, W. H. 1974. The adenohypophysis, p. 31–79. In R. H. Williams (ed.), Textbook of endocrinology, 5th ed. W. B. Saunders Co., Philadelphia.

5. Dimond, R. C., S. R. Brammer, R. L. Atkinson, Jr., W. J. Howard, and J. M. Earll. 1973. Chlorpromazine treatment and growth hormone secretory responses in acromegaly. J. Clin. Endocrinol. Metab. 36:1189–1195.

6. Dimond, R. C., L. Wartofsky, and S. W. Rosen. 1974. Heterogeneity of circulating growth hormone in acromegaly. J. Clin. Endocrinol. Metab. 39:1133–1137.

7. Earll, J. M., L. L. Sparks, and P. M. Forsham. 1967. Glucose suppression of serum growth hormone in the diagnosis of acromegaly. J. Am. Med. Assoc. 201:134–136.

8. Glick, S. M. 1969 The regulation of growth hormone secretion, p. 141–182. In W. F. Ganong and L. Martini (ed.) Frontiers in neuroendocrinology. Oxford University Press, New York.

9. Glick, S. M. 1973. Loss of antigen-antibody affinity with storage of antiserum at −20 C. J. Clin. Endocrinol. Metab. 37:461–462.

10. Glick, S. M., J. Roth, R. S. Yalow, and S. A. Berson. 1963. Immunoassay of human growth hormone in plasma. Nature (London) 197:784–787.

11. Glick, S. M., J. Roth, R. S. Yalow, and S. A. Berson. 1965. The regulation of growth hormone secretion. Recent Prog. Horm. Res. 21:241–283.

12. Goodman, A. D., R. Tanenbaum,and D. Rabinowitz. 1972. Existence of two forms of immunoreactive growth hormone in plasma. J. Clin. Endocrinol. Metab. 35:868–878.

13. Gorden, P., M. A. Lesniak, C. M. Hendricks, and J. Roth. 1973. "Big" growth hormone components from human plasma: decreased reactivity demonstrated by radioreceptor assay. Science 182:829–831.

14. Greenwood, F. C., W. M. Hunter, and J. S. Glover. 1963. The preparation of ^{131}I-labeled human growth hormone of high specific activity. J. Biol. Chem. 89:114–123.

15. Holmström, B., and K. Fhölenhag. 1975. Characterization of human growth hormone preparations used for the treatment of pituitary dwarfism: a comparison of concurrently used batches. J. Clin. Endocrinol. Metab. 40:856–862.

16. Laron, Z., A. Pertzelan, and S. Mannheimer. 1966. Genetic pituitary dwarfism with high serum concentration of growth hormone: a new inborn error of metabolism? Israel J. Med. Sci. 2:152–155.

17. Li, C. H. 1973. p. 257–261. In S. A. Berson and R. S. Yalow (ed.), Methods in investigative and diagnostic endocrinology, vol. 2A. North-Holland Publishing Co., Amsterdam.

18. Martin, J. B. 1973. Neural regulation of growth hormone secretion. N. Engl. J. Med. 288:1384–1393.

19. Mills, J. B., R. B. Ashworth, A. E. Wilhelmi, and A. S. Hartee. 1969. Improved method for the extraction and purification of human growth hormone. J. Clin. Endocrinol. Metab. 29:1456–1459.

20. Odell, W. D., and W. H. Daughaday (ed). 1971. Principles of competitive protein-binding assays. J. B. Lippincott Co., Philadelphia.

21. Raben, M. S. 1959. Human growth hormone. Recent Prog. Horm. Res. 15:71–114.

22. Reiland, J. 1971. Gel filtration. Methods Enzymol. 22:287–321.

23. Rodbard, D., and G. R. Frazier. 1975. Statistical analysis of radioligand assay data. Methods Enzymol. 37:3–22.

24. Roos, P., H. R. Fevold, and C. A. Gemzell. 1963. Preparation of human growth hormone by gel filtration. Biochim. Biophys. Acta 74:525–531.

25. Roth, J. 1975. Methods for assessing immunologic and biologic properties of iodinated peptide hormones. Methods Enzymol. 37:223–233.

26. Schalch, D. S., and M. L. Parker. 1964. A sensi-

tive double antibody immunoassay for human growth hormone in plasma. Nature (London) 203:1141–1142.

27. Skom, J. S., and D. W. Talmage. 1958. Nonprecipitating insulin antibodies. J. Clin. Invest. 37:783–786.

28. Utiger, R. D., M. L. Parker, and W. H. Daughaday. 1962. Studies of human growth hormone. I. A radioimmunoassay for human growth hormone. J. Clin. Invest. 41:254–261.

29. Yalow, R. S. 1974. Heterogeneity of peptide hormones. Recent Prog. Horm. Res. 30:597–633.

Chapter 24

Radioimmunoassay for Pituitary Gonadotropins: Luteinizing Hormone and Follicle-Stimulating Hormone

MANJULA S. KUMAR AND SHARAD D. DEODHAR

INTRODUCTION

In the past, gonadotropins were measured by bioassays which, besides being tedious, time-consuming, and expensive, did not distinguish between luteinizing hormone (LH) and follicle-stimulating hormone (FSH). The development of radioimmunoassays for these hormones (5, 7–9) provided substantial advantages such as precision, simplicity, and specificity. These assays have been applied extensively in studying the control of gonadotropins during physiological and pathophysiological states of human gonadal function, and they are widely used in clinical investigations.

The first radioimmunoassay described for gonadotropins was for human chorionic gonadotropins (HCG; 15). Later, Midgley (7) and Odell et al. (9) made use of the cross-reactivity of human LH and HCG and used antisera produced against HCG to measure levels of LH in the sera and urine of men and nonpregnant women. In subsequent studies, the antigenic similarities of LH, HCG, FSH, and thyrotropin (TSH) were demonstrated (7, 9, 12). Biochemical studies (4, 10) showed all these hormone molecules to be glycoproteins consisting of two peptide chains designated as alpha and beta subunits. The amino acid sequences for the alpha subunit are identical or very similar for all these hormones. The biological and immunological specificity appears to reside in the beta subunit.

This similarity of alpha subunit may be the cause of major problems of cross-reactivity in the radioimmunoassay of gonadotropins, particularly in FSH assay. The cross-reacting antibodies in the anti-FSH serum can be neutralized by preadsorption with HCG. Virtually all the reported FSH assays have utilized this technique of preadsorption with HCG.

More recently, the successful separation of the alpha and beta subunits resulted in the production of more specific antisera. Antisera produced against HCG beta subunit had been found to be very specific with practically no cross-reaction with LH (14).

TEST PROCEDURES

Preparation and characterization of antisera

Antisera to FSH and LH are available to qualified investigators from the National Institute of Arthritis, Metabolism, and Digestive Disease (NIAMDD), Bethesda, Md., and can also be purchased from Calbiochem, La Jolla, Calif., or other commercial sources. Whatever the source, the antisera should be characterized for specificity before use in the assay. Also, antibodies can be produced in rabbits if the purified hormone preparations are available.

The immunization procedure outlined by Vaitukaitis et al. (13) for HCG beta subunit seems to be particularly useful in developing antisera suitable for radioimmunoassay. The method is excellent, especially when the amount of purified antigen available is limited. In this procedure, 20 to 100 μg of antigen is dissolved in 0.15 M NaCl solution, and the solution is mixed with an equal amount of complete Freund's adjuvant and dried tubercle bacilli (2.5 mg/ml of total mixture). The mixture is homogenized for 5 to 10 min, and the emulsion is injected intradermally at more than 30 sites in young rabbits about 3 months old. Peak antibody titers are obtained at 53 to 107 days. Titer indicates the final dilution which should be used in the assay. It can be obtained by incubating the doubling dilution of antiserum with the labeled antigen and then precipitating the antibody-bound antigen by optimal dilution of goat anti-rabbit gamma globulin. Usually, the dilution of antiserum capable of binding 30 to 40% of labeled antigen is selected for the assay.

Detection and elimination of cross-reacting antibodies. Antibodies raised to even highly purified LH and FSH show a variable degree of cross-reaction with each other or with other glycoproteins like HCG and TSH. These cross-reacting antibodies must be checked and removed before the antiserum is used in the assay.

The cross-reactivity can be checked by studying the binding of labeled gonadotropin to its antibody in the presence of various concentrations of other purified hormones. For example, to check FSH antibodies, one should run inhibition curves (using labeled FSH) with highly purified FSH, LH, HCG, and TSH. Now, assuming the concentration at 50% incept of standard curve for FSH as 1, one can calculate the relative activity causing the same inhibition with other hormones. Figures 1 and 2 show the cross-reactions of anti-LH and anti-FSH (NIAMDD) with FSH, LH, and TSH.

A highly specific antiserum can be obtained by removing the cross-reacting antibodies by adsorption technique. For example, from FSH antiserum, antibodies cross-reacting with LH or HCG can be neutralized by adding a suffi-

cient amount of HCG. Solid immunoadsorbent for HCG can also be used for the same purpose.

Preparation of labeled hormone

For a sensitive radioimmunoassay, radiolabeled hormone of high specific activity is required. As for other protein hormones, labeling with iodine-125 has been the method of choice for gonadotropins. The relatively long half-life of ^{125}I allows the use of one preparation for 3 to 4 weeks. The basic reaction in the labeling procedure involves oxidation of labeled sodium iodide; this liberates ^{125}I which, in turn, binds to the tyrosine residue of the hormone. The separation of labeled hormone from unreacted io-

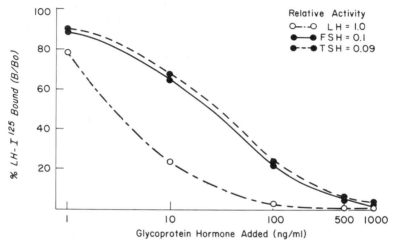

FIG. 1. *Cross-reaction of anti-LH (NIAMDD) with FSH and TSH. The relative activity is calculated as nanograms of LH/nanogram of FSH or TSH at 50% inhibition.*

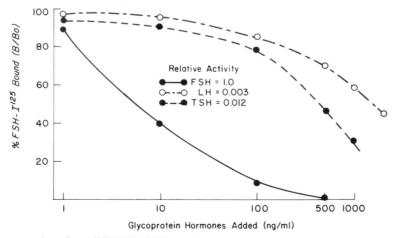

FIG. 2. *Cross-reaction of anti-FSH (NIAMDD) with LH and TSH. Relative activity is nanograms of FSH/nanogram of LH or TSH at 50% inhibition.*

dine is achieved by column chromatography. The following two methods have been successfully used for iodination of LH and FSH.

1. Iodination by Chloramine-T. This method for labeling human growth hormone was first described by Greenwood et al. (6), and since then the technique has been widely utilized for other hormones.

Requirements

1. Highly purified preparations of LH and FSH, such as LER 960 for LH and LER 1575-C for FSH, can be obtained from the NIAMDD. Each preparation is dissolved in 0.01 M phosphate-buffered saline, pH 7.0, to a concentration of 2 μg/10 μliters. Portions of 10 μliters (2 μg) are instantly frozen in 12 × 5 mm plastic vials and stored at −20 C.

2. High specific activity Na ^{125}I purchased from New England Nuclear Corp. or Amersham/Searle (2 mCi/20 μliters).

3. Chloramine-T (Eastman Kodak), 10 mg/ml in 0.5 M phosphate buffer, pH 7.5. This should be prepared fresh every time.

4. Sodium metabisulfite, 8 mg in 10 ml of 0.5 M phosphate buffer, pH 7.5.

5. Bovine serum albumin (BSA), 1 and 3% solutions in phosphate buffer.

6. Potassium iodide (KI), 1% solution.

Procedure

The following reagents are added with rapid mixing to a 12 × 75 mm plastic tube (Falcon Plastics) containing a 10-μliter (2-μg) sample of purified hormone: 25 μliters of 0.5 M phosphate buffer, pH 7.5, 5 μliters of Na^{125}I (0.5 mCi), 10 μliters of Chloramine-T, and, after rapid mixing for no longer than 20 s, 300 μliters of sodium metabisulfite.

The entire reaction mixture is applied to a column of Bio-Gel (Bio-Rad Laboratories) to separate the labeled protein from unreacted ^{125}I. The tube is washed once with 100 μliters of 1% KI and then with 200 μliters of phosphate buffer, and the contents are poured on the column. The details of chromatography are described later.

Although this method is widely used, it must be cautioned that Chloramine-T, being a strong oxidizing agent, is likely to damage the protein, which, in turn, may affect the biological and immunological activity of the hormone. To avoid this, a short reaction time is important. A reaction time of 15 to 20 s gives good preparations which can be used for 4 weeks; if purified on a column, they can be used for an additional period of 4 weeks.

2. Lactoperoxidase method of iodination. As mentioned, Chloramine-T is a strong oxidizing agent which can damage the proteins, leading to loss of biological and immunological activity. An alternative, gentler technique for iodination of gonadotropins described by Yukitaka et al. (16) does not affect the biological or immunological activity of the proteins, and yet comparable high specific activity preparations can be obtained. The preparations obtained by this technique are generally more stable than those prepared by the Chloramine-T method.

Requirements

1. Lactoperoxidase can be purchased from Calbiochem, La Jolla, Calif. Dissolve 2.5 μg in 1 ml of 0.4 M sodium acetate buffer, pH 5.6.

2. Hydrogen peroxide, 30% solution. Dilute with deionized water 1:15,000 to give the concentration of 500 ng/25 μliter.

Procedure

The following reagents are added to a tube (12 × 75 mm) containing 2 μg of the hormone/10 μliters, and the contents are rapidly mixed after each addition: 20 μliters of 0.4 M sodium acetate buffer, pH 5.6, 40 μliters (100 ng) of lactoperoxidase, 5 μliters (0.5 mCi) of Na^{125}I, and 25 μliters (500 ng) of H$_2$O$_2$ added twice at 10-min intervals.

The whole reaction mixture is then applied to the Bio-Gel column.

Purification by column chromatography. The labeled gonadotropins are purified by chromatography on a column of Bio-Gel P-10, 50 to 100 mesh (1 × 30 cm). The column is first equilibrated with 0.1 M phosphate buffer, pH 7.5. Before application of the reaction mixture on the column, 2 ml of 3% BSA is passed through to minimize the adsorption of protein on the column. The collecting tubes (13 × 125 mm, plastic) are coated with gelatin (5 mg/ml) solution which also contains 0.2 ml of 1% BSA. Thirty fractions of 1 ml each are collected, and 5-μliter samples from each tube are counted in a gamma counter. Usually, the protein peak comes in fractions 8 to 12, and the iodine peak follows later in fractions 20 to 25. The protein peak is stored at −20 C. After 4 weeks, the labeled protein may be repurified on a column and used for another 4-week period.

Preparation of standards

For gonadotropin radioimmunoassay, different reference preparations are being used and the results are expressed accordingly. The material which is currently distributed by NIAMDD is a crude pituitary extract (LER-907), and the results are expressed in terms of weight (ng/ml). The other preparation which has also been widely used is 2-IRP-HMG (Second International Reference Preparation of Human Menopausal Gonadotropins) which is distributed by the World Health Organization (WHO) in sealed ampoules (International Laboratory for Biological Standards, National Institute of Medical Research, Polly Hill, London, England). Each ampoule contains 40 IU of LH and 40 IU of FSH, and the results are expressed as mIU/ml. Recently, a more purified preparation for LH 64/108 has been made available by the WHO. Many laboratories also use other purified FSH and LH preparations for standardization and express results on a weight basis. This has made comparison of results between laboratories quite difficult.

2-IRP-HMG. Each ampoule contains 40 U of LH and 40 U of FSH. A stock solution is prepared by dissolving the lyophilized material of each ampoule in 10 ml of phosphate buffer-saline (0.05 M, pH 7.5, and 0.15 M NaCl) also containing 1% BSA to give a concentration of 4 U/ml. This is diluted further to give a concentration of 1 U/ml and then stored at −20 C in 1-ml amounts. Further dilutions using the same buffer are made as shown in Table 1.

LER 907. Reference preparation for LH and FSH (NIAMDD), 1 mg of the lyophilized material is dissolved in 10 ml of phosphate-buffered saline (0.05 M, pH 7.5, and 0.15 M NaCl) with 1% BSA to give a concentration of 100,000 ng/ml and then is stored at −20 C in 2-ml amounts. Further dilutions are made as shown in Table 2. The final dilutions of standards are stored in 0.5-ml amounts to avoid repeated thawing and freezing.

Assay procedure

A typical protocol for the LH or FSH assay using double antibody separation, as used in our laboratory, is outlined below.

Materials.
1. Antiserum (NIAMDD) LH, Batch no. 1; FSH, Batch no. 3.
2. Goat anti-rabbit antibody (Antibodies, Inc., Davis, Calif.).
3. Normal rabbit serum.
4. Phosphate-saline buffer, 0.05 M, 0.15 M NaCl, pH 7.4, with 1% BSA, 0.01% Merthiolate, and 0.02% ethylenediaminetetraacetate.

TABLE 1. *Dilutions for 2-IRP-HMG*

Sample	Standard concn (mU/ml)	Dilution	Stock solution (1,000 mU/ml)	Buffer (ml)	Final vol (ml)
A	100	1:10	1 ml of stock	9	5
B	50	1:2	4 ml of A	4	5
C	25	1:2	3 ml of B	3	6
D	10	1:10	1 ml of A	9	5
E	5	1:2	5 ml of D	5	5
F	2.5	1:2	5 ml of E	5	6
G	1.25	1:2	4 ml of F	4	8

TABLE 2. *Dilutions for LER (907)*

Sample	Standard concn (ng/ml)	Dilution	Stock solution (100,000 ng/ml)	Buffer (ml)	Final vol (ml)
A	1,000	1:100	0.1 ml	9.9	4
B	500	1:2	5 ml of A	5	5
C	250	1:2	5 ml of B	5	10
D	100	1:10	1 ml of A	9	5
E	50	1:2	5 ml of D	5	5
F	25	1:2	5 ml of E	5	5
G	12.5	1:2	5 ml of F	5	5
H	6.2	1:2	5 ml of G	5	5
I	3.1	1:2	5 ml of H	5	10

5. Labeled hormone prepared as described above. Labeling material obtained from NIAMDD: LH, LER-960; and FSH, LER-1575-C. The preparation is diluted to 10,000 to 12,000 counts/min.

6. Standards, 2-IRP-HMG. Diluted as described above.

7. Disposable plastic tubes, 12 × 75 mm (Falcon Plastics, no. 2052).

8. Eppendorf micropipette, 100- and 200-μliter size.

9. Biopette (0.1 to 1 ml), Schwarz/Mann.

Stage I incubation. Disposable plastic tubes (12 × 75 mm) are numbered in duplicate for nonspecific binding tube (NSB), zero standards, standards, serum controls, and unknowns, and the following reagents are added.

1. *Buffer:*
   a. 500 μliters to NSB tubes.
   b. 400 μliters to zero standard tubes.
   c. 200 μliters to each standard tube.
   d. 200 μliters to controls and unknown sample tubes.

2. 200 μliters of each standard is added to the respective tubes (1.25, 2.5, 5, 10, 50, 100, and 200 mIU/ml, respectively).

3. 200 μliters of serum sample for serum controls and unknown sera are added.

4. 100 μliters of antiserum (LH, 1:12,000 dilution; and FSH, 1:5,000 dilution) is added to all the tubes except to NSB tubes (maximal binding, approximately 30 to 40%).

5. To each tube 100 μliters of ^{125}I-labeled LH or ^{125}I-labeled FSH (10 to 12,000 counts/min) is added.

6. All the tubes are mixed well on a Vortex mixer and then incubated overnight (20 to 24 h) at room temperature.

Stage II incubation. After the first incubation, the following reagents are added the next morning.

1. 100 μliters of 1:25 dilution of normal rabbit serum to each tube.

2. 100 μliters of goat anti-rabbit gamma glob-

ulin (appropriate dilution determined for each batch to contain amount sufficient to precipitate antibody complex). Each batch of goat anti-rabbit gamma globulin should be titered in advance to give maximal binding for the first antibody dilution and normal rabbit serum dilution used.

All the tubes are mixed well and then incubated for 12 to 24 h at room temperature or 4 C. The next morning, any six tubes are counted to give the actual total counts added, and then all the tubes are centrifuged at 4,000 to 5,000 rpm for 30 min. The supernatant fluid is removed by aspiration or by decanting, and the tubes containing the precipitate are counted for 1 min in a gamma counter (Searle Analytical Co., Des Plaines, Ill.).

Calculations.

Maximal binding

$$= \frac{\begin{array}{c}\text{counts in zero standard tubes} - \\ \text{average counts in NSB tubes}\end{array}}{\begin{array}{c}\text{total counts added} \\ \text{(average of six precounts)}\end{array}} \times 100$$

Bound/bound zero (B/B_0)

$$= \frac{\begin{array}{c}\text{counts in standard or unknown} - \\ \text{average counts in NSB}\end{array}}{\begin{array}{c}\text{average counts in zero standard tubes} \\ - \text{average counts in NSB}\end{array}} \times 100$$

mIU/ml vs. B/B_0 are plotted on semilog graph paper. Unknowns are then read off the graph. Typical standard curves obtained by this procedure for LH and FSH are shown in Fig. 3 and 4, respectively.

The data can be calculated and expressed in a number of ways. Percentage of total bound can be calculated by dividing each tube counts per minute by the total counts used and multiplying by 100. Bound/free ratio can also be calculated and plotted accordingly.

Many laboratories employ 72 to 120 h of incubation at 4 C during the first step for LH and FSH assay. However, we have obtained identical results with incubation at room temperature for 24 h. Figures 3 and 4 show the two inhibition curves obtained for LH and FSH, respectively, by incubating for 72 h at 4 C and for 24 h at room temperature.

Separation of antibody-bound antigen from the free antigen

Of the several methods used for the separation of antibody-bound and free antigen in gonadotropin assays, the double antibody method is probably the most satisfactory. This method involves the precipitation of a soluble antigen-

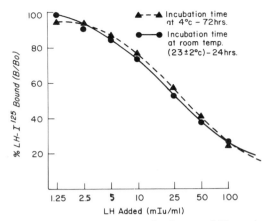

FIG. 3. *Inhibition curves for human LH as obtained by incubating the assay at 4 C for 72 h and at room temperature (23 ± 2 C) for 24 h.*

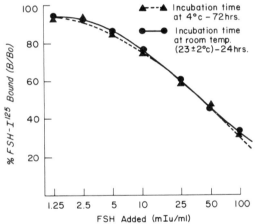

FIG. 4. *Inhibition curves for human FSH as obtained by incubating the assay at 4 C for 72 h and at room temperature (23 ± 2 C) for 24 h.*

antibody complex by using a second antibody at optimal dilution. If the first antibody is produced in rabbits, the second antibody to rabbit gamma globulin can be produced in sheep or goat. Commercial preparations are available from many sources, such as Calbiochem or Antibodies, Inc. The second antibody must be titered against the first antibody dilution and the normal rabbit serum concentration used in the assay. We have used 100 μliters of 1:25 dilution of normal rabbit serum in each assay tube, which gives a satisfactory amount of precipitate. A lower concentration of normal rabbit serum can also be used which, in turn, will require the use of a lesser amount of second antibody.

An alternate procedure is the use of solid phase radioimmunoassay where antibody is coated on the inner surface of polypropylene or

TABLE 3. *Assay performance for LH*

1. Sensitivity: Lowest detectable dose − 1.0 mIU/ml
2. Reproducibility: Variation within repeated estimates in different assays

Sample	No. of assays	LH (mIU/ml)	CV[a] (%)
A	10	42.3 ± 3.2	4.9
B	10	9.2 ± .46	7.5
C	10	2.8 ± .4	15

3. Accuracy: Closeness of measurements to the true value

Sample	Known amt added (mIU/ml)	No. of assays	Percent recovery[b]	CV (%)
1	1.0	5	96 ± 15	15
2	10	6	102 ± 6	6

[a] CV = coefficient of variation.
[b] Mean ± standard deviation.

TABLE 4. *Assay performance for FSH*

1. Sensitivity: Limit of detection − 1.0 mIU/ml
2. Reproducibility: Variation within repeated estimates in different assays

Sample	No. of assays	Mean ± SD	CV[a] (%)
A	10	44.1 ± 3.9	8.8
B	8	28.3 ± 1.99	7
C	10	5.3 ± 0.54	10

3. Accuracy: Closeness of measurements to the true value

Sample	Known amt added (mIU/ml)	No. of assays	Recovery[b]	CV (%)
1	5	5	86.4 ± 13.8	16
2	50	8	106 ± 12.7	12

[a] CV = coefficient of variation.
[b] Mean ± standard deviation.

polystyrene tubes or other solid disks (2, 3). The method is simple and rapid but is not as reproducible as the double antibody method and needs more antiserum than the double antibody method.

Dextran-coated charcoal has also been used for separation of bound and free antigen in LH assay (11). This method has been successfully utilized in assays of low-molecular-weight antigens. One drawback of this procedure has been that it is significantly affected by the protein concentration present in this system. The volume of unknown serum used and the protein concentration of the incubation mixture both appear to affect the adsorbing capacity of charcoal.

Validation of assay technique

Some of the important parameters of the reliability of the method are presented for LH and FSH in Table 3 and Table 4, respectively.

CLINICAL INDICATIONS

The normal levels for LH and FSH in men and women, as observed in our laboratory, are listed in Table 5.

The low levels of gonadotropins are detectable in plasma and urine (1) in early childhood, and these levels increase with age and stage of sexual development. Patients with gonadal dysgenesis have elevated FSH concentrations early in childhood and after age 9 to 11 years have elevated LH concentrations. Patients with idiopathic isosexual precocity have serum FSH and LH concentrations elevated for age but consistent with stage of sexual development (1).

Measurement of LH and FSH is valuable in the assessment of hypothalamic and pituitary function. Usually, a single determination is sufficient to distinguish between primary and secondary gonadal failure in the adult, as significantly elevated LH and FSH are found in the former case. In the secondary gonadal failure, however, these levels frequently fall in the low normal adult range, and it is usually not possible to distinguish these patients from normal individuals on the basis of a single LH-FSH measurement. Some provocative tests like

TABLE 5. *Normal range with standard 2-IRP-HMG (2nd International Reference Preparation of Human Menopausal Gonadotropins)*

Subject	No.	LH (mIU/ml)		FSH (mIU/ml)	
		Mean ± SD	Range	Mean ± SD	Range
Normal female					
Follicular phase	24	12.7 ± 5	3.7–26	10.7 ± 6	2.7–27
Luteinic phase	23	12.5 ± 9	2.3–38	6.4 ± 3.2	1.2–15
Normal male	29	11.6 ± 4	5.6–28	8.4 ± 4.2	3.7–20

clomiphene or LHRH stimulation are required for adequate assessment of hypothalamic or pituitary reserve.

The other areas where radioimmunoassay of LH and FSH are finding increasing applications are in monitoring ovulation induction and in the follow-up of patients with choriocarcinoma and hydatidiform mole before and after clinical treatment.

LITERATURE CITED

1. Blizard, R. M., R. Penny, T. P. Foley, Jr., et al. 1972. Pituitary-gonadal interrelationships in relation to puberty, p. 502–523. *In* B. B. Saxena, C. G. Beling, and H. M. Gandy (ed.), Gonadotropins. Wiley Interscience, New York.

2. Catt, K. J. 1968. Radioimmunoassay with antibody coated discs and tubes, p. 222. *In* E. Diczfalusy (ed.), Immunoassay of gonadotropins, Karolinska Symposia on Methods in Reproductive Endocrinology. Karolinska Institute, Stockholm.

3. Catt, K. J., H. D. Niall, G. W. Tregiar, and H. G. Burge. 1973. Disc solid phase radioimmunoassay of human luteinizing hormone. J. Clin. Endocrinol. Metab. 28:121–126.

4. De La Llosa, T., C. Courte, and M. Jutisz. 1967. On the mechanism of reversible inactivation of luteinizing hormone by urea. Biochem. Biophys. Res. Commun. 26:411.

5. Faiman, C., and R. J. Ryan. 1967. Radioimmunoassay for human follicle stimulating hormone. J. Clin. Endocrinol. Metab. 27:444–447.

6. Greenwood, F. C., W. M. Hunter, and J. S. Glover. 1963. The preparation of I^{131} labelled human growth hormone of high specific radioactivity. J. Biochem. 89:114.

7. Midgley, A. R., Jr. 1966. Radioimmunoassay: a method for human chorionic gonadotropin and human luteinizing hormone. Endocrinology 79:10–18.

8. Midgley, A. R. 1967. Radioimmunoassay for human follicle-stimulating hormone. J. Clin. Endocrinol. Metab. 27:295–299.

9. Odell, W., G. Ross, and P. Rayford. 1966. Radioimmunoassay for human luteinizing hormone. Metabolism 15:287–289.

10. Reichert, L. E., Jr., and R. A. Midgley, Jr. 1968. Preliminary studies of the effect of urea and chymotrypsin on the molecular, biological, and immunological properties of human follicle stimulating hormone and luteinizing hormone, p. 25. *In* E. Rosenberg (ed.), Gonadotropins. Seron-X-Inc., Los Altos, Calif.

11. Sand, T., and P. A. Torjesen. 1973. Dextran-coated charcoal used in the radioimmunoassay of human pituitary luteinizing hormone. Acta Endocrinol. 73:444–454.

12. Schlaff, S., S. W. Rosen, and J. Roth. 1968. Antibody to human follicle stimulating hormone: cross-reactivity with three other hormones. J. Clin. Invest. 47:1722–1729.

13. Vaitukaitis, J., J. B. Robbins, E. Nieschlag, and G. T. Ross. 1971. A method for producing specific antisera with small doses of immunogen. J. Clin. Endocrinol. Metab. 33:988–991.

14. Vaitukaitis, J. L., and G. T. Ross. 1973. Recent advances in evaluation of gonadotropic hormones. Annu. Rev. Med. 24:295–302.

15. Wilde, C. E., A. H. Orr, and K. D. Bagshawe. 1965. A radioimmunoassay for human chorionic gonadotropins. Nature (London) 205:191–192.

16. Yukitaka, M., J. L. Vaitukaitis, E. Nieschlag, and M. B. Lipsett. 1972. Enzymatic radioiodination of gonadotropins. J. Clin. Endocrinol. Metab. 34:23–28.

Chapter 25

Measurement of Chorionic Gonadotropin and Placental Lactogen in Human Body Fluids

M. J. LEVITT AND J. B. JOSIMOVICH

Human Chorionic Gonadotropin

INTRODUCTION

Human chorionic gondotropin (HCG) is a 40,000 molecular weight complex glycoprotein structurally related closely to human luteinizing hormone (HLH) and more distantly to human follicle-stimulating hormone (HFSH) and human thyroid-stimulating hormone (HTSH). It consists of an alpha subunit (peptide chain with attached carbohydrate residues) which is common to all four of the hormones and a beta subunit which is unique to HCG but is closely similar to the beta subunit of HLH (28, 38). Biologically inactive isolated HCG subunits are present in normal and pathological states (4, 6). HCG and HLH have very similar biological properties. As a product of the placenta, HCG is present normally only during pregnancy, when it serves to stimulate steroid production by the ovaries.

Three general categories of techniques exist for the measurement of serum HCG levels. The first two types, bioassays and radioligand receptor assays, actually measure the total amount of circulating HCG and HLH activity. The third type, radioimmunoassay, is suitable for precise survey in clinical research. All of these techniques require highly trained personnel and sufficient samples to establish and maintain expertise in their performance. A much simpler, although less sensitive, method for detecting HCG is the agglutination-inhibition test perfored on urine. This technique is suited for the routine laboratory and will be described in detail.

The urine HCG tests are designed primarily to confirm the diagnosis of pregnancy. They generally consist of antigen particles prepared by coating HCG onto gross particulate matter such as tanned sheep red cells (67) or latex particles (25). In the absence of added HCG, antibodies to HCG will cause either hemagglutination or latex particle agglutination. However, if a specimen containing sufficient HCG (or HLH) is also added, agglutination will be inhibited. Since the antibodies currently used are not specific for HCG, it is possible to get false-positive results due to HLH interference. To reduce the incidence of such results, the sensitivities of the tests are adjusted so that small levels of HLH are not detected. The result is that the tests will detect approximately 1 mIU of HCG in 1 ml of an undiluted urine specimen. The tests are approximately 75 to 95% reliable for the detection of normal pregnancy at 6 weeks of menstrual dates gestation (27), and possibly as low as 50% at any time in ectopic pregnancies (32).

To determine the lesser amounts of HCG that are present in earlier pregnancy, it is necessary to use more sensitive assays. Bioassays of urine or serum can detect pregnancy at less than 4 weeks of menstrual dates gestation (27), but these tests are so complex that they are no longer used widely (10, 18). They have been largely supplanted by radioligand receptor assays which are, in effect, bioassays performed in vitro (5, 14, 33, 34, 36, 45, 56). They measure the ability of a sample to inhibit the binding of radiolabeled HCG to receptors derived from gonadal tissue. These assays can be performed in as little as 1 h and have sufficient sensitivity to detect pregnancy as early as 8 days after ovulation (32, 46). However, since they also detect HLH, low values indicative of very early pregnancy may have to be repeated on a sample drawn the next day to rule out the possibility of a false-positive result due to the preovulatory surge in release of HLH (34, 45). Both in vivo and in vitro bioassays are poorly suited to the management of patients with trophoblastic or neoplastic disease since these conditions may be characterized by the presence of only isolated, inactive HCG subunits (3, 43).

Distinction between HCG and HLH can be made, under favorable circumstances, on the basis of immunological differences between the two hormones. Radioimmunoassays measure the amount of HCG present in a sample by the extent to which it inhibits the binding of radiolabeled HCG to an antibody preparation. If the antibodies are prepared against intact HCG, they will recognize antigenic sites on both hormones, and the radioimmunoassay will not be specific for HCG (39, 40). However, it is possible to select those antibody preparations which have a much higher affinity for HCG and use them in an HCG radioimmunoassay which has virtually no interference from HLH (14, 15, 37, 41, 45, 54, 65). More consistent specificity can be obtained by using only the beta subunit of HCG as the immunizing agent; in this case, the antibodies will be directed against fewer shared antigenic sites, and the radioimmunoassay will be virtually free from interference by HLH.

The beta subunit-specific radioimmunoassay for HCG (10, 11, 27, 30, 43, 48, 49, 51, 58, 60) is able to detect pregnancy as early as 8 days after ovulation with no false-positive results from the preovulatory release of HLH (29, 31, 37). The assay can detect the presence of small amounts of trophoblastic tissue which may remain after evacuation of a normal or molar pregnancy (19). The test is particularly valuable for assessing the success of chemotherapy for HCG-producing tumors, since it will detect isolated beta subunits that may be produced by neoplasms (19, 26, 40, 48, 57, 59).

To measure the isolated alpha subunit of HCG which may be present during pregnancy (1, 16, 21, 22, 43) and in trophoblastic (12, 43, 58) and neoplastic (17) disease, it is necessary to use antibodies prepared against this subunit (41, 61).

The beta subunit radioimmunoassay specific for HCG is clearly the preferable test to use in the management of the patient with gestational trophoblastic disease or with neoplastic disease characterized by the production of HCG. Radioligand receptor assays are suitable for the detection and management of most pregnancies, but are suspect when interference by HLH is possible, as in very early pregnancy or in the menopausal woman. For most pregnancies advanced beyond 4 weeks, the urinary immunological tests are satisfactory and give results that accurately reflect changes in serum levels of HCG. The ease and simplicity of these tests suggest that they will continue to be used widely.

CLINICAL INDICATIONS

Detection of HCG is the most sensitive indicator of the presence of small amounts of active trophoblastic tissue. Measurement of HCG is therefore indicated to confirm a diagnosis of pregnancy or to resolve clinical uncertainty as to whether trophoblast is present in a patient.

Pregnancy tests are indicated in any woman of child-bearing age with lower abdominal pain or abnormal vaginal bleeding; negative tests should be repeated on later specimens if symptoms continue. Pregnancy tests are also warranted before a woman of child-bearing age undergoes surgery or X-ray studies that could endanger embryonic or fetal development.

Detection of pregnancy within 4 weeks permits the patient to elect miniabortion (menstrual extraction) at the optimal time for this procedure (32). Molar pregnancies detected and treated by 10 weeks result in a spontaneous remission rate of 80 to 95%; later detection is associated with an increased incidence of actual invasive trophoblastic neoplasia (10, 23, 47).

During the first trimester of pregnancy, serial HCG determinations can aid in evaluating gestational progess (9). Measurements of HCG can indicate pregnancies characterized by poor placental function and thus assist in the diagnosis of ectopic pregnancy or threatened abortion.

Maternal levels of HCG after the first trimester are of little value in assessing fetal health directly, although a variety of maternal and fetal disorders may accompany a disturbance in placental metabolism (9). Maternal levels of HCG do not parallel placental or fetal growth and thus cannot be used to assess fetal development (51). Even fetal death in utero can occur without directly affecting maternal HCG levels (9).

Measurement of HCG is also warranted in unexplained cases of gynecomastia (7) or sexual precosity (42) since tumors producing HCG have been associated with these symptoms in men and children.

Patients with gestational trophoblastic disease should be monitored by serial HCG measurements for at least a year to detect a recurrence of the disease (10, 13, 19). These patients, and those with HCG-producing neoplasms, should have their chemotherapy modulated on the basis of their HCG levels. The HCG determinations may be performed and interpreted by experts at regional trophoblastic centers handling large numbers of cases (10, 13).

TEST PROCEDURE

Urine tests for the detection of pregnancy are sold as kits containing all the necessary reagents and supplies. A list of test names and manufacturers is given in Table 1. Each kit should be used according to the directions provided by the manufacturer. The following instructions are based on those provided with the Placentex kit; added commentaries are in parentheses. This kit is only suitable for testing urine samples.

Preparation of sample

The test may be performed on any urine specimen (however, first-voided morning specimens

TABLE 1. *Commercial urine pregnancy testing kits*

Name	Manufacturer
DAP test	Wampole Laboratories
Gravindex	Ortho Diagnostics
Hyland HCG slide test	Hyland Laboratories
Placentex	Roche Diagnostics
Pregnosticon	Organon, Inc.
Pregnosticon slide test	Organon, Inc.
Pregslide	Wampole Laboratories
Prepuerin	Burroughs-Wellcome Co.
Prequest	Parke-Davis & Co., Inc.
UCG test	Wampole Laboratories

provide greatest sensitivity and consistency). Grossly turbid urine specimens should be centrifuged (2,000 rpm for 5 min) prior to testing. Urine specimens kept at room temperature should be tested within 12 h of collection. Otherwise, they should be stored frozen (at -20 C).

Preparation of reagents

Provided in the kit are test tubes containing rabbit antiserum to HCG. Each tube is imprinted with a vertical black bar to facilitate viewing of the end point. These tubes should not be frozen; they should be stored in a refrigerator at 2 to 8 C and can be used before reaching room temperature.

Test performance

Using a provided disposable pipette, add sufficient patient urine (1 ml) to bring the fluid level in the antiserum tube to the top of the black bar. Mix the provided HCG antigen reagent consisting of a suspension of latex particles to which HCG is bound chemically; then add 2 drops with the provided dropper into the antiserum tube. Cap the tube and invert it three times to mix the reagents. Place the tube upright in a water bath or heating block preheated to 35 to 39 C. The tube should be placed in the heating device to approximately the level of the bottom of the black bar. After 90 min of incubation, hold the tube vertically and view the contents in a strong light. Viewed against the black bar, the appearance of agglutinated or flocculated latex particles at any time within 90 min is a negative test result. A milky or translucent suspension due to the inhibition of latex particle agglutination is a positive test result, indicating an HCG (and/or HLH) level of more than approximately 1 IU/ml.

Quantitation

An estimate of the amount of HCG may be obtained by testing serial twofold dilutions made with urine from a male as diluent. The highest dilution which is still positive indicates the approximate concentration of HCG in the original specimen. For example, a final positive result at a dilution of 1:8 indicates 8 IU/ml of HCG (and/or HLH) in the urine specimen.

Quality control

Each set of tests should include control specimens. (For a positive control, use an early pregnancy sample; for a negative control, use a specimen from a nonpregnant nonmenopausal normal woman.) Store the control specimens frozen (at -20 C) in small enough amounts that they are not thawed and refrozen (1 to 2 ml). The antigen reagent should be delivered only with the dropper provided, and the dropper tip should not touch the walls of the tube when dispensing reagent. Reagents from different kits should not be used since their strengths are adjusted for use only with the other reagents in the same kit. The presence in the specimen of 100 to 1,000 mg of protein per 100 ml may yield a false-positive result due to a nonspecific interference. Other false-positive results (for pregnancy) may result from high HLH levels in the urine of postmenopausal women. The reagents are provided completely in the Placentex kit.

INTERPRETATION

Hemagglutination-inhibition pregnancy tests give results that are clearly positive or negative, but latex agglutination-inhibition tests may give intermediate results; it is necessary to be consistent in judging tests with slight agglutination as either positive or negative. The urine pregnancy tests are subject to false-positive results due to high HLH levels or high protein concentration, and to false-negative results due to low sensitivity.

Laboratories performing radioligand receptor assays or radioimmunoassays must establish their own normal values since these depend upon the standard used, as well as individual variations in techniques (66).

Typical HCG values in a normal pregnancy are shown in Fig. 1. There is a sharp rise from barely detectable levels at 1 week after fertilization to a maximal level at 7 to 10 weeks. There follows a slower decline throughout the first trimester until a plateau is reached in the fourth month and maintained until term. Some laboratories report a second, small rise in HCG at approximately 36 weeks (63). There is a tendency for slightly higher HCG levels to occur near term in gestations involving a female fetus as compared with those involving a male fetus (2, 24, 68). HCG levels do not rise in proportion to placental mass throughout gestation; however, the levels in blood and urine do

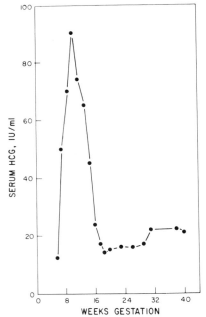

FIG. 1. *Serum HCG determined by immunoassay throughout pregnancy (after D. R. Mishell, Jr., L. Wide, and C. A. Gemzell, J. Clin. Endocrinol. 23:125, 1956). Urinary concentrations paralleled serum concentrations.*

change in proportion to the placental levels of HCG (51).

It is extremely important to note that on occasion a completely normal pregnancy may be accompanied by HCG levels outside the normal range. Pregnancy should never be terminated for suspected pathology solely on the basis of HCG values.

Poor placental function during early pregnancy will result in lower than normal values of HCG and may be indicative of ectopic pregnancy or threatened abortion (30, 31). Simultaneous findings of low human placental lactogen (HPL) values strengthen the diagnosis of threatened abortion (9). In contrast, molar pregnancies are characterized by high levels of HCG and low levels of HPL (9, 55). Elevation of HCG beyond 90 to 100 days can be diagnostic of molar pregnancy (10, 12, 13).

Pregnancy can be monitored more successfully with a combination of HCG and HPL determinations than by either measurement alone. Table 2 illustrates some complications of pregnancy that can be suggested by HCG and HPL values.

With the sole exception of the period up to 3 months after delivery or abortion (19), the presence of HCG in a nonpregnant patient is a diagnostic sign of trophoblastic disease or non-

trophoblastic neoplastic disease (3). Determinations of HCG are essential to determine whether all trophoblastic tissue has been removed by physical or chemical treatment. The recurrence of disease and functioning trophoblastic tissue is detected more readily by HCG measurements than by any other means (23).

Measurements of HCG provide a rational basis for the decisions when to begin and when to stop chemotherapy in patients with HCG-producing diseases (26). Use of the test can reduce the total dose of drug and length of hospital stay without any sacrifice in therapeutic effectiveness (19, 40).

Human Placental Lactogen

INTRODUCTION

HPL (alternatively known as human chorionic somatomammotropin, or HCS) is a 21,000 molecular weight single-chain simple protein very similar in structure to pituitary growth hormone. Although it displays growth hormone effects which contribute to the metabolic changes of late pregnancy, it is more potent as a lactogenic hormone which prepares the breasts for lactation (27).

Three general categories of techniques exist for the measurement of serum HPL levels. The first two types, radioimmunoassay (20, 27, 28) and hemagglutination inhibition (28), are suitable for precise survey in clinical research. These techniques require highly trained personnel for their performance and a sufficient volume of specimens so that expertise may be maintained. A much simpler, although less precise, technique for measuring HPL is the radial immunodiffusion test (50). This technique is suited for the routine laboratory and will be described in detail.

The radial immunodiffusion test is designed to obtain a rapid estimate of the amount of HPL in the serum of a pregnant woman as an indication of the extent of fetal-placental development. It involves the diffusion of a spot of HPL radially through a gel impregnated with antibodies to HPL. As the HPL diffuses, it becomes

TABLE 2. *Hormone levels in complications of pregnancy*

Gestation (weeks)	HCG	HPL	Indicated condition
0–15	↓	↓	Threatened abortion
3–17	↓	—	Ectopic pregnancy
12–25	↑	↓	Molar pregnancy
25–40	↑	↓	Toxemia
25–40	↑	↑	Diabetes mellitus

diluted until its concentration in relation to the antibody is such that a precipitating antigen-antibody complex will be formed. The diameter of the precipitin ring will be related to the distance the HPL diffuses prior to complex formation, and thus will be proportional to the amount of HPL present in the original spot. The actual amount of HPL can be established by comparison with the sizes of precipitin rings formed by known amounts of standard HPL treated similarly.

To measure low levels of HPL during early pregnancy, the more sensitive complex techniques are advisable. However, late pregnancy is the only period in which there appears to be much clinical value in measuring maternal serum levels of HPL. At that stage of pregnancy, radial immunodiffusion measurements can provide sufficient information on HPL levels to assist in the diagnosis of retarded fetal-placental development.

CLINICAL INDICATIONS

The primary indication for the determination of HPL is to suggest the presence of fetal-placental growth retardation during the third trimester of pregnancy (27).

Some groups have proposed that HPL measurements be used as a *general screening test* to detect pregnancies in which there is a high risk of intrauterine or perinatal death of the conceptus (35, 52, 53). As support, they cite evidence that perinatal mortality is reduced if premature delivery is initiated automatically (if other tests suggest fetal pulmonary maturity) in response to a low level of maternal serum HPL (49). The evidence, however, is not conclusive, since it is not known to what extent perinatal mortality would be reduced by premature delivery when the HPL level is normal. There remains serious doubt whether HPL measurements are a significant adjunct to traditional maternal care consisting of physical examination, measurement of weight and blood pressure, and determination of urine protein concentration.

Maternal serum HPL levels are not of value in determining whether fetal demise is imminent in high-risk pregnancies such as those involving hypertension, diabetes mellitus, malnutrition, or Rh isoimmunization (27). In these cases, HPL levels often fail to decline in proportion to the severity of the conditions. Even after fetal death, HPL levels can remain constant until a later decrease in protein anabolism occurs within the placenta, the tissue which produces the hormone.

Maternal serum HPL determinations can be of use in confirming a clinical suspicion of fetal growth retardation as indications for alteration in patient treatment or for premature delivery if fetal pulmonary maturity has been attained (62). In many hospitals, fetal growth retardation is confirmed by serial ultrasonographic measurements of fetal biparietal head diameter. Where such measurements are not available, a combination of finding low maternal serum HPL values in addition to low maternal urinary total estrogen excretions may suggest fetal growth retardation (27). In a more recent series of 66 high-risk patients studied at our hospital in the last trimester of pregnancy, all but one of the 17 with marked fetal growth retardation showed low maternal HPL levels. Similarly, of 17 with both low total estrogen excretion and low serum HPL levels, only 1 failed to show marked growth retardation. Conversely, only 1 of the 49 patients not showing both low serum HPL and low urinary estrogen levels had marked fetal malnutrition.

Other suggested uses for the measurement of serum HPL have not been widely adopted because other tests verify the clinical diagnoses more adequately:

1. Measurement of HPL in early pregnancy may be undertaken by radioimmunoassay (8). In those cases, serum or urinary chorionic gonadotropin measurements (see first section of this chapter) may more precisely give prognoses as to the eventual loss or retention of viability of the conceptus.

2. Low maternal serum HPL values, measured by radioimmunoassay, usually combined with high serum or urinary levels of chorionic gonadotropin may be found in cases of hydatidiform mole (20, 27, 44, 69). Ultrasonographic or X-ray studies are available in most hospitals and more accurately confirm the clinical diagnosis.

3. The followup of patients with trophoblastic neoplasia (hydatidiform mole, choriocarcinoma) would be theoretically possible by serial measurement of HPL in a patient's serum (69). It has been found, however, that a rising level of chorionic gonadotropin may precede a reappearance of HPL, making the measurement of the latter hormone the best method for following such patients (reference 69 and first section of this chapter).

4. Nontrophoblastic neoplasms may be associated with detectable amounts of HPL and chorionic gonadotropin in the patients' serum (e.g., certain pulmonary carcinomas; 64). The measurement of HPL in the sera of such patients would be readily performed in specialized hospital centers where more sensitive radioimmunoassays are available.

TEST PROCEDURE

The following instructions are based on those provided with the Plac-Gest kit manufactured by Lederle Laboratories; commentaries are added in parentheses. This radial immunodiffusion system consists of a plastic slide coated with agar gel containing rabbit antiserum to HPL.

1. Using the provided capillary pipette, dispense a standard quantity of patient serum into one of the circular wells cut in the gel. Similarly, dispense the provided HPL standards (3, 6, and 9 μg/ml) into other wells.

2. Incubate the slide in a horizontal position at room temperature for 18 to 20 h in a sealed chamber (or in the original plastic bag after resealing).

3. Immerse the slide in the provided Tris buffer for 2 h. (The purpose of this step is to wash out nonprecipitated proteins. Incomplete washing, as may occur if the slides are too crowded, will result in haziness around the precipitin ring, making precise measurement of ring diameter difficult. If the slide is placed vertically, agitation of the buffer may cause the gel to separate from the slide. If the slide is placed horizontally, it must be weighted down to hold it in the buffer.)

4. Immerse the slide in the provided cupric chloride solution for 30 min to fix the immunoprecipitate.

5. Immerse the slide in distilled water for 10 min.

6. Using the provided rule, measure the greatest diameter of each precipitin ring under fluorescent or other wide band of transmitted light. (Weak magnifying lenses, with or without micrometer lines, can be used to aid in measuring ring diameters.)

7. On the graph paper provided, plot the square of the diameter of the precipitin ring for each standard against the concentration of each standard. Draw a line through the points (it should be a straight line) to obtain a standard curve. Use the standard curve to determine the HPL concentration of the patient serum from the square of the diameter of the precipitin ring of this sample.

Control specimens can be included in each analysis by retesting frozen samples of sera of known HPL concentrations. Analytical results by radial immunodiffusion should be periodically checked by radioimmunoassay of the same specimens. The potencies of the kit standards can be compared against a standard HPL preparation obtainable from the Hormone Distribution Office, National Institutes of Health, Bethesda, Md. 20014.

REAGENTS

The following reagents are all provided in the Lederle Laboratories Plac-Gest Kit.

The Lederle Diagnostics Plac-Gest Kit, no. 2800-93, provides six slides with gel impregnated with antiserum to HPL. Also provided are:

0.5 ml of each of the three reference sera (I-III) as HPL standards

two 300-mg vials of cupric chloride dihydrate

two 1.2-g packets of Tris buffer

60 disposable capillary pipettes

one immunodiffusion measuring rule

graph paper for plotting HPL standards and deriving concentrations of the hormone in unknown sera.

INTERPRETATION

To use maternal serum HPL values to establish the presence of fetal-placental growth retardation, it is necessary to establish the lower limit of values for 95% of normal pregnant women. The necessary normal control serum samples can be obtained conveniently when patients have blood drawn for typing upon entry into the hospital labor suite. Serum HPL levels do not drop more than 10% during labor until the time of delivery of the placenta. Collection of blood for normal controls should exclude samples from patients already delivered, since the hormone disappears from the maternal circulation with an initial half-life of approximately 15 min.

As shown in Fig. 2, maternal serum HPL levels determined by radioimmunoassay increase steadily throughout normal pregnancies. After 30 weeks of gestation, the lower limit of normal is usually 4 μg/ml. The finding

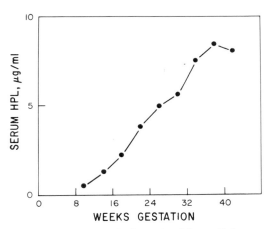

Fig. 2. *Serum HPL determined by radioimmunoassay throughout pregnancy in our laboratory.*

of low maternal serum HPL and low maternal urine total estrogen (or estriol) excretion gives a 94% assurance of failure of the fetus to grow at a normal rate.

LITERATURE CITED

1. Ashitaka, Y., R. Nishimura, Y. Endoh, and S. Tojo. 1974. Subunits of human chorionic gonadotropin and their radioimmunoassays. Endocrinol. Jpn. 21:429–435.

2. Boroditsky, R. S., F. I. Reyes, J. S. D. Winter, and C. Faiman. 1975. Serum human chorionic gonadotropin and progesterone patterns in the last trimester of pregnancy: relationship to fetal sex. Am. J. Obstet. Gynecol. 121:238–241.

3. Braunstein, G. D., J. L. Vaitukaitis, P. P. Carbone, and G. T. Ross. 1973. Ectopic production of human chorionic gonadotrophin by neoplasms. Ann. Intern. Med. 78:39–45.

4. Braunstein, G. D., J. L. Vaitukaitis, and G. T. Ross. 1972. The in vivo behavior of human chorionic gonadotropin after dissociation into subunits. Endocrinology 91:1030–1036.

5. Catt, K. J., M. L. Dufau, and T. Tsuruhara. 1972. Radioligand-receptor assay of luteinizing hormone and chorionic gonadotropin. J. Clin. Endocrinol. 34:123–132.

6. Catt, K. J., M. L. Dufau, and T. Tsuruhara. 1973. Absence of intrinsic biological activity in LH and hCG subunits. J. Clin. Endocrinol. 36:73–80.

7. Charles, M. A., R. Claypool, M. Schaaf, S. W. Rosen, and B. D. Weintraub. 1973. Lung carcinoma associated with production of three placental proteins. Arch. Intern. Med. 132:427–431.

8. Crosignani, P. G. 1974. Correlation of human chorionic gonadotropin (HCG) and somatotropin (HCS) with fetal nutrition, p. 203–217. In J. B. Josimovich, M. Reynolds, and F. Cobo (ed.), Lactogenic hormones, fetal nutrition and lactation. John Wiley & Sons, Inc., New York.

9. Crosignani, P. G., L. Trojsi, A. E. M. Attanasio, and G. C. L. Finzi. 1974. Value of HCG and HCS measurement in clinical practice. Obstet. Gynecol. 44:673–681.

10. Curry, S. L., C. B. Hammond, L. Tyrey, W. T. Creasman, and R. T. Parker. 1975. Hydatidiform mole. Diagnosis, management, and long-term followup of 347 patients. Obstet. Gynecol. 45:1–8.

11. Dattatreyamurty, B., A. R. Sheth, L. R. Joshi, and S. S. Rao. 1975. Changes in the ratio between serum and "specific" levels of human chorionic gonadotropin in different trimesters of pregnancy. Am. J. Obstet. Gynecol. 121:300–305.

12. Dawood, M. Y., S. S. Ratnam, and E. S. Teoh. 1974. Serum estradiol-17 beta and serum human chorionic gonadotropin in patients with hydatidiform moles. Am. J. Obstet. Gynecol. 119:904–910.

13. Delfs, E. 1975. Hydatidiform mole. An editorial comment. Obstet. Gynecol. 45:95–96.

14. Dufau, M. L., C. R. Mendelson, and K. J. Catt. 1974. A highly sensitive in vitro bioassay for luteinizing hormone and chorionic gonadotropin: testosterone production by dispersed Leydig cells. J. Clin. Endocrinol. 39:610–613.

15. Franchimont, P. 1970. A study of the cross-reaction between human chorionic and pituitary luteinizing hormones (HCG and HLH). Eur. J. Clin. Invest. 1:65–68.

16. Franchimont, P., H. Burger, and J. J. Legros. 1973. Impact of radioassay techniques on the field of sex hormones. Metabolism 22:1003–1011.

17. Franchimont, P., and A Reuter. 1974. Radioimmunoassay of HCG, alpha and beta subunits in cancer. Br. J. Cancer. 30:175.

18. Goldstein, D. P., F. Nudemberg, N. Lymeburner, L. Levesque, and C. Shore. 1973. The management of patients with gestational trophoblastic neoplasia based on the antigenic properties of human chorionic gonadotropin. J. Surg. Oncol. 5:1–8.

19. Goldstein, D. P., G. B. Pastorfide, R. Osathanondh, and T. S. Kosasa. 1975. A rapid solid-phase radioimmunoassay specific for human chorionic gonadotropin in gestational trophoblastic disease. Obstet. Gynecol. 45:527–530.

20. Grumbach, M. M., S. L. Kaplan, and A. Vinik. 1973. Human chorionic somatomammotropin (HCS). Measurement, p. 802–807. In S. A. Berson and R. S. Yallow (ed.), Methods in investigative and diagnostic endocrinology, vol. IIB. North Holland Publishing Co., Amsterdam.

21. Hagen, C., and A. S. McNeilly, 1975. The gonadotropic hormones and their subunits in human maternal fetal circulation at delivery. Am. J. Obstet. Gynecol. 121:926–930.

22. Hagen, C., A. S. McNeilly, and T. Chard. 1974. Measurement and identification of gonadotrophins and their subunits in human maternal and foetal circulation around term. J. Endocrinol. 63:28P.

23. Hilgers, R. D., and J. L. Lewis, Jr. 1974. Gestational trophoblastic neoplasms. Gynecol. Oncol. 2:460–475.

24. Hobson, B., and L. Wide. 1974. Chorionic gonadotrophin in the human placenta in relation to the sex of the foetus at term. J. Endocrinol. 60:75–80.

25. Horowitz, C. A., E. Jerome, R. Diamond, and P. C. J. Ward. 1973. Evaluation of a latex tube agglutination-inhibition pregnancy test. Am. J. Obstet. Gynecol. 116:626–632.

26. Jones, W. B., J. L. Lewis, Jr., and M. Lehr. 1975. Monitor of chemotherapy in gestational trophoblastic neoplasm by radioimmunoassay of the beta-subunit of human chorionic gonadotropin. Am. J. Obstet. Gynecol. 121:669–673.

27. Josimovich, J. B. 1973. Placental protein hormones in pregnancy. Clin. Obstet. Gynecol. 16:46–65.

28. Josimovich, J. B., and J. E. Zuckerman. 1971.

Methods for the measurement of human placental lactogen, p. 622–635. *In* F. W. Sunderman and F. W. Sunderman, Jr. (ed.), Laboratory diagnosis of endocrine disorders. Warren H. Green, St. Louis.

29. Kosasa, T., L. Levesque, D. P. Goldstein, and M. L. Taymor. 1973. Early detection of implantation using radioimmunoassay specific for human chorionic gonadotropin. J. Clin. Endocrinol. Metab. 36:622–624.

30. Kosasa, T. S., L. A. Levesque, D. P. Goldstein, and M. L. Taymor. 1974. Clinical use of a solid-phase radioimmunoassay specific for human chorionic gonadotropin. Am. J. Obstet. Gynecol. 119:784–791.

31. Kosasa, T. S., R. J. Pion, R. W. Hale, D. P. Goldstein, M. L. Taymor, L. A. Levesque, and T. Y. Kobara. 1975. Rapid hCG-specific radioimmunoassay for menstrual aspiration. Ostet. Gynecol. 45:566–568.

32. Landesman, R., and B. B. Saxena. 1974. Radioreceptorassay of human chorionic gonadotropin as an aid in miniabortion. Fertil. Steril. 25:1022–1029.

33. Lee, C. Y., and R. J. Ryan. 1973. Interaction of ovarian receptors with human luteinizing hormone and human chorionic gonadotropin. Biochemistry 12:4609–4615.

34. Lee, C. Y., and R. J. Ryan. 1975. Radioreceptor assay for human chorionic gonadotropin. J. Clin. Endocrinol. Metab. 40:228–233.

35. Letchworth, A. T., and T. Chard. 1972. Placental lactogen levels as a screening for fetal distress in neonatal asphyxia. Lancet 1:704–706.

36. Leyendecker, G., L. Wildt, and W. Nocke. 1973. Radiolog and receptor assay for the determination of LH and HCG activities utilizing rat ovarian receptors. Acta Endocrinol. (Copenhagen) Suppl. 173:62.

37. Mishell, Jr., D. R., R. M. Nakamura, J. M. Barberia, and I. H. Thorneycroft. 1974. Initial detection of human chorionic gonadotropin in serum in normal human gestation. Am. J. Obstet. Gynecol. 118:990–991.

38. Morgan, F. J. 1974. Glycoprotein hormones: gonadotrophins and thyrotrophins. Med. J. Aust. 2:931–934.

39. Nakamura, R. M., Y. Nagata, C. Osborn, and D. R. Mishell, Jr. 1974. Use of a post-menopausal serum pool as a reference preparation for RIA of gonadotrophins. Acta Endocrinol. (Copenhagen) 75:478–490.

40. Pastorfide, G. B., D. P. Goldstein, and T. S. Kosasa. 1974. The use of a radioimmunoassay specific for human chorionic gonadotropin in patients with molar pregnancy and gestational trophoblastic disease. Am. J. Obstet. Gynecol. 120:1025–1028.

41. Rabinowitz, D., R. Benveniste, and J. Bell. 1974. Heterogeneity of human luteinizing hormone. Israel J. Med. Sci. 10:1272–1279.

42. Romshe, C. A., and J. F. Sotos. 1975. Intracranial human chorionic gonadotropin-secreting tumor with precocious puberty. J. Pediatr.

86:250–252.

43. Rosen, S. W., B. D. Weintraub, J. L. Vaitukaitis, H. H. Sussman, J. M. Hershman, and F. M. Muggia. 1975. Placental proteins and their subunits as tumor markers. Ann. Intern. Med. 82:71–83.

44. Saxena, B. B., D. P. Goldstein, K. Emerson, Jr., and H. A. Selenkow. 1968. Serum placental lactogen levels in patients with molar pregnancy and trophoblastic tumors. Am. J. Obstet. Gynecol. 102:115–121.

45. Saxena, B. B., S. H. Hasan, F. Haour, and M. Schmidt-Gollwitzer. 1974. Radioreceptor assay of human chorionic gonadotropin: detection of early pregnancy. Science 184:793–795.

46. Saxena, B. B., and R. Landesman. 1975. The use of a radioreceptorassay of human chorionic gonadotropin for the diagnosis and management of ectopic pregnancy. Fertil. Steril. 26:397–404.

47. Segal, S., A. Adoni, and J. G. Schenker. 1975. Choriocarcinoma of the fallopian tube. Gynecol. Oncol. 3:40–45.

48. Sheth, N. A., J. N. Saruiya, K. J. Ranadive, and A. R. Sheth. 1974. Ectopic production of human chorionic gonadotropin by human breast tumours. Br. J. Cancer 30:566–570.

49. Spellacy, W. N., W. C. Buhi, and S. A. Birk. 1975. The effectiveness of human placental lactogen measurements as an adjunct in decreasing perinatal deaths. Am. J. Obstet. Gynecol. 121:835–844.

50. Spellacy, W. N., W. C. Buhi, and S. A. McCreary. 1974. Measurement of human placental lactogen with a simple immunodiffusion kit (Plac-Gest^R). Obstet. Gynecol. 43:306–309.

51. Spellacy, W. N., P. W. Conly, W. W. Cleveland, and W. C. Buhi. 1975. Effects of fetal sex and weight and placental weight on maternal serum progesterone and chorionic gonadotropin concentrations. Am. J. Obstet. Gynecol. 122:278–282.

52. Spellacy, W. N., E. S. Teoh, and W. C. Buhi. 1970. Human chorionic somatomammotropin (HCS) levels prior to fetal death in high-risk pregnancies. Obstet. Gynecol. 35:685–689.

53. Spellacy, W. N., E. S. Teoh, W. C. Buhi, S. A. Birk, and S. A. McCreary. 1971. Value of human chorionic somatomammotropin in managing high risk pregnancies. Am. J. Obstet. Gynecol. 109:588–598.

54. Sussman, H. H., B. D. Weintraub, and S. W. Rosen. 1974. Relationship of ectopic placental alkaline phosphatase to ectopic chorionic gonadotropin and placental lactogen. Cancer 33:820–823.

55. Tojo, S., M. Mochizuki, and A. Kanazawa. 1974. Comparative assay of HCG, HCT, and HCS in molar pregnancy. Acta Obstet. Gynecol. Scand. 53:369–373.

56. Tomoda, Y., T. Miwa, and N. Ishizuka. 1975. Radioligand receptor assay for urinary and serum hCG. J. Clin. Endocrinol. Metab. 40:644–651.

57. Tormey, D. C., T. P. Waalkes, D. Ahmann, C.

W. Gehrke, R. W. Zumwatt, J. Synder, and H. Hansen. 1975. Biological markers in breast carcinoma. I. Incidence of abnormalities of CEA, HCG, three polyamines, and three minor nucleosides. Cancer 35:1095–1100.

58. Vaitukaitis, J. L. 1973. Immunologic and physical characterization of human chorionic gonadotropin (hCG) secreted by tumors. J. Clin. Endocrinol. Metab. 37:505–514.

59. Vaitukaitis, J. L. 1974. Human chorionic gonadotropin as a tumor marker. Ann. Clin. Lab. Sci. 4:276–280.

60. Vaitukaitis, J. L., G. D. Braunstein, and G. T. Ross. 1972. A radioimmunoassay which specifically measures human chorionic gonadotropin in the presence of human luteinizing hormone. Am. J. Obstet. Gynecol. 113:751–758.

61. Vaitukaitis, J. L., and G. T. Ross. 1974. Subunits of human glycoprotein hormones. Their immunological and biological behavior. Israel. J. Med. Sci. 10:1280–1287.

62. Venning, E. H., and J. B. Josimovich. 1975. Hormonal physiology of the placenta. II. Polypeptide and steroid hormones, p. 78–95. In J. J. Gold (ed.), Gynecologic endocrinology. Harper and Row, New York.

63. Watanabe, N., M. Seki, K. Seki, and T. Yoshihara. 1974. Urinary follicle stimulating hormone, chorionic gonadotrophin and oestrogens during human pregnancy. Acta Endocrinol. (Copenhagen) 75:763–772.

64. Weintraub, B. D., and S. W. Rosen. 1971. Ectopic production of human chorionic somatomammotropin by non-trophoblastic cancers. J. Clin. Endocrinol. Metab. 32:94–101.

65. Weintraub, B. D., S. W. Rosen, J. A. McCammon, and R. L. Perlman. 1973. Apparent cooperativity in radioimmunoassay of human chorionic gonadotropin. Endocrinology 92:1250–1255.

66. W.H.O. Report of a Meeting. 1972. Assay of protein hormones related to human reproduction: problems of specificity of assay methods and reference standards. Acta Endocrinol. (Copenhagen) 71:625–637.

67. Wide, L. 1962. An immunological method for the assay of human chorionic gonadotrophin. Acta Endocrinol. (Copenhagen) 41(Suppl. 70):1–111.

68. Wide, L., and B. Hobson. 1974. Relationship between the sex of the foetus and the amount of human chorionic gonadotrophin in placentae from the 10th to the 20th week of pregnancy. J. Endocrinol. 61:75–81.

69. Yen, S. S. C., O. H. Pearson, and J. S. Rankin. 1968. Radioimmunoassay of serum chorionic gonadotropin and placental lactogen in trophoblastic disease. Obstet. Gynecol. 32:86–93.

Chapter 26

Radioimmunoassay of Thyroxine, Triiodothyronine, and Thyrotropin in Human Serum

P. REED LARSEN

INTRODUCTION

The determinations of the concentration of thyroxine (T_4), triiodothyronine (T_3), and thyrotropin (TSH) in human serum are often critical steps in the evaluation of the patient with suspected thyroid disease. In this chapter, techniques for quantitation of these hormones by use of radioimmunoassay are presented. The methods for measurement of the two thyroid hormones are quite similar and are presented first; a double-antibody immunoassay technique for TSH follows thereafter.

THYROXINE

Quantitation of serum T_4 concentrations by radioimmunoassay represents the most recent modification in methods for the measurement of this thyroid hormone in human serum. Historically, T_4, as estimated by protein-bound iodine (PBI), was the first hormone to be measured accurately in human serum. Since the development of this assay some 50 years ago, great progress has been made in overcoming the nonspecificity of the iodine determination used in this test. Over the past 10 years, competitive protein-binding analysis, or a modification thereof, has been widely used. Quantitation in this test was obtained by analyzing the displacement of labeled T_4 from a specific binding site on human thyroxine-binding globulin (TBG). The radioimmunoassay for T_4 represents a further improvement on this technique, though the principle of the test is the same. The advantages of radioimmunoassay over the competitive protein-binding technique are several: it has greater sensitivity (the test can be performed with as little as 2.5 μliters of serum if necessary), extraction of T_4 from unknown sera is not required, and the recovery of T_4 from serum is complete as opposed to a maximum of approximately 80% in the older technique. The last major advantage is that large numbers of samples can be processed in a single assay.

The two types of T_4 immunoassays in common use today differ only in the substance used to inhibit T_4 binding to endogenous protein and in the technique used for separation of bound and free hormone. The method to be described is a minor modification of one that has been used extensively in my laboratory since 1971 (10). Sodium salicylate is added to the assay buffer to inhibit T_4 binding, and a dextran-charcoal solution is added to separate bound and free hormone. The T_4 immunoassay initially reported by Chopra uses 8-anilino-1-naphthalene sulfonic acid (ANS) as an inhibitor of T_4-protein binding and a second antibody technique for precipitation of antibody-bound T_4 (2). This type of method is also widely used (1, 12). Both give comparable results though the question of possible nonspecificity, especially in hyperthyroid patients, was raised in early reports on the use of the ANS–double-antibody method (1, 2).

Clinical indications

Determination of serum T_4 is currently the method of choice in the screening of patients with suspected thyroid dysfunction. It is also valuable in the assessment of the effects of treatment for patients with either hypo- or hyperthyroidism. In most patients, a normal serum T_4 concentration is good evidence that thyroid dysfunction is not the cause of the patient's symptoms. The major difficulty in interpretation of the results is that the concentration of the major T_4-binding protein in the serum (TBG) varies under certain clinical circumstances. Despite this variation in bound T_4, the free hormone concentration is maintained in a narrow normal range by hypothalamic-pituitary feedback mechanisms. Since all methods for T_4 measure the total hormone in serum or plasma, the fact that it is the free thyroid hormone (<0.05% of the total) which is the active fraction may lead to confusing results. Thus, in the euthyroid patient with elevated TBG, total T_4 is increased, the fraction of T_4 that is free is diminished, and the free T_4 concentration is normal. To differentiate protein-related "abnormalities" in serum T_4 (and T_3) concentrations from alterations due to thyroid disease, some index of the concentration of unoccupied TBG binding sites is necessary. The usual technique is to determine the charcoal or resin uptake of labeled T_3 in the patient's serum. The combined use of these two tests is discussed extensively in many endocrinology texts and has been recently reviewed (9).

Radioimmunoassay of serum thyroxine

The method for immunoassay of T_4 currently used in my clinical laboratory is presented below. Before beginning, the technician should be familiar with the general theory of radioimmunoassay and be especially cognizant of the special problems presented by assay of a hormone where high-affinity endogenous binding proteins are present.

Preparation of solutions.

1. *Glycine-acetate buffer (GAB):* 60.04 g of glycine and 69.66 g of crystalline sodium acetate are added to 4 liters of distilled water; pH is adjusted to 8.6 with 10 N NaOH.

2. *Assay diluent:* Add 20 mg of bovine serum albumin (fraction V) plus 2 g of sodium salicylate and ~700,000 counts/min of ^{125}I-labeled T_4/100 ml of GAB required.

3. *Antibody solution:* Add anti-T_4 antiserum to assay diluent to yield desired final concentration for the antisera to be used.

4. *Charcoal-dextran mixture:* Dissolve 0.125 g of dextran in 200 ml of GAB; add 1.25 g of Norit charcoal and stir for 15 min. Store at 4 C.

5. *T_4-free serum:* Obtain a pool of Australia antigen-free human serum. Add ~3,000 counts/min of ^{125}I-labeled T_4 per ml and 7 g of Norit charcoal per 100 ml. Stir overnight at 4 C. Centrifuge at 40,000 × g for four 1-h periods to remove charcoal. Count 1 ml to ascertain that >95% of ^{125}I-labeled T_4 was removed.

6. *Standards:* Dissolve L-thyroxine (free acid) in 0.04 M NaOH at a concentration of 1 mg/ml. Dilute in 0.04 M NaOH to a concentration of 40 μg/ml. Determine absorption at 325 nm in a spectrophotometer, and check the concentration using the molar extinction coefficient of 6,207 in the following equation:

$$T_4 \text{ concentration (mg/ml)} = \text{optical density}$$
$$(1 \text{ cm}) \times 0.1252$$

Add T_4 to T_4-free serum at concentrations of 300 ng/ml, and make serial dilutions of this with T_4-free serum to result in T_4 concentrations of 260, 200, 160, 80, 40, 20, and 10 ng of T_4/ml. Prepare about 16 ml of each standard and also 48 ml of the T_4-free serum (equivalent to 0 standard). Store at −20 C in 0.15-ml amounts

(three assays) except for the 0 standard, which should be stored in 0.45-ml amounts.

7. *Quality control pools:* Obtain an Australia antigen-free pool of human serum. By addition of a suitable quantity of T_4-free serum, prepare about 30 ml of serum with a T_4 concentration of about 4 μg/100 ml. Using the T_4 solution prepared in step 6, add 0.4 μg of T_4 to one 10-ml amount and 0.8 μg of T_4 to a second. Thus, pool A = ~4 μg of T_4/100 ml, pool B = ~8 μg of T_4/100 ml, and pool C = ~12 μg of T_4/100 ml.

Assay procedure.

1. *Standard curve:* Add 20 μliters of each standard (including 0-T_4) in duplicate to 75 × 100 mm glass or plastic tubes. Also, add 20 μliters × 2 of the 0 standard for nonspecific binding (NSB) control tubes.

2. *Quality control:* Prepare 20- and 10-μliter amounts of each quality control in duplicate. To each tube containing 10 μliters, add 10 μliters of T_4-free serum.

3. *Unknowns:* Add 20 μliters of serum or plasma of each unknown per tube in duplicate.

4. *Assay diluent:* Prepare assay diluent as described. Add 1 ml to each of the two NSB tubes (step 1).

5. *Antibody solution:* Prepare antibody solution as described. Add 1 ml to each tube of standard, quality control, and unknown (not to NSB tubes).

Each tube now contains 20 μliters of serum plus either 1 ml of antibody solution or 1 ml of assay diluent (two tubes).

The assay may now be left overnight at 4 C or incubated at 37 C for 90 min and then cooled to 4 C.

Separation of bound and free.

1. Count 10 tubes at random for total count.

2. Place rack containing tubes in an ice-water bath.

3. Add 1 ml of dextran-charcoal solution to each assay tube up to the number of tubes that can be accommodated in a single spin of the refrigerated centrifuge available (e.g., 80 to 160 tubes). The addition of charcoal to all tubes should not require more than 5 min.

4. Vortex each tube briefly, incubate 45 min.

5. Centrifuge for 15 min in a refrigerated centrifuge.

6. Decant supernatant fluid and count supernatant fluid or charcoal with appropriate adjustments for geometry if required by the counter. Collect at least 2,000 counts per tube.

7. Plot standard curve. Calculate the T_4 con-

centrations of controls and unknowns using the standard curve.

8. The percent bound of NSB tubes should be ±8%. Recovery of T_4 should be 100 ± 10% in the quality controls. The precision of the assay (intra-assay coefficient of variation) should be <5%, and reproducibility (between-assay coefficient of variation) should be <10% at T_4 concentrations in the normal range.

Comments. Although the directions given above are self-explanatory, some further discussion of the charcoal technique for bound and free separation is necessary. In my experience, different lots of charcoal, even from the same manufacturer, appear to have different binding capacities for labeled T_4. Therefore, it is necessary to determine the appropriate concentration of charcoal for separation of bound and free for each new batch of charcoal purchased. This is readily ascertained by preparing several sets of four tubes each, two 0 standards and two nonspecific binding tubes. These are allowed to incubate overnight, and separation of bound and free is obtained by using serial dilutions of the dextran-charcoal suspension described above. The optimal charcoal concentration is that which results in the widest absolute difference between percent bound in the tubes containing antibody and no antigen and the tubes in which there is no antibody. Binding in the absence of antibody generally should not exceed 7%.

Reagents

T_4 antibody is available from various commercial outlets. I have no personal experience with any of these products, but suitable testing can be readily performed by use of this assay. Alternatively, T_4 antibody can be produced by immunization of rabbits with bovine thyroglobulin. The thyroglobulin is dissolved in 0.15 M sodium chloride at a concentration of 2 mg/ml. This solution is then mixed with an equal volume of complete Freund's adjuvant. A 1-ml amount of the emulsion is injected in 0.1-ml portions into the front toe pads of New Zealand white female rabbits. Subsequently, an additional 1 ml of this emulsion is injected subcutaneously 2 and 4 weeks later. Bleeding of the rabbits is begun 5 to 7 days after the last injection. The titer of T_4 antibody varies between 1:1,000 and 1:40,000 in various animals. The antibody should be tested for cross-reactivity as described previously (10). It is also necessary to compare the T_4 estimates obtained with this antibody and those obtained by a competitive protein-binding displacement assay or a refer-

ence preparation. This is to assure that the antibody does not cross-react with circulating non-T_4 iodocompounds, as apparently has occurred with some antisera (1, 2).

Reagents can be obtained from the following vendors: glycine, Mann Research Laboratories, Becton Dickinson & Co., New York, N.Y.; thyroxine (free acid), Sigma Chemical Co., St. Louis, Mo.; sodium salicylate, Fisher Scientific, Pittsburgh, Pa.; charcoal (Norit A), Fisher Scientific; dextran T-80, Pharmacia, Piscataway, N.J.; thyroglobulin (type 1), Sigma Chemical Co.; bovine serum albumin (Fraction V), Pentex, Miles Laboratories, Kankakee, Ill.; ^{125}I-labeled thyroxine, 70 mCi/mg, Abbott Laboratories, North Chicago, Ill.; Freund's adjuvant, Difco Laboratories, Detroit, Mich.

Interpretation

The mean and normal ranges for serum T_4 in various patients are presented in Table 1. Women receiving oral contraceptives or estrogen therapy, or who are pregnant, have elevated TBG and serum T_4 content and are presented separately, as are results in patients with decreased serum TBG. The lower boundary of the normal range is more easily defined than the upper in that patients with serum T_4 concentrations of less than 5 µg/100 ml due to primary thyroid disease almost universally have an elevation in serum TSH (8).

To interpret the test accurately for clinical purposes, some estimate of the unoccupied TBG binding sites such as a charcoal or resin uptake must be combined with a T_4 determination. By using the combination of these two tests, the following general pattern of interpretation can

TABLE 1. *Normal ranges for serum thyroxine and triiodothyronine concentrations in humans*

Group	Range (and mean)	
	T_4 (µg/100 ml)	T_3 (ng/100 ml)
Euthyroid adults		
TBG[a] normal	5.0–10.2 (7.6)	60–160 (111)
TBG increased	7.0–22 (14)	100–230 (171)
TBG reduced	1.5–5.0 (3.4)	24–100 (64)
Euthyroid infants		
Cord serum	7.5–14.1 (10.9)	16–80 (48)
Age 6 weeks	7.3–13.3 (10.3)	121–204 (163)
Hyperthyroid adults	7.0–>30 (21)	150–>1,000 (478)
Hypothyroid adults	0–5.0 (2.1)	0–140 (48)

[a] Thyroxine-binding globulin.

be made. Elevation of serum T_4 and the resin uptake indicates excess thyroid hormone production. A subnormal serum T_4 associated with a low normal or low charcoal uptake test indicates thyroid hypofunction. The combination of an elevated serum T_4 and reduced charcoal uptake is consistent with elevation in circulating TBG, and a reduction in TBG is associated with decreased serum T_4 and an increased charcoal uptake.

TRIIODOTHYRONINE

The concentration of T_3 in human serum is about 1/70th that of T_4. This is primarily due to the lower binding affinity of plasma thyroid hormone-binding proteins for T_3 than for T_4. Because of these low concentrations, it has only been in the past 5 years that accurate quantitation of serum T_3 has been achieved on a routine basis. The method described below is quite similar to the immunoassay method for T_4 and is a minor modification of my original method (7). Sodium salicylate is added to inhibit binding of labeled and unlabeled T_3 to the serum T_4-binding proteins, thus avoiding the necessity for extraction of thyroid hormones from the serum prior to quantitation. As with the T_4 assay, other laboratories have presented methods which use 8-anilino-1-naphthalene-sulfonic acid, thimerosal, or diphenylhydantoin for this purpose (3, 6, 11, 12). All appear to work equally well, and the results of most methods are similar to those which are reported here. A comparative review of the different techniques available and theoretical aspects of the assay has been published (8).

Clinical indications

Serum T_3 concentrations are almost universally elevated in patients with hyperthyroidism. Some hyperthyroid patients may even have elevated serum T_3 concentrations with a normal serum T_4, a condition sometimes called "T_3-thyrotoxicosis." Therefore, the diagnosis of hyperthyroidism cannot be excluded in a patient without establishing that serum T_3 is normal.

On the other hand, as demonstrated in Table 1, serum T_3 concentrations in patients with hypothyroidism appear to overlap considerably with the lower portion of the normal range. The reasons for the maintenance of serum T_3 concentrations in the normal range in some hypothyroid patients may be related to increases in the T_3 to T_4 ratio of the secreted thyroid hormones under this circumstance or to an increase in the fractional conversion of T_4 to T_3 in the periphery. Whatever the reason, serum T_3 concentrations are a poor discriminator for separating the hypothyroid from the euthyroid patient.

Radioimmunoassay of triiodothyronine

The method for the immunoassay of T_3 presented below is quite similar to that for T_4, and only the differences between the two methods need be emphasized here. As with the T_4 radioimmunoassay, it is critical that a constant amount of serum be present in each tube of the assay, standards and unknowns. Because the concentration of T_3 in human serum is so low, 100 μliters (as opposed to 20 μliters in the T_4 assay) is used. The 1- to 2-day delay in tracer addition also provides greater sensitivity. Because the concentration of protein (10% serum) in this assay is considerably higher than that of the T_4 assay, the charcoal concentration used is greater. The comments regarding optimization of dextran-charcoal concentration described for the immunoassay of T_4 are also applicable to the T_3 immunoassay. Nonspecific binding in the T_3 RIA is generally 8 to 10% with this system. With ^{125}I-labeled T_3 (and T_4), the nonspecific binding will increase slowly with increasing age of the tracer. This is due to the poor adsorption of I by the charcoal under the circumstances of the assay. Nonspecific binding greater than 12% of the total is unacceptable if it represents a significant percentage of the binding in the 0 tubes of the standard curve. With antibody at a 1:150,000 dilution, binding in the 0 tubes is approximately 50% and decreases to approximately 15% in the presence of 300 pg of T_3/tube.

Preparation of solutions.

1. *Glycine-acetate buffer (GAB):* See above, Radioimmunoassay of serum thyroxine.
2. *Assay diluent:* Add 20 mg of bovine serum albumin (fraction V) + 1 g of sodium salicylate/ 100 ml of GAB. Set aside ~5 ml for nonspecific binding (NSB) tubes.
3. *Tracer solution:* Determine number of tubes in the assay (see below). Prepare sufficient tracer solution to allow addition of 0.1 ml/ tube. Add 30,000 to 50,000 counts/min (200 pg or less) of ^{125}I-labeled T_3 per ml of assay diluent.
4. *Antibody solution:* Add anti-T_3 antiserum to assay diluent to yield desired final concentration.
5. *Charcoal-dextran mixture:* Dissolve 0.500 mg of dextran T-80 in 200 ml of GAB. Add 5 g of Norit charcoal and stir for 15 min. Store at 4 C.
6. *T_3-free serum:* May use T_4-free serum or

an alternative method. Obtain 500 ml Australia antigen-free human serum. Add 2,000 counts/min of ^{125}I-labeled T$_3$ per ml. Prepare a 30 × 3 cm column of Amberlite CG-400 resin in distilled water. Apply serum to column and collect all serum after the void volume; count 1 ml of the effluent serum to ascertain that >95% of ^{125}I-labeled T$_3$ is removed.

7. *Standards:* Dissolve L-triiodothyronine (free acid) in 0.04 M NaOH at a concentration of 1 mg/ml. Dilute in 0.04 M NaOH to a final concentration of 20 μg/ml. Determine absorption at 320 nm, and check the concentration using the molar extinction coefficient of 4,658 in the following equation:

$$T_3 \text{ concentration (mg/ml)} = \text{optical density} \\ (1 \text{ cm}) \times 0.1398$$

Add T$_3$ to T$_3$-free serum to make a final concentration of 3 ng/ml. Prepare serial dilutions of this solution with T$_3$-free serum to result in final T$_3$ concentrations of 2, 1.5, 1.0, 0.5, 0.25, 0.125, and 0.06 ng/ml. The T$_3$-free serum serves as a 0 standard. Prepare about 20 ml of each standard serum and store in 0.5-ml amounts along with 3-ml amounts of T$_3$-free serum at −20 C.

8. *Quality control pools:* Obtain about 100 ml of an Australia antigen-free pool of human serum. Using the T$_3$ prepared above, add 30 ng of T$_3$ to one 30-ml amount and 60 ng of T$_3$ to a second. Store in 1-ml portions at −20 C.

Assay procedure.

1. *Standard curve:* Add 0.1 ml of each standard to 75 × 100 mm glass or plastic tubes in duplicate. Also add 0.1 ml in duplicate of the T$_3$-free serum to two tubes for the determination of nonspecific binding (NSB).

2. *Quality control:* Add 100 μliters and 50 μliters of pool and pool + 1 ng of T$_3$/ml to each of two tubes (eight tubes). Add 50 and 25 μliters of pool + 2 ng of T$_3$ to tubes in duplicate. Make the total volume of each tube up to 100 μliters with appropriate quantities of T$_3$-free serum.

3. *Unknowns:* Prepare 100 and 50 μliters of each unknown in duplicate. Make up total serum volume to 100 μliters with T$_3$-free serum.

4. Prepare assay diluent as described. Add 0.8 ml to the two NSB tubes.

5. Prepare antibody solution as described. Add 0.8 ml to all other tubes. Each tube now contains 100 μliters of human serum and 0.8 ml of antibody solution or assay diluent. Store at 4 C.

6. Prepare tracer solution as described. Store at 4 C.

7. After ~24 h, add 0.1 ml of tracer solution to each tube and return to refrigerator.

Separation of bound and free.

1. After a second 24-h period, bound and free ^{125}I-labeled T$_3$ may be separated by addition of the charcoal-dextran mixture in the same way as described for the T$_4$ radioimmunoassay.

2. Calculation, recovery, precision, and reproducibility are the same as for the T$_4$ assay.

3. The assay procedure may be shortened by more rapid addition of tracer (after several hours) and incubation at 37 C for 90 min. Sensitivity will be reduced by about 50%.

Reagents

The sources of the various reagents used in this assay are the same as described for the T$_4$ radioimmunoassay. L-3,5,3'-Triiodothyronine (T$_3$) is obtained as the free acid from Sigma Chemical Co. The T$_3$ antibody can be purchased commercially, but it can also be developed in the laboratory. To accomplish this, it is necessary to synthesize a protein-T$_3$ conjugate. I have used the following modification of the method of Goodfriend et al. (4).

A 20-mg amount of sodium L-3,5,3'-triiodothyronine is dissolved in 0.1 ml of 0.4 M NaOH. Successive 0.1-ml amounts of distilled water are then added to make a total volume of 1 ml. To this is added 20 mg of crystalline bovine serum albumin and 10 μliters of ^{125}I-labeled T$_3$ in 50% propylene glycol for labeling purposes. Then 0.5 ml of a solution containing 400 mg of 1-ethyl-3-(3-dimethyl-amino-propyl)-carbodiimide HCl (Sigma Chemical Co.) is added. After addition of the "ethyl CDI," the solution became cloudy but cleared somewhat on shaking for 30 min, and 3.5 ml of water was added. The material was divided into two portions and dialyzed against distilled water, followed by 0.1 M phosphate buffer, pH 7.4, for 4 to 5 days. Calculations indicated that ~2 mol of T$_3$ was bound per mol of albumin. Although a portion of this material appeared to be insoluble, the entire solution was lyophilized after dialysis against distilled water. At the time of immunization, it was suspended in 0.15 M NaCl at a concentration of 2 mg/ml. The rabbits were immunized by injection of 1 mg in divided portions suspended in 50% Freund's adjuvant on the same schedule as used for the thyroglobulin immunization for production of T$_4$ antibodies. Titers obtained in such animals vary from 1:5,000 to 1:300,000. The testing of antibody for cross-reactivity, particularly against T$_4$, requires addition of large quantities of T$_4$ of high purity. This process is described in greater detail in the original reference (7). The cross-reactivity of the T_3 antibody produced in my laboratory by this method is ~1/1,000 on a weight basis.

Amberlite CG-400 can be obtained from Mallinckrodt, St. Louis, Mo.

Interpretation

The normal range for serum T_3 in euthyroid patients with normal TBG concentrations is 60 to 160 ng/100 ml. As with T_4, the normal range is determined both by thyroid hormone production and metabolism as well as by the binding protein levels. As can be seen in Table 1, if serum TBG is elevated, the normal range is shifted upwards; if it is reduced, comparable changes occur in the normal serum T_3 levels. Elevation of serum T_3 above the normal range is excellent evidence supporting the diagnosis of hyperthyroidism. A normal concentration of T_3 may be helpful in explaining maintenance of a euthyroid status in a patient with a reduction in serum T_4. This occurs not uncommonly in the patient who has been treated with ^{131}I therapy for Graves' disease.

THYROTROPIN

Although techniques for measuring the concentration of TSH in human serum have been available for at least a decade, it has only been recently that their full potential as diagnostic tests for the patient with thyroid dysfunction have been realized. The method for TSH radioimmunoassay is a standard double-antibody technique and has been modified little since its initial development by Odell, Wilbur, and Utiger (13). The major problem in the TSH immunoassay is in the definition of the normal range. The most common purpose of the assay of serum for TSH is to determine whether it is normal or elevated. At present, none of the assay methods appears to be sensitive enough to discriminate readily between normal and subnormal ranges. The problem of definition of the normal range appears to be a technical one. Studies in our own and other laboratories have shown that human serum causes displacement of labeled TSH from the antibody even when TSH is not present in the serum (14). The magnitude of this effect may differ slightly from patient to patient such that the "apparent" TSH in normal patients is quite variable. To obviate this difficulty, we have added a standard quantity of TSH-free serum to the standard curve and to all the unknown tubes. This results in a normal range which is lower than that published by some laboratories but appears to be more specific. Serum TSH concentrations of >2 μU but <5 μU are also likely to be physiologically significant, but they do not appear to be associated with clinical manifestations.

Clinical indications

In primary hypothyroidism, failure of thyroid hormone(s) to inhibit pituitary TSH release results in elevation of serum TSH. The patient may or may not be clinically hypothyroid, depending upon the capacity of the damaged thyroid gland to compensate under the influence of the increased TSH production. As pointed out in the section on T_3, increased T_3 secretion relative to T_4 may be a normal compensatory response for the thyroid gland under these circumstances. The relatively small percentage of patients with hypothyroidism on the basis of pituitary disease or hypothalamic failure can be readily distinguished from those with primary hypothyroidism by virtue of the association of a normal TSH with a subnormal serum T_4 concentration. The TSH assay is also required in the testing of patients for normal pituitary function following thyrotropin-releasing hormone (TRH) administration. The clinical use of this test has been reviewed recently (5).

Radioimmunoassay of thyrotropin

The immunoassay of TSH presented below is derived from the method of Odell, Wilber, and Utiger (13). Human chorionic gonadotropin (HCG) is added to all tubes since human TSH, HCG, and lutenizing hormone (LH) all share a common antigenic subunit—the alpha chain. Therefore, there is some degree of cross-reactivity between these various glycoprotein hormones. Addition of HCG eliminates the possibility that a markedly elevated LH, such as is present in menopausal females, or HCG, such as is present in pregnancy, might lead to an apparent increase in TSH.

For convenience, the immunoassay in my laboratory is usually run over a 5-day period. The assay is prepared on Monday, second antibody is added on Thursday, and the tubes are centrifuged on Friday and counted over the weekend. Various modifications of this schedule can be used with the general rule that the longer the incubation period (up to 2 weeks) the more sensitive will be the assay. Repeat of specimens which are too high for the standard curve with the use of dilutions in TSH-free serum can be performed. However, the clinical indication for this is not frequent. Serum TSH concentrations >60 μU/ml are clearly abnormal and clearly indicative of thyroid pathology. More precise quantitation may be of value in specific instances where effects of treatment are being monitored by use of this parameter. The quality control samples in the assay are necessary to provide month-to-month monitoring of the assay.

Preparation of solutions.

1. *Buffers:* Prepare 0.2 M phosphate buffer (dilute a solution of 2.769 g of NaH_2PO_4/100 ml with a solution containing 2.84 g of Na_2HPO_4/100 ml to obtain pH 7.5). Add 15 ml of 0.2 M sodium phosphate buffer to 285 ml of 0.15 M sodium chloride to make 0.01 M sodium phosphate-0.15 M saline buffer. Also prepare ~10 ml of 0.01 M phosphate-0.15 M saline with 2% bovine serum albumin.

2. *Assay diluent:* 0.01 M PO_4-0.15 M NaCl buffer with 2% normal rabbit serum, 0.02% Merthiolate.

3. *EDTA:* 0.1 M ethylenediaminetetraacetate in assay buffer.

4. *Human chorionic gonadotropin:* Make up solution containing 100 international units/ml in assay diluent.

5. *Standards:* Dissolve 1 ampoule (147 mU) of World Health Organization Standard (purified human TSH 68/38) in 5 ml of 2% bovine serum albumin-phosphosaline buffer. Divide into 1-ml portions and freeze (29.4 mU/ml). The stock solution for the standard curve is 294 μU/ml (a 1:100 dilution of the standard solution). Using assay diluent, prepare the following standards:

		Assay diluent		μU/ml
(1)	2.0 ml of 294 μU/ml standard	+	5.36 ml	= 80
(2)	1.2 ml of (1)	+	0.375 ml	= 60
(3)	0.8 ml of (1)	+	0.80 ml	= 40
(4)	0.8 ml of (3)	+	0.80 ml	20
(5)	0.8 ml of (4)	+	0.80 ml	= 10
(6)	0.8 ml of (5)	+	0.80 ml	= 5
(7)	0.4 ml of (6)	+	0.40 ml	= 2.5
(8)	0.4 ml of (7)	+	0.40 ml	= 1.25
(9)	0	+	2.00 ml	= 0

6. *Antiserum:* Dilute anti-human TSH antiserum to 10 times the desired final dilution in assay diluent.

7. *Tracer TSH:* Dilute commercially available ^{125}I-labeled TSH to 5,000 counts per min per 0.1 ml in assay diluent (specific activity, 70 mCi/mg or greater).

8. *TSH-free serum:* Obtain a pool of Australia antigen-negative serum from patients with active hyperthyroidism.

9. *Quality control pools:* Enrich two samples of a pool of normal Australia antigen-negative serum with standard TSH such that 10 and 30 μU of TSH per ml are added to the endogenous level.

Assay procedure.

Using 11 or 13 × 100 mm tubes, prepare the following.

1. *Standards (in triplicate):*

Solution	Volume (ml)
Standards 1, 2, etc.	0.1
TSH-free serum	0.2
EDTA	0.1
HCG	0.1
Assay diluent	0.3
Antibody	0.1
Tracer TSH	0.1
Total	1.0 ml

Also in triplicate

Standard 1	0.15
TSH-free serum	0.2
EDTA	0.1
HCG	0.1
Assay diluent	0.25
Antibody	0.1
Tracer TSH	0.1
Total	1.0 ml

2. *Nonspecific binding tubes:* Three tubes are prepared as for the standards, substituting 0.2 ml of assay diluent for the standard and the antibody.

3. *Quality controls:*

Pool	0.2	0.1	—	—	—	—
Pool + 10	—	—	0.2	0.1	—	—
Pool + 30	—	—	—	—	0.2	0.1
TSH-free serum	—	0.1	—	0.1	—	0.1
EDTA	0.1	0.1	0.1	0.1	0.1	0.1
HCG	0.1	0.1	0.1	0.1	0.1	0.1
Antibody	0.1	0.1	0.1	0.1	0.1	0.1
Assay diluent	0.4	0.4	0.4	0.4	0.4	0.4
Tracer TSH	0.1	0.1	0.1	0.1	0.1	0.1

4. *Unknowns:*

Unknown serum	0.2
EDTA	0.1
HCG	0.1
Antibody	0.1
Assay diluent	0.4
Tracer TSH	0.1

The tubes are incubated for 1 to 3 days at 4 C.

Separation of bound and free.

Then 50 to 100 μliters of goat anti-rabbit or sheep anti-rabbit gamma globulin antibody is added to all tubes. The quantity used depends on the titer of the antiserum. The tubes are then allowed to incubate overnight at 4 C.

After the second incubation, 1 ml of phosphate-saline buffer is added to all tubes, and they are centrifuged at 2,400 rpm in a refrigerated centrifuge for 40 min.

The supernatant fluid is decanted, and the bound (precipitate) and free (supernatant fluid) are counted. Alternatively, total counts may be obtained and percent bound is determined by counting only the bound fraction.

A standard curve can be plotted in the usual fashion using percent bound or bound/free, and the TSH concentration in the unknowns is determined.

If the quantity of TSH in the 0.2-ml sample exceeds 12 μU (serum concentration >60 μU/ml), the serum can be diluted 1:2, 1:4, etc., with TSH-free serum and precise quantitation is then obtained. It is necessary to have the same concentration of serum in all tubes in the assay. The nonspecific binding should not exceed 5 to 10% of the total. Recovery should be 90 to 110%, and reproducibility and precision should be 10% or less in terms of the coefficient of variation.

Reagents

Antibody to TSH for research purposes can be obtained upon application to the National Pituitary Agency. For routine chemical testing it is necessary to purchase antibody from commercial sources or to produce it in the laboratory. The latter can be performed by the following method. Human TSH is dissolved in 0.01 M phosphate buffer, pH 7.4, and mixed with an equal volume of Freund's adjuvant. Rabbits are immunized every 2 to 3 weeks for three immunizations consisting of 50 μg of TSH per rabbit distributed in 10 sites of 0.1 ml each. The antibody is then harvested as previously described on a twice-weekly basis. Titers of antibody between 1:30,000 and 1:400,000 have been produced in this way.

The remainder of the reagents are obtained from the following suppliers. Human TSH standard is obtained from the World Health Organization, London, England, and is standard 68/38. Human chorionic gonadotropin is APL-chorionic gonadotropin USP, Ayerst Laboratories, Inc., New York, N.Y. (usually available in most hospital pharmacies). EDTA, Merthiolate, and bovine serum albumin can be obtained from most general chemical houses.

Normal rabbit serum is available from Arnel Corp., Brooklyn, N.Y., or Grand Island Biological Co., Grand Island, N.Y. The goat anti-rabbit gamma globulin antiserum can be obtained from Antibodies Inc., Davis, Calif. Human TSH (6 U/mg) is obtained from Calbiochem, San Diego, Calif.

Interpretation

The normal range for TSH is from undetectable levels (usually less than 1 μU/ml with this assay) to 5 μU/ml. About 30% of normal subjects have undetectable quantities of TSH. TSH concentrations greater than this indicate the presence of primary thyroid dysfunction which, from a clinical point of view, probably requires treatment. In evaluation of the patient receiving thyroid hormone replacement therapy, TSH concentration may be used as an indication that adequate serum levels of thyroid hormone have been achieved.

ACKNOWLEDGMENTS

This work was supported by Public Health Service grant AM 18616 from the National Institute of Arthritis, Metabolism, and Digestive Diseases. The author is an Investigator of the Howard Hughes Medical Institute.

LITERATURE CITED

1. Beckers, C., C. Corvette, and M. Thalasso. 1973. Evaluation of serum thyroxine by radioimmunoassay. J. Nucl. Med. 14:317–320.
2. Chopra, I. J. 1972. A radioimmunoassay for measurement of thyroxine in unextracted serum. J. Clin. Endocrinol. 34:938–947.
3. Chopra, I. J., R. S. Ho, and R. Lam. 1972. An improved radioimmunoassay of triiodothyronine in serum: its application to clinical and physiological studies. J. Lab. Clin. Med. 80:729–739.
4. Goodfriend, T. L., L. Levine, and G. D. Fasman. 1964. Antibodies to Bradykinin and angiotensin: a use of carbodiimides in immunology. Science 144:1344–1346.
5. Hershman, J. M. 1974. Clinical application of thyrotropin-releasing hormone. N. Engl. J. Med. 290:886–890.
6. Hufner, M., and R. D. Hesch. 1973. A comparison of different compounds for TBG-blocking used in radioimmunoassay for triiodothyronine. Clin. Chim. Acta 44:101–107.
7. Larsen, P. R. 1972. Direct immunoassay of triiodothyronine in human serum. J. Clin. Invest. 51:1939–1949.
8. Larsen, P. R. 1972. Triiodothyronine: review of recent studies of its physiology and pathophysiology in man. Metabolismo 21:1073–1092.
9. Larsen, P. R. 1975. Tests of thyroid function. Med. Clin. North Am. 59:1063–1074.

10. Larsen, P. R., J. Dockalova, D. Sipula, and F. M. Wu. 1973. Immunoassay of thyroxine in unextracted human serum. J. Clin. Endocrinol. 37:177–182.

11. Lieblich, J., and R. D. Utiger. 1972. Triiodothyronine radioimmunoassay. J. Clin. Invest. 51:157–166.

12. Mitsuma, T., J. Colucci, L. Shenkman, and C. S. Hollander. 1972. Rapid simultaneous radioimmunoassay for triiodothyronine and thyroxine in unextracted serum. Biochem. Biophys. Res. Commun. 46:2107–2113.

13. Odell, W. D., J. F. Wilber, and R. D. Utiger. 1967. Studies of thyrotropin physiology by means of radioimmunoassay. Recent Prog. Horm. Res. 23:47–85.

14. Patel, Y. D., H. G. Burger, and B. Hudson. 1971. Radioimmunoassay of serum thyrotropin. J. Clin. Endocrinol. 33:768–774.

Chapter 27

Plasma Cortisol and Urinary Free Cortisol

GUSTAVO REYNOSO

INTRODUCTION

Clinical laboratory tests for plasma and urinary cortisol are designed to provide an estimate of the rate of secretion of cortisol by the adrenal cortex, with the ultimate goal of establishing whether or not, at the time of the examination, the patient had significant hypo- or hypercorticism. In the context of this chapter, hypercorticism and hypocorticism refer specifically to those functions of the adrenal cortex known to be mediated by cortisol itself. The androgenic or mineralocorticoid functions of the adrenal gland are not considered here.

Methods of estimating cortisol secretion rates include:

1. Direct calculation by *double-isotope derivative* procedures, a complicated, costly, and time-consuming procedure suitable for research purposes but seldom used for clinical diagnosis (1).

2. *Colorimetric methods* based on the Porter-Silber reaction for the dihydroxyacetone side chain of cortisol. This approach, although sensitive, is nonspecific, since the chromogenic reaction used is also given by cortisone, 11-deoxycortisol, and all the tetrahydro derivatives of steroids that share with cortisol the 17-21-dihydroxy-20-keto configuration (13). Because of the limitations and difficulties of measuring plasma cortisol by colorimetric methods, most laboratories still rely on the estimation of cortisol metabolites in the urine as the best approximation to the actual cortisol secretion rate. The popular urinary 17-hydroxy method based on the Porter-Silber reaction described above suffers, in urine, from the same limitations as in plasma. The widely used 17-ketogenic steroid test is, again, indirect and based on the oxidative cleavage of the side chain of the steroid molecule, with the production of 17-keto derivatives, and the subsequent development of the Zimmerman color reaction followed by estimation of the tetrahydro derivatives of cortisol (as well as all other 17-21-dihydroxy-20-keto compounds) as 17-keto steroids (7). Colorimetric methods, as discussed above, are intrinsically nonspecific, are subject to many interferences by contaminants, suffer from erratic recoveries,

and, even under ideal conditions, correlate only poorly with the clinical status of the patient (10).

3. *Fluorometric methods* depend on the development of the specific fluorescence of 11-hydroxycorticoids upon the addition of sulfuric acid to ethanolic solutions of steroids (15). Although less subject to interference by nonspecific chromogens than colorimetric methods, fluorescence methods are still nonspecific. Comparable acid fluorescence under the same analytical conditions is given, for instance, by cholesterol and corticosterone, both of which may be present in ethanolic extracts of plasma (16). Estrogens and spironolactones are known to interfere also, and there are nonsteroid fluorescent substances in the plasma and in the solvents used in the procedure. Drugs such as tetracyclines fluoresce upon the addition of sulfuric acid, etc. All of these steroid and nonsteroid fluorogenes contribute to nonspecific fluorescence and, therefore, to the limited reliability of the method. Procedures based on kinetic fluorescence, a method by which nonspecific is differentiated from specific fluorescence by the faster rate of development of the latter, while improving specificity, introduce problems of excessive variability, especially at the lower range, since readings are taken by extrapolating the time versus fluorescence curve back to zero time (14).

4. *Competitive protein binding and radioimmunoassay* procedures which have become available over the past 10 years offer the clinical laboratory the optimal combination of sensitivity, precision, and accuracy required for reliable estimates of plasma and urinary cortisol in most clinical situations. When the specificity of immunology is combined with the sensitivity of radiochemistry, as is done in radioligand assays, methods can be implemented in the clinical laboratory that bring to the cortisol determinations required for day to day clinical diagnosis the same standards of analytical excellence previously available only in the most specialized research laboratories. In my laboratory, a competitive protein-binding method using human transcortin as macromolecule and [³H]cortisol as radioligand has been routinely

231

in use for over 7 years. The method is described in detail here.

TEST PROCEDURES

Sample collection

Plasma is obtained in heparinized test tubes and centrifuged within 0.5 h. The cortisol in plasma is stable overnight in a refrigerator and indefinitely at freezer temperatures. For routine purposes, plasma cortisols are drawn at exactly 8 A.M. and at exactly 4 P.M. (A discussion on the timing of the samples is given in the section on Clinical Interpretation.) Urine determinations require a 24-h urine sample, collected without preservative but maintained cold at all times. It is important to ascertain the completeness of the urine collection by measuring the creatinine in a well-mixed portion of the urine sample. For mailed-in tests, a 10-ml portion, well mixed, is submitted without preservative in a screw-top, plastic container. A note on the total volume of the 24-h specimen should accompany the requisition.

Plasma cortisol (all determinations are carried out in duplicate)

1. Extraction of cortisol:
   a. Pipette 0.1 ml of unknown plasma and appropriate controls into test tubes containing 3.0 ml of ethanol.
   b. The tubes are mixed on a Vortex mixer for 30 s.
   c. Centrifuge at 2,500 rpm for 10 min.
   d. Transfer the supernatant fluid to another tube.
   e. An additional 3.0 ml of ethanol is added to each tube, and the contents are mixed for 30 s.
   f. Centrifuge again at 2,500 rpm for 10 min.
   g. Pour the supernatant fluid from the second extraction into the appropriate tubes containing the first extraction; Vortex.
   h. Pipette 0.6 ml of ethanol extract into appropriately labeled test tubes (in duplicate).
2. Pipette 0, 0.1, 0.2, 0.3, 0.4, 0.5, and 0.6 ml of the working standard into test tubes (0 to 6 ng). Label two extra tubes "NSB" (nonspecific binding).
3. Extract 1.0 ml of urine containing no cortisol once with 5 ml of petroleum ether and three times with 5 ml of methylene chloride. (Cortisol-free urine is obtained from a normal subject who has been fully suppressed by dexamethazone. See Clinical Interpretation.) The second and third extracts of methylene chloride are mixed, and 0.5 ml of this mixture is added to each standard tube including the NSB tubes.

4. Dry all tubes under N_2 at 45 C.
5. Prepare [³H]cortisol-0.5% plasma (the amount used in my laboratory; the actual amount in each case must be determined from a titration curve; see below) solution by mixing 100 μliters of pooled plasma and 20 μliters of [³H]cortisol with 20 ml of 0.01 M phosphate buffer, pH 7.4.
6. Add 1.0 ml of [³H]cortisol-0.5% plasma to all standard tubes and unknowns; 1.0 ml of [³H]cortisol in buffer containing no plasma is added to the two NSB tubes.
7. Shake the tubes for 1 min at room temperature; then place in a 45 C water bath for 5 min.
8. Remove the tubes from the water bath, shake for 1 min, and incubate for 10 min in an ice-water bath.
9. Add 40 mg of florisil to each tube.
10. Shake the tubes on a shaker (180 strokes per min) in the cold for 7 min.
11. Pipette 0.5 ml of supernatant fluid into counting vials containing 10 ml of liquid scintillation fluid.
12. Pipette 0.5 ml of [³H]cortisol-plasma buffer (step 5) into a counting vial to be used as a "Total."
13. The vials are placed in the liquid scintillation counter and counted for 5 min or 10,000 gross counts.

Calculations. Manual: Determine the disintegrations per minute (dpm) of each vial from the counts and the method of quench correction in use in the laboratory. Plot the percent bound of standards versus the nanograms of standard curve, and multiply the nanograms × 10 to obtain microgram percentage of cortisol. Report the average of the duplicates.

Urinary free cortisol (all determinations are carried out in duplicate)

The urine specimen is first washed with petroleum ether to remove interfering progesterone. Urinary free cortisol is then extracted by use of methylene chloride and measured by competitive protein-binding radioassay.

1. Wash 1 ml of urine with 5 ml of petroleum ether using a Vortex mixer. Centrifuge and aspirate the upper layer.
2. A recovery control is run with each urine. Pipette 1 ml of urine and add 20 μliters of intermediate cortisol standard. Treat this as an unknown. The extract contains 1 ng of added cortisol per 0.5 ml of extract.
3. The urinary-free cortisol is extracted twice with 5 ml of methylene chloride. Vortex 30 s and centrifuge at 2,500 rpm for 3 min.
4. Combine the extracts.
5. Pipette 0.5 ml of the combined extracts into 16 × 100 mm tubes.

6. Prepare an extract of a "0" urine and pipette 0.5 ml into each of 16 tubes.

7. Pipette 0 to 0.6 ml of working cortisol standard into the tubes containing the "0" urine extract. The two remaining tubes are the NSB tubes.

8. Proceed as in steps 4 to 13 of the plasma cortisol procedure.

Calculations. Manual: Plot percent bound versus nanograms of cortisol per tube.

$$\text{ng (from standard curve)} \times 20 \times \text{sample volume in liters} = \mu g/24 \text{ h}$$

REAGENTS

Macromolecules

It is the affinity of the macromolecule for the ligand that ultimately defines the specificity and sensitivity of any radioligand assay. Published methods for plasma and urinary cortisol rely on the use of naturally occurring transcortin, the cortisol-binding globulin (CBG) of plasma, or on the use of antibodies. Methods using nonhuman transcortin have been published (5). Radioimmunoassay methods require the prior preparation of conjugates of cortisol with another macromolecule such as albumin, since steroids are not, by themselves, very antigenic. Once the conjugate has been prepared, it is then purified and injected into an animal. The resulting antiserum will show specificity against the haptene, in this case, cortisol. Radioimmunoassay methods for cortisol have been developed over the past several years. It is likely that they will continue to improve to the point that they can be adapted for general use in clinical laboratories (3).

The method described here uses human transcortin from high-titer pregnancy plasma. Transcortin (CBG) is a glycoprotein with a molecular weight around 50,000 and α_2 mobility on electrophoresis. It has a single steroid-binding site per molecule of protein. The site is not specific for cortisol. Other steroids that bind to the site include progesterone, 17-hydroxyprogesterone, cortisone, corticosterone, and 11-deoxycortisol. Lesser affinities are shown for testosterone and aldosterone. The affinity for the steroids is temperature dependent. At 37 C, for instance, the affinity for progesterone is greater than for cortisol. At 4 C, the greatest affinity shown is for cortisol, a fact that contributes to the specificity of the method described here, since all incubations are carried out at 4 C (2).

To determine the optimal amount of CBG to be used in the assay, one must titrate the plasma or serum to be used as source. Standard quality control sera (Hyland Laboratories, Lederle Laboratories, etc.) often contain high titers of CBG. The lyophilized control serum should be diluted as per instructions before being titrated. The optimal amount is defined as that titer (dilution) of macromolecule that will result in binding of 50% of a trace amount of radioactive cortisol, under the conditions of the assay, and in the absence of nonradioactive cortisol.

The method for constructing a titration curve is described below, and an actual curve from my laboratory is shown in Fig. 1.

1. Prepare a solution of tritiated cortisol in buffer (see below) to contain approximately 40,000 counts/min of [³H]cortisol per ml.

2. Into each of six test tubes, pipette 10.0 ml of [³H]cortisol solution and 10, 20, 40, 50, 75, or 100 μliters of high-titer pregnancy plasma.

3. Pipette 0.2 ml of the nonradioactive cortisol standard solution ("working standard") into each of seven 16 × 100 mm tubes. Label this series "curve B" or "2 μg."

4. To another series of seven 16 × 100 mm tubes, add *no* cold standard. Label this series "curve A" or "0 μg."

5. To all 14 tubes, add 0.5 ml of an extract of urine that contains no cortisol (zero extract; see Test Procedures).

6. Evaporate all 14 tubes to dryness under a stream of nitrogen. Tubes are placed on a water bath at 45 C.

7. To each tube from series A and B (above) is added 1.0 ml of the corresponding solution from step 2, except that the first tube that is labeled "zero" receives 1.0 ml of [³H]cortisol-buffer solution from step 1. (No plasma in this tube.) All the other six tubes in each series are labeled 0.1%, 0.2%, etc., to 1.0%.

8. In all 14 tubes perform the cortisol assay (steps 7 to 13) as described above.

9. Plot percentage of [³H]cortisol bound versus titer of plasma in each tube. Construct a smooth curve by connecting all points in each series.

Interpretation of titration curve. The optimal dilution of CBG to be used in the assay is given by that dilution of plasma that will bind 50% of radioactive cortisol in curve A. In most cases, this dilution of plasma will also show the greatest difference between curves A and B (8). Often, where such is not the case, we have in fact used the dilution that does give the greatest depression between curves, even though this may not be exactly 50% zero binding. Once this decision has been made, the chosen dilution of CBG is used for all standards and all unknowns.

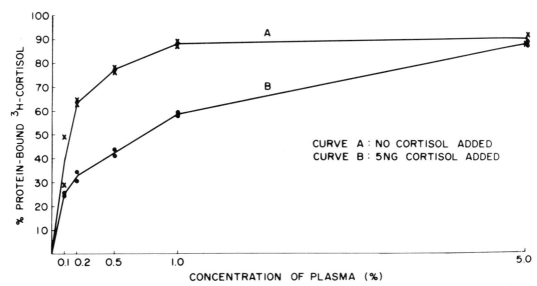

Fig. 1. *Titration curve for the cortisol-binding globulin of plasma. Curve A is in the absence of nonradioactive cortisol. Curve B shows the results when 2 ng of "cold" cortisol is added to each tube. Data on this experiment indicate that a solution of 0.2% plasma would be optimal for the assay.*

Other reagents

Nonradioactive cortisol standards, reagent grade (Schwarz/Mann or Sigma Chemical Co.).

Stock standard: Dissolve 10.0 mg of cortisol in 100 ml of 100% ethanol. Store at −20 C.

Intermediate standard (1 μg/ml): Dilute 1.00 ml of the stock standard to 100 ml with 100% ethanol. Store at −20 C.

Working standard (10 ng/ml): Dilute 1.00 ml of the intermediate standard to 100 ml with 100% ethanol. Store at −20 C.

Ethanol, 100% reagent grade.

Tritiated cortisol, highest specific activity available: Dilute 1 mCi to 20 ml with ethanol; 20 ml of the above will result in the proper quantity of tritiated cortisol per ml. The ethanol solution is kept in a freezer at −20 C. (High specific activity [³H]cortisol is obtained from New England Nuclear Corp., item #NET396.)

Florisil, 60/100 mesh (Sigma Chemical Co.).

Disposable test tubes, 16 × 150 and 16 × 100 mm borosilicate glass only.

Water bath, 45 C.

Shaker, 180 to 240 strokes per min.

Petroleum ether, 30–60 C.B.P., pesticide grade (Fisher or Burdick-Jackson).

Methylene chloride, pesticide quality, or distilled in glass (Fisher or Burdick-Jackson).

Buffer: Dissolve 1.38 g of $NaH_2PO_4 \cdot H_2O$ in 900 ml of distilled water. Adjust pH to 7.4 with NaOH. Dilute to 1 liter and refrigerate.

Scintillation fluid: Scintisol, complete (Isolabs), or Scentiverce (Fisher).

Standardization

A method of standardization based on the logit transformation of the data is shown in Fig. 2. For manual reporting only the upper curve (percent bound versus concentration) is necessary. The logit transformation (lower two figures) is used for quality control purposes. If the data are reduced by a computer, then the logit-log curve is used for actual reporting, since the value of the unknown is calculated from the equation for the regression line of the log of the concentration (standard) over the logit of the bound radioactivity (11).

Sensitivity

Sensitivity will vary from laboratory to laboratory depending on the initial slope of the standard curve and in the ability of the analyst to reproduce B/T (bound radioactivity over total radioactivity) at the lower end of the standard curve, with statistical significance. In my laboratory, 2.0 ng in the final assay mixture can routinely be distinguished from zero (see Fig. 2).

Specificity

As mentioned before, the binding site in CBG is not specific for cortisol. Practically, however, the interferences are few, and can usually be eliminated by differential solvent extraction. In a series of experiments in my laboratory, it was shown that two extractions of urine (or plasma) recover better than 97% of the cortisol. Previous washing of the sample with petroleum ether removes, in two steps, 96% of [³H]progesterone. Another interfering substance, 11-deoxycortisol, can be removed with carbon tetrachloride (90% of 11-[³H]deoxycortisol removed in a single washing). Pharmacologically administered cortisone, on the other hand, cannot be distinguished from cortisol by this method.

Precision and accuracy

The reproducibility of the standard curve in terms of initial B/T, slope, and intercepts is shown in Table 1. Also shown is the accuracy of the method, in terms of the results obtained by serial analysis of a sample of known concentration. The mean difference between replicate analysis in the range of 5 to 40 µg for deciliter (usual clinical range) is 6 ± 4%.

CLINICAL INTERPRETATION

Indications for the test

Measurements of plasma and urinary free cortisol are indicated whenever Cushing syndrome or adrenocortical insufficiency, organic or functional, primary or secondary, is suspected. Because of the well-known circadian rhythm of cortisol secretion, no single determination, either in plasma or in urine, is likely to be of much clinical significance.

It is now well accepted that cortisol is secreted intermittently by the adrenal gland, under similarly episodic stimuli from the pituitary (17). Cortisol secretion is nearly zero between 11 P.M. and midnight. Between 2 A.M. and 8 A.M., there are about six short bursts of cortisol secretion. These bursts of activity result in the highest concentrations of plasma cortisol being found in the blood between 6 and 8 o'clock in the morning. Two more bursts of secretion occur later in the morning or early afternoon, but afterwards the plasma concentration decreases steadily until it reaches the nadir previously described late at night. Steroid hormones other than cortisol are also known to be secreted episodically (12). In order, then, to estimate cortisol secretion rates within the limitations imposed by the episodic nature of the secretion and the correspondingly changing plasma levels, it is necessary to measure the plasma concentration several different times during the day. Although some controversy remains in research circles as to how many points, and at what specific times, are really required, for clinical purposes the contro-

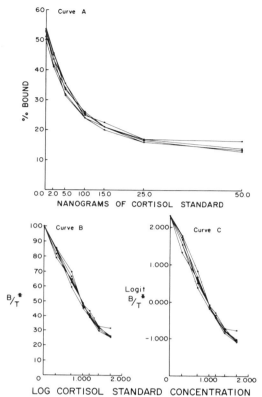

FIG. 2. *Standardization and data reduction method for cortisol competitive binding assay. The upper curve is based on the titration curve from Fig. 1. Unknowns can be calculated from any of the three curves, but for manual methods usually the upper curve is used. The lower two curves are used for quality control purposes or for computer calculation of the data.*

versy is somewhat less. It is generally accepted that two samples, one in the morning between 6 and 8 A.M., to catch the peak level of early secretion, and another late in the afternoon, or evening, are all that is required.

But the plasma levels alone may be misleading, since there are variations in the circadian rhythm from patient to patient, variations that may contribute to alterations in the morning and afternoon levels without significantly altering the overall rate of secretion over the complete 24-h period. Because of this, it is desirable to measure, in addition to the morning and afternoon plasma cortisols, the total urinary free cortisol in a simultaneously collected 24-h urine sample.

Although urinary free cortisol represents less than about 1% of the total cortisol secreted per day, its estimation is important not only for the

Table 1. *Quality control data for the competitive binding assay for cortisol*

Tube	% B/B_o	Slope	90% Intercept	50% Intercept	Control
1	53.33	−1.15	.24	1.63	10.27
2	49.95	−1.22	.27	1.64	12.79
3	53.38	−1.15	.24	1.62	12.0
4	52.59	−1.12	.22	1.57	11.57
5	48.97	−1.18	.24	1.55	8.97
6	51.51	−1.16	.22	1.47	10.93
7	51.06	−1.19	.25	1.57	13.04
8	51.86	−1.20	.25	1.57	12.24
9	48.44	−1.28	.26	1.46	13.8
10	47.30	−1.19	.21	1.34	10.19
11	49.28	−1.21	.26	1.60	10.79
12	49.64	−1.08	.19	1.47	12.78
13	45.28	−1.24	.24	1.43	9.77
Mean	50.71	−1.18	.24	1.53	11.47
Variance	8.310	0.0020	.0005	0.0080	1.940
Standard deviation	2.880	0.0480	.0210	0.0870	1.390
Standard error	0.7700	0.0130	.0060	0.0240	0.3850

[a] The target value for the serum control in the last column is 12 μg.

TABLE 2. *Plasma cortisol and uninary free cortisol in 38 patients with normal adrenal function*

Determination[a]	Plasma cortisol			Urinary free cortisol
	8 A.M. (μg)	4 P.M.		
		(μg)	Percent	
Mean ..	17.0	8.3	49.5	50.4
SD	5.2	2.8	11.8	18.2
SEM ..	0.86	0.46	1.96	3.06
Range .	6.66–27.4	2.7–13.9	25.9–73.1	14.0–86.8

[a] SD = Standard deviation; SEM = standard error of the mean.

reasons given above but also, and just as importantly, because, being "free" cortisol, it correlates rather well with the concentration of the free plasma fraction and, therefore, with cortisol-mediated functions in the target tissues.

The routine that has evolved in clinical laboratories, and that I recommend, consists of measuring, in every patient, the plasma cortisol twice, at 8 A.M. and 4 P.M., and the simultaneously collected total urinary free cortisol. In my laboratory all three determinations are considered a single test.

Normal levels

Values for 8 A.M. and 4 P.M. plasma cortisol and for urinary free cortisol in 38 patients with normal adrenal function recently studied in my laboratory (9) are shown in Table 2. These values agree well with others reported in the liter-

ature (6). In contrast, in 21 patients with signs and symptoms of hypercorticism, the 8 A.M. cortisol ranged from 9.3 to 38.9 μg (mean 24.1), the 4 P.M. cortisol was between 3.8 and 29 (mean 16.8), and the total urinary free cortisol was between 60 and 244 with a mean of 152, or about three times the mean of the normal population.

As can be seen in Table 2, proper differentia-

TABLE 3. *Plasma cortisol and urinary free cortisol in 22 patients with signs and symptoms of hypercorticism*

Group	No. of patients	Percent
A. Increased urinary free cortisol Increased morning cortisol Afternoon cortisol greater than 60% of morning value	6	27
B. Increased urinary free cortisol Normal morning cortisol Afternoon cortisol greater than 60% of morning value	6	27
C. Increased urinary free cortisol Increased morning cortisol Afternoon cortisol less than 60% of morning value	4	19
D. Increased urinary free cortisol Normal morning cortisol Afternoon cortisol less than 60% of morning value	6	27

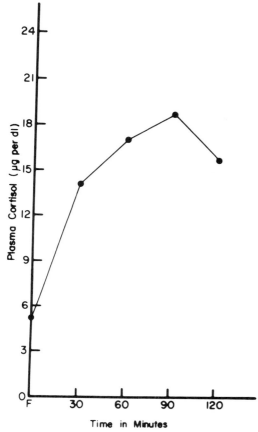

FIG. 3. *Cortrosyn tolerance. Serial determinations of plasma cortisol in a patient originally suspected of adrenal insufficiency. The prompt response following cortrosyn administration indicates normal adrenal glands, although the possibility of centrally mediated hypocorticism remains in this case.*

tion between patients with and without hyper-corticism can be accomplished with the use of these tests. Although overlaps do exist, these are minimal for the urinary fraction. A patient with total urinary free cortisol of less than 100 μg per 24 h is unlikely to have significant hypercorticism. The simultaneously determined plasma values further assist in the differentiation of normal from abnormal, particularly in the diagnosis of early Cushing's syndrome, where the only alteration may be a loss of circadian rhythm with lack of the normal decrease in the afternoon cortisol (4).

Table 3 shows the pattern of distribution of abnormalities in 22 patients with diagnosed hypercorticism. As shown, the full set of abnormalities was seen in only 6 of the 22 patients (group A). In groups B and C, the abnormal

urine test was accompanied by at least one abnormal plasma value. In group D (6 patients), the only initial abnormality was the elevated urine fraction. It is in this last group of patients that functional tests of suppression and stimulation are most important, but in no patient, not even in the apparently obvious ones, should the diagnosis of Cushing's syndrome be established without performing at least some suppression tests.

In the diagnosis of adrenal insufficiency, the overlaps are even greater since normal individuals can and often do have low levels of urinary free cortisol. Again, the diagnosis is established not by any single test but by the pattern of response of the patient to a battery of stimulation and suppression stimuli designed to evaluate whether the potential abnormality is likely to be primarily functional or primarily organic and, further, if organic, whether peripheral (adrenal gland) or central (pituitary gland or hypothalamus, etc.).

An example of a cortrosyn test in a patient with initial diagnosis of adrenal insufficiency is shown in Fig. 3. Examples of other functional tests are shown in Fig. 4 and 5.

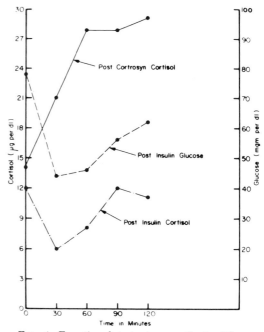

FIG. 4. *Functional tests in a patient with suspected adrenal insufficiency. The post-cortrosyn rise in plasma cortisol indicates normal adrenal gland function. The good response following insulin-induced hypoglycemia is consistent with normal hypothalamic-pituitary response. Addison's disease was ruled out in this case.*

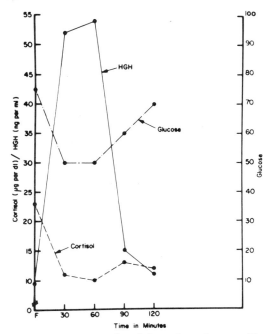

FIG. 5. *Insulin-induced hypoglycemia test. The prompt response by human growth hormone (HGH) indicates normal hypothalamic-pituitary function. Failure of plasma cortisol to increase is consistent with hypoadrenalism of adrenal gland origin (primary cortical disease).*

In appropriate circumstances, such as in the differential diagnosis of adrenal tumors, such suppression and stimulation tests can be performed directly in adrenal vein blood with the aid of adrenal vein catheterization.

It is because of the development of radioligand methods for cortisol, such as the one described in this chapter, with their improved specificity, sensitivity, accuracy, and precision, that stimulation and suppression tests, including tests in adrenal vein blood, are now available in day to day clinical medicine.

ACKNOWLEDGMENTS

Most of the work reported here was carried out in our laboratory of Radiochemistry under the direction of my associate Stanley J. Konopka, and with the technical support of Cheryl Lawrence and Margaret Keane. Their support is gratefully appreciated.

LITERATURE CITED

1. Bietins, I. Z., M. H. Shaw, A. Kowarski, and C. J. Migeon. 1970. Comparison of competitive protein-binding radioassay of cortisol to double isotope dilution and Porter Silber meth-

ods. Steroids 15:765-776.
2. Doe, R. P., and U. S. Seal. 1967. Corticosteroid finding globulin, radioisotopes in medicine, in vitro studies. AEC Symp. Ser. 13:339-350.
3. Farmer, R. W., and C. E. Pierce. 1974. Plasma cortisol determinations: radioimmunoassay and competitive protein-binding compared. Clin. Chem. 20:411-414.
4. Melby, J. C. 1971. Assessment of adrenocortical function. N. Engl. J. Med. 285:735-739.
5. Murphy, B. E. P. 1967. Some studies of the protein-binding of steroids and their application to the routine micro and ultramicro measurement of various steroids in body fluids by competitive protein-binding radioassay. J. Clin. Endocrinol. Metab. 27:973-990.
6. Newsome, H. H., A. S. Clements, and E. J. Borum. 1972. The simultaneous assay of cortisol, corticosterone, 11-deoxycortisol and cortisone in human plasma, J. Clin. Endocrinol. 34:473-482.
7. Norymberski, J. K., R. D. Stubbs, and H. F. West. 1953. Assessment of adrenocortical by assay of 17-ketogenic steroids in urine. Lancet 1:1276-1281.
8. Reynoso, G. 1972. Competitive protein-binding and radioimmunoassay, p. 55-69. American Society of Clinical Pathology, Chicago.
9. Reynoso, G. 1975. Simultaneous determination of plasma cortisol and urinary free cortisol in the evaluation of adrenal function. Radioassay News 2(11):86-87.
10. Reynoso, G., T. M. Chu, O. Holyoke, and G. P. Murphy. 1972. Adrenalectomy and hypophysectomy in advanced prostatic carcinoma. Cancer 29:941-945.
11. Rodbard, D., P. S. Rayford, J. A. Cooper, and G. T. Rosa. 1968. Statistical quality control of radioimmunoassay. J. Clin. Endocrinol. 28:1412-1418.
12. Rosenfeld, R. S., L. Hellman, H. Roffwarg, E. D. Weitzman, D. K. Fukushima, and T. F. Gallagher. 1971. Dehydroisoandrosterone is secreted episodically and synchronously with cortisol by normal man. J. Clin. Endocrinol. 33:87-92.
13. Silber, R. H., and R. D. Busch. 1956. An improved procedure for the determination of hydrocortisone in human plasma. J. Clin. Endocrinol. 16:1333-1336.
14. Stewart, C. P., F. Albert-Recht, and L. M. Osman. 1961. The simultaneous fluorimetric microdetermination of cortisol and corticosterone in plasma. Clin. Chim. Acta 6:696-701.
15. Sweat, M. L. 1954. Sulfuric acid-induced fluorescence of corticosteroids. Anal. Chem. 26:773-776.
16. Sweat, M. L., and R. E. Phillips. 1965. Fluorescence analysis of steroids, p. 289-291. G. K. Turner Associates, Palo Alto, Calif.
17. Weitzman, E. D., D. Fukushima, C. Nogeire, H. Roffwarg, T. F. Gallagher, and L. Hellman. 1971. Twenty-four hour pattern of the episodic secretion of cortisol in normal subjects. J. Clin. Endocrinol. 33:14-22.

Chapter 28

Radioimmunoassay of Estradiol-17β

ROSS MACKENZIE

INTRODUCTION

The most reliable assays for serum estrogens available at present are radioimmunoassays using highly specific antisera. All natural estrogens are steroid hormones containing a phenolic A-ring, and an important implication of this fact is that they may be extracted from acid, neutral, or mildly alkaline aqueous solutions by solvents such as ether. Strong alkalis, however, are capable of extracting the estrogens from the ether phase into the aqueous alkaline phase. The antiserum used in my laboratory was raised in New Zealand white rabbits by use of a conjugate of 6-oxo-estradiol with bovine serum albumin.

The initial efforts at radio receptor assay of plasma estradiol involved the use of the normal sex steroid-binding globulin (SSBG) or uterine cytosol as the macromolecule. Such methods require careful purification of the extracted hormone before assay. The first antisera were raised against estrogens conjugated to protein in the 17 or 3 positions. Such antisera had relatively low specificity, and chromatographic purification of the extracts was required before assay. Later experiments (1, 4) have demonstrated that antisera raised against estrogens conjugated at position 6 (Fig. 1) have good sensitivity and specificity, adequate to permit radioimmunoassay of estradiol-17β without chromatography.

The synthesis of the conjugate is quite complex and expensive, and the original literature should be consulted for details. The first step is the synthesis or purchase of 6-oxo-estradiol. From this, an oxime is prepared and is coupled to bovine serum albumin by carbodiimide condensation. The last reaction is carried out in pyridine which is later removed by dialysis. The lyophilized or frozen conjugate seems quite stable. A 1-mg amount may be injected intramuscularly into rabbits or sheep. My limited experience suggests that one may expect a lifetime supply of serum in a single bleeding from an animal after 6 months. Animals showing no response at 3 months are commonly considered not to be worth the trouble of further injection and are replaced.

Once serum is obtained, it must be checked for specificity and sensitivity. The specificity is measured by testing steroids other than estradiol for their competence to compete with tritiated estradiol-17β for antibody-binding sites. Good examples are available in the literature (1). It is also helpful to assay male sera and pediatric sera to ascertain that these do not give unreasonable results.

The tracer used in the method described is tritiated estradiol, and this involves liquid scintillation counting. There is some evidence (5) that tyramine compounds of estradiol may be labeled by the method of Hunter and Greenwood (3), and the compound thus obtained may be used as a tracer. Such methods may increase the sensitivity of the procedure but, unless tritiated estradiol is also used, there is no correction for extraction efficiency.

REAGENTS

Standard

Stock: Estradiol, 1 mg/100 ml. Dissolve 1 mg in 100 ml of absolute alcohol.

Working: Estradiol, 5 pg/μliter. Dilute 25 μliters of stock standard to 50 ml with alcohol.

Antiserum

The antiserum is diluted so that about 50% of the label is bound in a "zero" standard. This dilution is determined by direct experiment. A suitable diluent is phosphate-buffered saline, pH 7.4.

Anesthetic ether

Anesthetic ether is obtained from freshly opened cans and should be used ice-cold. Ether which has been in contact with air for some time contains peroxide, and such ether is unsuitable for this assay. All precautions must be taken to avoid fire hazard when quite large quantities of ether are used. Naked flame, glowing electrical heating elements, and electric sparks at switches are extremely hazardous. Ether vapor is heavy and rolls off the working surfaces and along the floor. Exercise extreme caution.

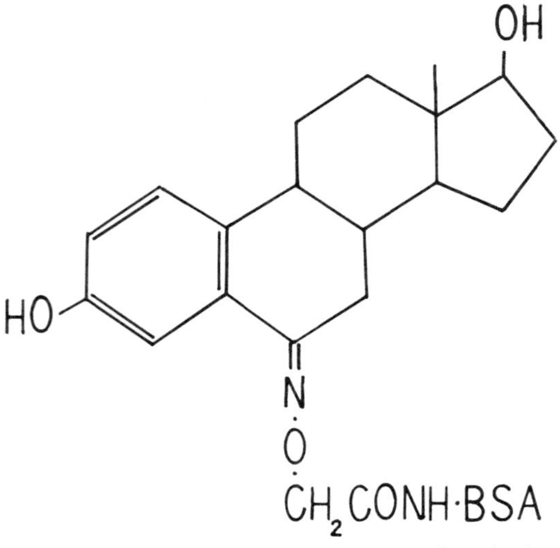

FIG. 1. *6-Oxo-estradiol oxime coupled to bovine serum albumin.*

Boric acid buffer

Concentrated hydrochloric acid is diluted fourfold with water and is then saturated with boric acid crystals.

"Dextran charcoal" 10%

Weigh out 5.0 g of activated charcoal such as Norit A. Mix it with 50 ml of high quality distilled water and centrifuge lightly. Decant the fines and repeat the process until, on centrifugation at the speed used in the assay, the supernatant fluid is crystal clear. After decanting for the last time, make the volume up to 50 ml with phosphate-buffered saline, and add about 60 mg of either dextran-40 or polyvinylpyrrolidone. Mix. This reagent must be stirred constantly during the pipetting process so that sedimentation does not take place in the bulk container. If sedimentation is allowed to occur, the tubes pipetted earlier will contain more charcoal than those pipetted later. The efficacy of the reagent must be checked when the charcoal is purchased by making up the suspension as directed and testing it out on a tube which resembles the highest standard used *except* that it contains phosphate-buffered saline instead of antiserum. Under these conditions, the charcoal should adsorb about 98% of the radioactivity.

Tritiated estradiol

Estradiol-*2,4,6,7-³H* is suitable. Dilute 1 mCi to 100 ml with ethanol. A sample from this stock is diluted suitably each time the assay is run.

TEST PROCEDURES

1. To 5 ml of serum in a 100-ml tube, add about 1,500 counts/min of tritiated estradiol and 5 ml of water.

2. Extract twice with 20 ml of ice-cold anesthesic ether. Agitation may be for 15 min on a tilt-top table.

3. Combine the ethereal extracts and reduce the volume to about 20 ml on a hot-water bath under a hood.

4. Extract the estrogens into 2 ml of 1.0 M NaOH. Remove and save the aqueous phase. Re-extract the ether with another 2 ml of 1.0 M NaOH. Combine the aqueous extracts and discard the ether. On a tilt-top table, 15 min is an adequate extraction time.

5. To the aqueous extract add 1 ml of boric acid buffer. Adjust the pH carefully to 9.0 using a pH meter.

6. Re-extract the estrogens from the aqueous phase with 20 ml of ether. Separate and save the aqueous phase. Repeat the extraction once and combine the ether extracts.

7. Dry the combined extracts and then add 1 ml of absolute ethanol, washing down the walls of the tube with it.

8. Remove 100 μliters and add to scintillation cocktail in a counting vial. This is to determine recovery.

9. Two samples of 400 μliters are taken for assay. These are dried down in plastic tubes with a stream of nitrogen or oil-free air.

10. Standard tubes containing 0, 50, 100, 150, 200, and 250 pg in alcohol are prepared and dried down.

11. To each tube add 500 μliters of dilute antiserum.

12. To each tube add 100 μliters of tritiated estradiol tracer.

13. Incubate for 18 h at 4 C.

14. To each tube add 50 μliters of "dextran charcoal."

15. Mix all tubes by shaking the rack containing them.

16. Centrifuge all tubes in a refrigerated centrifuge at 4 C. Typically, 3,000 rpm for 2 min is adequate.

17. Decant each tube completely into a scintillation vial containing a suitable phosphor.

18. Count each sample until 10,000 counts accumulate and estimate the counts per minute.

19. Plot the counts versus the standard concentration.

20. Compute the concentration of hormone in each unknown tube. Division of this by the recovery factor gives the concentration of estradiol in 2 ml of serum.

21. The results are reported in terms of picograms per milliliter.

A very convenient method (2) of ether extraction is to place the tube containing the two phases in a vertical position in dry ice in a styrofoam container. After 5 min, the ether phase may be decanted into another tube while the aqueous phase remains frozen.

The overall recovery of the method may be expected to be about 60%. When the procedure is carried out on water or on surgically castrated females, the estradiol levels will be found to be indistinguishable from zero.

Normal range

Children under puberty ... <10 pg/ml
Women .... 15–400 pg/ml
Men .... 20–60 pg/ml

CLINICAL INTERPRETATION

Estradiol-17β is the definitive estrogen found in the blood of women of reproductive age. In men, the definitive hormone is testosterone, and the blood of men contains much more testosterone, by a factor of 20 times, as compared with women. Estradiol levels in the sexes show a considerable overlap between the range found in men and the range found in women. This is because the level in women varies during the menstrual cycle. It is low at the beginning and the end of the cycle; in between, it exhibits two peaks, one at midcycle just before rupture of the follicle and another at the midpoint of the luteal phase.

Women who show persistently low estradiol levels accompanied by high levels of follicle-stimulating hormone (FSH) in the blood may be presumed to suffer from primary ovarian failure. Those who have low levels of both estradiol and FSH commonly have a pituitary or hypothalamic cause for amenorrhea. Measurement of estradiol and FSH levels may, therefore, prove useful in the establishment of the endocrine status of women in whom menstruation fails to take place after discontinuation of contraceptive tablets. The role of estradiol measurements in the assessment of postmenopausal women and their requirement for intermittent estrogen therapy is not yet clear, and opinion is divided on this count. If the conflicting views are resolved in the future, estradiol assays may be crucial for rational prevention of osteoporosis as well as the maintenance of normal vaginal structure and function.

LITERATURE CITED

1. den Hollander, F. C., B. K. van Weeman, and G. F. Woods. 1974. Specificities of antisera against estrogens linked to albumin at different positions (C_6, C_{11}, C_{16}, C_{17}). Steroids 23:549–560.
2. England, B. G., G. D. Niswender, and A. R. Midgely. 1974. Radioimmunoassay of estradiol-17β without chromatography. J. Clin. Endocrinol. Metab. 38:42–50.
3. Hunter, W. M., and F. C. Greenwood. 1962. Preparation of iodine-131-labelled human growth hormone of high specific activity. Nature (London) 194:495–496.
4. Jeffcoate, S. L., and J. E. Searle. 1972. Preparation of a specific antiserum to estradiol-17β coupled to protein through the B-ring. Steroids 19:181–192.
5. Lindberg, P., and L. E. Edgrist. 1974. The use of 17β-oestradiol-6 (O-carboxy-methyl) oxime-[^{125}I] tyramine as a tracer for the radioimmunoassay of 17β-oestradiol. Clin. Chim. Acta 53:169–174.

Chapter 29

Quantification of Progesterone by Competitive Protein Binding and Immunological Radioisotope Assays

J. A. DEMETRIOU

INTRODUCTION

Over the past decade, methods for the determination of progesterone have changed from the difficult and time-consuming double isotope derivative (24) and gas chromatography (28) techniques to the relatively easy and rapid competitive protein binding (CPB) assay (5, 6, 11, 15, 17–19, 22, 23, 29) and radioimmunoassay (RIA) method (3, 8, 30). An initial CPB method first described by Murphy (19) was subsequently applied to measure daily progesterone levels during the menstrual cycles of normal women (10, 20).

Since the publication of the simple CPB method (19), numerous modifications have improved accuracy, specificity, sensitivity, precision, and speed. Yoshimi and Lipsett (29) substituted gel filtration for Florisil (19) to separate the free and bound fractions. Sources of binding protein used for the assays have been from women in the last trimester of pregnancy (19), or receiving estrogen and dexamethasone (29). Dog (18, 20) or pregnant guinea pig sera have also been utilized (22). A variety of solvents has been examined to effect the selective extraction of progesterone and to reduce the levels of other cross-reacting steroids (5, 11, 17, 19). Other investigators have used paper (18), thin-layer (11, 15), and Celite-column (25) chromatography to eliminate the interfering steroids.

The CPB (5) and RIA (30) methods selected for presentation are simple, practical, and rapid assays. The CPB method has the advantage of the ready availability of late pregnancy serum, whereas sources of progesterone-specific antisera are rather limited. On the other hand, column chromatographic fractionation of the plasma extract, coupled with the progesterone antiserum, provides a very specific method. However, the chromatographic technique could also be applied in the CPB assay to improve the specificity of this method.

From the standpoint of ease of performance, speed, and expense, the CPB method is the most practical technique for use as a routine laboratory test. Admittedly, the selective sol-vent extraction with nonpolar solvents, such as hexane or petroleum ether, provides a method of qualified specificity, but the clinical validity of progesterone levels with this rapid method in comparison with an added chromatographic step has been demonstrated by Johansson (11).

Two excellent symposia dealing with both competitive protein binding and immunological steroid assays appeared in the past 5 years (7, 21). In addition, a review of analytical methods for progesterone and metabolites deals with both plasma and urinary determinations commonly used in the hospital laboratory (16).

CLINICAL INDICATIONS

Progesterone assays were initially done to establish the blood levels of this hormone during the normal menstrual cycle and the relationship to luteinizing hormone (13, 20). Subsequent measurements of progesterone during the menstrual cycle included other hormones, such as follicle-stimulating hormone (2, 4). Studies on 17α-hydroxyprogesterone (1, 27) and estradiol-17β (1) have provided the basis for the utilization of plasma progesterone levels as an indication of ovulation (9, 13), the diagnoses of inadequate corpus luteum function in women with short luteal phases (26), and the induction of ovulation by injections of human chorionic gonadotropins (12).

Measurements of plasma progesterone levels have been utilized clinically for the investigation of: the occurrence of ovulation, induction of ovulation by therapeutic means, ovulatory and anovulatory dysfunctional bleeding, corpus luteum insufficiency during short luteal phases, problems of fertility, and suppression of progesterone levels during the luteal phase by oral contraceptives.

Single progesterone determinations are generally of little value diagnostically, but presumptive evidence of ovulation has been reported by performing a progesterone assay between 11 and 4 days prior to the onset of menses (9). Levels of 300 ng/100 ml or greater accompanied by a secretory endometrium were considered presumptive evidence of ovulation.

Serial determinations are recommended to afford sufficient data in the assessment of most progesterone-related clinical conditions. However, in some cases 17α-hydroxyprogesterone, luteinizing hormone, follicle-stimulating hormone, or estrogen determinations on the same specimens or at specific times of the menstrual cycle may be required to make a diagnosis. The major advantage of progesterone assays is that one measures the active hormone instead of a metabolite, such as pregnanediol.

TEST PROCEDURES

CPB assay (5)

In duplicate, pipette 0.6 ml of serum or plasma into 15-ml Teflon-stoppered test tubes. Add 10 μliters of 2 N NaOH (with a Hamilton syringe) to each tube, and mix for 2 to 3 s with a Vortex-type mixer. Add 3.0 ml of hexane to each tube, cap tightly, shake for 10 min, and then centrifuge for 2 to 3 min at 1,500 rpm. Transfer 2.5-ml amounts of hexane (or 0.25 ml for pregnant subjects) to 10 × 75 mm disposable glass test tubes. This portion of the test should be completed within 30 min after addition of the sodium hydroxide because of increased variation in values with longer standing times. Ten specimens in duplicate can be processed in this time.

Add 1.5 ml of hexane to 20 test tubes (10 × 75 mm) to be used for the standard curve (hexane prevents adsorption of progesterone to glass during the drying step). Accurately pipette in duplicate 0.00, 0.02, 0.04, 0.06, 0.09, 0.10, 0.20, 0.50, and 1.00 ml of working standard II (10 ng/ml) into the first 18 tubes. Pipette 0.20 ml of working standard I (100 μg/ml) into the last tube. Remove solvent by evaporation under nitrogen in a 45 C water bath.

Add 1.0 ml of ³H-labeled corticosterone–late pregnancy serum to each tube, plus two additional tubes to be used for the total-count tubes. Mix contents of tubes for 5 to 10 s (Vortex-type mixer); incubate all tubes for 5 min in a 45 C water bath and again mix for 5 to 10 s. Place tubes in an ice bath and allow to stand for 10 min. Add 40 mg of Florisil with a measuring spoon to each tube, with the exception of the total-counts tube (Florisil can be added via a specially bored Teflon plug on a separatory funnel). Mix each tube for exactly 30 s on a Vortex-type mixer and immediately return to the ice bath. With an automatic dilution unit (1:10-ml L/I Autodilutor), dispense 0.5 ml of supernatant fluid into counting vials along with 10 ml of liquid scintillation solution. The processing of the specimens should be completed within 30 min after the addition of the Florisil.

The vials containing a biphasic solution are shaken 20 to 30 times and allowed to stand for at least 2 h at 4 C before counting. Samples are counted to a standard error of ± 1%. Counts per minute and nanograms of progesterone are plotted on graph paper, counts per minute on the ordinate and nanograms on the abscissa. A French curve is used to fit the points. Alternatively, logit-log graph paper may be used to give a straight-line plot. Calculation of results is performed with the following equation:

$$\text{reading} \times \frac{1}{R} \times \frac{1}{V} \times 100$$

$$= \text{ng of progesterone/100 ml}$$

where reading = nanograms from curve; R = recovery = 81%; and V = volume (0.5-ml serum volume for normal subjects and 0.05-ml serum volume for pregnant women. The assay is performed on serum or heparinized plasma. Although serum progesterone is stable for several days at room temperature, it is recommended that specimens be stored at 4 or −10 C if the analysis is delayed. Serum is the preferred specimen because fibrin clots in heparinized plasma frequently contribute to the formation of emulsions during ether extraction (25). Serum progesterone levels were also reported to be slightly higher, although not statistically, than for plasma.

Progesterone assays in amniotic fluid, urine, or other body fluids are feasible, but clinical indications for the assessment of hormone levels in these fluids have not been reported.

Control pools consist of progesterone solutions that have been prepared to contain 250, 750, and 1,250 ng/100 ml. To three 500-ml volumetric flasks, individually add 250, 750, and 1,250 μliters of progesterone standard (5 μg/ml) prepared in distilled ethanol. Evaporate alcohol under a nitrogen stream in a 45 C water bath. Add 100 ml of 3% bovine serum albumin in isotonic saline to each flask, mix, and incubate for 10 min at 45 C. Cool and dilute to 500 ml with the albumin solution. Store at 4 C.

Reagents for CPB assay.

Hexane, practical grade 95% (Matheson Coleman and Bell): With this grade of hexane, the recovery of added radioactive progesterone to plasma at a plasma to solvent ratio of 1:5 was 81 ± 3%. No effect on extraction efficiency was observed when many different lots were examined.

Progesterone standard solutions: A stock standard is prepared in ethanol to contain 100 μg/ml. From this stock standard, working standard solutions of 100 ng/ml (I) and 10 ng/ml

(II) are prepared in ethanol monthly. All solutions are stored at 4 C.

[1,2-³H]corticosterone from New England Nuclear Corp. or Amersham-Searle is used as the isotopic tracer. The benzene in the vials is evaporated under a nitrogen stream, and the radioactive steroid is dissolved in redistilled ethanol to give a final concentration of 25 μCi/ml.

Late pregnancy serum: 1.5-ml amounts of pooled serum from women in the last trimester of pregnancy are stored in plastic vials at -10 C.

Protein binding solution, 0.05 μCi/ml: Add 1.0 ml of [³H]corticosterone to a 500-ml volumetric flask and evaporate to dryness under a nitrogen stream. Add 1.0 ml of late pregnancy serum, and incubate with mixing for 5 min at 45 C. Cool the flask and add distilled water to the 500-ml mark; cap, mix by gentle inversion, and again incubate at 45 C for 5 min. This solution is stored at 4 C and is stable for 1 month. The concentration of late pregnancy serum to be used should be established by titration of each new lot.

Florisil (Floridin Co.), 60 to 100 mesh: 100 g is allowed to stand in 10 volumes of distilled water for 1 h. The Florisil is stirred vigorously and allowed to settle for 30 s; the fines are removed by decantation. This procedure is repeated with 10 volumes of water (about 10 times) until the granules clearly settle in 30 s. The washed Florisil is dried in a flat porcelain tray for 24 h in a 100 C oven and then is stored in a tightly capped bottle.

Sodium hydroxide (2 N): Store in a Pyrex bottle.

Liquid scintillation solution: Prepare by dissolving 8 g of BBOT (2,5-bis 2'-(5-tert-butylbenzoxazoyl)-thiophene, Packard Instrument Co.) with 1,980 ml of toluene in a 2-liter volumetric flask. Triton X-100 (Rohm and Haas) is added to bring the volume to 2 liters, and the contents are mixed. This solution is stored in a brown bottle. Counting efficiency for tritium is 46%.

Bovine serum albumin, fraction V: 30% solution from Nutritional Biochemical Corp. A 3% solution is prepared by diluting 1:10 with normal saline solution.

Radioimmunoassay (30)

To 2 ml of plasma or deionized distilled water (method blank), and scintillation vials is added 10 μliters of [³H]progesterone (2,000 dpm, 3 pg) as an internal standard to assess recovery. This volume of plasma is suitable for the assay of specimens for men and women (days 1 to 14 of cycle and postmenopausal). Volume require-

ments are 0.2 and 0.1 ml when specimens are obtained in the luteal phase or from pregnant subjects, respectively. Plasma is extracted twice with 10 ml of diethyl ether by use of a Vortex mixer.

Extracts are transferred to a conical test tube, and the solvents are evaporated under a nitrogen stream at 40 C. Several drops of ether are used to wash the extract to the point of the tube, and the extract is again dried.

If chromatography is to be included, then the dried extract is dissolved in a few drops of benzene-methanol (95:5), colored yellow with a small amount of azobenzene. The extract is transferred to a 7-cm column of Sephadex LH 20, previously equilibrated in benzene-methanol (95:5), in a 23-cm disposable Pasteur pipette. Elution is performed with the same solvent mixture, and the yellow fraction containing progesterone is collected in a tube or vial. The solvent is removed by evaporation under nitrogen.

Sample extracts or the chromatographic fractions are redissolved in 1 ml of acetone. Volumes of 10 μliters (only 1 μliter for pregnant subjects) in triplicate are transferred to 10 × 75 mm disposable glass test tubes, and the solvent is evaporated under a nitrogen stream. The remainder, or a sample of the acetone, is subjected to liquid scintillation counting to correct for recovery.

Progesterone (1 pg/μliter of acetone) is added in triplicate to glass tubes to give a standard curve of 0, 10, 25, 50, 100, 150, and 200 pg. The solvent is evaporated under nitrogen.

To each tube of standards and unknowns, 10 μliters of antiserum is added, Vortex-mixed, and allowed to equilibrate for 30 min at room temperature. After addition of 100 μliters of [³H]progesterone (20,000 dpm, 30 pg), the solutions are Vortex-mixed and equilibrated for a suitable period of time, either 5 min at 37 C followed by 10 min at 4 C or, if convenient, at 4 C overnight. To each tube is added 1 ml of dextran-charcoal (maintained in suspension by a magnetic stirrer and in an ice bath), and the contents are mixed. After standing for exactly 15 min at 4 C, the tubes are centrifuged (15 min, 8 C, 2,000 rpm). The supernatant fluid is carefully decanted into a vial with 10 ml of scintillation fluid, capped, mixed vigorously, and set at 4 C for 1.5 h before counting.

The disintegrations per minute of the standard-curve tubes are plotted on the ordinate and the mass of progesterone is plotted on the abscissa. Using a French curve, draw a curve that best joins the plotted points. The following formula is used to calculate the nanograms of progesterone per 100 ml:

$$S = \left[\frac{T}{\alpha} \times \frac{D\beta}{d} - M\right] \frac{1}{10V}$$

where α is the sample taken for radioimmunoassay and T is the reading from the standard curve in picograms; D is the dpm added for recovery, and d is the dpm in a sample β of the unknown. M is the mass of internal standard, and V is the volume of plasma in milliliters.

Reagents for RIA.

Diethyl ether, benzene, methanol, and acetone are all reagent grade and are redistilled before use.

Sephadex LH-20: Pharmacia, Uppsala, Sweden.

Phosphate-buffered-saline (PBS): 9 g of sodium chloride, 9 g of sodium azide, and 1 g of gelatin are dissolved in 305 ml of 0.2 M disodium hydrogen phosphate and 195 ml of 0.2 M bovine serum albumin (Sigma Chemical Co., St. Louis, Mo.).

Sodium dihydrogen phosphate: After adjusting to pH to 7.0, the solution is diluted to 1 liter with deionized distilled water.

[1,2,6,7-³H]progesterone from New England Nuclear Corp., supplied in benzene, is dried under nitrogen and redissolved in benzene-ethanol, 95:5 (vol/vol), to a concentration of 10 mCi/ml.

[³H]progesterone-PBS: 100 μliters of [³H]progesterone is dried and redissolved in 10 ml of PBS to give a solution containing 20,000 dpm/100 μliters.

Antiserum: Although the authors used an antiserum prepared in their laboratory from 11α-hydroxyprogesterone-bovine serum albumin conjugate, suitable antisera are available from several commercial sources: Endocrine Sciences, Tarzana, Calif.; Nuclear Medical Systems, Newport Beach, Calif.; and others. The dilution of antiserum with buffer to be used in the assay is adjusted to yield approximately 50% binding of the [³H]progesterone in the assay.

Dextran-coated charcoal: Norit A charcoal, repeatedly washed with distilled water to remove fines and dried, is used. To 500 ml of PBS is added 125 mg of Dextran T-70 (Pharmacia) and 1.25 g of charcoal. The solution is stored and used at 4 C. A suspension is maintained in an ice bath with a magnetic stirrer when used for the assay.

Liquid scintillation solution: Prepare by dissolving 6 g of PPO (2,5-diphenyloxazole) in 1 liter of toluene and adding 500 ml of Triton X-100.

INTERPRETATION

The development of rapid and sensitive competitive protein binding and immunological radioisotopic assays for plasma progesterone has afforded techniques for the assessment of gonadol and placental hormonal functions and relationships. Although radioimmunoassays provide greater sensitivity than competitive protein binding methods, especially in the measurement of progesterone levels in children, male subjects, and during the follicular phase of the menstrual cycle, larger amounts of specimen can afford comparable sensitivity with the latter method. Specificity, when measuring increased levels of hormone, can be attained with the use of a highly specific antiserum for progesterone.

Alternatively, selective solvent extraction, hexane or petroleum ether, coupled with a single chromatographic method, can afford specificity with either radioisotopic technique.

The diagnostic value of progesterone levels in male subjects has not been established, but could have application in the diagnosis of steroid-producing tumors or in adrenal hyperplasia. Normally, plasma levels in males are low and comparable to the amount of hormone present in the serum of ovariectomized women or during the follicular phase (Table 1). In general, about twice the level of progesterone in males has been reported with methods that do not utilize chromatographic purification of the serum extract. Approximately 10% interference is due to testosterone (10).

The major use of progesterone assays has been in the establishment of blood levels during normal menstrual cycles and their relationship to follicle stimulating hormone, luteinizing hormone, estradiol, 17-hydroxyprogesterone levels, ovulation, body temperature measurements, and genital tissue morphology. From a study of 20 cycles, Johansson (10) reported an average cycle of 29 ± 2.7 days and a luteal phase of 14 ± 1 day. A significant rise of progesterone level occurred 14 to 16 days from the

TABLE 1. *Plasma progesterone (ng/100 ml) in men*

Method and authors	Mean ± SD
Competitive protein binding	
Yoshimi and Lipsett (29)	33 ± 17
Martin et al. (18)	25 ± 16
Reeves et al. (23)	43 ± 11
Pichon and Milgrom (22)	46 ± 14
Radioimmunoassay	
Furuyama and Nugent (8)	22 ± 10
Abraham et al. (3)	23 ± 6
Youssefnejadian et al. (30)	23 ± 7

TABLE 2. *Plasma progesterone (nanograms/100 ml) in women*

Method and authors	Follicular phase (±SD)	Luteal phase (±SD)
Competitive protein binding		
Johansson (10)	32 ± 25	1,000 – 2,000
Martin et al. (18)	100 ± 20	820 ± 740
Cargille et al. (4)	40 ± 5	940 ± 93
Radioimmunoassay		
Furuyama and Nugent (8)	26 ± 19	828 ± 634
Abraham et al. (1) ..	55 ± 10	856 ± 466
Youssefnejadian et al. (30)	42 ± 19	770 ± 190

onset of menses, with a peak of 1,200 to 1,600 ng/100 ml at 5 to 9 days. Normal values reported for normal follicular and luteal phases are shown in Table 2.

Other investigators have utilized the midcycle peak of luteinizing hormone levels in blood to relate daily variations in progesterone levels (1, 4). An increase in progesterone occurs simultaneously with the luteinizing hormone peak, followed by a sharp elevation in levels over a 3- to 4-day period and then a plateau at levels between 1,000 and 2,000 ng/100 ml. This secondary rise correlated with the formation of a functioning corpus luteum.

Short luteal phases or menstrual cycles of less than 25 days have been reported (11, 26). This condition is characterized by the finding of a normal or low luteinizing hormone peak and levels of 200 to 300 ng/100 ml of progesterone. Strott et al. (26) postulated that this defect was due to low preovulatory follicle-stimulating hormone levels with resulting abnormal follicular development and subsequent inadequate luteinization.

Another application of plasma progesterone determinations has been to establish the occurrence and time of ovulation (9, 13, 31). A rise in luteinizing hormone, accompanied by an increase in progesterone concentration to a level of 100 to 200 ng/100 ml, followed by a rapid decrease in luteinizing hormone, but with a continued increase in progesterone levels, was reported to indicate the formation of a corpus luteum (13, 31). A single determination of serum progesterone at a concentration of 300 ng/100 ml or greater, 11 to 4 days prior to menses, accompanied by a secretory endometrium, was considered to be presumptive evidence of ovulation (9).

Plasma progesterone assays have been of interest in the assessment of initiation and maintenance of pregnancy, fetal well-being, and pathological manifestations of pregnancy. A recent study of progesterone levels in patients with the diagnoses of toxemia of pregnancy, hypertension, fetal growth retardation, diabetes, and Rh-immunization reported no constant changes relative to the clinical condition, and that progesterone values in high-risk pregnancies were inconclusive (14). The limited value of progesterone assays may be due in part to the large intra-individual variations and wide normal range during the latter part of pregnancy.

LITERATURE CITED

1. Abraham, G. E., W. D. O'Dell., R. S. Swerdloff, and K. Hopper. 1972. Simultaneous radioimmunoassay of plasma FSH, LH, progesterone, 17-hydroxyprogesterone and estradiol-17β during the menstrual cycle. J. Clin. Endocrinol. 34:312–318.
2. Abraham, G. E., R. E. Swerdloff, D. Tulchinsky, K. Hopper, and W. D. O'Dell. 1971. Radioimmunoassay of plasma 17-hydroxyprogesterone. J. Clin. Endocrinol. 33:42–46.
3. Abraham, G. E., R. Swerdloff, D. Tulchinsky, and W. D. O'Dell. 1971. Radioimmunoassay of plasma progesterone. J. Clin. Endocrinol. 32:619–624.
4. Cargille, C. M., G. T. Ross, and T. Yoshimi. 1969. Daily variations in plasma follicle stimulating hormone, luteinizing hormone and progesterone in the normal menstrual cycle. J. Clin. Endocrinol. 29:12–19.
5. Demetriou, J. A., and F. G. Austin. 1971. A rapid competitive protein binding assay for plasma progesterone. Clin. Chim. Acta 33:21–32.
6. deSouza, M. L. A., H. O. Williamson, L. O. Moody, and E. Diczfalusy. 1970. Further assessment of the reliability of progesterone assays by competitive protein binding. Acta Endocrinol. 64(Suppl. 147):171–183.
7. Diczfalusy, E. 1970. Steroid assay by protein binding. Karolinski Symposia, 2nd Symposium. Bogtrykkeriet Forum, Copenhagen.
8. Furuyama, S., and C. A. Nugent. 1971. A radioimmunoassay for plasma progesterone. Steroids 17:663–674.
9. Israel, R., D. R. Mishell, Jr., S. C. Stone, I. H. Thornycroft, and D. L. Moyer. 1972. Single luteal phase serum progesterone assay as an indicator of ovulation. Am. J. Obstet. Gynecol. 112:1043–1046.
10. Johansson, E. D. B. 1969. Progesterone levels in peripheral plasma during the luteal phase of the normal human menstrual cycle measured by a rapid competitive protein binding technique. Acta Endocrinol. 61:592–606.
11. Johansson, E. D. B. 1970. A simplified procedure for the assay of progesterone. Acta Endocrinol. 64(Suppl. 147):188–200.

12. Johansson, E. D. B., and C. Gemzell. 1969. The relation between plasma progesterone and total urinary oestrogens following induction of ovulation in women. Acta Endocrinol. 62:89–97.

13. Johansson, E. D. B., and L. Wide. 1969. Periovulatory levels of plasma progesterone and luteinizing hormone in women. Acta Endocrinol. 62:82–88.

14. Lindberg, B. S., B. A. Nilsson, and E. D. B. Johansson. 1974. Plasma progesterone levels in normal and abnormal pregnancies. Acta Obstet. Gynecol. Scand. 53:329–335.

15. Lipsett, M. B., P. Doerr, and J. A. Bermudez. 1970. An improved method for the assay of progesterone by competitive protein binding. Acta Endocrinol. 64(Suppl. 147):155–165.

16. Lucis, O. J. 1974. Progesterone and metabolites, p. 45–78. In A. S. Curry and S. V. Hewett (ed.), Biochemistry of women: methods for clinical investigation. CRC Press, Cleveland, Ohio.

17. Lurie, A. O., and R. J. Patterson. 1970. Progesterone in nonpregnancy plasma: an assay method for the clinical chemistry laboratory. Clin. Chem. 16:856–860.

18. Martin, B. T., B. A. Cooke, and W. P. Black. 1970. Evaluation of a rapid method for the measurement of plasma progesterone by competitive protein binding. J. Endocrinol. 46:369–377.

19. Murphy, B. E. P. 1967. Some studies of the protein binding of steroids and their application to the routine micro and ultramicro measurement of various steroids in body fluids by competitive protein binding radioassay. J. Clin. Endocrinol. 27:973–990.

20. Neill, J. D., E. D. B. Johansson, J. K. Datta, and E. Knobil. 1967. Relationship between the plasma levels of luteinizing hormone and progesterone during the normal menstrual cycle. J. Clin. Endocrinol. 27:1167–1173.

21. Peron, F. G., and B. V. Caldwell (ed.). 1970. Immunological methods in steroid determination. Appleton-Century Crofts, New York.

22. Pichon, M. F., and E. Milgrom. 1973. Competitive protein binding assay of progesterone without chromatography. Steroids 21:335–346.

23. Reeves, B. D., M. L. A. deSouza, I. E. Thompson, and E. Diczfalusy. 1970. An improved method for the assay of progesterone by competitive protein binding. Acta Endocrinol. 63:225–241.

24. Riondel, A., J. F. Tait, S. A. S. Tait, M. Got and, B. Little. 1965. Estimation of progesterone in human peripheral blood using ^{35}S-thiosemicarbazide. J. Clin. Endocrinol. 25:229–242.

25. Stone, S., R. M. Nakamura, D. R. Mishell, Jr., and I. H. Thorneycroft. 1971. A modified technique for the assay of progesterone blood using celite column chromatography. Steroids 17:411–422.

26. Strott, C. A., C. M. Cargille, G. T. Ross, and M. B. Lipsett. 1970. The short luteal phase. J. Clin. Endocrinol. 30:246–251.

27. Strott, C. A., T. Yoshimi, G. T. Ross, and M. B. Lipsett. 1969. Ovarian physiology: relationship between LH and steroidogenesis by the follicle and corpus luteum; effect of HCG. J. Clin. Endocrinol. 29:1157–1167.

28. van der Molen, H. J., and D. Groen. 1965. Determination of progesterone in human peripheral blood using gas-liquid chromatography with electron capture detection. J. Clin. Endocrinol. 25:1625–1639.

29. Yoshimi, T., and M. B. Lipsett. 1968. The measurement of plasma progesterone. Steroids 11:527–540.

30. Youssefnejadian, E., E. Florensa, W. P. Collins, and I. F. Sommerville. 1972. Radioimmunoassay of plasma progesterone. J. Steroid Biochem. 3:893–901.

31. Yussman, M. A., and M. L. Taymor. 1970. Serum levels of follicle stimulating hormone and luteinizing hormone and of plasma progesterone related to ovulation by corpus luteum biopsy. J. Clin. Endocrinol. 30:396–399.

Chapter 30

Routine Analysis of Circulating Testosterone

HOWARD R. NANKIN AND PHILIP TROEN

INTRODUCTION

The most common method for evaluating testosterone production is to measure circulating titers in blood. The procedure includes concentrating and extracting testosterone from serum or plasma. The testosterone is usually purified to remove other structurally similar steroids which may alter assay results. Before extraction, we use saturated ammonium sulfate precipitation of testosterone bound to rather specific serum proteins as a partial purification method to remove other serum steroids which are similar to testosterone but do not bind to these proteins (3, 4, 11). Other laboratories utilize thin-layer chromatography (2) or columns (1) to isolate testosterone after extraction. We prefer ammonium sulfate purification to the other two on the basis of convenience, lower blank, and the ability to process more sera at a time. Some laboratories do not purify the specimens (7). The specificity of the latter types of assays depends on the antibody used. With an antibody which binds only testosterone, no purification would be needed; however, such an antibody has not been reported. With our antibody, testosterone results were the same when purification by ammonium sulfate precipitation was compared with sera further purified by column chromatography (4). For the assay, the purified extracted specimen is incubated with precisely measured amounts of radioactive testosterone and a substance which binds testosterone. Early radioassays utilized the testosterone-binding protein present in high titers in blood drawn from pregnant women. More recently, antibodies to testosterone generated in laboratory animals have become popular. Antibody technique (radioimmunoassay) is more sensitive, more reproducible, and more specific than the protein binding assays. During the incubation, the added radioactive testosterone and the testosterone in the purified extracted specimen compete for binding sites on the antibody. After equilibrium is accomplished, antibody-bound testosterone is separated, and bound radioactivity is measured with an automatic scintillation counter. The proportion of radioactive testosterone bound is

used to calculate the concentration of circulating testosterone by using a standard curve and making appropriate corrections for recovery and the serum volume used. The details are given below.

CLINICAL INDICATIONS

The steroid hormone testosterone produced by the testis causes maleness. The fetal testis produces testosterone by the end of the second month of gestation, and, by the fourth month of gestation, as a result of testosterone, the external genitalia of a male fetus are completed. For the first 12 to 13 years of life, boys have low circulating levels of testosterone, which increase gradually during the period of pubertal development and reach adult concentrations after maturation is complete. Testosterone is responsible for all of the androgenic changes associated with sexual development, including growth spurt, increased muscle mass, increase in penis size, sexual hair, prostatic growth, and deepening of the voice. Some time during the seventh decade, testicular function gradually begins to decrease, and the production of testosterone is reduced. The pituitary gland regulates testis production of testosterone by producing and secreting luteinizing hormone. Luteinizing hormone titers are very low prior to puberty, increase gradually to adult levels after maturation is complete, and become high as testis function changes with advancing age.

There is some testosterone circulating in girls and women. The concentrations are low prepubertally. After puberty, the circulating levels of testosterone increase, but in normal women concentrations are only 7 to 8% of those found in men. If a female fetus, prepubertal girl, or woman is exposed to excessive amounts of testosterone, virilization ranging from hirsutism to frank maleness can occur. If the exposure occurs in utero, the external genitalia can appear masculine.

In adult men 95% of testosterone is produced by the testis, with a small adrenal contribution. In men and women other steroid hormones can be converted to testosterone in the body. In women, about 50% of testosterone originates by peripheral conversion of Δ^4 androstenedione and dehydroepiandrosterone produced by the adrenal and ovary. Some testosterone is directly produced by the latter two endocrine glands, probably as by-products of formation of adrenal hormones and ovarian hormones.

Circulating testosterone is largely bound to proteins. Only a small percentage of circulating male hormone is free and metabolically active. Protein-bound testosterone is proportionally greater in prepubertal boys and girls and in adult women than it is in men. During pregnancy, as a result of high titers of estrogen, testosterone-binding protein is extremely high. In some instances of women with virilization, when the concentration of testosterone is within normal limits, it can be shown that testosterone-binding protein is reduced, thus making more metabolically active testosterone available in the free form to produce the clinical changes. For problems such as this, it is helpful to get an estimate of testosterone-binding protein in the same serum sample used for testosterone determination. In other virilized patients with both normal serum testosterone and testosterone-binding protein, the clinical effects ascribed to increased testosterone are explained by increased metabolic clearance. The latter situation appears to be rare.

Complicating the routine analysis of testosterone are diurnal rhythms in men and in women. The higher testosterone titers occur in early morning in both sexes. In men, titers fall by 30 to 50% by midafternoon. In women the drop is less, approximately 20% by midafternoon. Just preceding and following ovulation, levels tend to be about 10% higher than during other phases of the menstrual cycle. Consequently, it is important to establish normal ranges of testosterone in men and women during a 1- or 2-h time interval and attempt to draw specimens during that period. For example, 7:00 to 9:00 A.M. is convenient for most laboratories.

TEST PROCEDURE

See flow charts (Fig. 1 and 2) and protocol chart (Table 1).

A detailed description of the procedure used in our laboratory follows (4). For details concerning purification of radioactive (tritiated) testosterone, testosterone standard, buffer preparation, dextran/charcoal preparation, complete or partial kits, antibody production and dilution, glassware washing, redistillation of liquids, and equipment, see section on Reagents and equipment.

Assay

Prepare an assay protocol listing patients, volume of serum used, tube numbers, background, and standard curve modeled after the outline provided by Odell, Rayford, and Ross (6). Add 1,000 counts/min, equal to about 2,500 dpm, of tritiated testosterone in 100 μliters of ethanol, to each conical tube and to four scintillation counting vials for total recovery counts added. This will permit a correction for losses during analysis. Place tubes in a vacuum oven (37 C, negative pressure scale set to 26) to evaporate ethanol. Add 10 ml of scintillation fluid (Insta-gel, Packard Instrument Co.) to each vial and store at 4 C until completion of assay. Frozen patient sera are thawed. We use 0.2 ml for men and 0.5 ml for women and children. Each serum is run in duplicate. Samples of serum pools obtained from men and women are run in each assay to quantitate interassay variation and quality control results. Serum is added to dried conical tubes, mixed in a Vortex mixer for 10 s (speed 5), placed in a water bath (32 C) for 1 h, and then kept at 4 C overnight to allow complete equilibration of added tracer. This can probably also be adequately accomplished in 2 h at 32 C. The specimens are now ready for purification.

Add redistilled water to specimens: 1.8 ml to male sera and 4.5 ml to female or children sera. Dilution of serum with water by at least 10:1 is essential to get reproducible purification. Add equal volumes of saturated ammonium sulfate to each conical tube: 2 ml to male sera and 5 ml to female sera. Mix specimens on a Vortex mixer for 10 s at speed 5. Allow conical tubes to sit at 4 C for 10 min (we keep them in a refrigerated centrifuge) and then spin them at 2,000 rpm for 20 min. A white pellet forms on the tube bottom. The supernatnat fluid is aspirated and discarded. Redistilled water is again added to the specimens (1.8 and 4.5 ml for male and female sera, respectively), and the tubes are mixed on a Vortex mixer to dissolve the white pellet, followed by addition of saturated ammonium sulfate solution (2.0 and 5.0 ml, respectively). The specimens are mixed, kept at 4 C for 10 min, and centrifuged at 2,000 rpm for 20 min; the supernatant fluid is again aspirated and discarded. This process precipitates only those steroids bound to the circulating binding protein.

The precipitated mixture is dissolved in 2 ml of 0.1 M NaOH (Hartman-Leddon Co., #1309) and mixed on a Vortex mixer. The alkalinized distilled water retains polar steroids. Thus, estrogens are retained in the water and the androgens are next extracted with 5 ml of a 2:5 (vol/vol) mixture containing benzene (J. T. Baker Co., #9155) and petroleum ether (J. T. Baker Co., #3-9268). Seal conical tubes with Teflon stoppers, put another test tube rack over tube tops, and put on a shaker for 10 min (we use gentle mixing; Fig. 1). Allow tubes to sit upright for a minimum of 20 min and then place in a 0 C freezer for approximately 40 min. The aqueous layer freezes; the organic layer remains a liquid.

At this point, 13 × 100 mm disposable culture tubes (Corning, #99445) are numbered. The organic layer in the conical tubes is next transferred to each corresponding culture tube by pouring off the organic layer, and the culture tubes are placed in a vacuum oven. Evaporation requires 2 to 3 h at 37 C with a vacuum set at 26 units. This is a convenient stopping point, and we leave specimens overnight at room temperature in the vacuum oven set at 10 units of negative pressure.

Scintillation counting vials (Packard Instrument Co.) are numbered for the assay and for the recovery counts, and 10 × 75 mm disposable assay tubes (Kimble, #6605010) are numbered with numbered labels (self-sticking, $1^{1/2}$ × $^{5/8}$ inch; Professional Tape Co.). About 25,000 dpm (or about 10,000 counts/min assuming 40% counting efficiency) of [³H]testosterone, diluted to 100 μliters in ethanol, is added to each assay tube and to four counting vials (to check total assay counts per minute added). Testosterone standard is added to assay tubes 13 to 32; each point is done in duplicate. The testosterone standard is diluted in ethanol so that 1 μliter contains 1 pg. We use the following points: 15, 25, 50, 75, 100, 150, 200, 300, 400, and 500 pg. Four assay tubes, no. 1 to 4, have no antibody and no dextran/charcoal and are used to quantitate total counts transferred to scintillation vials; tubes 5 to 8 have no anti-testosterone antibody but are treated with dextran-coated charcoal and are the hot background tubes to be subtracted from all succeeding tubes; and assay tubes 9 to 12 have *no* standard but the same dilution of specific anti-testosterone serum as utilized in all the other assay tubes. The final four assay tubes are made up in identical fashion to tubes 9 to 12 as a check for pipetting accuracy (Table 1). Then place assay tubes in a 37 C vacuum oven using 26 on the vacuum scale for 240 min or until dry.

The dried culture tubes are taken from the vacuum oven the next morning, and 0.5 ml of 0.1% bovine serum albumin (BSA) buffer is added to each tube. Complete mixing is insured by mixing tubes on a Vortex mixer for 10 s at

1. Add recovery counts (about 1,000 counts/min) to conical tubes and dry.
2. Add serum to tubes and allow to equilibrate overnight at 4 C.
3. Add water and saturated ammonium sulfate twice to tubes.
4. Dilute in 0.1 M NaOH.
5. Extract with benzene/petroleum ether.
6. Transfer organic phase to 13 × 100 mm disposable test tubes and dry.
7. Add 0.5 ml of 0.1% BSA buffer, transfer 0.2 ml to recovery count vial, and transfer 0.2 ml to a 10 × 75 mm tube (step 2 of radioimmunoassay, Fig. 2).
8. Add scintillation fluid to recovery vials and count. This will determine procedural losses of testosterone.

FIG.1. *Flow chart of testosterone purification and extraction.*

TABLE 1. *Radioimmunoassay protocol chart: assay tube contents*[a]

Tubes	Trace (counts/ min of [³H]testosterone)	Buffer (ml)	Antibody (ml)	Standard	Unknowns (ml)
1–4	10,000	1	—	—	—
5–8	10,000	1	—	—	—
9–12	10,000	0.8	0.2	—	—
13–33	10,000	0.8	0.2	Yes	—
33–All unknowns	10,000	0.6	0.2	—	0.2
Final 4	10,000	0.8	0.2	—	—

[a] Add dextran-coated charcoal to tube 5 and all subsequent tubes. Pour contents of tubes 1 to 4 into scintillation vial to assess total counts transferable. Take 1 ml of supernatant fluid (dextran/charcoal binds free testosterone) containing antibody-bound testosterone and add to counting vials (tube 5 to end).

setting 6. Then 0.2 ml from each culture tube is added to the respective counting vial for calculation of recovery, and 0.2 ml is added to the respective dry assay tube. Next, 10 ml of scintillation fluid is added to each of the recovery counting vials. These vials are each counted for 10 min with the vials containing the total recovery counts added, using the appropriate settings for tritium in a liquid scintillation counter. For each patient serum, recovery will be about 15% (range, 10 to 20% usually) of the total recovery counts initially added.

The following reagents are added: (i) to assay tubes 1 to 8, 1 ml of 0.1% BSA buffer, (ii) to assay tubes 9 through 32, 0.8 ml of 0.1% BSA buffer, and (iii) to assay tubes 33 through the last tube, 0.6 ml of 0.1% BSA buffer. To tubes 9 and beyond, add 0.2 ml of antiserum (diluted in

0.1% BSA buffer). We use 0.2 ml of a serum diluted 1:14,000. The final dilution is 1:70,000. Other antibodies may be used at different dilutions. The final four tubes receive no antibody (pipetting check).

The tubes are mixed on a Vortex mixer (setting 4) and incubated overnight at 4 C. In general, the equilibrium reached after overnight incubation at 4 C gives a more precise result, but shorter intervals at higher temperatures have been considered satisfactory for clinical use (10, 11).

The next step is separation of antibody-bound testosterone from free testosterone. Several different techniques are available. We have experience with the double antibody technique and dextran-coated charcoal. The latter method is quicker and more sensitive than the double antibody technique in our experience. Keep the dextran/charcoal solution at 4 C and stir constantly on a magnetic stirrer. Add 1.0 ml of the dextran/charcoal solution to assay tubes 5 onward (not tubes 1 to 4), mix on a Vortex mixer, and place in a refrigerated centrifuge set at 4 C. After 15 min from the addition of dextran/charcoal, spin at 2,500 rpm for 15 min. Take a sample of 1.0 ml of the supernatant fluid from each tube and place in its respective counting vial. Pour contents of assay tubes 1 to 4 (total counts transferred) into respective counting vials. Add scintillation fluid to all vials and mix on a Vortex mixer; count using the same settings as the recovery vials (Fig. 2).

Calculation

Calculation of results includes recovery and unknowns. Counts in recovery vials are compared with the total number of counts origi-

1. Label 10 × 75 mm tubes and add 10,000 counts/min (or about 25,000 dpm) of tritiated testosterone to each tube.
2. Add known amounts of testosterone to standard curve tubes and dry.
3. Add 0.2 ml of testosterone in 0.1% BSA buffer (step 7 of purification and extraction, Fig. 1) to each respective assay tube.
4. Add buffer to all assay tubes; add 0.2 ml of properly diluted antibody to assay tube 9 through the remaining tubes and mix.
5. Allow to incubate.
6. Separate testosterone bound to antibody from free testosterone using dextran-coated charcoal.
7. Take a 1-ml sample of supernatant fluid and add to scintillation vials; add scintillation fluid and count in liquid scintillation counter.

FIG. 2. *Flow chart of testosterone radioimmunoassay.*

nally added to serum unknowns. This count should routinely be at least four times the background count of the scintillation counter for accuracy. Since about 50% of T is precipitated by ammonium sulfate and of the remainder 20% is used for recovery and 20% is used for unknown quantification, the recovery counts usually average 15% (range, 10 to 20%). Procedural loses account for lower recovery.

Counts for all the assay tubes are handled as follows. All counts are expressed as counts per minute. The hot background tubes, 5 to 8, are averaged, and the value is subtracted from each of the other tubes. Then tubes 9 to 12 are averaged to yield the 100% values (B_0). Those tubes, 9 to 12, represent the total number of counts which can be bound by the antibody in the absence of any testosterone. The count bound to antibody (B) for each successive tube is divided by the B_0 average, B/B_0, and the result is expressed as a percent. The standard curve is plotted on logit (log log) paper (9). The vertical (ordinate) is the percent ($B/B_0 \times 100$), and the horizontal (abscissa) is the dose in picograms, increasing dose from left to right and decreasing percent from top to bottom. Logit plot is usually linear between 10 and 90%, and a straight line can be fitted. There may be one or two obviously wrong points (outlyers) per assay, and these points should be revised or discarded. Other methods of assay plotting can be used (arithmetic, Scatchard, etc.). The unknowns are read off the standard curve, multiplied by the reciprocal of the percent recovered (example 100/15), and multiplied by the reciprocal of the volume used to yield result per milliliter (example: 1.0/0.2 for men, 1.0/0.5 for women); if expressed in nanograms per 100 ml, they are multiplied by 100 and divided by 1,000 (or just divide picograms per milliliter by 10) to get nanograms per 100 ml.

We make a further correction in calculating unknown results. Since recovery counts (RC) contribute to the total counts (TC) added for each unknown count (UC), we use the following equation to find the True UC: UC/TC + RC = True UC/TC. Since TC equals about 10,000 counts/min and recovery is usually between 300 and 600 counts/min, without this correction the answer would be a few percent lower (higher counts are recognized as less testosterone in picograms on the standard curve).

We plot each standard curve to characterize the slope and correct for outlyers. The results are calculated by use of a computer program (8). If a computer program does not correct for obviously spurious points, it is necessary to do this in advance.

Quality control

Analysis of a pool of the same serum specimen analyzed in 20 consecutive tubes in the same testosterone assay and calculated as 10 specimens done in duplicate should give an intra-assay coefficient of variation (CV) of less than 10%. The CV is equal to 1 standard deviation/mean. The same serum divided into portions and frozen, and run in duplicate in consecutive assays, should give a CV of less than 18% for interassay precision. Frozen samples from pools of male and female sera are each run in duplicate in every testosterone assay. We keep these values together and constantly update quality control records. If replicate tubes of the same unknown vary by more than 25%, the serum is rerun in a later assay. Another technique to assure that an assay is valid is to add known amounts of testosterone to serum and then analyze the original concentration of testosterone and the concentration in the tubes with added testosterone. For example, 50 pg of testosterone is added to four of eight conical tubes, recovery counts are added to all eight conical tubes, and all the tubes are dried. Then 0.2-ml samples of one male serum are added to all eight conical tubes, mixed, and allowed to equilibrate overnight at 4 C. All eight tubes are then assayed in the same testosterone radioimmunoassay. The four tubes with 50 pg added should average about 50 pg/0.2 ml (45 to 55) more than the four tubes without added testosterone.

When setting up an assay, serum from 10 to 15 normal adult men and 10 to 15 normal adult women should be analyzed for testosterone content. Groups of normal women usually have testosterone averages of 30 to 40 ng/100 ml, and groups of normal men usually average concentrations of 550 to 650 ng/100 ml. See Interpretation section below.

REAGENTS AND EQUIPMENT

Glassware

All glassware used for testosterone analysis is soaked in Coleo (Colgate-Palmolive Co.) for 16 to 24 h. This is followed by a rinse in tap water and then a second soak of 1 N HCl (J. T. Baker Co., #3-9535) for 2 h or longer. Glassware is then rinsed in distilled water, rinsed in redistilled methanol (J. T. Baker Co., absolute methanol, #9070), and air-dried.

Solvents

Distilled water, methanol, and ethanol (Publicker Industries Inc.) are all redistilled in our laboratory.

Tritiated testosterone

High specific activity tritiated testosterone (New England Nuclear Corp., Net 187) is purified by column chromatography. Into a methanol-rinsed, clean 30-ml biuret (30 cm × 1 cm inner diameter) with Teflon stopcock, a glass wool plug is inserted and pressed to the bottom with a glass rod. The biuret is rinsed with methanol. Sephadex LH-20 (Pharmacia) is mixed with methanol for 1 h or longer. The supernatant methanol is decanted from the beaker containing the Sephadex LH-20. Elution solvent is made by mixing chloroform (Fisher, #C-574), n-heptane (Curtis), and ethanol (200:200:2.5). The solvent is saturated with water and shaken in a separatory funnel, and the excess water (on top) is removed. Then two volumes of the elution solvent is added to the beaker containing methanol and Sephadex LH-20. The Sephadex is kept suspended with a magnetic stirrer (Corning #351). Gradually, Sephadex is added to the biuret, allowing the extra solvent to flow out at the bottom. After the packing is complete, the solvent solution (about 200 ml) washes the column continuously for 2 to 3 h. The column will shrink. By use of a disposable microsampling pipette (Corning, #7099-S), 50 μliters (about 50 μCi of tritiated testosterone) is removed and placed in a test tube. The test tube is dried with a vacuum oven (National Appliance Co., #5831), or nitrogen gas can be used. The tube is rinsed with elution solvent, and the testosterone is transferred to the top of the column. The elution solvent reservoir is connected, and the fraction collector (Gilson; many types are available) is started. The fraction collector measures the eluent and adds 98 drops (or 1 ml) to each tube. In this system, testosterone usually comes off between fractions (tubes) 34 and 54. From each of tubes 25 to 61, 1 μliter of eluent is removed, and the radioactivity is counted in a liquid scintillation counter to localize the radioactive testosterone peak. The tubes containing tritiated testosterone are identified. The five tubes at the beginning and end of the peak are discarded, and the eluent in the remaining tubes, comprising the clearly identifiable peak, is pooled. The pooled solution is vacuum-dried and then diluted with 1 ml of ethanol, and a 1-μliter sample is counted. The tube is sealed and stored at 4 C.

Antibody

The antigen required to stimulate antibody production involves linking testosterone to a large protein (BSA, ICN Pharmaceuticals, #10152) at carbon 3, 6, or 7. Commercially prepared antigen can be purchased (Steraloids). A series of immunizations is administered to several animals (usually female New Zealand rabbits), and the resultant antibody is checked for titer and specificity (1–3). It is a cumbersome technique, though worthwhile both financially and for reproducibility, if many samples are to be assayed. Anti-testosterone serum can be purchased (11; Endocrine Sciences), or complete kits can be obtained (BIO-RIA, Serono, Micro-Medic). It has been our practice to produce our own antibody, and we have no experience with purchased antibody or kits.

The titer of antiserum to be used is important. We have adjusted our assay so that 0.2 ml of a 1:14,000 dilution (final tube dilution, 1:70,000) of rabbit antiserum binds about 30% of tritiated testosterone (tubes 9 to 12). Binding more than 50% of label usually gives poorer results since weaker affinity antibodies may be involved in binding testosterone. Varying antiserum concentration also changes the standard curve. Making serum more dilute makes the assay more sensitive and allows lower values to be determined more precisely. Generally, the usable range of the standard curve is reduced. Another factor to be considered is the blank. When we utilized 0.2 ml of 1:60,000 dilution (final dilution, 1:300,000) of anti-testosterone serum, our standard curve was steep and usable between 10 and 100 pg. The blank (ether-extracted serum or distilled water) averaged 4 pg (range, 0 to 10 pg), and often male sera were too high and had to be rerun. Using more concentrated antiserum we have no detectable blank, and the usable standard curve ranges from 15 to 500 pg, reducing greatly reruns of patient sera.

Standard testosterone

Testosterone standard is made in our laboratory by thrice recrystallizing testosterone (Steraloids, A 6950). The technique is listed below:

1. Have ready:
   a. sand bath, turned on, containing beaker of water sitting in it
   b. solvents — dichloromethane (methylene dichloride, CH_2Cl_2, Fisher, #D-123), benzene (J. T. Baker Co.), ethyl acetate ($CH_3COOC_2H_5$, Fisher, #ΔE-130), n-heptane (Curtis), and n-hexane (C_6H_{14}, Fisher, ΔH-301)
   c. disposable pipettes (Pasteur disposable pipettes; Fisher, #13-678-5B) for each solvent
   d. ice
2. Weigh testosterone (10 mg) into a test tube with a conical tip.

3. Dissolve crystals in a minimal amount of dichloromethane (usually 0.1 ml). Do this by adding the dichloromethane dropwise and dipping the test tube into 37 C water.
4. When testosterone is dissolved, add about 3 ml of n-heptane. Place tube on ice. Slow formation of crystals is important. If crystals form immediately, dry all solvents under nitrogen gas and repeat above, adding 0.120 ml of dichloromethane followed by 3 ml of n-heptane. If crystals have not formed after 30 min, gently scratch inside tube with clean disposable pipette and wait 1 h. If crystals do not appear, probably too much dichloromethane was added. Gently dry all solvents under nitrogen gas and repeat, using less dichloromethane.
5. After crystals have formed, centrifuge the test tube.
6. Draw off and discard the supernatant fluid.
7. Gently dry crystals by blowing with nitrogen gas.
8. Dissolve crystals in a minimal amount of benzene (usually 1 ml) in same manner as in step 3.
9. Add about 1 ml of n-heptane. Form crystals in same manner as in step 4.
10. Repeat steps 5 to 7.
11. Dissolve crystals in a minimal amount of ethyl acetate (usually 1 ml) in same manner as in step 3.
12. Add about 1 ml of n-heptane, as in step 3.
13. Repeat steps 5 to 7.
14. Dissolve crystals in a minimal amount of dichloromethane in the same manner as in step 3.
15. Add about 1 ml of n-hexane in the same manner as in step 4.
16. Repeat steps 5 to 7. Weigh crystals and store at 4 C in a desiccator.
17. Samples can be dissolved in ethanol and used as needed.
18. Purity may be checked by thin-layer chromatography or melting-point determination. We routinely compare new testosterone standard with existing standard by comparing curves in three consecutive testosterone radioimmunoassays.

Dextran/charcoal

Charcoal (Norit A, Pfanstiehl Laboratories) and Dextran T-70 (Grade D, Schwarz/Mann, #901803) are mixed, 1 g and 100 mg, respectively, dissolved in 400 ml of PBS (see below), well shaken, and stored at 4 C.

Buffers

Two buffers are used: buffer 1, PBS for dextran/charcoal; and buffer 2, 0.1% BSA buffer for radioimmunoassay.

Buffer 1, PBS (phosphate-buffered saline), consists of: (A) 0.5 M (Fisher, #S-369) monobasic sodium phosphate ($NaH_2 PO_4 \cdot H_2O$), 69 g diluted to 1 liter with sterile redistilled water and stored at 4 C; (B) 0.1 M (Fisher, #S-374) anhydrous dibasic sodium phosphate (Na_2HPO_4), 14.2 g diluted to 1 liter, shaken, and stored at 4 C; and (C) 1.05 M (Fisher, #S-671) sodium chloride (NaCl), 61.425 g, plus Merthiolate (Thimerosal; Lilly), 0.75 g, both added to 1 liter, shaken, and stored as above. For PBS, combine 5 ml of A, 50 ml of B, 100 ml of C, and 595 ml of redistilled water.

Buffer 2, 0.1% BSA buffer (0.1% bovine serum albumin buffer), consists of the following:

(A) Na_2HPO_4, 9.47 g, is added to 1 g of sodium azide (NaN_3; Fisher, #S-227) and diluted with 1 liter of redistilled water

(B) Potassium dihydrogen phosphate (Fisher, #P-382), KH_2PO_4, 9.08 g, plus 1 g of NaN_3 is diluted with 1 liter of redistilled water

(C) Ethylenediaminetetraacetate (EDTA; Fisher, #S-311), 37.2 g, is dissolved in 800 ml of deionized distilled water by mixing with a magnetic stirrer for 1 h. The pH is adjusted to 7.5 to 7.7 with 10 N NaOH, and the mixture is diluted to 1,000 ml with deionized distilled water.

To make 100 ml of buffer for radioimmunoassay, 64 ml of solution A, 16 ml of solution B, and 20 ml of solution C are mixed, and 100 mg of BSA is added. This is 0.1% BSA buffer.

Serum pools

From our routine laboratory extra sera drawn for routine studies are collected. These sera are divided into male and female pools (about 500 ml of each). Portions of the pools are then placed in separate small test tubes (0.5 ml for men, 1.2 ml for women), sealed, and stored at −20 C. Intra- and interassay precision and quality control can be obtained with these serum pools. New serum pools are analyzed in 10 consecutive assays before they are utilized as controls.

Saturated ammonium sulfate

Ammonium sulfate (Fisher, #A 702) stock is made by adding excess crystals to redistilled water to exceed solubility. This can be sealed and stored at 4 C.

Equipment

Refrigerated centrifuge, International Electric Co. (IEC) model PR-6, fitted with IEC #259 head, IEC #384 cups, and IEC #989 adapters for conical tubes. For 10 × 75 mm disposable tubes, IEC #1021 cups can be used. Six cups can be spun at a time, each cup holding 28 disposable culture tubes.

Liquid scintillation counter.

Mechanical shaker (Eberbach #6000) with a carrier top (Eberbach #6040).

Benchtop mixer (Vortex-Genie, Fisher #12-812-VI).

Accurate dispensing pipettes with disposable tips (Biopette #0010-19 for 50, 100, 150, and 200 μliters, and #0010-20 for 0.1 to 1.0 ml, Schwarz/Mann).

Other essential equipment includes 15-ml conical-shaped centrifuge tubes (Fisher #5-538-20A) with Teflon stoppers (Kimble #2402785).

INTERPRETATION

Testosterone has a diurnal rhythm with highest titers in the morning and also is released in episodic fashion, so blood specimens should be obtained during a limited time interval (7:00 to 9:00 A.M. is convenient). For enhanced precision, two or three specimens (either at 30-min intervals or on consecutive days) may be obtained from all patients and controls. If single specimens are utilized, the normal ranges are broader.

For clinical purposes, single specimens suffice; for research, multiple specimens are preferred. Normal ranges should be obtained by use of blood from 10 or more men (clinically normal ages 20 to 50 years with *normal sperm counts*) and 10 or more regularly menstruating women. Older men and menopausal women have lower testosterone titers. The specimens should be analyzed in duplicate over multiple assays. Since interassay precision is less constant than within assay precision, it is wrong to determine the normal ranges for all subsequent testosterone specimens in a single assay.

The normal ranges for testosterone in our laboratory are as follows: men, 300 to 1,000 ng/100 ml with a mean of 645 ng/100 ml; women, 20 to 50 ng/100 ml with a mean of 33 ng/100 ml. Children and menopausal females commonly have testosterone titers below 40 ng/100 ml.

Interpretation of a given testosterone concentration must include the clinical features, gonadotropin titers, and other diagnostic studies. It is always preferable to confirm an abnormal result with additional specimens.

"Low" testosterone titers in a man could mean pituitary or testicular failure. "High" testosterone titers in a virilized woman help in documenting the hormonal abnormality, and testosterone levels can be obtained sequentially to document progression or benefit of therapy. Testosterone titers can be followed during endocrine testing. In men or boys, 4,000 international units of human chorionic gonadotropin daily for 4 days should result in a 100% increase of testosterone in men on day 5, and normal prepubertal and pubertal boys usually have a testosterone titer of more than 250 ng/100 ml on day 5. In boys with clinically *nonpalpable* testes, this test is most useful. If serum testosterone does not increase with four injections of human chorionic gonadotropin, it is safe to assume that such boys have anorchia, and they can be spared an exploratory operation. In virilized women adrenal suppression and ovarian stimulation are done. Sometimes these endocrine studies help localize the major source for the elevated testosterone. During sleep, testosterone titers are normally elevated above daytime concentrations in pubertal boys. Such a finding helps one to reassure a young man and his family that normal maturation is anticipated.

When stimulation, suppression, diurnal rhythm, or night-time sampling studies for testosterone are performed on patients, the same studies should be performed on normal controls. With this information a response in a patient can then be evaluated. Since these studies and assay techniques are complicated and since some variation of results can occur between different laboratories, it is generally not a good practice to utilize criteria and results of other groups to characterize what is normal and abnormal for your laboratory.

LITERATURE CITED

1. Barberia, J. M., and I. H. Thorneycroft. 1974. Simultaneous radioimmunoassay of testosterone and dihydrotestosterone. Steroids 23:757–766.
2. Dufau, M. L., K. J. Catt, T. Tsuruhara, and D. Ryan. 1972. Radioimmunoassay of plasma testosterone. Clin. Chim. Acta 37:109–116.
3. Ismail, A. A. A., G. D. Niswender, and A. R. Midgley, Jr. 1972. Radioimmunoassay of testosterone without chromatography. J. Clin. Endocrinol. Metab. 34:177–184.
4. Nankin, H. R., R. Pinto, D. Fan, and P. Troen. 1975. Daytime titers of testosterone, LH, estrone, estradiol, and testosterone binding protein: acute effects of LH and LH releasing hormone in men. J. Clin. Endocrinol. Metab. 41:271–281.
5. Nieschlag, E., and D. L. Loriaux. 1972. Radioimmunoassay for plasma testosterone. Z. Klin. Chem. Klin. Biochem. 10:164–168.
6. Odell, W. D., P. L. Rayford, and G. T. Ross. 1967. Simplified, partially automated method for radioimmunoassay of human thyroid-stimulating, growth, luteinizing, and follicle stimulating hormones. J. Lab. Clin. Med. 70:973–980.
7. Pirke, K. M. 1973. A comparison of three methods of measuring testosterone in plasma: competitive protein binding, radioimmunoassay without chromatography and radioimmunoassay including thin layer chromatography. Acta Endocrinol. 74:168–176.
8. Rodbard, D., and J. E. Lewald. 1970. Computer analysis of radioligand assays and radioimmunoassay data. Karolinska Symposia, Research Methods in Reproductive Endocrinology, Geneva, March, 1970. Acta Endocrinol. 64:79–103.
9. Rodbard, D., P. L. Rayford, J. Cooper, and G. T. Ross. 1968. Statistical quality control of radioimmunoassays. J. Clin. Endocrinol. Metab. 28:1412–1418.
10. Weinstein, A., H. R. Lindner, A. Friedlander, and S. Bauminger. 1972. Antigenic complexes of steroid hormones formed by coupling to protein through position 7: preparation from Δ^4-3-oxosteroids and characterization of antibodies to testosterone and androstenedione. Steroids 20:789–812.
11. Wong, P-Y., D. E. Wood, and T. Johnson. 1975. Routine radioimmunoassay of plasma testosterone, and results for various endocrine disorders. Clin. Chem. 21:205–210.

Chapter 31

Digoxin Radioimmunoassay

BRUCE S. RABIN

INTRODUCTION

Heart failure is an extremely common disorder of cardiac function which occurs when the heart is no longer capable of delivering an adequate supply of oxygenated blood to the tissue. One of the important causes of heart failure is the inability of heart muscle to contract normally. Digitalis is a pharmacological agent which produces an improvement in the contractility of the heart muscle cells (12). There are several derivatives of digitalis which are used in the clinical management of patients, some of which are effective for short periods of time and others for long periods. The properties of two of the most commonly used oral digitalis preparations are shown in Table 1.

In addition to myocardium, the digitalis preparations affect other tissue. The resultant side effects include anorexia, food aversion, nausea, vomiting, diarrhea, mental confusion, and visual abnormalities. With high concentration of these drugs, toxic effects also occur on myocardial tissue. This toxicity primarily involves interference with the generation of the electrical impulses which initiate contraction of the heart and a blocking effect on the electrical stimulus for myocardial contraction. Without an assay to determine the concentration of the digitalis drug in a patient's serum, one must depend upon signs of clinical toxicity to determine when an adequate but not excessive amount of the drug is being given (10).

CLINICAL INDICATIONS

Digoxin is the most commonly used of the digitalis group of drugs. It may be administered both orally and intravenously. Its effect usually occurs within 1 to 2 h after oral administration, and the maximal effect is seen 6 to 8 h after administration. As it is rapidly eliminated, withholding a dose is a useful means of treating toxicity. However, the concentrations in serum do fluctuate widely because of its rapid elimination.

Digoxin is primarily excreted by the kidney, and the urinary excretion of digoxin decreases as renal impairment increases in severity (2). A decrease in the creatinine clearance very closely parallels a decrease in the clearance of digoxin by the kidney. This is an important consideration in adjusting the concentration of digoxin given to patients with renal disease. An assay for the amount of digoxin present in the serum is exceedingly useful in such patients. Thus, in patients with normal renal function, approximately two-thirds of the digoxin given after 24 h is excreted, whereas patients with severe renal insufficiency may require approximately one-third less of the drug to have the same amount of digoxin present at 24 h. Digoxin retention can only be determined adequately by assays for the amount of digoxin in a patient's serum.

In addition to problems of excreting digoxin, there are also problems of absorbing digoxin. Patients who have malabsorption syndromes do not adequately absorb digoxin when it is administered orally (7). Here again, an assay to determine serum digoxin concentration is a very important part of the management of these patients.

One difficulty in using a drug which is rapidly absorbed and rapidly eliminated is determining at what time after administration of the drug the serum concentration should be assayed, particularly when such concentrations are being used as an indication of drug toxicity. It has been found that within the first 4 h after oral administration of digoxin the serum concentrations fluctuate rapidly and are not reflective of a steady-state situation (13). High serum concentrations may not represent the drug concentration at the myocardium and are therefore not indicative of toxicity (6). The optimal time for determining the serum digoxin concentration is just prior to giving the daily dose. Although samples can be assayed earlier than this, they should not be assayed within the first 6 h after drug administration (13).

TEST PROCEDURES

The radioimmunoassay procedure for determining serum concentrations of digoxin has greatly increased knowledge regarding use of this drug. The radioimmunoassay procedures for serum digoxin are essentially identical to all

TABLE 1. *Properties of digitalis preparations*

Property	Digoxin	Digitoxin
Initial dose	1.0 mg	0.75 mg
Dose needed to obtain therapeutic effect ..	2.5 mg	1.5 mg
Average maintenance dose	0.25 mg	0.1 mg
Percent of adminis-tered dose absorbed from gastrointes-tinal tract	70–80	90–100
Maximal effect after oral administration	6–8 h	8–12 h
Duration of effect ...	1–3 days	4–7 days
Time needed for elimi-nation	3–6 days	12–14 days

Tube no.	Digoxin standard	Digoxin as ng/ ml of serum
5, 6	2 μliters	0.4
7, 8	5 μliters	1.0
9, 10	10 μliters	2.0
11, 12	15 μliters	3.0
13, 14	25 μliters	5.0
15, 16	50 μliters	10.0

other radioimmunoassay procedures. Antiserum to digoxin can be produced by coupling digoxin to a protein carrier. Digoxin can be labeled by tritium (in the 12 alpha position) or by radioactive iodine (3-O-succinyl digoxigenin tyrosine ^{125}I).

There are several commercially available procedures for performing the radioimmunoassay of digoxin. The principal difference between these procedures is the means of separating the bound from the unbound digoxin. A method for performing one such assay is as follows.

Materials

1. Digoxin (^{125}I) radioimmunoassay kit (Schwarz/Mann), containing digoxin standard solution, digoxin derivative (^{125}I), and digoxin antiserum.
2. Normal human plasma which is free from radioactivity and digoxin.
3. Phosphate-buffered saline (PBS) solution, pH 7.4.
4. Dextran-coated charcoal (DCC) stock suspension.
5. DCC working suspension, a 1:10 dilution of stock suspension. Maintain under magnetic stirring during subsequent use.
6. Polystyrene tubes, disposable, 12 × 75 mm.
7. Micropipettes, 2-, 5-, 10-, 15-, 50-μliter capacities.
8. Cornwall syringe with metal holder and tubing adapter.
9. Counting system for gamma radiation.

Preparation of the standard curve

1. Pipette 50 μliters of serum or plasma into 16 numbered tubes. Maintain the tubes at room temperature.
2. Add 1.0 ml of PBS to each tube.
3. Add digoxin standard solution as follows:

(If desired, samples of the digoxin standard solution can be diluted with 30% ethanol so that 10-μliter samples are taken in place of the 2- and 5-μliter samples indicated above. For the 0.4-ng level, dilute 10 μliters of standard with 40 μliters of 30% ethanol; for the 1.0-ng level, dilute 20 μliters of standard with 20 μliters of 30% ethanol. Do not prepare a dilution for these levels that will necessitate an addition to the assay in excess of 10 μliters).

4. Add 10 μliters of digoxin derivative (^{125}I) to tubes 1 to 16. Mix well.
5. Add 10 μliters of digoxin derivative (^{125}I) to 1.5 ml of PBS in each of two polystyrene tubes numbered 17 and 18.
6. Add 10 μliters of digoxin antiserum to tubes 3 to 16.
7. Mix each tube well after each of the above additions. Shake the rack of tubes to mix all reagents thoroughly.
8. Incubate at room temperature for 30 min from the time of the last addition, in step 6.
9. Add 0.5 ml of DCC working suspension to tubes 1 to 16. The reagent is "squirted" into each tube to obtain a uniform suspension of charcoal in the reaction mixture, using a Cornwall syringe and metal holder with tubing adapter.
10. Keep at room temperature for 5 min from the time of the last addition, in step 9.
11. Centrifuge at about 2,500 rpm in the cold (about 4 C) for 20 min or for a time that gives adequate packing of the charcoal.
12. Decant each clear supernatant fluid into a correspondingly numbered polystyrene tube. Maximal transfer is obtained by hitting the rims together. Discard the charcoal residues.
13. Count in the γ counter for 1 to 10 min those tubes into which the supernatant fluids have been decanted.
14. Include in the counting sequence tubes 17 and 18. The counts in these tubes should be 3,000 to 7,000 counts/min; these tubes give the total count per assay.

Clinical assays

1. Add 50 μliters of patient serum or plasma to each of two tubes. Keep the tubes at room temperature.
2. Add 1.0 ml of PBS to each tube.

3. Add 10 μliters of digoxin derivative (^{125}I) to each tube.

4. Add 10 μliters of digoxin antiserum to each tube. Mix well.

5. Incubate at room temperature for 30 min.

6. Add 0.5 ml of DCC working suspension to each tube, as above.

7. Keep at room temperature for 5 min from the time of the last addition, in step 6.

8. Centrifuge at the same speed and for the same time used for the standards.

9. Decant each clear supernatant fluid into a correspondingly numbered plastic tube. Discard the charcoal residues.

10. Count each tube containing the decanted solution for the same period as the standards.

A protocol for the assay of digoxin is shown in Table 2.

Calculations

The "blank," or "background," is the average count found in tubes 1 and 2.

Preparation of the standard curve:

1. The counts found in tubes 3 to 16 are corrected by subtracting the "blank" counts.

2. The average of the counts found in tubes 17 and 18, the total count per assay, is corrected by subtracting the blank counts.

3. Percent bound = $\dfrac{\text{standard count (B1)}}{\text{total count (B2)}} \times 100$.

4. The percent bound for tubes 3 and 4, "trace binding," indicates the binding of digoxin derivative (^{125}I) in the absence of digoxin standards.

5. Plot percent bound against nanograms per milliliter of serum on semilog paper with nanograms per milliliter as the logarithmic function.

Under Clinical assay:

1. The counts found in step 10 are corrected for the "blank" counts, as above.

2. Percent bound = $\dfrac{\text{serum sample count (C1)}}{\text{total count (B2)}} \times 100$.

3. Determine nanograms per milliliter of serum from the standard curve.

The data can be plotted as percent bound versus the log of the standard concentration. This produces a curve that is partially linearized. More complete linearization of the standard curve can be obtained with logitlog paper by plotting each percent bound as a percentage of the trace binding (counts per minute bound in the presence of standard as a percentage of the counts per minute bound in the absence of standard) as a logit function versus concentration as a logarithmic function.

When tritium-labeled rather than iodine-labeled digoxin is used in the assay, there are various factors which can interfere with the test (5). Included among these are hemoglobin released from lysed red blood cells and bilirubin present in the plasma of patients with jaundice. These factors cause quenching of the counts and must be corrected for. With quenching, the energy given off by the beta emitter is partially absorbed by the coloration caused by hemoglobin or bilirubin. Counts are therefore lost to counting by the photomultiplier tube. The observed activity of the isotope is therefore less than its true activity.

When this occurs during the radioimmunoassay for digoxin, the value of digoxin reported becomes elevated. Also, chemiluminescence which may occur with the plasma of uremic patients presents a problem with the tritium assay. No quenching or chemiluminescence problems occur when radioactive iodine is used as the marker. Other problems which occur may affect both types of tests. These involve alteration of the labeled digoxin with aging, the presence of radioactive isotopes in the patients serum (4, 5), and effects induced by different

TABLE 2. *Protocol for radioimmunoassay of digoxin*

Tube no.	Serum (μliters)	Buffer (ml)	Standard (μliters)	^{125}I (μliters)	A$_b$[a] (μliters)	DCC (ml)
1,2	50	1.0	—	10	—	0.5
3,4	50	1.0	—	10	10	0.5
5,6	50	1.0	2	10	10	0.5
7,8	50	1.0	5	10	10	0.5
9,10	50	1.0	10	10	10	0.5
11,12	50	1.0	15	10	10	0.5
13,14	50	1.0	25	10	10	0.5
15,16	50	1.0	50	10	10	0.5
17,18	—	1.5	—	10	—	—
19,20[b]	50	1.0	—	10	10	0.5

[a] Incubate for 30 min at room temperature before adding dextran-coated charcoal (DCC).

[b] Patient sample.

lots of normal serum used in the assay (3).

A newer technique which has proved fairly easy and reproducible utilizes plastic tubes which are coated with the anti-digoxin serum. All incubations are performed in the tube, and the reactions occur on the tube wall. Therefore, no centrifugation is needed. Modifications of this have been introduced by using insoluble glass particles that are coded with the anti-digoxin serum.

REAGENTS

Reagents for the digoxin radioimmunoassay can be purchased from the commercial sources listed below (8). Kits containing either the iodinated or tritium-labeled digoxin are available.

Schwarz/Mann, Orangeburg, N.Y. 10962 (separation by dextran-coated charcoal)

Corning Biologic Products, Medfield, Mass. 02052 (antiserum bound to glass beads)

Clinical Assays Inc., Cambridge, Mass. 02142 (antiserum bound to plastic tube)

Kallestad Laboratories, Chaska, Minn. 55318 (separation by solid phase)

Burroughs-Wellcome, Greenville, N.C. 27834 (separation by double antibody technique)

INTERPRETATION

By using the radioimmunoassay procedure for determining digoxin concentration, ranges of concentration where therapeutic effect is obtained and where toxic effects are produced have been determined. As a general rule, patients with a digoxin concentration below 2.0 ng/ml do not have evidence of toxicity. Concentrations of digoxin greater than 2.7 ng/ml generally do have manifestations of toxicity, and patients with the intermediate concentrations have equivocal toxicity (1, 9–11).

LITERATURE CITED

1. Beller, G. A., T. W. Smith, W. H. Abelmann, E. Haber, and W. B. Hood, Jr. 1971. Digitalis intoxication, a prospective clinical study with serum level correlations. N. Engl. J. Med. 284:989–997.
2. Bloom, P. M., and W. B. Nelp. 1969. The relationship of the excretion of tritiated digoxin to renal function. Am. J. Med. Sci. 251:133–144.
3. Burnett, G. H., R. L. Conklin, G. W. Wasson, and A. A. MacKinney. 1973. Variability of standard curves in radioimmunoassay of plasma digoxin. Clin. Chem. 19:725–726.
4. Butler, V. P. 1971. Digoxin radioimmunoassay. Lancet 1:186.
5. Cerceo, E., and C. A. Elloso. 1972. Factors affecting the radioimmunoassay of digoxin. Clin. Chem. 18:539–543.
6. Doherty, J. E., W. H. Perkins, and W. J. Flanigan. 1967. The distribution and concentration of tritiated digoxin in human tissues. Ann. Intern. Med. 66:116–124.
7. Heizer, W. D., S. E. Goldfinger, T. W. Smith, and E. Haber. 1970. Reduced serum digoxin levels in patients with malabsorption syndromes. Am. J. Cardiol. 25:101.
8. Kubasik, N. P., N. S. Norkus, and H. E. Sine. 1974. Comparison of commercial kits for radioimmunoassay. II. The radioimmunoassay of serum digoxin using iodinated tracer. Clin. Biochem. 1:307–312.
9. Park, H. M., I. Chen, G. T. Manitasas, A. Lowey, and E. L. Saenger. 1972. Clinical evaluation of radioimmunoassay of digoxin. J. Nucl. Med. 14:531–533.
10. Smith, T. W. 1971. Measurement of serum digitalis glycosides, clinical implications. Circulation 43:179–182.
11. Smith, T. W., V. P. Butler, and E. Haber. 1969. Determination of therapeutic and toxic serum digoxin concentrations by radioimmunoassay. N. Engl. J. Med. 281:1212–1216.
12. Smith, T. W., and E. Haber. 1970. Digoxin intoxication: the relationship of clinical presentation to serum digoxin concentration. J. Clin. Invest. 49:2377–2386.
13. Walsh, F. M., and J. Sode. 1975. Significance of non-steady-state serum digoxin concentrations. Am. J. Clin. Pathol. 63:446–456.

Chapter 32

Introduction

ERWIN NETER

With the introduction of modern immunization, sanitation, and chemotherapy, it was assumed that infectious diseases and infestations would be readily controlled. To a significant degree this aim has been accomplished. From a global point of view, however, many of these maladies still exist. In addition, certain infections, such as gonorrhea, are encountered with increasing frequency in countries with a high standard of living. Further, in part because of the very triumphs of medicine, nosocomial and host-conditioned infections play an ever-increasing role. Thus, the subject of the immune response of patients to microbial and parasitic agents continues to be of importance. The extraordinary advances made in the field of immunology have a striking effect on the methodology used for immunological diagnosis and will influence it even more in the future.

In this section experts discuss immune response to a large number of microbial agents. For reasons beyond the control of the Editors it was not possible to include the chapters on the immune response to *Streptococcus pneumoniae* and *Haemophilus influenzae*. In view of the fact that the subjects of syphilis serology, serodiagnosis of fungal diseases, and serodiagnosis of parasitic diseases were competently discussed in the *Manual of Clinical Microbiology*, the authors of these chapters, with the approval of the Editors of both *Manuals*, were invited to up-date their chapters for inclusion in the present volume. This arrangement in no way precludes publication of their chapters in a new edition of the *Manual of Clinical Microbiology*.

Chapter 33

Immune Response to Streptococcal Infection

GEORGE C. KLEIN

INTRODUCTION

Group A beta-hemolytic streptococci produce several intracellular and extracellular antigens which stimulate the production of antibodies by the infected patient. Many of these antibodies can be detected with an appropriate serological test. In most of the serological tests in use at the present time, soluble extracellular antigens are used, and the most familiar of these is streptolysin O, an enzymelike toxin. The following enzymes also serve as useful streptococcal extracellular antigens: deoxyribonuclease B (DNase B), hyaluronidase, nicotinamide adenine dinucleotidase, and streptokinase. One of the few intracellular antigens which has been used is a group A streptococcal polysaccharide sometimes referred to as group A carbohydrate. The serological tests and the antibodies which they detect are antistreptolysin O (ASO), antideoxyribonuclease B (ADN-B), antihyaluronidase (AH), antinicotinamide adenine dinucleotidase (ANAD), antistreptokinase (ASK), and antistreptococcal polysaccharide A (ASPAT).

Space does not permit a description of the procedure for all these tests; therefore, the two most suitable tests from an all-round standpoint have been selected. These are the ASO and ADN-B tests. The ASO test was selected because (i) it has good reproducibility, (ii) the antigen is produced by most strains of group A streptococci, (iii) the antigen is available commercially, and (iv) it is the best known test. The ADN-B test was chosen because (i) it has good reproducibility, (ii) the antigen is produced by most strains of group A streptococci, (iii) it is the test of choice for streptococcal pyoderma and its complications, and (iv) the antigen is available commercially.

Reagents for the AH test are available commercially, and there is good antibody response in skin infection; however, the antibody response in patients with pharyngitis and the reproducibility of the test are not as good. Reagents for the ANAD, ASK, and ASPAT tests are not available commercially. In addition, the ANAD response is not as good as the ADN-B in patients with pyoderma and its complications. The ASK test is not as suitable because anti-body response occurs less frequently and reproducibility is not as good. Procedures have been published for these tests: AH (6), ANAD (9), ASK (2), and ASPAT (4).

ANTISTREPTOLYSIN O TEST

The ASO test is the most popular of the tests mentioned above, and the most frequently used type of ASO test is a neutralization test often referred to as a hemolytic test. The test is based on the ability of reduced streptolysin O to act as a hemolysin and lyse erythrocytes. Thus, the erythrocytes serve as an indicator of whether the hemolytic property of the streptolysin O antigen has been neutralized by being combined with ASO (antibody) or is free to lyse the erythrocytes in the absence of ASO. The test is performed by preparing various dilutions of the patient's serum, adding a constant volume of streptolysin O to each dilution, and then incubating the mixture to allow for combination of antigen and antibody. This is followed by the addition of a constant volume of erythrocytes to the streptolysin O-serum mixture and reincubation. If ASO is present in the serum in sufficient amount, it will combine with the streptolysin O and prevent lysis of the erythrocytes. The end point of Todd's ASO neutralization test was the highest dilution of serum showing no hemolysis (26). This is also the end point of most of the ASO neutralization tests in use at the present time. An end point of 50% hemolysis has been recommended but is not widely used (17). A significant disadvantage of the neutralization test is that substances other than ASO can neutralize the hemolytic property of reduced streptolysin O, resulting in "false-positive" titers. Examples are serum beta-lipoprotein produced in liver disease (5) and products of the growth of certain bacteria, notably *Bacillus cereus* and *Pseudomonas* sp., in serum specimens (18). In addition, the oxidation of streptolysin O from the reduced state eliminates its hemolytic effect on erythrocytes (21), which results in "false-positive" titers. It should be pointed out that, although oxidation of streptolysin O negates its hemolytic ability, it does not interfere with its ability to combine with ASO (7).

Another type of ASO test, used less frequently than the neutralization test, is the particle agglutination test. In this type of test, the streptolysin O is coated onto particles such as latex, treated erythrocytes, or certain bacterial cells. The coated particles are mixed with the patient's diluted serum on a slide. The particles agglutinate in a few minutes if ASO is present in the serum. The reason that erythrocytes can be used as a particle carrier for the streptolysin O in this type of test without being lysed is because the streptolysin O is in the oxidized state and thus nonhemolytic. The chief advantage of this type of test is that serum lipoproteins, bacterial growth products, or oxidized streptolysin O do not cause "false-positive" titers. The Streptozyme test is a well-known particle agglutination test in which erythrocytes are coated with a mixture of unpurified streptococcal extracellular antigens including streptolysin, deoxyribonucleases, nicotinamide adenine dinucleotidase, hyaluronidase, streptokinase, and probably others. It appears to be a good screening test (14) and in time may prove to be of value as a quantitative test, but more work is needed on this aspect. Streptozyme titers cannot be converted into Todd units or ASO titers.

The method recommended by most of the commercial suppliers of ASO reagents in the United States is that of Rantz and Randall (23). This is a neutralization test carried out in tubes. The following serum dilutions are added: 1:12, 1:50, 1:100, 1:125, 1:166, 1:250, 1:333, 1:500, 1:625, 1:833, 1:1,250, and 1:2,500. The chief disadvantage of this method is that the dilution intervals are not equally spaced on a logarithmic scale. The ASO tests which we recommend are described below. These tests use a serum dilution scheme in which the intervals between successive dilutions are equally spaced on a logarithmic scale at 0.15-log intervals (15). This is a metrically and serologically advantageous feature not found in the Rantz-Randall dilution scheme. These tests also differ from the Rantz-Randall test in that the diluent used is a barbital-buffered saline solution (pH 7.2) containing 0.1% gelatin. The gelatin retards spontaneous lysis of the erythrocytes and acts as an enzyme stabilizer for the streptolysin O (A. Gillen and H. A. Feldman, Fed. Proc. 13:494, 1954).

The microtitration test has the following advantages over the tube test: (i) smaller amounts of serum and reagents required, (ii) more tests performed per man hour, and (iii) lower cost per test. Reproducibility of the microtitration ASO test in our laboratory was 98.1% (13).

Clinical indications

An elevated ASO titer usually indicates a recent infection with group A beta-hemolytic streptococcus and as such can be an aid to the physician in the diagnosis of acute rheumatic fever and acute glomerulonephritis.

In patients with acute rheumatic fever, streptococcal antibody tests are, in general, a more reliable indicator of recent streptococcal infection than throat cultures (31). This is because by the time that acute rheumatic fever is suspected the streptococci may have been eliminated by antibiotic therapy, or even without antibiotics they may be so few in number that they do not show up on routine culture.

The ASO test is not as useful as the ADN-B or AH tests in suspected cases of acute glomerulonephritis, if the disease is a sequela of streptococcal pyoderma rather than pharyngitis. This is because very low levels of ASO are produced in streptococcal skin infections (8).

The advantage of the ASO test is that it has been the most widely used of the streptococcal antibody tests and thus is the most familiar. Some pitfalls of the ASO test are (i) the low titers associated with skin infection and their sequelae, (ii) "false-positive" titers associated with liver disease, (iii) "false-positive" titers caused by the growth of certain bacteria in the serum specimen, and (iv) "false-positive" titers caused by oxidation of the streptolysin reagent.

Antistreptolysin O microtitration test

Materials.

1. Microtitration equipment: 0.025- and 0.05-ml calibrated dropper pipettes; 0.05-ml microdiluters; disposable U plates; test reading mirror.
2. Vibrator mixer (paper jogger).
3. Serological pipettes (0.2, 1, 2, and 5 ml) and long-tip measuring pipettes (0.2 or 0.5 ml).
4. Test tubes (13 × 100 mm) and supports (racks), 15-ml conical centrifuge tube.
5. Buffered diluent, streptolysin O, cold distilled water, erythrocyte suspension, reference (control) serum of known titer.

Procedure.

1. Initial serum dilutions of 1:10, 1:60, and 1:85 are prepared in test tubes, and subsequent dilutions are carried out in U plates. Label tubes with specimen number and dilution.
2. Mix the sera and prepare a 1:10 dilution of each by adding 0.1 ml of serum (with a 0.2-ml pipette) to 0.9 ml of diluent. Mix thoroughly.
3. Prepare a 1:60 dilution by adding 0.2 ml of

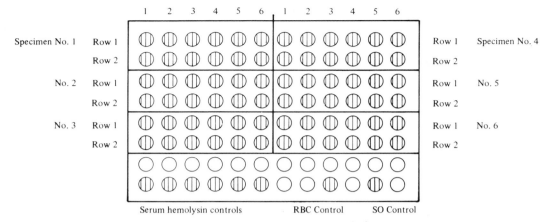

FIG. 1. *Antistreptolysin O microtitration U plate setup.*

the 1:10 dilution of serum to 1.0 ml of diluent. Mix thoroughly.

4. Prepare a 1:85 dilution by adding 0.2 ml of the 1:10 dilution of serum to 1.5 ml of diluent. Mix thoroughly.

5. Mark off disposable U plates into sections so that each specimen is assigned two rows (1:60 row and 1:85 row) with six wells per row. Include two rows for a reference (control) serum in each run (not each plate). Label six wells on the bottom row of each plate as serum hemolysin controls. Label a well for the streptolysin O control and a well for the erythrocyte control on the bottom row of one of the plates in each run (not each plate). See Fig. 1.

6. Use a calibrated pipette dropper to add 0.05 ml of diluent to the second through sixth well of each row assigned to the specimens and reference serum. Add diluent to the control wells as follows: 0.025 ml to the serum hemolysin control, 0.05 ml to the streptolysin control, and 0.075 ml to the erythrocyte control.

7. Add 0.1 ml of the 1:60 serum dilution to the first well of the first row and 0.1 ml of the 1:85 serum dilution to the first well of the second row. Also add 0.05 ml of the 1:60 serum dilution to the serum hemolysin control well. Use long-tip measuring pipettes to add the initial serum dilutions to the U plate wells.

8. Dilute each row by the microdilution technique using the 0.05-ml microdiluters. For each specimen, the serum dilutions in the first row are 1:60, 1:120, 1:240, 1:480, 1:960, and 1:1,920, and in the second row, 1:85, 1:170, 1:340, 1:680, 1:1,360 and 1:2,720. The intervals between dilutions are evenly spaced at 0.15 log.

9. Rehydrate the streptolysin O immediately before use with cold (2 to 6 C) distilled water. Stopper and let stand for a few seconds to dissolve. Mix end over end gently to avoid aera-

tion. *Caution:* Extended agitation may cause oxidation and inactivation of the streptolysin O. Keep the streptolysin cold during use by placing the vial in a beaker of ice water. Use the streptolysin within 20 min after rehydration.

10. Add 0.025 ml of streptolysin O with a calibrated pipette dropper to all wells except the hemolysin and the erythrocyte control wells.

11. Place the plates on a vibrator and mix for 15 to 20 s.

12. Place an empty U plate on top of each plate to serve as a cover to reduce evaporation from the wells. Incubate the plates at 37 C for 15 min. Keep a large pan of water in the incubator at all times to provide a moist atmosphere to reduce evaporation from the plates.

13. Remove the plates from the incubator, and add 0.025 ml of a 2.5% suspension of sheep or rabbit erythrocytes to all wells. Human erythrocytes are not suitable because they adhere to the side of the U plate wells and make it difficult to determine the end point. Do not use the same pipette dropper that was used to add the streptolysin.

14. Place the plates on a vibrator and mix for 15 to 20 s.

15. Cover the plates and incubate at 36 to 37 C for 15 min.

16. Remove the plates from the incubator and mix on the vibrator for 15 to 20 s to resuspend the erythrocytes.

17. Cover the plates and incubate at 36 to 37 C for an additional 30 min.

18. Remove the plates from the incubator and centrifuge for approximately 1 min at 200 to 250 × g to pack the erythrocytes.

Read and report the results as described below.

Antistreptolysin O tube test

Materials.

1. Test tubes (13 × 100 mm) and supports (racks) with 12 spaces per row.
2. Serological pipettes (0.2, 1, and 5 ml).
3. Buffered diluent, erythrocyte suspension, cold distilled water, streptolysin O, and reference (control) serum of known titer.

Procedure.

1. Arrange the test tubes in a rack with two rows of six tubes for each specimen. Include a reference (control) serum of known titer in each run. Label the tubes with the specimen number and the dilution number. The dilutions in the first row will be 1:60, 1:120, 1:240, 1:480, 1:960, and 1:1,920, and in the second row, 1:85, 1:170, 1:340, 1:680, 1:1,360, and 1:2,720. This dilution scheme has the advantage of having evenly spaced log intervals (0.15 log) between dilutions.
2. For each specimen, label initial serum dilution tubes 1:10, 1:60, and 1:85 and a hemolysin control tube. Also label a streptolysin control and an erythrocyte control for each run.
3. To the 1:10, 1:60, and 1:85 initial serum dilution tubes, add 1.8, 2.0, and 3.0 ml of diluent, respectively. Add 1.0 ml of diluent to all of the serum specimen tubes except the first one in each row (1:60, 1:85). Add diluent to the control tubes as follows: 0.5 ml to the serum hemolysin control, 1.0 ml to the streptolysin control, and 1.5 ml to the erythrocyte control.
4. Mix the sera and prepare a 1:10 dilution of each specimen by adding 0.2 ml of serum to 1.8 ml of diluent and mixing thoroughly. The temperature of the serum and the diluent should be approximately the same to minimize differences in the volumes measured. The 1:10 dilution may be inactivated in a water bath at 56 C for 30 min if so desired.
5. Prepare a 1:60 dilution by adding 0.4 ml of the 1:10 dilution to 2.0 ml of diluent. Mix thoroughly.
6. Prepare a 1:85 dilution by adding 0.4 ml of the 1:10 dilution to 3.0 ml of diluent. Mix thoroughly.
7. Add 1.0 ml of the 1:60 dilution to the first and second tubes (1:60, 1:120) in row one. Also add 1.0 ml of the 1:60 dilution to the specimen hemolysin control. Mix the contents of the second tube (1:120) thoroughly, and transfer 1.0 ml to the third tube (1:240). Mix thoroughly and continue to make serial dilutions through the sixth tube (1:1,920). Discard 1.0 ml after mixing the contents of the sixth tube.
8. Add 1.0 ml of the 1:85 dilution to the first and second tubes (1:85, 1:170) of row two. Carry

out serial dilutions through the sixth tube (1:2,720) as above.
9. Rearrange the specimen tubes into one row of 12 tubes as follows: 1:60, 1:85, 1:120, 1:170, 1:240, 1:340, 1:480, 1:680, 1:960, 1:1,360, 1:1,920, and 1:2,720.
10. Rehydrate the streptolysin O just before use with cold (2 to 6 C) distilled water. Stopper and let stand for a few seconds to dissolve. Mix end-over-end gently to avoid aeration. *Caution:* Extended agitation may cause oxidation and inactivation of the streptolysin O. Keep the streptolysin cold during use by placing the vial in a beaker of ice water.
11. Add 0.5 ml of streptolysin O to all tubes except the serum hemolysin control and the erythrocyte control. Shake the rack to mix the contents of the tubes.
12. Incubate in a water bath at 36 to 37 C for 15 min.
13. Add 0.5 ml of 2.5% suspension of sheep, rabbit, or human O erythrocytes to all tubes. Shake the rack to mix the contents of the tubes.
14. Incubate in a water bath at 36 to 37 C for 15 min.
15. Shake the rack to resuspend the erythrocytes and reincubate at 37 C for 30 min.
16. Centrifuge the tubes for 2 min at 250 to 300 × *g* to pack the erythrocytes.

Reading antistreptolysin O tests

Light source. Use a fluorescent lamp and a test reading mirror for the microtitration test. Use a fluorescent lamp and a white background for the tube test.

Validity. The test must be repeated on all specimens in the run if:

1. The titer of the reference (control) serum differs from the expected value. A one-dilution increment difference is not allowed for the reference serum.
2. The streptolysin control does not show complete homolysis of the erythrocytes.
3. The erythrocyte control shows any hemolysis.

If there is hemolysis in the serum hemolysin control, the test on that specimen is not valid unless there is at least one well or tube above the 1:60 dilution in the test which has no hemolysis. Hemolysis in a specimen hemolysin control tube or well indicates the presence of a natural hemolysin for erythrocytes in the patient's serum. This hemolysin is usually diluted out above 1:85 so that most of the time it does not interfere with the determination of the end point of the ASO titer above this dilution.

End point. The highest serum dilution with no visible hemolysis is the end point.

Titer. The titer is the end-point dilution factor, i.e., the dilution factor of the highest serum dilution with no visible hemolysis.

Unit. The units are equivalent to the titer when streptolysin O produced in the United States is used.

Reporting

Report the titer in terms of Todd units (TU) or international units (IU); e.g., ASO titer = 240 TU or 240 IU. The number of units will be the same as the titer when streptolysin O produced in the United States is used.

The titer should be expressed in Todd units if the potency of the streptolysin O used in the test has been adjusted against the Todd Standard or in international units if the World Health Organization International Standard has been used. The units are equivalent for practical purposes (24). There appears to be a mistaken belief among some serologists that the Todd unit is associated with a particular dilution scheme or method such as the Rantz-Randall method. This is not true. As pointed out above, it is determined by the standard used to adjust the potency of the streptolysin O used in the test.

Reagents

Buffered diluent.

Stock barbital solution

Barbital (diethylbarbituric acid)	3.2 g
Sodium barbital (sodium diethylbarbiturate)	1.6 g
Sodium chloride	42.5 g
Distilled water .... to 1,000 ml	

Heat to boiling with constant stirring. Cool to room temperature and determine the pH. It should be 7.2 ± 0.05. Store at room temperature in a screw-cap flask. Discard at the first sign of microbial growth.

Stock gelatin solution

Gelatin (bacteriological grade)	1.25 g
Distilled water	1,000 ml

Use gelatin designated for use in bacteriological culture media. Heat to boiling with constant stirring to prevent scorching the gelatin. Cool to room temperature. Store in a refrigerator (2 to 6 C) in a screw-cap flask. Discard at first sign of microbial growth.

Working solution of buffered diluent

Prepare a working solution of buffered diluent as needed by adding 1 part of stock barbital solution to 4 parts of stock gelatin solution, e.g., 20 ml of barbital solution to 80 ml of gelatin solution. Store in a refrigerator (2 to 6 C) in a screw-cap flask. Discard at the first sign of microbial growth. A stock phosphate buffer solution, pH 7.2, may be substituted for the stock barbital solution; however, it should be diluted with the stock gelatin solution.

Red blood cell suspension (2.5%). Use citrated or defibrinated rabbit, sheep, or human O erythrocytes for the tube technique and rabbit or sheep erythrocytes for the microtitration technique. Human erythrocytes are not suitable for the microtitration technique because they adhere to the sides of the U plate wells and make it difficult to determine the end point. Rabbit erythrocytes undergo spontaneous lysis more readily than do sheep or human erythrocytes. The type of erythrocytes used can have an effect on the titer (10).

Prepare a 2.5% suspension of the erythrocytes by either the spectrophotometric method or the following centrifuge method.

1. Pipette 3 to 4 ml of citrated blood into a 12- or 15-ml graduated centrifuge tube. Add 4 to 5 volumes of diluent to each volume of blood. Centrifuge at 300 to 350 × *g* for 5 min.

2. Remove the supernatant fluid and the layer of white blood cells from the packed red blood cells. Add diluent to within 1 or 2 ml of the top of the centrifuge tube. Resuspend the erythrocytes by mixing gently. Centrifuge at 300 to 350 × *g* for 5 min. Discard the supernatant fluid and repeat the wash.

3. After the second washing, resuspend the cells in fresh diluent and centrifuge at 300 to 350 × *g* for 10 min. The supernatant fluid should be colorless; if not, the erythrocytes are too fragile and should not be used. Record the volume of packed erythrocytes. Remove the supernatant fluid. Prepare a 2.5% suspension by adding 3.9 ml of diluent to each 0.1 ml of packed erythrocytes.

4. Check the accuracy of the erythrocyte suspension in a calibrated centrifuge tube by centrifuging at 300 to 350 × *g* for 10 min.

5. Store the erythrocyte suspension in a refrigerator (2 to 6 C). Discard at the first sign of hemolysis or microbial growth.

Source of reagents and materials.

Streptolysin O: Difco, Detroit, Mich.; Grand Island Biological Co., Grand Island, N.Y.; Lederle Diagnostics, Pearl River, N.Y.; Sylvana Co., Millburn, N.J.; and others.

ASO kit containing barbital gelatin diluent: Beckman Instruments, Fullerton, Calif.

Barbital and sodium barbital: Fisher Scientific Co.

Microtitration equipment: Cooke Engineering Co., Alexandria, Va.

Disposable U plates: Linbro Scientific Co., New Haven, Conn.; Cooke Engineering Co.

Vibrator mixer: paper jogger model JIA, Syntron Co., Homer City, Pa.; vertical vibrator, Arthur H. Thomas Co., Philadelphia, Pa.

Interpretation

An elevated ASO titer is not in itself diagnostic for acute rheumatic fever or acute glomerulonephritis; however, when combined with clinical findings it is of great value in arriving at a diagnosis because it documents the streptococcal infection which precedes these complications. Although the ASO titer is elevated in 80 to 85% of patients with acute rheumatic fever, it is within the normal range for the other remaining 15 to 20%; therefore, a diagnosis of acute rheumatic fever can never be ruled out on the basis of the ASO test alone (31). A second test such as the ADN-B or AH will frequently show an elevated titer for patients with normal or borderline ASO titers.

A rise in ASO titer may occur as early as 1 week, but the titer does not reach its peak until 3 to 5 weeks after infection (19). Usually, the titer starts falling during the second month after infection, but the rate of decline varies considerably from patient to patient. The titer returns to preinfection levels within 6 months to 1 year (25). Antibiotic therapy may depress the magnitude of the antibody response and hasten its rate of decline (22).

A rise in titer of two (0.3 log) or more dilution increments between acute- and convalescent-stage specimens is considered to be significant regardless of the magnitude of the titer. Usually, the patient is not seen early enough to obtain both acute and convalescent serum specimens, and a rise in titer cannot be demonstrated. In this situation an "upper limit of normal" value can be used as a base line for determining the significance of the titers of these specimens. The "upper limit of normal" value is the titer which is not exceeded by 85% of a population with no apparent recent streptococcal infection. The "upper limit of normal" value varies with age, season of the year, and geographical area. It is highest in a population of school age children and in young adults in military service or in college. It is thought to be higher for all age groups in northern latitudes (3). Ideally, each laboratory should establish its own "upper limit of normal" range. We have found the "upper limit of normal" for ASO in the Atlanta, Ga., area to be as follows: preschool age, 85; school age, 170; and adult, 85 (12). Thus, an ASO titer of 240 or greater in a school age patient or 120 or greater in a preschool age or adult patient is suggestive of a recent group A streptococcal infection, but there is no clear-cut demarcation between a "normal" and a low elevated titer in the absence of a demonstrable rise in titer.

ANTIDEOXYRIBONUCLEASE B TEST

Streptococci produce at least four DNases, and most of these are shared between the various groups of streptococci. However, DNase B is found only among group A beta-hemolytic streptococci and a few strains of groups C and G, thus making it the DNase of choice for the detection of group A infections. Group A streptococci also produce DNase A, C, and D in addition to B. The DNases are antigenically distinct, and the antibodies produced against them are specific (28).

The ADN-B test is a neutralization test employing an enzyme, streptococcal DNase B, as the antigen. The test is performed by adding a constant volume of DNase B to various dilutions of the patient's serum. The mixture is incubated to allow for combination of DNase with its antibody. A constant volume of deoxyribonucleic acid (DNA) is added to the DNase-serum mixture and the test is reincubated. The DNA serves as an indicator of whether the DNase has been neutralized by being combined with antibody (ADN-B) or is free to depolymerize the DNA substrate. Alcohol was added to the early ADN-B tests to determine whether the DNA had been depolymerized (31). The DNA was coagulated and formed a clot if it had not been depolymerized. In the test described below under microtitration test, methyl green dye is used to determine whether the DNA has been depolymerized. The methyl green retains its color when combined with polymerized DNA but the color fades if the DNA is depolymerized (16).

The microtitration test described below has the advantage over a tube test of requiring smaller amounts of reagents and less time to perform. The method can be used as a tube test (12 × 75 mm tubes) by increasing the amounts, e.g., 0.2 ml of serum dilution, 0.2 ml of DNase B, and 0.4 ml of DNA-methyl green (DNA-MG) substrate. The same dilution scheme is used. The tubes are incubated in a water bath instead of an incubator at the same temperature and for the same length of time as for the microtitration method.

Clinical indications

The ADN-B test appears to be the best single test for the serological detection of streptococcal infection (8). Not only can it be used for confirming a recent streptococcal infection when acute rheumatic fever or acute glomerulonephritis is suspected, but it is also useful for Sydenham's chorea (30). It is a better test than the ASO test for patients with acute glomerulonephritis due to streptococcal pyoderma (29).

The ADN-B test has the advantage over the ASO test of not being subject to "false-positive" titers caused by: (i) bacterial growth in the serum specimen, (ii) liver disease, and (iii) oxidation of the antigen. A disadvantage is that it is not as well known and has not been as widely used as the ASO test.

Microtitration test

Materials.

1. Microtitration equipment: 0.025- and 0.05-ml calibrated dropper pipettes; 0.025-ml microdiluters; disposable U plates; test reading mirror.

2. Vibrator mixer (paper jogger).

3. Serological pipettes (0.2, 1, 2, and 5 ml) and long-tip measuring pipettes (0.2 or 0.5 ml).

4. Test tubes (13 × 100 mm) and supports (racks); 15-ml conical centrifuge tube.

5. Buffered diluent, DNase B, DNA-MG, reference (control) serum.

Procedure.

1. Prepare initial serum dilutions of 1:10, 1:60, and 1:85 in test tubes and then subsequent dilutions in U plates. Label tubes with the specimen number and dilution.

2. Mix the sera and prepare a 1:10 dilution of each by adding 0.1 ml of serum (with a 0.2-ml pipette) to 0.9 ml of diluent. Mix thoroughly.

3. Prepare a 1:60 dilution by adding 0.2 ml of the 1:10 dilution of serum to 1.0 ml of diluent. Mix thoroughly.

4. Prepare a 1:85 dilution by adding 0.2 ml of the 1:10 dilution of serum to 1.5 ml of diluent. Mix thoroughly.

5. Mark off disposable U plates into sections so that each specimen is assigned two rows (1:60 row and 1:85 row) with six wells per row. Include two rows for reference (control) serum in each run (not each plate). Label six wells on the bottom row of each plate as serum DNase controls. Label a well for the DNase B (antigen) control and a well for the DNA-MG control on the bottom row of one of the plates in each run (not each plate).

6. Use a calibrated pipette dropper to add 0.025 ml of diluent to the second through sixth well of each row assigned to the specimens and reference serum. Add diluent to the control wells as follows: 0.025 ml to the serum DNase and the DNase B (antigen) well; 0.05 ml to the DNA-MG well.

7. Add 0.05 ml of the 1:60 serum dilution to the first well of the first row and 0.05 ml of the 1:85 dilution to the first well of the second row. Also add 0.025 ml of the 1:60 serum dilution to the serum DNase control wells. Use long-tip 0.2- or 0.5-ml measuring pipettes to add the 1:60 and 1:85 serum dilutions to the U plate wells.

8. Dilute each row using 0.025-ml microdiluters. The serum dilutions in the first row are 1:60, 1:120, 1:240, 1:480, 1:960, and 1:1,920, and in the second row, 1:85, 1:170, 1:340, 1:680, 1:1,360, and 1:2,720. The intervals between dilutions are evenly spaced at 0.15 log.

9. Prepare a working solution of DNase B in a 15-ml conical centrifuge tube by diluting the stock solution with buffered diluent. Mix thoroughly and use a 0.025-ml calibrated pipette dropper to add 0.025 ml to all wells except the DNA-MG and serum DNase control wells. The working solution of DNase B should be prepared fresh for each run. The rehydrated stock solution of DNase B will keep for several weeks at 2 to 6 C.

10. Place the plates on the vibrator mixer for 15 to 20 s to mix.

11. Place an empty U plate on top of each plate to serve as a cover to reduce evaporation from the wells. Incubate the plates at 37 C for 15 min. Keep a large pan of water in the incubator at all times to provide a moist atmosphere to reduce evaporation from the plates.

12. Remove the plates from the incubator, and add 0.05 ml of DNA-MG substrate to all wells. The DNA-MG should be removed from the refrigerator before making the serum dilutions so that it will be at room temperature when added to the test.

13. Place the plates on a vibrator mixer and mix for 30 to 40 s.

14. Seal the tops of the plates with transparent plastic tape and incubate for 3 h at 45 C. The plates may be incubated at 37 C for 4 h if a 45 C incubator is not available; however, a more concentrated solution of DNase B must be used. See determination of DNase B working solution below under Reagents.

15. Remove the plates from the incubator and place a piece of thin white translucent paper, such as onionskin, over the top of the plate before reading. This softens the light and makes it easier to see the color. Read the plate on a test reading mirror illuminated by a fluorescent lamp. The end point is the highest dilution of serum showing a definite green color. The titer is the dilution factor of this endpoint dilution. The DNase B (antigen) control should be colorless, and the DNA-MG control and the serum DNase controls should be green. If any of the serum DNase controls are colorless, it means that the serum has an elevated

DNase level, and the test is not valid unless there are wells above the 1:60 dilution which have a green color. The reference (control) serum should show the correct titer.

Reagents.

Buffered diluent.

Stock imidazole buffer solution

Imidazole	17.0 g
Calcium chloride (CaCl$_2 \cdot$H$_2$O)	1.47 g
Magnesium sulfate, anhydrous (MgSO$_4$)	0.6 g
Distilled water	900 ml

Dissolve ingredients and adjust pH to 8.0 with 1 N hydrochloric acid. Bring the volume up to 1,000 ml with distilled water. Store at room temperature.

Gelatin solution

Gelatin (bacteriological grade)	1.25 g
Distilled water	1,000 ml

Use gelatin designated for bacteriological culture media. Heat to boiling with constant stirring to prevent scorching the gelatin. Cool and store in a refrigerator (2 to 6 C) in a screw-cap flask. Discard at the first sign of microbial growth.

Working solution of buffered diluent

Prepare a working solution of buffered diluent as needed by adding 1 part of stock imidazole solution to 4 parts of gelatin solution, e.g., 50 ml of imidazole solution plus 200 ml of gelatin solution. Store in a refrigerator (2 to 6 C), and discard at the first sign of microbial growth.

DNase B. Streptococcal DNase B is prepared as described by Wannamaker (27) with the following modifications: HDCL broth (11) is used instead of Pfanstiehl dialysate broth as the culture medium, and the buffer for starch block electrophoresis consists of 0.2 M tris(hydroxymethyl)-aminomethane and 0.6 M glycine instead of 0.1 μM glycine alone. The DNases may also be separated by acrylamide gel electrophoresis (20). The lyophilized DNase B is stored under vacuum at 2 to 5 C.

The working dilution of DNase B is determined by means of a reference serum of known titer. It should be determined each time a new lot number of DNase B or DNA-MG is used for the first time or if the incubation time or temperature of the test is changed. The reference serum is diluted in the usual way by the microtitration technique except that it is not necessary to carry out the dilutions more than two or three increments above the known titer of the reference serum. The stock solution of DNase B is diluted in increments of 1 ml in test tubes. *Do not make dilutions of DNase B with microdiluters because the enzyme is inhibited by ferrous metals.* Add 0.025 ml of the test dilution of DNase B to 0.025 ml of the diluted reference serum in U plates, and carry out the test in the usual manner. The proper working dilution of the DNase B is the dilution which gives a definite green color with the known titer of the reference serum but no color with the next highest dilution of the reference serum. Occasionally, it may be necessary to use a working dilution between two test dilutions, e.g., 1 ml of DNase B stock solution to 5.5 ml of diluent instead of 1 ml + 5 ml or 1 ml + 6 ml.

DNA-MG substrate. DNA-MG substrate is prepared as described by Klein et al. (11) except that 0.1 g of DNA is added to 80 ml of distilled water instead of 1 g of DNA (typographical error). The DNA-MG may be lyophilized and stored under vacuum at 2 to 6 C. The rehydrated DNA-MG may be kept at 2 to 6 C for several weeks.

Source of reagents and materials

ADN-B test kit: Beckman Instruments, Inc., Fullerton, Calif.

DNA highly polymerized from calf thymus: Worthington Biochemical Corp., Freehold, N.J.; Calbiochem, La Jolla, Calif.

Methyl green dye (C.I. 42590): Fisher Scientific Co., Pittsburgh, Pa.

Imidazole (best grade): Sigma Chemical Co., St. Louis, Mo.; Calbiochem.

Microtitration equipment: Cooke Engineering Co., Alexandria, Va.

Disposable U plates: Linbro Scientific Co., New Haven, Conn.; Cooke Engineering Co.

Vibrator mixer: paper jogger model J1A, Syntron Co., Homer City, Pa.; vertical vibrator, Arthur H. Thomas Co., Philadelphia, Pa.

Interpretation

An elevated ADN-B titer is indicative of a recent beta-hemolytic streptococcal infection and as such is a valuable aid to the physician in suspected cases of acute rheumatic fever, acute glomerulonephritis, and Sydenham's chorea.

A rise in ADN-B titer usually occurs later than the rise in ASO titer and does not reach its peak until 4 to 6 weeks after infection (1). Also, the ADN-B titer tends to remain elevated for a longer period of time (1). This makes the test more valuable than the ASO test in Sydenham's chorea because of the long latent period between streptococcal infection and development of chorea. Antibiotic therapy may suppress the magnitude and cause a more rapid decline of the titer.

An elevated DNase level in the patient's serum can cause a "false-negative" ADN-B titer, because ADN-B is specific for streptococcal DNase B and does not neutralize serum DNase. Fortunately, elevated serum DNase is seldom encountered in patients with streptococcal infection; however, it is markedly elevated in acute hemorrhagic pancreatitis. An enzyme poison can cause a "false-positive" titer by inactivating the DNase B; therefore, it is important to use clean glassware for the collection of serum specimens and for the test.

A rise in titer of two (0.3 log) or more dilution increments between acute and convalescent specimens is considered to be significant regardless of the magnitude. "Upper limit of normal" values can be used as a base line for determining the significance of a titer in the absence of a demonstrable rise. The ADN-B "normal" values, like the ASO values, vary with age of the subject, season of the year, and geographical area. Values for the peak streptococcal season in the Atlanta area are as follows: preschool age, 60; school age, 170; and adult, 85 (12). Therefore, titers are usually significant if they are 85 or greater in a preschool age patient, 240 or greater in a school age patient, and 120 or greater in an adult patient.

LITERATURE CITED

1. Ayoub, E. M., and L. W. Wannamaker. 1962. Evaluation of streptococcal desoxyribonuclease B and diphosphopyridine nucleotidase antibody tests in acute rheumatic fever and acute glomerulonephritis. Pediatrics 29:527–538.
2. Christensen, L. R. 1949. Methods for measuring the activity of components of the streptococcal fibrinolytic system and streptococcal deoxyribonuclease. J. Clin. Invest. 28:163–172.
3. Coburn, A. F., and R. H. Pauli. 1935. Limited observations on the antistreptolysin titer in relation to latitude. J. Immunol. 29:515–521.
4. Goedvolk-De Groot, L. E., N. Michel-Bensink, M. M. Van Es-Boon, A. H. Van Vonno, and M. F. Michel. 1974. Comparison of the titers of ASO, anti DNase B and antibodies against the group polysaccharide of group A streptococci in children with streptococcal infections. J. Clin. Pathol. 27:891–896.
5. Hallen, J. 1963. Non-specific streptolysin O inhibition in diseases of the liver and billiary system. Acta Pathol. Microbiol. Scand. 57:301–306.
6. Harris, Z. N., and S. Harris. 1949. Studies in the relation of the hemolytic streptococcus to rheumatic fever. V. Streptococcal antihyaluronidase titers in the sera of patients with rheumatic fever, streptococcal. Am. J. Med.

Sci. 217:174–186.
7. Hodge, B. E., and H. F. Swift. 1933. Varying hemolytic and constant combining capacity of streptolysins; influence on testing for antistreptolysins. J. Exp. Med. 58:277–287.
8. Kaplan, E. J., B. F. Anthony, S. S. Chapman, E. M. Ayoub, and L. W. Wannamaker. 1970. The influence of the site of infection on the immune response to group A streptococci. J. Clin. Invest. 49:1405–1414.
9. Kellner, A., E. B. Freeman, and A. S. Carlson. 1958. Neutralizing antibodies to streptococcal diphosphopyridine nucleotidase in the serum of experimental animals and human beings. J. Exp. Med. 108:299–309.
10. Klein, G. C., B. V. Addison, J. S. Boone, and M. D. Moody. 1968. Effect of type of red blood cells on antistreptolysin O titer. Appl. Microbiol. 16:1761–1763.
11. Klein, G. C., C. N. Baker, B. V. Addison, and M. D. Moody. 1969. Micro test for streptococcal antideoxyribonuclease B. Appl. Microbiol. 18:204–206.
12. Klein, G. C., C. N. Baker, and W. L. Jones. 1971. "Upper limits of normal" antistreptolysin O and antideoxyribonuclease B titers. Appl. Microbiol. 21:999–1001.
13. Klein, G. C., E. C. Hall, C. N. Baker, and B. V. Addison. 1970. Antistreptolysin O test. Comparison of micro and macro technics. Am. J. Clin. Pathol. 53:159–162.
14. Klein, G. C., and W. L. Jones. 1971. Comparison of the Streptozyme test with the antistreptolysin O, antideoxyribonuclease B, and antihyaluronidase tests. Appl. Microbiol. 21:257–259.
15. Klein, G. D., M. P. Moody, C. N. Baker, and B. V. Addison. 1968. Micro antistreptolysin O test. Appl. Microbiol. 16:184.
16. Kurnick, N. B. 1950. The determination of desoxyribonuclease activity by methyl green; application to serum. Arch. Biochem. 29:41–53.
17. Liao, S. J. 1951. A modification of the antistreptolysin test. J. Lab. Clin. Med. 38:648–659.
18. Lofgren, S. 1944. Bacterial contamination of blood samples as a source of error in antistreptolysin titration. Acta Pathol. Microbiol. Scand. 21:768–774.
19. McCarty, M. 1954. The antibody response to streptococcal infections, p. 130–142. In M. McCarty (ed.) Streptococcal infections. Columbia University Press, New York.
20. Marker, S. C., and E. D. Gray. 1972. Simple method for the preparation of streptococcal nucleases. Appl. Microbiol. 23:368–371.
21. Neill, J. M., and T. B. Mallory. 1926. Studies on the oxidation and reduction of immunological substances. IV. Streptolysin. J. Exp. Med. 44:241–260.
22. Rantz, L. A., P. J. Boisvert, and W. W. Spink. 1946. Hemolytic streptococcal sore throat; antibody response following treatment with penicillin, sulfadiazine and salicylates. Science 103:352.
23. Rantz, L. A., and E. Randall. 1945. A modifica-

tion of the technic for determination of the antistreptolysin titer. Proc. Soc. Exp. Biol. Med. **59**:22–25.

24. Spaun, J., M. M. Bentzon, S. Olsen Larsen, and L. F. Hewitt. 1961. International standard for antistreptolysin O. Bull. WHO **24**:271–279.

25. Stollerman, G. H., A. J. Lewis, I. Schultz, and A. Taranta. 1956. Relationship of immune response to group A streptococci to the course of acute, chronic and recurrent rheumatic fever. Am. J. Med. **20**:163–169.

26. Todd, E. W. 1932. Antigenic streptococcal hemolysin. J. Exp. Med. **55**:267–280.

27. Wannamaker, L. W. 1958. Electrophoretic studies of the extracellular products of group A streptococci. J. Exp. Med. **107**:783–795.

28. Wannamaker, L. W. 1964. Streptococcal deoxyribonucleases, p. 140–165. *In* J. W. Uhr (ed.), The streptococcus, rheumatic fever and glomerulonephritis. The Williams & Wilkins Co., Baltimore.

29. Wannamaker, L. W. 1970. Differences between streptococcal infections of the throat and of the skin. N. Engl. J. Med. **282**:78–85.

30. Wannamaker, L. W. 1970. Serum antibodies to streptococci in rheumatic fever, glomerulonephritis and chorea. Zentralbl. Bakteriol. Paristenkd. Infektionskr. Hyg. Abt. I Orig. **214**:331–378.

31. Wannamaker, L. W., and E. M. Ayoub. 1960. Antibody titers in acute rheumatic fever. Crication **21**:598–614.

Chapter 34

Immune Response to *Neisseria meningitidis*

MALCOLM S. ARTENSTEIN,[1] BRENDA L. BRANDT, EDMUND C. TRAMONT,
AND WENDELL D. ZOLLINGER

INTRODUCTION

A discussion of the immunological response of humans to infection with *Neisseria meningitidis* must, of necessity, begin with a description of the antigens of the bacterium which are used in the serological assays. The surface of the meningococcus contains three major classes of antigens: (i) a polysaccharide capsule, (ii) cell wall proteins, and (iii) cell wall lipopolysaccharides. Capsular polysaccharides have served as the basis for classifying meningococci into serogroups, of which nine are currently recognized: A, B, C, D, X, Y, Z, 29E, and 135. These capsular antigens are specific in relation to one another, although immunologically similar antigens have been identified in some other bacterial species. Cell wall protein antigens are not unique for a given meningococcal serogroup; rather, immunologically similar proteins have been identified in different serogroups (8) and have been used in subtyping schemes (4). Lipopolysaccharides of meningococci have received only limited study as serological tools, but at least several specific determinants have been recognized (14). These, as well as cell wall proteins, cross-react to some extent with strains of *N. gonorrhoeae* (11). Although each of these classes of antigens has been used in studies of human immune responses, clinical experience has been limited to use of polysaccharide antigens and whole viable bacteria, and, therefore, the methods to be described will be limited to these two antigens.

Infection of humans with meningococci may present a variety of clinical forms: the asymptomatic carrier state, meningitis, bacteremia, fulminant shock (Waterhouse-Friderichsen syndrome), chronic meningococcemia, and many different localized organ infections (pneumonia, pericarditis, ophthalmitis). An immunological response has been observed in each syndrome in which studies have been carried out, and no clear-cut difference in serological response appears to characterize a syndrome. Immunization with polysaccharide vaccines stimulates a humoral antibody response and has proven effective in preventing systemic disease caused by serogroup C and A meningococci (3, 12).

Four serological tests will be described in detail because of their general utility and ease of performance in diagnosing meningococcal infection: passive hemagglutination (HA), latex agglutination, serum bactericidal, and indirect fluorescent-antibody tests. Other tests either lack sufficient specificity (complement fixation) or sensitivity (gel diffusion) or are too complex or expensive for any but a research laboratory (radioactive bactericidal test, radioactive binding assay) and will not be discussed further.

PASSIVE HEMAGGLUTINATION TEST

Passive HA is a relatively simple, specific serological test for detection of antibody response to infection or polysaccharide immunization. The test is based upon the ability of antibodies to agglutinate erythrocytes coated with polysaccharide antigen. Peak serum antibody titers occur 1 to 3 weeks after infection or immunization. After natural infection, antibody titers fall rapidly within 2 months (2), but after vaccination antipolysaccharide titers remain near the peak level for many years (1).

Passive HA polysaccharide antibody responses are highly specific, and, therefore, the laboratory must know the serogroup of the infecting organism or must use each polysaccharide as an antigen. To do the latter would, therefore, require performing four to nine different assays on the patients' sera. Preliminary studies have indicated the feasibility of adsorbing multiple serogroup antigens onto erythrocytes to make a polyvalent particle, but this procedure has not been carried through to the stage of clinical usefulness.

There are two disadvantages in passive HA (polysaccharide) testing of which the physician should be aware. (i) Infants and young children may produce low titers of antipolysaccharide antibody after infection or vaccination and passive HA may fail to detect the response (9). More sensitive assays (such as radioactive binding) must be used in this age group. (ii) Group B polysaccharide is poorly immunogenic

[1] Deceased.

in humans, and even natural systemic infection may fail to induce significant anti-B antibodies (13). However, some batches of group B antigen may show antibody titers in many normal human sera, and increasing titers are seen with increasing age (2).

Sensitization of erythrocytes

The optimal concentration of polysaccharide to use for sensitization of the erythrocytes must be determined for each batch of polysaccharide by performing a grid titration of the antigen against a human serum with high antibody content. Serial twofold dilutions of the antigen are used to sensitize small amounts of erythrocytes which are then tested against serial twofold dilutions of the serum. The lowest concentration of antigen which gives maximum titer and the best pattern is used for the test (20 to 40 μg/ml is often optimal).

Sensitization is carried out by diluting the stock solution of polysaccharide in phosphate-buffered saline (PBS) to the optimal concentration and mixing with an equal volume of erythrocytes which were previously washed three times by gently suspending the cells in PBS to a concentration of about 4% (vol/vol) and centrifuging at $500 \times g$ for 10 min. The mixture is incubated at 37 C for 30 min with occasional stirring.

The sensitized erythrocytes are washed three times in buffer to remove excess antigen and then resuspended in buffer to 0.5% (vol/vol). Bovine serum albumin is then added from a 10% stock solution to a final concentration of 0.5% (wt/vol). Cells are stored as a 0.5% suspension at 4 C and should be used within 24 h after sensitization.

Test procedure

Serum is heat-inactivated at 56 C for 30 min, and then 10 to 12 serial twofold dilutions are made in PBS by use of disposable Microtiter U plates (Linbro Chemical Co., Inc., New Haven, Conn.) and 0.05-ml diluters (Cooke Engineering Co., Alexandria, Va.). One drop (0.05 ml) of sensitized erythrocytes is then added to each well. The plates are gently rotated by hand to mix reagents and then are placed at room temperature for 1 to 2 h. Patterns of agglutination are read on a 1+ to 4+ scale, with a 3+ or 4+ agglutination considered positive. A positive and a negative control serum should be included in each test as well as an antigen control which contains no serum and which should show no agglutination.

Reagents

PBS: Contains 66.6 ml of 0.15 M Na_2HPO_4, 33.3 ml of 0.15 M KH_2PO_4, and 8.5 g of NaCl per liter of buffer. The pH should be 6.9.

Bovine serum albumin, 10%: Made up in PBS with the use of Fraction V powder (Research Products Division, Miles Laboratories, Inc., Kankakee, Ill.).

Human group O, Rh-negative erythrocytes: Cells are collected in Alsever's solution (Microbiological Associates, Inc., Bethesda, Md.) and can be used for up to 3 weeks if kept at 4 C.

Polysaccharide antigen: Prepared from meningococcal culture supernatant fluids as follows.

A. Growth of organisms

1. Mueller-Hinton agar is used as the solid medium. Liquid cultures are grown in a medium containing (per liter of medium) 10 g of Casamino Acids (technical grade), 120 mg of KCl, 10.3 g of Na_2HPO_4, and 25 ml of a $40\times$ glucose-magnesium sulfate solution (2.4 g of $MgSO_4 \cdot 7H_2O$ and 20 g of glucose per 100 ml), which is autoclaved separately and added after the medium has cooled. Final pH should be 7.5.

2. Meningococci of the desired serogroup are streaked on an agar plate and grown overnight at 37 C in a CO_2 incubator or candle jar. This culture is used to inoculate 50 ml of liquid medium in a 250-ml Erlenmeyer flask (optical density [OD] at 650 nm, 0.2 to 0.3), and the suspension is incubated aerobically at 35 to 37 C on a rotary shaker (150 rpm) for 4 to 6 h. About 20 ml of this culture is then used to inoculate 500 ml of medium in a 2-liter flask, and this suspension is then grown under the same conditions for 14 to 16 h.

B. Preparation of the polysaccharide antigens (11)

1. Kill the bacteria by addition of phenol to a final concentration of 0.5%.

2. After 1 h, remove the bacteria by centrifugation ($13,000 \times g$, 15 min) and collect the supernatant fluid.

3. Add Cetavlon (hexadecyltrimethylammonium bromide; Eastman Organic Chemicals, Rochester, N.Y.) to a concentration of 0.1% (wt/vol).

4. Collect the precipitate by centrifugation ($5,000 \times g$, 15 min).

5. Dissolve the precipitate in 10 ml of 0.9 M $CaCl_2$.

6. Centrifuge out any insoluble material ($13,000 \times g$, 15 min).

7. To the supernatant fluid, add absolute ethanol to a final concentration of 25% (vol/vol), and place at 4 C for 2 h.

8. Remove the precipitate by centrifugation and discard.

9. Add ethanol to the supernatant fluid to a final total concentration of 80% (vol/vol), and collect the resulting precipitate by centrifugation.

10. Dissolve the precipitate in 10 ml of normal saline, centrifuge ($25,000 \times g$, 30 min), and discard any insoluble material. This is the stock solution of polysaccharide and is stored frozen.

Interpretation

Passive HA antibody response to infection or immunization occurs in well over 90% of subjects. However, individual responses vary greatly in magnitude. Thus, mean maximal increases in titer have been 32- to 128-fold. Occasional normal subjects fail to respond, and interpretation of results of immunization of patients suspected of having immunodeficiency disease must take this into account. Antibody measured by the passive HA assay is primarily of the immunoglobulin M (IgM) class although small amounts of IgG have been noted. Passive HA cannot be used for determination of immune status in a population because most normal adults have negligible titers (1:4 or less), but the great majority of such persons have been shown to have serum bactericidal antibodies and are immune (5).

LATEX AGGLUTINATION TEST (10)

The latex test is based upon the same principle as passive HA except for the nature of the insoluble particle. This test has the advantage that the latex suspension is commercially available and standardized. However, the test is somewhat less sensitive than passive HA.

Sensitization of latex

One volume of latex particles (Latex 0.81, Difco Laboratories, Detroit, Mich.) is added to an equal volume of polysaccharide diluted in PBS (pH 7.2 ± 0.1) and mixed gently for 30 min at 37 C. The optimal amount of polysaccharide antigen is determined by performing a grid titration as described for the passive HA test. The suspension is pelleted by centrifugation at $2,000 \times g$ for 15 min, the supernatant fluid is discarded, and the sensitized latex particles are suspended in 15 times the original volume of PBS. Once sensitized, latex particle suspensions may be stored at 4 C for the following periods of time: A and Y antigens, 2 months; B and C antigens, 8 months.

Test procedure

Serial twofold dilutions of fresh or inactivated serum (0.025 ml) in PBS are made in V-bottom microtiter plates (Linbro Chemical Co., Inc.). To each well is added an equal volume of sensitized latex particles. The plates are sealed, gently rotated to mix the reagents, and then incubated. When A, B, or C polysaccharides are used, the incubation times are 4 to 5 h at 37 C or 16 h (overnight) at room temperature; tests utilizing Y polysaccharide are incubated for 16 h (overnight) at room temperature.

Agglutination patterns are recorded on a 1+ to 4+ scale, and 1+ can be considered positive since the end points are so distinct.

An unsensitized suspension of latex particles should be tested with each serum at a 1:2 dilution to rule out nonspecific agglutination (seldom a problem). Known positive and negative control sera must be included on each test day.

Antigens

Crude meningococcal polysaccharide antigens are prepared by suspending a 6-h chocolate agar culture (early exponential growth phase) in PBS for 2 h. (MacFarland BaSO4 standard no. 10). The suspension is then centrifuged at $2,000 \times g$ for 15 min, the bacterial pellet is discarded, and the supernatant fluid is sterilized by filtration (0.20 or 0.45-μm membrane filter; Millipore Corp., Bedford, Mass.) and stored at -20 C. A new batch of antigen should be prepared each month. Polysaccharide antigen may also be prepared as described for the passive HA test. Polysaccharide preparations which do not contain small amounts of protein will not readily adhere to latex particles.

Interpretation

Interpretation of results is essentially the same as with passive HA.

SERUM BACTERICIDAL TEST

The serum bactericidal test is especially helpful in studies of patients with immune deficiencies and patients with recurrent meningitis or other unusual syndromes because of the positive correlation with immunity (5). The test is cumbersome, however, and must contain numerous controls to assure validity. The test measures the ability of serum to kill viable bacteria and requires an exogenous source of complement if antibody is to be measured accurately. Because viable bacteria are used, safety precautions must be instituted in the laboratory, and results must await overnight incubation. Sterile reagents and technique must be used throughout the procedure since the end point is the growth of viable bacteria as colonies.

Preparation of bacteria

Organisms for the bactericidal test are prepared by growing *N. meningitidis* for 16 h at 37 C in a CO_2 atmosphere on Mueller-Hinton agar. Growth from this culture is transferred with a loop into a 250-ml screw-cap nephelometer flask containing 25 ml of Mueller-Hinton broth. Enough organisms are added so that an initial OD of approximately 0.130 can be read at 650 nm in a Bausch & Lomb Spectronic 100 spectrophotometer. The flask is then incubated at 37 C in a shaking water bath until an OD of 0.600 is reached (1.5 to 2 h). The organisms are removed from the medium by centrifugation at $5,000 \times g$ for 10 min in a refrigerated centrifuge (Sorvall). The organisms are next washed once with 25 ml of cold Gey's balanced salt solution containing 0.1% gelatin (GBSS). The pelleted organisms are then suspended in 1 ml of GBSS. A sample of this suspension is adjusted to an OD of 0.495 to 0.505 at 650 nm with GBSS as the diluent. This suspension contains approximately 3×10^8 bacteria/ml and is further diluted 1:7,000. The growth of the organisms should be so regulated that the bacterial suspension is prepared just prior to use and is kept in an ice bath until needed.

Test procedure

The reaction mixture consists of 0.1 ml of serum dilution, 0.2 ml of GBSS, 0.1 ml of organisms, and 0.1 ml of complement. The test is performed in sterile 12×75 mm plugged test tubes. A 0.2-ml amount of serum previously diluted 1:5 in GBSS is added to the first tube; four serial twofold dilutions are made for the acute or prevaccination sera and seven are made for the postinfection or postimmunization sera with GBSS as the diluent. To 0.1 ml of serum dilution is added a further 0.2 ml of GBSS; this mixture is heated at 46 C for 30 min. After heat inactivation, the tubes are placed in an ice-water bath. To each tube is added 0.1 ml of organism suspension and then 0.1 ml of complement. The reactants are agitated on a Vortex mixer and placed in a shaking water bath at 37 C for 1 h. After the incubation period, the number of viable bacteria is determined as colony-forming units by transferring 20-µliter samples of each reaction mixture to Mueller-Hinton agar with an Eppendorf microliter pipette (Brinkman Instruments, Inc., Westbury, N.Y.). This sampling is performed

in triplicate as follows. Three 20-µliter drops are placed across the top of the agar plate, and the plate is tipped so that the drops run down the plate spreading the inoculum. The agar dish is then placed on a flat surface and the inoculum is allowed to dry.

The following controls are included in each assay: (i) a 0- and 60-min plate count on a sample containing only organisms and GBSS (0.1 ml of organisms and 0.4 ml of GBSS); (ii) a complement control to determine whether the complement alone kills the organisms (0.1 ml of organisms, 0.1 ml of complement, 0.3 ml of GBSS); (iii) a known positive serum control; and (iv) a negative serum control.

Incubate the Mueller-Hinton agar plates used for the viability counts at 37 C in a 10% CO_2 atmosphere or a candle extension jar for 16 h. Colony counts are recorded, and the results of triplicate samples are averaged. With the bacterial inoculum described above, approximately 200 colonies are present in the 20-µliter samples plated from control tubes. Serum antibody titer is the greatest dilution in which at least a 50% decrease in mean number of colonies is observed compared with the zero-time organism control.

Reagents

Mueller-Hinton Broth and Agar (Difco Laboratories).

Gey's Balanced Salt Solution for Ambient Atmosphere without Phenol Red (Microbiological Associates, Inc., Bethesda, Md.).

Gelatin, 10%: Prepared in distilled water with the use of Bacto-Gelatin (Difco Laboratories).

Complement: Undiluted "baby" rabbit serum (less than 4 weeks of age) is used as the complement source (Rockland Farms, Gilbertsville, Pa.). Each lot of complement must be tested against the strain or strains of *N. meningitidis* used as the test antigen to determine whether the complement alone has antibodies which kill the organism. Each lot of complement is filter-sterilized (0.45-µm membrane filter) and divided into small volumes (3 ml) which are stored at -70 C for subsequent use. The complement is thawed just prior to use in the test and must be kept in an ice-water bath so it does not lose its activity.

Interpretation

Whole viable organisms are used for this assay; therefore, antibodies detected are those which are directed against one or more of the surface antigens. In particular, since protein cell wall antigens may differ among strains even of the same serogroup, it is usually necessary to use the strain isolated from a given patient in testing his serological response. For studies involving polysaccharide vaccination, almost any strain of the homologous serogroup is satisfactory for use. Both IgG and IgM antibodies participate in the meningococcal bactericidal reaction. In performing this assay, serial dilutions of sera must be tested routinely because IgA antibodies in some sera block the bactericidal activity of IgM and IgG (7). Normal responses range from 4- to 256-fold antibody increase when paired sera are tested.

INDIRECT FLUORESCENT-ANTIBODY TEST (2, 5)

Serological testing for antibodies to meningococci by indirect immunofluorescence is quite feasible for a laboratory equipped for immunofluorescence procedures of any kind. In this assay meningococci fixed to slides are exposed to human serum. After removal of unabsorbed Ig's by washing, specific antibodies attached to the organisms are detected with fluorescein-conjugated anti-human globulin antibodies. Since the whole organism is the antigen, the homologous isolate is preferred when testing individuals. If standard laboratory strains are used as antigens, antibody response after natural colonization will often be detected (2). After polysaccharide immunization, the only positive response can be measured with strains of the same serogroup as the vaccine. The IFA assay has the advantage that the specific Ig class of the antibody can be readily determined by using fluorescein-conjugated anti-H chain antisera as reagents.

Test procedure

Eight twofold dilutions of serum and two controls can be conveniently tested on Teflon-coated slides with 10 equal 7-mm circles (Reboz Surgical Instruments, Washington, D.C.). The controls are (i) the organism alone to control for autofluorescence (seldom a problem) and (ii) the fluorescein-conjugated antiserum and bacteria but without human serum to control for "nonspecific" fluorescent staining.

Meningococci are grown for 5 to 6 h on chocolate agar at 37 C under 10% CO_2 (early logarithmic growth phase), washed once in distilled water, and suspended to a concentration of approximately 10^8 organisms (absorbance 0.100, Bausch & Lomb Spectronic 100) in Dulbecco's PBS, pH 7.2 ± 1 (Grand Island Biological Co., Grand Island, N.Y.). A 0.01-ml volume is air-dried onto each circumscribed area of the slide. Such slides are fixed with gentle heat and may

be stored in a desiccator jar for as long as 5 days. The fixed antigen is overlaid with each of the human serum dilutions and incubated for 20 to 30 min at 37 C in a moist chamber. Slides are then washed in three changes of PBS (5 min each), reincubated for 20 to 30 min with fluorescein-conjugated anti-human rabbit antiserum (whole or heavy chain specific; Behring Diagnostics, Sommerville, N.J., or Hyland Laboratory, Costa Mesa, Calif.; fluorescein/protein molar ratio ⩽5), rewashed as before, and mounted in buffered glycerol (9 parts glycerol, 1 part PBS; pH 7.8 ± 0.1).

The fluorescein-conjugated antisera are standardized by testing various dilutions of the antisera (1:10, 1:20, 1:50, etc.) for nonspecific fluorescent staining and reactivity. That dilution giving a strong reaction with a known high-titered human serum and no nonspecific staining is chosen. Fluorescence due to the presence of "natural" antibodies may be removed by absorbing the conjugated antiserum with meningococcal organisms. Growth from one agar plate of appropriate meningococci is removed and added directly into the conjugated antiserum. The mixture is shaken on a rotary shaker for 4 to 16 h at 4 C and then centrifuged at $2,000 \times g$; the supernatant serum is filtered through a 0.45-μm membrane filter (Millipore Corp., Bedford, Mass.). Any fluorescence microscope equipped with BG 12 excitation filter and barrier filters No. 53 and 44 or 50 and 41 may be used.

Fluorescence is scored on dispersed organisms only:

4+ = brilliant fluorescence of all organisms in the field

3+ = well-defined fluorescence of all organisms in the field

2+ = low-intensity but definite fluorescence of 75% or more of the organisms in the field

1+ = occasional organisms with low-intensity fluorescence

− = no fluorescence, low-grade background fluorescence, or fluorescent clumps with no evidence of fluorescence of isolated organisms.

Interpretation

A 2+ or greater reaction is considered positive. Paired sera are necessary for proper interpretation; fourfold or greater increases in titer are considered significant. Most normal sera give positive reactions at dilutions of 1:2 to 1:32, depending upon the bacterial strain used in the assay. Titer increases of 4- to 128-fold are observed after infection or vaccination.

LITERATURE CITED

1. Artenstein, M. S. 1971. Meningococcal infections. 5. Duration of polysaccharide vaccine induced antibody. Bull. WHO 45:291–293.
2. Artenstein, M. S., B. L. Brandt, E. C. Tramont, W. C. Branche, Jr., H. D. Fleet, and R. L. Cohen. 1971. Serologic studies of meningococcal infection and polysaccharide vaccination. J. Infect. Dis. 124:277–288.
3. Artenstein, M. S., R. Gold, J. G. Zimmerly, F. A. Wyle, H. Schneider, and C. Harkins. 1970. Prevention of meningococcal disease by group C polysaccharide vaccine. N. Engl. J. Med. 282:417–420.
4. Gold, R., and F. A. Wyle. 1970. New classification of *Neisseria meningitidis* by means of bactericidal reactions. Infect. Immun. 1:479–484.
5. Goldschneider, I., E. C. Gotschlich, and M. S. Artenstein. 1969. Human immunity to the meningococcus. I. The role of humoral antibodies. J. Exp. Med. 129:1307–1326.
6. Gotschlich, E. C., T. Y. Liu, and M. S. Artenstein. 1969. Human immunity to the meningococcus. III. Preparation and immunochemical properties of the group A, group B and group C meningococcal polysaccharides. J. Exp. Med. 129:1349–1365.
7. Griffiss, J. M. 1975. Bactericidal activity of meningococcal antisera: blocking by IgA of lytic antibody in human convalescent sera. J. Immunol. 114:1779–1784.
8. Kasper, D. L., J. L. Winklehake, B. L. Brandt, and M. S. Artenstein. 1973. Antigenic specificity of bactericidal antibodies in antisera to *Neisseria meningitidis*. J. Infect. Dis. 127:378–387.
9. Monto, A. S., B. L. Brandt, and M. S. Artenstein. 1973. Response of children to meningococcal polysaccharide vaccine. J. Infect. Dis. 127:394–401.
10. Tramont, E. C., and M. S. Artenstein. 1972. Latex agglutination test for measurement of antibodies to meningococcal polysaccharides. Infect. Immun. 5:346–351.
11. Tramont, E. C., J. C. Sadoff, and M. S. Artenstein. 1974. Cross-reactivity of *Neisseria gonorrhoeae* and *Neisseria meningitidis* and the nature of antigens involved in the bactericidal reaction. J. Infect. Dis. 130:240–247.
12. Wahdan, M. H., F. Rizk, A. M. El-Akkad, A. A. ElGhoroury, R. Hablas, N. I. Girgis, A. Amer, W. Boctar, J. E. Sippel, E. C. Gotschlich, R. Traiau, W. R. Sanborn, and B. Cvjetanovic. 1973. A controlled field trial of a serogroup A meningococcal polysaccharide vaccine. Bull. WHO 48:667–673.
13. Wyle, F. A., M. S. Artenstein, B. L. Brandt, E. C. Tramont, D. L. Kasper, P. L. Altieri, S. L. Berman, and J. P. Lowenthal. 1972. Immunologic response of man to group B meningococcal polysaccharide vaccines. J. Infect. Dis. 126:514–522.
14. Zollinger, W. D., C. L. Pennington, and M. S. Artenstein. 1974. Human antibody response to three meningococcal outer membrane antigens: comparison by specific hemagglutination assays. Infect. Immun. 10:975–984.

Chapter 35

Immune Response to *Neisseria gonorrhoeae*

D. S. KELLOGG AND A. BALOWS

Immune responses to pathogenic microorganisms may be perceived either in the clinic through signs and symptoms associated with a patient or in the laboratory through an examination of various fluids and cells from the patient. The clinical character of the immune response to *Neisseria gonorrhoeae,* as judged by clinical description, has not changed appreciably over at least the past 50 years. Those changes that might have occurred would be difficult to distinguish from changes related to increased incidence and physician awareness of gonorrhea, widespread availability and use of antibiotics, improved nutritional and public health conditions, and changes in social and sexual behavior.

In the laboratory the immune response to *N. gonorrhoeae* has been detected through the use of serological tests. The desirability of a serological test for gonorrhea has been uppermost in the thinking concerning this disease for many years. Several serological tests have been available for gonorrhea for years; however, they are not considered useful. Therefore, the need has been not for a serological test per se but for a test or tests with particular characteristics. These characteristics will depend on: (i) how the test is to be used, i.e., in private versus public health medicine, (ii) what we would be willing to accept in terms of sensitivity versus specificity, (iii) cost per test, (iv) what degree of technical and interpretive complexity is appropriate, and, finally, (v) what type of action ensues as a consequence of a given serological result. A test which has all of these desirable features, regardless of the intended use, is unlikely to be developed, and more than one type of test will probably be needed to cover the potential uses adequately.

An impressive body of information on the gonococcus has been developed since it was identified as the causal agent of gonorrhea. This information was accumulated over a considerable period under the influence of various economic, social, military, and medical necessities. Consequently, much of the research dealt with improved cultivation of the gonococcus from diagnostic specimens, therapy with new drugs, improved treatment regimens, and epidemiological considerations. The advent of penicillin as an effective therapeutic agent abruptly and drastically reduced support for and research on the gonococcus for over 20 years. However, since about 1970 there has been a positive coalescence of many factors, resulting in the rapid development of needed basic information concerning immune responses to gonococcal infections.

Immune responses to gonococcal infections have been detected in both cellular and humoral test systems. Cellular responses to gonococci were demonstrated with a lymphocyte transformation system (12). Specific transformations were detected in a population of males attending a venereal disease clinic. Significant cellular response was principally found in those males who had had three or more previous gonococcal infections. Individually, the differences between normal subjects and patients with a single, current gonococcal infection were not of diagnostic value. The potential epidemiological value is unknown.

Several types of serological procedures have been developed for detecting humoral responses to *N. gonorrhoeae* (3-5, 7, 10, 13-23). These procedures, listed in Table 1 in a general order of increasing sensitivity to antibody nitrogen, range from precipitin to radioimmunoassay types. In terms of micrograms of antibody nitrogen detected, there is a roughly 1,000-fold difference in sensitivity from top to bottom (8). These differences may be increased or decreased slightly according to the laboratory personnel's technical expertise. The listed tests do not comprise all of the proposed procedures or modifications thereof. For example, there are many complement-fixation procedures or modifications; however, most of them either were of no greater apparent usefulness than those listed or were less adequately evaluated with documented sera. Modifications of these procedures could materially alter, in particular, their specificities.

These modifications would be principally of the antigens used or the antibodies detected, since the procedures detecting their interactions are less amenable to change. Additionally, a given antigen may be used in different

TABLE 1. *Serological tests*

Category	Reference	Sensitivity (%)		Specificity (%)		Antigen character	Special equipment needed
		F	M	F	M		
Precipitin	Reising and Kellog (20)	62	73	72	100	Phenol extract	None
	Chacko and Nair (4)	75	81	94	94	Lipopolysaccharide fraction	None
Flocculation	Lee and Schmale (13)	86	68	88	88	Precipitated gonococcal protoplasm	None
	Wallace et al. (21)	78	77	96		Phenol extract	None
	Reising (19)	79	49	95	93	Sonically treated cell supernatant	None
Complement fixation	Magnusson and Kjellander (15)	53	37	94		Heated (60 C) gonococcal cells	None
	Peacock (18)	73	50	97	97	Gonococcal protoplasm	Useful (autotiter)
	Danielsson et al. (7)	36	20	95		Pooled gonococcal cells	None
Passive hemagglutination	Logan et al. (14)	88	77	85	96	Gonococcal protoplasm	Useful (autotiter)
	Ward and Glynn (22)	84	46	96	98	Lipopolysaccharide fraction	None
Indirect fluorescent antibody	Welch and O'Reilly (23)	79	56	97	—	Selected gonococcal cells	Necessary (special microscope)
	Kearns et al. (10)	—	83	—	83	Selected gonococcal cells	
Radioimmunoassay	Buchanan et al. (3)	86	44	81	86	Gonococcal pili	Radioactivity detection

procedures for practical reasons as well as for increased sensitivity or specificity. Certain characteristics of test procedures are apparently unrelated to antigen characteristics. Aggregation-type tests (precipitin, flocculation) are most responsive to antibody globulins of the immunoglobulin M (IgM) class, whereas non-aggregation tests appear to be responsive to antibodies of all three globulin classes. Complement fixation is an exception in the latter group in that antibodies of the IgA class are not detected under the usual conditions of test performance.

The antigenic material used in these tests varied considerably in the character of the antigens themselves, their methods of preparation, and their sources. In most instances, their physical structure, chemical character, quantity, and avidity are unknown. Cultivation techniques for the source of the antigens, the organisms themselves, are naturally quite different in some respects. Finally, the gonococcal strains used were selected under different crite-

ria. This last point is very important to the effectiveness of any procedure for detecting antibodies in a variety of human sera when the known antigenic variability of the gonococcus is considered. None of these antigens could be considered well characterized, and most are mixtures of the whole spectrum of gonococcal antigens. Two examples of gonococcal strain importance are evident in the hemagglutination procedure of Ward and Glynn (22) in which three strains gave sensitivities which varied between 27 and 84% and in the indirect fluorescent-antibody procedure of Welch and O'Reilly (23) in which 12 strains gave sensitivities between 25 and 95%.

The antibodies detected by these procedures were made in response to some or all of the approximately 15 antigens that have been demonstrated for gonococci as of 1965 (6). The tests measured the total response of the host with an unknown distribution of the response to the individual antigens. Potentially, antigens that were strong antibody stimulators could have dominated the antibody response. If these antigens were shared with other organisms in the human microflora, they might well stimulate secondary-type responses during an episode of gonorrhea. The response would be early, and the titer attained presumably would be the highest. Such responses may have been the reason for such disparate results between serological procedures of comparable sensitivity when run on the same sera but with a different antigen mixture.

Antibodies against *N. gonorrhoeae* have been detected in the Ig classes IgG, IgM, IgA, and secretory IgA. Human volunteer studies demonstrated that antibodies could be produced against *N. gonorrhoeae* in the three main Ig classes: IgG, IgA, and IgM (5). The degree of response in each class varied widely between individuals who were infected in a quantitatively similar manner with the same strain of gonococcus. Although current knowledge about reagent specificities casts some doubt on the degree of specificity in each class of reagent, the different responses to an essentially similar exposure indicate that variability of response depends on host as well as gonococcal antigen factors. Secretory IgA antibodies have been detected in urethral and vaginal secretions from culturally proven gonorrhea in both males and females, respectively (10, 16). In four of six female patients, secretory antibody titers rapidly resolved after therapy.

Under the usual conditions of exposure and infection, antibody response is detectable approximately 1 week after infection is initiated. Although the antibody titers vary according to the serological test used, the titers tend to remain elevated for weeks and in some instances months after effective treatment. This was true whether the patients were from high or low prevalence groups for gonorrhea. Nearly all of the sensitivity data in Table 1 have been derived from patients in high gonorrhea prevalence groups (30 to 40%) such as venereal disease clinic populations. The sensitivities vary between 62 and 88% for female sera and from 56 to 77% for male sera. Specificities vary between 72 and 97% for females and 86 to 97% for males. Specificities of these tests were developed through examination of sera from a variety of nongonorrheal patients, including children, tuberculosis sanitorium residents, and patients with chronic bronchitis or dermatoses. As such, these specificities are measures of test specificity in a distinctly different population from that used for the development of sensitivity data. Few studies have been performed on sera from persons in low prevalence groups, but the results so far indicate that the specificity is about

the same as that of the high prevalence groups. This would indicate that current procedures would develop a relatively high ratio of false positives per unit of true positives.

Examinations of sera from animal models, such as male chimpanzees, whose urethral infections mimic those of man, have shown an antibody response similar to that found in man (2). Furthermore, chimpanzees can be immunized with either whole gonococcal cell bacterins or cell fractions against challenge levels of gonococci much greater (on the order of 6 to 8 logs) than those encountered during natural human exposure (1, 11).

Although current serological procedures are capable of detecting antibodies against *N. gonorrhoeae*, certain problems invalidate their diagnostic usefulness. Some of these follow. The 7-day development period for detectable antibody response reduces the utility of these tests in epidemiological studies of gonorrhea distribution, because the infected individual is infectious and may be sexually active during this period. The prolonged retention of antibody titers after cure of the disease has negated the usefulness of serological tests as diagnostic tools. This has been particularly true for that segment of the population which appears to have had a considerable role in the maintenance and distribution of the disease — the high prevalence group. The sensitivities of the current tests have been generally at the same level. At least for the more sensitive tests, it would appear that more sensitivity is not a major issue. Considering the 1,000-fold theoretical difference in the tests' sensitivities to antibody nitrogen, present tests may in fact have detected nearly 100% of those individuals who had made an antibody response at the time serum was drawn.

The often prevailing inverse relationship between sensitivity and specificity usually determines the practical limits of sensitivity for each test. Specificity, on the other hand, is a weak aspect of most tests in two regards: first, specificity to the gonococcus over other microorganisms, and second, specificity to the presence of a gonorrheal infection. Too many responses are obtained in serological tests with sera from persons who have neither a current gonococcal infection nor a history of a recent gonococcal infection. Assuming that accurate historical data have been obtained from the patient, these reactions could be due to antibodies produced against antigens shared by the gonococcus with other microorganisms in the human microflora, such as saprophytic *Neisseria* and enteric organisms (9). The accuracy and completeness of the patient's historical data has been a very uncertain area, and this uncertainty has un-doubtedly been responsible for some incorrect assignments to the false-positive category. Se-rologically reactive sera in the absence of a culturally documented gonococcal infection may be a result of a missed infection or a re-sponse to antibodies remaining from a previ-ously treated and cured gonococcal infection. To be of diagnostic, as opposed to epidemiological, value a serological test would need to differen-tiate between current and past infection.

Serological tests for gonococcal antibodies have deficiencies in specificity and/or sensitiv-ity noted previously in this chapter; these greatly limit their applicability as diagnostic support systems. Since no single test fits the needs of either private or public health medi-cine, we have not described any test in detail. All of the discussed tests have been published in the scientific literature and are referenced in this chapter.

If serological tests have these drawbacks, what are their potential uses? First, there are two perspectives regarding their use — as an adjunct to the diagnosis of gonorrhea by the private physician and as a part of a national venereal disease control effort. Given the cur-rent character of serological tests, the major potential use appears to be in the national con-trol effort. For the private physician, the deci-sion concerning presence or absence of a gonor-rheal infection must be based on culture re-sults. Sensitivities and specificities of existing serological tests are such that some infections will be missed and some persons will be falsely designated as having gonorrhea. Nevertheless, with an appropriate test under particular cir-cumstances, it might be quicker to perform a serological test and have an indication of the situation before the cultural information is re-ceived. This would not necessarily be an eco-nomical approach. Additionally, and more im-portantly, neither a positive nor a negative ac-tion with regard to the patient can legitimately be taken solely on the basis of a serological test result.

How current serological tests could be most effectively applied to a national venereal dis-ease control effort is not clear. The most likely application would be in screening large or di-verse low prevalence segments of the popula-tion to develop information concerning preva-lence groups or areas. A more specialized form of screening would be the serotyping of strains. Strain identification would be important in de-termining which infected persons constitute a public health problem in terms of carrying and/or distributing gonorrhea. Other potential uses are in examining the impact of treatment, in

epidemiological studies, in clinically categoriz-ing particular syndromes, and in epidemiologi-cal studies of contacts.

The future of serological tests for gonorrhea rests principally upon additional research into the immune response to gonorrhea. Improving the specificity of serological tests is a primary concern. Research on the separation and purifi-cation of antigens should lead to a reduction in nonspecific serological reactions. Elucidation of the immune responses to specific antigens may yield the specificity to presence of disease that would be most useful diagnostically. The types of antibody responses made to different anti-gens may permit stages in the response to gon-orrhea to be identified. Current and future studies with primates should produce addi-tional information about the development of immunity to gonorrhea. Such information, with that developing in the typing of gonococcal strains, should enable us to identify the princi-pal gonococcal strains and the persons involved in maintaining the present epidemic of gonor-rhea.

LITERATURE CITED

1. Arko, R. J., S. J. Kraus, W. J. Brown, T. M. Buchanan, and U. S. G. Kuhn. 1974. Neis-seria gonorrhoeae: effects of systemic immu-nization on resistance of chimpanzees to ure-thral infection. J. Infect. Dis. **130**:160–163.

2. Brown, W. J., and C. T. Lucas. 1973. Gonorrhea in the chimpanzee — serological testing. Br. J. Vener. Dis. **49**:441–445.

3. Buchanan, T. M., J. Swanson, K. K. Holmes, S. J. Kraus, and E. C. Gotschlich. 1973. Quanti-tative determination of antibody to gonococcal pili. Changes in antibody levels with gonococ-cal infections. J. Clin. Invest. **52**:2896–2909.

4. Chacko, C. W., and C. M. Nair. 1969. Sero-diagnosis of gonorrhea with a microprecipitin test using a lipopolysaccharide antigen from N. gonorrhoeae. Br. J. Vener. Dis. **45**:33–39.

5. Cohen, I. R., D. S. Kellogg, and L. C. Norins. 1969. Serum antibody response in experimen-tal human gonorrhea. Br. J. Vener. Dis. **45**:325–327.

6. Danielsson, D. 1965. The demonstration of N. gonorrhoeae with the aid of fluorescent anti-bodies. 3. Studies by immunofluorescence and double diffusion — in gel technique on the an-tigen relationship between strains of N. gon-orrhoeae. Acta Pathol. Microbiol. Scand. **64**:243–266.

7. Danielsson, D., N. Thryesson, V. Falk, and J. Barr. 1972. Serologic investigation of the im-mune response in various types of gonococcal infection. Acta Derm.-Venereol. **52**:467–475.

8. Gill, T. J. 1970. Methods for detecting antibody. Immunochemistry **7**:997–1000.

9. Grados, O., and W. H. Ewing. 1970. Antigenic relationship between Escherichia coli and

Neisseria meningitidis. J. Infect. Dis. 122:100–103.

10. Kearns, D. H., R. J. O'Reilly, L. Lee, and B. G. Welch. 1973. Secretory IgA antibodies in the urethral exudate of men with uncomplicated urethritis due to Neisseria gonorrhoeae. J. Infect. Dis. 127:99–101.

11. Kraus, S. J., W. J. Brown, and R. J. Arko. 1975. Acquired and natural immunity to gonococcal infection in chimpanzees. J. Clin. Invest. 55:1349–1356.

12. Kraus, S. J., G. H. Perkins, and R. C. Geller. 1970. Lymphocyte transformation in repeated gonococcal urethritis. Infect. Immun. 2:655–658.

13. Lee, L., and J. D. Schmale. 1970. Identification of a gonococcal antigen important in the human immune response. Infect. Immun. 1:207–208.

14. Logan, L. C., P. M. Cox, and L. C. Norins. 1970. Reactivity of two gonococcal antigens in an automated microhemagglutination procedure. Appl. Microbiol. 20:907–909.

15. Magnusson, B., and J. Kjellander. 1965. Gonococcal complement fixation test in complicated and uncomplicated gonorrhea. Br. J. Vener. Dis. 41:127–131.

16. O'Reilly, R. J., L. Lee, and B. G. Welch. 1976. Secretory IgA antibody responses to Neisseria gonorrhoeae in the genital secretions of infected human females. J. Infect. Dis. 133:113–125.

17. O'Reilly, R. J., B. G. Welch, and D. S. Kellogg. 1973. An indirect fluorescent-antibody technique for the study of uncomplicated gonorrhea. II. Selection and characterization of the strain of Neisseria gonorrhoeae used as antigen. J. Infect. Dis. 127:77–83.

18. Peacock, W. L., Jr. 1971. An automated complement fixation procedure for detecting antibody to N. gonorrhoeae. Health Serv. Ment. Health Admin. Rep. 86:706–710.

19. Reising, C. 1971. Microflocculation assay for gonococcal antibody. Appl. Microbiol. 21:852–853.

20. Reising, G., and D. S. Kellogg. 1965. Detection of gonococcal antibody. Proc. Soc. Exp. Biol. Med. 120:660–663.

21. Wallace, R., B. B. Diena, H. Yugi, and L. Greenberg. 1970. The bentonite flocculation test in the assay of Neisseria antibody. Can. J. Microbiol. 16:655–659.

22. Ward, M. E., and A. A. Glynn. 1972. Human antibody response to lipopolysaccharides from Neisseria gonorrhoeae. J. Clin. Pathol. 25:56–59.

23. Welch, B. G., and R. J. O'Reilly. 1973. An indirect fluorescent antibody technique for the study of uncomplicated gonorrhea. I. Methodology. J. Infect. Dis. 127:69–76.

Chapter 36

Agglutinin Titration (Widal) for the Diagnosis of Enteric Fever and Other Enterobacterial Infections

ROLF FRETER

INTRODUCTION

With the development of improved procedures for the isolation of salmonellae from patients, diagnostic methods based on the detection of agglutinins in patients' sera, i.e., the various modifications of the "Widal test," have lost much of their former importance. Paradoxically, the rather enormous volume of literature covering every conceivable parameter which might affect the outcome and interpretation of this test (reviewed in 15 and 19) also has contributed to its eclipse. These studies have emphasized the shortcomings and the numerous variables that affect serological tests for enteric fevers, yet they have failed to stimulate the development of generally accepted standards of procedure and interpretation. The methods outlined below are therefore only guidelines. Interpretation of the Widal test depends to a considerable extent on the experience accumulated by individual laboratories for their own geographical area. For this reason, a change in locally established procedures should be contemplated only if a laboratory has clearly established that its current techniques are inadequate.

TEST PROCEDURE

The O (somatic) and H (flagellar) antigens of *Salmonella typhi* and *S. enteritidis* serotypes Paratyphi A, Paratyphi B, and Paratyphi C, i.e., the classical agents of enteric fever, have the compositions shown in Table 1.

Suspensions of O and H antigens of these bacteria are available from a number of manufacturers. Alternatively, they may be prepared as described by Edwards and Ewing (6). Serial twofold dilutions of patient's serum are prepared in 0.9% saline, starting with a 1:10 dilution. These are mixed with equal volumes of the bacterial suspension. The first tube of each series will then have a final serum dilution of 1:20. As reviewed by Olitzki (15), the traditional incubation temperature is 50 to 52 C, with 2 h of incubation for H agglutination and 20 to 24 h for O agglutination. At the end of the incubation period, the tubes should be shaken *gently*. H agglutination forms large floccular aggregates which are easily broken up by agitation. O agglutination results in a small granular aggregate. Use of a magnifying glass (a microscope ocular held against the eye is effective) often results in the detection of O agglutination at two- to fourfold higher serum dilutions than can be observed with the unaided eye. Agglutination should be compared with a negative control tube containing only saline and antigen. Such controls should be prepared separately for each antigen because different suspensions may show spontaneous agglutination because of varying degrees of roughness. The highest serum dilution which shows agglutination can be detected easily by comparison with the saline control and may be designated as the serum titer. More complex methods of computing agglutinin titers have been described (9), but convincing data to show the superiority of these in the interpretation of the Widal test are not available. Consistency among different workers of a given laboratory in observing procedural details probably is more important than are methodological niceties. It is important, therefore, that sera from successive bleedings of a given patient should be stored in a freezer and that all sera should be titrated at the same time.

Obviously, the antigens of certain serotypes or bioserotypes (e.g., Paratyphi C) may be omitted from the test in areas where these serotypes are not prevalent. Some instructions (e.g., those supplied by Difco Laboratories with their antigens) call for the use of *S. typhi* O antigen only, but retain the use of separate H antigens for the various serotypes. One must presume that this is done because *S. typhi* shares O antigen 12 with serotypes Paratyphi A and B (see Table 1). Consequently, one may expect to detect some agglutinins for *S. typhi* O antigens in patients infected with cross-reacting serotypes. However, such cross-reactions may be expected to result in titers lower than the agglutination titers with homologous antigens. Since most of the published data were obtained in titrations with homol-

TABLE 1. *Composition of O and H antigens of Salmonella*

Organism	O antigens	H antigens	
		Phase 1	Phase 2
S. typhi	9, 12	d	—
S. enteritidis			
bioser. Paratyphi A ...	1, 2, 12	a	—
ser. Paratyphi B	1, 4, 5, 12	b	1, 2
bioser. Paratyphi C ...	6, 7	c	1, 5

ogous antigens, omission of some Paratyphi serotype O antigens from the test will make interpretation difficult.

A standard antiserum of known agglutinin titer should be titrated at about weekly intervals along with the patients' sera as a quality control of the antigen suspensions used.

INTERPRETATION

A large number of variables affect the agglutinin titer in febrile illness. Consequently, those who lack extensive personal experience should consult the excellent and detailed discussion in Topley and Wilson (19) before attempting to interpret the results of Widal tests. Briefly, agglutinin titers against the typhoid and paratyphoid organisms in patients' sera are affected by:

1. The stage of the disease. Agglutinin titers usually begin to rise during the second week of enteric fever.

2. The presence of "normal" agglutinins in the patient's population group. Not only the geographical area from which a person originates is of importance here, but also a patient's age and other individual circumstances. For example, Vogel et al. (17) have shown that narcotics addicts have higher than average agglutinin titers to *S. typhi* O and H antigens.

3. The effect of previous vaccination. Administration of typhoid or TAB vaccine causes a rise in both O and H agglutinins. The latter may persist at elevated titer for several years. In contrast, the rise in O agglutinins after vaccination is more transient, lasting for only a few months. However, as reviewed elsewhere (19, see also 4 and 15), O and H agglutinins to typhoid or paratyphoid antigens also may rise during *unrelated* febrile illness, especially in vaccinated individuals. Using a sensitive hemagglutination method, Neter et al. (14) showed that during enteric infections there is frequently a fourfold or higher antibody response to unrelated bacteria from the patients' intestinal flora (in addition to a still greater antibody response to the etiological

agent). The finding by Koomen and Morgan (10) that there was no rise of typhoid or paratyphoid agglutinins in 14 patients with influenza A and in 18 patients with undiagnosed febrile illness does not justify their sweeping conclusion that "fever, as a nonspecific stimulus does not produce an elevation in circulating antibody level to certain bacterial and virus antigens in the human host, and the antibody response is specific for homologous or very closely related antigens." The issue is complicated by the fact that some of those who found rising agglutinins in "unrelated" febrile illness had to define their diagnosis on the basis of failure to culture the causative organism—a rather imprecise criterion. In view of the unsettled status of this problem it may be preferable to avoid the use of agglutinin tests as an aid in the diagnosis of enteric fever in vaccinated individuals.

4. The effect of antibiotics. Effective treatment early in the disease appears to prevent further rise in antibody titers (reviewed in 19).

5. The effect of technical details. In 1937, Gardner (9) published a study in which 64 patient sera had been distributed among four laboratories, and the agglutinin titers had been determined against standardized antigens of *S. typhi* by methods which were identical in all conceivable details (including the shape of the tubes). Fourfold or greater (often considerably greater) discrepancies in titers between laboratories were found in 29% of the titrations with standarized H antigens and in 36% of the standarized O antigen titrations. When local methods and antigen suspensions were used by the various participating laboratories, these discrepancies rose to 76% and 70%, respectively. Additional evidence of a similar nature is quoted by Schroeder (16).

In view of the above-mentioned variables, which are known to affect agglutinin titers to salmonellae, one cannot justify the practice of defining a "minimum titer" above which the Widal test should be considered "positive." Therefore, the *only* usable information to be gained from the Widal test is the observation of an *increase* in titer among sera from successive bleedings of a given patient. If such increases in titer are fourfold or greater, they may be regarded as consistent with a diagnosis of enteric fever. Obviously, this type of serological evidence is insufficient by itself to *establish* a diagnosis. The demonstration of a rise in agglutinin titer is most valuable, therefore, if it motivates the physician to submit several appropriate specimens for the isolation of the causative microorganism, the only finding which would establish the diagnosis with certainty.

RAPID SLIDE TEST

In 1936, Welch and Mickle (18) developed a rapid slide method which has since been described in essentially unmodified form in most of the standard laboratory handbooks (1, 5, 8, 11) and in the manufacturers' literature. These authors (18) compared 1,100 sera by the new method and by the standard tube test and reported good agreement between these tests in terms of detecting "positive" or "negative" sera. Unfortunately, their criterion for a positive reaction appears to have been the finding of agglutination at *any* serum dilution between 1:20 and 1:320. However, their data show considerable discrepancies between the two tests in terms of the actual agglutinin titers determined for a given serum. It is therefore impossible to decide from the available data whether or not the slide test would give results comparable to the standard tube method when the Widal test is interpreted in the only proper manner, i.e., in terms of a rise in agglutinin titer during the patient's illness. I have been unable to find later critical studies on this point. Despite its venerable age, the rapid slide method must therefore be regarded as an experimental screening test, and laboratories that use this method without having collected extensive evidence of their own should state so in their reports.

OTHER ANTIGENS OF SALMONELLA

In 1955, Eisenberg et al. recommended titrations of patients' sera for agglutinins against *Salmonella* O antigens of groups C and E, in order to detect infections with salmonellae other than the *typhi-paratyphi* organisms (7). These authors presented no data to validate this approach. Olitzki (15) and Neter (13) reviewed some studies in which rising agglutinins to such salmonellae were detected in patients by direct agglutination or by hemagglutination. Most of the standard laboratory handbooks (1, 5, 8, 11) and manufacturers' literature describe the use of additional salmonella antigens in the Widal test, and commercial antigen preparations are available. However, to my knowledge, critical studies determining the significance and specificity of agglutinins to "other" salmonellae are not available. Moreover, McCullough and Eisele (12) found, in extensive studies of experimental infections of human volunteers with a number of serotypes of *S. enteritidis* (other than the paratyphoid group), that only a minority of volunteers who developed clinical disease showed a fourfold or greater rise in agglutinins to the homologous microorganism. Only with serotype Pullorum was there a fourfold or greater agglutinin response in 19 of 25 volunteers who developed clinical disease. However, this bacterium was so avirulent for humans that enormous oral doses had to be given to induce experimental infection, and this procedure must therefore be regarded as a special instance of oral vaccination.

It seems reasonable to assume that infection with *any* bacterium will often result in some sort of agglutinin response. The experience with the classical Widal test as applied to the *typhi-paratyphi* group, reviewed above, shows quite clearly, however, that extensive studies of the clinical significance and specificity of such agglutinin responses are required before they can be utilized for diagnostic purposes. In the absence of such data, the determination of agglutinins in patients' sera to salmonellae other than the *typhi-paratyphi* group must be regarded as an experimental procedure, and the results should be reported as such.

ANTI-Vi AGGLUTININS

As reviewed in references 15 and 19, there is a large volume of literature linking the presence of Vi agglutinins to the typhoid carrier state. However, Bokkenheuser et al. (2) demonstrated, in extensive laboratory and statistical studies, that the high incidence of false-positive and false-negative reactions makes this test considerably less useful than has been assumed formerly.

HEMAGGLUTINATION

Neter and co-workers are primarily responsible for demonstrating that the use of antigen-coated erythrocytes in agglutinin titrations constitutes a convenient and highly sensitive method for the determination of serological responses to enterobacterial infections (reviewed in 13). In spite of this evidence, the method has not been adopted in routine use and must therefore be considered experimental. Recent data from several laboratories (e.g., 3) suggest that this test may become especially useful in the diagnosis of bacillary dysentery.

LITERATURE CITED

1. Bailey, W. R., and E. G. Scott. 1974. Diagnostic microbiology, 4th ed., p. 341–346. C. V. Mosby, St. Louis.
2. Bokkenheuser, V., P. Suit, and N. Richardson. 1964. A challenge to the validity of the Vi test for the detection of chronic typhoid car-

riers. Am. J. Public Health 54:1507–1513 (and earlier papers by the senior author quoted therein).

3. Caceres, A., and L. J. Mata. 1974. Serologic responses of patients with Shiga dysentery. J. Infect. Dis. 129:439–443.

4. Das, K. K., and M. V. Sant. 1972. Hemagglutination test as an aid in the laboratory diagnosis of enteric fever. Indian J. Pathol. Bacteriol. 15:104–112.

5. Davidson, I., and J. B. Henry. 1974. Todd-Sanford clinical diagnosis by laboratory methods, 15th ed., p. 1223–1224. W. B. Saunders, Philadelphia.

6. Edwards, P. R., and W. H. Ewing. 1972. Identification of Enterobacteriaceae, 3rd ed. Burgess Publishing Co., Minneapolis.

7. Eisenberg, G. M., A. J. Palazzolo, and H. F. Flippin. 1955. Clinical and microbiologic aspects of salmonellosis. N. Engl. J. Med. 253:90–94.

8. Frankel, S., S. Reitman, and A. C. Sonnenwirth. 1970. Gradwohl's clinical laboratory methods and diagnosis, 7th ed., p. 1482–1488. C. V. Mosby, St. Louis.

9. Gardner, A. D. 1937. An international experiment on the Widal reaction. J. Hyg. 37:124–142.

10. Koomen, J., Jr., and H. R. Morgan. 1954. An evaluation of the anamnestic serum reaction in certain febrile illnesses. Am. J. Med. Sci. 228:520–524.

11. Levinson, S. A., and R. P. MacFate. 1969. Clinical laboratory diagnosis, 7th ed., p. 656–658. Lea and Febiger, Philadelphia.

12. McCullough, N. B., and C. W. Eisele. 1951. Experimental human salmonellosis. IV. Pathogenicity of strains of Salmonella pullorum obtained from spray-dried whole egg. J. Infect. Dis. 89:259–265 (and earlier papers of this series quoted therein).

13. Neter, E. 1965. Indirect bacterial hemagglutination and its application to the study of bacterial antigens and serologic diagnosis. Pathol. Microbiol. 28:859–877.

14. Neter, E., O. Westphal, O. Lüderitz, and E. A. Gorzynski. 1965. The bacterial hemagglutination test for the demonstration of antibodies to enterobacteriaceae. Ann. N.Y. Acad. Sci. 66:141–156.

15. Olitzki, A. 1972. Enteric fevers, p. 330–387. S. Karger, Basel.

16. Schroeder, S. A. 1968. Interpretation of serologic tests for typhoid fever. J. Am. Med. Assoc. 206:839–840.

17. Vogel, H., C. E. Cherubin, and S. J. Millian. 1970. Febrile agglutinins in narcotic addicts. Am. J. Clin. Pathol. 53:932–935.

18. Welch, H., and F. L. Mickle. 1936. A rapid slide test for the serological diagnosis of typhoid and paratyphoid fevers. Am. J. Public Health 26:248–255.

19. Wilson, G. S., and A. A. Miles. 1964. Topley and Wilson's principles of bacteriology and immunity, 5th ed., p. 1841–1848. The Williams & Wilkins Co., Baltimore. (The 6th edition, 1975, reprints a condensed version of this chapter without adding new information.)

Chapter 37

Immune Response to *Vibrio cholerae*

JOHN C. FEELEY AND WALLIS E. DeWITT

INTRODUCTION

Several methods have been used to measure the immune response of humans to infection with *Vibrio cholerae*. Early literature on the subject has been reviewed extensively by Pollitzer (33); more recent work has been aptly summarized by Barua (1).

The most practical and easily performed methods for this purpose involve the measurement of antibodies against somatic O antigens of *V. cholerae* by agglutination or vibriocidal antibody assays. Another approach of value involves the measurement of antibody ("antitoxin") against the heat-labile enterotoxin (11, 18) produced by this organism. Relevant studies pertinent to these procedures are discussed below.

Agglutination test

A variety of procedures and antigens have produced conflicting results (33). There is now almost universal agreement that O antibodies are best measured in agglutination tests by use of a suspension of living vibrios as the agglutinogen (15, 21, 23, 25, 37). Unlike the results with *Salmonella*, O agglutination with *V. cholerae* occurs rapidly, whereas H agglutination is a slowly developing reaction that is often difficult to detect and does not take place under the test conditions specified below (15). Furthermore, H antigens of *V. cholerae* are weak antigens and lack the specificity of O antigens since both *V. cholerae* and noncholera vibrios may share common H antigens (8, 35). Boiled suspensions can be used to measure O agglutinins (10), but their agglutinability is greatly reduced. In fact, a study by Vella and Fielding (37) has shown that live antigens are more sensitive than antigens killed by a large number of methods.

When live antigens are used, a fourfold or greater rise in titer has been found to occur approximately 90 to 95% of the time between acute- and convalescent-phase serum specimens obtained from persons with bacteriologically confirmed cases of cholera (2, 4, 6, 7, 14, 23, 34, 36). A variety of techniques have been used (1); the method used in this laboratory (see

below) is a tube agglutination test, described earlier (28). A microtiter agglutination test method amenable to assay of small serum samples (e.g., finger-prick blood) has been described (6). Our laboratory favors the vibriocidal procedure (see below) for the microtiter system because it is easier to read end points.

Vibriocidal test

Vibriocidal tests depend on the bactericidal effect of O antibody in the presence of complement on *V. cholerae*. Again, a number of techniques have been used. Dilutions of serum are allowed to react with a standardized inoculum of *V. cholerae* in the presence of excess guinea pig complement; after an incubation period to allow killing of the bacteria, the various dilutions of serum and appropriate controls are subcultured on agar (2, 17, 34) or in broth (4, 14, 28, 38) to assess the bactericidal effect. The procedure requires careful standardization and can be made extremely sensitive by using a small inoculum. The procedures in use in this laboratory are (i) a tube test (28) that is a modification of the broth assay system of Muschel and Treffers (31) and (ii) a microtiter test nearly identical to that described by Benenson et al. (4) which is based on the tube test procedure (28) with volumes reduced to microtiter amounts.

Like the agglutination test, the vibriocidal test can be expected to demonstrate an antibody rise in sera from 90 to 95% of patients with bacteriologically confirmed cases of cholera (2, 4, 14, 34). Authors who have made such a comparison have found a very high, in fact nearly perfect, correlation between the results of living vibrio agglutination tests and vibriocidal tests in detecting diagnostic rises in antibody levels with paired acute-convalescent sera (14, 34). The vibriocidal test is significantly more sensitive than the agglutination test; therefore, it detects a greater background of antibody levels in normal or acute-phase sera and gives higher titers with convalescent-phase sera (14, 22, 34).

The vibriocidal antibody test has been extensively used for serological surveys, and acquisition of significant levels of antibody, either through natural exposure or as a result of vaccine, has been correlated with apparent immunity to cholera on a population basis (29).

A radiobacteriolytic method based on release of ^{51}Cr from labeled V. cholerae cells (in lieu of assay for "killing") in the presence of antibody and complement has recently been described (9) and deserves further study.

Indirect hemagglutination test (for antibacterial antibody)

Indirect hemagglutination (IHA) tests with V. cholerae have been examined by a number of workers in the past. In general, they have not been found to have advantages over vibriocidal or agglutination tests for this purpose. For example, Barua and Sack (2) found the IHA test less sensitive than the Vibrio agglutination test with live antigens. Our own experience (unpublished data) has been similar.

Antitoxic antibody

The heat-labile enterotoxin produced by V. cholerae is antigenic and elicits an antibody response ("antitoxin") in many patients who are convalescing from the disease.

Antitoxin levels may be assayed by in vivo toxin neutralization assays such as the ligated rabbit ileal loop (27, 32), the infant rabbit model (18, 19), or the rabbit skin permeability factor (PF) test (11, 12). In vitro neutralization tests in which Y1 adrenal cell cultures (13) or Chinese hamster ovary cell cultures (24) are used are also feasible. The best standardized in vivo procedures are the skin PF assay (11, 12) and the much more laborious ileal loop assay (27, 32). A standard antitoxin unit has been proposed by Craig (11, 12), and standard antitoxin calibrated according to Craig's unitage is available from the Geographic Medicine Branch, National Institute of Allergy and Infectious Diseases. The in vitro cell culture assays have not been extensively used for this purpose with cholera antitoxin but should be readily amenable to standardization since they are sensitive and reproducible assays for cholera enterotoxin.

Antitoxin levels may also be measured in vitro by passive hemagglutination tests (20, 26). Good correlations with toxin neutralization antitoxin assays have been obtained (20, 26); stable preserved sensitized erythrocytes can be used in the test (26), and it can be performed in microtiter configuration (20, 26).

A significant antitoxin response was detected in the ileal loop model (27, 32) and the PF test with sera from convalescent patients with bacteriologically confirmed cases of cholera (5).

Pierce et al. (32) in a study of 16 patients by the ileal loop method found the antitoxin response to be variable and frequently of small magnitude but persisting at elevated levels for 12 to 18 months. Unlike the vibriocidal antibody response, it was diminished by prompt antimicrobial therapy. Benenson et al. (5) reported a diagnostic rise in 73% of bacteriologically proven cases by the PF test. Hochstein et al. (26) found a response in 9 of 15 cholera patients for whom paired sera were available using a hemagglutination test. Measurement of antitoxin response would appear, therefore, somewhat less sensitive than the agglutination or vibriocidal tests. However, it may offer certain diagnostic advantages in some cases since, unlike vibriocidal or agglutinating antibody, antitoxin is not stimulated by most currently available cholera vaccines (16, 30).

Detailed test procedures for antitoxin assays are not described below because of the requirements for technical experience and for special reagents not generally available (e.g., toxin, standard antitoxin). Based on our experience, we would recommend the skin PF test (12) and the indirect hemagglutination test (20, 26) as the most suitable and most easily standardized in vivo and in vitro procedures at this time for most laboratories that wish to assay antitoxin.

CLINICAL INDICATIONS

A retrospective diagnosis of cholera can be established with a high degree of certainty by titration of paired acute- and convalescent-phase sera by agglutination or vibriocidal tests. Acute-phase sera should be collected 0 to 3 days and convalescent sera 10 to 21 days after onset of illness. Demonstration of a fourfold or greater rise in titer is diagnostic, provided recent (within 2 weeks) cholera immunization can be ruled out. Titration of single convalescent sera is usually not worthwhile, except that the absence of vibriocidal or agglutinating antibody 10 to 28 days after illness would raise serious doubts about the likelihood of a diagnosis of cholera. Since vibriocidal and agglutinating antibody titers reach a peak between 10 and 21 days after onset and decline within 3 weeks, falling titers may also be useful, again assuming that immunization shortly prior to illness can be excluded.

Antitoxin titrations could be helpful in cases where there are cholera immunization histories, since antitoxin occurs with low frequency in the normal adult population (12) and is not induced by currently available cholera vaccines.

Unexplained elevated levels of antibody

measured by the more sensitive vibriocidal antibody tests are found in most adults in the United States (22), and increasing levels develop with advancing age from childhood in Bangladesh even in the absence of known or suspected cholera infection (29). Antigenic cross-reactions detectable by agglutination or vibriocidal tests are known or reported to occur with *Brucella* sp. (15, 22), *Yersinia enterocolitica* serotype 9 (3), *Citrobacter* sp. (22), and possibly other enteric organisms (33). Except in known cholera endemic areas, one must assume that these naturally occurring antibodies are due to exposure to antigens other than *V. cholerae*.

REAGENTS

Only the macroscopic tube agglutination and microtiter vibriocidal assays are described below. Either procedure is an acceptable method for retrospective serodiagnosis of cholera.

V. cholerae (either classical or E1 Tor biotype) occurs mainly as two serotypes: Ogawa (O antigen formula = AB) and Inaba (O antigenic formula = AC). A third and very rare serotype, "Hikojima" (ABC), also occurs.

Because of differences in type-specific antigens B and C, it has been the practice of most laboratories, including ours, to use both serotypes as test antigens. Antibodies with anti-A, -B, and -C specificities operate in both tests. Since the dominant antibody response generally is group specific (anti-A), experience indicates that both serotypes are not necessary except in very rare cases. When a single antigen is used, the Ogawa serotype is preferred for two reasons: (i) it often gives greater cross-reactivity with anti-Inaba sera than Inaba antigen gives with anti-Ogawa sera (J. C. Feeley, unpublished data), and (ii) the Ogawa serotype shows a lower level of cross-reactivity with *Brucella* (15, 22), *Citrobacter* (22), and *Y. enterocolitica* (3).

Antigens

Stock cultures of *V. cholerae* serotype Ogawa (strain VC12) and serotype Inaba (strain VC13) are maintained in the freeze-dried state. After reconstitution and purity checks, the cultures are maintained on Trypticase agar (Trypticase [BBL], 1%; NaCl, 1%; agar, 1.5%) slants at 4 C with monthly transfers. It is our practice to make no more than three transfers before opening a new freeze-dried culture. These cultures are used for both vibriocidal and agglutination tests.

Veronal-buffered saline

Veronal-buffered saline (VBS) is prepared by dissolving 83.0 g of NaCl and 10.19 g of Na-5,5 diethyl-barbiturate in 1,500 ml of distilled water in a 2,000-ml volumetric flask. Then 34.58 ml of exactly 1 N HCl is added, and the volume is brought up to 2,000 ml. The solution is stored in a refrigerator and discarded after 2 weeks. For use in the test, fivefold dilution is made in sterile distilled water (pH should be 7.3), and the unused portion is discarded daily. Addition of Mg^{2+} (31) is unnecessary because of the high concentration of guinea pig serum in the test.

Complement

Pooled nonvibriocidal guinea pig serum is used. Individual guinea pig sera are pretested for naturally occurring vibriocidal activity against *V. cholerae* at the same concentration used in the tests; then 25 to 30 nonvibriocidal sera are pooled, distributed in 5- to 10-ml amounts, and stored at −70 C. Activity is retained for at least 6 months. In our experience, approximately 5% of normal guinea pig sera have natural vibriocidal activity, although this may vary with different animal colonies. Commercial freeze-dried guinea pig complement sometimes may be used. In this case, the diluent supplied by the manufacturer should not be used since it contains a preservative; VBS (pH 7.3) should be used instead. Other animal sources of complement have been unsatisfactory.

Source of reagents

The above cultures may be obtained from the Bacterial Immunology Branch, Bacteriology Division, Center for Disease Control, Atlanta, Ga. 30333. Other cultures can be used but have not been evaluated extensively.

Positive control sera can be prepared by immunization of rabbits with *V. cholerae*, preferably using both serotypes separately and making a pool of serum. If a single serotype is used, it should be Inaba, since anti-Inaba serum is slightly more cross-reactive with the Ogawa serotype than vice versa. The serum should be stored frozen at −20 C in small amounts. No preservative should be added since live organisms are used as antigens in both vibriocidal and agglutination tests.

A reference preparation of cholera convalescent human serum (catalog no. G-005-501-572) can be obtained from the Research Resources Branch, National Institute of Allergy and Infectious Diseases, Bethesda, Md. 20014. This serum has been subjected to collaborative vibriocidal assays by several laboratories, including the Center for Disease Control, which have used this test, and the serum has been found useful for standardization of the procedure.

Normal rabbit or human serum can be used as a negative control. However, many healthy human subjects but only a few normal rabbits can be expected to have detectable levels of naturally occurring antibody by the vibriocidal test.

All other reagents, media, etc., are available from commercial sources.

TEST PROCEDURES

Tube agglutination test

Serum preparation. Serum may be tested with or without inactivation at 56 C for 30 min with no detectable difference, although some slight lysis of the live antigen suspension may be noted in low dilutions with noninactivated sera having high titers. Serum should not contain a preservative since it might cause lysis of the rather light antigen suspension used.

Antigen preparation. The test strains (Ogawa only or Ogawa and Inaba) are inoculated with one loopful of growth from a 16- to 18-h (overnight) culture on Trypticase agar into 100 ml of Trypticase broth (Trypticase, 1%; NaCl, 1%) in a 250-ml Erlenmeyer flask. Then they are incubated at 35 C without shaking for 4 to 6 h or until a turbidity of 1 opacity unit of the U.S. Opacity Standard (obtained from Bureau of Biologics, Food and Drug Administration, Bethesda, Md. 20014) is achieved or exceeded. If the culture is too turbid, it should be diluted in sterile Trypticase broth until the turbidity level is the same as that of the opacity standard by visual comparison. At this point, the antigen suspension may be used immediately or placed in an ice-water bath for up to 4 h.

Test protocol.

1. For each serum (unknowns and controls) to be tested, set up a row of six to eight 13 × 100 mm tubes for each serotype antigen to be used.

2. Add 0.9 ml of 0.85% NaCl to the first tube and 0.5 ml of 0.85% NaCl to the remaining tubes.

3. Add 0.1 ml of serum to the first tube, mix, and serially transfer 0.5-ml volumes to successive tubes in the row, discarding 0.5 ml from the last tube.

4. Add 0.5 ml of each antigen to each tube containing serum dilutions and to an antigen control tube containing 0.5 ml of saline.

5. Shake the rack and incubate in a 37 C water bath for 1 h. Tests may be read at this time or, preferably, after overnight refrigeration at 4 C. Agglutination is easier to read after overnight refrigeration, and end points will often be one dilution higher.

6. After the tubes warm to room temperature (to allow condensation film to evaporate), tap each tube gently and observe for agglutination. A black background attached behind the hood of a fluorescent lamp is useful.

7. Record the titer as the dilution factor of the highest final dilution (after antigen is added, the first tube dilution is 1:20) showing definite agglutination. Antigen control and negative serum control should show no agglutination, and the positive control serum should react within ±1 dilution of its expected titer.

Microtiter vibriocidal antibody test

Serum preparation. Sterile serum is preferred, but not absolutely essential. Visibly contaminated sera are unsatisfactory. Sera are not inactivated, but inactivation at 56 C for 30 min rarely affects the titer except for low levels of naturally occurring antibody in certain normal sera. Since an excess of complement is used in the system, inactivation of complement in the test serum is not an important consideration.

Antigen preparation. The afternoon prior to the test, the test strain(s) should be inoculated on heart infusion agar (HIA) slants and incubated at 35 C. Uninoculated HIA slants should also be placed in the incubator to prewarm. After 16 to 18 h of incubation, the prewarmed slants should be inoculated with one loopful from the overnight culture and then incubated for 4 h at 35 C. Chilled VBS (pH 7.3) is used to wash growth from slants, and the turbidity is photometrically adjusted to the equivalent of 10 opacity units/ml (U.S. Opacity Standard). For preparation of a suspension of 1 opacity unit/ml, the standardized suspension is diluted 1:10 in chilled VBS. The suspension should be promptly mixed with complement, as described below.

Complement. Guinea pig complement should be diluted 1:5 in chilled VBS. Equal volumes of complement and of 1 opacity unit/ml bacterial suspension are mixed. The mixture should be maintained in an ice-water bath and used within 30 min.

Test protocol.

1. Use round-bottom microtiter plates. Prepare an initial 1:5 dilution of each serum in microtiter wells by placing one loopful (0.025 ml) of each serum in 0.1 ml (4 × 0.025-ml drop) of VBS.

2. For each serum to be tested (unknown and control), allow a row of 8 to 10 wells for each antigen used. Add 0.025 ml (1 drop) of VBS to each of these wells.

3. Add one loopful (0.025 ml) of serum di-

luted 1:5 (step 1) to the first well, rotate the loops, and transfer serially to successive wells in the row, discarding one loopful from the last well.

4. Set up two complement controls for each test culture in 13×100 mm tubes to be used to follow growth photometrically. Add 0.5 ml of VBS to each tube. For each culture also include a complement control well containing 0.025 ml of VBS (to be used for visual grading of growth).

5. Add 1 drop (0.025 ml) of complement-bacteria mixture to each well as appropriate and 0.5 ml to the complement-photometer control tubes.

6. Seal the plates with sealing tape and incubate plates and complement control tube(s) in a 37 C water bath for 1 h.

7. After incubation, add 0.15 ml of Brain Heart Infusion broth to plate wells and 3.0 ml to complement-photometer tubes. Reseal the plates and return them to the water bath along with one complement control tube for each culture. Place the other complement control tube in an ice bath (this will be used as a photometer blank).

8. Allow growth to proceed until the optical density of the complement control tube reaches 0.15 at 580 nm in a Coleman Junior spectrophotometer in which the refrigerated tube is used as a blank. This is near the end of, but still within, the logarithmic phase of growth and usually requires 2 to 2.5 h. (It is advisable to determine a growth curve for the particular conditions [media, complement, etc.] prevailing in the laboratory.) Growth should not be

continued beyond this point.

9. Read the plates by placing them on a test reading mirror with transmitted light against a black background. Crystal clear yellowish wells (growth inhibited) are readily distinguished from turbid wells in which growth has occurred. The titer is recorded as the dilution factor of the highest dilution (after bacteria-complement mixture is added, the first well is diluted 1:20) in which growth was visibly inhibited as compared with the complement control well. This can best be judged after overnight refrigeration, because then both turbidity and buttons of sedimented bacteria are readily visible. The positive control serum should react within ±1 dilution of its expected titer. The negative control should show no bactericidal effect.

Note: If desired, an anticomplementary control in which hemolysin-sensitized sheep erythrocytes are used to detect anticomplementary sera can be included. In hundreds of sera tested, an anticomplementary reaction was never encountered, and the procedure was eliminated. A method is described by Benenson et al. (4). Because of the excess complement in the system and the high dilutions of sera at which end points are detected, this is an unlikely problem.

INTERPRETATION

Some concept of the normal range of agglutination and vibriocidal titers experienced in the normal population of healthy individuals in the United States is given in Table 1. A more extensive treatment of the problem of naturally

TABLE 1. *Distribution of anti-Ogawa titers in sera of healthy individuals in the United States*

Test	Year of collection	No. of sera	No. with titers of							
			<20	20	40	80	160	320	640	>640
Agglutination[a] ...	1962	133	113	9	6	1	3	0	1	0
Vibriocidal[b]	1967–68	441	309		95[c]		16	10	7	4

[a] Feeley et al., unpublished data.
[b] Based on Gangarosa et al. (22).
[c] Includes 20 to 80 range.

TABLE 2. *Antibody response of cholera patients as measured by agglutination and vibriocidal tests[a]*

Day of disease	No. of sera tested	Agglutination		Vibriocidal	
		GMAT[b]	Range	GMAT	Range
1–4	39	23	<32–512	362	<32–16,380
5–10	24	223	<32–4,096	11,590	512–262,144
11–22	27	178	32–2,048	23,170	512–131,072

[a] Adapted from Feeley (14).
[b] GMAT = geometric mean antibody titer. For purposes of calculation, titers of <32 were arbitrarily assumed to be 16.

acquired antibody has been presented by Gangarosa et al. (22). Data illustrative of the agglutinating and vibriocidal antibody responses of cholera patients are shown in Table 2.

As stated earlier under Clinical Indications, paired or serial sera are necessary for establishment of a certain retrospective diagnosis of cholera. Barring the possible demonstration of a significant change in titer by either agglutination or vibriocidal tests that is chronologically related to onset of illness, the only significant interpretation possible with a single serum specimen is that the absence of vibriocidal or agglutinating antibody 10 to 28 days after illness raises serious doubts about the likelihood of cholera.

Other aspects of interpretation of serodiagnostic methods are discussed under Clinical Indications.

LITERATURE CITED

1. Barua, D. 1974. Laboratory diagnosis of cholera, p. 85–126. *In* D. Barua and W. Burrows (ed.), Cholera. W. B. Saunders Co., Philadelphia.
2. Barua, D., and R. B. Sack. 1964. Serological studies in cholera. Indian J. Med. Res. 52:855–866.
3. Barua, D., and Y. Watanabe. 1972. Vibriocidal antibodies induced by *Yersinia enterocolitica* serotype IX. J. Hyg. 70:161–169.
4. Benenson, A. S., A. Saad, and W. H. Mosley. 1968. Serological studies in cholera. 2. The vibriocidal antibody response of cholera patients determined by a microtechnique. Bull. WHO 38:277–285.
5. Benenson, A. S., A. Saad, W. H. Mosley, and A. Ahmed. 1968. Serological studies in cholera. 3. Serum toxin neutralization – rise in titre in response to infection with *Vibrio cholerae*, and the level in the "normal" population of East Pakistan. Bull. WHO 38:287–295.
6. Benenson, A. S., A. Saad, and M. Paul. 1968. Serological studies in cholera. 1. Vibrio agglutinin response of cholera patients determined by a microtechnique. Bull. WHO 38:267–276.
7. Beran, G. W. 1964. Serological studies on cholera. 1. Antibody levels observed in vaccinated and convalescent persons. Am. J. Trop. Med. Hyg. 13:698–707.
8. Bhattacharya, F. K., and S. Mukerjee. 1974. Serological analysis of the flagellar or H agglutinating antigens of cholera and NAG vibrios. Ann. Microbiol. (Paris) 125A:167–181.
9. Blachman, U., W. R. Clark, and M. J. Pickett. 1973. Radiobacteriolysis: a new technique using chromium-51 for assaying anti-*Vibrio cholerae* antibodies. Infect. Immun. 7:53–61.
10. Burrows, W., A. N. Mather, V. G. McGann, and S. M. Wagner. 1946. Studies on immunity to Asiatic cholera. II. The O and H antigenic structure of the cholera and related vibrios. J. Infect. Dis. 79:168–197.
11. Craig, J. P. 1971. Cholera toxins, p. 189–254. *In* S. Kadis, T. C. Montie, and S. J. Ajl (ed.), Microbial toxins, vol. IIA. Academic Press Inc., New York.
12. Craig, J. P., E. R. Eichner, and R. B. Hornick. 1972. Cutaneous responses to cholera toxin in man. I. Responses in unimmunized American males. J. Infect. Dis. 125:203–215.
13. Donta, S. T., and D. M. Smith. 1974. Stimulation of steroidogenesis in tissue culture by enterotoxigenic *Escherichia coli* and its neutralization by specific antiserum. Infect. Immun. 9:500–505.
14. Feeley, J. C. 1965. Comparison of vibriocidal and agglutinating antibody responses in cholera patients. Proc. Cholera Res. Symp. U.S. Public Health Serv. Publ. No. 1328, p. 220–222.
15. Feeley, J. C. 1969. Somatic O antigen relationship of *Brucella* and *Vibrio cholerae*. J. Bacteriol. 99:645–649.
16. Feeley, J. C., and C. O. Roberts. 1969. Immunological responses of laboratory animals to cholera vaccine, toxin, and toxoid. Tex. Rep. Biol. Med. 27:213–226.
17. Finkelstein, R. A. 1962. Vibriocidal antibody inhibition (VAI) analysis: a technique for the identification of the predominant vibriocidal antibodies in serum and for the detection and identification of *Vibrio cholerae* antigens. J. Immunol. 89:264–271.
18. Finkelstein, R. A. 1973. Cholera. Crit. Rev. Microbiol. 2:553–623.
19. Finkelstein, R. A., and P. Atthasampunna. 1967. Immunity against experimental cholera. Proc. Soc. Exp. Biol. Med. 125:465–469.
20. Finkelstein, R. A., and J. W. Peterson. 1970. *In vitro* detection of antibody to cholera enterotoxin in cholera patients and laboratory animals. Infect. Immun. 1:21–29.
21. Gallut, J., and G. Brounst. 1949. Sur la mise en évidence des agglutines cholériques. Ann. Inst. Pasteur (Paris) 76:557–559.
22. Gangarosa, E. J., W. E. DeWitt, J. C. Feeley, and M. R. Adams. 1970. Significance of vibriocidal antibodies with regard to immunity to cholera. J. Infect. Dis. 121(Suppl.):S36–S44.
23. Goodner, K., H. L. Smith, Jr., and H. Stempen. 1960. Serologic diagnosis of cholera. J. Albert Einstein Med. Cent. 8:143–147.
24. Guerrant, R. L., L. L. Brunton, T. C. Schnaitman, L. I. Rebhun, and A. G. Gilman. 1974. Cyclic adenosine monophosphate and alteration of Chinese hamster ovary cell morphology: a rapid, sensitive in vitro assay for the enterotoxins of *Vibrio cholerae* and *Escherichia coli*. Infect. Immun. 10:320–327.
25. Heiberg, B. 1935. On the classification of *Vibrio cholerae* and the cholera-like vibrios. Nyt Nordisk Forlag-Arnold Busck, Copenhagen.
26. Hochstein, H. D., J. C. Feeley, and W. E. DeWitt. 1970. Titration of cholera antitoxin in human sera by microhemagglutination with formalinized erythrocytes. Appl. Microbiol. 19:742–745.

27. Kasai, G. J., and W. Burrows. 1966. The titration of cholera toxin and antitoxin in the rabbit ileal loop. J. Infect. Dis. **116**:606–614.

28. McIntyre, O. R., and J. C. Feeley. 1964. Passive serum protection of the infant rabbit against experimental cholera. J. Infect. Dis. **114**:468–475.

29. Mosley, W. H. 1969. The role of immunity in cholera. A review of epidemiological and serological studies. Tex. Rep. Biol. Med. **27**(Suppl. 1):227–241.

30. Mosley, W. H., and A. Ahmed. 1969. Active and passive immunization in the adult rabbit ileal loop model as an assay for production of antitoxin immunity by cholera vaccines. J. Bacteriol. **100**:547–549.

31. Muschel, L. H., and H. P. Treffers. 1956. Quantitative studies on the bactericidal actions of serum and complement. I. A rapid photometric growth assay for bactericidal activity. J. Immunol. **76**:1–10.

32. Pierce, N. F., J. G. Banwell, R. B. Sack, R. C. Mitra, and A. Mondal. 1970. Magnitude and duration of antitoxic response to human infection with *Vibrio cholerae*. J. Infect. Dis. 121(Suppl.):S31–S35.

33. Pollitzer, R. 1959. Cholera. WHO Monogr. Ser. No. 43, p. 266–270.

34. Sack, R. B., D. Barua, R. Saxena, and C. C. J. Carpenter. 1966. Vibriocidal and agglutinating antibody patterns in cholera patients. J. Infect. Dis. **116**:630–640.

35. Sakazaki, R., K. Tamura, C. Z. Gomez, and R. Sen. 1970. Serological studies on the cholera group of vibrios. Jpn. J. Med. Sci. Biol. **23**:13–20.

36. Smith, H. L., Jr., and K. Goodner. 1965. Antibody patterns in cholera. Proc. Cholera Res. Symp. U.S. Public Health Serv. Publ. No. 1328, p. 215–219.

37. Vella, E. E., and P. Fielding. 1963. Note on the agglutinability of cholera suspensions. Trans. R. Soc. Trop. Med. Hyg. **57**:112–114.

38. Verwey, W. F., Y. Watanabe, J. C. Guckian, H. R. Williams, Jr., P. E. Phillips, S. S. Rocha, Jr., and E. B. Bridgeforth. 1969. Serological responses of human volunteers to cholera vaccine. Tex. Rep. Biol. Med. **27**(Suppl. 1):243–274.

Chapter 38

Immune Response to *Yersinia* and *Pasteurella*

STEN WINBLAD

INTRODUCTION

The species of *Yersinia, Pasteurella,* and *Francisella* separated from the former common group called pasteurellae have several common characteristics. They often cause infections in animals as well as in humans, and often vectors are the carriers of the infecting agent. Another common characteristic is the involvement of the lymphatic nodes in the early stages of the infection, resulting in enlargement of the regional lymph nodes as, for example, "buboes" in the plague. Furthermore, a marked increase in titer of antibodies is easily demonstrated shortly after the infection. Some of these microorganisms, for example, *Y. pestis* and *F. tularensis,* are too dangerous to work with in ordinary laboratories, and therefore the diagnosis of these infections must often be based on the immunological response.

YERSINIA ENTEROCOLITICA (YERSINIOSIS ENTEROCOLITICA)

The immunological response to infections with *Y. enterocolitica* is best demonstrated by agglutinins in the patient's serum (23). The Widal reaction method is without doubt the best way to follow the antibody response. Strains of *Y. enterocolitica* are differentiated by the O-lipopolysaccharide antigen into about 28 O serotypes (16–18, 20; G. Wauters, Thesis, Vander, Louvain, Belgium). Furthermore, differentiation may be based on fermentation reactions (biotypes) or according to their source, from humans or water. The different O serotypes agree very well with the specific biotypes (10). The O serotypes are, however, from an epidemiological point of view, the most important characteristics. H agglutinins also exist but are not suitable for classification (15). The O serotypes 3, 8, and 9 dominate in human infections. O serotype 1 is observed in chinchillas, and O serotype 2, in hares and goats. O serotype 3 is the etiological organism from human cases of yersiniosis enterocolitica in Europe, Africa, Asia (Japan), Canada, and many other countries. O serotype 8 has, so far, been observed only in the United States, where cases caused by infection with O serotype 3 seem to

be rare. Infection with O serotype 9 is predominantly observed in Finland, Hungary, the Netherlands, and the Scandinavian countries.

The antigen for immunological diagnosis must be chosen from a geographical viewpoint. In Europe serotype 8 does not play any role. In the United States serotype O-8 must be the antigen of choice, but serotypes O-3 and O-9 may also be used. Agglutinin reactions on the model of the "Widal" reaction are to be preferred. Passive hemagglutinin reaction shows antibodies cross-reacting with common O antigens from other gram-negative microorganisms. In the Widal agglutination the O antigen of *Y. enterocolitica* seems to be very specific and rarely gives a cross-reaction phenomenon.

Clinical indications

Immunological methods should be combined with attempts to isolate these organisms from feces or from extirpated appendices or mesenteric lymph nodes. The agglutinins have the advantage of immunological specificity and seldom give cross-reactions against other gram-negative bacteria. For that reason, high agglutinin titers are very significant. Agglutinins are, however, low in titer or nondetectable during the first 5 to 6 days of the intestinal symptoms but develop very soon thereafter in high titers (Fig. 1). During the first days of illness, attempts should be made to cultivate the bacteria.

The clinical panorama of yersiniosis enterocolitica is illustrated in Fig. 2 (21). Small children get acute gastroenteritis (5), usually of short duration and often connected with fever. Older children and youths react with symptoms of appendicitis, but no real appendicitis is found upon operation. Instead, a state of acute terminal ileitis, lymphadenitis mesenterica, or only pseudoappendicitis is observed. People of older ages react with acute enteritis, sometimes complicated with erythema nodosum (19), fever, or arthritis. Such symptoms are often of long duration (4). Cases with myocarditis (2) and acute glomerulonephritis have also been observed. Practically all cases of acute terminal ileitis in Sweden seem to have been caused by infections with *Y. enterocolitica,* proved either by positive culture from stools or appendix or by a significant immune response against the *Y. enterocolitica* antigen (14). The agglutinin test is also very useful for diagnosing cases of pseudoappendicitis (during the convalescent state), enteritis, erythema nodosum, or acute arthritis.

Test procedure

Agglutinin against O antigen. The serum complement is inactivated by heating the serum to 56 C for 30 min.

Tube method. Patient serum is mixed as shown in Table 1 with resulting dilutions of 1:10 to 1:5,120. The solution may be either saline or Veronal buffer at pH 7.4. (Diemal-Na, 10.2 g; NaCl, 83.29 g; distilled water, 1.5 liters; $CaCl_2$, 85 g; $MgCl_2 \cdot 6H_2O$, 500 g; 1 N HCl, 31.3 ml; and distilled water to 2 liters. This solution is autoclaved for 30 min at 120 C and then is diluted

TABLE 1. *Agglutination technique (serum dilution 1:10 to 1:20, etc.) for yersiniosis enterocolitica*

Prepn	Amt (ml)						
	Tube 1	Tube 2	Tube 3	Tube 4	Tube 5	Tube 6	etc.
Buffer solution or saline	0.45	0.25	0.25	0.25	0.25	0.25	...
Serum, undiluted	0.05						
Serum dilutions transferred .		0.25	0.25	0.25	0.25	0.25	
O-antigen dilutions	0.25	0.25	0.25	0.25	0.25	0.25	

1:4 with distilled water before use.) The antigen is also suitably diluted for easy estimation of the Widal reaction. The reaction is read after being incubated overnight in a water bath at 52 C. It is advisable to observe the granular sedimentation before shaking the tubes. This test is suitable for blood serum but is not applicable to synovial fluid, spinal fluid, or urine. Controls must always be maintained against a serum of high agglutinin titer and a negative serum; also include a tube without serum, to avoid overlooking spontaneous agglutination of the antigen.

This is the method of choice for testing agglutinins against antigens O-3 and O-8. Agglutinins against O-9 are best observed by using OH antigen prepared with formalinized bacteria (1). This method is exactly the same as the agglutination method for *Y. pseudotuberculosis.*

Reagents. It is essential to avoid rough transformation of these strains. The O antigen of choice for serotype O-3 is strain My O (strain "Winblad," Pasteur Institut number Ye 134). Strain Py 311 (Pasteur Institut number Ye 106) and strain "Sonnenwirth," in the Atlanta collection A 9466 (Pasteur Institut number Ye 636), are recommended for the O-8 antigen. The following strains representing the antigen for O-9 are recommended: N 5385 from Malmö, Sweden (Pasteur Institut number 336), or Fy 4 Ahvonen, Finland 169/68 (Pasteur Institut number 347). All strains for antigen preparation can be obtained from the Center for Disease Control, Atlanta, Ga., from the Institut Pasteur collection of *Yersinia* strains, or from

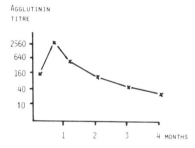

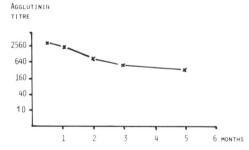

FIG. 1. *Agglutinin titers in yersiniosis enterocolitica. Top: acute terminal ileitis (appendix and feces cultivation positive). Bottom: erythema nodosum and enteritis (feces cultivation positive).*

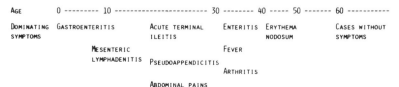

FIG. 2. *Clinical panorama of human yersiniosis enterocolitica (serotype 3).*

the Bacteriological Laboratory, Malmö General Hospital, S-214 01 Malmö, Sweden.

Preparation of Widal O antigen. The strain is cultivated on 10 blood agar plates for 2 days at room temperature. The culture is then suspended in saline. The collected bacterial suspension is centrifuged, and the sediment is washed once in saline and then resuspended in 10 ml of saline. The suspension is autoclaved at 120 C for 1 h; alternatively, it may be heated in boiling water for 1 h. The suspension is then centrifuged and washed once in saline. This washing is very important as it helps to prevent a zone phenomenon in the reaction. The sediment is collected in 5 ml of saline and diluted in a suitable dilution for the Widal agglutination. Collection of the strains from blood agar plates must be done with care. Laboratory infections, though seldom observed, can be avoided by proper technique.

Preparation of the Widal OH antigen. This is useful for testing agglutinins against *Y. enterocolitica* O-9 and *Y. pseudotuberculosis*. The strain is cultivated on 10 blood agar petri plates. After incubation for 2 days at room temperature, the culture is suspended in saline. The suspension is centrifuged, and the sediment is washed once in saline and resuspended in 10 ml of saline to which is added 0.5 ml of 40% formalin. Sterility is controlled by observing that no growth appears after 1 day at room temperature. The suspension is then centrifuged, and the sediment is washed once again in saline; thereafter, it is resuspended in 5 ml of saline and suitably diluted for the "Widal" agglutination. It should be observed that the reaction temperature for the OH agglutination will be 37 C overnight.

Interpretation

In cases of acute yersiniosis enterocolitica, for example, gastroenteritis in children, acute form of terminal ileitis, pseudoappendicitis, and acute enteritis, it is possible to observe increasing agglutinins in paired samples of serum.

In cases in which it had not been possible to obtain serum in the acute stage, an agglutinin titer of 1:160 or higher may be interpreted as significant, indicating actual infection. A titer of 1:1,280 or higher is always diagnostic of an acute and actual infection with *Y. enterocolitica*. The decrease from high agglutinin titers takes a long time, and titers of 1:40 or 1:80 may persist for several months or for years. For this reason, caution should be used in interpreting these low titers as significant for an actual disease. So far as agglutinins against *Y. enter-*

ocolitica serotype 9 are concerned, cross-antigenicity between this serotype and brucellae has to be kept in mind (3).

Investigators in the United States should work with the three antigens O-3, O-8, and O-9, of which antigen O-8 is probably the most important. For investigations in other parts of the world, the antigen against O-8 is of no importance, but antigens O-3 and O-9 are recommended.

After observing a case with a high agglutinin titer, it is often helpful to complete the suspected diagnosis by the cultivation of *Y. enterocolitica* from feces. In this way, the diagnosis of yersiniosis will be proved beyond any doubt.

YERSINIA PSEUDOTUBERCULOSIS (YERSINIOSIS PSEUDOTUBERCULOSIS)

The immunological response to infection with *Y. pseudotuberculosis* is most suitably observed by the development of specific agglutinins in a Widal reaction. Antibodies detected with passive hemagglutination and complement fixation have also been described. Different O serotypes of *Y. pseudotuberculosis* exist, namely, Ia, Ib, IIa, IIb, III, IV, and V. Of these different serotypes, types Ia and Ib have most often been observed as human pathogens. The other serotypes are only observed in animal infections. Serotypes II and IV have cross-antigenicity with *Salmonella* B and D groups (7, 9).

Clinical indications

Typical human infections with *Y. pseudotuberculosis* I (Ia, Ib) are described by Knapp and Masshoff as a mesenterical lymphadenitis in children and young people (8). The agglutinin levels against this microorganism are, however, very high in the acute symptomatic stage, in contrast to *Y. enterocolitica* infections, in which there are no detectable antibodies during the first stage of the disease.

Test procedure

Agglutinins against *Y. pseudotuberculosis* are titrated by the same technique as described above for *Y. enterocolitica* O-9. The reaction should be read after overnight incubation at 37 C.

Reagent

The antigen should be prepared from strains of *Y. pseudotuberculosis* I, as described above for OH antigen of *Y. enterocolitica* O-9. The antigen should first be suspended in formalin for 18 h at 37 C. Thereafter, the suspension should be centrifuged, washed with saline, and resuspended in saline to a concentration suitable for a Widal reaction.

Knapp and Steuer (9) observed that living cultures may be more practical than killed O antigen. Such living cultures may be supplied as drops from a broth culture or from a buffered suspension of living bacteria. Because of the danger of laboratory infection, it is recommended that the bacterial suspension be sterilized with formalin.

Interpretation

Cultivation of *Y. pseudotuberculosis* from stools has not been successful. The only practical way to isolate the bacteria is from extirpated mesenteric lymph nodes or abscesses. Agglutination reactions are a useful diagnostic test. A titer of 1:160 or higher is indicative of an actual infection.

YERSINIA PESTIS (PLAGUE)

Because of the danger of laboratory infection, culturing should be done only in laboratories with special facilities. The immunological response of patients, therefore, is the only practical way to investigate suspected cases. Passive agglutination with sensitized sheep red blood cells is recommended as the best way to study antibody development. Fraction I is the antigen of choice.

Clinical indications

Immunological diagnosis can be used in those parts of the world in which infection with *Y. pestis* is endemic or in travelers returning from these areas.

Test procedure

The best description of this technique is in the article by Rust et al. (12). Serum samples may be stored in a refrigerator with sodium acid at a concentration of 0.2% as preservative. The sera must be inactivated before use and absorbed by incubating a mixture of 9 volumes of serum with 1 volume of a 5% suspension of nonsensitized tanned pyruvaldehyde-treated erythrocytes for 30 min at 56 C. After centrifugation and removal of the sensitized red blood cells, the sera are ready for use.

Hemagglutinin titration can be performed in U-bottom plates with microtitration equipment. Rust et al. (12) recommend the preparation of a sufficient number of replicate, twofold dilutions of each test serum, in a final volume of 0.05 ml. This may be done in duplicate.

In the first set, 0.05 ml of FR-I-sensitized sheep erythrocytes is added to one and the corresponding amounts of nonsensitized sheep erythrocytes are added to other dilution series. The mixtures should be incubated overnight at 25 C. The end point of each titration is defined as the highest serum dilution that yields 4+ agglutination; i.e., the bottom of the well is covered uniformly with erythrocytes. Rabbit antiserum against FR-I may be used as the positive control and normal serum as the negative control.

Reagent

It is recommended that laboratories not specializing in this area use FR-I-sensitized sheep red cells from Walter Reed Army Institute of Research, Walter Reed Army Medical Center, Washington, D.C. 20012. A high degree of standardizing of HA reagents for plague serology is required.

Interpretation

An antibody titer of 1:256 or higher may be considered as evidence of a specific immunological response to plague infection.

PASTEURELLA MULTOCIDA

The only important human infections caused by pasteurellae are those due to *P. multocida*, which often follow a cat scratch or bite.

P. multocida is not a suitable antigen for agglutinin reactions, since the strains have a tendency to change to the rough form and thus agglutinate spontaneously. When it is of interest to investigate the immunological response to infection with *P. multocida* in humans, passive hemagglutination with an extract of heated strains as antigen may be used. However, experience with this test is too limited to describe it here. The diagnosis of this infection is usually based on the cultivation of the microorganism from the lesion.

FRANCISELLA TULARENSIS (TULAREMIA)

Documentation of the antibody response to *F. tularensis* is a very good diagnostic method.

Clinical indications

The agglutination test may be done as a Widal reaction in those geographical areas where tularemia is endemic, namely, Russia, northern Scandinavia, the Balkans, Canada, and the middle and southern states of the United States. There are seasonal variations in the occurrence of this infection. Mosquitos infected by blood from sick or dead hares are known to transmit *F. tularensis*. During the season when lingonberries or other berries are harvested, infection with *F. tularensis* is frequently seen in northern Scandinavia. The infection occasionally may be airborne (11). Localized infection of the skin, with enlargement of the regional nodes, is the predominant feature.

Procedures

The agglutination technique is the same as that described above for *Y. enterocolitica*, antigen 9 (OH), or *Y. pseudotuberculosis*.

Reagent

The best culture medium for *F. tularensis* is PTM agar of Gaspar et al. (6). The base consists of 2.6% tryptose broth with thiamine (Difco), 0.5% cysteine hydrochlorate, and 0.2% natrium thioglycolate, all mixed without heating in distilled water of pH 7.2. Agar is added to a final concentration of 1%. The mixture is heated with streaming vapor for 5 min and is then autoclaved at 121 C for 20 min. After cooling to room temperature, 30% sterile glucose solution is added until the final concentration is 1%. Thereafter, defibrinated rabbit blood is added to yield a final concentration of 5%. The culture medium in petri dishes (15 cm in diameter) is incubated at 37 C for 24 h to assure sterility. The plates are inoculated with *F. tularensis* and incubated at 37 C. If incubation is carried out in a humid milieu, good growth is obtained after 1 day of incubation or, if the humidity is not correct, after 2 days.

The best strain is the LVS strain that can be ordered from Fort Detrick, Frederick, Md. The strain can be preserved in agar tubes. Before preparing the antigen for the Widal test, the culture from one tube should be suspended in 2.5 ml phosphate-buffered saline (PBS), pH 7.2, sufficient to inoculate a PTM agar plate. After 2 h of aerobic incubation at 37 C, the bacteria should be suspended in 15 ml of 0.5% phenol-PBS. This suspension must be heated at 100 C for 1 h, and sterility is ascertained by culture on PTM agar plates.

The antigen suspension is at a suitable dilution with a concentration of 2×10^{10} bacterial/ml. This antigen suspension should be diluted with PBS-Merthiolate to a final concentration of 1:10,000.

Interpretation

Agglutinins in titers of 1:40 to 1:80 or higher are considered to be diagnostic of an actual infection. Pairs of serum samples are recommended in an attempt to follow the antibody titers. Cross-reactions with *Y. enterocolitica* or *Y. pseudotuberculosis* have not been observed, but cross-reaction with *Brucella abortus* has been described (13).

LITERATURE CITED

1. Ahvonen, P. 1972. Human yersiniosis in Finland. Ann. Clin. Res. 4:30–38.
2. Ahvonen, P., L. Hiisi-Brummer, and K. Aho. 1971. Electrocardiographic abnormalities and arthritis in patients with Yersinia enterocolitica infection. Ann. Clin. Res. 3:69–75.
3. Ahvonen, P., E. Jansson, and K. Aho. 1969. Marked cross-agglutination between Brucellae and a subtype of Yersinia enterocolitica. Acta Pathol. Microbiol. Scand. 75:291–295.
4. Arvastson, B., K. Damgaard, and S. Winblad. 1971. Clinical symptoms of infection with Yersinia enterocolitica. Scand. J. Infect. Dis. 3:37–40.
5. Bergstrand, C. G., and S. Winblad. 1974. Clinical manifestations of infection with Yersinia enterocolitica in children. Acta Paediatr. Scand. 63:875–877.
6. Gaspar, A. J., H. B. Tresselt, and M. K. Ward. 1961. New solid medium for enhanced growth of Pasteurella tularensis. J. Bacteriol. 82:564–569.
7. Knapp, W. 1956. Die Agglutinationsreaktion in der Serodiagnostik menschlicher Infektionen mit Pasteurella pseudotuberculosis. Z. Immunitaetsforsch.113:262–277.
8. Knapp, W., and W. Masshoff. 1954. Zur Ätiologie der abscendierenden reticulocytären Lymphadenitis. Dtsch. Med. Wochenschr. 79:1266.
9. Knapp, W., and W. Steuer. 1956. Untersuchungen über den Nachweis komplementbindende und agglutinierender Antikörper gegen Pasteurella pseudotuberculosis in Sera infizierter und immunisierter Menschen und Tiere. Z. Immunitaetsforsch. 113:370–374.
10. Niléhn, B. 1969. Studies on Yersinia enterocolitica with special reference to bacterial diagnosis and occurrence in human acute enteric disease. Acta Pathol. Microbiol. Scand. Suppl. 206.
11. Olin, G. 1942. The occurrence and mode of transmission of Tularemia in Sweden. Acta Pathol. Microbiol. Scand. 19:220–247.
12. Rust, J. H., Jr., S. Berman, W. H. Habig, J. D. Marshall, Jr., and D. C. Cavanaugh. 1972. Stable reagent for the detection of antibody to the specific fraction I antigen of Yersinia pestis. Appl. Microbiol. 23:721–724.
13. Shoichiro, O., S. Tadashi, and H. Morio. 1974. Serological studies on Francisella tularensis, Francisella novicida, Yersinia philomiragia, and Brucella abortus. Int. J. Syst. Bacteriol. 24:191–196.
14. Sjöström, B. 1973. Surgical aspects of infection with Yersinia enterocolitica. Contrib. Microbiol. Immunol. 2:137–140.
15. Wauters, G., L. Le Minor, and A. M. Chalon. 1971. Antigénes somatiques et flagellaires des Yersinia enterocolitica. Ann. Inst. Pasteur (Paris) 120:631–642.
16. Wauters, G., L. Le Minor, A. M. Chalon, and J. Lassen. 1972. Supplément au schéma antigénique de "Yersinia enterocolitica". Ann.

Inst. Pasteur (Paris) **122**:951–956.

17. Winblad, S. 1967. Studies on serological typing of Yersinia enterocolitica. Acta Pathol. Microbiol. Scand. Suppl. 187, p. 115.

18. Winblad, S. 1968. Studies on O-antigen factors of "Yersinia enterocolitica". Symp. Ser. Immunobiol. Stand. **9**:337–342.

19. Winblad, S. 1969. Erythema nodosum associated with infection with Yersinia enterocolitica. Scand J. Infect. Dis. **1**:11–16.

20. Winblad, S. 1973. Studies on the O-serotypes of Yersinia enterocolitica. Contrib. Microbiol. Immunol. **2**:27–37.

21. Winblad, S. 1973. The clinical panorama of human Yersiniosis enterocolitica. Contrib. Microbiol. Immunol. **2**:129–132.

22. Winblad, S., B. Niléhn, and N. H. Sternby. 1966. Yersinia enterocolitica (Pasteurella X) in human enteric infections. Br. Med. J. **2**:1363–1366.

Chapter 39

Immune Response to *Francisella*

MERRILL J. SNYDER

INTRODUCTION

The difficulty and hazards of cultivating *Francisella tularensis* in the routine laboratory have influenced the use of serological testing for conventional laboratory confirmation of tularemic infection. Since bacteriological methods are essentially unavailable, serological results assume greater importance. The bacterial agglutination test in which formalinized whole cells are used has had wide and long application in the clinical diagnostic laboratory (6). However, other immunological techniques have been evaluated and, in special laboratories, can be employed in the study of the immune response to this organism—microagglutination (10), precipitation (1), flocculation (9), agar-gel precipitation (15), hemagglutination of antigen-coated erythrocytes (2, 3), bactericidal assay (14), passive neutralization (11), immunofluorescence (7), opsinization (8), and skin test (4, 5). The last in conjunction with the agglutination test has been used extensively in epidemiological surveys.

The emphasis upon humoral antibody in the immunological approach to diagnosis is in conflict with the demonstrations that cell-associated immune factors have major importance in the acquired resistance to this obligate intracellular parasite. The light shed by studies of these host cell-*F. tularensis* interrelationships brightens our hope for fundamental understanding of immunopathogenesis and for new laboratory techniques to measure response at the cellular level.

CLINICAL INDICATIONS

A serum specimen for agglutination should be taken as soon as and whenever the clinical diagnosis of tularemia is considered. The most common clinical presentation of tularemic infection is ulceroglandular disease. Patients with pulmonic and typhoidal tularemia have rare and frequently unsuspected infections. The history of tick bite or exposure to rabbits and other sick-looking wild animals should alert the physician to the possibility of *F. tularensis* infection. Very small numbers of virulent organisms (<50) can cause either the ulceroglandular or pulmonic form of the disease. The serological results can be used to support and, under the proper circumstances, confirm the diagnosis. Uncommon cross-reactions with *Brucella* and *Proteus* OX 19 antibody have been reported, but almost invariably homologous titers exceed heterologous. *F. tularensis* agglutinins remain elevated for years after exposure, and a single positive finding may be the consequence of a past infection rather than the present illness. A rising titer in subsequent serum specimens, as always, aids interpretation.

TEST PROCEDURE

Dilutions of serum, usually 1:10 to 1:2,560, are made in 0.5 ml of physiological saline by the twofold serological dilution technique in 12 × 75 mm test tubes. An equal quantity of tularemia antigen containing 3×10^9 formalinized *F. tularensis* cells, usually avirulent strain B38 of Francis, is added to each tube and mixed by shaking. The tubes are incubated at 37 C for 2 h and then placed in a refrigerator at approximately 4 C overnight (18 h). The tubes are read with a suitable light source without magnification by gently shaking or flipping and observing for agglutination. Readings are recorded as "complete" agglutination when the background liquid is clear, as "partial" when clearly visible agglutinated particles are suspended in a cloudy fluid, as "questionable" when one is uncertain of the presence of particles, and as "negative" when a homogeneous cloudy suspension without clumps is seen. Readings of finer gradation or based upon the size of the clumps are unwarranted. The titer is reported as the greatest final dilution of serum showing definite and unquestionable agglutination of the antigen.

Suitable positive low-titered (<1:160) and high-titered (>1:160) human sera as well as negative serum should be included with each test.

Antigen is usually prepared from *F. tularensis* strain B38 of Francis, ATCC 6223, grown on glucose-cysteine-blood agar at 37 C for 24 h. Growth is harvested with physiological saline containing 0.5% formaldehyde (1.35% Formalin), washed four times by centrifuging and resuspending in fresh 0.5% formaldehyde-saline solution, and finally resuspended for use at a turbidity representing 3×10^9 cells/ml.

Strain 38 is avirulent and therefore is recommended for use, although antigens prepared from virulent strains such as Schu S-4 give a somewhat greater sensitivity to the test. Use of phenol instead of formaldehyde reduces the sensitivity of the antigen. Not all commercial antigens are of equal sensitivity, although they are prepared in accord with recommendations of the National Institutes of Health (Circular E-677 revised).

Satisfactory antigens are available commercially from many sources including Lederle Laboratories, Difco Laboratories, and BioQuest Division of Becton, Dickinson & Co. Reference serum can be obtained from the Center for Disease Control, Atlanta, Ga.

INTERPRETATION

The broad experience with tularemia in volunteers infected by the intracutaneous and respiratory route has furnished valuable information about antibody response in individuals in whom both dose and time of infection are known (12, 13). Persons without previous experience with tularemia or tularemia vaccine demonstrate circulating antibody by agglutination in 3 weeks (range, 14 to 31 days) and by hemagglutination in 2 weeks (range, 10 to 21 days) after infection. Mean peak agglutination titer of 1:640 (maximum titer, 1:2,560) is reached by the 5th week after inoculation, whereas mean peak hemagglutination titer of 1:10,240 (maximum titer, 1:80,000) is attained by the 4th week postinfection. Responses to pulmonary and intradermal challenge are similar.

The heterologous agglutination against *Brucella* was seen in approximately 25% of these volunteers; others have reported from 18 to 40% cross-reactions in studies of naturally acquired infection. Vaccinees who were subsequently challenged displayed a greater incidence of cross-reaction to *Brucella* antigen. In no case was the titer of *Brucella* agglutinins equal to or higher than the titer to tularemia antigen.

Titers greater than 1:40 to 1:80 are of diagnostic significance but may be an indication of previous infection. Since peak antibody titer may not be reached until at least 1 month into the disease, demonstration of a rise in titer in serially obtained specimens at 7- to 10-day intervals provides the clinician with additional diagnostic assurance. The difficulties occasioned by cross-reactions with *Brucella*

and *Proteus* OX 19 can be eliminated by parallel testing with these antigens whenever serum is tested for tularemia agglutinins.

LITERATURE CITED

1. Alexander, M. M. 1950. A quantitative antibody response of man to infection or vaccination with *Pasteurella tularensis*. J. Exp. Med. 92:51–57.
2. Alexander, M. M., G. G. Wright, and A. G. Baldwin. 1950. Observations on the agglutination of polysaccharide-treated erythrocytes by tularemia antisera. J. Exp. Med. 91: 561–566.
3. Charkes, N. D. 1959. Hemagglutination test in tularemia. Results in 56 vaccinated persons with laboratory-acquired infection. J. Immunol. 83:213–220.
4. Foshay, L. 1932. Tularemia. Accurate and earlier diagnosis by means of the intradermal reaction. J. Infect. Dis. 51:286–291.
5. Foshay, L. 1936. The nature of the bacterial-specific intradermal antiserum reaction. J. Infect. Dis. 59:330–339.
6. Francis, E., and A. C. Evans. 1926. Agglutination, cross-agglutination and agglutinin absorption in tularemia. Public Health Rep. 41:1273–1295.
7. Franek, J. 1965. Use of fluorescent antibodies for the rapid diagnosis of infections caused by *B. anthracis* and *P. tularensis*. J. Hyg. Epidemiol. Microbiol. Immunol. 9:160–168.
8. Friedwald, W. F., and G. A. Hunt. 1939. The diagnosis of tularemia. Am. J. Med. Sci. 197:493–502.
9. Hunter, C. A., R. Burdorff, and B. Colbert. 1958. Flocculation tests for tularemia. J. Lab. Clin. Med. 51:134–140.
10. Massey, E. D., and J. A. Mangiafico. 1974. Microagglutination test for detecting and measuring serum agglutinins of *Francisella tularensis*. Appl. Microbiol. 27:25–27.
11. Pannell, L., and C. M. Downs. 1953. Studies on the pathogenesis and immunity of tularemia. I. The demonstration of a protective antibody in mouse serum. J. Infect. Dis. 92: 195–204.
12. Saslaw, S., and S. Carhart. 1961. Studies with tularemia vaccines in volunteers. III. Serologic aspects following intracutaneous or respiratory challenge in both vaccinated and nonvaccinated volunteers. Am. J. Med. Sci. 241:689–699.
13. Saslaw, S., and H. N. Carlisle. 1961. Studies with tularemia vaccines in volunteers. IV. Brucella agglutinins in vaccinated and nonvaccinated volunteers challenged with Pasteurella tularensis. Am. J. Med. Sci. 242:166–172.
14. Stanziale, W. G. 1957. *In vitro* bactericidal activity of blood for *Pasteurella tularensis*. J. Immunol. 78:156–159.
15. Vosti, K. L., M. K. Ward, and W. D. Tigertt. 1962. Agar gel precipitation analyses in laboratory-acquired tularemia. J. Clin. Invest. 41:1436–1445.

Chapter 40

Immune Response to *Brucella*

NORMAN B. McCULLOUGH

INTRODUCTION

Genus Brucella

The genus *Brucella* consists of facultatively intracellular parasites infecting a wide range of animals, including humans. They are aerobic, gram-negative rods, or coccobacilli, without capsules, flagella, or exotoxins. An endotoxin is present in S (smooth) cultures.

Infection in humans is due almost entirely to *B. abortus* (nine biotypes), *B. suis* (four biotypes), and *B. melitensis* (three biotypes). *B. neotomae* and *B. ovis* have not been incriminated in human disease. To date, *B. canis* has been responsible for a dozen recognized cases of human infection.

B. abortus, *B. suis*, *B. melitensis*, and *B. neotomae* occur in nature in the S form. They all contain two main cell wall antigens, A (abortus) and M (melitensis), in varying ratios which determine the specificity of the antibody response. *B. ovis* and *B. canis* lack the A and M antigens and occur in nature as rough, or rough mucoid, forms. Their surface antigens are the same as or similar to those of the R (rough) forms of the other members of the genus. Other subsurface antigens likewise are shared throughout the genus (3).

Immune response

Hosts infected with members of the genus elaborate an array of antibodies (immunoglobulins M, G, A [IgM, IgG, IgA]) against the surface antigens of the organisms, demonstrated as bactericidins, agglutinins, precipitins, opsonins, and complement-fixing antibodies. As in other diseases, macroglobulins (19S, IgM) appear early in infections followed by 7S (IgG) antibody which usually becomes dominant. In some instances of chronic disease, IgM may be produced for an extended period.

In addition to the humoral response, the host also develops delayed-type hypersensitivity to the organism or to some of its components together with an accompanying cell-mediated immunity. This latter response largely determines the course of the infection (7).

Humoral response

The only test in wide use clinically in the United States for determining the presence and amount of antibody to *Brucella* is the agglutination test. A complement-fixation test has been in limited use in the past and may detect antibody a bit earlier in the disease than the agglutination test. It is, however, subject to all the variation described below for the agglutination test, and from a practical standpoint the agglutination test is preferable.

Brucella species and biotypes containing the A and M (S) antigens are indistinguishable in the agglutination test. Hence, theoretically, any smooth *Brucella* strain could be used for production of antigen to detect antibodies to *B. abortus*, *B. suis*, or *B. melitensis*. A different antigen preparation is necessary to determine the response to *B. canis* since the surface antigens are different.

S → R variation

An understanding of S → R variation in *Brucella* is necessary to appreciate the problems involved in preparation of a dependable antigen. Most *Brucella* strains exhibit considerable S → R variation on artificial media. Cloned dissociants do not revert to the S form readily if at all. Further, they rapidly outgrow the S form. Unless continuous clonal selection of S colonies is practiced, a culture soon becomes a mixture of dissociants with loss of virulence and change in antigenicity. This change is largely inapparent to the eye unless the plate is viewed through a low-power stereoscopic microscope with reflected 45° incident transmitted light (4). (A mirror is placed between the light source and the microscope.) Cultures grown on Trypticase-soy agar or tryptose agar and incubated for 4 days are most suitable for identification of colony types. There are a number of intermediate colony types ranging between the S and R types (6). Those most closely resembling the S type were designated by Huddleson as smooth intermediate (SI) types. The first observable change was designated SI$_1$. Under incident lighting, S colonies are a blue-green color throughout. SI$_1$ colonies are similar but larger with a yellowish cast in the center. Other intermediates depart further from the S color value and appear granular. S and SI₁ colony types only are suitable for production of antigen to detect antibody against smooth strains of *Brucella*. Intermediate forms beyond the SI₁ have changed antigenicity.

In addition to visual inspection, agglutinability in neutral acriflavine (trypaflavine), 1:1,000 (aqueous solution), is helpful in recognizing dissociants (5) beyond the SI₁ range. This test can be done as a spot or slide test by emulsifying a portion of a colony in a drop of the acriflavine solution. Dissociants should agglutinate promptly. If no agglutination is apparent macroscopically, the specimen should be examined under a low-power stereoscopic microscope. The recognition of S and SI₁ colony types and proper maintenance of cultures require considerable practice and continuing diligence. However, this is vital to the preparation of a suitable antigen.

Twenty to thirty years ago, a number of studies emphasized the tremendous variability of agglutination titers done in different laboratories or with different antigens on the same serum specimens. The situation was ridiculous. A National Research Council Committee (NRC Committee) on the Public Health Aspects of Brucellosis considered the problem and recommended a standard antigen and technique for the agglutination test for human brucellosis (12). These recommendations are just as pertinent today as when published.

The Committee recommended the tube antigen prepared from *B. abortus* strain 1119 by the Bureau of Animal Industry as the standard antigen. This antigen had a long history of dependable use and was, and still is, the official antigen for veterinary use. That organization had learned that it was necessary to center maintenance of the culture and standardization of the product in a single organization to assure a uniformly satisfactory antigen.

B. abortus strain 1119 is more antigenically stable than most wild strains of *Brucella*, thus reducing the labor and attention of maintaining it in suitable phase. Further, it is an SI₁ colony type of markedly reduced pathogenicity, which lessens the hazard to personnel handling it.

The Committee also recommended that, because of variability in results, commercially available slide tests and other rapid tests of all varieties be used only as screening tests and that only the standard antigen and test be used to determine the titer; that the serum not be inactivated by heat prior to testing since this

significantly reduces the titer of some sera; and that incubation be carried out for 48 h at 37 C. The latter provision reduces the occurrence of prozones and "blocking" reactions and yields higher titers for some sera.

The standard antigen was made available commercially for some time but unfortunately was withdrawn from the market as the incidence of human brucellosis dropped. It is suggested that those who do not have access to this antigen through a state laboratory or otherwise make their own. *B. abortus* strain 1119 in suitable form for use as seed should be obtained from a central source such as the U.S. Department of Agriculture National Animal Disease Center, Ames, Iowa, each time it is needed rather than attempting to maintain the organism in acceptable antigenic form.

Blocking antibody

Sera from some patients contain blocking antibody. These antibodies usually occur only in low titer and do not confuse the interpretation of the agglutination test if the full range of serum dilutions is carried out (10). Occasionally, a patient may have a high titer of blocking antibody. Blocking antibody can be detected and measured by the Coombs technique, but I prefer a more simple direct blocking test to detect such antibody.

B. canis infection

There is no designated standard serological test for human brucellosis due to *B. canis*. The agglutination test antigen used for detecting antibodies in dogs has been used similarly with human serum. A number of methods for preparation of antigen have been proposed (2, 9).

If a laboratory has only an occasional request, it is suggested that the specimen be sent to the state laboratory or to the Center for Disease Control, Atlanta, Ga.

Since *B. canis* occurs naturally as a rough mucoid colony type, the problem is to produce a stable antigen which does not agglutinate spontaneously. There seems to be no single method which unfailingly yields a satisfactory product.

I have prepared satisfactory antigen according to the method described. However, an occasional lot must be discarded due to spontaneous agglutination. The strain used for preparation of antigen is *B. canis* RM-66 (ATCC 23365). This strain originated from L. E. Carmichael's laboratory, Cornell University, Ithaca, N.Y.

Delayed hypersensitivity

A variety of reagents derived from *Brucella* organisms, including saline suspensions of killed whole cells, have been used in the intradermal test to detect dermal hypersensitivity. The simplest to prepare, whole-cell suspension, is unsatisfactory from two standpoints. Minimal allergic responses may be confused with nonspecific inflammatory reactions to the material. More importantly, in subjects with positive reactions there is a considerable incidence of necrosis and sloughing of the involved tissue. The use of whole-cell suspensions in the intradermal test is not recommended.

Various filtrates and lysates (1, 5, 10), as well as a soluble protein prepared by a method similar to that used for making purified protein derivative from the tubercle bacillus, have been used experimentally with reported satisfactory results. In the United States, Brucellergen (5), a preparation of *Brucella* protein nucleate developed by I. F. Huddleson at Michigan State University and made available commercially, was widely used for many years. It is highly specific for detecting delayed hypersensitivity to *Brucella* (in the intradermal test), is well standardized, and has fewer undesirable side effects than most of the preparations mentioned above. This product is no longer commercially available. A markedly lowered incidence of human brucellosis in the United States, together with revised Food and Drug Administration requirements pertaining to the product, led to its withdrawal from the market. Nevertheless, this is still the reagent of choice for the intradermal test for determining delayed hypersensitivity to *Brucella* in humans.

CLINICAL INDICATIONS

The agglutination test should be the first test done when the physician suspects that a patient may have brucellosis. If the standard antigen and technique are used, with extremely rare exceptions, antibodies will be demonstrable in the blood if the patient has the disease. If antibody is completely lacking, the probability that the patient has brucellosis becomes very small indeed (11).

If antibodies are not demonstrated and the physician still considers brucellosis likely, a test for blocking antibody should be done.

The physician should be alert to the possibility of infection with *B. canis* and the need to request specifically an agglutination test with the appropriate antigen.

Determination of the presence or absence of dermal hypersensitivity is not helpful in making or excluding a diagnosis of brucellosis (11). The test does have a use in epidemiological surveys to determine the relative incidence of exposure to brucellosis.

TEST PROCEDURES

Rapid slide test

The rapid slide test is not a recognized standard test, but since it is widely used the procedure is included here. As mentioned earlier, the NRC Committee recommended that such tests be used only as screening tests and that all specimens yielding positive results at any dilution be retested to determine the titer by means of the standard antigen and standardized technique as described in the section immediately following this one.

A number of antigens are available commercially for use in the rapid slide test. The test is performed by mixing serum and antigen in ruled squares on a glass slide. A convenient size of slide is one measuring 9 by 14 inches (23 by 31 cm). A series of 1.5-inch (3.8-cm) ruled squares are made with a diamond-point pencil. This results in rows of six squares across the 9-inch width.

Using a 0.2-ml serological pipette with 0.001-ml graduations, deliver 0.08, 0.04, 0.02, 0.01, and 0.005 ml of test serum to the squares in one row on the glass slide, proceeding from left to right. Mix the contents of the antigen vial by shaking. Using a dropper provided by the manufacturer, or a serological pipette, place one drop (0.03 ml) of antigen on each quantity of serum on the slide. These serum-antigen ratios are said to yield results approximating those obtained in the test tube method at dilutions of 1:20, 1:40, 1:80, 1:160, and 1:320, and this is the basis of reporting the titer. The serum-antigen mixture in each square is thoroughly mixed with a wooden applicator or toothpick. A single applicator is used for each specimen, and the squares are mixed from right to left (smallest amount of serum to largest amount) to reduce the effect of carry-over by the applicator. The slide is then picked up and held over a light source to provide maximal visibility of any agglutination which may occur. The slide is slowly rotated and tilted by hand for 3 min. The results are then read macroscopically.

The degree of agglutination is recorded for each square as 4+ (complete agglutination), 3+, 2+, 1+, or negative. The test is reported as negative if all mixtures fail to agglutinate. If agglutination occurs, the titer is usually reported as the dilution (in the tube test) corresponding to the mixture with 2+ agglutination. An alternative method is to take 4+ as the end point for reporting the titer, but to report also the lesser reactions at their corresponding dilutions.

The variability in results obtained in screening tests of this nature is great. As a quality control measure each time unknown sera are tested, it is mandatory that appropriate positive and negative control sera be included in the test batch.

Technique of performing the agglutination test (12)

Blood drawn from the patient is allowed to clot, and the serum is separated by centrifugation. The serum is not inactivated. Using 10 test tubes (13 × 100 mm) for each specimen, add isotonic sodium chloride solution containing 0.5% phenol (phenolized saline) to each tube: 0.9 ml to tube 1 and 0.5 ml to all others. Add 0.1 ml of serum to tube 1 using a serological pipette of 1-ml capacity calibrated to 0.1 ml. Draw up and expel the mixture from the pipette seven or eight times, and transfer 0.5 ml to the next tube. Repeat the process through the tenth tube, discarding the last 0.5 ml. To each tube, add 0.5 ml of standard antigen and mix the contents in each tube by shaking. Tube 1 now represents a 1:20 dilution of serum, and the dilution doubles in each succeeding tube through 1:10,240 for the tenth tube. Always run an antigen control, using a 1:2 dilution in phenolized saline. Incubation is carried out in a water bath for 48 h at 37 C.

The titer is recorded as the highest dilution of serum showing complete clumping of the antigen and clearing of the fluid. In addition, dilutions showing partial agglutination are recorded as such. This also applies in tests with no tubes showing complete agglutination.

Blocking antibody test

The blocking antibody test makes use of a known positive serum (human) with a sharp and well-established end-point titer. Prepare a dilution of the known positive serum equal to that in the second tube immediately preceding (in a doubling dilution series) the end-point tube. (If the end-point tube represents a dilution of 1:160, then make a dilution of 1:40.) A 0.25-ml amount of this serum dilution contains the amount of antibody present in the end-point tube. Using the patient's serum, prepare serum dilutions as usual except that in tube 1 put 0.8 ml of saline and 0.2 ml of the patient's serum. Now discard 0.25 ml from each tube. Start with the highest dilution first so as not to change the concentrations in the various tubes. Now add to each tube 0.25 ml of the prepared dilution of the known positive serum. Add the antigen, mix, and incubate as usual. (The final dilutions are 1:20 through 1:10,240.)

If no blocking antibody is present, all tubes should show agglutination. If blocking antibody is present, there should be a prozone followed by tubes showing agglutination. The dilution of the patient's serum in the tube just prior to the first tube showing complete agglutionation is reported as the blocking antibody titer.

B. canis agglutination test

The *B. canis* agglutination test is done with an antigen made from *B. canis*. Serum dilutions are made in isotonic sodium chloride solution containing Merthiolate, 1:10,000, as a preservative (do not use phenolized saline). Otherwise, the test is incubated and read as usual. Control tests using known positive and negative sera should be done every time unknowns are run, in addition to an antigen control in saline.

Intradermal test

The intradermal test is performed and read similarly to a tuberculin test. Using a sterile 1-ml tuberculin syringe and a 26-gauge needle, inject 0.1 ml of Brucellergen intradermally on the volar surface of the forearm. Read the test at 48 h. A positive reaction consists of erythema, edema, and induration at the injection site. Any reaction less than 0.5 cm in diameter is considered a negative test. Most sensitized individuals give a 1.0-cm or greater reaction. Those highly sensitive may have a systemic reaction.

If there is no visible reaction or the reaction is less than 0.5 cm in diameter, the test is reported as negative. If the reaction area is 0.5 cm in diameter or larger, it is reported as positive. The reaction area should be measured in two diameters and the size in millimeters should also be reported.

Since Brucellergen is no longer available commercially, an alternative is the use of a heat-killed suspension of *Brucella* cells. Such preparations are not available in the United States either, but are more easily prepared than Brucellergen. A heat-killed suspension of *B. abortus* cells in physiological saline containing 2×10^9 cells per ml is most commonly used. The test is performed and read as described above with the use of 0.1 ml of the suspension.

As mentioned earlier, I do not recommend the use of this preparation in humans. It may be used as a research tool to determine dermal sensitivity in laboratory animals. Even here, if extensive testing is to be done, it is preferable to prepare and standardize Brucellergen rather than to employ such a crude preparation.

REAGENTS

Preparation of standard antigen

Commercially prepared media such as Trypticase-Soy, Tryptose, and Albimi Brucella agars, although excellent for culture of *Brucella* from small inocula, are less suitable for growth of large amounts of cells. The two media most satisfactory from the standpoint of yield and economy are potato infusion agar and liver infusion agar. The veterinary product designated as the standard antigen is grown on potato infusion agar. I believe that there is less dissociation on liver infusion agar and prefer that medium.

Potato infusion agar (1, 5)

Sound raw potatoes are peeled, and 250 g are thinly sliced into 1,000 ml of distilled water with minimal exposure to air. The mixture is infused overnight in a covered container at 60 C and filtered through a single layer of cotton gauze. The filtrate is made up to original volume with distilled water, and the following ingredients are added: sodium chloride, 5 g; peptone (Bacto or equivalent), 10 g; beef extract, 5 g; and agar, 25 g. (The concentration of agar is a factor in adherence of the agar to the wall of the culture bottle. Various laboratories use from 20 to 30 g per liter.)

The mixture is heated to dissolve the agar (flowing steam), and 20 ml of glycerol is added. The medium is adjusted to pH 7.4 (after autoclaving the pH should be 6.8) and filtered while hot through two thin pads of nonabsorbent cotton. Finally, 10 g of glucose is added and the medium is dispensed in 32-oz Pyrex culture bottles to provide a 0.25-inch (6.35-cm) thick layer on one side of the bottle when solidified. Bottle closures must allow oxygen exchange. After sterilization at 120 C for 30 min, the bottles are placed in a horizontal position while the medium solidifies. The bottles of medium should be held in an incubator for 24 to 48 h to allow evaporation of water of condensation prior to seeding.

Liver infusion agar (5)

Liver infusion is prepared by grinding 1 lb (454 g) of fresh beef liver, free from fat, adding 500 ml of distilled water, and allowing the mixture to infuse for 24 h at 4 to 8 C. The mixture (covered) is placed in flowing steam for 1.5 h. It should be stirred once or twice to assure uniform heating. It is then filtered through a fine-mesh wire gauze. It should be used promptly for preparation of medium. (Excessive heating reduces the growth-promoting properties.)

To prepare 1 liter of medium, the following ingredients are required: agar, 20 g; peptone (Bacto or equivalent), 5 g; sodium chloride, 5 g; liver infusion, 500 ml; and distilled water, 500 ml. The ingredients are mixed, and the container is placed in flowing steam for 1 h. The mixture is cooled to 60 C, and the pH is adjusted to 7.2 (after sterilization it should be 6.6 to 6.8). The medium is now ready for dispensing into culture bottles and sterilization as described for potato infusion agar.

With either medium, 48-h slant cultures (25 × 200 mm tubes) of *B. abortus* strain 1119 are used as seed. The cultures are rigorously examined for purity macroscopically and microscopically by smear and stain. The growth is suspended in sterile isotonic sodium chloride solution (saline) to give a suspension equal in density to tube no. 2 McFarlane nephelometer. To each culture bottle, 4 or 5 ml of seed suspension is added. The culture bottles are rotated to allow uniform distribution, inverted, and incubated in a horizontal position for 72 h at 37 C.

Each culture bottle is examined macroscopically, and representative bottles are examined microscopically by smear and stain for purity. Any water of condensation is removed by suction. This is important as soluble material may affect the sensitivity of the product.

Approximately 40 ml of sterile isotonic saline is added to each culture bottle, and the growth is suspended by gentle agitation. The bacterial suspension should be removed promptly by suction to prevent absorption of soluble factors from the agar. The pooled suspension is centrifuged and the supernatant fluid is discarded. The sediment (paste) is transferred to sterile, tared, 500-ml wide-mouthed bottles and weighed. At this point, cultures are made on Trypticase-soy or tryptose agar for examination for purity and colony type after 4 days of incubation. Stained smears should also be made and examined microscopically for purity before proceeding. To each bottle is added two parts of sterile phenolized saline. The suspension is homogenized on a shaking machine for 4 h and then placed in flowing steam at 100 C for 25 min to kill the bacteria. (Some prefer heating the suspension at 60 C for 1 h.)

To each 1 g of paste, add an additional 17 ml of phenolized saline, and homogenize. The cell volume is then determined by placing exactly 1 ml of suspension in each of four Fitch-improved Hopkins tubes to which 4 ml of distilled water has been added. The tubes are centrifuged for 75 min at 2,750 rpm (30-cm centrifuge head), and the amount of sediment is read. If the average reading is 0.045 ml, then the suspension is 4.5%. If not, it is adjusted to that level by adding more cells or diluent and redetermining the cell volume.

Amounts of 20 ml of this concentrated suspension may be placed in vials, tested for purity and sterility, and stored in a refrigerator at 4 C. To make test antigen, the suspension is diluted by adding the contents of each vial to 1,980 ml of sterile phenolized saline to provide a suspension of 0.045% cells.

Each newly prepared lot of antigen should be tested on a battery of sera of known titer for performance. Sera of a range of end-point titers should be used. If necessary, further adjustment of the cell volume is made to provide the proper sensitivity. Addition of more cells reduces the sensitivity; dilution increases it.

An alternative method of standardization is to adjust the final diluted product to a density yielding 78% light transmission as measured in a spectrophotometer at a wavelength of 65 nm. Here again, the sensitivity should be checked as above and adjusted if necessary.

Preparation of B. canis antigen

Examine the culture carefully for purity. Prepare seed culture by inoculating an appropriate number of Trypticase-soy agar slants. Incubate at 37 C for 18 to 24 h. Suspend the growth in sterile isotonic saline. Use the suspension immediately to seed Pyrex culture bottles containing Trypticase-soy agar layered on one side. Incubate at 37 C for 24 to 40 h. Growth should be visible but not grossly mucoid. Longer incubation results in more mucoid material and greater instability in the final product. Harvest in sterile isotonic saline (do not use phenolized saline). Pool the harvest and mix well. Remove a sample of the suspension, and culture it on Trypticase-soy agar or tryptose agar plates for purity check after growth. A stained smear should also be examined microscopically for purity. Immediately heat the suspension for 1 h at 60 C to kill the bacteria. Collect the bacterial cells by centrifugation (aseptic technique) and resuspend in sterile isotonic saline to the same density as for regular antigen. Add Merthiolate, 1 part per 10,000, as a preservative. For use, dilute to a density comparable to that of the standard antigen.

Preparation of Brucellergen (5)

Since preparation of Brucellergen involves use of virulent cultures of *Brucella*, standardization on infected rabbits, sterility testing, and tests of tolerance and effectiveness on humans prior to use, few laboratories will want to accept the risks of producing this reagent. A concise summary of the method of production and standardization is presented.

In large culture bottles containing liver infusion agar, a smooth strain of *B. abortus, B. suis,* or *B. melitensis* is grown at 37 C for 72 h. The growth is washed from the medium with sterile distilled water, and the cells are recovered by centrifugation and extracted with anhydrous ether for two successive 5-day periods to remove lipids. The extracted cells are collected on a filter and dried in vacuo over H_2SO_4 at 37 C. The dried cells are ground in a ball mill. The powder is suspended in distilled water, with 2 liters of water for each 10 g of powder. The suspension is adjusted to pH 7 (1 N NaOH) and allowed to stand in a cold room (6 to 8 C) for 12 to 15 h; the insoluble material is removed by centrifugation. The protein nucleate in the clear supernatant fluid is precipitated at a pH of 3.9 by addition of a 1:2 dilution of reagent-grade glacial acetic acid and is allowed to stand in the cold room for 24 h. The precipitate is separated by decantation and centrifugation and is resuspended in cold distilled water, with 1 liter of water for each 10 g of initial ball mill powder. The precipitate is redissolved by use of 1 N NaOH with adjustment of the pH to 6.8. Insoluble material is removed by centrifugation. The preceding step of precipitation at pH 3.9 and resolution at pH 6.8 is repeated two more times. The last precipitate obtained is dissolved at pH 6.8 and adjusted to a concentration of approximately 1% (vol/vol). Phenol is added to a concentration of 0.5%. The product is sterilized by filtration through sintered glass. This 1% solution is a stock solution ready for standardization. Store in a cold room.

Standardization of Brucellergen (5)

Rabbits are sensitized by infecting them intravenously with a virulent culture of *Brucella*; 1 ml of a 1:100 dilution of the growth obtained from a 48-h agar slant culture (liver agar) is used. About 30 days are required for development of dermal hypersensitivity. Rabbits may be used repeatedly at 2-week intervals for intradermal tests.

The 1% stock solution is adjusted with 1 N HCl until it becomes visibly cloudy. Progressive dilutions of this suspension from 1:1,000 to 1:32,000 are made in sterile phenolized saline. Each dilution is tested by injecting 0.1 ml intradermally into the shaved skin of the abdomen of sensitized rabbits. The tests are read at 48 h. A positive reaction is characterized by erythema and induration. The first progressive dilution producing a reaction 5 mm in diameter is taken as the dilution to be used for diagnostic purposes. This is usually the 1:8,000 or 1:10,000 dilution. Noninfected rabbits are used as controls. All dilutions greater than 1:1,000 should give no reaction in the controls.

The stock solution is diluted to the desired level with sterile phenolized saline and is then ready for sterility testing, filling into vials, final sterility check, and tests for tolerance and effectiveness on known positive and negative individuals.

INTERPRETATION

Agglutination test

When the NRC Committee-recommended standard antigen and procedure for the agglutination test are used, most patients with acute brucellosis proved by culture display antibody titers of 1:320 or higher (8, 10–12). In the general population this titer provides presumptive confirmation of a clinical diagnosis of brucellosis. In an occupational group exposed repeatedly to *Brucella*, such as abbatoir workers, 40% of clinically well individuals carry titers of this magnitude. In these cases, the agglutination titer is of little help to the clinician.

There are three species of bacteria which give significant cross-reactions with smooth *Brucella* and may possibly cause confusion. These are *Vibrio cholera*, *Franciscella tularensis*, and *Yersinia enterocolitica*.

Prior treatment with *Brucella* vaccines renders the agglutination titer impossible to interpret for years. A Brucellergen skin test, positive or negative, may engender antibodies in a small percentage of people. These are usually present in low titer and disappear in a few months. I observed one such incident in which the titer rose to 1:2,500.

If blocking antibodies are present, the reported titer is given the same significance as discussed above for the titer of ordinary antibodies.

The number of human infections due to *B. canis* is too small to provide data on average agglutination titers. The presence of even low titers in an undiagnosed febrile illness calls for an intensive effort to culture the organism from the patient.

Finally, the agglutination test can only provide backing for a presumptive diagnosis of brucellosis. Isolation of the organism is necessary for confirmation.

Intradermal test (5, 10)

The test results are interpreted similarly to those of a tuberculin test. The intradermal test is highly specific. A positive reaction denotes delayed dermal hypersensitivity to cellular components of members of the genus *Brucella*. It does not distinguish between present and past infection. Positive tests can be demonstrated for years after clinical or subclinical illness. There have been no recent surveys, but 20 years ago from 10 to 25% of the general population gave positive reactions. Certainly, a considerable percentage would react at present if tested. Further, about 5% of the patients with brucellosis proved by culture do not develop dermal hypersensitivity. Accordingly, the test is not helpful as a diagnostic aid in the ill patient. The NRC Committee recommended that its use in clinical medicine be discontinued (11). From a clinical standpoint, there is no reason to reverse that recommendation at the present time. If the incidence of brucellosis continues to drop by lessened exposure and removal of reactors by death, the possible role of the test in clinical medicine may need to be reconsidered.

LITERATURE CITED

1. Alton, G. G., and L. M. Jones. 1967. Laboratory techniques in Brucellosis. WHO Monogr. Ser. No. 55.
2. Carmichael, L. E. 1967. Canine brucellosis: isolation, diagnosis, transmission. Proc. U.S. Livestock Sanit. Assoc. 71:517–527.
3. Diaz, R., L. M. Jones, and J. B. Wilson. 1968. Antigenic relationship of the gram-negative organism causing canine abortion to smooth and rough brucellae. J. Bacteriol. 95:618–624.
4. Henry, B. S. 1933. Dissociation in the genus *Brucella*. J. Infect. Dis. 52:374–402.
5. Huddleson, I. F. 1943. Brucellosis in man and animals. The Commonwealth Fund, New York.
6. Huddleson, I. F. 1952. Studies in Brucellosis III. Michigan Agric. Exp. Stn., Mem. 6.
7. McCullough, N. B. 1970. Microbial and host factors in the pathogenesis of brucellosis, p. 324–345. *In* S. Mudd (ed.), Infectious agents and host reactions. W. B. Saunders Co., Philadelphia.
8. McCullough, N. B. 1971. Brucellosis, p. 202–205. *In* H. F. Conn and R. B. Conn (ed.), Current diagnosis, 3rd ed. W. B. Saunders Co., Philadelphia.
9. Moore, J. A., B. N. Gupta, and G. H. Connor. 1968. Eradication of *Brucella canis* infection from a dog colony. J. Am. Vet. Med. Assoc. 153:523–527.
10. Spink, W. W. 1956. The nature of Brucellosis. Univ. of Minnesota Press, Minneapolis.
11. Spink, W. W., N. B. McCullough, L. M. Hutchings, and C. K. Mingle. 1952. Diagnostic criteria for human brucellosis. Report No. 2 of the

National Research Council Committee on Public Health Aspects of Brucellosis. J. Am. Med. Assoc. 149:805–808.

12. Spink, W. W., N. B. McCullough, L. M. Hutchings, and C. K. Mingle. 1954. A standardized antigen and agglutination technic for human brucellosis. Report No. 3 of the National Research Council Committee on Public Health Aspects of Brucellosis. J. Clin. Pathol. 24:496–498.

Chapter 41

Serological Response to *Bordetella pertussis*

CHARLES R. MANCLARK

INTRODUCTION

The efficacy of pertussis vaccine to prevent whooping cough was demonstrated by the British Medical Research Council (11–13). These studies established the value of the mouse potency test for measuring vaccine potency and showed that agglutinin titers of human vaccinees correlated with clinical protection. Immunization with pertussis vaccine or recovery from pertussis disease may not always result in the production of agglutinins, and immunity may exist in the absence of demonstrable agglutinins; however, infection does not occur in the presence of agglutinins of high titer (15). The production and/or presence of agglutinins is indirect evidence of vaccine potency in vaccinees and is more closely related to the protective power of the vaccine than other antibody (23). Agglutination tests are of value in epidemiological studies to evaluate the immunological experience of a survey population with *Bordetella pertussis* infection, disease, or vaccine, but they are of limited utility in the evaluation of individual clinical cases.

CLINICAL INDICATIONS AND APPLICATIONS

The basis of immunity in pertussis is not understood. Evidence suggests that immunity is not mediated by serum antibodies (3, 4, 10) and that agglutinogens are not protective antigens (17). Secretory antibodies may be involved (6), but, by default rather than based on specific knowledge, pertussis immunity is generally considered to be mediated by cellular mechanisms.

Pertussis immune globulin (human) is used for the passive immunization of children exposed to pertussis infection, but opinion varies as to its efficacy (1, 7). The product is licensed, produced, and sold in the United States, and an agglutination test is one of the procedures used to obtain potency estimates in the control testing of the product.

A variety of methods for performing agglutination tests on pertussis antiserum have been proposed (5, 8, 9, 14, 22). Although the tests differ in their specifics, they have certain common characteristics. Nearly all the methods employ a variety of expedients to insure maximal contact of antigen and antibody. Such techniques as using concentrated reactants, shaking, water-bath convection, or prolonged incubation have been shown to be useful.

Assays for pertussis antibody have their greatest application in epidemiological studies of pediatric sera. It follows that the ideal agglutination tests can be done with small serum volumes, require a minimum of manipulative procedures, and demand no critically timed steps to determine accurately titration end points with the large numbers of sera usually employed in epidemiological studies.

The choice of the diagnostic antigen is important, and most methods recommend that the antigen be prepared from a young, actively growing phase 1 culture of representative and/or broad antigenic coverage. To evaluate the response to vaccine, it is possible and practical to use the vaccine strain as a diagnostic agglutinating antigen, provided it is shown to be both typical and antigenically stable. To evaluate exposure to natural infection or response to vaccines for which the origins and antigenic content are unknown, mixtures of *B. pertussis* strains to insure broad antigenic coverage are recommended.

Comparisons of results obtained by different test methods are difficult because diagnostic antigens differ qualitatively and quantitatively, as do test methods, incubation times, and end-point determinations. The reproducibility obtained by an individual method is best controlled by an antiserum of known titer. Unless titrations are comparable and reproducible, meaningful comparisons of test results cannot be made, and the concept of using significant increases in titer (viz., fourfold) as a measure of vaccine or disease experience is of no value (19).

The following procedure has been used in epidemiological studies involving large numbers of serum specimens and has been useful for titering pertussis immune globulin (human) and clinical sera from individual patients. It is a microagglutination test requiring 0.1 ml of the patient's serum. Reproducibility has been improved by using working antigen prepared from stock concentrates of two *B. pertussis* strains of demonstrated stability, specificity, and broad antigenic coverage. Reproducibility is further controlled by a standard antipertussis serum.

TEST PROCEDURE

Twofold serial dilutions of the antisera to be tested (paired sera should be tested simultaneously) are made in microagglutination plates with eight rows of 12 round-bottom wells (U plates). Saline and sera are delivered with 0.05-ml pipettes and are diluted with 0.05-ml calibrated diluters. Place 0.05 ml of saline (0.15 M NaCl) diluent in all except the first well of each row. Add 0.1 ml of the test antisera to the first wells of each row. Using the diluter, remove 0.05 ml from the first well to the second of that row, mix, then remove 0.05 ml from the second to the third well (using same diluter), and repeat to the twelfth well; then discard 0.05 ml. Repeat for each antiserum to be tested, using one row per antiserum.

In addition, each titration should contain an antigen control of saline and antigen and a titration done with a reference or standard antiserum of known titer.

After all antiserum dilutions have been made, 0.05 ml of working antigen is added to each well and mixed. The plates are covered with plastic seals and incubated overnight at 35 C. Results are read with obliquely transmitted light at 5 to 10 diameters magnification. A negative test will appear as a thick yellowish button of cells. Complete agglutination or a 4+ reaction appears as a folded sheet of cells covering the bottom of the well. A 1+ reaction is defined as a thin sheet of cells with slight button formation and is taken as the titration end point.

REAGENTS

Typical phase 1 *B. pertussis* strains 134 and 165, shown to be stable in saline and neutral acriflavine (2), are grown separately on Mishulow's charcoal agar (16), harvested in 1:10,000 thimerosal-saline, and pooled. Stock suspensions containing 400 opacity units (OPU; 1 OPU is approximately 6 × 10⁸ bacteria) per ml are stored at 4 C and are comprised of equal amounts of strains 134 and 165. Working suspensions (20 OPU) are made each day of use. Freeze-dried cultures of *B. pertussis* strains 134 and 165 are available from the author. The serotypes and the titers of their agglutinogens are given in Table 1.

TABLE. 1. *Bordetella pertussis serotypes and titers of their agglutinogens*

Strain	Agglutinogen	Titer
B. pertussis 134, serotype 1.2.3.5.6	1	1:1,000
	2	1:960
	3	1:320
	5	1:64
	6	1:960
B. pertussis 165, serotype 1.2.3.4.6	1	1:512
	2	1:960
	3	1:160
	4	1:672
	6	1:240

Mishulow's charcoal agar (16)

Bacto-peptone (Difco)	10 g
Sodium chloride	5 g
Soluble starch	10 g
Yeast extract (Difco)	3.5 g
Agar	20 g
Beef-heart for infusion (Difco)	90 g
Charcoal, Norit-A	4 g
Distilled water	1,000 ml

Add 1 liter of distilled water to 90 g of beef-heart for infusion (90 g of beef-heart for infusion is equivalent to about 1 lb of fresh tissue) and infuse at room temperature, with stirring, for 1 h. Filter. Heat to 80 C for 5 min, and refrigerate overnight. Filter again to remove precipitates. Add other ingredients of the medium except charcoal, melt agar, and adjust to pH 7.5 ± 0.1 with NaOH. Add 4 g of Norit-A charcoal, mix, and sterilize at 121.6 C for 15 min.

Other materials

The following materials can be obtained from Cooke Engineering Co., Alexandria, Va., or from Canalco, Rockville, Md.

   Disposable U plates (round or hemispherical bottoms in wells, Cooke no. 220-24)
   Disposable pipettes, 0.05 ml (Cooke No. 220-36)
   Calibrated diluter, 0.05 ml (Cooke No. 220-34)

Pressure Sensitive Film for sealing titration plates is Falcon Plastics #3044 (Bio-Quest Division, Becton, Dickinson & Co., Cockeysville, Md.).

INTERPRETATION

A significant change in titer (≥fourfold) in an individual patient must be considered as evidence of recent exposure to pertussis vaccine or pertussis infection. In the absence of recent vaccine immunization, a significant increase in antibody titer is supportive but not diagnostic of pertussis infection.

High agglutinin titers have been correlated with protection from disease (11, 15, 17, 20, 21). Agglutinin titers of 1:320 or greater were correlated with protection in the British Medical Research Council studies (13), and this has been supported by most other workers as a useful index. Conversely, it has been reported that protection may occur in infants with low agglutinin responses (3, 4, 10, 18, 20).

These discrepancies in the relationship of agglutinin titer to protection from disease are due in part to differences in the various agglutination methods. The recommended procedure employs a stable antigen of known composition and reactivity. The assay is monitored with a reference antiserum control.

The method is uncomplicated, and titration end points are easily determined and reproduced. Experience with large numbers of sera has shown that some nonspecific agglutination does occur, but this is no greater than that obtained with other agglutination procedures. No definitive study has been done to relate agglutinin titers obtained by this method to clinical protection from pertussis. Until such a study is done, it would seem reasonable to accept the 1:320 agglutinin titer reported in the Medical Research Council trials (13) as correlative evidence of clinical protection from pertussis disease.

LITERATURE CITED

1. Balagtas, R. C., K. E. Nelson, S. Levin, and S. P. Gotoff. 1971. Treatment of pertussis with pertussis immune globulin. J. Pediatr. 79:203–208.

2. Braun, W., and A. E. Bonestell. 1947. Independent variation of characteristics in *Brucella abortus* variants and their detection. Am. J. Vet. Res. 8:386–390.

3. Brown, G. C., V. K. Volk, R. Y. Gottshall, P. L. Kendrick, and H. D. Anderson. 1964. Responses of infants to DPT-P vaccine used in nine injection schedules. Public Health Rep. 79:585–602.

4. Butler, N. R., B. D. R. Wilson, P. F. Bensen, J. A. Dudgeon, J. Ungar, and A. J. Beale. 1962. Response of infants to pertussis vaccine at one week and to poliomyelitis, diphtheria, and tetanus vaccine at six months. Lancet 2:112–114.

5. Evans, D. G., and F. T. Perkins. 1953. An agglutinin-production test in the study of pertussis vaccine. J. Pathol. Bacteriol. 66:479–488.

6. Geller, B. D., and M. Pittman. 1973. Immunoglobulin and histamine-sensitivity response

7. Kabat, E. A. 1963. Uses of hyperimmune human gamma globulin. N. Engl. J. Med. 269:247–254.

8. Kendrick, P. 1933. Rapid agglutination technique applied to *H. pertussis* agglutination. Am. J. Public Health 23:1310–1312.

9. Kendrick, P. L., R. Y. Gottshall, H. D. Anderson, V. K. Volk, W. E. Bunney, and F. H. Top. 1969. Pertussis agglutinins in adults. Public Health Rep. 84:9–15.

10. Martin de Pan, R. M. 1958. Vaccination of the newborn infant against pertussis. J. Pediatr. 53:180–186.

11. Medical Research Council. 1951. Prevention of whooping cough by vaccination. Br. Med. J. 1:1463–1471.

12. Medical Research Council. 1956. Vaccination against whooping cough: relation between protection in children and results of laboratory tests. Br. Med. J. 2:454–462.

13. Medical Research Council. 1959. Vaccination against whooping cough: final report to Whooping Cough Immunization Committee. Br. Med. J. 1:994–1000.

14. Miller, J. J., and R. J. Silverberg. 1939. The agglutinative reaction in relation to pertussis and prophylactic vaccination against pertussis with description of a new technique. J. Immunol. 37:207–221.

15. Miller, J. J., Jr., R. J. Silverberg, T. M. Saito, and J. B. Humber. 1943. An agglutinative reaction for *Haemophilus pertussis*. II. Its relation to clinical immunity. J. Pediatr. 22:644–651.

16. Mishulow, L., L. S. Sharpe, and L. L. Cohen. 1953. Beefheart charcoal agar for preparation of pertussis vaccines. Am. J. Public Health 43:1466–1472.

17. Munoz, J., and B. Hestekin. 1963. Antigens of *Bordetella pertussis*. III. Protective antigen. Proc. Soc. Exp. Biol. Med. 112:799–805.

18. Preston, N. W. 1970. Pertussis agglutinins in the child. International Symposium on Pertussis, Bilthoven 1969. Symp. Ser. Immunobiol. Stand. 13:121–125.

19. Preston, N. W., and T. N. Stanbridge. 1975. Whooping cough vaccination. Lancet 1:1089.

20. Provenzano, R. W., L. H. Wetterlow, and C. L. Sullivan. 1965. Immunization and antibody response in the newborn infant. I. Pertussis inoculation within twenty-four hours of birth. N. Engl. J. Med. 273:959–965.

21. Sako, W. 1947. Studies on pertussis immunization. J. Pediatr. 30:29–40.

22. Wilkins, J., F. F. Williams, P. F. Wehrle, and B. Portnoy. 1971. Agglutinin response to pertussis vaccine. I. Effect of dosage and interval. J. Pediatr. 79:197–202.

23. Wilson, G. S., and A. A. Miles. 1975. Topley and Wilson's principles of bacteriology, virology, and immunology, 6th ed., p. 2157. The Williams & Wilkins Co., Baltimore.

of mice to live *Bordetella pertussis*. Infect. Immun. 8:83–90.

Chapter 42

Immune Response to *Pseudomonas*

WALLIS L. JONES AND EDITH A. HAMBIE

INTRODUCTION

Infections due to various *Pseudomonas* organisms may be seen in many hospitalized patients. Many of these infections and their complications are due to *Pseudomonas aeruginosa* organisms or their by-products and are found frequently in patients with severe burns (2, 3, 4, 7), cystic fibrosis (5), and neoplastic disease (6), as well as patients receiving immunosuppressive therapy.

Immunization therapy comprising a heptavalent *Pseudomonas* vaccine has been used in patients with severe burn injury. Antibody levels were tested by passive hemagglutinating assay, hemagglutination after 2-mercaptoethanol inactivation, radial immunodiffusion, and bacterial agglutination (2, 3). Hemagglutination and hemagglutination-inhibition procedures were used in studies to detect antibodies to O antigens of *P. aeruginosa* strains in patients with cystic fibrosis (5) and neoplastic diseases (6).

At the present time, *Pseudomonas* immunological tests are not routinely done by the clinical immunology laboratory. The only *Pseudomonas* test carried out at this laboratory is an indirect hemagglutination test for the detection of antibodies to *P. pseudomallei* for the disease called melioidosis. The indirect hemagglutination test described is a modification by Alexander et al. (1) of the procedure described by Ileri (8).

Melioidosis is an infectious disease endemic to Southeast Asia (10). It may range from a mild subacute state to a rapidly fatal septicemic form. Unfortunately, severe fulminating forms of the disease may occur years after exposure.

ANTIGEN PREPARATION

Three strains of *P. pseudomallei* consisting of smooth strains of 8202, China 3, and 292 are used. Each strain is inoculated into a protein-free broth (9), pH 7.0 to 7.2, and incubated at 37 C for 2 weeks. The cultures are then autoclaved at 121 C for 15 min. Cellular material is removed by centrifugation. The supernatant fluid is removed and phenol is added to 0.5% by volume. This material is then stored at 4 C and

has been found to be stable up to 3 years (1). The optimal dilution for each antigen prepared is determined by block titration against a reference serum preparation. These are then pooled together in equal volumes.

MATERIALS

Reagents

Sheep red blood cells.
P. pseudomallei antigen.
Phosphate-buffered saline (PBS), pH 7.2: 100 ml of 0.15 M NaCl, 23.9 ml of 0.15 M KH_2PO_4, and 76.0 ml of 0.15 M Na_2HPO_4.
Antisera: positive and negative controls.
Phenol, liquefied.
Bovine serum albumin, 0.06% (0.06 g of bovine albumin powder, reagent grade), in 100 ml of PBS, pH 7.2 (PBS-BSA).

Equipment

Tubes, serological 12 × 75 mm.
Centrifuge.
Centrifuge tubes, graduated.
Pipettes.
Flasks.
Water bath, 37 C, 56 C.
Racks.

TEST PROCEDURES

Preparation of 10% sheep red blood cell suspensions

1. Wash sheep red blood cells three times in PBS, pH 7.2, for 5 min at 600 × g.
2. Pack the cells for 10 min at 600 × g and make a 10% suspension (9 volumes of pH 7.2 PBS to 1 volume of packed cells).

Sensitization of cells

1. Make the optimal dilution of antigen in PBS, pH 7.2. This optimal dilution has been predetermined by appropriate block titrations of reference antiserum and antigen.
2. Pipette into a graduated centrifuge tube 1 volume of 10% sheep red blood cells and 10 volumes of antigen dilution in PBS, pH 7.2.

315

Into a separate graduated centrifuge tube, pipette 1 volume of 10% sheep red blood cells and 10 volumes of PBS, pH 7.2.

3. Incubate both tubes for 1 h at 37 C.

4. Centrifuge the tubes for 5 min at 600 × g; remove and discard the supernatant fluid.

5. Wash the cells in two to three times their volume with PBS-BSA.

6. Centrifuge and discard supernatant fluids, and resuspend the cells in 10 times the original volume of sheep red blood cells using PBS-BSA. This results in a 1% concentration of sensitized and nonsensitized cells. The cells are now ready for use in the test.

Indirect hemagglutination test

1. Set up two rows of tubes for each serum specimen, 10 tubes for the test serum itself and a 4-tube row as a heterophile control.

2. Make a starting dilution of 1:10 for each test serum. Inactivate at 56 C for 30 min.

3. Add 1 ml of this starting dilution to the first tube for each test to be run.

4. Add 0.5 ml of PBS-BSA to all other tubes in each row.

5. Add 0.5 ml of PBS-BSA to each of two tubes labeled as cell controls for the sensitized and nonsensitized cells.

6. Make serial dilutions of each serum in 0.5-ml amounts. Discard 0.5 ml from the last tube in each row.

7. Into the test row (10 tubes) for each serum specimen and the proper cell control tube, add 0.1 ml of the sensitized cells. Into the second row (4 tubes) and the proper cell control tube, add 0.1 ml of the nonsensitized cells.

8. Shake all tubes thoroughly.

9. Incubate tubes at 25 C for 2 h.

10. Read and record as positive or negative as seen in hemagglutination patterns. The titer is the end-point dilution factor of the highest dilution showing distinct agglutination with sensitized cells.

Absorption of heterophile agglutinins

If the heterophile test is positive, i.e., agglutination in the second row of tubes, the test serum must be absorbed to remove these agglutinins and the test must be repeated. Sera need not be absorbed in those instances where significantly higher titers are obtained with sensitized cells than with nonsensitized cells.

1. Add 0.2 ml of inactivated serum to 0.6 ml of saline.

2. Add 0.2 ml of the 10% red cell suspension, prepared as described in "Preparation of 10% sheep red blood cell suspensions," to the 0.8 ml of diluted serum. This results in a 1:5 dilution of absorbed serum. Incubate at room temperature for 10 min, centrifuge, and save the supernatant fluid.

3. Make a 1:10 dilution from the 1:5 dilution of treated serum and proceed with test as above. The heterophile reaction with nonsensitized cells should be eliminated.

INTERPRETATION

An antibody titer of 40 or greater is considered to be serological evidence of infection in the indirect hemagglutination test (1). As in all serological tests, a rising titer is of greater significance where it can be demonstrated. Alexander et al. (1) reported that antibodies were usually detected by the second week of disease, and high antibody titers were present by the third week. Antibodies were detected in one case 7 years after infection (1). Cross-reactions have been noted in the sera of patients with *P. aeruginosa* and *P. stutzeri* infections as well as in a few persons with infections caused by microorganisms other than *Pseudomonas*. Typhus and leptospirosis patients have shown low titers to the indirect hemagglutination test (1).

LITERATURE CITED

1. Alexander, A. D., D. L. Huxsoll, A. R. Warner, V. Shepler, and A. Dorsey. 1970. Serological diagnosis of human melioidosis with indirect hemagglutination and complement fixation tests. Appl. Microbiol. **20**:825–833.

2. Alexander, J. W., and M. W. Fisher. 1970. Immunological determinants of *Pseudomonas* infections of man accompanying severe burn injury. J. Trauma **10**:565–574.

3. Alexander, J. W., M. W. Fisher, and B. G. MacMillan. 1971. Immunological control of *Pseudomonas* infection in burn patients: a clinical evaluation. Arch. Surg. **102**:31–35.

4. Crowder, J. G., M. W. Fisher, and A. White. 1972. Type specific immunity in *Pseudomonas* diseases. J. Lab. Clin. Med. **79**:47–54.

5. Diaz, F., L. L. Mosovich, and E. Neter. 1970. Serogroups of *Pseudomonas aeruginosa* and the immune response of patients with cystic fibrosis. J. Infect. Dis. **121**:269–274.

6. Diaz, F., and E. Neter. 1970. *Pseudomonas aeruginosa*: serogroups and antibody response in patients with neoplastic diseases. Am. J. Med. Sci. **259**:340–345.

7. Fisher, M. W., H. B. Devlin, and F. J. Gnabasik. 1969. New immunotype schema for *Pseudomonas aeruginosa* based on protective antigens. J. Bacteriol. **98**:835–836.

8. Ileri, S. Z. 1965. The indirect hemagglutination test in the diagnosis of melioidosis in goats. Br. Vet. J. **121**:164–170.

9. Rice, C. E., H. Koust, and R. C. Duthie. 1951.

Studies by complement fixation methods of malleins produced in broth and synthetic media. I. Relations immunizing activities in horses and rabbits. Can. J. Comp. Med. 15:284–291.

10. Strauss, J. M., A. D. Alexander, G. Rapmund, E. Gan, and A. Dorsey. 1969. Melioidosis in Malaysia. III. Antibodies to *Pseudomonas pseudomallei* in the human population. Am. J. Trop. Med. Hyg. 18:703–707.

Chapter 43

Immune Response to *Listeria*

SANDRA A. LARSEN, GERALDINE L. WIGGINS, AND WILLIAM L. ALBRITTON

INTRODUCTION

The immune response to infections with *Listeria monocytogenes* includes both humoral and cell-mediated components. The role of each in immunity to infections with this organism in humans is poorly defined.

Gray and Killinger in their 1966 review of *Listeria* and listeric infections stated that, although legions of articles have been published on the serological diagnosis of listeriosis, most have contributed little but an expanded bibliography (15).

There have been agglutination tests for both O and H antigens, with and without 2-mercaptoethanol reduction (1, 5, 10, 17, 22, 24, 32, 33), precipitation tests (19, 32, 37), complement-fixation tests (11, 32), hemagglutination tests, both direct and indirect (6, 20, 29, 30, 32), skin tests (8, 9, 12, 28), growth tests (26), antigen-fixation tests (21), mobility-inhibition tests (4), and indirect fluorescent-antibody techniques (3) developed for the diagnosis of listeriosis in humans and animals. Unfortunately, most of the findings cannot be compared because of the diversity of methods used and the failure of many earlier investigators to take into account the serological cross-reactions of *L. monocytogenes* with other organisms, especially *Staphylococcus aureus* and *Streptococcus faecalis* (16, 17, 20, 25, 27, 31, 39, 40).

In 1965, Osebold, Aalund, and Chrisp (23) found that treatment of *L. monocytogenes* cells with trypsin increased the antigen's sensitivity and eliminated some cross-reactions. Their further studies (1, 22) of the immune response of animals and humans to listeric infections indicated that the test might be applicable to the diagnosis of listeriosis in humans, and these findings concurred with those of Armstrong and Sword (2). In 1972, Larsen and Jones (17) used a modification of the method described by Osebold, Aalund, and Chrisp (22, 23) to test a number of sera which had been collected from bacteriologically confirmed cases of listeriosis. From these initial investigations, the sensitivity of the test looked promising. Since 1972, the test as described below under Test Procedure has been offered as a diagnostic service in our laboratory. A microagglutination test described in 1974 (16) has been successfully used for large-scale screening; however, positive results are confirmed by the tube agglutination test.

CLINICAL INDICATIONS

The clinical syndrome of listeriosis in humans is varied and may be manifested by abortion, conjunctivitis, endocarditis, meningoencephalitis, pneumonitis, pyoderma, septicemia, or urethritis (14). Although many *Listeria* infections occur in infants and in patients with underlying diseases, an increasing number of cases of listeriosis have recently been reported in previously healthy urban residents in all age groups (7, 18).

As with all febrile agglutination tests, both an acute and a convalescent serum (at an interval of 2 to 3 weeks) are desirable for the interpretation of the test. If these two sera are available, then the test may be applicable to all clinical situations with the exception of neonates and patients with underlying immunosuppressive diseases or therapy.

We have been unable to detect agglutinins in newborns with bacteriologically confirmed listeriosis (Table 1). This phenomenon was also noted by Seeliger and Potel (34) with other test procedures. Whether or not the failure of the newborn to make agglutinins in response to infection with *L. monocytogenes* is due to a delay in maturation of the immune response to the somatic antigens of *Listeria* as suggested for *Salmonella* somatic antigens by Smith et al. (35) remains to be determined.

In our earlier report (17) and in additional studies (Table 1), we found that sera from cancer patients or from other patients with suppressed immunity reacted poorly in this test. Tripathy and Mackaness (38) previously reported that administration of cancer chemotherapeutic agents suppressed the immune response of mice infected with *L. monocytogenes*.

In addition to this lack of applicability to all clinical situations, two other pitfalls detract from its usefulness as a routine test. One is the high geometric mean agglutination titers (GMAT) to serotype 1a among presumably nor-

TABLE 1. *Geometric mean agglutination titers (GMAT) with L. monocytogenes and S. aureus antigens of sera from normal persons and patients with L. monocytogenes isolates*

Type of serum and group identification	No. of sera in group	GMAT		
		L. monocytogenes		*S. aureus*
		Serotype 1a	Serotype 4b	
Convalescent sera from patients with isolates of L. monocytogenes				
Neonates				
1a/1b	6	<12.5	<12.5	<12.5
4b isolate	8	<12.5	<12.5	<12.5
Mothers of neonates with				
1a/1b isolate	9	147.0[a]	39.7	17.0
4b isolate	8	70.7	70.7	<12.5
Nonimmunosuppressed patients				
2 mo–1 yr				
1a/1b isolate	2	17.7	<12.5	<12.5
4b isolate	2	<12.5	<12.5	<12.5
1–60 yr				
1a/1b isolate	6	56.1	31.5	14.0
4b isolate	14	78.0	60.9	12.5
61+ yr				
1a/1b isolate	5	57.4	18.9	<12.5
4b isolate	3	79.3	50.0	19.8
Immunosuppressed patients				
22–58 yr				
1a/1b isolate	11	<12.5	<12.5	<12.5
4b isolate	5	<12.5	<12.5	<12.5
Sera from normal persons				
Neonates	29	<12.5	<12.5	<12.5
Mothers of neonates	25	67.8	27.2	12.5
Other age groups				
3–12 mo	12	16.7	<12.5	<12.5
1–10 yr	98	64.0	15.1	<12.5
11–20 yr	35	88.8	21.3	<12.5
21–30 yr	21	84.8	25.0	<12.5
31–40 yr	18	65.5	12.5	<12.5
41–50 yr	25	52.9	14.0	<12.5
51–60 yr	25	35.8	<12.5	<12.5
Total: 1–60 yr	222	64.0	16.0	<12.5
61+ yr	25	18.9	<12.5	<12.5

[a] For calculations, log of 6.25 was used for titers less than 12.5 and log of 12.5 was used for titers less than 25 when starting dilution was 1:25.

mal individuals (Table 1). These titers may truly reflect specific antibodies to *L. monocytogenes,* although these individuals have exhibited no clinical manifestations of the disease or infection, or they may represent cross-reacting antibodies not removed by absorption with *S. aureus.* The other pitfall is the failure of some bacteriologically confirmed cases of listeriosis in otherwise normal individuals to show fourfold rises in agglutination titers between acute and convalescent sera.

Even though this agglutination test has many drawbacks, in our laboratory, other tests, i.e., hemagglutination and H agglutination,

were found to be no more effective and often not as effective as this test at detecting *Listeria* antibodies in humans. The preferred method for diagnosis of listeric infection remains the isolation of the suspect bacterium.

REAGENTS

Antigens

Three test antigens and one absorption antigen are needed for the performance of the test. The two *L. monocytogenes* strains that are used for *Listeria* antigen preparation are serotype 1a, NCTC 7973, H. P. R. Seeliger, ATCC 19111, and serotype 4b, F4, J. Donker-Voet. These antigens represent strains with factors found in the majority of the strains isolated from patients in the United States. The two *S. aureus* strains necessary for absorption and/or antigen are Bacterial Immunology Branch (BIB) KC 28, Center for Disease Control (CDC) 1641y, and BIB KC 59, CDC 4282. Either of the *S. aureus* strains can be used in serum absorption provided that the other strain is used as the test antigen. *Caution:* These strains of *S. aureus* do not remove immunoglobulin G nonspecifically when prepared for use in this test; however, other strains of *S. aureus* with increased amounts of protein A may do so (13).

Antigen preparation. The antigens of *L. monocytogenes* and *S. aureus* are prepared by the method of Osebold, Aalund, and Chrisp (23) as modified by Larsen and Jones (17).

1. Cultures of the above strains in 5 ml of tryptose broth (Difco) are incubated for 18 to 24 h at 35 C.

2. These cultures are used to seed 32-oz (ca. 1 liter) prescription bottles containing 250 ml of tryptose agar (Difco) which has solidified on the flat surface of the bottle.

3. The inoculated bottles are incubated for 48 h at 35 C.

4. Cells are harvested from the agar surface in a minimal amount of 0.15 M NaCl (0.85% saline) and steamed for 1 h at 100 C.

5. Cell suspensions are washed twice in Sørensen's phosphate-buffered saline (PBS), pH 7.3.

6. After the second wash, cells are resuspended in the pH 7.3 PBS to a concentration that, when diluted 1:20, will read 50 to 53% optical transmission (T) at 430 nm on a Coleman Junior spectrophotometer (cuvette size, 10 × 75 mm).

7. The concentrated suspensions are treated with crude trypsin (Difco 1-300) for 15 min at 35 C by adding one part of 1% trypsin in pH 7.3 PBS to nine parts of the suspension.

8. Cells are washed twice in saline and resuspended to a concentration that will read 50 to 53% T when diluted 1:20.

9. These undiluted suspensions are the concentrated stock antigens and may be preserved with thimerosal (Merthiolate) at a final concentration of 1:10,000.

Source of reagents for antigen production. *L. monocytogenes* can be obtained from BIB, CDC (both strains) or the American Type Culture Collection (7973, 1a).

S. aureus strains are available from the BIB, CDC.

Tryptose Broth, Tryptose Agar, and Trypsin

1-300 are available from Difco Laboratories, Detroit, Mich.

Sørensen's PBS (36), pH 7.3, is prepared as follows.

Stock solutions A: 0.2 M solution of monobasic sodium phosphate (27.8 g in 1,000 ml of 0.85% saline).

Stock solution B: 0.2 M solution of dibasic sodium phosphate (53.65 g of $Na_2HPO_4 \cdot 7H_2O$ or 71.7 g of $Na_2HPO_4 \cdot 12H_2O$ in 1,000 ml of 0.85% saline). Mix 23.0 ml of solution A with 77.0 ml of solution B and dilute to 200 ml with 0.85% saline. Check pH and adjust if necessary with either solution A or solution B.

Thimerosal is available as Ethylmercurithiosalicylic Acid Sodium Salt from Fisher Scientific Co.

Control sera

Antisera for use as control sera can be produced in New Zealand white rabbits by using antigens prepared as above, but without trypsin treatment and diluted 1:20 in saline.

The inoculation schedule is essentially that of Seeliger (32). Rabbits are injected with antigen in graduated doses from 0.5 to 5.0 ml at 3- to 4-day intervals.

A week after the last injection, rabbits are exsanguinated. Serum is separated from the clot and stored either at refrigerator temperature or frozen.

Rabbits should be pre-bled, and those exhibiting a titer of greater than 1:2 with the trypsinized antigens should not be used.

L. monocytogenes antisera produced in rabbits can also be purchased from Difco.

TEST PROCEDURE

This test is designed for use with serum only.

Serum preparation

Human sera should be absorbed with either of the *S. aureus* antigens to remove cross-reactive agglutinins.

1. Mix 0.4 ml of human serum with 2.1 ml of the concentrated *S. aureus* antigen: a 1:6.25 dilution.

2. Incubate serum plus *S. aureus* at 50 C for 2 h and then overnight at 4 C.

3. Separate serum from cells by centrifugation; then decant and test.

Test protocol

Human sera. Since each serum must be tested with three antigens, three rows of six (12 × 75 mm) tubes are necessary.

1. To the first tube in each row, add 0.5 ml of serum absorbed as above.

2. To tubes 2 through 6 add 0.25 ml of 0.85% saline.

3. Transfer 0.25 ml of serum from tube 1 to tube 2, mix thoroughly, and continue serial dilutions through tube 6. Discard the last 0.25 ml from each row.

4. Dilute stock antigens in saline to read 50 to 53% T on a Coleman Junior spectrophotometer at 430 nm. This is usually a 1:20 dilution; however, with time, some antigens lyse and must be used at a slightly higher concentration.

5. Add 0.25 ml of diluted antigen to each tube, e.g., row 1, *L. monocytogenes* serotype 1a; row 2, *L. monocytogenes* serotype 4b; and row 3, *S. aureus* (the strain not used for absorption).

6. Shake the rack and incubate it in a 50 C water bath for 2 h.

7. Refrigerate the rack of tubes overnight.

8. After the tubes have warmed to room temperature, tap each tube and read against a black background near the hood of a fluorescent lamp.

9. Record titers as the highest dilution with a 2+ or stronger agglutination.

Controls. Sera from bacteriologically confirmed and serotyped cases of human listeriosis are particularly helpful in establishing antigen titers, but are somewhat difficult to obtain. Rabbit control sera for each of the two *L. monocytogenes* antigens can be successfully substituted for human sera.

The same procedure as above for the human sera is followed, except that additional dilution tubes are needed to reach an end point. Absorption of rabbit sera is not necessary, and sera are tested only against the homologous antigen. In addition, a negative control for the antigen containing only antigen and diluent is prepared.

Controls should be run each time the test is performed. If there is a drop in the end-point titer, recheck the % T of the diluted antigen. A lower % T indicates autolysis of the antigen, and the concentration of the diluted antigen should be adjusted to read 50 to 53% T. The control test should be repeated; if end-point titer remains low, the stock antigen should be discarded.

Granulation in the negative control usually indicates contamination, and stock antigen should be discarded.

INTERPRETATION

Table 1 shows the distribution of the GMAT for sera of convalescent patients from whom *L. monocytogenes* was isolated as well as a control group of sera from persons not suspected of having listeriosis. All sera were examined according to the above procedure including absorption with *S. aureus*.

Sera from neonates from whom *L. monocytogenes* had been isolated and sera from normal neonates were negative at the first dilution tested with all of the antigens. Mothers of neonates from whom the organism had been isolated had GMAT which were significantly different (*t* test) from the GMAT of sera from mothers of babies suspected of having congenital infections other than listeriosis. Titers of the sera of "normal" mothers with the 1a antigen ranged from <25 to 200 and with the 4b antigen from <25 to 100, whereas titers of sera from mothers of neonates with *Listeria* isolates ranged from 12.5 to 400 with the 1a antigen and 12.5 to 200 with the 4b antigen. The mothers of neonates with listeriosis and 1a or 1b isolates showed results significantly different ($P < 0.02$) from those of the control group with the 1a antigen only. The mothers of neonates with 4b isolates had significantly different GMAT from those of the control group of mothers with the 4b agglutination antigen ($P < 0.005$). One of two mothers within this group, for whom both acute and convalescent sera were available, showed a fourfold rise in titer.

When sera from a control group of normal subjects aged 3 months to 90 years was tested, the GMAT had reached 64 in the 1- to 10-year group, with titers ranging from <12.5 to 400, and was highest in the 11- to 20-year group (88.8), with titers ranging from <12.5 to 400 with the 1a antigen. The GMAT then dropped to 18.9 in the ≥61-year group with the 1a antigen, with titers ranging from <12.5 to 200. The range with 4b antigen in the 3-month to 90-year group was <12.5 to 200. The highest GMAT with the 4b antigen was 25 in the normal group aged 21 to 30 years.

When the serum titers of nonimmunosuppressed patients (1 to 60 years) with *Listeria* isolates were compared with those of normal controls of the same age, those patients with 1a/1b isolates had GMAT which were significantly different from the GMAT of the controls with the 4b antigen only ($P < 0.05$). Those patients with 4b isolates also had GMAT significantly different from the controls with the 4b antigen only ($P < 0.001$). Titers from this group of patients ranged from <12.5 to 400 with both the 1a and 4b antigens. Three of 10 patients within this group demonstrated fourfold rises in titer between acute and convalescent sera.

Sera from confirmed cases in patients aged ≥61 years with 1a/1b isolates had GMAT which were significantly different from the controls, with the antigen representing the same major factors as the infecting organism ($P < 0.02$). Patients with 4b isolates had GMAT that were significantly different from the GMAT of the control group with both the 1a antigen ($P < 0.025$) and the 4b antigen ($P < 0.01$). Titers from this group of patients ranged from 25 to 400 with the 1a antigen and from <12.5 to 200 with the 4b antigen.

In confirmed cases in immunosuppressed patients, the titers were all <25 with both test antigens except for two patients whose titers were 50 with only one test antigen. Of these patients, 13 had cancer (predominantly Hodgkin's disease) and 3 had renal transplants. A single patient in this group for whom both acute and convalescent sera were available failed to show a rise in titer.

In summary, although there are significant differences in the GMAT between the patient and control groups, the ranges of titers within the two groups overlap considerably. Therefore, a high-titered single serum in certain select groups (mothers of neonates and elderly patients with symptoms indicative of listeriosis) may be suggestive, and a fourfold or greater rise in titer may be considered presumptive for listeriosis; however, a confident diagnosis of listeriosis requires isolation of the organism.

LITERATURE CITED

1. Aalund, O., J. W. Osebold, F. A. Murphy, and R. A. DiCapua. 1966. Antibody heterogeneity in experimental listeriosis. J. Immunol. 97:150–157.

2. Armstrong, A. S., and C. P. Sword. 1967. Antibody responses in experimental infections with *Listeria monocytogenes*. J. Immunol. 98:510–520.

3. Bakulov, I., and V. M. Kotlyarov. 1968. Nopryamoi metod fluorestsiruyushchikh antitel pri diagnostike listerioza. Veterinariya (Moscow) 45:19–21.

4. Berger, J. 1970. Mobility inhibition test in serological diagnosis of listeriosis. Dtsch. Tieraerztl. Wochenschr. 77:459–463.

5. Brandis, H., H. Werner, and A. Viebahn. 1971. Erfahrungen mit der chemischen Immunoglobulin-Differenzierung bei der Serodiagnostik der Listeriose. Klin. Wochenschr. 49:989–992.

6. Burenkova, N. A. 1959. Procedure of preparing listeriosis antigen for the indirect haemagglutination test. Zh. Mikrobiol. Epidemiol. Immunobiol. 30:136–138.

7. Busch, L. A. 1971. Human listeriosis in the United States 1967–1969. J. Infect. Dis. 123:328–332.

8. Dedie, K. 1958. Weitere experimentelle und untersuchungbefunde zur Listeriose bei Tieren p. 99–109. *In* E. Roots and D. Strauch (ed.),

9. Degen, R., and C. Goldenbaum. 1965. Katamnestische Untersuchungen von 29 Kindern mit geheilter Neugeborene-Listeriose. Dtsch. Med. Wochenschr. 90:1898.

10. Despierres, M. 1971. Diagnostic serologique des listerioses a l'aide d'une reaction d'agglutination sur gelose. Ann. Inst. Pasteur (Paris) 121:503–526.

11. Elischerova, K., and S. Stupalova. 1972. Listeriosis in professionally exposed persons. Acta Microbiol. Acad. Sci. Hung. 19:379–384.

12. Eveleth, D. F., A. I. Goldsby, F. M. Bolin, G. C. Holm, and J. Turn. 1953. Field trials and laboratory tests with Listeria bacterins. Proc. Am. Vet. Med. Assoc., p. 154–155.

13. Forsgren, A., and J. Sjoquist. 1966. Protein "A" from *S. aureus*. I. Pseudoimmune reaction with human γ-globulin. J. Immunol. 97:822–827.

14. Gray, M. L. 1964. Listeriosis: a round table discussion. Health Lab. Sci. 1:261–272.

15. Gray, M. L., and A. H. Killinger. 1966. *Listeria monocytogenes* and listeric infections. Bacteriol. Rev. 30:309–382.

16. Larsen, S. A., J. C. Feeley, and W. L. Jones. 1974. Immune response to *Listeria monocytogenes* in rabbits and humans. Appl. Microbiol. 27:1005–1013.

17. Larsen, S. A., and W. L. Jones. 1972. Evaluation and standardization of an agglutination test for human listeriosis. Appl. Microbiol. 24:101–107.

18. Medoff, G., L. J. Kunz, and A. N. Weinberg. 1971. Listeriosis in humans: an evaluation. J. Infect. Dis. 123:247–250.

19. Muraschi, T. F., and V. N. Tompkins. 1963. Somatic precipitinogens in the identification and typing of *Listeria monocytogenes*. J. Infect. Dis. 113:151–154.

20. Neter, E., H. Anzai, and E. A. Gorzynski. 1960. Identification of an antigen common to *L. monocytogenes* and other bacteria. Proc. Soc. Exp. Biol. Med. 105:131–134.

21. Njoku-Obi, A. N. U. 1963. Serologic aspects of listeriosis: the antigen-fixation test, p. 223–226. *In* M. L. Gray (ed.), Second symposium on listeric infections, Montana State College, Bozeman.

22. Osebold, J. W., and O. Aalund. 1968. Interpretation of serum agglutinating antibodies to *Listeria monocytogenes* by immunoglobulin differentiation. J. Infect. Dis. 118:139–148.

23. Osebold, J. W., O. Aalund, and C. E. Chrisp. 1965. Chemical and immunological composition of surface structures of *Listeria monocytogenes*. J. Bacteriol. 89:84–88.

24. Osebold, J. W., and M. T. Sawyer. 1955. Agglutinating antibodies for *Listeria monocytogenes* in human serum. J. Bacteriol. 70:350–351.

25. Potel, J. 1956. Wo stehen wir im Wissen uber die Listeriose? Medizinische 28:977–982.

26. Potel, J., and L. Degen. 1960. Zur Serologie und Immunobiologie der Listeriose. I. Metteilung:

Listeriosen Beiheft I, Zentralbl. Veterinaermed. Paul Paray Verlag, Berlin.

die Wachstumsprobe. Zentralbl. Bakteriol. Parasitenkd. Infektionskr. Abt. I Orig. **180:** 61–67.

27. Rantz, L. A., E. Randall, and A. Zuckerman. 1956. Hemolysis and hemagglutination by normal and immune serums of erythrocytes treated with a non-species specific bacterial substance. J. Infect. Dis. **98:**211–222.

28. Reichertz, P., and H. P. R. Seeliger. 1962. Untersuchungen zur Frage der Beziehung Zwischen Serumantikorpen und Hautreaktionen bei Verdachtsfallen von Listeriose. Z. Klin. Med. **157:**331–349.

29. Sachse, H., and J. Potel. 1957. Uber Kreuzreaktionen zwischen Hamosensitinen aus Streptokokken und Listerien. Z. Immunitaetsforsch. Exp. Ther. **114:**472–485.

30. Schierz, G., and A. Burger. 1966. Untersuchungen zur Serodiagnostik der Listeria-Infektion des Menschen. II. Herstellung und Anwendung eines spezifischen Listeria-Antigen. Z. Med. Mikrobiol. Immunol. **152:**300–310.

31. Seeliger, H. P. R. 1955. Serologische Kreuzreaction zwischen *Listeria monocytogenes* und Enterokokken. Z. Hyg. Infektionskr. **141:**15–25.

32. Seeliger, H. P. R. 1961. Listeriosis. Hafner Publishing Co., Inc., New York.

33. Seeliger, H. P. R., and P. Emmerling. 1970. Zum Vorkommen 2-Mercaptoathanol-resistenter und empfindlicher Listeria-Agglutinine in Human- und Tierseren. Z. Med. Mikrobiol. Immunol. **155:**218–227.

34. Seeliger, H. P. R., and J. Potel. 1969. Listeriose, p. 1023–1032. *In* A. Grumbach and O. Bonin (ed.), Die Infektionskrankheiten des Menschen und ihre Erreger, vol. 2, 2nd ed. George Thieme Publishers, Stuttgart.

35. Smith, R. T., D. V. Eitzman, M. E. Catlin, E. O. Wirtz, and B. E. Miller. 1964. The development of the immune response. Characterization of the response of the human infant and adult to immunization with Salmonella vaccines. Pediatrics **23:**163–183.

36. Sørensen, S. P. L. 1909. Supplement to the paper. Enzyme studies (II) concerning the measurement and significance of the hydrogen ion concentration in enzymatic processes. Biochem Z. **22:**352–356.

37. Szatalowicz, F. T., D. C. Dlenden, and M. S. Khan. 1970. Occurrence of listeria antibodies in select occupational groups. Can. J. Public Health **61:**402–406.

38. Tripathy, S. P., and G. B. Mackaness. 1969. The effect of cytoxic agents on the primary immune response to *Listeria monocytogenes*. J. Exp. Med. **130:**1–16.

39. Welshimer, H. J. 1960. Staphylococcal antibody production in response to infections with *Listeria monocytogenes*. J. Bacteriol. **79:**456–457.

40. Welshimer, H. J. 1963. Some serological reactions observed with *Listeria monocytogenes*, p. 237–243. *In* M. L. Gray (ed.), Second symposium on listeric infections, Montana State College, Bozeman.

Chapter 44

Immune Response to *Corynebacterium diphtheriae* and *Clostridium tetani*

JOHN P. CRAIG

INTRODUCTION

The exotoxins of *Corynebacterium diphtheriae* and *Clostridium tetani* are among the most highly antigenic proteins. Toxoids prepared from these toxins regularly evoke high levels of neutralizing antitoxins which are highly protective against the risk of disease in humans. Indeed, these two toxoids are among the most effective prophylactic immunogens in general use today. Moreover, good methods for the assay of these antitoxins have existed for decades. In spite of these facts, the measurement of the immune response during the natural course of disease in the *individual patient* has played almost no role in the diagnosis or management of these infections. Indeed, regular clinical laboratories seldom maintain the capability for titrating diphtheria or tetanus antitoxin levels. Instead, these methods have been used almost exclusively as research tools for epidemiological investigation in the case of diphtheria or in the study of immunogenicity of toxoids in both diseases. The reasons for this are fourfold: (i) the pathogenesis of these two intoxications demands that an immediate decision for or against specific immunotherapy be made on clinical grounds or, in the case of diphtheria, with the assistance of direct bacteriological examination; (ii) the assay methods now available are too time-consuming to be used as admission procedures to aid the clinician in deciding on the need for immunotherapy; (iii) in all cases in which there are reasonably good clinical grounds for suspecting either of these diseases, specific immunotherapy is begun at once, rendering convalescent determinations of little value; and (iv) in tetanus, and also in some individuals with diphtheria, the pathogenetic dose of toxin is less than the immunogenic dose. Therefore, even in untreated cases, if such existed, determination of serum antitoxin levels during convalescence would not be a reliable retrospective diagnostic tool (19). For these reasons, there are also almost no data on the immune response in untreated patients, and the natural sequence of immunological events in these diseases is virtually unknown. In communities in which laboratories capable of titrating antitoxins exist, virtually all recognized cases of tetanus and diphtheria receive therapeutic antitoxin.

DIPHTHERIA

The best evidence concerning the immune response to infection with diphtheria bacilli was derived from epidemiological studies carried out before the introduction of toxoid. These studies employed the Schick test, which was the earliest method of estimating diphtheria antitoxin levels on a routine bases. In the 1920s, the majority of children in New York and Baltimore had experienced immunizing infections with diphtheria by the age of 15 years (7, 29). Since few of these had clinical disease, Frost (7) reached the inevitable conclusion that enough toxin is liberated during inapparent infection to evoke an immune response in most individuals. This is especially interesting in view of the fact that some individuals with clinically manifest disease may not develop detectable antitoxin. More recently, Nyerges et al. (20) have provided immunological evidence that a high proportion of children can be shown to evince an antitoxin response during disease even when antitoxin therapy is used. It is also generally accepted that diphtheria almost never occurs in individuals with preexisting antitoxin levels of 0.01 antitoxin unit (AU) or more.

Several methods are now available for the determination of diphtheria antitoxin levels in body fluids. The Schick test, although not a laboratory procedure, still remains today a reliable, roughly quantitative measure of antitoxic immunity. Details of its application are provided below. The most reliable methods of measuring diphtheria antitoxin levels depend upon the neutralization of toxin, with rabbit or guinea pig skin as the indicator. The method first described by Jensen (12) is detailed below. This is recommended as the most direct and relevant method for a clinical laboratory, and the method least fraught with problems of technique, interpretation, and reproducibility.

The basic method of passive hemagglutination (HA) of protein-coated red blood cells (2, 24, 25) is now widely used for the detection of diphtheria antitoxin in sera (6, 14, 22, 26–28). Diphtheria toxin is adsorbed to formalinized and tannic acid-treated sheep or horse red blood cells. These cells are then agglutinated by specific diphtheria antitoxin. In one modification, the tanned cells are also treated with bis-diazobenzidine (3) to improve adsorption of toxin. A number of workers have used various modifications of passive hemagglutination methods in serological surveys and in animal and human studies on the immunogenicity of toxoids (17, 26, 27). There is good statistical correlation between titers obtained by the passive HA method and by toxin neutralization in rabbit skin, indicating that in the main the passive HA test is detecting specific antitoxin (22, 26, 27, 28). However, most workers agree that in individual sera there may be marked discrepancies, up to eightfold, which render the interpretation of the passive HA test very risky in the individual patient (4, 14). It must be remembered that passive HA is an indirect and inferential method, not dependent upon actual neutralization of the biological effect of a toxin, but rather upon immunological recognition. Therefore, if an accurate measurement of antitoxin titer in an individual body fluid is desired, an in vivo test is recommended. Moreover, the use of an animal as an indicator system obviates many of the technical variables inherent in an in vitro technique. For these reasons, I have selected the rabbit intracutaneous method for detailed description below as the method of choice.

Tissue culture methods have also been used extensively in the titration of diphtheria antitoxin. These methods are based on the fact that diphtheria toxin causes readily observable changes in several cell lines as a result of its inhibitory effect on protein synthesis (10, 13, 15, 21, 23). Specific antitoxin neutralizes this effect. As one might expect, tissue culture methods show closer agreement than does passive HA with the rabbit skin neutralization method, since both tissue culture and skin methods depend upon actual neutralization of the biological activity of the toxin. The technique described by Miyamura et al. (18), employing VERO cells and depending upon color change as the end point, would appear at the present time to be the simplest and most satisfactory method available, if a tissue culture method is desired. Again, however, the establishment of a tissue culture system for a procedure which is rarely done in a clinical laboratory would seem inadvisable, and the rabbit skin method is probably fraught with far fewer problems.

TETANUS

As in diphtheria, the most reliable and relevant method of antitoxin determination involves in vivo neutralization of toxin. In this case, the mouse neutralization assay is the most widely used (1). The method is described in detail below.

Passive HA has been used extensively in serological surveys as well as in studies on the immunogenicity of toxoids (16, 17, 26–28). The same problems apply here as in the case of diphtheria passive HA. The test is highly sensitive, and there is probably better correlation between neutralization and passive HA titers than in the case of diphtheria (8, 9). However, discrepancies between neutralization and passive HA titers in individual sera are frequent (11, 14). It is therefore recommended that in a clinical laboratory, where values in individual patients are important, the more reliable mouse neutralization test be employed. There is no tissue culture method available for the titration of tetanus toxin or antitoxin.

CLINICAL INDICATIONS

There are few indications for the determination of diphtheria or tetanus antitoxin levels in a clinical laboratory.

Probably the most frequent need for these assays today is in connection with studies on immunocompetence. The response to diphtheria or tetanus toxoid in individuals suspected of immunodeficiency disorders is gaining wider use. Although the Schick test has been used for this purpose, it is only very roughly quantitative and has the disadvantage of requiring injections of the subject and repeated observations. The rabbit intracutaneous assay for diphtheria antitoxin and the mouse neutralization test for tetanus are the assays of choice. With these assays the actual neutralizing capacity of the antibody can be measured as precisely as desired.

It has been suggested that the measurement of diphtheria antitoxin by a rapid passive HA method on admission can provide the clinician with information which may be helpful in deciding whether to give antitoxin (20). If the clinical diagnosis is in doubt, the presence of high levels of diphtheria antitoxin would militate against a diagnosis of diphtheria and obviate the need for immunotherapy. This could be of value in reducing unnecessary cases of serum sickness. This concept deserves further study. It is not clear what level of antitoxin should be considered high enough to eliminate the need for antitoxin treatment. A value of 0.4 AU/ml or over was suggested. The fact that individual discrepancies between passive HA and neutralizing antibody titers are not rare makes one worry about withholding antitoxin treatment on the basis of a single passive HA assay. At the moment, there is no known assay system which can provide evidence of *neutralizing* diphtheria antitoxin in less than 2 or 3 days.

TEST PROCEDURES

Schick test

Although the Schick test is not a laboratory procedure, it must be considered along with other indicators of the immune response to diphtheria toxin antigen. The Schick test is capable of dividing the population into two broad categories, designated Schick positive and Schick negative, based on their response to approximately $1/50$ of a guinea pig minimal lethal dose (MLD) of diphtheria toxin (roughly 0.5 ng). It is generally agreed that most persons who are Schick positive possess a serum antitoxin level of less than 0.01 AU/ml, whereas most persons who are Schick negative possess levels of 0.01 AU/ml or over. However, although this generalization can be applied to epidemiological studies involving large groups, many individual exceptions are found when serum antitoxin titers as determined by the rabbit intracutaneous method are compared with Schick test results (5).

Schick test reagents must be obtained from laboratories which are licensed to produce biological materials for human use. Under no circumstances should materials prepared in an unlicensed laboratory be used for testing in humans.

The Schick test is of no value in determining the need for diphtheria antitoxin in the treatment of diphtheria. The results of the test are available no earlier than 18 to 24 h after application of the test, and the decision regarding specific immunotherapy must be made as soon as the diagnosis of diphtheria is entertained.

The Schick test is performed by injecting 0.1 ml of the appropriate dilution of diphtheria toxin (approximately $1/5$ guinea pig MLD per ml) intracutaneously on the flexor surface of one arm, and 0.1 ml of the same material which has been heated for 30 min at 70 C on the other arm. Some suppliers of Schick test materials provide a dilution of fluid diphtheria toxoid as control material instead of heated toxin. In such cases, the dose of control toxoid often contains much more toxin-derived antigen than

does the Schick toxin. This has the advantage of providing the subject with a small booster dose of diphtheria toxoid, but the disadvantage of not being a true "control."

The importance of including a control injection needs to be stressed. Most toxins used in the preparation of Schick test reagents are not highly purified. They may contain a variety of corynebacterial antigens immunologically unrelated to the toxin, and these may evoke skin responses which are usually delayed in type and which may be confused with the skin response to diphtheria toxin. A smaller number of individuals develop immediate-type wheal and flare reactions to either or both toxin and control materials, but these reactions disappear within a few hours. Therefore, they pose no problem in interpretation of the Schick test.

To gain the most information from a Schick test, the reactions should be examined daily, and the diameter of redness and the diameter and intensity of induration should be recorded. Readings on the 2nd and on the 5th and 7th days are essential. The findings in the four categories of response are shown in Table 1. Certain qualitative differences in response are important and can be recognized by the careful observer, but cannot be presented in a table.

Typically, the redness produced by the toxin in a nonimmune person appears at about 18 h as a rosy blush 8 to 12 mm in diameter, growing more intensely red and reaching a maximal size of 10 to 25 mm in 3 to 5 days. A central blanched area of necrosis may develop. The redness fades very slowly, often leaving an area of increased pigmentation for 1 year or more. Although the positive Schick test may be accompanied by slight to moderate edema, the marked induration of a typical reaction of delayed hypersensitivity does not appear, and redness alone is the major feature.

In the typical pseudoreaction, the redness and induration appear on *both* arms. These usually resemble positive tuberculin reactions, and they wax and wane with identical time-

TABLE 1. *Schick test responses*

Schick reaction	Reaction				Interpretation	
	Toxin		Control		Circulating antitoxin	Sensitivity to bacterial antigens
	36 h	120 h	36 h	120 h		
Positive ...	±	+	0	0	0	0
Negative ..	0	0	0	0	+	0
Pseudoreaction	+	0	+	0	+	+
Combined reaction .	+	+	+	0	0	+

courses. The peak of the reaction is at 48 to 72 h. However, if the control material contains more antigen than does the toxin, the maximal reaction size may be greater at the control site.

In individuals with adequate circulating and tissue antitoxin but possessing no sensitivity to other corynebacterial antigens, no reaction whatsoever will be seen on either arm from the second day on. It is important to recognize that the in vivo combination of toxin and antitoxin does *not* give rise to a visible skin response except for the occasional immediate reaction which occurs during the first few hours after administration. Such reactions are spent within the first hour and do not interfere with the interpretation of the Schick test.

Combined reactions are the most difficult to interpret, and, indeed, a clear-cut determination of the status of antitoxic immunity cannot be made in a few individuals. A very marked reaction of delayed hypersensitivity to nontoxin antigens may persist for more than 1 week and mask the reaction to toxin. Usually, a decision can be made at 2 to 3 weeks. In a true pseudo-reaction both lesions will have faded simultaneously. In a combined reaction evidence of toxin-mediated necrosis will persist longer than the lesion of delayed sensitivity.

The amount of antigen in the usual Schick test materials will exert a substantial booster effect in individuals possessing low levels of antitoxin, and even in some Schick-positive individuals who nonetheless have been previously primed with toxin or toxoid. On the average, individuals who possess detectable antitoxin levels at the time of Schick testing (0.001 AU/ml or above) develop about 10-fold rises in circulating antitoxin titer in response to the Schick test, even when the control material contains only the same amount of toxin antigen as does the test toxin (unpublished data).

Rabbit intracutaneous method for the titration of diphtheria antitoxin

The method first described by Jensen (12) is probably the simplest and most reliable. The backs of two adult white rabbits are clipped as closely as possible with an electric clipper fitted with a head designed for clipping rabbit fur. The small animal clipper with "Angra" head supplied by John Oster, New York, N.Y., is satisfactory. During moulting, many rabbits are found to have irregular, patchy areas of dense and rapid hair growth. If, during clipping, it is found that a rabbit has more than a few such patches, it is best to reject that animal and select another because these areas are unsuitable for injection. The margins of such patches are indurated and reddened. During clipping, it is necessary to restrain the rabbit on an operating board with all four legs sufficiently taut to prevent struggling. Mark off the clipped area in approximately 15-mm squares in a grid using a black felt pen. Sixty to 100 squares can easily be accommodated on the back of a 2.5- to 4-kg rabbit. Depilation is unnecessary and, in fact, undesirable because it causes generalized erythema and dryness and cracking of rabbit skin which makes the reading of the lesions produced by diphtheria toxin more difficult. If rabbits free from areas of heavy hair growth are selected, the amount of growth at 3 days will be slight and can be removed just before reading by a light clipping.

Potencies of antitoxins are expressed in units. It is therefore necessary to determine the proper test dose of the sample of diphtheria toxin selected by titrating it against a sample of standard antitoxin. The most satisfactory toxin dose for this type of antitoxin titration is the Lr/20,000 dose. An Lr dose of diphtheria toxin is defined as that amount of toxin which, when mixed with 1 AU of diphtheria antitoxin and injected intracutaneously, will elicit a minimal area of redness. The Lr/20,000 is the amount of toxin which will elicit the same minimal area of redness in the presence of 1/20,000 AU. It is important to remember that the fixed reference point in all these assays is the antitoxin unit, which was originally arbitrarily assigned to an antitoxic serum, and against which all subsequent antitoxins have been calibrated. The toxin, which is much more labile than antibody, is always measured in reference to the antitoxin.

Diphtheria toxin batches vary so greatly in potency that no guide can be offered for initial titration. Crude culture filtrates or partially purified preparations are as satisfactory as highly purified toxins for antitoxin titrations. One Lf (limit of flocculation) dose of toxin is roughly equal to one Lr. Therefore, if the Lf potency of the toxin is provided, the general magnitude of toxic potency can be predicted. In any case, when the assay is being newly established in a laboratory, it will be necessary to carry out preliminary screening titrations in order to establish the approximate potency of the toxin to be used.

Use borate-buffered saline, pH 7.5, containing 0.1% gelatin as the diluent for both toxin and antitoxin as well as the sera to be tested. Diphtheria toxin is heat-labile, and although it is not rapidly deactivated at room temperature, it is best to carry out all procedures in ice baths to maintain constant conditions. A convenient procedure is to keep a supply of pans 4 to 5 inches deep containing 1 inch of water in the freezing compartment of a refrigerator. By adding another inch of water, an ice bath for test tube racks is quickly produced, obviating the need for a supply of crushed ice. Test tube racks containing toxin-antitoxin mixtures can be returned to these ice trays after incubation at 37 C, and the mixtures can be kept at 0 to 4 C throughout the injection period.

For the screening test, prepare 10 serial three- to fivefold dilutions of toxin encompassing the expected Lr/20,000 end point. To a series of 10 Wassermann tubes add 0.5 ml of standard diphtheria antitoxin containing 0.001 AU/ml. To these tubes add 0.5 ml of each appropriate toxin dilution. Mix by gentle shaking and incubate at 37 C for 1 h; then transfer to an ice bath. Inject each of the toxin-antitoxin mixtures in 0.1-ml volumes intracutaneously in duplicate on the backs of each of two rabbits. Each injection site will thus receive 1/20,000 AU. If strict objectivity is desired, a randomized pattern should be prepared on paper, and the mixtures should be injected accordingly. Use disposable 26-gauge, $3/8$-inch, intradermal bevel needles on glass tuberculin syringes. Inject with bevel downward. Plastic syringes may be used, but the removal of air bubbles during filling may be troublesome. Failure to expel all air from syringes and needles hilts leads to inaccurate injection volumes.

Read at 3 days. Only slight differences will be noted if the reading is done at 2 or 4 days. Record the diameter of redness to the nearest millimeter.

Determine the mean erythema diameter for each mixture. On graph paper plot diameters on the ordinate against the log of the toxin dose on the abscissa. The amount of toxin which yields a mean erythema diameter of 8 mm can be considered the preliminary Lr/20,000 dose. If the proper range of toxin doses has been chosen, diameters of erythema should range from 0 to 20 mm or more. If complete neutralization has not been achieved with a lower toxin dose or lesions at least 15 mm in diameter with higher doses, repeat the screening test after raising or lowering the range. Diphtheria toxin evokes palpable swelling as well as redness, but the diameter of induration or edema is difficult to estimate, whereas the margin of erythema is usually discrete and easily measurable.

After the Lr/20,000 screening test has been completed, repeat the test using 0.1 or 0.15 log increments of toxin instead of the three- to fivefold increments. The amount of toxin yielding a mean erythema diameter of 8 mm in this test can be considered the final Lr/20,000 dose to be used for antitoxin titrations. Once this value has been determined for a given batch of

properly aged toxin, it will remain stable as long as the undiluted toxin sample is kept refrigerated. Fresh dilutions should be made from the neat stock once a week because diluted toxin samples are not stable. Newly prepared toxin usually loses potency more rapidly during the first few months as a result of spontaneous change to toxoid.

All human and animal sera to be injected in rabbit skin should be inactivated at 56 C for 30 min. Some human sera contain components that produce redness and induration which may resemble the lesion elicited by diphtheria toxin. These are usually destroyed by inactivation, but not in all instances. Therefore, a serum control of the highest concentration of the serum tested should be included in each test. When the Lr/20,000 dose of toxin is used, any serum dilution which yields a lesion less than 8 mm in diameter can be considered to contain more than 0.001 AU/ml, and dilutions which yield lesions more than 8 mm in diameter to contain less than 0.001 AU/ml. The accuracy desired will determine the serum dilution increments employed. For survey purposes, 10-fold serum diutions are usually employed, and all persons possessing more than 0.01 AU/ml are considered the equivalent of Schick negative. In the rare clinical situations in which the determination of diphtheria antitoxin levels is critical, however, twofold serum dilutions would probably be required.

Prepare the desired serial dilutions of inactivated test sera in borate-gelatin buffer and dispense 0.3 to 0.4 ml of each dilution into chilled Wassermann tubes. Dispense an extra tube of the highest serum concentration. To the serum control tube, add an equal volume of diluent. To all other tubes, add an equal volume of diphtheria toxin containing 20 Lr/20,000 doses per ml. (This is the Lr/20,000 concentration determined above; 0.05 ml of this material will contain 1 Lr/20,000 dose.) Include an Lr/20,000 titration in each rabbit test to insure that the test dose on that day is actually at or near the Lr/20,000 test dose of toxin and diluent. The Lr/20,000 titration of that day will determine the actual end point in the day's test. For example, if the test dose which was assumed to be one Lr/20,000 actually yielded a 6-mm lesion in the Lr/20,000 titration, then 6 mm should be the cut-off value in the antitoxin titrations.

Since all determinations are done on each of two rabbits, the diameters elicited by a given toxin-serum mixture can be averaged. The antitoxin content of an unknown serum is expressed as a range. For example, if a serum dilution of 1:2 completely neutralized the Lr/20,000 dose of toxin, but 1:4 yielded redness 10 mm in diameter, and the test dose that day evoked a lesion 8 mm in diameter in the presence of 1/20,000 AU of standard antitoxin, then the antitoxin titer of that serum would be >1/500 but <1/250 AU/ml (>1/10,000 but <1/5,000 AU per 0.05 ml).

It is important to titrate all the sera from a single patient on the same set of rabbits. In spite of adequate serum and toxin controls, rabbits may differ markedly in their susceptibility to diphtheria toxin; this can be reflected in differences in end points.

The rabbit intracutaneous test may be useful in estimating immune competence by determining antitoxin levels following the administration of diphtheria toxoid. Although Schick tests are sometimes used for this purpose, the rabbit skin test is much superior because it allows for more precise measurement of the antitoxin level. Moreover, the Schick test is designed to detect very low levels of diphtheria antitoxin (0.01 AU/ml). To assess immune competence properly, one must be able to recognize a higher range of titers.

Titration of tetanus antitoxin by the mouse toxin-neutralization test

The procedure is based upon the capacity of tetanus antitoxin to protect mice from death following the subcutaneous injection of tetanus toxin. The following procedure is based upon the method of Barile et al. (1).

The sample of tetanus toxin to be used must first be titrated against a Standard Tetanus Antitoxin to determine the $L^+/1,000$ toxin dose. The $L^+/1,000$ dose is the least amount of tetanus toxin which, when mixed with 1/1,000 AU of antitoxin and injected subcutaneously into mice in a volume of 0.5 ml, causes the death of all mice by 96 h.

Use female 15- to 18-g mice; males tend to fight. Any strain can be used, but strain and source should not be changed once the titration procedure has been established. Preliminary estimation of the $L^+/1,000$ dose of toxin can be made in groups of four to six mice. In all mouse tests, pool all mice needed for the test, including all controls, and distribute randomly into the groups required.

Phosphate-buffered saline, 0.067 M, pH 7.4, containing 0.2% gelatin is used as the diluent for all reagents.

For the initial screening test to estimate the $L^+/1,000$ dose of toxin, add constant volumes of standard antitoxin containing 0.004 AU/ml to a series of 8 to 10 tubes. Prepare a series of three- to fivefold dilutions of tetanus toxin, and add an equal volume to each tube of antitoxin. Shake gently and incubate for 1 h at 37 C; then keep the mixtures at 4 to 8 C until time of injection.

Inject 0.5 ml of each toxin-antitoxin mixture subcutaneously in the right inguinal fold of the mice using 26-gauge, 3/8-inch needles. Each injection contains 0.001 AU. Observe for 96 h, and record the number of deaths. The smallest dose of toxin which kills all mice is the approximate $L^+/1,000$. (The corresponding toxin dilution contained 4 $L^+/1,000$ per ml.)

To ascertain a more precise $L^+/1,000$, repeat the test using narrower increments of toxin and 12 mice per toxin dose. Since tetanus toxin produces very precise and reproducible results in mice, good results may be obtained by using a very narrow range of doses. Five percent increments over a twofold range can usually be used successfully. For example, the following progression in micrograms of toxin per mouse has been used: 16, 17, 18, 19, 20, 20.5, 21, 21.5, 22, 22.5, 23, 23.5, 24.

For serum titrations test sera should be inactivated at 56 C for 30 min. Constant volumes of 2- to 10-fold dilutions of serum are dispensed into Wassermann tubes. To each tube, add an equal volume of toxin containing 4 $L^+/1,000$ doses per ml. Run a concurrent $L^+/1,000$ titration of the toxin against standard antitoxin in the same pool of mice. One group of mice should receive the toxin test dose mixed with an equal volume of diluent. For serum titrations, groups of four mice per serum dilution give satisfactory results. The test is considered satisfactory if the concurrent $L^+/1,000$ dose of toxin is within 25% of the test dose.

The results are interpreted as follows: if all mice are protected by undiluted serum but all die at 1:10 dilution, 0.25 ml of the undiluted serum contained >0.001 AU, and 0.25 ml of the 1:10 dilution contained <0.001 AU. Thus, the serum contained >0.004 but <0.04 AU/ml. For purposes of calculation, such a serum can be assigned a value equal to the logarithmic mean of the values or 0.12 AU/ml. For more precise titration, narrowing increments of test sera can be used. Also, the level of testing can be shifted by using multiples or fractions of the $L^+/1,000$ dose of toxin.

As in the case of diphtheria, determination of serum tetanus antitoxin is of no value in determining the need for prophylactic or therapeutic antitoxin in the management of tetanus. This decision must be made on clinical grounds and certainly cannot await the outcome of a 4-day mouse test.

The determination of antitoxin level in serum collected before antitoxin therapy may be of retrospective academic interest in situations in which the diagnosis of tetanus was in doubt, but in which antitoxin was administered. A pretreatment antitoxin titer >0.01 AU/ml would speak strongly against a diagnosis of tetanus. On the other hand, tetanus is usually considered a nonimmunizing disease because the pathogenetic dose is much less than the immunogenic dose of this antigen. Therefore, the absence of antitoxin in serum collected *after* recovery from an illness in an untreated individual does not rule out the possibility that the illness was tetanus.

REAGENTS

Diphtheria and tetanus toxins are not available commercially. Samples can sometimes be obtained upon request from pharmaceutical companies which are engaged in the manufacture of diphtheria and tetanus toxoids.

Standard antitoxins

Samples of International Standard Diphtheria and Tetanus Antitoxins are supplied to qualified laboratories by the Bureau of Biologics, Food and Drug Administration, Rockville, Md. The Bureau supplies a single small vial containing low-titer antitoxin preserved in glycerol. This sample is to be used by the receiving laboratory in preparing and substandardizing its own stock. Therefore, it is necessary to purchase antitoxins from pharmaceutical houses or state laboratories which prepare diphtheria and tetanus antitoxins for prophylactic or therapeutic use. The approximate potency of these antitoxins is recorded on the vial, but they must be precisely standardized against the official standard preparation before they can be used as a reference reagent. Tetanus immune globulin of human origin can be purchased from several pharmaceutical companies and then standardized against the standard reagent.

Schick test materials

It is regrettable that there is no longer a commercial source of Schick toxin in the United States. Schick test outfits may be purchased from the Biologic Laboratories of the Department of Public Health of the Commonwealth of Massachusetts, Jamaica Plain, Mass. 02130. The outfits are provided free of charge to qualified residents of the Commonwealth of Massachusetts.

Borate-gelatin buffer

H_3BO_3, 0.5 M	100 ml
NaCl, 1.5 M	80 ml
Gelatin, 5%	20 ml
NaOH to	pH 7.5
Water to	1,000 ml

LITERATURE CITED

1. Barile, M. F., M. C. Hardegree, and M. Pittman. 1970. Immunization against neonatal tetanus in New Guinea. 3. The toxin-neutralization test and the response of guinea pigs to the toxoids as used in the immunization schedules in New Guinea. Bull. WHO 43:453–459.
2. Boyden, S. V. 1951. The adsorption of proteins on erythrocytes treated with tannic acid and subsequent hemagglutination by antiprotein sera. J. Exp. Med. 93:107–120.
3. Butler, W. T. 1963. Hemagglutination studies with formalinized erythrocytes. Effect of bisdiazo-benzidine and tannic acid treatment on sensitization by soluble antigen. J. Immunol. 90:663–671.
4. Chatterjee, S. C. 1964. A comparative study of the haemagglutination and bioassay procedures for the assay of guinea pig anti-diphtheria and antitetanus sera. Indian J. Med. Res. 52:1241–1249.
5. Craig, J. P. 1962. Diphtheria: prevalence of inapparent infection in a nonepidemic period. Am. J. Public Health 52:1444–1452.
6. Fisher, S. 1952. The estimation *in vitro* of small amounts of diphtheria antitoxin by means of a haemagglutination technic. J. Hyg. 50:445–455.
7. Frost, W. H. 1928. Infection, immunity and disease in the epidemiology of diphtheria with special reference to studies in Baltimore. J. Prev. Med. 2:325.
8. Fulthorpe, A. J. 1957. Tetanus antitoxin titration by haemagglutination. J. Hyg. 55:382–401.
9. Fulthorpe, A. J. 1958. Tetanus antitoxin titration by haemagglutination at a low level of test. J. Hyg. 56:183–189.
10. Greaves, M. D., C. W. Potter, and M. G. McEntegart. 1971. A comparison of the sensitivity of cell cultures to diphtheria toxin by the dye-uptake method. J. Med. Microbiol. 4:519–527.
11. Hardegree, M. C., M. F. Barile, M. Pittman, C. J. Maloney, F. Schofield, and R. Maclennan. 1970. Immunization against neonatal tetanus in New Guinea. 4. Comparison of tetanus antitoxin titres obtained by hemagglutination and toxin neutralization in mice. Bull. WHO 43:461–468.
12. Jensen, C. 1933. Die intrakutane kaninchen methode zur auswertung von diphtherie toxin und antitoxin. Acta Pathol. Microbiol. Scand., Vol. 10, Suppl. 14.
13. Kriz, B., B. Vysoka-Burianova, K. Zacek, J. Teply, and V. Burian. 1967. The titration of diphtheria antitoxins on tissue culture. Cesk. Epidemiol. 16:72–80.
14. Landy, M., R. J. Trapani, R. Formal, and I. Klugler. 1955. Comparison of a hemagglutination procedure and the rabbit intradermal neutralization test for the assay of diphtheria antitoxin in human sera. Am. J. Hyg. 61:143–154.

15. Lennox, E. S., and A. S. Kaplan. 1957. Action of diphtheria toxin on cells cultivated *in vitro*. Proc. Soc. Exp. Biol. Med. **95**:700–702.

16. Levine, L., and L. Wyman. 1964. A nationwide serum survey of the US military recruits, 1962. V. Serologic immunity to tetanus. Am. J. Hyg. **80**:314–319.

17. Levine, L., L. Wyman, E. Broderick, and J. Ipsen. 1960. A field study in triple immunization (diphtheria, pertussis, tetanus): estimation of 3 antibodies in infant sera from single heel puncture using agglutination techniques. J. Pediatr. **57**:836–843.

18. Miyamura, K., S. Nishi, A. Ito, R. Murata, and R. Kono. 1974. Micro cell culture method for determination of diphtheria toxin and antitoxin titres using VERO cells. I. Studies on factors affecting the toxin and antitoxin titration. J. Biol. Stand. **2**:189–201.

19. Mueller, J. H. 1948. The diphtheria bacilli and the diphtheroids: *Corynebacterium diphtheriae*, p. 209. *In* R. J. Dubos (ed.), Bacterial and mycotic infections of man. Philadelphia.

20. Nyerges, G., G. Nyerges, M. Surjan, J. Budai, and J. Csapo. 1963. A method for the rapid determination of diphtheria antitoxin in clinical practice. Acta Paediatr. Acad. Sci. Hung. **4**:399–409.

21. Placedo-Sousa, C., and D. G. Evans. 1957. The action of diphtheria toxin on tissue cultures and its neutralization by antitoxin. Br. J. Exp. Pathol. **38**:644–650.

22. Scheibel, I. 1956. A comparative study on intracutaneous and haemaglutination procedures for assaying diphtheria antitoxin, with special reference to the avidity of the antitoxin.

Acta Pathol. Microbiol. Scand. **39**:455–468.

23. Schubert, J. H., G. L. Wiggins, and G. C. Taylor. 1967. Tissue culture method for the titration of diphtheria antitoxin in human sera. Health Lab. Sci. **4**:181–188.

24. Stavitsky, A. B. 1954. Micromethods for the study of proteins and antibodies I. Procedure and general applications of hemagglutination and hemagglutination and hemagglutination-inhibition reactions with tannic acid and protein-treated red blood cells. J. Immunol. **72**:360–367.

25. Stavitsky, A. B. 1954. Micromethods for the study of proteins and antibodies. II. Specific applications of hemagglutination and hemagglutination-inhibition reactions with tannic acid and protein-treated red blood cells. J. Immunol. **72**:368–375.

26. Surjan, M., and G. Nyerges. 1962. Haemagglutination procedure for the assay of tetanus antitoxin of children's sera. Z. Immunitaetsforsch. Exp. Therap. **124**:390–400.

27. Surjan, M., and G. Nyerges. 1962. Diphtheria antitoxin titration of human sera by haemagglutination. Z. Immunitaetsforsch. Exp. Ther. **124**:401–410.

28. Tasman, A., J. D. Van Ramshorst, and L. Smith. 1960. Determination of diphtheria and tetanus antitoxin with the aid of haemagglutination. Antonie van Leeuwenhoek J. Microbiol. Serol. **26**:413–429.

29. Zingher, A. 1923. The Schick test performed on more than 150,000 children in public and parochial schools in New York (Manhattan and the Bronx). Am. J. Dis. Child. **25**:392–405.

Chapter 45

Immune Response to Mycobacteria

HUGO L. DAVID AND MERLE J. SELIN

INTRODUCTION

In 1890, Koch (12) reported that when tuberculous animals are infected with the tubercle bacillus the small inoculation wound heals at first but that on the next or second day "the area becomes indurated and assumes a dark color, and these changes do not remain limited to the inoculating point, but spread to involve an area 0.5 to 1.0 cm in diameter. In the succeeding days, it becomes evident that the altered skin is necrotic. It finally sloughs, leaving a shallow ulcer that usually heals quickly and permanently, and the regional lymph nodes do not become infected." The description of this phenomenon, later to be known as the Koch phenomenon, marks the beginning of immunological studies in tuberculosis. It can be divided into three components: an accelerated inflammatory reaction, the healing of the ulcer, and the failure of the bacilli to spread to the lymphatic nodes and beyond. The first component is a hypersensitivity reaction that progresses to reach its maximal intensity within 48 to 72 h (delayed hypersensitivity), and the two latter components are indicative of acquired resistance against tuberculosis. This chapter deals exclusively with the inflammatory reaction of delayed hypersensitivity.

ACCELERATED INFLAMMATORY REACTION

The accelerated inflammatory reaction is elicited not only by living tubercle bacilli but also by dead bacilli, by subcellular fractions thereof, and by concentrated cell-free filtrates of autoclaved cultures of the tubercle bacilli (12). Koch called the latter tuberculin "Koch's Old Tuberculin." In this section, we shall discuss the tuberculins and the tuberculin reaction.

The tuberculin reaction is the prototype of delayed hypersensitivity reactions, also called cellular sensitivity reactions and tuberculin-like reactions. When tuberculin is administered either intradermally, as proposed by Mantoux (3), or by contact, as proposed by Von Pirquet (3), to individuals who are sensitized to tubercle bacilli, it elicits a well-defined area of induration that develops to its maximal degree in 48 to 72 h. The diameter of the area of induration, usually expressed in millimeters, is proportional to the individual's degree of sensitivity. Highly sensitized individuals may exhibit severe local reactions with necrosis and systemic reactions with fever, myalgia, and hypotension.

Figures 1 and 2 illustrate the relationship between the intensity of skin reactions elicited by tuberculin and increasing amounts of heat-killed tubercle bacilli used to sensitize experimental animals. The data show that there is a threshold amount of tubercle bacilli below which hypersensitivity detectable by the skin reaction is not induced and that very large amounts of the inducing antigen may interfere with the immunological response (tolerance).

Tuberculins

Long and Seibert (15) found that the active components of tuberculin, which elicit the delayed hypersensitivity reactions, are proteins. Siebert (22) partially purified the active proteins either from heated culture filtrates according to Koch or from unheated culture filtrates. The products prepared from unheated filtrates are antigenic and induce false-positive reactions on repeated testing (21); the products from heated filtrates are less antigenic, and, therefore, heated culture filtrates were preferred in the preparation of a large batch of a purified protein derivative (PPD) to be used as a standard diagnostic tuberculin (PPD-S) by Seibert (23) in cooperation with the U.S. Public Health Service (USPHS).

The strain of the tubercle bacillus used in the preparation of PPD-S was Dorset's DT strain of *Mycobacterium tuberculosis* obtained from the laboratories of the Bureau of Animal Industry, Washington, D.C. This strain can be obtained from the Trudeau Institute culture collection (strain TMC 119) and the Mycobacteriology Branch, Center for Disease Control, culture collection (strain DT-612).

Other PPD preparations have been prepared according to Seibert's procedure, either with the same strain used to make PPD-S or other strains. These other products are called PPD-

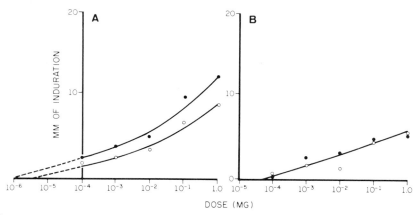

FIG. 1. *Dose response of the induction reaction. Guinea pigs were sensitized intramuscularly with the indicated doses of heat-killed whole cells of M. tuberculosis and of M. avium. Five weeks later, the animals were tested with 25 TU of PPD-Tuberculin (●) and 25 U of PPD-B (○). (A) Homologous reactions; (B) heterologous reactions.*

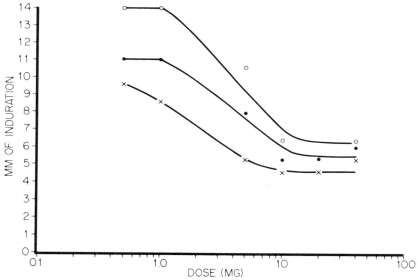

FIG. 2. *Dose response of the M. tuberculosis induction reaction. The experiment was performed as described in Fig. 1. The same phenomenon was observed in animals sensitized with M. avium (not represented). Animals tested with (○) 50 TU, (●) 25 TU, and (×) 12.5 TU of PPD-Tuberculin.*

Tuberculin, the designation PPD-S being reserved to designate the International Standard, made by Seibert. The International Standard is deposited officially in the Bureau of Biologics, National Institutes of Health, Bethesda, Md., and in the Statens Serum Institute, Copenhagen, Denmark.

Tuberculin reaction

In what follows, tuberculin refers to purified products (PPDs) and not to the crude preparations (Koch's Old Tuberculin). Tuberculin is a very specific product in the sense that it elicits delayed reactions exclusively in individuals infected with mycobacteria, but not necessarily only with tubercle bacilli (6, 13, 17). Because tuberculin consistently elicits some reactions in animals infected with other mycobacteria (11), the need to define what constitutes a specific reaction becomes clear. Conceptually, but not necessarily historically, the definition of a specific reaction unfolded in three stages.

A high percentage of positive reactors among tuberculosis patients is detected by the intradermal injection of as little as 0.00002 mg of PPD-S (expressed as protein nitrogen in this preparation), and this amount of protein is designated one tuberculin unit (1 TU; 14). Extensive studies on minimal tuberculosis lesions in nurses showed that "tuberculin reaction 5 or more mm in diameter, of definite induration, to a dosage of 0.0001 mg of PPD-S [0.0001 mg of PPD-S is equivalent to 5 TU] would serve as a highly satisfactory definition of a specific tuberculosis reaction" (9, 10). Very extensive epidemiological investigations conducted by the USPHS (18), using not only PPD-S but also PPDs prepared from mycobacteria other than tubercle bacilli, revealed that infections with a number of mycobacteria consistently induced cross-reactions (see below, Delayed hypersensitivity induced by mycobacteria other than the tubercle bacillus), which led to the redefinition of the initial Goddard et al. (see above) definition of what constitutes a specific tuberculin reaction. The current definition is that a definite induration of 10 mm or more in the Mantoux test (see below, Tuberculin testing procedures) is a positive tuberculin reaction. The definition no longer includes the term "specificity" because persons highly sensitized against other mycobacteria may reveal a 10-mm induration reaction when tuberculin is injected with what will be the heterologous PPD-Tuberculin.

TUBERCULIN TESTING PROCEDURES

The most accurate and reliable method of skin testing is the Mantoux text. It consists of intracutaneous injection of 0.1 ml of PPD-Tuberculin containing the bioequivalent of 5 TU (that amount of PPD-Tuberculin that elicits the same reaction as 0.0001 mg of PPD-S). Lower doses or higher doses have no demonstratable usefulness in ordinary practice. The following interpretation is recommended (2):

10 mm or more of induration = positive reaction

5 to 9 mm of induration = doubtful reaction (Some may be specific, but they are most likely cross-reactions.)

0 to 4 mm of induration = negative reaction

Other methods of skin testing are the tine test, the Mono-Vacc test, the Heaf or Sterneedle test, and the Hypospray-Jet Gun. The advantages and disadvantages of each are summarized in Table 1.

DEVELOPMENT OF HYPERSENSITIVITY

Tuberculosis is essentially an airborne infection, and the human is the chief reservoir of *M. tuberculosis* in nature. Wells, Riley, and their associates (20, 26, 27) demonstrated that the droplets that dry while settling to a size of about 2 to 3 μm (droplet nuclei) are the main vehicles for the transmission of tubercle bacilli. Generally, the airborne particle is deposited in an alveolus in the well-ventilated middle or lower lobe of the right lung, just beneath the pleura. At the site of the implantation, a nonspecific exudative inflammatory reaction occurs. During the infection, the character of the cellular response changes, and the exudative reaction is replaced by a productive reaction that appears to evolve from it (5). These changes occur within 4 to 12 weeks, and they relate to the appearance of delayed hypersensitivity and to the development of acquired resistance against tuberculosis (see the Koch phenomenon described in the Introduction). In the tuberculin-positive host, the lymphogenous dissemination stops, and most of the bacilli that become implanted in various organs die or remain dormant.

The time course of delayed hypersensitivity in experimental animals is illustrated in Fig. 3. The data show that after a lag period of 1 to 2 weeks the degree of hypersensitivity increases rapidly to attain a maximum in about 5 weeks.

Delayed hypersensitivity induced by mycobacteria other than the tubercle bacillus

Tuberculin was known to cause nonspecific reactions. The nature of these reactions became apparent when other mycobacterioses began to be recognized (7). Affronti (1) prepared PPD antigens from two strains of *M. kansasii* and from two strains of the Battey bacilli *(M. avium-intracellulare)*. These PPDs were prepared by Seibert's method and were shown to elicit a reaction in all sensitized animals irrespective of the inducing antigens used, but the size of the hypersensitivity reaction was consistently greater with the homologous PPD. Further investigations confirmed the notion that infected animals react more strongly to the PPD antigens homologous to the organism used to induce hypersensitivity (8). After these earlier observations, PPD preparations were made by the USPHS from different species of the mycobacteria, and some of these PPDs are listed in Table 2. By analogy to the tuberculin, these antigens were standardized to contain 5 working units of PPD. In the absence of agreed-upon international standards, the working unit is that amount of PPD that will elicit in the homologous animal a reaction the same size that 1 TU of PPD-S will elicit in animals sensitized with tubercle bacilli.

A question often raised is whether these

TABLE 1. *Advantages and disadvantages of various skin testing procedures*

Test	Advantages	Disadvantages
Tine	1. Anybody can do it	1. Requires dried Old Tuberculin a. Highly concentrated b. Not a pure product c. False-positive reactions
	2. No equipment necessary	2. Multiple puncture a. Dose not measured b. Operators apply different amounts of pressure
	3. Convenient for private physicians	3. Verification with Mantoux necessary
	4. Good for screening out nonreactors	4. Expensive 5. Results difficult to interpret
Mono-Vacc	1. Anybody can do it	1. Uses liquid Old Tuberculin a. Highly concentrated b. Not a pure product c. False-positive reactions
	2. No equipment necessary	2. Multiple puncture a. Dose not measured b. Operators apply different amounts of pressure
	3. Convenient	3. Verification with Mantoux necessary
	4. Less frightening to children	4 Expensive
	5. Good for screening out nonreactors	5. Results difficult to interpret
Heaf or Sterneedle	1. No training necessary	1. Highly concentrated
	2. Less frightening to children	2. Multiple dose puncture a. Dose not measured b. Dip in solution or paint injection site
	3. Good for screening	3. Verification with Mantoux necessary
	4. Easier to classify interpretation as grades 1, 2, 3, and 4 rather than precision measurement	4. Results difficult to interpret
	5. Best screening test using PPD, 5 TU	5. Retesting with Mantoux may be necessary

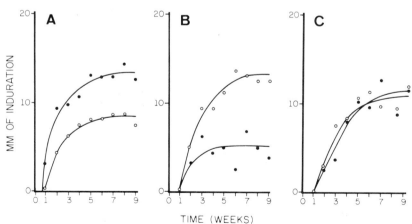

FIG. 3. *Time course of development of delayed hypersensitivity. Guinea pigs were sensitized intramuscularly with (A) 1 mg of heat-killed whole cells of M. tuberculosis, (B) 1 mg of heat-killed whole cells of M. avium, and (C) 1 mg of both. The intensity of the skin reactions towards the homologous and heterologous eliciting antigens was measured at weekly intervals by injecting 25 units of the PPDs:* ●, *PPD-Tuberculin;* ○, *PPD-B.*

TABLE 2. *Source of organism from which mycobacterial sensitin was prepared*

Antigen	Species	Runyon group	Strain	Source
PPD-Y	*M. kansasii*	I	Bostrom 035	Pollack
PPD-G	*M. scrofulaceum*	II	Gause 210	Keltz
PPD-B	*M. intracellulare*	III	Boone 100616	Corpe
PPD-F	*M. fortuitum*	IV	Martin 383	Runyon
PPD-Platy	*M. marinum*	I	Platy 613	Shepherd
PPD-S	*M. tuberculosis*		Dorset	Seibert
PPD-T[a]	*M. bovis*		Otto 606	Weybridge

[a] Stabilized with 5 ppm of Tween 80.

PPDs are of diagnostic value. The question has not been resolved satisfactorily, mainly because the nature of cross-reactions is not fully understood. However, it appears that there is good agreement between the skin reaction and the causative agent of disease in children, and there is less agreement between skin reactions and the causative agent of infection (or disease) in adults, possibly because the opportunity to be infected by a variety of mycobacteria increases with age.

In dealing with the problem of cross-reactions, one must take into consideration the following factors:

1. Cross-reactions imply the presence of common antigenic determinants in the inducing antigens (in nature, living mycobacterial species).

2. The PPD antigens are partially purified products, and, therefore, cross-reactions may be elicited either by unwarranted components in the products called PPDs or by common antigenic determinants in the specific protein molecules that elicit the homologous reaction.

INDICATIONS FOR TESTING

Tuberculin testing is essential for (i) detecting tuberculosis infection in contacts of persons with active cases of tuberculosis, (ii) detecting possible "epidemics" of tuberculosis in schools or institutions, and (iii) differentiating pulmonary diseases. Tuberculin testing should be used, however, as part of a planned program, whether it is for an individual or a group. It must not be used as a single diagnostic test; it must be coordinated with other tests and interpreted by an experienced physician on the basis of all factual findings pertinent to his opinion of a diagnosis.

INTERPRETATION OF TESTS

A positive tuberculin test means only that the individual has become hypersensitive through infection or vaccination with attenuated or dead bacilli. It does not convey the extent of the infection or the degree of its activity. A genuinely and persistently negative test in all ages is very strong evidence against the presence of active tuberculosis except under the conditions mentioned below.

A negative tuberculin reaction during the acute stage of pertussis (19), measles, scarlet fever, or infectious mononucleosis should be regarded as unreliable (4). Cortisone in large doses may also impair reactivity. When the matter is of diagnostic importance, no negative tuberculin test should be regarded as proof of a lack of hypersensitivity until it has been demonstrated that the individual's skin possesses the normal reactivity to nonspecific irritants. The capacity of the skin to react may be suppressed by advanced age or by terminal or severe acute illness, and rapidly progressive tuberculosis may cause specific desensitization through massive release of antigen.

TESTS FOR SERUM ANTIBODIES

Tests for serum antibodies are not at present suitable for use in the diagnostic laboratory (16, 24, 25).

LITERATURE CITED

1. Affronti, L. F. 1959. Purified protein derivatives (PPD) and other antigens prepared from atypical acid-fast bacilli and *Nocardia asteroides*. Am. Rev. Tuberc. Pulm. Dis. **79**:284–295.

2. American Lung Association. 1974. The tuberculin skin test. A supplement to diagnostic standards and classification of tuberculosis and other mycobacterial diseases. Committee on Diagnostic Skin Testing of the American Thoracic Society, American Lung Association, New York.

3. Aronson, J. D., D. Zacks, and J. J. Poutas. 1933. The comparative sensitiveness of the Pirquet and the intracutaneous tuberculin test. Am. Rev. Tuberc. **27**:465–473.

4. Bentzon, J. W. 1953. The effect of certain infectious diseases on tuberculin allergy. Tubercle **34**:34–41.

5. Canetti, G. 1955. The tubercle bacillus in the pulmonary lesion of man. Springer Publishing Co., Inc., New York.

6. Christie, A., and J. C. Peterson. 1945. Pulmonary calcification in negative reactors to tuberculin. Am. J. Public Health 35:1131–1147.

7. Edwards, L. B., P. Q. Edwards, and C. E. Palmer. 1959. Sources of tuberculin sensitivity in human populations. Acta Tuberc. Scand. 47:77–97.

8. Edwards, L. B., L. Hopwood, L. F. Affronti, and C. E. Palmer. 1961. Sensitivity profiles of mycobacterial infection. Bull. Int. Union Tuberc. 32:384–394.

9. Edwards, L. B., and C. E. Palmer. 1958. Epidemiologic studies of tuberculin sensitivity. I. Preliminary results with purified protein derivatives prepared from atypical acid-fast organisms. Am. J. Hyg. 68:213–231.

10. Goddard, J. C., L. B. Edwards, and C. E. Palmer. 1949. Studies of pulmonary findings and antigen sensitivity among student nurses. IV. Relationship of pulmonary calcification with sensitivity to tuberculin and to histoplasmin. Public Health Rep. 64:820–846.

11. Green, H. H. 1946. Weybridge PPD tuberculins. Vet. J. 102:267–278.

12. Koch, R. 1890. Weitere Mitteilungen uber ein Heilmittel gegen Tuberkulose. Dtsch. Med. Wochenschr. 16:1029.

13. Long, E. R. 1939. The tuberculin test. Am. Rev. Tuberc. 40:607–639.

14. Long, E. R., J. D. Aronson, and F. B. Seibert. 1934. Tuberculin surveys with the purified protein derivative. The determination of optimum dosage. Am. Rev. Tuberc. 30:733–756.

15. Long, E. R., and F. B. Seibert. 1926. The chemical composition of the active principle of tuberculin. I. A non-protein medium suitable for the production of tuberculin in large quantity. Am. Rev. Tuberc. 13:393–397.

16. Minden, P., J. K. McClatchy, E. J. Bardana, Jr., and R. S. Farr. 1972. Antigens and antibodies in tuberculosis. In E. C. Chamberlayne (ed.), Status of immunization in tuberculosis. Fogarty International Center Proceedings No. 14. Department of Health, Education, and Welfare Publication No. (NIH) 72-68. U.S. Public Health Service, Washington, D.C.

17. Palmer, C. E. 1945. Non-tuberculous pulmonary calcification and sensitivity to histoplasmin. Public Health Rep. 60:513–520.

18. Palmer, C. E., L. B. Edwards, L. Hopwood, and P. Q. Edwards. 1959. Experimental and epidemiologic basis for the interpretation of tuberculin sensitivity. J. Pediatr. 55:413–429.

19. Pieroni, R. E., D. L. Stevens, A. Stojanovic, and L. Levine. 1972. Investigation of the responsiveness of BCG-vaccinated children with whooping-cough to tuberculin. Int. Arch. Allergy 42:583–589.

20. Riley, R. L., and F. O'Grady. 1961. Airborne infection: transmission and control. The MacMillan Co., New York.

21. Seibert, F. B. 1932. Chemical composition of the active principle of tuberculin. J. Infect. Dis. 51:383–406.

22. Seibert, F. B. 1934. The isolation and properties of the purified protein derivative of tuberculin. Am. Rev. Tuberc. 30:713–725.

23. Seibert, F. B., and J. T. Glenn. 1941. Tuberculin purified protein derivative. Preparation and analyses of a large quantity for standard. Am. Rev. Tuberc. 44:9–25.

24. Shubert, J. H., and C. A. Brasher. 1967. An appraisal of serologic tests for tuberculosis using agar gel and complement-fixation procedures. Am. Rev. Respir. Dis. 96:745–750.

25. Sonnenwirth, A. C., and E. Neter. 1970. Serology, p. 1467–1585. In S. Frankel, S. Reitman, and A. C. Sonnenwirth (ed.), Gradwohl's clinical laboratory methods and diagnosis, vol. 2. C. W. Mosby Co., St. Louis.

26. Wells, W. F. 1948. On the mechanics of droplet nuclei infection. I. Apparatus for the quantitative study of droplet nuclei infection of animals. Am. J. Hyg. 47:1–10.

27. Wells, W. F. 1948. On the mechanics of droplet neuclei infection. II. Quantitative experimental airborne tuberculosis in rabbits. Am. J. Hyg. 47:11–28.

Chapter 46

Immune Response to Aerobic Pathogenic *Actinomycetaceae*

MORRIS A. GORDON AND EL SHEIKH MAHGOUB

INTRODUCTION

Diagnostic serology of infections attributed to members of the aerobic pathogenic *Actinomycetaceae*, with the exception of tests for actinomycetoma, has not been developed to the point of offering practical laboratory procedures. Reliable immunodiffusion tests have, however, been established for systemic nocardiosis in dogs and for nocardial mastitis of cattle (7). None of the serological tests for mycetoma is widely employed, but the best-developed method is the Ouchterlony double-immunodiffusion procedure (1, 6). Complement fixation has been used in cases of mycetoma caused by *Streptomyces somaliensis* (2), but it is more complicated and apparently less specific than immunodiffusion. More recently, counter-immunoelectrophoresis has been advocated as superior to immunodiffusion for routine use in following up patients on treatment and for confirmation of weakly positive immunodiffusion reactions (3). There is no established serological survey method for mycetoma.

A lucid description of all aspects of mycetoma, including serology and mycology, is given by Mahgoub and Murray (5); serological methods, including preparation of antigens, are detailed in an appendix thereto. Serological diagnosis of mycetoma was reviewed by Mahgoub (4). The most extensive and definitive study on the use of immunodiffusion in diagnosis of mycetoma is that by Murray and Mahgoub (6). Earlier work employing different (polysaccharide) antigens was done by Bojalil and Zamora (1).

CLINICAL INDICATIONS

A serological test should be used clinically when either actinomycetoma or eumycetoma is suspected, or when a diagnosis of mycetoma has been made without conclusive differentiation between actinomycetoma and eumycetoma, or in following up patients undergoing therapy.

The greatest potential advantage of a serological diagnosis of mycetoma lies in the possibility of early detection of the infection, preceding extensive tissue destruction. The lesion generally begins as a small, firm, painless, subcutaneous tumorlike mass or induration, but diagnosis at this early stage is rare. Most frequently, the diagnosis is made, by either histopathology or fungal culture, during the second or third year of development of the infection, and it may be made as late as 20 years after the start of infection. A second advantage of serological tests is that they differentiate actinomycetic from eumycetic etiology. This is extremely important, since actinomycetic mycetoma usually responds to chemotherapy, whereas eumycetoma does not.

Definitive diagnosis of either form of mycetoma may be made by histopathological examination or by culture. However, a biopsy may induce dissemination of the microorganism in the tissues, and culture methods are time-consuming and may yield erroneous results because of contamination or unfamiliarity of laboratory workers with the etiological agents.

TEST REAGENTS AND PROCEDURES

The immunodiffusion and counterimmunoelectrophoresis tests are performed on blood serum, which may be preserved by addition of 1:10,000 thimerosal. Successful results have been obtained with the following procedures (5):

For preparation of soluble antigens for immunodiffusion, actinomycetes are cultured on glucose nutrient agar plates for 2 weeks at 37 C and then killed by overnight immersion in 10% Formol-saline. The growth is washed six times with distilled water and then is scraped off and suspended, with an equal volume of no. 12 Ballotini beads, in 0.9% saline. The mixture is shaken for 3 h at 4 C in a Mickle shaker at maximal amplitude and then stored at 4 C for 1 or 2 days. After centrifugation to sediment the beads and cell debris, the supernatant fluid is combined with twice its volume of acetone and a small volume of sodium acetate and is stored in a refrigerator for 1 or 2 days. The resulting precipitate is collected by centrifugation, dried over phosphorus pentachloride, and dissolved in 0.9% saline to a concentration of 50 mg/ml.

Cytoplasmic antigens of the actinomycetes (*Nocardia brasiliensis, Actinomadura pelletieri, A. madurae, S. somaliensis*, etc.) for counterimmunoelectrophoresis may be prepared as follows (2). The organisms are grown on glucose nutrient agar. Growth is scraped off, and an even suspension in normal saline is made by grinding it in a Ten Broeck tube. Particles are broken further by an MSE ultrasonic disintegrator (MSE, Inc., Westlake, Ohio) for 20 min. The suspension is collected in dialysis bags, left in a refrigerator for 48 to 72 h to dialyze against distilled water, and then spun at 9,400 × *g* at 4 C. The supernatant fluid is decanted, collected in dialysis bags, and transferred to a tray containing flakes of polyethylene glycol 6,000 to reduce the volume. The concentrated material is then lyophilized. The antigen is reconstituted in 1:10,000 thimerosal in distilled water (usually about 40 to 60 mg/ml) and titrated against a known positive serum before use.

The same method can be applied to molds (*Madurella mycetomii, Aspergillus nidulans,* etc.), except that the mold is grown either in a stirred or floating culture and homogenized first in an MSE homogenizer instead of a Ten Broeck tube.

Control antisera may be prepared by intravenous injection of rabbits with a 2% (vol/vol) suspension of the formolized material prepared by Mickle-cell disintegration. Animals are given 1 ml of the suspension twice weekly for 3 weeks and are then bled for antibody titration. If the titer is low or negative, the series may be repeated for another 3 weeks. The serum is harvested when strong precipitin lines appear.

A satisfactory medium for the immunodiffusion test is 1% Oxoid Ionagar, buffered to pH 8.6 with 6.7 g of boric acid and 13.4 g of sodium borate·$10H_2O$ per liter. This medium has the advantages of being clear and self-sterilizing. Amounts of 4 ml of the medium are poured into 50-mm petri dishes. Six antiserum wells, each 9 mm in diameter (made with a no. 5 corkborer), are spaced around a 9-mm central antigen well, with a distance of 14 mm between the centers of adjacent wells. Although reactions may be discernible after only 48 h, plates are kept at 25 C (constant temperature box) in moist chambers for 1 week before being considered negative.

The medium employed for counterimmunoelectrophoresis is 1% Oxoid Ionagar No. 1 in normal saline with 1:10,000 thimerosal. A suitable buffer is barbitone-acetate at pH 7.2 (5.4 g of sodium barbitone, 4.3 g of sodium acetate, 58.2 ml of 0.1 N HCl, made up to 1 liter

with distilled water). Buffer should be prepared on the day it is used. In a successful application of this technique, antigen and antibody wells were 5 mm in diameter and 5 mm apart. A constant electromotive force of 6 V/cm was applied for 2 h at about 30 C.

Results may be immediate, but the following staining procedure, applicable to both immunodiffusion and counterimmunoelectrophoresis, often reveals more precipitation lines and produces a permanent record of the test. When lines are well developed (usually after 48 to 72 h), the slides or plates are transferred to a tank containing physiological saline (pH 7.2) and washed for 48 h to destroy nonspecific reactions. The whole agar medium is then removed to a microscope slide, covered with filter paper, dried at 42 C for 1 h, stained with 0.05% naphthalene black in 50% methanol-10% acetic acid-40% water for 3 to 6 min, and differentiated in the solvent alone.

INTERPRETATION

Immunodiffusion tests differentiate actinomycetoma from eumycetoma (maduromycosis; 6). They also differentiate the several specific etiological agents of actinomycetoma, except that there is some cross-reactivity between *A. madurae* and *A. pelletieri*. The intensity and number of precipitin lines are directly related to the size of the patient's lesion, and the lines gradually disappear as the patient responds to medical treatment (4).

Appearance of any precipitin band is considered indicative of active infection. Although there may sometimes be cross-reaction among the actinomycetes, the homologous reaction is stronger, showing either more or more prominent bands of precipitation (6). The test may also be used to verify the etiological role of an unusual actinomycete or mold which may have been isolated from the lesions.

False-negative results may occur if the antigen is too strong or too weak relative to the antiserum; dilution or concentration may be necessary.

Although the emphasis here is on actinomycetes as the etiological agents of mycetoma, the methods described are equally applicable to the detection and diagnosis of mycetoma caused by molds.

LITERATURE CITED

1. Bojalil, L. E., and A. Zamora. 1963. Precipitin and skin tests in the diagnosis of mycetoma due to *Nocardia brasiliensis* (28270). Proc. Soc. Exp. Biol. Med. 113:40–43.
2. Gumaa, S. A., and E. S. Mahgoub. 1973.

Evaluation of the complement fixation test in diagnosis of actinomycetoma. J. Trop. Med. Hyg. **76:**140–142.

3. Gumaa, S. A., and E. S. Mahgoub. 1975. Counterimmunoelectrophoresis in the diagnosis of mycetoma and its sensitivity as compared to immunodiffusion. Sabouraudia **13:**309–315.

4. Mahgoub, E. S. 1975. Serologic diagnosis of mycetoma, p. 154–161. *In* Pan American Health Organization Proceedings of the Third International Conference on the Mycoses, Sâo Paulo, Brazil, 27–29 August, 1974. Pan Am. Health Organ. Sci. Publ. No. 304.

5. Mahgoub, E. S., and I. G. Murray. 1973. Mycetoma. William Heinemann Medical Books, London.

6. Murray, I. G., and E. S. Mahgoub. 1968. Further studies in the diagnosis of mycetoma by double diffusion in agar. Sabouraudia **6:**106–110.

7. Pier, A. C., J. R. Thurston, and R. E. Fichtner. 1975. Serologic and immunologic tests for nocardiosis in animals, p. 162–167. *In* Pan American Health Organization Proceedings of the Third International Conference on the Mycoses, Sâo Paulo, Brazil, 27–29 August, 1974. Pan Am. Health Organ. Sci. Publ. 304.

Chapter 47

Tests for Syphilis

RONALD M. WOOD

INTRODUCTION

Infection with *Treponema pallidum*, the etiological agent of syphilis, produces in the host antibodies of two known types: (i) nontreponemal antibodies, or reagin, which react with lipid antigens, and (ii) treponemal antibodies, which react with *T. pallidum* and closely related strains.

REAGIN TESTS

Serological testing in the management of syphilis traditionally has been based on the detection of reagin by use of antigens prepared from normal tissues, most commonly beef heart. An example of a reliable, inexpensive, and easily performed reagin test is the Venereal Disease Research Laboratory (VDRL) slide technique which can be used qualitatively and quantitatively for detecting reagin in serum and cerebrospinal fluid. The procedure is given below.

In the original rapid plasma reagin (RPR) test (36), the basic VDRL antigen modified by the incorporation of choline chloride permits the testing of plasma without preliminary heating. An extension of this principle is seen in the plasmacrit test (1), unheated serum reagin test (33, 35), RPR (teardrop) card test (34), RPR (circle) card test (32), and automated reagin test (27, 48). Commercial reagents are now under development and evaluation for other rapid reagin tests which are designed to react at a level comparable to the VDRL test (5; R. W. March, G. E. Stiles, and P. S. Forgione, Abstr. Annu. Meet. Am. Soc. Microbiol., 1974, p. 73).

VDRL slide test with serum (17, 18, 46)

Principle. A buffered saline suspension of cardiolipin-lecithin-cholesterol antigen is mixed with the patient's serum, agitated on a mechanical rotator, and examined microscopically for degrees of flocculation. If any reactivity is obtained in the undiluted serum, the test is repeated on serum dilutions to determine the relative amount of reagin present.

Equipment.

1. Rotating machine, adjustable to 180 rpm,

circumscribing a circle 1.9 cm in diameter on a horizontal plane.

2. Hypodermic needles, without bevels: 18, 19 or 20, and 23 gauge.

Glassware.

1. Slides or plates with paraffin or ceramic rings approximately 14 mm in diameter. Glass slides with concavities or glass rings are not satisfactory for this test.

2. Syringe, Luer-type, 1- or 2-ml, or observation tube with rubber bulb.

3. Bottles, 30-ml, round, flat-bottomed, glass-stoppered, narrow mouth.

Reagents. Serologically standardized antigen and buffered saline are commercially available from several manufacturers.

1. VDRL antigen is an alcoholic solution containing 0.03% cardiolipin, 0.9% cholesterol, and sufficient purified lecithin (usually 0.21 ± 0.01%) to produce a standard reactivity. Each lot of antigen has been serologically standardized. Store antigen at room temperature in sealed ampoules or in screw-capped (Vinylite liners) brown bottles. If precipitate forms, discard the antigen.

2. VDRL buffered saline containing 1.0% sodium chloride, pH 6.0 ± 0.1: formaldehyde, neutral, reagent grade, 0.5 ml; secondary sodium phosphate ($Na_2HPO_4 \cdot 12H_2O$), 0.093 g; primary potassium phosphate (KH_2PO_4), 0.170 g; sodium chloride (A.C.S.), 10.0 g; distilled water, 1,000.0 ml. Check pH of solution and store in screw-capped or glass-stoppered bottles.

3. Saline, 0.9%.

Controls. To control serological procedures adequately and to maintain a standard level of reactivity from day to day, the following control sera are recommended: titered reactive serum (TR), tested quantitatively; weakly reactive serum (W), tested qualitatively; and nonreactive serum (N), tested qualitatively. Each antigen suspension should be checked quantitatively with the TR and qualitatively with the W and N controls before acceptance for test purposes. A log of control results as well as reagent lot numbers is recommended as an aid in locating and correcting test difficulties. Sterile preserved control sera are available from commercial sources, or controls may be prepared as follows.

Prepare controls by collecting two pools of serum (one of reactive serum and one of nonreactive serum) from routine syphilis serology specimens. Sterilize pools by filtration and, if desired, add sodium azide (final concentration 1:1,000). Prepare controls of desired reactivity by combining reactive and nonreactive serum and mixing well. Establish the pattern of reactivity for each control by testing several times in duplicate with a reference serum of known reactivity. Distribute in portions sufficient for each day's testing and store at −20 C or at 4 C. Serum stored in this way will maintain its reactivity for several months.

Preparation of antigen suspension. The temperature of buffered saline and antigen should be in the range of 73 to 85 F (23 to 29 C) at the time the antigen suspension is prepared.

1. Pipette 0.4 ml of buffered saline to the bottom of a 30-ml, round glass-stoppered bottle. Be sure the saline completely covers bottom in a thin layer.

2. Add 0.5 ml of antigen (from the lower half of a 1.0-ml pipette graduated to the tip) directly onto the saline while continuously but gently rotating the bottle on a flat surface. Add antigen drop by drop, rapidly, allowing 6 s for each 0.5 ml of antigen. The pipette tip should remain in the upper third of bottle, and rotation should not be vigorous enough to splash saline onto the pipette. The proper speed of rotation is obtained when the center of the bottle circumscribes a 5-cm diameter circle approximately three times per second.

3. Blow the last drop of antigen from the pipette without touching the pipette to the saline.

4. Continue rotation of the bottle for 10 s.

5. Add 4.1 ml of buffered saline from a 5-ml pipette.

6. Place the top on the bottle and shake bottom to top and back approximately 30 times in 10 s.

7. Antigen suspension then is ready for preliminary testing (see below) before use. The suspension may be used for a period of 1 day.

8. Double this amount of antigen suspension may be prepared at one time by using doubled quantities of antigen and saline. Use a 10-ml pipette for delivering the 8.2-ml volume of saline. If larger quantities of antigen suspension are required, prepare two or more batches. Test each batch of antigen suspension, and pool those showing proper reactivity with control sera. Test the pool with control sera.

9. Mix the antigen suspension gently each time it is used. Do not force it back and forth

through the syringe and needle since this procedure may cause loss of reactivity.

Testing accuracy of delivery needles. The proportion of antigen suspension to serum is important in all flocculation tests. An improper ratio of antigen suspension to serum may lead to inaccurate results. Needles used for dispensing antigen suspensions for slide tests should be checked to determine the size of the drop *each time* tests are performed. Check needles for correct delivery as follows.

Fill a 1-ml pipette graduated in 0.01 ml with *reagent to be dispensed* and attach the needle to be calibrated. Hold the pipette *vertically* and count the number of drops in 0.5 ml. The amount delivered should check within ± 1 drop per 0.5 ml of reagent. Needles must be calibrated and checked frequently. The reagent drop size rather than the needle gauge is the important factor. Needles must be checked with the reagent to be used and adjusted so that the proper number of drops is obtained.

Preliminary testing of antigen suspension. Check each antigen suspension against control sera before it is used for each day's test. The suspension should give expected results with titered reactive, weakly reactive, and nonreactive control sera. The antigen control (suspension in saline) should be smooth in appearance, with antigen particles well dispersed.

Do not use antigen suspension which does not meet the control pattern.

Preparation of patient's serum. Heat serum, obtained from centrifuged, clotted blood, in a water bath at 56 C for 30 min. Allow to cool to room temperature before testing. Recentrifuge any serum showing particulate debris. Sera to be tested more than 4 h after the original heating period should be reheated at 56 C for 10 min.

Procedure for VDRL slide qualitative test. For uniform results, the temperature of the room where VDRL slide tests are performed should be in the range of 23 to 29 C.

1. Pipette 0.05 ml of heated serum into one ring of a paraffin-ringed or ceramic-ringed slide.

2. Add one drop ($1/60$ ml) of antigen suspension onto each serum with a calibrated 18-gauge needle.

3. Rotate slides for 4 min. Mechanical rotators that circumscribe a 1.9-cm diameter circle should be set at 180 rpm.

4. Read the test microscopically immediately after rotation with a low-power objective, at $100\times$ magnification, using as much light as possible. Report results as follows: medium and large clumps, reactive (R); small clumps, weakly reactive (W); no clumps or very slight

roughness, nonreactive (N).

Zonal reactions occasionally occur in serological tests. In such cases, a strongly reactive serum may show a weak or atypical reaction in undiluted serum. A completely negative reaction due to a prozone in very strongly reactive sera is extremely rare. Test quantitatively any serum suspected of giving a prozone reaction.

Procedure for VDRL slide quantitative test (45). Retest quantitatively to an end-point titer all sera that show any reactivity in the qualitative VDRL slide test. Test dilutions of the serun as follows: 1:1 (undiluted), 1:2, 1:4, 1:8, 1:16, and 1:32.

1. Measure 0.05 ml of 0.9% saline onto the second through the sixth rings. Do not spread the saline. Saline may be delivered from a large needle or calibrated dropper that delivers 0.05 ml; these should be checked daily for accuracy of delivery.

2. Using a safety pipetter device with disposable tip (that delivers 0.05 ml or 50 μliters), measure 0.05 ml of serum to the first and second rings. Avoid contamination of the instrument with serum.

3. Use the same pipetter and tip to prepare serial two-fold dilutions by drawing the serum-saline mixture up and down in the tip five or six times. Avoid excess bubbles. (Use a clean plastic tip for each serum tested.)

4. Mix the serum and saline in ring 2 (1:2 dilution); transfer 0.05 ml of the 1:2 dilution to ring 3, and continue to mix and transfer, discarding 0.05 ml from the sixth ring. Additional serial dilutions may be set up for strongly reactive sera. (If the 0.05 ml of serum dilution has now spread within the entire area of a paraffin ring, spread this with the pipetter tip before proceeding to the next ring.)

5. Add 1 drop (1/60 ml) of VDRL antigen suspension to each ring with the calibrated 18-gauge needle (used for antigen suspension in the qualitative test).

6. Complete tests in the manner described for the VDRL slide qualitative test with serum.

7. Report results in terms of the highest serum dilution that produces a reactive (not weakly reactive) result.

Interpretation of results. A reactive or weakly reactive test result indicates the presence of reagin, which almost invariably is formed in treponemal infection, but which may be produced by a variety of other conditions (29, 40). Medical practice considers a reactive result in the presence of clinical symptoms as confirmatory evidence of syphilitic infection. However, in the absence of clinical findings, test reactivity can represent any of the following: (i) latent syphilis; (ii) a biological false-positive

reaction, either temporary or chronic; or (iii) a technical or clinical error. The simplest step open to the physician is to request VDRL testing on a repeat specimen. The titer on the second specimen can then be compared with that of the first: a drop to nonreactive suggests a prior technical problem, or a temporary biological false-positive condition in the patient; a rise in titer suggests the likelihood of syphilis; a stable titer remains inconclusive, requiring further medical follow-up as well as serological testing for treponemal antibodies.

Pitfalls and sources of error. It is important for physicians and laboratory workers to be familiar with those conditions other than syphilis which can cause reagin reactivity. Acute or chronic infections such as malaria, leprosy, infectious mononucleosis, and upper respiratory diseases, as well as collagen and immunological diseases such as rheumatoid arthritis and lupus erythematosus (23, 29, 40), can produce false-positive reagin tests. Other less well-known physiological conditions contributing to this problem include: tissue regeneration, pregnancy, heroin addiction, and the use of certain drugs for hypertension (23, 29, 40). Reliable test results require strict attention to details of technique, including proper identification of specimens, accurate measurement, temperature control, correct timing, and use of principles of quality control. Additional information on test interpretation, biological false-positive reactions, and sources of error can be found in many publications (23, 29, 40).

VDRL slide test with spinal fluid (12, 46)

Equipment.

1. Rotating machine (refer to VDRL test with serum).

2. Hypodermic needle, without bevel: 21 or 22 gauge.

Glassware. Agglutination slides, $2^{1}/_{4} \times 3$ inches (5.7×7.6 cm), with 12 concavities, each measuring 16 mm in diameter and 1.75 mm in depth.

Reagents (refer to VDRL test with serum).

1. VDRL antigen.

2. VDRL buffered saline.

3. Saline, 0.9% and 10.0%.

Controls. Although this test is performed with spinal fluids, it is more convenient to prepare controls from a high-titered reactive serum.

1. Select serum with a VDRL slide test titer of 1:80 or greater.

2. Prepare additional dilutions of serum with 0.9% saline, selecting those that produce reactive, minimally reactive, and nonreactive results in the VDRL slide spinal fluid test.

3. Dispense quantities of reactive and non-reactive sera sufficient for one testing period into properly labeled tubes and stopper tightly with paraffin-coated corks. Store in a freezer.

4. For daily use, remove one set of reactive and nonreactive sera, thaw and mix thoroughly, and prepare the proper dilutions in 0.9% saline. Control sera are tested without preliminary heating in the slide test.

Preparation of sensitized antigen suspension.

1. Prepare antigen suspension as described for the VDRL slide test.

2. Add one part of 10% saline to one part of VDRL slide test suspension.

3. Mix well and allow to stand at least 5 min, but not more than 2 h, before use.

VDRL slide qualitative test with spinal fluid.

1. Pipette 0.05 ml of control serum diluted to produce reactive (R), minimally reactive (R_m), and nonreactive (N) results into each of three concavities of an agglutination slide.

2. Pipette 0.05 ml of spinal fluid into one concavity of the slide.

3. Add one drop (0.01 ml) of sensitized antigen suspension to each control and spinal fluid with a calibrated 21- or 22-gauge needle.

4. Rotate slides for 8 min on a mechanical rotator at 180 rpm.

5. Immediately after rotation, read tests microscopically at 100× magnification and report the results as follows: definite clumping, reactive (R); no clumping or very slight roughness, nonreactive (N).

VDRL slide quantitative test with spinal fluid. Quantitative tests are performed on all spinal fluids found to be reactive in the qualitative test.

1. Prepare spinal fluid dilutions as follows. Pipette 0.2 ml of 0.9% saline into each of five or more tubes. Add 0.2 ml of unheated spinal fluid to tube 1, mix well, and transfer 0.2 ml to tube 2. Continue mixing and transferring 0.2 ml from one tube to the next until the last tube is reached. The respective dilutions are 1:2, 1:4, 1:8, 1:16, 1:32, etc.

2. Test each spinal fluid dilution and undiluted spinal fluid as described for the VDRL slide qualitative test with spinal fluid.

3. Report results in terms of the greatest spinal fluid dilution that produces a reactive result.

TREPONEMAL TESTS

Tests for syphilis employing treponemal antigens are of most value in testing sera from patients presenting diagnostic problems. Such individuals most frequently have reactive reagin tests in the absence of clinical or historical evidence of syphilis, but they may have nonreactive reagin tests and clinical signs of late syphilis. A reactive treponemal test is considered good evidence of past or present syphilitic infection, provided that other treponematoses can be ruled out.

The *T. pallidum* immobilization (TPI) test determines the presence of immobilizing antibodies in the serum of patients with syphilis or other treponematoses (30). The test antigen is the virulent Nichols strain of *T. pallidum* freshly harvested from rabbit testicular syphilomas. Motile treponemes suspended in Nelson's medium are exposed to the patient's serum and active guinea pig complement during overnight incubation at 37 C in an atmosphere of 95% nitrogen and 5% carbon dioxide. These organisms are observed by dark-field microscopy for loss of motility as compared with organisms in serum controls treated in a similar fashion but exposed to inactivated complement (30).

The TPI test has undergone extensive clinical and laboratory evaluation, and has been accepted as the treponemal test of reference. Because of its specificity, it is most useful in evaluating diagnostic problem cases. Like other treponemal tests, the TPI test remains reactive over long periods of time, it is not useful in assessing therapy, and it does not distinguish between the treponematoses. The TPI test is insensitive in early syphilis. It is the test of choice for spinal fluids, especially for detecting neurosyphilis when reagin tests give nonreactive or equivocal results (23, 29).

Fluorescent treponemal antibody absorption test (46, 47, 49)

Following the development of the TPI test, many other procedures were devised to overcome the complexities of the TPI test and make reliable treponemal testing available to most medical laboratories. Although some of these procedures (TPCF, RPCF) were widely used, they were found to lack sensitivity and reproducibility (23, 40). The most promising and useful technique to date is an indirect fluorescence procedure originally described by Deacon et al. in 1957 (10). The fluorescent treponemal antibody absorption (FTA-ABS) test, an improved procedure utilizing absorption of sera with Reiter sorbent was first published by the VDRL in 1968 (47).

Because of problems experienced in some laboratories with apparent loss of treponemes from acetone-fixed slides in the FTA-ABS test, Wood and his associates (49) developed an alternate method of fixation employing methanol. Fresh methanol-fixed slides give reactions in the FTA-ABS test comparable to those obtained with acetone. Methanol-fixed slides may give slightly lower plus readings on some sera than does acetone, but this does not appear to affect the reportable reactivity.

The FTA-ABS test employing either acetone- or methanol-fixed slides (46) is described below. The procedure is well standardized, and commercial reagents are available from several manufacturers.

Principle. Nonviable *T. pallidum* (Nichols strain) cells are allowed to react with patient's serum which has been treated to remove substances reacting nonspecifically with *T. pallidum* (11, 19). Specific antitreponemal antibodies present in the serum combine with the treponemal antigens and are detected by the addition of antihuman globulin labeled with fluorescein isothiocyanate.

Equipment.

1. Incubator, adjustable, 35 to 37 C.
2. Dark-field fluorescence microscope assembly.
3. Bibulous paper.
4. Slide board or holder.
5. Moist chamber. Any convenient cover for slides may be made into a moist chamber by placing wet paper inside cover.
6. Loop, bacteriological, standard 2-mm, 26-gauge, platinum.
7. Small dropper bottle.
8. Polyethylene bottle with faucet, 5-gallon size.

Glassware.

1. Microscope slides, 1×3 inch (2.5×7.6 cm), frosted end, approximately 1 mm thick with two etched circles 10 mm in diameter. (Pre-etched slides are available commercially). Slides should be cleaned by soaking in 70% alcohol for 1 h and wiping dry, or by washing in detergent, rinsing well, and wiping dry.
2. Cover slips, no. 1, 22×50 mm or 22×22 mm. Cover slips should be cleaned by soaking in 70% alcohol for 1 h and wiping dry.
3. Disposable capillary pipettes, 5.75 inches (14.6 cm) in length.
4. Dish, staining, with removable glass tray. Inside dimension: $3^5/_8 \times 2^3/_4 \times 2^1/_2$ inches in height ($9.2 \times 7.0 \times 6.4$ cm). Coplin staining jars may be used when few slides are involved.
5. Glass rods, approximately 100×4 mm, both ends fire-polished.

Reagents. All reagents for the FTA-ABS test are available commercially.

1. Antigen for this test is *T. pallidum* Nichols strain. Lyophilized antigen suspensions are reconstituted according to the manufacturers' directions. A satisfactory reconstituted antigen suspension should contain a minimum of 7 to 10 organisms per high dry field (for methanol-fixed slides) or a minimum of 30 organisms per high dry field (for acetone-fixed slides). The suspension should be free from extraneous material such as tissue fragments, fibrin, etc. Antigen suspensions stored in a refrigerator may be used for 2 weeks if the antigen does not become badly clumped or contaminated and if satisfactory results are obtained with control sera.

2. Reiter sorbent is a standardized extract of nonpathogenic Reiter treponemes. Sorbent stored at 6 to 10 C can be used indefinitely if it does not become contaminated and if satisfactory results are obtained with controls.

3. Fluorescein-labeled antihuman globulin. Store rehydrated conjugate in convenient quantities (0.3 ml or more) at -20 C or lower. High-titered antihuman globulin can be reconstituted to volume and diluted 1:10 in sterile phosphate-buffered saline (containing Merthiolate in a concentration of 1:5,000) or sterile phosphate-buffered saline containing 2% Tween 80 before freezing. When thawed for use, do not refreeze but store undiluted at 6 to 10 C for not more than 1 week.

4. Phosphate-buffered saline. Formula per liter: NaCl, 7.65 g; Na_2HPO_4, 0.724 g; KH_2PO_4, 0.21 g. The pH should be 7.2 ± 0.1. If a change in pH is noted or if the solution is contaminated by molds or bacteria, discard it and prepare a fresh solution. Store in a large polyethylene bottle.

5. Tween 80. To prepare a solution of 2% Tween 80 in phosphate-buffered saline, heat the two reagents in a water bath at 56 C for 15 to 30 min. To 98 ml of buffered saline, add 2 ml of Tween 80, measuring from the bottom of a pipette, and rinse out the pipette. The pH should be 7.0 to 7.2. This solution keeps well at refrigerator temperature but should be discarded when found to contain precipitate. Prepare a fresh solution with each fresh preparation of phosphate-buffered saline.

6. Mounting medium. To prepare the mounting medium, add 1 part buffered saline (pH 7.2 ± 0.1) to 9 parts glycerol (reagent grade).

7. Absolute methanol, A.C.S. reagent grade. To prepare a 10% solution of methanol, add 1 part absolute methyl alcohol to 9 parts distilled water. Prepare a fresh solution on the day of use. Do not use the solution for more than one fixation period or for more than 20 slides per 200 ml.

8. Acetone, A.C.S. reagent grade. Not more than 60 slides should be fixed with 200 ml of acetone. Store acetone-fixed smears at -20 C or

below. Fixed, frozen smears are usable indefinitely, provided that satisfactory results are obtained with the controls. Do not thaw and refreeze antigen smears.

9. Oil, immersion, low fluorescence, nondrying.

Preliminary testing of antigen suspension. Mix antigen suspension well according to the manufacturers' directions to insure an even distribution of treponemes. Determine by darkfield examination that treponemes are adequately dispersed before making smears for the FTA test.

Compare a new lot of antigen, or an antigen of unknown quality, with an antigen of known reactivity using control sera and individual sera of graded reactivity before incorporating it into the routine test procedure. A satisfactory antigen preparation should give comparable results with control sera and individual sera. It should not stain nonspecifically with a diluted conjugate of known quality.

Preliminary testing of Reiter sorbent. Compare a new lot of sorbent with a sorbent of known activity using control sera and individual sera of graded reactivity before use in routine test procedures. A satisfactory sorbent should give comparable results with control sera and individual sera. It should not cause nonspecific staining of antigen with a diluted conjugate of known quality.

Preliminary testing of fluorescein-labeled antihuman globulin conjugate.

1. Determine the titer of each new lot of fluorescein-labeled conjugate before use in routine testing.

2. Prepare serial twofold dilutions of the new conjugate in phosphate-buffered saline containing 2% Tween 80 to include two to three dilutions greater than the manufacturer's titer.

3. Test each conjugate dilution with the reactive (4+) control serum diluted 1:5 in phosphate-buffered saline in accordance with the FTA-ABS technique.

4. Test each conjugate dilution with antigen as a check on nonspecific staining (antigen smear treated with 0.03 ml of buffered saline in place of serum).

5. A reference conjugate is tested at its previously determined dilution with the reactive (4+) control serum, the minimally reaction (1+) control serum, and the nonspecific staining control for the purpose of controlling reagents and test conditions.

6. Read the control slides to insure that reagents are working properly and test conditions are satisfactory. Then examine the slides with the new conjugate, starting with the lowest dilution of conjugate. Record readings in pluses.

7. The end point of the titration is the highest dilution giving maximum (4+) fluorescence. The working titer of the new conjugate is one doubling dilution below the end point.

8. The new conjugate should not stain nonspecifically at three doubling dilutions below the working titer of the conjugate.

9. Using the reference conjugate at its working dilution and the new conjugate at the titer determined by the titration, test the following sera in parallel: (i) 3 control sera, unabsorbed and absorbed; (ii) 10 sera of graded reactivity, absorbed. Results obtained with the two conjugates should be comparable.

Controls. The following controls must be included in each test run.

1. Reactive control serum (syphilitic human serum). Reactive control serum should show 4+ fluorescence in unabsorbed test and may show slightly reduced fluorescence in absorbed test. (i) Unabsorbed: using a 0.2-ml pipette, measuring from the bottom, add 0.05 ml of reactive control serum to a tube containing 0.2 ml of buffered saline. Mix at least eight times with the same pipette. (ii) Absorbed: using another 0.2-ml pipette, measuring from the bottom, add 0.05 ml of reactive control serum to a tube containing 0.2 ml of Reiter sorbent. Mix at least eight times with the same pipette.

2. Minimally reactive control serum (syphilitic human serum). The minimally reactive control serum should show 1+ fluorescence. Control serum showing 2 to 3+ fluorescence in the unabsorbed test and 1+ fluorescence in the absorbed test may be used. (i) Unabsorbed: same as for the reactive control. (ii) Absorbed: same as for the reactive control.

A dilution of the reactive control serum, showing 1+ fluorescence, may also be used. (i) Unabsorbed: dilute the reactive control serum in phosphate-buffered saline to the predetermined titer showing 1+ fluorescence.

3. Nonspecific control serum (a nonsyphilitic human serum known to demonstrate nonspecific reactivity to *T. pallidum*, Nichol's strain, at a 1:5 or higher dilution). (i) Unabsorbed: same as for reactive control. (ii) Absorbed: same as for reactive control.

4. Control of nonspecific staining by conjugate. (i) Unabsorbed: 0.03 ml of buffered saline in place of serum. (ii) Absorbed: 0.03 ml of Reiter sorbent in place of serum.

Preparation of sera. Heat the test and control sera in a water bath at 56 C for 30 min. Previously heated sera should be reheated for 10 min at 56 C on the day of testing.

Procedure for FTA-ABS test with serum.

1. Prepare antigen smears on day of test by spreading 0.005 ml or one loopful of *T. pallidum* antigen from a standard 2-mm, 26-gauge

platinum wire loop within each circle on grease-free slides. Allow to air-dry.

2. Immerse in or cover slides with freshly prepared 10% methanol for 20 s. Remove the slides and blot them dry with bibulous paper. If acetone fixation is preferred, fix smears in acetone for 10 min and allow them to air-dry thoroughly.

3. Arrange 12 × 75 mm test tubes in suitable racks so that there is one tube for each serum to be tested. Add tubes for dilutions of control sera prepared as described under Controls.

4. For each serum to be tested, pipette 0.2 ml of standardized Reiter sorbent into a test tube. Using a 0.2-ml pipette, measuring from the bottom of the pipette, add 0.05 ml of the test serum into each tube. Mix at least eight times with the same pipette. The test should be performed within 30 min after dilutions are made. If it is necessary to test a specimen after this period, make a new serum dilution.

5. Cover the *T. pallidum* smears with 0.03 ml of the serum-sorbent mixture to be tested. Include controls as described above.

6. Place the slides in a moist chamber to prevent evaporation of serum.

7. Place the moist chamber containing the slides in an incubator at 35 to 37 C for 30 min.

8. Rinse the slides with running buffered saline for approximately 5 s. Soak them in two changes of buffered saline for a total of 10 min. (At the end of 5 min of the soaking period, rinse the slides by dipping them in and out of buffered saline 10 times.) Follow with a brief rinse of running distilled water to remove salt crystals.

9. Blot the slides with bibulous paper to remove all water drops.

10. On the day of use, dilute fluorescein-labeled antihuman globulin to its working titer in phosphate-buffered saline containing 2% Tween 80.

11. Place approximately 0.03 ml of diluted fluorescein conjugate on each smear. Spread the conjugate with a glass rod in a circular pattern so that smears are completely covered. A disposable pipette, calibrated needle, or dropper may be used for dispensing conjugate.

12. Repeat steps 6, 7, 8, and 9.

13. Place a small drop of mounting medium on each smear, apply a cover slip, and place the slides in a covered slide holder.

14. Slides should be examined immediately or may be stored in a darkened room for several hours before reading. Exposure to light will cause fading of fluorescence and make readings, particularly those in the moderately fluorescent (2+) zone, difficult to read.

15. Smears are studied microscopically, by use of ultraviolet light and a high-power dry objective. The total magnification should approximate 400×. A combination of BG 12 (primary) filter and Zeiss 50/-(II/0) or OG 1 (secondary) filter has been found to be satisfactory for routine use.

16. Nonreactive smears should be checked by switching from ultraviolet to white light to verify the presence of treponemes.

17. Using the minimally reactive (1+) control slide as the reading standard, record the intensity of fluorescence of the treponemes according to the chart given in Table 1.

Control pattern illustration.

Reactive control serum:
1:5 in buffered saline .... R 4+
1:5 in sorbent .... R 3-4+

Minimally reactive control serum:
1:5 in buffered saline .... R 2-3+
1:5 in sorbent .... MR 1+

Or

Minimally reactive control serum:
Predetermine dilution in
   buffered saline of the reactive
   control serum .... MR 1+

Nonspecific control serum
1:5 in buffered saline .... R 2+
1:5 in sorbent .... N

Control of nonspecific staining by conjugate
buffered saline .... N
sorbent .... N

Interpretation. Reactive: confirms presence of treponemal antibodies, but does not indicate stage or activity of infection.

Nonreactive: no treponemal antibodies de-

TABLE 1. *Fluorescence intensity of treponemes*

Reading	Intensity of fluorescence	Report
4+	Very strong	Reactive (R)
3+	Strong	Reactive (R)
2+	Moderate	Reactive (R)
1+	Equivalent to minimally reactive (1+) control	Reactive (R)[a]
<1+	Weak but definite, less than minimally reactive (1+) control	Borderline (B)[a]
– to ±	None to barely visible	Nonreactive (N)

[a] Retest all specimens with intensity of fluorescence of 1+ or less. When a specimen initially read as 1+ is retested and is subsequently read as 1+ or greater, the test is reported as "reactive." All other results on retest are reported as "borderline." It is not necessary to retest nonfluorescent (nonreactive) specimens.

tected. If early infection is suspected, repeat serological testing may be helpful.

Borderline: results are inconclusive and cannot be interpreted. May indicate a very low level of treponemal antibody, or may be due to nonspecific factors. Further follow-up and repeat serological testing may be helpful.

The FTA-ABS test is most often used to determine whether a reactive reagin test is due to latent syphilis or to some condition other than syphilis. It may also be used on patients with nonreactive reagin tests but with clinical evidence of syphilis (40). It is more sensitive than the TPI test in all stages of syphilis, especially in the very early and very late stages. Once the FTA-ABS test becomes reactive, it tends to remain so for long periods of time, regardless of therapy. Extensive evaluation by several investigators (11, 43, 49) indicates good agreement between the FTA-ABS and TPI tests in patients presenting diagnostic problems. Although the specificity of the FTA-ABS test is considered to be extremely good, the possibility of false-positive reactions in some patient groups should be considered. False-positive reactions have been reported in patients with diseases associated with increased or abnormal globulins (3, 28), in patients with lupus erythematosus and antinuclear antibodies (21, 24), and during pregnancy (4, 7). The majority of these reactions are in the borderline to minimally reactive range.

Pitfalls and sources of error. The FTA-ABS test does not distinguish between syphilis and other treponematoses such as pinta, yaws, and bejel. It is not useful in measuring the effectiveness of therapy. The technical procedure, although simple and reliable in the hands of well-trained laboratory workers, involves subjective readings of degrees of fluorescence and requires careful standardization and checking of reagents and controls.

Treponema pallidum hemagglutination tests

A *T. pallidum* hemagglutination (TPHA) test for the serological diagnosis of syphilis was described by Rathlev (37, 38). The procedure was modified by Tomizawa and Kasamatsu (41) and Tomizawa, Kasamatsu, and Yamoya (42) through the use of an absorbing reagent to remove cross-reacting antibodies. The reagents for the test in the form of a kit are manufactured by Fuju Zoki Laboratories, Tokyo, Japan. A TPHA test kit is also manufactured by Wellcome Reagents Ltd., Beckenham, England. The two test kits differ in their reagents as well as their techniques. The Fuji Zoki kit uses tanned sheep red cells and an absorbing diluent containing components of Reiter treponemes

and ox and sheep red cells; no inactivation of test sera is necessary, and results are read after 4 h. The Wellcome kit differs in that it uses tanned turkey cells and a simple buffered diluent; serum is inactivated, and test results are read after 1 h or overnight if necessary. The difference in the two test kits was found by Garner and Clark (16) to make little difference in the test results.

The TPHA test uses treponemal antigen and, like other tests using *T. pallidum* as antigen, should be of value in distinguishing between specific treponemal reactions and biological false-positive reactions. Although the TPI and FTA-ABS tests currently remain the accepted confirmatory tests, the TPHA test promises the advantages of economy, specificity, and sensitivity, while requiring inexpensive equipment and less technical skill than either the TPI or the FTA-ABS tests (20).

The test lends itself to automation, and such a procedure (the AMHA-tp test) has been described by Cox, Logan, and Norins (8) and Logan and Cox (26).

There is general agreement among authors that the TPHA test is somewhat less sensitive than the FTA-ABS test in early primary syphilis, but at other stages of the disease it has a high reactivity and is comparable to the FTA-ABS test (6, 9, 14, 25, 39, 44). Treatment of the disease does not necessarily result in lower reactivity; consequently, quantitation of the test is of limited value in following treatment (20).

There are conflicting reports in the literature on the ability of the TPHA tests to distinguish between specific treponemal and biological false-positive reactions. Young and Henrichsen (51) found a specificity of 99.7%, and Sequeira and Eldridge (39) found a specificity of 99.8%. On the other hand, Garner et al. (15) found 11.3% of 274 biological false-positive sera to show false-positive TPHA reactions, and Blum et al. (2) reported that 8.8% of 306 sera showed false-positive TPHA tests. Cox, Logan, and Stout (9) reported that false-positive TPHA reactions were given by 3 of 100 patients with infectious mononucleosis. Ovcinnikov and Timcenko (31) found that 7% of cancer patients and 12% of patients with various skin diseases gave positive TPHA results in the absence of indications of syphilis. Garner (13), in studying reproducibility, recommended careful checking of each lot of TPHA antigen with sera of known reactivity to detect any variation in sensitivity and specificity. Further evaluation of the TPHA tests is needed in the diagnostic problem area.

Detection of T. pallidum by the fluorescent-antibody dark-field technique (22)

Principle. The diagnosis of infectious syphilis can be made by the demonstration of *T. pallidum* from external lesions or from the aspirate of regional lymph nodes. The organisms may be demonstrated by conventional dark-field or by fluorescent-antibody dark-field (FADF) techniques. In either method, it is essential that specimens be taken for examination prior to the beginning of therapy.

In the conventional dark-field method, *T. pallidum* is differentiated from other treponemes by its characteristic morphology and motility. In the FADF method, *T. pallidum* is differentiated from other treponemes by the use of specific absorbed conjugates. In the past, use of the FADF test has been limited to those laboratories preparing their own conjugates Reagents are now commercially available (Bioquest Laboratories, Cockeysville, Md.).

Collection of material. Material should be collected by the physician, who should attempt to obtain tissue serum from the deeper layers of the lesion, avoiding if possible red blood cells and tissue debris.

Remove any crust or scab from the surface of the lesion. Clean with a gauze sponge moistened with water or saline only. Do not use antiseptics or detergents. Abrade the lesion with a sponge, needle, or suitable instrument to provoke slight bleeding. When the lesion is oozing, blot successively with gauze until relatively clear serum appears. Press a glass slide against the oozing lesion until an adequate amount of serum adheres to the slide. Material should be confined within a small area of the slide, approximately 10 mm in diameter. Air-dry the slide, label it, and insert it in a container provided for transportation to the laboratory, together with the appropriate laboratory request form.

Treat lesions of the body cavities in a similar manner to those of the surfaces. Obtain serum with a fine pipette and express it onto the surface of the slide, using a wire loop if necessary. Remove vaginal, cervical, or anal discharges by the usual preliminary cleansing.

In the event that a regional node is to be aspirated, prepare for aseptic skin puncture. Perform local infiltration of an anesthetic solution down to the surface of the node, if necessary. With the node stabilized by external pressure, puncture with a large-gauge needle on a syringe holding approximately 0.5 ml of sterile normal saline. Inject saline and move the needle tip about within the substances of the node. Apply suction until the needle tip is withdrawn from the node capsule. Release the plunger traction and withdraw the needle through the skin. Prepare slides from aspirated material in the needle shaft, in the manner described above.

Scarify or incise suspected secondary skin lesions to produce bleeding, and treat the serum as above.

Examination of slides by the FADF technique. Equipment and glassware are the same as described above for the FTA-ABS procedure.

Reagents.

1. FTA-ABS antigen, *T. pallidum*, Nichols strain, for use as a positive control.

2. Fluorescein-labeled anti-*T. pallidum* conjugate, prepared by labeling the globulin fraction of high-titered syphilitic serum of human origin with fluorescein isothiocyanate. Conjugate must be absorbed with Reiter treponemes to remove antibodies reacting with spirochetes other than *T. pallidum* and titrated to determine the optimal dilution for use (22). Store stock conjugate in a refrigerator in the dark.

3. Other reagents: phosphate-buffered saline, Tween 80, mounting fluid, and immersion oil are as described above for the FTA-ABS procedure.

Procedure.

1. Heat-fix the smears to be tested by flaming the smears three times over a Bunsen burner. After fixation, smears can be stored at 4 to 6 C for several days before examination. Be sure to allow the smears to come to room temperature before proceeding with the staining procedure.

2. Mark off an area of the smear approximately 10 mm in diameter to be stained.

3. Dilute the conjugate according to a previously determined titer with equal parts of 2% Tween 80 in phosphate-buffered saline and sterile normal rabbit serum.

4. Apply the diluted conjugate to test and control smears.

5. Incubate the slides in a moist chamber at 35 to 37 C for 30 min.

6. Rinse the slides under running phosphate-buffered saline (pH 7.2) and soak them in buffered saline for 10 min with a change of saline at the end of 5 min.

7. Rinse the slides briefly under running distilled water. Blot the smears dry with bibulous paper. Place a small amount of phosphate-buffered glycerol (pH 7.2) on each smear and apply a cover slip.

8. Examine smears using ultraviolet light and high-power dry objective with total magnification of approximately 400 to 450×. A combination of BG 12 (primary) filter and Zeiss 50/-(II/0) or OG 1 (secondary) filter has been found

satisfactory. Examine smears for spirochetes with morphology characteristic of *T. pallidum* which show fluorescence of 2+ or greater.

9. Report the presence or absence of spirochetes resembling *T. pallidum,* as seen by the FADF technique.

Interpretation of results. The presence in suspicious lesions of spirochetes detected by FADF examination is presumptive evidence of syphilitic infection. Recent studies (21, 50) indicate that this procedure is as accurate as the traditional examination by dark-field microscopy, and it does not depend on the presence of motile treponemes of typical morphology. The test is applicable to specimens sent through the mails.

Pitfalls and sources of error. A reliable FADF test is dependent on thorough examination of microscopic smears so that even small numbers of treponemes will be detected. A high-titered conjugate, adequately absorbed to eliminate cross-reactions with saprophytic spirochetes, is essential.

LITERATURE CITED

1. Andujar, J. J., and E. E. Mazurek. 1959. The plasmacrit (PCT) test on capillary blood. Am. J. Clin. Pathol. 31:197–204.
2. Blum, G., P. D. Ellner, L. R. McCarthy, and T. Papachristos. 1973. Reliability of the treponemal hemagglutination test for the serodiagnosis of syphilis. J. Infect. Dis. 127:321–326.
3. Bradford, L. L., D. L. Tuffanelli, J. Puffer, M. L. Bissett, H. L. Bodily, and R. M. Wood. 1967. Fluorescent treponemal absorption and *Treponema pallidum* immobilization tests in syphilitic patients and biologic false positive reactions. Am. J. Clin. Pathol. 47:525–532.
4. Buchanan, C. S., and J. R. Haserick. 1970. FTA-ABS test in pregnancy: a probable false positive reaction. Arch. Dermatol. 102:322–325.
5. Caputo, M. J. 1975. Clinical evaluation of the Hyland Syphilocheck (TM) Test. Hyland Technical Discussion No. 27. Hyland Laboratories, Costa Mesa, Calif.
6. Coffey, E. M., L. L. Bradford, L. S. Naritomi, and R. M. Wood. 1972. Evaluation of the qualitative and automated quantitative micro-hemagglutination assay for antibodies to *Treponema pallidum*. Appl. Microbiol. 24:26–30.
7. Cohen, P., G. Stout, and N. Ende. 1969. Serologic reactivity in consecutive patients admitted to a general hospital: a comparison of the FTA-ABS, VDRL, and automated reagin tests. Arch. Intern. Med. 124:364–367.
8. Cox, P. M., L. C. Logan, and L. C. Norins. 1969. Automated, quantitative microhemagglutination assay for *Treponema pallidum* antibodies. Appl. Microbiol. 18:485–489.
9. Cox, P. M., L. C. Logan, and G. W. Stout. 1971. Further studies of a quantitative automated microhemagglutination assay for antibodies to *Treponema pallidum*. Public Health Lab. 29:43–50.
10. Deacon, W. E., V. H. Falcone, and A. Harris. 1957. A fluorescent test for treponemal antibodies. Proc. Soc. Exp. Biol. Med. 96:477–480.
11. Deacon, W. E., J. B. Lucas, and E. V. Price. 1966. Fluorescent treponemal antibody absorption (FTA-ABS) test for syphilis. J. Am. Med. Assoc. 198:624–628.
12. Duncan, W. P., H. N. Bossak, and A. Harris. 1961. VDRL slide spinal fluid test. Am. J. Clin. Pathol. 35:93–95.
13. Garner, M. F. 1973. Reproducibility of the qualitative and quantitative *Treponema pallidum* hemagglutination (TPHA) test. WHO Document WHO/VDT/RES/73.306.
14. Garner, M. F., J. L. Backhouse, G. Daskalopoulos, and J. L. Walsh. 1972. *Treponema pallidum* haemagglutination test for syphilis. Comparison with the TPI and FTA-ABS tests. Br. J. Vener. Dis. 48:470–478.
15. Garner, M. F., J. L. Backhouse, G. Daskalopoulos, and J. L. Walsh. 1973. *Treponema pallidum* haemagglutination (TPHA) test in biological false positive and leprosy sera. J. Clin. Pathol. 26:258–260.
16. Garner, M. F., and M. E. Clark. 1975. The *Treponema pallidum* hemagglutination (TPHA) test. WHO Document WHO/VDT/RES/75.332.
17. Harris, A., A. A. Rosenberg, and E. R. Del Vecchio. 1948. The VDRL slide flocculation test for syphilis. II. A supplementary report. J. Vener. Dis. Inf. 29:72–75.
18. Harris, A., A. A. Rosenberg, and L. M. Riedel. 1946. A microflocculation test for syphilis using cardiolipin antigen. Preliminary report. J. Vener. Dis. Inf. 27:169–174.
19. Hunter, E. F., W. E. Deacon, and P. E. Meyer. 1964. An improved test for syphilis — the absorption procedure (FTA-ABS). Public Health Rep. 79:410–412.
20. Johnston, N. A. 1972. *Treponema pallidum* hemagglutination test for syphilis. Evaluation of a modified micro-method. Br. J. Vener. Dis. 48:474–478.
21. Jokinen, E. J., A. Lassus, and E. Linder. 1969. Fluorescent treponemal antibody (FTA) reaction in sera with antinuclear factors. Ann. Clin. Res. 1:77–80.
22. Jue, R., J. Puffer, R. Wood, G. Schochet, W. Smartt, and W. Ketterer. 1967. A comparison of fluorescent and conventional darkfield methods for the detection of *Treponema pallidum* in syphilitic lesions. Am. J. Clin. Pathol. 47:809–811.
23. King, A. 1964. Recent advances in venereology. Little, Brown and Co., Boston.
24. Kraus, S. J., J. R. Haserick, and M. A. Lantz. 1970. Fluorescent treponemal antibody-absorption test reactions in lupus erythematosus: atypical beading pattern and probable false-positive reactions. N. Engl. J. Med. 282:1287–1290.
25. Le Clair, R. A. 1971. Evaluation of a qualitative hemagglutination test for antibodies to *Treponema pallidum*. J. Infect. Dis. 123:668–670.
26. Logan, L. C., and P. M. Cox. 1970. Evaluation of a quantitative automated microhemagglutin-

ation assay for antibodies to *Treponema pallidum*. Am. J. Clin. Pathol. 53:163–166.

27. McGrew, B. E., M. J. F. Du Cros, G. W. Stout, and V. H. Falcone. 1968. Automation of a flocculation test for syphilis. Am. J. Clin. Pathol. 50:52–59.

28. Mackey, D. M., E. V. Price, J. M. Knox, and A. Scotti. 1969. Specificity of the FTA-ABS test for syphilis: an evaluation. J. Am. Med. Assoc. 207:1683–1685.

29. Miller, S. E. 1966. The laboratory diagnosis of venereal infections, p. 757–790. *In* S. E. Miller (ed.), A textbook of clinical pathology, 7th ed. The Williams & Wilkins Co., Baltimore.

30. Nelson, R. A., Jr., and M. M. Mayer. 1949. Immobilization of *Treponema pallidum* in vitro by antibody produced in syphilitic infection. J. Exp. Med. 89:369–393.

31. Ovcinnikov, N. M., and G. F. Timcenko. 1974. The haemagglutination test (TPHA) in the serodiagnosis of syphilis. WHO Document WHO/VDT/RES/74.315, WHO/VDT/74.394.

32. Portnoy, J. 1963. Modifications of the rapid plasma reagin (RPR) card test for syphilis for use in large scale testing. Am. J. Clin. Pathol. 40:473–479.

33. Portnoy, J., H. N. Bossak, V. H. Falcone, and A. Harris. 1961. Rapid reagin test with unheated serum and new improved antigen suspension. Public Health Rep. 76:933–935.

34. Portnoy, J., J. H. Brewer, and A. Harris. 1962. Rapid plasma reagin card test for syphilis and other treponematoses. Public Health Rep. 77:645–652.

35. Portnoy, J., and W. Garson. 1960. New and improved antigen suspension for rapid reagin test for syphilis. Public Health Rep. 75:985–988.

36. Portnoy, J., W. Garson, and C. A. Smith. 1957. Rapid plasma reagin test for syphilis. Public Health Rep. 72:761–766.

37. Rathlev, T. 1965. Hemagglutination test utilizing antigens from pathogenic and apathogenic *Treponema pallidum*. WHO Document WHO/VDT/RES/77.65.

38. Rathlev, T. 1967. Hemagglutination test utilizing pathogenic *Treponema pallidum* for the sero-diagnosis of syphilis. Br. J. Vener. Dis. 43:181–185.

39. Sequeira, R. J. L., and A. E. Eldridge. 1973. Treponemal haemagglutination test. Br. J. Vener. Dis. 49:242–248.

40. Sparling, P. F. 1971. Medical progress. Diagnosis and treatment of syphilis. N. Engl. J. Med. 284:642–653.

41. Tomizawa, T., and S. Kasamatsu. 1966. Hemagglutination tests for diagnosis of syphilis. A preliminary report. Jpn. J. Med. Sci. Biol. 19:305–308.

42. Tomizawa, T., S. Kasamatsu, and S. Yamaya. 1969. Usefulness of hemagglutination test using *Treponema pallidum* antigen (TPHA) for the serodiagnosis of syphilis. Jpn. J. Med. Sci. Biol. 22:341–350.

43. Tuffanelli, D. L., K. D. Wuepper, L. L. Bradford, and R. M. Wood. 1967. Fluorescent treponemal-antibody absorption tests: studies of false-positive reactions to tests for syphilis. N. Engl. J. Med. 276:258–262.

44. Uete, T., S. Fukazawa, K. Ogi, and Y. Takeuchi. 1971. Clinical evaluation of the *Treponema pallidum* haemagglutination test. Br. J. Vener. Dis. 47:73–76.

45. U.S. Department of Health, Education, and Welfare. 1975. VDRL slide quantitative test on serum (safety pipetor method). Memorandum to State and Territorial Public Health Laboratory Directors. Center for Disease Control, Atlanta, Ga.

46. U.S. Department of Health, Education, and Welfare, National Communicable Disease Center, Venereal Disease Branch. 1969. Manual of tests for syphilis. U.S. Government Printing Office. Washington, D.C.

47. Venereal Disease Research Laboratory. 1968. Technique for the fluorescent treponemal antibody-absorption (FTA-ABS) test. Health Lab. Sci. 5:23–30.

48. Venereal Disease Research Laboratory. 1970. Provisional technic for the automated reagin (AR) test. Center for Disease Control, Atlanta, Ga.

49. Wood, R. M., Y. Inouye, W. Argonza, L. Bradford, R. Jue, Y. Jeong, J. Puffer, and H. L. Bodily. 1967. Comparison of the fluorescent treponemal antibody absorption and *Treponema pallidum* immobilization tests on serums from 1182 diagnostic problem cases. Am. J. Clin. Pathol. 47:521–524.

50. Yobs, A. R., L. Brown, and E. F. Hunter. 1964. Fluorescent antibody technique in early syphilis. Arch. Pathol. 77:220–225.

51. Young, H., C. Henrichsen, and D. H. H. Robertson. 1974. The *Treponema pallidum* hemagglutination test as a screening procedure for the diagnosis of syphilis. WHO Document WHO/VDT/RES/74.313, WHO/VDT/74.391.

Chapter 48

Serological Diagnosis of Leptospirosis

A. D. ALEXANDER

INTRODUCTION

Leptospirosis is an acute, febrile, septicemic disease attributable to any one of a large number of serologically distinct members of the spirochetal species *Leptospira interrogans* (10). The other currently recognized species, *L. biflexa*, comprises the nonpathogenic leptospires commonly found in natural waters. The various pathogenic leptospires are not readily distinguishable on the basis of morphological, biochemical, and cultural characteristics. They do, however, have distinct antigenic properties as disclosed in agglutination and agglutinin-adsorption tests. These properties are important for serological diagnosis and provide the basis for their classification by serovars (synonym: serotype)—the basic taxon. Currently, over 150 known pathogenic serovars have been arbitrarily assembled into 16 serogroups on the basis of common cross-reacting agglutinogens (21).

Leptospires occur naturally in a wide variety of feral and domestic mammals. In natural hosts, the spirochetes nest in kidneys and are shed in the urine. Humans are accidental hosts. Infections are usually related to occupational or recreational activities which entail either direct contact with animal urine (e.g., abattoir workers, miners, sewer cleaners, or fish workers in rat infested surroundings) or contact with natural waters and soils contaminated with animal urine (e.g., rice field workers, cane field workers, swimmers in ponds and streams about which livestock are pastured, etc.; 9). The organisms invade hosts through abrasions in the skin or through mucosa of the nose, pharynx, eye, and esophagus.

The clinical manifestations of leptospirosis are variable and include inapparent infections, flulike illnesses, "aseptic" meningitis, and, less frequently, an icteric-hemorrhagic form with severe liver and kidney involvement. Diagnosis is usually established in the laboratory by the demonstration of the organisms or by serological tests. The laboratory procedures for cultivation and identification of leptospires are described in a companion volume (2). The onset of leptospirosis is usually abrupt, following an incubation period generally of 10 to 12 days

(range 3 to 30 days). Leptospiremia occurs at the time of disease onset and persists for about 1 week. Antibodies are usually detectable by the end of the first week of disease and reach maximal levels by the third or fourth week. Thereafter, antibody levels gradually recede but may be detectable for years (19).

MICROSCOPIC AGGLUTINATION TEST

The microscopic agglutination test is most often used and is generally accepted as the standard reference test for demonstration of leptospiral antibodies (1). It has excellent sensitivity for the diagnosis of recent as well as past infections in humans and animals. However, the test has limitations because of its high serological specificity. Consequently, to ensure detection of antibodies which may be provoked by any of the large number of serovars, it is necessary to use a battery of different serovar antigens which cover most of the known cross-reactions of leptospires. The following 15 serovars have been recommended (1):

copenhageni	*grippotyphosa*	*autumnalis*
poi	*wolffi*	*bratislava*
canicola	*borincana*	*pomona*
castellonis	*szwajizak*	*tarassovi*
pyrogenes	*djatzi*	*patoc*

Additional serovars recommended for supplementary tests are *shermani, panama, celledoni, djasiman, cynopteri,* and *louisiana. L. biflexa,* serovar *patoc,* is used because it frequently cross-reacts with leptospiral antibodies in human sera irrespective of the infecting serovar. The proposed list of antigens may be modified according to local experience and needs. Substitution of local isolates of the same or related type could provide a more sensitive test. In the continental United States, approximately 23 different pathogenic serovars have been disclosed in nonhuman animal hosts. However, relatively few serovars have been associated with infections in humans and domestic animals (8). Therefore, *at this time* the use of the following eight serovars as antigens would serve to detect all but rare cases of leptospirosis:

copenhageni	grippotyphosa
canicola	wolffi
pomona	djatzi
autumnalis	patoc

Sera that are found to be negative with the above eight antigens should be retested with the larger battery of antigens in those cases where leptospirosis is highly suspected on the basis of clinical and epidemiological findings. Extended testing is available at the Leptospira Laboratory, Bacterial Immunology Branch, Center for Disease Control, Atlanta, Ga.

Preparation of antigen

Young cultures of leptospires in fluid medium are used as antigens. Organisms are grown in fluid medium containing rabbit serum (e.g., Stuart's medium) or serum albumin plus fatty acid. Formulas for media are given in the *Manual of Clinical Microbiology* (18). Media are inoculated with mature culture in amounts comprising 5 to 10% of the fresh culture volume and incubated at 30 C. Usually, suitable antigens are obtained after 4 to 7 days. Cultures for use as antigens are examined microscopically by dark-ground illumination for homogeneity, purity, and density. Some strains tend to form small clumps of cells or microcolonies, which can be confused with agglutination, but which can often be avoided by frequent sequential transfers of cultures. If microcolonies are not too numerous, they may be removed from otherwise suitable cultures by centrifugation at 1,500 to 2,000 × g for 15 to 30 min. A culture density of approximately 2×10^8 organisms per ml is desirable (21). It can be determined nephelometrically or by microscopic counts in a Petroff-Hausser chamber. Density can also be estimated by microscopic examination of a 0.01-ml drop under a 22 × 22 mm cover slip. A count of 100 to 200 leptospires per high dry field (450 magnification) will provide an antigen of satisfactory density. Overly dense antigens may be diluted with medium or physiological salt solution.

Antigens may be used live or Formalin-treated. To prepare Formalin-fixed antigens, reagent-grade, neutral Formalin is added to a final concentration of 0.3% by volume to 4- to 7-day-old cultures previously checked for purity, density, and homogeneity. The Formalin-treated antigen is kept at room temperature for 1 to 2 h and then centrifuged for 10 min at 1,000 to 1,500 × g to remove clumped cells and extraneous material. Formalin-treated antigens are usually stable for 1 to 2 weeks if stored at 4 C. Stored antigen should be checked microscopically for appearance and homogeneity before

each use. Fixed as well as live antigens may be tested for sensitivity by titration with standard homologous antisera.

Preparation of standard antisera

Antisera for most test serovars are available commercially (Difco Laboratories, Detroit, Mich.). Alternatively, antisera may be prepared in rabbits by injecting successive doses of 0.5, 1.0, 2.0, and 4 ml of live antigen into the marginal ear vein at 5- to 7-day intervals. Five- to seven-day cultures in Fletcher's semisolid medium containing rabbit sera are used as a source of inoculum. Seven days after the last injection, homologous serum agglutinin titers are measured. If the titer is 1:6,400 or greater, blood is removed by cardiopuncture. Otherwise, an additional 4-ml antigen dose is administered. The separated serum is distributed into vials and can be stored in the frozen state (−20 to −30 C), in the freeze-dried state, or by the addition of glycerol (equal volume) or Merthiolate (1:10,000 concentration).

The use of live cultures has obvious potential infection hazards in the technical procedure as well as in the maintenance of infected rabbits who may become renal shedders of leptospires. For this reason many laboratories use as inocula cultures inactivated by Formalin, by heat (56 C for 30 min), or by repeated freezing and thawing. Antisera prepared with killed antigens usually have lower titers than those elicited with viable organisms.

Agglutination test

Test sera are diluted with physiological salt solution or phosphate-buffered, pH 7.4 physiological salt solution. An initial serum dilution of 1:50 is prepared by adding 0.2 ml of serum to 9.8 ml of diluent; from this, serial fourfold dilutions to 1:3,200 are prepared. Each dilution is added in 0.2-ml amounts in a series of agglutination tubes or wells in plastic trays; an equal volume of antigen is then added to each tube or well in the serum dilution series, giving final dilutions of 1:100 to 1:6,400. The antigen-serum mixtures are shaken, incubated at room temperature for 2 to 3 h, shaken again, and examined for agglutination.

Small drops from the reaction mixtures are placed on a slide with a dropper or loop, spread to flatten, and examined microscopically (10× objective and 15× ocular) by dark-ground illumination without the use of cover slips.

The microscopic agglutination test has been adapted for use with microtitration techniques (4). Twofold serum dilutions are prepared in microdilution plastic plates with flat-bottom wells with the use of 0.05-ml microdiluters. Antigens are added in equivalent volume with disposable microliter pipettes. Plates are covered, gently shaken, kept at room temperature for 2 h, and then read after gentle shaking. Reactions in the well may be examined directly under a dark-field microscope by the use of a long-working-distance 10× objective.

Two types of reactions are manifest with live antigens: agglutination and so-called "lysis." Agglutinated cell aggregates are generally spherical with occasional leptospires extruding from the surface. Some antigens may agglutinate along their longitudinal axis, giving a frayed rope appearance. When "lysis" occurs, there are few or rare freely moving leptospires, and small refractile granules are seen. The granules are tightly packed, clumped cells.

"Lysis" does not occur when Formalin-fixed antigens are used. Agglutination is manifest as relatively large, irregularly outlined clumps which have a lacy appearance. Fixed antigens are less sensitive than live antigens and tend to react more broadly with diverse serovars.

Positive and negative control sera should be included in each test. Reference to reactions in controls is helpful in determining the degree of reaction, and in distinguishing agglutinated clumps from microcolonies when the latter are present. Prozone phenomena may occur, especially with high-titer sera. Reactions are graded on the following basis:

4+ = 75% or more cells agglutinated

3+ = 50 to 75% of cells agglutinated; many clumps present in each field

2+ = 25 to 50% of cells agglutinated; at least one specific clump in each field

1+ = occasional small clump or small stellate aggregations.

The recommended end titer reaction (21) is defined "as the highest final dilution of serum in the serum-antigen mixture in which 50% or more of the cells are agglutinated" (3+ or 4+ reactions). Titers of 1:100 or greater are considered to be significant. Titers may range as high as 1:25,600 or greater. Since leptospiral agglutinins may persist for months and even years after infection, the presence of antibodies in a single serum may not necessarily reflect current illness but may have been incited at an earlier time. Generally, a titer of 1:1,600 or greater in a single specimen provides strong presumptive evidence of recent infection. Preferably, tests should be done on paired acute and convalescent serum samples. A demonstrable fourfold or greater rise in titer is significant.

The microscopic agglutination test has important drawbacks which limit its usefulness for the small diagnostic laboratory. It is laborious and time-consuming; it involves handling of live cultures with attendant risk to personnel and maintenance of a large number of serovars. A variety of alternative serological procedures have therefore been proposed (17). Two procedures that have been widely used in lieu of microscopic agglutination tests are the macroscopic agglutination (slide or plate) test (7, 12) and a "genus-specific" hemolytic or erythrocyte-sensitizing substance test (5, 6). A third test, complement fixation, carried out with an *L. biflexa* antigen has had favorable application in Rumania and Great Britain (13, 17).

MACROSCOPIC (SLIDE) AGGLUTINATION TEST

Slide test antigens consist of a standard suspension of Formalin-treated washed cells in a suitable buffer. Commercially available antigens are prepared according to the method of Galton et al. (7) for antigens from Difco or that of Stoenner and Davis (12) for antigens from Fort Dodge Laboratories, Fort Dodge, Iowa. The former are prepared from 12 or more different serovars and are used singly or are pooled into groups of three. Commercially produced Stoenner and Davis antigens are available only for 5 serovars and therefore have less serovar coverage than available pools of slide test antigens, which incorporate at least 12 different serovars. The test is conducted on a glass slide or plate by mixing a drop of serum with a drop of antigen. The serum-antigen mixtures are shaken for a few minutes on a rotary shaker and then examined for agglutination by indirect light with a black background. Pooled antigens are usually stable for 9 months or longer. Older preparations may give nonspecific reactions. Nonspecific reactions resulting from clumpy antigens may frequently be eliminated by vigorous shaking of antigens prior to use. It is important to use positive and negative control sera in the performance of this test. The test is simple to perform and had good sensitivity and specificity for detecting antibodies in humans and animals with recent or current disease. It cross-reacts more broadly than the microscopic agglutination test but is less sensitive than the latter in detecting antibodies for retrospective studies, e.g., in serological surveys (20). Paired acute and convalescent sera can be tested with pooled or individual antigens to demonstrate titer conversions. Slide test titers are lower than microscopic agglutination test titers and generally range to 1:160.

HEMOLYTIC AND INDIRECT HEMAG-GLUTINATION TESTS

The hemolytic test (5) is conducted with one antigen consisting of a 50% ethyl alcohol-insoluble, 95% ethyl alcohol-soluble extract from leptospiral cells. The antigen is not available commercially at present. L. biflexa strains (e.g., serovars codice, andamana, or patoc) are commonly used as a source of the extracted antigen which can be stored for years in the freeze-dried state without loss of activity. The antigen is very light. To prevent evacuation of antigen during freeze-drying, a binder, human albumin in a concentration of 2%, is added to stock solutions. The optimal antigen dilution for sensitizing sheep red blood cells is predetermined by checkerboard titration with a standard reference antiserum; pooled rabbit antiserum from diverse serovars may be used as the standard reference serum. The antigen-sensitized cells are washed and resuspended to a concentration of 1%, and are than added together with guinea pig complement to serial dilutions of sera. The reaction mixtures are incubated at 37 C for 1 h. A positive reaction is manifested by lysis of sensitized erythrocytes. Details on the preparation, standardization of antigen, and conduct of the test are given by Cox (5). Titers of 1:100 and greater are usually considered to be significant. In the extensive test series reported by Cox et al. (6), convalescent serum titers were generally greater than 1:1,000 and ranged as high as 1:100,000. Microtiter techniques can be used for the hemolytic test.

The test can detect antibodies in human sera irrespective of the infecting serotypes, but it may lack sensitivity for detecting antibodies in animal sera, and its use for this purpose is not recommended. It has limited usefulness as a serological survey tool (16). The hemolytic test is particularly useful for diagnosis of cases in endemic areas of multiple leptospirosis and for testing large numbers of samples. The test is relatively laborious for testing few samples and consequently has rarely been used in the United States. The test has been simplified by the use of sensitized erythrocytes which have been fixed with either glutaraldehyde (3) or pyruvic aldehyde (14, 15). The fixed antigens are used in an indirect hemagglutination procedure with human O red blood cells. The indirect hemagglutination test is being extensively evaluated at the Center for Disease Control, Atlanta, Ga. (14). To date, the test has been found to have excellent genus specificity and excellent sensitivity for detecting antibodies in the early stages of disease (14). Titers ranged

from 1:100 to 1:51,200. The test may become negative a few weeks after convalescence (11). Its usefulness for detecting antibodies in animal sera has not been reported. The test would appear to be a promising tool for the small diagnostic laboratory if reagents become available.

COMPLEMENT-FIXATION TEST WITH L. BIFLEXA ANTIGEN

The complement-fixation test, like the hemolytic test, utilizes an L. biflexa antigen and has genus-specific activity (13, 17). The antigen consists of a washed, Merthiolate-killed suspension of leptospires, concentrated to about 2% of the original culture volume in physiological saline. It is preserved by the addition of sodium azide (final concentration, 1:1,000) and is kept at 4 C. Turner (17) has found this test to be useful in detecting current and recently past infections in humans. Titers in proved cases range from 1:128 to 1:5,120. The test is not suitable for testing animal sera.

Optimal dilution of antigen is predetermined by conventional checkerboard titration with a standard antiserum (e.g., pooled rabbit antiserum as in the hemolytic test). The complement-fixation test antigen is not available commercially.

CLINICAL USEFULNESS

Serological tests for leptospirosis are used not only for diagnosis of cases in humans but even more frequently for diagnosis of cases in domestic animals, particularly dogs, cattle, and swine. Tests are also used for epidemiological investigations which frequently entail retrospective determination of antibodies which may have been provoked many months previously. The microscopic agglutination test, when used with a judicious selection of antigens, serves all of these purposes. Moreover, the test frequently provides clues on the identity of the infecting serovar. It is stressed, however, that the determination of the infecting serovar can only be definitely established by isolation and typing of the organism. The identification of the infecting serovar is obviously important for epidemiological investigations, but it has little or no importance for the clinician in management and treatment of human cases. Consequently, a laboratory diagnosis of leptospirosis per se would serve the primary needs of the clinician and could be fulfilled by the use of the relatively simple slide test with pooled antigens or with a genus-specific test.

The slide test could also serve the serological diagnostic needs in veterinary medicine. Its usefulness for seroepidemiological surveys has limitations because of test sensitivity in detecting antibodies of long duration. Nevertheless, the slide test can still be advantageously used for serological surveys if an index of the percentage of missed positives is derived by testing an appropriate portion of the negative sample population with the conventional microscopic agglutination test.

The genus-specific hemolytic and complement-fixation tests are not recommended for use with animal sera. When used for seroepidemiological surveys, the sensitivity of the test should be monitored by parallel tests with the microscopic agglutination tests, as suggested above for slide test antigens. Unfortunately, the current serological procedures rarely establish a diagnosis before the first week of disease. There is still a critical need for a rapid, laboratory diagnostic test.

LITERATURE CITED

1. Abdussalam, M., A. D. Alexander, B. Babudieri, K. Bogel, C. Borg-Peterson, S. Faine, E. Kmety, C. Lataste-Dorolle, and L. H. Turner. 1972. Research needs in leptospirosis. Bull. WHO 47:113–122.

2. Alexander, A. D. 1974. *Leptospira*, p. 347–354. *In* E. H. Lennette, E. H. Spaulding, and J. P. Truant (ed.), Manual of clinical microbiology, 2nd ed. American Society for Microbiology, Washington, D.C.

3. Baker, L. A., and C. D. Cox. 1973. Quantitative assay for genus-specific leptospiral antigens and antibody. Appl. Microbiol. 25:697–698.

4. Cole, J. R., Jr., C. R. Sulzer, and A. R. Pursell. 1973. Improved microtechnique for the leptospiral microscopic agglutination test. Appl. Microbiol. 25:976–980.

5. Cox, C. D. 1957. Standardization and stabilization of an extract from *Leptospira biflexa* and its use in the hemolytic test for leptospirosis. J. Infect. Dis. 101:203–209.

6. Cox, C. D., A. D. Alexander, and L. C. Murphy. 1957. Evaluation of the hemolytic test in the serodiagnosis of human leptospirosis. J. Infect. Dis. 101:210–218.

7. Galton, M. M., D. R. Powers, A. D. Hale, and R. G. Cornell. 1958. A rapid macroscopic slide screening test for the serodiagnosis of leptospirosis. Am. J. Vet. Res. 19:505–512.

8. Geistfeld, J. G. 1975. Leptospirosis in the United States, 1971–1973. J. Infect. Dis. 131:743–745.

9. Hoeden, J. van der. 1958. Epizootiology of leptospirosis. Adv. Vet. Sci. 4:277–339.

10. International Committee on Systematic Bacteriology. 1974. Subcommittee on the Taxonomy of *Leptospira*. Minutes of the Meeting, 30 August–4 September 1973, Jerusalem, Israel. Int. J. Syst. Bacteriol. 24:381–382.

11. Jones, W. L. 1974. Immunoserological tests other than syphilis, p. 455–460. *In* E. H. Lennette, E. H. Spaulding, and J. P. Truant (ed.), Manual of clinical microbiology, 2nd ed. American Society for Microbiology, Washington, D.C.

12. Stoenner, H. G., and E. Davis. 1967. Further observations on leptospiral plate antigens. Am. J. Vet. Res. 28:259–266.

13. Sturdza, N., M. Elian, and G. Tulpan. 1960. Diagnosis of human leptospirosis by the complement-fixation test with a single antigen. Arch. Roum. Pathol. Exp. 19:572–582.

14. Sulzer, C. R., J. W. Glosser, F. Rogers, W. L. Jones, and M. Trix. 1975. Evaluation of an indirect hemagglutination test for the diagnosis of human leptospirosis. J. Clin. Microbiol. 2:218–221.

15. Sulzer, C. R., and W. L. Jones. 1974. Leptospirosis. Methods in laboratory diagnosis (revised edition). Department Health, Education, and Welfare Publication No. (CDC) 74-8275.

16. Tan, D. S. K. 1969. Sensitized-erythrocyte-lysis (SEL) test as an epidemiological tool for human leptospirosis serological surveys. Bull. WHO 40:899–902.

17. Turner, L. H. 1968. Leptospirosis. II. Serology. Trans. R. Soc. Trop. Med. Hyg. 62:880–889.

18. Vera, H. D., and M. Dumoff. 1974. Culture media, p. 881–929. *In* E. H. Lennette, E. H. Spaulding, and J. P. Truant (ed.), Manual of clinical microbiology, 2nd ed. American Society for Microbiology, Washington, D.C.

19. Wolff, J. W. 1954. The laboratory diagnosis of leptospirosis. Charles C Thomas, Publisher, Springfield, Ill.

20. Wolff, J. W., and H. J. Bohlander. 1966. Evaluation of Galton's macroscopic slide test for the serodiagnosis of leptospirosis in human serum samples. Ann. Soc. Belge. Med. Trop. 46:123–132.

21. World Health Organization. 1967. Current problems in leptospirosis. Report of a World Health Organization Expert Group. WHO Tech. Rep. Ser. No. 380.

Chapter 49

Serology of Mycoplasmic Infections

GEORGE E. KENNY

INTRODUCTION

The organisms classified in order *Mycoplasmatales* are small organisms (0.3 to 0.5 μm) which are surrounded by a unit membrane without evidence of a cell wall (24). The fact that they are membrane-bound is most important to their immunlogical reactivity: the organisms can be readily killed and/or their growth can be inhibited by specific antiserum, a reaction which takes place at the membrane surface. The external antigens, which are probably most important in the immune response, are membrane components or membrane associated in contast to the cell wall and capsular materials found on bacteria.

Some 50 species are included in the three genera presently classified in the *Mycoplasmatales*. Most of these are found in various animals. Nine species have been isolated from humans (Table 1). These species are divided into three genera at present: *Mycoplasma*, *Ureaplasma*, and *Acholeplasma*.

The organisms in the *Mycoplasmatales* are strikingly heterogeneous antigenically (17). The human species can be divided into at least four serological groups (Table 1) between which essentially no cross-reactions are observed even though tests are used which can detect as many as 10 antigens (17). The major antigen of *M. pneumoniae* is found in the lipid fraction of the organism (18), which contains a variety of serologically active glyceroglycolipids (1, 27). In contrast, the major complement-fixing antigens of *M. hominis* are not lipids (14) but appear to be protein in nature. Thus, techniques used for a particular species cannot be extrapolated to other organisms unless the antigens of the organism are known to be similar.

PATHOGENESIS FOR HUMANS

The only clearly demonstrated pathogen is *M. pneumoniae*, which is the major etiological agent of primary atypical pneumonia (3). Although both *U. urealyticum* and *M. hominis* frequently have been isolated from persons with nonspecific urethritis, the ubiquity of these organisms in normal persons (23) argues against their being major pathogens. More important, the case for a large role in nonspecific urethritis has been further weakened by recent data which indicate a major role for chlamydiae in this disease (11). However, it does appear that both *M. hominis* and *U. urealyticum* may be opportunists, particularly in postpartum infections in which both agents have been isolated from the uterus and even occasionally from the blood (8, 9, 12, 13, 21).

SEROLOGICAL TESTS

Serological procedures for detection of antibody of *M. pneumoniae* will be stressed because of the importance of this agent and because reasonable procedures are available. Provisional methods are described for *M. hominis* and *U. urealyticum* because much less information is available both on antigenic structure and immune response with these organisms. Three general approaches to the measurement of antibody to the *Mycoplasmatales* have been employed: complement fixation, metabolic inhibition testing, and fluorescent antibody. Metabolic inhibition testing is unique to the *Mycoplasmatales* in that the effect of antiserum on the growth of the organisms is assessed by the failure of the inhibited organisms to produce an acidic or basic end product of the metabolism of major substrates: arginine, glucose, or urea, as appropriate for the organism (Table 1).

Two general methods of determining antibody to *M. pneumoniae* are in broad use: complement fixation with the use of either whole organism or lipid antigen and metabolic inhibition testing. Both tests appear to measure antibody to the lipid determinants of the organism and the two tests correlate well (32). The advantage of the complement-fixation test is that the methodology used is identical to that commonly used in most laboratories with microtitration equipment. The test, however, does require the use of a relatively expensive antigen from a commerical source or the preparation of the lipid antigen in the laboratory. The metabolic inhibition test is difficult to use in the laboratory which does not routinely culture mycoplasmata, but it has the advantage that tests can be performed without propagating

TABLE 1. *Characteristics and nomenclature of organisms in the Mycoplasmatales found in humans*

Species	Sero-logical group[a]	Glu-cose fer-men-ta-tion	Argi-nine utili-zation	Urea utili-za-tion	Habitat
Mycoplasma hominis	1	−	+	−	Genital tract, oral cavity
M. salivar-ium	1	−	+	−	Periodontal crevices, oral cavity
M. orale (M. pharyn-gis)	1	−	+	−	Oral cavity
M. orale type I	1	−	+	−	Oral cavity
M. buccale (M. orale type 2)[b]	1	−	+	−	Oral cavity
Mycoplasma faucium (M. orale type 3)[b]	1	−	+	−	Oral cavity
M. fermen-tans	2	+	+	−	Genital tract (mouth, rarely)
M. pneumo-niae	5	+	−	−	Throat, lungs
Ureaplasma urealyti-cum (T-strains)[c]	?	−	−	+	Genital tract (mouth oc-casionally)
Achole-plasma laidlawii	4	+	−	−	Skin, oral cavity; orig-inally found in sewage

[a] Groups are divided serologically as described previously (16). Numbers for each group are assigned arbitrarily and are not intended as final designations.
[b] See reference 5.
[c] See reference 34.

large quantities of test antigen. Metabolic inhibition testing may give false-positive reactions when antibiotics are present in the sera.

Complement-fixation testing with the lipid antigen of M. pneumoniae

The use of lipid antigen for complement-fixation testing for *M. pneumoniae* antibodies is preferred over the use of whole organism antigen, because the lipid preparation is less anticomplementary and greater differences in titer are found between acute and convalescent serum (18).

Preparation of lipid antigen. Lipid antigen is prepared by extracting the organisms with 2:1 chloroform-methanol and partitioning the emulsion with aqueous 0.1 M KCl (18). In de-

tail, 5 ml of 100-fold concentrated *M. pneumoniae* organisms (approximately 10 mg of organisms cultivated as described elsewhere [16]) is placed in a separatory funnel, and the following reagents are added in order with vigorous shaking after each addition: 50 ml of methanol, 100 ml of chloroform, and 37.5 ml of 0.1 M KCl. This mixture is allowed to stand in a separatory funnel until two clear phases separate (separation of phases may be accelerated by chilling and then permitting the mixture to stand at room temperature). The lower phase (chloroform) is then removed and evaporated to dryness (a rotary evaporator is helpful but not necessry since the chloroform phase can be evaporated in a hood). After the chloroform is evaporated, the antigen is solubilized in 5 ml of ethanol by scraping the drying container with a glass rod or rubber policeman. Dissolving the lipids may be accelerated by placing the flask in a 56 C water bath. The ethanolic solution will appear turbid, and this turbidity will increase upon storage in the cold (storage at −20 C is recommended).

The above procedure was devised for simplicity and is not designed as a method for purifying lipids (see 1, 19, 27 for such methods). The organic solvents are present in great excess, and as much as 10 times the protein content of organisms could be fractionated without any danger of overloading the fractionation procedure provided that volume of the concentrated antigen is not increased. Similarly, the extraction of the lipid is rapid and does not require more than several minutes of shaking at each step. Finally, the lipid antigen is extraordinarily stable; thus, its activity will not be impaired by any of the recommended steps.

For use, the alcohol extract is complexed to bovine albumin: 1 part of alcohol extract is mixed with 3 parts of bovine albumin (fraction V or better grade) in the diluent used for complement-fixation testing. Both reagents should be heated to 56 C before mixing to facilitate complexing. The complexed antigen may be stored at 4 C or frozen. If it has been stored in the cold, it should be heated at 56 C for 15 min to solubilize the lipids.

Serological testing. This material can then be used as antigen in any standard complement-fixation test. To standardize the system, block (chessboard) titration should be set up in which twofold dilutions of antigen ranging from 1:2 to 1:1,024 are tested against similar twofold dilutions of a human serum. The end point of the titration is the highest dilution of antigen which gives complete fixation with 4 units of antibody (block titrations with *M. pneumoniae* lipid antigen give reasonably "square" block titrations; i.e., neither excess antigen nor antibody markedly increases the titer of the other reagent). In the event that human antisera cannot be obtained for initial testing, animal antisera may be used with the caution that the antigen titers, though similar within two- or fourfold, are not identical to those obtained with human antisera. When a good human antiserum (titer 1:256 or greater) is obtained, it should be used to control the antigen titrations and the daily tests. Once the antigen titer has been determined for a batch of complexed material, this titer will be stable either in a freezer or at 4 C (provided that the material is warmed to 56 C briefly before each use). This material may be used in any standardized complement-fixation system. The anticomplementary control must contain the same concentration of bovine albumin as the test antigen to guard against the test measuring antibovine antibody. Under the conditions of this test, very few sera have been found anticomplementary because of antibovine albumin antibody. A daily antigen titration against four antibody units should be included in each test. Four antigen units are used in the test versus two "full" complement units.

Significance of serological test results for diagnosis of M. pneumoniae infections

Since isolation of *M. pneumoniae* from patients with primary atypical pneumonia is time-consuming (positive results require 1 to 4 weeks), and isolation is carried out only in certain specialized laboratories, serological testing is frequently requested not only for diagnostic purposes on individual cases but as an epidemiological tool to assess the incidence of *M. pneumoniae* infections in the community (7). Although antibody decreases following infection, the decrease is slow, and accordingly the presence of antibody cannot be used to indicate recent infection. On the other hand, high titers, 1:256 or greater, are suggestive of recent infection. Accordingly paired sera (one at onset and one 3 weeks later) are commonly tested, and a fourfold or greater titer rise is indicative of recent infection. Fourfold titer rises correlate well with infection: 58% of pneumonia patients with *M. pneumoniae* isolates showed fourfold titer rises and 65% of those with fourfold titer rises yielded *M. pneumoniae* isolates (7). Thus, excellent correlation is found between isolation of the organism and serological test results. However, some caution should be employed. Patients with pancreatitis show antibody increases to *M. pneumoniae* lipid antigen (22, 25);

arguments have been made on epidemiological grounds that this antibody is not induced by infection with *M. pneumoniae* (22). Several surprising cross-reactions between glycolipids are known: the lipid antigen of *M. neurolyticum* (a rodent *Mycoplasma* species) cross-reacts with *M. pneumoniae* (15), and a galactose-containing glyceroglycolipid from spinach works well as a complement-fixing antigen for diagnosis of *M. pneumoniae* infections (19). Galactolipids have broad distribution in plants, and these glycolipids may prove to be a future inexpensive source of serological test antigens for *M. pneumoniae* infection. Although cold agglutinins are frequently seen in *M. pneumoniae* infections, about half of the positive patients showing increase, they also occur in other diseases without any relationship to *M. pneumoniae* (7).

Metabolic inhibition test for measurement of mycoplasmic antibody

The metabolic inhibition test measures the ability of antibody to stop growth of the organism. The end point of the test is the inability of the organism to produce a normal end product (acid, ammonia, or reduction of tetrazolium), which is demonstrated as a color change in the pH or redox indicator in the growth medium (28–30, 32, 35).

The microtests described by Purcell et al. (29, 30) and Taylor-Robinson et al. (35) are recommended. These tests are suitable for measurement of antibodies to glycolytic organisms, arginine-utilizing organisms, and urea-hydrolyzing organisms (Table 1).

Medium. The medium used is 7 parts Difco PPLO broth, 2 parts unheated horse serum, and 1 part fresh yeast extract (25%).

The medium contains 1,000 units of penicillin per ml, 0.5 mg of thallium acetate per ml (omit thallium acetate for *Ureaplasma*), and 0.001% phenol red.

Substrates to be added to the medium from concentrated stock solutions and the final pH of the medium for the various groups of organisms (Table 1) are as follows: for glycolytic species, add 1% glucose, pH 7.8; for arginine-utilizing species, add 1% arginine, pH 7.2; and for *Ureaplasma* (T-strains), add 1% urea, pH 7.2.

Equipment.

Microtiter plates (U-shaped), 96 wells (Cooke Engineering Co., Alexandria, Va.).
Microtiter loops (Cooke Engineering Co.).
Droppers, 0.025 ml (Cooke Engineering Co.).
Incubator, 37 C.
Freezer, −70 C.

Cellophane tape, 3.25 inches wide (Cooke Engineering Co.).

Cultivation of organisms. Organisms are cultivated to the top of log phase (until the pH begins to change) in the appropriate medium (described above). Portions of 1 ml are stored at −70 C.

Titration of organisms. Suspensions of frozen mycolasmata are titrated for color-changing units (CCU) by preparing 10-fold serial dilutions of organisms in the *appropriate* medium and dropping 0.05 ml of each dilution into separate wells on the microtiter plate; then 0.15 ml of medium is added to each hole. The end point of the titration is the highest dilution or organism which will produce a color change of 0.5 pH unit, which is 1 CCU. This titer will remain constant in the vials in a properly functioning freezer, but this should be checked by titrating vials of organisms over time.

Assay of antibody. Samples of medium (0.025 ml) are dropped into holes 2 to 12. One drop (0.025 ml) of test serum (heat-inactivated at 56 C for 30 min) diluted 1:5 in medium is dropped into wells 1 and 2. Serial dilutions are carried on from tubes 2 through 12 (final dilutions are 1:5 to 1:10,240 in this example, though other dilution sequences may be employed depending on the titers obtained in trial runs). A suspension of organisms containing 10^3 to 10^4 CCU per 0.05 ml (10^2 to 10^3 for *Ureaplasma*) is prepared in medium, and 0.05 ml is dropped into each well. An additional 0.125-ml sample of medium is dropped into each hole to bring the final volume to 0.2 ml per well. Control wells are prepared which contain organisms (0.05 ml of organisms and 0.15 ml of medium). Serum alone (0.025 ml of serum and 0.175 ml of medium) is used for a control, though contamination by means of the serum should not be a large problem with properly collected, processed, and stored serum.

End point. The test is read when the organism controls show a 0.5 pH unit change on the color indicator. The highest dilution of serum which gives a color change of no more than 0.25 pH unit (50% suppression) is deemed the end point. Sera which contain bacteria resistant to the antimicrobial agents employed will give a false-negative answer, but this can be detected by the serum control.

Complement. For T strains, the use of 10% unheated guinea pig serum (do not use commercial complement unless you know that it does not contain antimicrobial agents [4]) has been recommended (29). This is included in the final 0.125 ml of medium placed into the cups.

Significance of results and problems with metabolic inhibition tests

Fourfold antibody rises to *M. pneumoniae* infections can be readily demonstrated by metabolic inhibition testing. The tests have certain difficulties in that the end point is influenced by the number of organisms (4, 28), and the end point changes from day to day. Nevertheless, the procedure is adequate for measuring antibody changes between paired sera when tested simultaneously. An additional problem is the fact that antibiotic treatment of the patient may result in sufficient levels of serum antibody that inhibition of growth of the organism can occur via antibiotic and not antibody. This difficulty has been circumvented by use of antibiotic-resistant variants in the case of *M. pneumoniae* (26). The tetrazolium-reduction-inhibition test correlates very well with the complement-fixation test using lipid antigen (33). The role of accessory factors such as complement in the test is controversial and has been difficult to establish (4, 28, 32). In the case of *M. pneumoniae*, killing of the organism is totally complement-mediated and resembles complement-mediated lysis of sheep red blood cells (6). However, in the metabolic inhibition test all that is required is inhibition of the growth of the organism to give a positive result; thus, the mycoplasmacidal tests cannot be equated with the metabolic inhibition tests. Some progress has been made at adapting the mycoplasmacidal test to a practical laboratory procedure, but the test is still complex (2).

Testing of sera for M. hominis and U. urealyticum antibody

Testing of human sera for measurement of antibody increase to both *M. hominis* and *U. urealyticum* has been carried out by the appropriate metabolic inhibition tests (29–30, 32, 35). Complement-fixation testing has been used for detection of *M. hominis* antibody, but considerable complications arise because of strain variation (10). For *U. urealyticum* the only usable test is the metabolic inhibition test because it has not yet proven practical to prepare a sufficient amount of organism for complement-fixation testing. However, *U. urealyticum* shows extensive antigenic variation (20). Complement fixation for *M. hominis* is carried out with whole organism antigen. The major complement-fixing antigens are heat-labile (14), and thus care should be used in handling the antigen in contrast to the drastic treatment that *M. pneumoniae* lipid antigen will withstand.

Cold agglutinin test

Patients infected with *M. pneumoniae* frequently show the presence of cold agglutinins (antibodies which agglutinate human red cells in the cold but not at 37 C). This response is not specific to *M. pneumoniae*, but an increase in antibodies is found in 34 to 68% of *M. pneumoniae* infections (7).

The cold agglutinin test of Schmidt et al. (31) is recommended.

Materials.

A 1.0% suspension of washed human group O erythrocytes in physiological saline.
Physiological saline.

Equipment.

Test tubes (micro).
Refrigerator.
Incubator or water bath, 37 C.

Procedure.

1. Blood to be tested for cold agglutinins should be stored at room temperature before separation of the clot. Storage at 4 C will result in absorption of the cold agglutinins onto the red cells, though warming to 37 C will release the antibodies (31).

2. Twofold serial dilutions of serum are prepared in saline and dispensed in 0.1-ml volumes into test tubes.

3. A 0.1-ml volume of 1.0% human group O erythrocytes are added to each tube.

4. The tests are incubated at 4 C for 1 h.

5. Tests are read immediately upon removal from the cold. A positive test will result in a shield pattern of red cells which will form on the bottom of the tube and is difficult to disrupt by gentle shaking. The reversibility of the agglutination is tested by incubation at 37 C for 15 to 30 min.

6. The highest dilution of antibody which agglutinates the red cells and which is reversible at 37 C is termed the end point.

A fourfold or greater rise in cold agglutinins is suggestive of an *M. pneumoniae* infection though a variety of other diseases also produce a fourfold rise. The large number of false-positive reactions plus the relative small percentage of *M. pneumoniae* infections which show fourfold rises indicate that this is not the method of choice. High titers (greater than 1:32) may indicate infection with *M. pneumoniae*, but are frequently present in the absence of such infection. The test may be useful for other diseases, however.

LITERATURE CITED

1. Beckman, B. L., and G. E. Kenny. 1968. Immunochemical analysis of serologically active lipids of *Mycoplasma pneumoniae*. J. Bacteriol. 96:1171–1180.

2. Brunner, H., W. D. James, R. L. Horswood, and R. M. Chanock. 1972. Measurement of *Mycoplasma pneumoniae* mycoplasmacidal antibody in human serum. J. Immunol. 108:1491–1498.

3. Chanock, R. M., L. Hayflick, and M. F. Barile. 1962. Growth on artificial medium of an agent associated with atypical pneumonia and its identification as a PPLO. Proc. Natl. Acad. Sci. U.S.A. 48:41–49.

4. Fernald, G. W., W. A. Clyde, and F. W. Denny. 1967. Factors influencing growth inhibition of *Mycoplasma pneumoniae* by immune sera. Proc. Soc. Exp. Biol. Med. 126:161–166.

5. Freundt, E. A., D. Taylor-Robinson, R. H. Purcell, R. M. Chanock, and F. T. Black. 1974. Proposal of *Mycoplasma buccale* and *Mycoplasma faucium* nom. nov. for *Mycoplasma orale* "types" 2 and 3 respectively. Int. J. Syst. Bacteriol. 24:252–255.

6. Gale, J. L., and G. E. Kenny. 1970. Complement dependent killing of *Mycoplasma pneumoniae* by antibody: kinetics of the reaction. J. Immunol. 104:1175–1183.

7. Grayston, J. T., H. M. Foy, and G. E. Kenny. 1969. The epidemiology of Mycoplasma infections of the human respiratory tract, p. 651–682. *In* L. Hayflick (ed.), The Mycoplasmatales and L-phase of bacteria. Appleton-Century-Crofts, New York.

8. Harwick, H. J., J. B. Iuppa, R. H. Purcell, and F. R. Fekety, Jr. 1967. *Mycoplasma hominis* septicemia associated with abortion. Am. J. Obstet. Gynecol. 99:725–727.

9. Harwick, H. J., R. H. Purcell, J. B. Iuppa, and F. R. Fekety, Jr. 1970. *Mycoplasma hominis* and abortion. J. Infect. Dis. 121:260–268.

10. Hollingdale, M. R., and R. M. Lemcke. 1970. Antigenic differences within the species *Mycoplasma hominis*. J. Hyg. 68:469–477.

11. Holmes, K. K., H. H. Handsfield, S. P. Wang, B. B. Wentworth, M. Turck, J. Anderson, and E. R. Alexander. 1975. Etiology of nongonococcal urethritis. N. Engl. J. Med. 292:1199–1205.

12. Jones, D. M. 1967. *Mycoplasma hominis* in pregnancy. J. Clin. Pathol. 20:633–635.

13. Jones, D. M., and P. J. L. Sequeira. 1966. The distribution of complement-fixing and growth-inhibiting antibody to *Mycoplasma hominis*. J. Hyg. 64:441–449.

14. Kenny, G. E. 1967. Heat-lability and organic solvent-solubility of Mycoplasma antigens. Ann. N.Y. Acad. Sci. 143:676–681.

15. Kenny, G. E. 1971. Serological cross-reaction between lipids of *Mycoplasma pneumoniae* and *Mycoplasma neurolyticum*. Infect. Immun. 4:149–153.

16. Kenny, G. E. 1974. Mycoplasma, p. 333–337. *In* E. H. Lennette, E. H. Spaulding, and J. P. Truant (ed.) Manual of clinical microbiology. American Society for Microbiology, Washington, D.C.

17. Kenny, G. E. 1975. Antigens of the Mycoplasmatales and Chlamydiae, p. 449–478. *In* M. Sela (ed.), The antigens, vol. 3. Academic Press Inc., New York.

18. Kenny, G. E., and J. T. Grayston. 1965. Eaton PPLO (*Mycoplasma pneumoniae*) complement fixing antigen: extraction with organic solvents. J. Immunol. **95**:19–25.

19. Kenny, G. E., and R. M. Newton. 1973. Close serological relationship between glycolipids of *Mycoplasma pneumoniae* and glycolipids of spinach. Ann. N.Y. Acad. Sci. **225**:54–61.

20. Lin, J. S., and E. H. Kass. 1973. Serotypic heterogeneity in isolates of human genital T-mycoplasmas. Infect. Immun. **7**:499–500.

21. Lamey, J. R., H. M. Foy, and G. E. Kenny. 1974. Infection with *Mycoplasma hominis* and T-strains in the female genital tract. Obstet. Gynecol. **44**:703–708.

22. Leinikki, P., P. Pantzar, and H. Tykkä. 1973. Antibody response in patients with acute pancreatitis to *Mycoplasma pneumoniae*. Scand. J. Gastroenterol. **8**:631–635.

23. McCormack, W. M., P. Braun, Y.-H. Lee, J. O. Klein, and E. H. Kass. 1973. The genital mycoplasmas. N. Engl. J. Med. **288**:78–89.

24. Maniloff, J., and H. J. Morowitz. 1972. Cell biology of the mycoplasmas. Bacteriol. Rev. **36**:263–290.

25. Mårdh, P.-A., and B. Ursing. 1974. The occurrence of acute pancreatitis in *Mycoplasma pneumoniae* infection. Scand. J. Infect. Dis. **6**:167–171.

26. Niitu, Y., S. Hasegawa, and H. Kubota. 1974. Usefulness of an erythromycin-resistant strain of *Mycoplasma pneumoniae* for the fermentation-inhibition test. Antimicrob. Agents Chemother. **5**:111–113.

27. Plackett, P. B., P. Marmion, E. J. Shaw, and R. M. Lemcke. 1969. Immunochemical analysis of *Mycoplasma pneumoniae*. III. Separation and chemical identification of serologically active lipids. Aust. J. Exp. Biol. Med. Sci. **47**:171–195.

28. Purcell, R. H., R. M. Chanock, and D. Taylor-Robinson. 1969. Serology of the mycoplasmas of man, p. 221–264. *In* L. Hayflick (ed.), The Mycoplasmatales and L-phase of bacteria. Appleton-Century-Crofts, New York.

29. Purcell, R. H., D. Taylor-Robinson, D. Wong, and R. M. Chanock. 1966. Color test for the measurement of antibody to T-strain mycoplasmas. J. Bacteriol. **92**:6–12.

30. Purcell, R. H., D. Taylor-Robinson, D. C. Wong, and R. M. Chanock. 1966. A color test for the measurement of antibody to the nonacid-forming human *Mycoplasma* species. Am. J. Epidemiol. **84**:51–66.

31. Schmidt, N. J., E. H. Lennette, J. Dennis, and P. S. Gee. 1966. On the nature of complement-fixing antibodies to *Mycoplasma pneumoniae*. J. Immunol. **97**:95–99.

32. Senterfit, L. B., and K. E. Jensen. 1966. Antimetabolic antibodies to *Mycoplasma pneumoniae* measured by tetrazolium reduction inhibition. Proc. Soc. Exp. Biol. Med. **122**:786–790.

33. Senterfit, L. B., J. D. Pollack, and N. L. Somerson. 1972. Antibodies to *Mycoplasma pneumoniae*: correlation of complement-fixation and tetrazolium reduction inhibition tests. Proc. Soc. Exp. Biol. Med. **140**:1294–1297.

34. Shepard, M. C., C. D. Lunceford, D. K. Ford, R. H. Purcell, D. Taylor-Robinson, S. Razin, and F. T. Black. 1974. *Ureaplasma urealyticum* gen. nov. sp. nov: proposed nomenclature for the human T (T-strain) mycoplasmas. Int. J. Syst. Bacteriol. **24**:160–171.

35. Taylor-Robinson, D., R. H. Purcell, D. C. Wong, and R. M. Chanock. 1966. A colour test for the measurement of antibody to certain *Mycoplasma* species based upon the inhibition of acid production. J. Hyg. **64**:91–104.

Chapter 50

Serodiagnosis of Fungal Diseases

LEO KAUFMAN

INTRODUCTION

Meticulous consideration of symptoms and epidemiological circumstances may result in an accurate clinical diagnosis of a mycotic disease; however, such diagnoses should be confirmed by standard cultural and histological laboratory procedures. Unfortunately, the diagnosis of a mycotic infection cannot always be proven by culture or histology, despite repeated efforts to isolate a fungus from patients or to demonstrate its presence in biopsy and autopsy material. In such situations, immunological procedures can be used to provide rapid and presumptive evidence of infection. Immunological reactions often provide the first clues to the existence of a fungus infection. Positive serological results can yield information on the effects of chemotherapy and, in many cases, lead to increased efforts for the isolation and identification of the etiological agent.

A positive serological reaction, particularly at a high titer, even though on a single specimen, can be diagnostically significant. A low titer (1:8 or less) may reflect early infection, a cross-reaction, or residual antibody from a previous infection. Many of the diagnostic antigens used in medical mycology are crude mixtures of multiple antigenic factors, some of which are shared by fungi of different genera and between fungi and other microorganisms. When a serum titer is low or cross-reactions are encountered, a prudent diagnosis rests upon (i) results of serological tests performed with a battery of antigens (including those representing antigenically related species), (ii) examination of serial serum specimens for titer changes, and (iii) information as to the acquisition of hypersensitivity. Some individuals suffering with a systemic mycosis are immunologically unresponsive. Others may not demonstrate antibody levels against a fungus because serum is taken before antibody levels are built up. Consequently, one must always bear in mind that negative immunological results do not exclude a diagnosis of mycotic infection. Knowledge of the patient's clinical history is helpful in interpreting serological data.

DETECTION OF HYPERSENSITIVITY

Most patients affected with coccidioidomycosis and histoplasmosis develop a hypersensitive state that is readily and reliably demonstrated by coccidioidin or spherulin and histoplasmin skin tests. The hypersensitive state has been demonstrated in individuals suffering from blastomycosis, candidiasis, and cryptococcosis, but not with sufficient frequency or specificity to warrant widespread use of these skin test antigens.

The skin test is administered by intradermally injecting 0.1 ml of an appropriate dilution of antigen into the volar surface of the forearm. In sensitized persons, an area of induration and erythema develops at the injection site. The cocidioidin test should be read at 24 to 36 h for maximal reaction, and the histoplasmin test, at 48 to 72 h. The largest diameter of induration, not erythema, is recorded. An induration 5 mm or more in diameter is considered a positive reaction.

The skin test is most useful in defining endemic areas for a disease. It has limited value as a diagnostic tool, since it does not distinguish between a past or present infection. In general, a positive reaction is of diagnostic value only if a negative reaction had been obtained before the onset of clinical symptoms. Except in infants, a positive reaction with no past history has little diagnostic value. A negative reaction is of greater significance because it shows definite absence of the disease, except when the patient is in the very early stages of infection, is in the terminal stages, or suffers from a defective cellular immune system. In such cases, the test is negative even though disease may be present.

For certain diseases, especially coccidioidomycosis, physicians rely upon the skin test to assess the prognosis. A reversion to a negative test indicates a state of anergy and a poor prognosis. In a healthy person, a positive coccidioidin skin test implies resistance to infection. Whether a positive histoplasmin skin test in a healthy subject implies such a state is not known.

Because fungi share common antigens, skin tests with several antigens, such as coccidioidin and histoplasmin, should be performed simultaneously. Interpretation is thus facilitated in instances when only one antigen produces a positive reaction or possibly when one elicits a larger area of induration than the other. The magnitude of the reaction, however, does not necessarily indicate the homologous reaction. Proper interpretation of tests with multiple antigens must be balanced with the clinical picture and other laboratory data.

COLLECTION, PRESERVATION, AND SHIPMENT OF SPECIMENS

Specimens for serological tests must be taken aseptically, and 10 ml of blood should be drawn. After the blood has clotted and the serum has separated, the serum is removed aseptically and preserved by adding Merthiolate to make a final concentration of 1:10,000.

It is convenient to maintain a 1% stock solution of Merthiolate in the laboratory. This is prepared by dissolving 1.4 g of sodium borate in distilled water, adding 1.0 g of Merthiolate, and adjusting the solution to a final volume of 100 ml with distilled water. Use 0.1 ml of the stock solution per 10 ml of serum or other clinical specimen. Specimens so treated do not require refrigeration during shipment.

Spinal fluid specimens should be aseptically taken when meningeal involvement is suspected. No preservative should be added if the material will be cultured before serological examination, but preservative may be added if the specimen is not to be cultured. Preferably, the specimen should be frozen or refrigerated if it is to be shipped to a laboratory for culture. This will curtail bacterial growth should contamination occur during transit.

All specimens should be enclosed in heavy-walled tubes secured with a tight-fitting screw-cap, cork, or soft-rubber stopper. The stoppers should be held in place with adhesive tape or sealed with paraffin. Specimens should be sent by airmail or air express to assure prompt arrival.

DETECTION OF CIRCULATING ANTIBODIES AND ANTIGENS

Antibody responses are useful indices in determining the diagnosis and the prognosis of a mycosis. Dependable diagnoses can frequently be made from a single serological test. Low titers or cross-reactions in the complement-fixation (CF) test are, however, difficult to interpret. In such cases, serum specimens taken 3 weeks apart should be studied. Ideally, to es-

tablish a diagnosis and to monitor the course of an infection properly, sera should be taken early in the course of illness, at its height, during convalescence, and several weeks after recovery. Fourfold or greater rises in titer are usually acceptable diagnostic signs of disease, although cross-reactions with heterologous antigens may appear early in illness and may cause confusion. Usually, cross-reacting antibody titers remain stable or move at a lower rate than the homologous titer as the disease progresses. False serodiagnoses may be avoided through the use of reference sera in immunodiffusion (ID) tests.

Aspergillosis

CF and ID tests for aspergillosis have been developed and evaluated. Many workers have shown the ID test to be an effective and specific method for establishing a diagnosis of aspergillosis (13, 16, 66, 67, 82). The CF test, although reportedly less specific than the ID test, was found useful for detecting active or very recent aspergillosis (65, 92). Studies in my laboratory indicate that the CF test is less sensitive than the ID test, but it does demonstrate good specificity. Sera analyzed by CF should be tested with a battery of *Aspergillus* spp. antigens.

Clinical indications. Patients with allergic bronchopulmonary disease, patients with suspected pulmonary aspergilloma, or fungus ball, and those receiving immunosuppressive therapy should be tested for *Aspergillus* precipitins. Allergic bronchopulmonary aspergillosis should be considered in patients with asthma, transient pulmonary infiltrates, and peripheral eosinophilia. This disease represents a hypersensitivity state characterized by both immediate and arthus-type skin test reactions at the site of aspergillin injection and the formation of precipitins. Pulmonary aspergilloma, or fungus ball, occurs when *A. fumigatus* or other *Aspergillus* species colonize open-healed cavities of tuberculosis, sarcoidosis, or carcinoma. Invasive aspergillosis includes those cases where aspergilli have been shown to actually penetrate tissue.

The greatest number of aspergillosis cases may be detected by the use of *A. fumigatus, A. flavus,* and *A. niger* precipitinogens (45) in separate tests performed at the same time. Precipitins can be found in over 90% of fungus ball cases and 70% of the cases of allergic bronchopulmonary aspergillosis. They are found less frequently in patients with invasive disease. The ID test, however, may be helpful in diagnosing systemic aspergillosis (13, 29, 60) and should be applied in suspected invasive aspergillosis. Some *Aspergillus* antigens contain C-substance. This substance is capable of reacting with the C-reactive protein frequently found in patients with inflammatory diseases. It forms a precipitate which may be erroneously interpreted as being due to *Aspergillus* antibodies.

Test. Immunodiffusion (ID) test for antibody. The micro-ID test of Busey and Hinton (8) is recommended. In addition to reference *Aspergillus* antigens and antisera, phenolized agar is required.

A. *Phenolized medium.*

Noble agar (or equivalent)..	1.0 g
Phenol	0.25 ml
Veronal (barbital) buffer, 0.1 ionic strength, pH 8.6 (LKB Produkter, AB, Stockholm, Sweden)	25.0 ml
Distilled water	to 100 ml

Heat to boiling until agar is completely dissolved.

B. *Equipment.*

1. Plexiglas matrix (3 mm) with 17 patterns of 7 wells each (L. L. Pellet Co., Dallas, Tex.).
2. Plastic petri dish, 15 × 90 mm.
3. Spatula, 1-mm tip (flattened).
4. Pasteur pipettes.
5. Viewing box for reading plates.

C. *Procedure.*

1. Pipette 6.5 ml of agar into a petri dish and allow it to harden.
2. Overlay 3.5 ml of hot agar, and immediately place the matrix in the liquid agar.
3. Plates may be used within 30 min or stored in a moist chamber at 4 C for up to 1 week.
4. Each pattern is numbered on the bottom of the dish (not template).
5. Excess agar is removed from wells down to the first layer with a spatula.
6. Reference serum is placed in the top and bottom wells of each pattern, and unknown or test sera are placed in the four lateral wells. Reference antigen is placed in the center well of each pattern, and reactants are incubated in a moist chamber for 48 h at 25 C.
7. The matrix is removed by gently pressing the sides of the petri dish against the matrix. The agar is washed with distilled water to remove excess reactants and is overlaid with distilled water and examined for lines of identity with reference sera.

D. *Controls.*

Positive control sera must be included in each test. Three or more distinct precipitin lines should be formed when *A. fumigatus* reference antiserum is allowed to react with *A. fumigatus* antigen. One or more distinct precipitin lines should be formed when *A. flavus* or *A.*

niger reference antiserum is allowed to react with homologous antigen.

Nonspecific bands due to C-reactive protein reacting with C-substance in certain *Aspergillus* spp. antigens will not fuse with the reference bands to give lines of identity. The nonidentity lines due to C-reactive protein may be identified and at the same time eliminated by soaking the agar with 5% sodium citrate for 45 min before making the final readings.

Reagents. Standardized and reproducible *A. fumigatus, A. flavus,* and *A. niger* antigens with either no or minimal C-substance can be prepared from 5-week-old stationary Sabouraud broth cultures grown at 31 C. The culture filtrates are acetone-precipitated and concentrated eight times. The carbohydrate content of these antigens is determined by the anthrone test and adjusted with distilled water to contain 1,000 to 1,500 μg/ml (13). After standardization, all *Aspergillus* antigens should be checked for the presence of C-substance with sera known to contain C-reactive protein.

Aspergillosis test reagents may be obtained from the following commercial sources:

Greer Laboratories, Inc., Lenoir, N.C. 28645.

Hollister-Stier Laboratories, Spokane, Wash. 99220.

Microbiological Associates, Inc., Bethesda, Md. 20014.

Interpretation. In the ID test only sera that produce a line or lines of identity with a reference serum from a proven case of human aspergillosis are considered positive. The demonstration of one or more precipitating antibodies indicates infection, fungus ball, or allergy due to an *Aspergillus* species. Although one or two precipitins could occur with any clinical form of aspergillosis, the presence of three or more was invariably associated with either a fungus ball or invasive disease.

The ID test, when used with reference sera, is 100% specific. Occasionally, bands of nonidentity are detected that are associated with aspergillosis cases. These should make one suspect aspergillosis, but a specific diagnosis cannot be made in the absence of reference bands. One cause of nonspecific bands is C-reactive protein. Such precipitates do not produce lines of identity and will disappear after treatment with sodium citrate. Sera that produce lines that are not identical with the specific reference lines and which remain after citrate treatment warrant further study.

Sera from most patients with fungus ball and allergic bronchopulmonary aspergillosis do not have to be concentrated to demonstrate precipitin bands. Some (nonconcentrated) sera from patients with invasive disease are precipitin positive. Precipitin-negative sera from patients with suspected invasive aspergillosis—particularly from immunosuppressed patients—should be retested after they are concentrated three to four times.

Blastomycosis

Two tests, CF and ID, are widely used in the serodiagnosis of blastomycosis. The CF is less sensitive and specific than the ID test, but because of its widespread use it will be discussed in this section.

Clinical indications. Serological tests for blastomycosis should be sought when a patient manifests signs of respiratory infection which progresses gradually with fever, loss of weight, cough, and purulent sputum. The tests should also be performed when skin lesions are apparent, since the disease may spread to a localized subcutaneous or cutaneous site.

Blastomycosis has no pathognomonic symptoms or radiological features. Diagnosis by histological or cultural studies, though ideal, may take time or be negative. The ID test for blastomycosis is specific, and a positive reaction can result in immediate treatment of the patient without the need for parallel tests with coccidioidin and histoplasmin. The test has a sensitivity of approximately 80% and detects more blastomycosis cases than the CF test. Negative tests, however, do not exclude a diagnosis (52).

The CF test suffers from a lack of specific antigens and insensitivity. Studies with sera from culturally or histologically proven cases of blastomycosis indicate that approximately 50% of the case sera react in the CF test with yeast type antigens and that positive reactions also occur with sera from patients with disease other than blastomycosis, such as coccidioidomycosis, histoplasmosis, and paracoccidioidomycosis. In documented serologically positive cases of blastomycosis, the CF test may have prognostic value.

The ID test is of value in interpreting CF results with sera, from patients with suspected blastomycosis, that react solely with the *Blastomyces dermatitidis* antigen or with the *B. dermatitidis* antigen and heterologous antigens. A positive ID test with such a serum indicates *B. dermatitidis* infection.

Test I. Immunodiffusion (ID) test.

The micro-ID procedure of Busey and Hinton (8) is recommended. In addition to reference *B. dermatitidis* antigens and antisera, phenolized agar is required.

A. *Phenolized medium.*

Sodium chloride .... 0.9 g

Sodium citrate
(Na$_3$C$_6$H$_5$O$_7 \cdot 2$H$_2$O) ..... 0.4 g
Phenol .... 0.25 ml
Glycine .... 7.5 g
Distilled water .... to 100 ml

Autoclave the mixture at 15 lb of pressure for 10 min. The final pH of the medium should be 6.3 to 6.4.

B. *Equipment.*

Same as for aspergillosis ID test.

C. *Procedure.*

Same as for aspergillosis ID test except that sera are preincubated for 45 min at 37 C before antigen is added. Reactants are incubated for 48 h at 37 C.

D. *Controls.*

Positive control sera must be included in each test. The *B. dermatitidis* antiserum must react with the homologous reference antigen to form either specific A or A and B precipitin bands. The *B. dermatitidis* antigen must react with the homologous reference antiserum to yield two precipitin bands, one close to the antigen well designated "A" and the other close to the serum well designated "B."

Reagents. Suitable reproducible antigens are prepared from 1-week-old brain heart infusion (Difco) broth cultures of yeast-form *B. dermatitidis* cells shaken at 150 to 160 rpm and maintained at 37 C. The culture filtrates are acetone-precipitated, and the precipitate is dissolved in a volume of phosphate-buffered saline, pH 7.2, equal to one-tenth of the original filtrate volume (52).

B. dermatitidis CF antigens and antisera may be obtained from Microbiological Associates, Inc.

Interpretation. Blastomycosis case sera reacting with yeast-filtrate antigen(s) frequently give rise to one (A) or two (A and B) precipitin lines. Sera containing A or A and B precipitins from patients or animals with proven blastomycosis are used as references. Only sera that produce lines of identity with either A or A and B reference bands are considered positive for blastomycosis. A positive reaction denotes recent or current infection by *B. dermatitidis*. In a recent study with sera from 113 proven cases of blastomycosis, the test permitted the serodiagnosis of 80% of the subjects. Some blastomycosis case sera are not easily diagnosed by currently available serological procedures. Some sera are CF and ID negative or CF positive but ID negative. Patients with sera in those categories should be studied intensively for cultural or histological evidence of blastomycosis. In addition, several serum specimens should be drawn from them at 3-week intervals and examined by CF and ID tests with *B. dermatitidis, Coccidioides immitis,* and *Histoplasma capsulatum* antigens to detect either the appearance of CF antibodies, significant changes in homologous titer levels, or the development of precipitin bands diagnostic for blastomycosis, coccidioidomycosis, and histoplasmosis.

In established cases of blastomycosis, a decline in number or the disappearance of precipitin lines is evidence of a favorable prognosis. The serological response, however, is often not as rapid as the clinical response.

Test II. Complement-fixation (CF) test.

The standardized Center for Disease Control Laboratory Branch Complement Fixation (LBCF) test (63, 88) is recommended when sera are titrated for complement-fixing antibodies. Either the macro- or micro-CF tests, with an optimal dilution of a suspension of ground yeast-form antigen of *B. dermatitidis* (27), may be used. Five 50% units of complement are used in the LBCF test with the optimal concentration of antigen and test serum. The antigen-antibody-complement mixture is incubated for 15 to 18 h at 4 C. Sensitized sheep red blood cells are added, and the mixtures are incubated for 30 min at 37 C. The percentages of hemolysis in the controls and in the tests are read. When controls are satisfactory, sera demonstrating 30% hemolysis or less at a particular dilution are recorded as positive. Anticomplementary sera are those showing less than 75% hemolysis in the serum control without antigen. In the microtest the initial 1:8 dilutions of heat-inactivated sera are prepared by using conventional pipettes and are transferred to the microplates. Ensuing dilutions are made with microloops.

Detailed directions for performing the LBCF test are given in references 63 and 88.

As controls, human blastomycosis case sera demonstrating a homologous CF titer of 1:16 or greater should be tested each time the blastomycosis CF test is performed.

Reagents. Yeast-form *B. dermatitidis* antigens for use in the CF test are prepared from 6- to 8-day-old cultures grown on brain heart infusion agar (27). The harvested cells are broken and adjusted to an optical density between 0.3 and 0.7 on a Coleman Junior spectrophotometer set at 540 nm. An LBCF box titration of this antigen with one or more known positive human sera should be performed. The antigen should have a CF titer of 1:32 or higher.

Interpretation. Titers of 1:8 or greater with the *B. dermatitidis* antigen are considered positive. When reactions occur solely with the *B. dermatitidis* antigen, one is inclined to suspect blastomycosis. This antigen, however, frequently reacts in low titers with sera from patients who show no evidence of blastomycosis and also with sera from persons with confirmed coccidioidomycosis and histoplasmosis. With such sera, a serological diagnosis would be based upon the reactions of several serum specimens taken 3 to 4 weeks apart. High titers or rising titers indicate that the patient probably has blastomycosis. If precipitins are demonstrated in the blastomycosis ID test, the testing of several serum specimens by CF is unnecessary. Because less than 50% of the sera from persons with proven blastomycosis react in the CF test, a negative CF reaction has little value and does not exclude the existence of active blastomycosis. Although the CF test for blastomycosis may have a limited diagnostic value, it frequently is of prognostic value in the study of culturally proven serologically positive cases.

Candidiasis

Agglutination, latex agglutination (LA), ID, and counterelectrophoresis (CEP) tests are valuable in the diagnosis of systemic candidiasis (14, 69, 71, 83–87). In contrast, the serodiagnosis of candidiasis by CF tests has proven to be of little value because of positive responses by healthy subjects or by individuals with superficial candidiasis and without systemic involvement (87). The quantitative LA and the ID and CEP tests appear to give the most reliable results insofar as systemic candidiasis is concerned. The ID and CEP procedures yield results which are apparently comparable (14).

Clinical indications. LA, ID, or CEP candidiasis serological tests should be applied to sera from patients with persistent candidemia, pneumonitis, endocarditis, wound or intra-abdominal abscess, and indwelling urinary or intravenous catheters. Debilitated patients and those receiving immunosuppressive or prolonged courses of antibiotic therapy should also be tested for candida antibodies.

Serological tests are frequently used to ascertain the clinical significance of *Candida* spp. isolates. The detection of precipitins or the recognition of fourfold changes in agglutinin titers is considered presumptive evidence of systemic candidiasis. They also can indicate colonization or transient candidemia. The ID test has a sensitivity of 88%, and the LA test detects about 90% of the proven candidiasis cases. The ID test is most specific, with extrageneric cross-reactions occurring only with *Torulopsis glabrata* antisera. In contrast, the LA test shows more nonspecific reactions. Sera from patients with cryptococcosis, torulopsosis, and tuberculosis have reacted with this test. The LA test is quantitative and appears to have prognostic value. Where candidiasis is suspected and ID reactions are negative with *C. albicans* antigens, the test should be performed with *C. krusei* antigen to rule out infection with this species (84).

The CEP test yields results essentially similar to those of the ID test but in a shorter period of time.

Test I. Immunodiffusion (ID) test (84).

A. *Medium: 0.9% agar.*

Sodium chloride . . . .   0.9 g
Sodium citrate
  ($Na_3C_6H_5O_7 \cdot 2H_2O$) . . . . .   0.4 g
Phenol . . . .   0.25 ml
Glycine . . . .   7.5 g
Special Noble agar (or
  equivalent) . . . .   0.9 g
Distilled water . . . . to 100 ml

Autoclave at 15 lb for 10 min.

B. *Equipment.*

1. ID template for cutting wells, outer diameters of 6 and 8 mm. Pattern consists of three serum wells (8 mm) and two antigen wells (6 mm) placed laterally; the reactant reservoirs are placed at a distance of 10 mm.

2. Petri dishes, 140 mm in diameter, with covers.

3. Suction flask with rubber tubing and Pasteur pipette.

4. Glass slides, 50 × 75 mm.

5. Humid chamber. (Petri dishes containing water-soaked filter paper may be used as humid chambers.)

C. *Procedure.*

1. Onto each slide, pipette 7.0 ml of hot molten agar.

2. Cover the slides with petri dish halves and allow the agar to solidify for approximately 20 min at room temperature.

3. Using a template, cut out five wells.

4. Remove agar plugs from the wells by suction with a Pasteur pipette connected to a vacuum source.

5. With separate Pasteur pipettes, add specimens to the wells as follows:

   a. Fill the center 8-mm well with the positive reference anti-*C. albicans* antiserum.

   b. Fill the upper 8-mm well with serum from a patient, and fill the lower 8-mm well with serum from another patient.

   c. Finally, fill the two 6-mm wells with *C. albicans* antigen.

6. After adding all specimens to slides, incubate them in a humid chamber at room temperature for 72 h.

D. *Controls.*

A positive control serum containing at least three precipitins should be included in the test each time it is performed.

Reagents. Whole-cell antigens are prepared from 48-h dextrose-peptone-yeast extract broth cultures grown at 37 C. A 1:4 suspension of the yeast cells is disrupted in a Braun MSK homogenizer and centrifuged for 30 min at 3,000 × *g*. The supernatent homogenate antigens are collected and concentrated to yield a total biuret protein concentration of 1.0 g/100 ml. Merthiolate is added to the antigen. The optimal antigen dilution is determined by testing various antigen dilutions (1:1 to 1:8) prepared with phosphate-buffered saline, pH 7.2, against a positive reference *C. albicans* antiserum. The optimal antigen dilution is the highest dilution demonstrating distinct A, B, and C precipitin bands (84).

Satisfactory ID antigens may be obtained from Hollister-Stier Laboratories as a 1:10 extract of *C. albicans* in 50% glycerol-saline solution.

Interpretation. Candidiasis case sera reacting with homogenate antigens of *C. albicans* in the ID test may produce between one and seven precipitates. The production of one or more lines by a patient's serum interacting with antigen constitutes a positive reaction. Systemic candidiasis should be strongly suspected when the study of serial serum specimens demonstrates serological conversion (i.e., when negative antibody tests become positive) or shows increases in the number of precipitins. In addition to diagnosing systemic candida infections, positive reactions may reflect colonization by *Candida* spp. or infection due to *T. glabrata*.

Test II. Latex agglutination (LA) test (84).

A. *Equipment and reagents.*

1. Glycine-buffered saline, pH 8.4 (GBS).

2. Glycine-buffered saline, 0.1% bovine serum albumin (GSB-BSA).

3. Polystyrene latex particle suspension, 0.81 μm (Difco).

4. *C. albicans* homogenate antigen.

5. Rotary shaker.

6. Glass slides, 50 × 75 mm (marked with 12 circles with 1.5-cm diameters).

B. *Procedure.*

1. Prepare a standardized suspension of sensitized latex particles.

2. Inactivate sera at 56 C for 30 min.

3. Prepare 1:4 dilutions of serum in GBS-BSA.

4. Include a negative control and a positive control serum known to give a 2+ reaction.

5. With a 0.1-ml pipette, add 0.02 ml of the optimally sensitized latex suspension to each of the circles on a slide.

6. With separate 0.1-ml pipettes, add 0.04 ml of each 1:4 dilution of the patient's serum, the 1:4 dilution of the negative control serum, and

the positive reference serum to the latex on the slide.

7. Rotate the slide at 150 rpm for 5 min on a rotary shaker.

8. Read macroscopically: positive control must show 2+ agglutination (small but definite clumps with slightly cloudy background); negative control must show no agglutination. Check reactions of the patient's sera diluted 1:4 and record as positive all specimens showing agglutination equal to or greater than the 2+ positive reference serum.

9. All specimens positive in the screening test should be diluted 1:8 to 1:64 and tested. If an end point is not reached, dilute the specimen to 1:1,024.

10. Record the titer of each specimen as the end-point dilution factor of the highest serum dilution that gives a 2+ agglutination.

C. *Controls.*

A positive control serum showing 2+ agglutination (small but definite clumps with slightly cloudy background) and a negative control serum must be included each time the test is performed.

Reagents. See Reagents under Candidiasis, Test I. Perform box titration by diluting the 1.0 g/100 ml protein homogenate antigen in GBS, pH 8.4, and attaching the diluted antigens to 0.81-μm latex particles. The sensitized particles are tested against positive human serum controls. Select the highest dilution of antigen showing 2+ agglutination with the highest dilution of positive serum (diluted in GBS-BSA) and no reaction with normal human serum.

Antigen may be purchased from Hollister-Stier Laboratories as a 1:10 extract of *C. albicans.* This antigen should be dialyzed to remove glycerol, concentrated, and box-titrated to obtain the optimal dilution for sensitizing latex particles.

Interpretation. A serum titer of 1:8 or greater is considered presumptive evidence of systemic candidiasis. Patients whose sera are LA positive at 1:4 and demonstrate precipitins in the ID test are regarded as having possible early cases or as colonized; a patient whose serum shows only a 1:4 LA titer may have early disease, be colonized, or show a nonspecific reaction. A serological conversion from negative to positive (1:4) for agglutinins or a fourfold or greater increase in titer between serum specimens is considered presumptive evidence of infection. The sera of patients colonized by *Candida* spp. or *T. glabrata* may frequently show titers. Fourfold declines in titer may denote the success of antifungal therapy or the elimination of colonization due to removal of contaminated intravascular catheters or prosthetic valves.

Coccidioidomycosis

The CF and tube precipitin (TP) tests are valuable aids in the diagnosis and prognosis of coccidioidomycosis (80). The two tests measure at least two different antigen-antibody systems. The TP test is most effective in detecting early primary infection or an exacerbation of existing disease. It is most frequently used in endemic areas. The CF procedure is the most widely used serological test for coccidioidomycosis, and its reacting antibodies persist for longer periods than those reactive in the TP test. Smith et al. (80) found that the combination of the CF and TP tests yielded positive results in over 90% of the primary symptomatic cases of coccidioidomycosis. Screening tests (32, 34), such as the latex particle agglutination (LPA) and ID tests which yield results comparable to the TP and CF tests, can be used by those laboratories not in a position to perform the TP or CF tests.

Clinical indications. Serological tests for coccidioidomycosis should be considered whenever patients display symptoms of pulmonary or meningeal infection and have lived or have traveled in endemic areas. These tests should be used particularly when such patients demonstrate sensitivity to a coccidioidin skin test.

Precipitins may be detected within 1 to 3 weeks after the onset of primary infections in a large percentage of cases in which CF tests have not yet become positive. They are diagnostic but not prognostic. Precipitins are rarely detected 6 months after infection. They could reappear if the infection spreads or relapse occurs. The CF test becomes positive later than the precipitin test, and it is most effective in determining disseminated disease. The CF titer results parallel the severity of the infection (80); titers rise as the disease progresses and decline as the patient improves.

Qualitative data similar to those obtained in the TP and CF tests may be obtained from the screening LAP and ID procedures, respectively.

Test I. Tube test for precipitins.

The TP test is performed with three dilutions of coccidioidin and constant amounts of serum (80). The dilutions of antigen are used to obviate the possible occurrence of a false-negative result due to inhibition of the precipitin reaction by excess antigen.

A. *Reagents and equipment.*

1. Undiluted serum containing Merthiolate diluted 1:10,000.

2. *C. immitis* precipitin antigen (coccidioidin), undiluted and diluted 1:10 and 1:40 with a final concentration of 1:10,000 Merthiolate.

3. Saline buffered at pH 7.0 with 0.7 M phos-

phate buffer containing Merthiolate at a concentration of 1:10,000 for use as diluent and control.

4. Culture tubes without lip, 7 × 70 to 75 mm.

B. *Procedure*.

1. Add 0.2 ml of serum to each of four tubes.

2. Add 0.2 ml of undiluted, 1:10, and 1:40 antigen concentrations, respectively, to serum in each of three of the tubes.

3. Add 0.2 ml of control to serum in the last tube.

4. Mix thoroughly.

5. Incubate at 37 C and read daily for 5 days by sharply flicking the bottom of the tube while holding the top of the tube between thumb and forefinger.

6. A button or a flake of precipitate in any of the first three tubes is diagnostic. The TP test may be applied to sera and pleural fluids.

Reagents. The antigens for both the TP and CF tests are filtrates of mycelial cultures of multiple or single isolates of *C. immitis*. Coccidioidin is prepared by a variety of procedures, the most widely known of which employs filtrates from cultures grown in a modified Bureau of Animal Industry tuberculin medium (81).

The preparation of coccidioidin in this medium usually requires incubation for 8 weeks or more at room temperature. Coccidioidins are also prepared in Trypticase-yeast extract-dextrose broth inoculated with a single isolate of *C. immitis* and incubated for 8 weeks at 28 C (27). Antigens can be prepared within 1 week by the toluene lysis technique of Pappagianis et al. (64).

Heating coccidioidin at 60 C for 30 min destroys the antigen responsible for the CF activity but has no effect on the precipitinogens (33, 64).

The LPA test uses latex particles sensitized with coccidioidin heated at 60 C for 30 min. LPA kits may be obtained from Hyland Laboratories, Los Angeles, Calif.

Interpretation. Early coccidioidomycosis is usually detected by the TP and the LA tests. A positive TP test, indicated by the appearance of a precipitated button or flake in any dilution, is considered diagnostic. In about 80% of all infections, the TP test becomes positive within 2 weeks of the onset of symptoms. It is diagnostic but not prognostic. Precipitins are rarely detected 6 months after infection.

The LPA test is highly sensitive but not as specific as the TP test; approximately 6 to 10% false-positive reactions may occur with the LPA test. The LPA test may become positive before the TP test, however. A positive LPA reaction

must be confirmed by a TP or CF test. The LPA results can be obtained in 4 min (12, 33).

Test II. Complement-fixation (CF) test.

The standardized LBCF test with coccidioidin is recommended for titering sera from suspected cases of coccidioidomycosis. Details for performing the test may be found in references 63 and 88. In addition, see the blastomycosis tests described in this chapter. The microadaptation of the CF test for coccidioidomycosis gives results comparable to those of the macrotest (50).

The CF tests may be performed on serum, cerebrospinal fluid (CSF), plasma, and pleural and joint fluids.

Coccidioidin is prepared as described for the TP test. The CF antigen is destroyed by heating at 60 C for 30 min; consequently, this antigen should not be heated. The CF antigen may be purchased from Microbiological Consulting Service, Long Beach, Calif. 90815, or Microbiological Associates, Inc., Bethesda, Md. 20014.

Spherulin, an extract of the tissue form of *C. immitis*, appears to have promise as a CF antigen (75). Its specificity as a serological test antigen has not been determined. Spherulin is available from Berkeley Biologicals, Berkeley, Calif. 94710.

Interpretation. Any CF titer with coccidioidin should be considered presumptive evidence for *C. immitis* infection. The ID test (32) gives results that correlate with those observed with the CF test. Titers of 1:2 and 1:4 in the CF test usually indicate early, residual, or meningeal coccidioidomycosis (80). However, sera demonstrating such titers have also been obtained from patients not known to have coccidioidomycosis. The parallel use of CF and ID tests is an effective means for specifically diagnosing coccidioidomycosis in patients with low levels of complement-fixing antibodies. Studies indicate that sera positive in the CF test at the 1:2 to 1:8 range and also positive in the ID test reflect active or recent *C. immitis* infections (49). Obviously, when low titers are obtained, a diagnosis of coccidioidomycosis must be based on subsequent serological tests and preferably on clinical and mycological studies. Generally, CF titers greater than 1:16 are indicative of disseminating disease. Negative serology does not exclude a diagnosis of coccidioidomycosis. About one-fourth of all patients with coccidioidal meningitis have a negative CF test in spinal fluid, and sera from many patients with chronic cavitary coccidioidomycosis are negative.

The coccidioidin skin test is considered a valuable screen for serological testing. Conversion from a negative to a positive skin test reaction is pathognomonic and is the earliest immunological response to infection.

Smith and his co-workers (80) did not obtain positive serological results in patients with primary coccidioidomycosis and negative skin tests unless the patients had impending or concomitant disseminating disease. Unlike the serological reactions sometimes noted after administration of the histoplasmin skin test (10, 54), coccidioidin skin tests do not elicit a homologous humoral antibody response (91).

Cryptococcosis

Conventional methodology for the diagnosis of cryptococcosis is time-consuming and in many cases inadequate. Until recently, individuals suffering from cryptococcosis were considered to be essentially immunologically inert. Previous immunological tests had only limited successful applications (9, 42), and even then results were difficult to interpret. Recent work on serological procedures for cryptococcosis has resulted in the development of diagnostically and prognostically useful tests. These procedures are an indirect fluorescent-antibody (IFA) technique (89, 90), a charcoal particle agglutination test (25), and a tube agglutination (TA) test for cryptococcal antibodies (26), and a latex (LA) slide agglutination test for cryptococcal antigen (6). The antibody tests are of value in detecting early cryptococcosis and in determining a prognosis. They are, however, less specific than the LA test. Because the LA test is very specific, has both diagnostic and prognostic value, and is widely used, this procedure is described.

Clinical indications. Serological tests for *Cryptococcus neoformans* antigens or antibodies or both should be considered with patients who have symptoms of pulmonary or meningeal infection. Cutaneous, skeletal, and visceral involvement occurs as the result of dissemination. The disease may be primary, but many cases are associated with various debilitating diseases such as Hodgkin's disease, leukemia, or diabetes.

The IFA and TA antibody tests are reactive with less than 50% of the sera from proven cases. The IFA test has a specificity of about 79%, whereas the TA test has a specificity of about 95%. Although the IFA test is not entirely specific, it is valuable in detecting those cases of cryptococcosis that are negative for *C. neoformans* agglutinins and antigens. Gordon and Vedder (26) used the TA test to detect cryptococcal antibodies and found it to be diagnostically reliable. Agglutinins were detected in the early stages of central nervous system infection and in infections with no central nervous system involvement.

The LA test (6) has been successfully used for the specific detection of cryptococcal antigen in sera and CSF from humans with proven cryptococcosis. The test is valuable in diagnosing active nonmeningeal and meningeal cryptococcosis, particularly the latter. Of 39 patients recently studied with culturally proven meningeal cryptococcosis, 36 (92%) had spinal fluids positive for cryptococcal antigen by the LA test. The test is also more sensitive in diagnosing cryptococcal meningitis than the India ink test. False-positive reactions are rare and occur only with some sera from patients with severe rheumatoid arthritis. Cryptococcal antigen may also be detected by a quantitative CF procedure (4).

Kaufman and Blumer (48) observed that the serological diagnosis of cryptococcosis is best accomplished through the concurrent use of three tests: the LA test for antigen and the IFA and TA tests for *C. neoformans* antibodies.

Test I. Latex agglutination (LA) test for cryptococcal antigen.

A. *Equipment and reagents.*

1. Glycine-buffered saline, 0.1% bovine serum albumin (GSB-BSA), pH 8.4.

2. Polystyrene latex particle suspension, 0.81 μm (Difco).

3. Latex optimally sensitized with rabbit anti-*C. neoformans* globulin (LI).

4. Latex sensitized with rabbit normal (preimmune) globulin (LN).

5. Sera:

    a. Positive reference human cryptococcosis case serum with known antigen titer.

    b. Negative control human serum.

    c. Human serum positive for rheumatoid factor (negative for *C. neoformans* antigen).

    d. Patient's serum, cerebrospinal fluid, or urine specimen.

6. Water bath, 56 C.

7. Rotary shaker.

8. Glass slides, 50 × 75 mm (marked with 12 circles, 1.5 cm in diameter).

9. Microtitration droppers, 0.025 and 0.05 ml.

B. *Procedure.*

1. Inactivate sera and CSF specimens at 56 C for 30 min. Urine specimens should be inactivated by heating in boiling water for 10 min.

2. Place positive and negative control sera and the patient's specimen in a test-tube rack in the order to be tested.

3. With a 0.025-ml microtitration dropper, add a 0.025-ml drop of LI reagent to each of the circles on a slide.

4. With a 0.05-ml dropper, add 0.05-ml drops

of positive and negative control sera and up to 10 patients' undiluted specimens to the drops of the LI reagent in separate circles. Mix the drops.

5. Place the slide on a rotating shaker and rotate at 125 ± 25 rpm for 5 min.

6. Read the test immediately and macroscopically over a dark background for agglutination: positive control must show 2+ agglutination (small but definite clumps with slightly cloudy background); negative control must show no agglutination. Check reactions of the patients' sera and record as positive all specimens showing agglutination equal to or greater than 2+ positive reference serum.

7. All specimens positive in the screening test should be tested with the LN control reagent to rule out false-positive reactions due to rheumatoid factor. Include rheumatoid factor-positive serum as a control.

8. All specimens positive with the LI reagent and negative with the LN reagent should be diluted serially to make 1:2, 1:4, and 1:8 dilutions, etc. Dilutions are prepared in GBS-BSA.

9. Record the titer of each specimen as the highest dilution that gives a 2+ agglutination.

10. Results of tests in which sera react with both the LI and LN reagents should be considered equivocal.

C. *Controls.*

A positive control serum showing 2+ agglutination (small but definite clumps with a slightly cloudy background) and a negative control serum must be included each time the test is performed. Rheumatoid factor in a patient's serum may interfere with the test. To avoid false-positive results due to rheumatoid factor, sera positive with the LI reagent should always be tested with LN reagent.

Reagents. A properly standardized suspension of latex particles having an optical density of 0.30 ± 0.02 when diluted 1:100 is sensitized with an optimal dilution of 4% rabbit anti-*C. neoformans* globulin. Similarly, such a standardized suspension is sensitized with a dilution (same as for LI) of preimmune 4% rabbit globulin obtained from the rabbit(s) later used to produce the anti-*C. neoformans* globulin.

Kits for the detection of *C. neoformans* antigen in clinical specimens are made by the Industrial Biological Laboratories, Inc., Rockville, Md.

Interpretation. The LA test for *C. neoformans* antigen has both diagnostic and prognostic value. A positive reaction in serum or CSF at any titer is usually indicative of active cryptococcosis. The detection of antigen in the CSF is indicative of cryptococcosis of the central nervous system (21). The antigen titer is usu-ally proportional to the extent of infection, with increasing titers reflecting progressive infection and a poor prognosis and declining titers indicating response to chemotherapy and progressive recovery. Failure of the titer to fall during therapy suggests inadequate treatment (15).

LA tests in which serum specimens react with both LI and LN reagents should be considered equivocal. Since cryptococcosis and arthritic conditions may occur concomitantly, tests with both LI and LN reagents should be performed. A fourfold or greater titer with the LI reagent suggests cryptococcosis, but additional specimens should be examined for titer change.

The controlled LA test appears to be highly specific. Some workers, however, have reported occasional false-positive reactions at low dilutions, particularly in CSF (3). A negative reaction should not exclude a diagnosis of cryptococcosis, especially when only a single specimen has been tested and the patient shows symptoms consistent with those of cryptococcosis.

Test II. Indirect fluorescent-antibody (IFA) test for *C. neoformans* antibody.

A. *Procedure.*

Heat-killed *C. neoformans* cells representing serotype A (89) are heat-fixed to a slide and covered with a 1:20 dilution of the heat-inactivated serum specimen. After incubation, the preparation is washed, air-dried, and treated with anti-human globulin conjugated to fluorescein isothiocyanate. A positive reaction is indicated by the cells staining to an intensity of 2+ or greater.

Test III. Tube agglutination (TA) test for *C. neoformans* antibody.

Formalin-killed whole yeast cells heated at 56 C for 30 min are used in the agglutination test (26). The cells are adjusted to a concentration of 15 million cells/ml, and 0.5-ml volumes of serial twofold dilutions of serum (inactivated at 56 C for 30 min) are mixed with equal volumes of antigens. The mixtures are shaken for 2 min, incubated at 37 C for 2 h, and then refrigerated at 4 C for 72 h, during which time readings are taken at 24-h intervals. The serum titer is the highest dilution that shows any degree of agglutination.

The antibody tests are performed only on serum. Positive and negative controls must always be included in a daily run.

Reagents for the antibody tests are not commercially available.

Interpretation. A positive antibody test is suggestive of infection by *C. neoformans*. A positive test could also reflect a past infection or a cross-reaction. Antibodies may be detected in the early course of the disease. As the disease progresses, abundant antigens may be produced and detected with concurrent exclusion of antibody. The antibody test may have prognostic value. With effective chemotherapy, the antigen titer declines, and antibody may become demonstrable.

Histoplasmosis

Serological evidence is often the prime factor responsible for a definitive diagnosis of histoplasmosis. Such evidence can be obtained through CF, ID, and LA tests, used singly or in some combination. Of these procedures, the most widely used is the CF test. Properly performed, either as a tube or a microtitration procedure (50), it can yield information of diagnostic and prognostic value. As many as 96% of the culturally proven cases of histoplasmosis may be positive by the CF test (43). Unfortunately, CF tests are complex and expensive and should be performed only by highly trained technicians.

Clinical indications. Serological tests for histoplasmosis should be applied to clinical specimens (serum, plasma, peritoneal fluid, or CSF) from patients with respiratory illness, hepatosplenomegaly, signs of extrapulmonary systemic infection, or meingeal involvement. The patient's history of residence, travel, and occupation may also be used as a guide for applying these tests. The CF test is very sensitive and has been positive with sera from over 90% of the histoplasmosis cases studied. With currently available antigens, however, the test is not entirely specific. Cross-reactions may occur with sera from patients with blastomycosis, coccidioidomycosis, and other fungus infections. In addition, positive reactions cannot be obtained with anticomplementary specimens. The histoplasmosis ID test (62) and the CF test with histoplasmin will react with about 85% of histoplasmosis case sera. The CF test with yeast-form antigen has the greatest sensitivity (43). The CF test with the yeast-form antigen should be used in the diagnostic laboratory (53), and, where possible, it should be supplemented with either the ID or CEP test with histoplasmin (23, 55). There is a greater than 90% agreement between results obtained with the ID and CEP tests. The latter tests are very useful for examining anticomplementary sera, and, because of their greater specificity, they provide a more accurate diagnosis with those sera that cross-react in CF tests.

The histoplasmin LA test is satisfactory for detecting acute primary infections, but may be negative with sera from persons with chronic histoplasmosis (1). Because of the transitory nature of these agglutinins, the LA test cannot be considered a replacement for the CF test, especially with the intact yeast-form antigens (30).

Test I. Complement-fixation (CF) test.

The standardized LBCF test with *H. capsulatum* yeast-form cells and histoplasmin antigens is recommended for titering sera from persons with suspected cases of histoplasmosis. Details for performing the test may be found in references 63 and 88. In addition, see the CF test under Blastomycosis. The microadaptation of the CF test for histoplasmosis gives results comparable to those of the macrotest (50).

Reagents. Two antigens are used in the Center for Disease Control LBCF test (88). One is a suspension of Merthiolate-treated intact yeast-form cells of *H. capsulatum* (76), and the other is a soluble mycelial filtrate antigen, histoplasmin, harvested after growth of the fungus for approximately 6 months in Smith's Asparagine Medium (27). The optimal dilution for the use of each antigen is determined by a block titration with low- and high-titered positive human case sera. These antigens may be purchased from Microbiological Associates, Inc.

Interpretation. Antibodies in primary pulmonary infections are generally demonstrable within 2 to 4 weeks after exposure to the fungus or frequently by the time symptoms appear. These are usually antibodies to the yeast form of the fungus. Antibodies to histoplasmin usually develop later in primary pulmonary cases, but titers are considerably lower than those with the yeast antigen. Histoplasmin titers are usually higher in sera from certain chronic cases. CF test results can be difficult to interpret, because cross-reactions or nonspecific reactions with the yeast or histoplasmin antigens are often encountered. In such instances, titers usually range between 1:8 and 1:16 and occur mainly with the yeast-form antigen. However, many sera from culturally proven cases of histoplasmosis give titers of only 1:8. Consequently, titers of 1:8 and 1:16 with either antigen are generally considered to provide only presumptive evidence of histoplasmosis. Titers above 1:16 or rising titers offer strong presumptive evidence of histoplasmosis. The probability of infection increases in proportion to the height of the CF titer. Nonetheless, one cannot rely solely on CF titers above 1:16 as a means of diagnosis, since false-positive reactions of that magnitude may occur in patients with other diseases. Titer movement is often of great assistance in diagnosing histoplasmosis. Fourfold changes in titer in either direction are significant indicators of disease progression or regression. Occasionally, in some patients, positive titers that slowly decline are obtained for a long time after the patient has been cured. Reactions with heterologous antigens may complicate the interpretation of results when only a single serum specimen has been tested. For example, in some situations, the first serological response noted in an individual suffering from histoplasmosis may be obtained only with the *B. dermatitidis* antigen. Some patients with histoplasmosis responses may even show antibody to all of the antigens (*H. capsulatum, B. dermatitidis,* and *C. immitis*), to only some of them, or to none. Furthermore, a lack of immunological response does not exclude histoplasmosis, particularly when only a single specimen has been tested and when the clinical pictures strongly suggests pulmonary mycotic disease. In disseminated or terminal histoplasmosis, a state of energy may exist, and immunological responses may be negative. The CF test is more frequently positive with sera from patients with chronic active pulmonary histoplasmosis than with sera from primay acute pulmonary histoplasmosis (1, 30).

As indicated above, the test antigens may cross-react in blastomycosis, coccidioidomycosis, and other fungal diseases. If cross-reactions are observed or suspected, the laboratorian should base the interpretation of results upon study of serial specimens in CF and ID tests, the clinical picture, and other laboratory tests.

Test II. Immunodiffusion (ID) and counterelectrophoresis (CEP) tests.

A. *ID test.*

The micro-ID procedure is recommended for detecting *H. Capsulatum* precipitins. See the description of the ID procedure under Blastomycosis. The procedure should be modified so that antigen and unknown sera and control sera with H and M precipitins are added immediately and the reactants are allowed to diffuse while the reactants are incubating in a moist chamber for 24 h at 25 C.

B. *CEP test.*

The histoplasmosis CEP procedure (55) is performed as follows: 10 ml of an equal mixture of 0.85% agarose and 0.85% Ionagar no. 2, dissolved in 0.01 M Veronal buffer, pH 7.2, is applied to a 3.25 × 4 inch (8.2 by 10.2 cm) projector slide cover glass, and 5-mm wells are cut into the agar. Each antigen well is 3 mm from each of two serum wells. Sera are placed in the anodic wells of each pair, and histoplasmin is placed in the cathodic wells. A control serum containing H and M antibodies is placed in the well adjacent to the serum to be tested. Electrophoresis is performed at room temperature with 0.05 M Veronal buffer, pH 7.2, in each chamber. A constant current of 25 mA is applied across the narrow dimension of the slide for 90 min. After electrophoresis, the slides are removed and read for lines of identity. ID and CEP test results are valid only when control reference sera showing H and M bands are positive.

Reagents. Histoplasmin is made as described for the CF test. The mycelial-form filtrate antigen is concentrated 5 to 10 times and titered to determine the optimal dilution that demonstrates well-defined H and M bands when allowed to react with a proven human histoplasmosis case serum.

Interpretation. The ID or CEP test is a useful screening procedure or adjunct in the serological diagnosis of histoplasmosis. The results usually obtained are qualitative. The ID test was first applied to the diagnosis of histoplasmosis in 1958 by Heiner (28). He demonstrated six precipitin bands when concentrated histoplasmin antigen interacted with serum from patients having histoplasmosis. Two of these bands had diagnostic value. One, designated "h", was uninfluenced by skin testing and was consistently found in the serum of patients with active histoplasmosis. The second, designated "m," was found in acute and chronic histoplasmosis and also appeared after normal sensitized individuals had been skin-tested with histoplasmin. Although the "h" band is usually associated with the "m" band, the "m" band frequently occurs alone. The "m" band has been considered presumptive evidence of infection with *H. capsulatum* (77). Finding only "m" antibodies in sera may be attributed to active or inactive disease or to skin testing (8, 93).

To interpret the ID and CEP reactions properly, laboratory workers must know whether the patient whose serum is being analyzed was recently skin-tested. If the patient has not had a recent histoplasmin skin test, detection of an "m" band may serve as an indicator of early disease, since this band appears before the "h" factor and disappears more slowly. The demonstration of both the "m" and "h" bands is highly suggestive of active histoplasmosis, regardless of other serological results.

Test III. Latex agglutination (LA) test.

The LA test is useful for detecting acute histoplasmosis. Commercially prepared antigen in the form of histoplasmin-sensitized latex particles is available from Wilson Diagnostics, Inc., Glenwood, Ill. 60425, or Hyland Laboratories, Los Angeles, Calif. 90039. When the test is performed, serial twofold dilutions of sera ranging from 1:4 to 1:512 are prepared in tubes, and optimally diluted antigen is added. The tubes are shaken, incubated for 2 h in a water bath at

37 C, and refrigerated overnight. The centrifuged reactants are then examined for strong agglutination (1, 30).

Interpretation. The LA test yields results in 24 h and may even be used with anticomplementary sera. Although the test may be negative with sera from persons with chronic histoplasmosis, it is an excellent aid in the diagnosis of acute histoplasmosis (1).

Hill and Campbell (30) considered an LA titer of 1:16 or greater to be significant, whereas Bennett (1) considered titers of 1:32 or greater strong evidence for active or very recent disease. A positive LA test should be confirmed by a CF test.

Caution. Recent investigations indicate that levels of CF antibodies, precipitins, and agglutinins to *H. capsulatum* antigens may be significantly increased in histoplasmin-sensitized individuals after a single histoplasmin skin test (2, 10, 58, 61). This makes subsequent changes in CF titers uninterpretable. For this reason, patients with suspected active histoplasmosis should not be skin-tested. A comprehensive study by Kaufman et al. (54) confirmed the antibody-inducing action of the skin test. For the most part, these antibody responses were detected in serum specimens drawn 15 days after skin testing. Preferably, blood should be drawn for serological studies before skin testing, but, obviously, the specimen can be taken within 2 or 3 days after the skin test, because antibodies do not develop that soon. Furthermore, one must bear in mind that it is the serum reaction with the histoplasmin antigen that is affected, although effects on the yeast titer have also been reported (58). A single histoplasmin skin test produced no serological response in nonsensitized individuals.

Paracoccidioidomycosis

CF and ID tests are useful in diagnosing paracoccidioidomycosis and in following the response to treatment (18, 72, 73).

Clinical indications. Serological tests for paracoccidioidomycosis should be performed for patients displaying symptoms of chronic disease with lung involvement, or ulcerative lesions of the mucosa (oral, nasal, intestinal) and of the skin. In addition, patients with paracoccidioidomycosis often have lymphoadenopathy. A history of travel or residence in Latin America also suggests paracoccidioidomycosis.

The CF test will detect antibodies in 80 to 96% of patients with paracoccidioidomycosis (19, 73). Complement-fixing antibodies are diagnostic. The CF test results with pooled filtrate antigens of the yeast form of *Paracoccidioides brasiliensis,* however, are not always specific, and cross-reactions may be obtained with sera from patients with other diseases. These cross-reactions, however, are infrequent and occur mainly at the 1:8 level. The ID test (72) with concentrated yeast filtrate antigens has a sensitivity of 94% with sera from patients with paracoccidioidomycosis. A 79% correlation was reported between the results obtained in the ID test and those obtained with the CF test. The ID test used with reference sera is entirely specific (44). An initial serodiagnosis of paracoccidioidomycosis can be obtained in over 95% of the cases by the concomitant use of the ID and CF tests (73, 74).

Test I. Complement-fixation (CF) test.

The standardized LBCF test with *P. brasiliensis* yeast-filtrate antigens is recommended for titering sera from suspected cases of paracoccidioidomycosis. Details for performing the test may be found in references 63 and 88. In addition, see the CF test under Blastomycosis.

Reagents. Paracoccidioidin antigens for CF and ID tests are produced from yeast-form shake cultures of three isolates of *P. brasiliensis* (B339, B341, and B1183) grown singly at 35 C in a Trypticase soy broth dialysate medium supplemented with glucose, ammonium sulfate, and vitamins (72). The 4-week culture filtrates of each isolate are dialyzed, concentrated 10 times, and mixed in equal volumes. The optimal dilution for each antigen pool is determined by titration with low- and high-titered CF-positive human paracoccidioidomycosis case sera or in ID tests with precipitin-positive sera. This antigen presently is not commercially available.

Interpretation. CF titers of 1:8 or greater are considered presumptive evidence of paracoccidioidomycosis. Titers may range from 1:8 to 1:4,096, depending upon the severity and extent of infection. Low CF titers are usually associated with localized disease or patients having reticuloendothelial involvement, whereas high CF titers are found in patients with pulmonary lesions or disseminating disease. Serial CF determinations are of prognostic value. Declines in titer indicate effective therapy, whereas clinical relapses are accompanied by increases in humoral antibodies. Complement-fixing antibodies at low levels may persist long after the patient is cured.

The sera of patients with paracoccidioidomycosis may contain one to three precipitins to *P. brasiliensis* as detected in ID tests with paracoccidioidin. The highest number of precipitin bands usually occurs in patients with lung involvement or disseminated disease. Precipitating antibodies, like those that react in the CF test, are long lasting. However, at least one of the three precipitins that might occur in blood could disappear after successful treatment (74).

Sporotrichosis

Serological tests can be used in establishing a diagnosis of sporotrichosis. These tests are especially helpful in the diagnosis of the extracutaneous or systemic form of sporotrichosis when distinct clinical features are lacking. Two tests, the TA and LA tests, are reliable and sensitive. Comparable sensitivity is not obtained in CF and ID tests with *Sporothrix schenckii* antigens. The slide LA and the TA tests are preferred because they are both highly sensitive and specific. The former provides results in minutes, whereas the TA test requires overnight incubation (7).

Clinical indications. Serological tests for sporotrichosis may be applied to sera from patients with skin lesions, subcutaneous nodules, bone lesions, lymphoadenopathy, or pulmonary disease. The disease should be suspected in patients who handle thorny plants, timber, or sphagnum moss.

Because of its sensitivity (94%), high specificity, and ability to provide results in 5 min, the LA test is highly recommended for routine use in the clinical laboratory. The TA test has a comparable sensitivity, but sera being tested for sporotrichosis may show false-positive reactions with 1:8 and 1:16 dilutions of sera from patients with leishmaniasis (7).

Test. Latex agglutination (LA) test for *S. schenckii* antibody.

A. *Equipment and reagents.*

1. Glycine-buffered saline (pH 8.4), 0.1% bovine serum albumin (GSB-BSA).

2. A spectrophotometrically standardized suspension of 0.81-μm polystyrene latex particles sensitized with an optimal dilution of *S. schenckii* (yeast-form) culture filtrate antigen.

3. Sera:
   a. Positive reference human anti-*S. schenckii* antiserum with known titer.
   b. Negative control human serum.
   c. Patients' sera.

4. Water bath, 56 C.

5. Rotary shaker.

6. Test tubes, 12×75 mm.

7. Glass slides, 50×75 mm.

8. Serological pipettes, 0.1, 0.5, and 1.0 ml.

B. *Procedure.*

1. Inactivate all sera at 56 C for 30 min.

2. Prepare enough 50×75 mm slides (12 circles per slide) to accommodate the specimens to be tested. Ten sera plus negative and positive control specimens can be screened on each slide.

3. Place positive and negative control sera and the patients' sera in a test-tube rack in the order to be tested. These specimens should be diluted 1:4 with GBS-BSA.

4. With a 0.1-ml pipette, add 0.02 ml of the optimally sensitized latex suspension to each of the circles on a slide.

5. With separate 0.1-ml pipettes, add 0.04 ml of each 1:4 dilution of the patients' sera and the positive and the negative controls onto the slide. Mix the drops with applicator sticks.

6. Place the slide on a rotating shaker and rotate at 150 rpm for 5 min.

7. Immediately read test macroscopically over a dark background for agglutination: positive control serum must show 2+ agglutination (small but definite clumps with slightly cloudy background); negative control must show no agglutination. Check reactions of patients' sera and record as positive all specimens showing agglutination equal to or greater than 2+ positive reference serum.

8. All specimens positive in the screening test should be diluted serially with GBS-BSA to make 1:8, 1:16, 1:32, and 1:64 dilutions of each serum for titration.

9. The test is performed as in steps 2 to 7. One slide will accommodate the four dilutions of each of two sera plus the positive and negative control sera.

10. Record as positive all dilutions that show agglutination equal to or greater than the 2+ positive reference serum.

If the reaction of a 1:64 dilution is greater than 2+, the specimen must be diluted through four more serial dilutions (1:128 to 1:1,024), and the testing procedure must be repeated until an end point is reached. The titer of each specimen is the highest serum dilution that gives a 2+ agglutination.

C. *Controls.*

Positive and negative control sera must be included each time the test is performed.

Reagents. A properly standardized suspension of latex particles having an optical density of 0.30 ± 0.02 when diluted 1:100 is sensitized with an equal volume of an optimal dilution of yeast-form *S. schenckii* culture filtrate antigens. The optimal quantity of filtrate is the highest dilution that produces a clear 2+ agglutination with the highest reactive dilution of rabbit *S. schenckii* reference antiserum or human sporotrichosis case serum (7). *S. schenckii* antibody test reagents presently are not commercially available.

Interpretation. Slide latex agglutinin titers of 1:4 or greater are considered presumptive evidence of sporotrichosis. Sera from patients with localized cutaneous, subcutaneous, disseminated subcutaneous, or systemic sporotrichosis may show titers ranging from 1:4 to 1:128. The test has limited prognostic value, since antibody levels may show little change during and after convalescence.

IN VITRO AND IN VIVO IDENTIFICATION OF FUNGI BY FLUORESCENT-ANTIBODY TECHNIQUES

Fluorescent-antibody (FA) procedures provide mycologists with a valuable adjunct to conventional diagnostic tests. Not only do they enable the rapid gathering of presumptive diagnostic data, but they also permit the rapid screening of clinical material designated for isolation and cultural studies. Above all, with fungus cultures these procedures permit rapid identification, whereas ordinary procedures might take 2 weeks or longer. The technique may be applied to viable and nonviable fungi in culture as well as to clinical materials or tissue sections.

I have found that a combination of a 5113 Corning glass primary filter, 3 mm thick, and a Wratten 2A secondary filter, 2 mm thick, is satisfactory for use with the fungi. Some workers use a BG-12, 3 mm thick, primary filter with the secondary filter. Recent studies indicate that an American Optical interference exciter filter used in combination with a Schott GG-9 ocular filter gives excellent results with FA-stained fungi (40). The following information pertains to those FA procedures that have been developed to a practical level.

Actinomyces species and related organisms

Immunofluorescence procedures readily permit the detection and identification of the principal etiological agents of actinomycosis in humans. FA reagents have been produced for the specific staining of the serotypes of *Actinomyces israelii*, *A. naeslundii*, and *Arachnia (Actinomyces) propionica* either in smears of tissue and exudates or in culture (5, 20, 56).

Blastomyces dermatitidis

Specific FA preparations for *B. dermatitidis* have been developed (39) by adsorbing rabbit anti-yeast-form *B. dermatitidis*-labeled antiglobulins with yeast-form cells of *H. capsulatum* and *Geotrichum candidum*. These yeast-form specific conjugates make possible the rapid and accurate detection of *B. dermatitidis* in culture and in clinical materials. FA techniques still cannot be used to identify the mycelial form of this fungus.

Candida species

Numerous investigators have studied the application of the FA technique to the detection and identification of *C. albicans* and other *Candida* species. All found that the *Candida* species are closely related antigenically. Attempts to isolate species-specific FA preparations useful for the definitive identification of *C. albicans* in clinical materials and cultures have failed. To date, no single specific reagent is available for use in the clinical laboratory. Some workers have reported the successful use of a combination of reagents to identify *Candida* cultures (22, 24, 38). In spite of the lack of species-specific FA reagents, some reagents that demonstrate broad intrageneric cross-staining qualities can be used for screening clinical specimens for the presence of *Candida* sp. (35).

Coccidioides immitis

FA reagents specific for the tissue form of *C. immitis* have been developed (36). Such conjugates have been produced from antisera of rabbits infected with viable *C. immitis* cultures. These reagents generally stain the walls of endospores and the contents of spherules. Cross-staining of heterologous fungal antigens by the conjugates is eliminated by dilution or adsorption with yeast-form cells of *H. capsulatum*. Alternatively, specific conjugates can be prepared from antisera of rabbits immunized with suspensions of Formalin-killed arthrospores of *C. immitis*. Cross-staining can be eliminated by adsorption with yeast-form cells of *H. capsulatum*.

The specific conjugates are used to detect *C. immitis* in a variety of specimens from humans and animals with coccidioidomycosis. They can be used in the diagnostic laboratory for the rapid and specific demonstration of the tissue form of *C. immitis* in clinical materials from laboratory animals injected with suspected *C. immitis* cultures.

Cryptococcus neoformans

Eveland et al. (17) successfully used unadsorbed *C. neoformans* conjugates to study the distribution of *C. neoformans* and its polysaccharide products in Formalin-fixed tissue. Similarly, Marshall et al. (59) stained histopathological sections from human cases of cryptococcosis with Mayer's mucicarmine stain and FA preparations. They observed that the conjugate, although nonspecific for *C. neoformans*, stained the yeast cells more intensely and rapidly than did mucicarmine. An effective and practical diagnostic FA reagent of higher specificity is produced by the adsorption of *C. neoformans* conjugate with cells of *C. diffluens* and *Candida krusei* (68).

Histoplasma capsulatum

A specific FA reagent for *H. capsulatum* is produced by adsorbing conjugated homologous antiglobulins with cells of *B. dermatitidis* (51). This conjugate is used to identify yeast-form cells of *H. capsulatum* in culture and in impression smears made from tissues from humans with histoplasmosis and from experimentally infected mice. Several workers have investigated the applicability of FA reagents to the rapid detection of *H. capsulatum* in human clinical specimens (11, 57). The direct FA procedure has been recommended as a rapid screening procedure for *H. capsulatum* and for staining of sputum smears as an adjunct to conventional cultural criteria.

Investigations have demonstrated the existence of five *H. capsulatum* serotypes (46). Of these serotypes, only one, the 1:4 type, consistently failed to react with the available FA reagent. Recent studies indicate that this serotype is closely related to *H. capsulatum* var. *duboisii* and *B. dermatitidis*. A diagnostically useful polyvalent reagent has been developed (47) for the detection and identification of *H. capsulatum*, regardless of serotype. Adsorption of labeled antibodies produced against the most complete *H. capsulatum* serotype (1:2:3:4) with cells of *C. albicans* yielded a reagent that intensely stained only *H. capsulatum*, *H. capsulatum* var. *duboisii*, and *B. dermatitidis*. Despite its cross-staining, the *C. albicans*-adsorbed reagent can be used diagnostically by employing the *B. dermatitidis*-specific FA reagent along with the polyvalent conjugate. Both of these FA reagents stain isolates of *B. dermatitidis*, whereas only the polyvalent conjugate stains *H. capsulatum*. *H. capsulatum* and *H. capsulatum* var. *duboisii* cannot, thus far, be differentiated from each other by use of FA reagents.

Paracoccidioides brasiliensis

FA reagents for the diagnosis of paracoccidioidomycosis have been developed (79). Tissue-form specific reagents are produced from antisera of rabbits immunized with suspensions of Formalin-killed yeast-form cells of *P. brasiliensis*. Cross-reactions are eliminated by multiple adsorptions with selected heterologous fungi. These reagents are used in the direct FA procedure to demonstrate *P. brasiliensis* cells in smears of clinical materials. These conjugates are especially useful in clinical materials in which *P. brasiliensis* cells are few and when morphologically typical cells are not present.

Sporothrix schenckii

Good quality reagents for the detection of the tissue form of *S. schenckii* both in clinical materials and in culture have been developed (37). Such reagents are produced from antiserum obtained by immunizing rabbits with suspensions of whole, Formalin-killed yeast cells of *S. schenckii*. Cross-reactions are readily eliminated by dilution, without compromising staining qualities. Although, as a rule, few *S. schenckii* cells are found in lesion exudates, they are usually readily detected with the FA tests. In a few cases, particularly if the patient is already under therapy, a number of fields may have to be searched before the fungi are found.

Comments on the application of fluorescent-antibody reagents to clinical materials

The FA technique is most effective for detecting fungus antigens in cultures, pus, exudates, blood, tissue impression smears, and spinal fluid specimens. It is, however, more difficult to use with sputum and tissue sections. Not only does one have to cope with tissue elements that autofluoresce, but for some reason the staining capacity of the conjugate is impaired in sputa and tissue sections. This impairment may be due to lack of surface interaction between antigen and antibody, as shown by the fact that enzymatic and chemical digestion of sputum specimens results in more effective staining of fungus elements (57, 70, 78). Such treatment may also be applied to tissue sections (40). FA work with tissue sections has shown that fungus elements are stained more intensely in thin sections (4 μm) than in thicker sections (41). Glass slides, 1 mm or less in thickness, are recommended.

Direct FA staining permits the rapid detection of fungi in paraffin sections of Formalin-fixed tissue. In addition, one can also identify fungi in tissue sections that were previously stained with hematoxylin and eosin, the Brown and Brenn, and the Giemsa stains. The conjugates, however, will not stain fungi in tissues stained previously by the Gomori methenamine-silver nitrate, the periodic acid-Schiff, or the Gridley procedures (40).

Prolonged storage of Formalin-fixed tissues, either wet or in paraffin blocks, does not appear to have adverse effects on the antigens of fungi contained therein. Therefore, the FA procedure may also be used in making a retrospective immunohistological diagnosis. Although fluorescein-labeled *H. capsulatum* antiglobulins regularly stain *H. capsulatum* in sections of fixed tissue with active histoplasmosis, they do not regularly stain *H. capsulatum* in healed calcified lesions (31).

LITERATURE CITED

1. Bennett, D. E. 1966. The histoplasmin latex agglutination test. Clinical evaluation and a re-

view of the literature. Am. J. Med. Sci. 251:175–183.

2. Bennett, D. E. 1966. Laboratory diagnosis of histoplasmosis: a review. South. Med. J. 59:922–926.

3. Bennett, J. E., and J. W. Bailey. 1971. Control for rheumatoid factor in the latex test for cryptococcosis. Am. J. Clin. Pathol. 56:360–365.

4. Bennett, J. E., H. F. Hasenclever, and B. S. Tynes. 1964. Detection of cryptococcal polysaccharide in serum and spinal fluid: value and diagnosis and prognosis. Trans. Assoc. Am. Physicians 77:145–150.

5. Blank, C. F., and L. K. Georg. 1968. The use of fluorescent antibody methods for the detection and identification of Actinomyces species in clinical material. J. Lab. Clin. Med. 71:283–293.

6. Bloomfield, N., M. A. Gordon, and D. F. Elmendorf, Jr. 1961. Detection of Cryptococcus neoformans antigen in body fluids by latex particle agglutination. Proc. Soc. Exp. Biol. Med. 114:64–67.

7. Blumer, S. O., L. Kaufman, W. Kaplan, D. W. McLaughlin, and D. E. Kraft. 1973. Comparative evaluation of five serological methods for the diagnosis of sporotrichosis. Appl. Microbiol. 26:4–8.

8. Busey, J. F., and P. E. Hinton. 1965. Precipitins in histoplasmosis. Am. Rev. Respir. Dis. 92:637–639.

9. Campbell, C. C. 1967. Serology in the respiratory mycoses. Sabouraudia 5:240–259.

10. Campbell, C. C., and G. B. Hill. 1964. Further studies on the development of complement-fixing antibodies and precipitins in healthy histoplasmin sensitive persons following a single histoplasmin skin test. Am. Rev. Respir. Dis. 90:927–934.

11. Carski, T. R., G. C. Cozad, and H. W. Larsh. 1962. Detection of Histoplasma capsulatum in sputum by means of fluorescent antibody staining. Am. J. Clin. Pathol. 37:465–469.

12. Chick, E. W., G. L. Baum, M. L. Furcolow, M. Huppert, L. Kaufman, and D. Pappagianis. 1973. The use of skin tests and serologic tests in histoplasmosis, coccidioidomycosis, and blastomycosis. Am. Rev. Respir. Dis. 108:156–159.

13. Coleman, R. M., and L. Kaufman. 1972. Use of the immunodiffusion test in the serodiagnosis of aspergillosis. Appl. Microbiol. 23:301–309.

14. Dee, T. H., and M. W. Rytel. 1975. Clinical application of counterelectrophoresis in detection of candida serum precipitins. J. Lab. Clin. Med. 85:161–166.

15. Diamond, R. D., and J. E. Bennett. 1974. Prognostic factors in cryptococcal meningitis. Ann. Intern. Med. 80:176–181.

16. English, M. P., and A. H. Henderson. 1967. Significance and interpretation of laboratory tests in pulmonary aspergillosis. J. Clin. Pathol. 20:832–834.

17. Eveland, W. C., J. D. Marshall, A. M. Silberstein, F. B. Johnson, L. Iverson, and D. J.

Winslow. 1957. Specific immunochemical staining of Cryptococcus neoformans and its polysaccharide in tissue. Am. J. Pathol. 33:616–617.

18. Fava Netto, C. 1965. The immunology of South-American blastomycosis. Mycopathologia 26:349–538.

19. Fava Netto, C. 1972. The serology of paracoccidioidomycosis: present and future trends. Proceedings of the First Pan American Symposium Paracoccidioidomycosis. Sci. Publ. Pan Am. Health Organ. No. 254, p. 209–213.

20. Gerencser, M. A., and J. M. Slack. 1967. Isolation and characterization of Actinomyces propionicus. J. Bacteriol. 94:109–115.

21. Goodman, J. S., L. Kaufman, and M. G. Koenig. 1971. Diagnosis of cryptococcal meningitis. Value of immunologic detection of cryptococcal antigen. N. Engl. J. Med. 285:434–436.

22. Gordon, M. A. 1962. Differentiation and classification of yeasts by the Coons fluorescent antibody technique, p. 207–219. In G. Dalldorf (ed.), Fungi and fungous diseases. Charles C Thomas, Publisher, Springfield, Ill.

23. Gordon, M. A., R. E. Almy, C. H. Greene, and J. W. Fenton. 1971. Diagnostic mycoserology by immunoelectroosmophoresis: a general, rapid, and sensitive microtechnic. Am. J. Clin. Pathol. 56:471–474.

24. Gordon, M. A., J. C. Elliott, and T. W. Hawkins. 1967. Identification of Candida albicans, other Candida species and Torulopsis glabrata by means of immunofluorescence. Sabouraudia 5:323–329.

25. Gordon, M. A., and E. Lapa. 1971. Charcoal particle agglutination test for detection of antibody to Cryptococcus neoformans: a preliminary report. Am. J. Clin. Pathol. 56:354–359.

26. Gordon, M. A., and D. K. Vedder. 1966. Serologic tests in diagnosis and prognosis of cryptococcosis. J. Am. Med. Assoc. 197:961–967.

27. Harrell, W. K., H. Ashworth, L. E. Britt, J. R. George, S. B. Gray, J. H. Green, H. Gross, and J. E. Johnson. 1970. Procedural manual for production of bacterial, fungal, and parasitic reagents. Biological Reagents Section, Center for Disease Control, Atlanta, Ga.

28. Heiner, D. C. 1958. Diagnosis of histoplasmosis using precipitin reactions in agar gel. Pediatrics 22:616–627.

29. Henderson, A. H., M. P. English, and G. Stewart-Smith. 1967. Fungal infections. Lancet 1:502.

30. Hill, G. B., and C. C. Campbell. 1962. Commercially available histoplasmin sensitized latex particles in an agglutination test for histoplasmosis. Mycopathol. Mycol. Appl. 18:169–176.

31. Hotchi, M., J. Schwarz, and W. Kaplan. 1972. Limitations of fluorescent antibody staining of Histoplasma capsulatum in tissue sections. Sabouraudia 10:157–163.

32. Huppert, M., and J. W. Bailey. 1965. The use of immunodiffusion tests in coccidioidomycosis. Am. J. Clin. Pathol. 44:364–368.

33. Huppert, M., and J. W. Bailey. 1965. The use of

immunodiffusion tests in coccidioidomycosis. Am. J. Clin. Pathol. 44:369-373.

34. Huppert, M., E. T. Peterson, S. H. Sun, P. Chitjian, and W. Derrevere. 1968. Evaluation of a latex particle agglutination test for coccidioidomycosis. Am. J. Clin. Pathol. 49:96-102.

35. Kaplan, W. 1973. Direct fluorescent antibody tests for the diagnosis of mycotic diseases. Ann. Clin. Lab. Sci. 3:25-29.

36. Kaplan, W., and M. K. Clifford. 1964. Production of fluorescent antibody reagents specific for the tissue form of Coccidioides immitis. Am. Rev. Respir. Dis. 89:651-658.

37. Kaplan, W., and M. S. Ivens. 1960. Fluorescent antibody staining of Sporotrichum schenckii in cultures and clinical materials. J. Invest. Dermatol. 35:151-159.

38. Kaplan, W., and L. Kaufman. 1961. The application of fluorescent antibody techniques to medical mycology—a review. Sabouraudia 1:137-144.

39. Kaplan, W., and L. Kaufman. 1963. Specific fluorescent antiglobulins for the detection and identification of Blastomyces dermatitidis yeast-phase cells. Mycopathol. Mycol. Appl. 19:173-180.

40. Kaplan, W., and D. E. Kraft. 1969. Demonstration of pathogenic fungi in formalin-fixed tissues by immunofluorescence. Am. J. Clin. Pathol. 52:420-437.

41. Kaufman, L. 1965. The application of fluorescent antibody techniques for the detection and identification of mycotic disease agents. Mycopathol. Mycol. Appl. 26:257-263.

42. Kaufman, L. 1966. Serology of systemic fungus diseases. Public Health Rep. 81:177-185.

43. Kaufman, L. 1970. Serology: its value in the diagnosis of coccidioidomycosis, cryptococcosis, and histoplasmosis. Proc. Int. Symp. Mycoses. Sci. Publ. Pan Am. Health Organ. No. 205, p. 96-100.

44. Kaufman, L. 1972. Evaluation of serological tests for paracoccidioidomycosis: preliminary report. Proc. Pan Am. Health Organ. No. 254, p. 221-223.

45. Kaufman, L. 1973. Value of immunodiffusion tests in the diagnosis of systemic mycotic diseases. Ann. Clin. Lab. Sci. 3:141-146.

46. Kaufman, L., and S. Blumer. 1966. Occurrence of serotypes among Histoplasma capsulatum strains. J. Bacteriol. 91:1434-1439.

47. Kaufman, L., and S. Blumer. 1968. Development and use of a polyvalent conjugate to differentiate Histoplasma capsulatum and Histoplasma duboisii from other pathogens. J. Bacteriol. 95:1243-1246.

48. Kaufman, L., and S. Blumer. 1968. Value and interpretation of serological tests for the diagnosis of cryptococcosis. Appl. Microbiol. 16:1907-1912.

49. Kaufman, L., and M. J. Clark. 1974. Value of the concomitant use of complement fixation and immunodiffusion tests in the diagnosis of coccidioidomycosis. Appl. Microbiol. 28:641-643.

50. Kaufman, L., E. C. Hall, M. J. Clark, and D. McLaughlin. 1970. Comparison of macrocomplement and microcomplement fixation techniques used in fungus serology. Appl. Microbiol. 20:579-582.

51. Kaufman, L., and W. Kaplan. 1961. Preparation of a fluorescent antibody specific for the yeast phase of Histoplasma capsulatum. J. Bacteriol. 82:729-735.

52. Kaufman, L., D. W. McLaughlin, M. J. Clark, and S. Blumer. 1973. Specific immunodiffusion test for blastomycosis. Appl. Microbiol. 26:244-247.

53. Kaufman, L., J. H. Schubert, and W. Kaplan. 1962. Fluorescent antibody inhibition test for histoplasmosis. J. Lab. Clin. Med. 58:1033-1038.

54. Kaufman, L., R. T. Terry, J. H. Schubert, and D. McLaughlin. 1967. Effects of a single histoplasmin skin test on the serological diagnosis of histoplasmosis. J. Bacteriol. 94:798-803.

55. Kleger, B., and L. Kaufman. 1973. Detection and identification of diagnostic Histoplasma capsulatum precipitates by counterelectrophoresis. Appl. Microbiol. 26:231-238.

56. Lambert, F. W., J. M. Brown, and L. K. Georg. 1967. Identification of Actinomyces israelii and Actinomyces naeslundii by fluorescent-antibody and agar-gel diffusion techniques. J. Bacteriol. 94:1287-1295.

57. Lynch, H. J., and K. L. Plexico. 1962. A rapid method for screening sputums for Histoplasma capsulatum employing the fluorescent-antibody technic. N. Engl. J. Med. 28:811-814.

58. McDearman, S. C., and J. M. Young. 1960. The development of positive serologic tests with Histoplasma capsulatum antigens following single histoplasmin skin tests. Am. J. Clin. Pathol. 34:434-438.

59. Marshall, J. D., L. Iverson, W. C. Eveland, and A. Kase. 1961. Application and limitations of the fluorescent antibody stain in the specific diagnosis of cryptococcosis. Lab. Invest. 10:719-728.

60. Murray, I. G. 1966. Aspergillosis. Lancet 1:1373.

61. Nicholas, W. M., J. A. Wier, L. R. Kuhn, C. C. Campbell, L. B. Nolte, and G. B. Hill. 1961. Serologic effects of histoplasmin skin testing. Am. Rev. Respir. Dis. 83:276-279.

62. Pan American Health Organization. 1972. Manual of standardized serodiagnostic procedures for systemic mycoses. Part I. Agar immunodiffusion tests. Pan American Health Organization, Washington, D.C.

63. Pan American Health Organization. 1974. Manual of standardized serodiagnostic procedures for systemic mycoses. Part II. Complement fixation tests. Pan American Health Organization, Washington, D.C.

64. Pappagianis, D., C. E. Smith, G. S. Kobayashi, and M. T. Saito. 1961. Studies of antigens from young mycelia of Coccidioides immitis. J. Infect. Dis. 108:35-44.

65. Parker, J. D., G. A. Sarosi, I. L. Doto, and F. E. Tosh. 1970. Pulmonary aspergillosis in the

South Central United States. Am. Rev. Respir. Dis. 101:551–557.

66. Pepys, J. 1969. Hypersensitivity diseases of lungs due to fungi and organic dusts. Monogr. Allergy 4:21.

67. Pepys, J., R. W. Riddell, K. M. Citron, Y. M. Clayton, and E. I. Short. 1959. Clinical and immunological significance of *Aspergillus fumigatus* in the sputum. Am. Rev. Respir. Dis. 80:167–180.

68. Pidcoe, V., and L. Kaufman. 1968. Fluorescent-antibody reagent for the identification of *Cryptococcus neoformans*. Appl. Microbiol. 16:271–275.

69. Preisler, H. D., H. F. Hasenclever, A. A. Levitan, and E. S. Henderson. 1969. Serologic diagnosis of disseminated candidiasis in patients with acute leukemia. Ann. Intern. Med. 70:19–30.

70. Reep, B. R., and W. Kaplan. 1972. The use of n-acetyl-1-cysteine and dithiothreitol to process sputa for mycological and fluorescent antibody examinations. Health Lab. Sci. 9:118–124.

71. Remington, J. S., J. D. Gaines, and M. A. Gilmer. 1972. Demonstration of *Candida* precipitins in human sera by counterimmunoelectrophoresis. Lancet 1:413–415.

72. Restrepo, M. A. 1966. La prueba de immunodiffusion en el diagnostic de la paracoccidioidomycosis. Sabouraudia 4:223–230.

73. Restrepo, M. A. 1967. Comportamiento immunologico de zo pacientes con paracoccidioidomycosis. Antioquia Med. 17:211–230.

74. Restrepo, M. A., and L. H. Moncada F. 1970. Serologic procedures in the diagnosis of paracoccidioidomycosis. Proc. Int. Symp. Mycoses Sci. Publ. Pan Am. Health Organ. No. 205, p. 101–110.

75. Scalarone, G. M., H. B. Levine, D. Pappagianis, and S. D. Chaparas. 1974. Spherulin as a complement-fixing antigen in human coccidioidomycosis. Am. Rev. Respir. Dis. 110:324–328.

76. Schubert, J. H., and L. Ajello. 1957. Variation in complement fixation antigenicity of different yeast phase strains of *Histoplasma capsulatum*. J. Lab. Clin. Med. 50:304–307.

77. Schubert, J. H., H. L. Lynch, and L. Ajello. 1961. Evaluation of the agar-plate precipitin test for histoplasmin. Am. Rev. Respir. Dis. 84:845–849.

78. Shamiyeh, B., and E. L. Shipe. 1964. Chlorox digestion of sputum for detection of *Histoplasma capsulatum* yeast cells by fluorescent antibody techniques. Public Health Lab. 22:198–199.

79. Silva, M. E., and W. Kaplan. 1965. Specific fluo-rescein-labeled antiglobulin for the yeast form of *Paracoccidioides brasiliensis*. Am. J. Trop. Med. Hyg. 14:290–294.

80. Smith, C. E., M. T. Saito, R. R. Beard, R. McF. Keep, R. W. Clark, and B. U. Eddie. 1950. Serological tests in the diagnosis and prognosis coccidioidomycosis. Am. J. Hyg. 52:1–21.

81. Smith, C. E., E. G. Whiting, E. E. Baker, H. G. Rosenberger, R. R. Beard, and M. T. Saito. 1948. The use of coccidioidin. Am. Rev. Tuberc. 57:330–360.

82. Stallybrass, F. C. 1963. The precipitin test in human systemic aspergillosis. Mycopathol. Mycol. Appl. 21:272–278.

83. Stallybrass, F. C. 1964. *Candida* precipitins. J. Pathol. Bacteriol. 87:89–97.

84. Stickle, D., L. Kaufman, S. O. Blumer, and D. McLaughlin. 1972. Comparison of a newly developed latex agglutination test and an immunodiffusion test in the diagnosis of systemic candidiasis. Appl. Microbiol. 23:490–499.

85. Taschdjian, C. L., G. B. Dobkin, L. Caroline, and P. J. Kozinn. 1964. Immune studies relating to candidiasis. Paper II. Sabouraudia 3:129–139.

86. Taschdjian, C. L., P. J. Kozinn, and L. Caroline. 1964. Immune studies in candidiasis. Paper III. Sabouraudia 3:312–320.

87. Taschdjian, C. L., P. J. Kozinn, A. Okas, L. Caroline, and M. A. Halle. 1967. Serodiagnosis of systemic candidiasis. J. Infect. Dis. 117:180–187.

88. U.S. Public Health Service. 1965. Standardized diagnostic complement fixation method and adaption to micro test. U.S. Public Health Serv. Publ. No. 1228.

89. Vogel, R. A. 1966. The indirect fluorescent antibody test for the detection of antibody in human cryptococcal disease. J. Infect. Dis. 116:575–580.

90. Vogel, R. A., T. F. Sellers, and P. Woodward. 1961. Fluorescent antibody techniques applied to the study of human cryptococcosis. J. Am. Med. Assoc. 178:921–923.

91. Wallraff, E. B., R. M. Van Liew, and S. Waite. 1967. Skin reactivity and serological response to coccidioidin skin tests. J. Invest. Dermatol. 48:553–559.

92. Walter, J. E., and K. D. Jones. 1968. Serologic tests in diagnosis of aspergillosis. Dis. Chest 53:729–735.

93. Wiggins, G. L., and J. H. Schubert. 1965. Relationship of histoplasmin agar-gel bands and complement-fixation titers in histoplasmosis. J. Bacteriol. 89:589–596.

Chapter 51

Serodiagnosis of Parasitic Diseases

I. G. KAGAN AND L. NORMAN

INTRODUCTION

Serological tests for the diagnosis of parasitic diseases have been used since the turn of the century, and excellent summaries and bibliographies of parasitic antigen-antibody reactions have been published (43, 86, 87, 130, 139, 140, 174). If diseases are not readily detected by stool or blood examinations, tests for the presence of specific antibodies can be of great assistance in diagnosis. Serological tests are of particular value in echinococcosis (hydatid disease; 57, 60, 62, 69), trichinosis (55, 65, 78), amebiasis (4, 21, 31), and toxoplasmosis (44, 51) because in these diseases antibody levels are often high. Serological tests also aid in the diagnosis of more occult infections such as visceral larva migrans (59), cysticercosis (12, 113), and filariasis (56). In such diseases as schistosomiasis (30, 72), toxoplasmosis (165), amebiasis (49, 90), malaria (84), and Chagas' disease (101), serological tests have been effectively applied to epidemiology as well.

At present, immunodiagnostic tests have been developed for at least 24 infestations with protozoa, trematode, cestode, and nematode species (63). Figure 1 shows the present status of 18 tests for the more common parasitic diseases. They are classified according to whether they are extensively evaluated and used, are partially evaluated, or are still research tools. The tests include complement fixation (CF); the particle agglutination tests—bentonite flocculation (BF), indirect hemagglutination (IHA), and latex agglutination (L); indirect immunofluorescence (IF); and the gel diffusion tests—double diffusion (DD), immunoelectrophoresis (IE), and countercurrent electrophoresis (CEP). The methods described in this review are those used at the Center for Disease Control (CDC) for routine diagnostic serology and for epidemiological surveys. A list of the antigens recommended for each test is included. Since only a few parasitic antigens can be purchased commercially, a brief summary of the major methods for preparing these antigens is presented as well as a table of the sources of commercially available reagents.

AMEBIASIS

The CF test for amebiasis, although the oldest serological test, has generally been superseded by other techniques, particularly IHA (73), DD (89, 90), and IF (4, 15, 53). CEP (97) and IE (21) are being evaluated and used. All of these tests are very sensitive and specific with sera of patients with invasive amebiasis. The sensitivity of the tests decreases with sera from patients with amebic dysentery because tissue invasion is minimal. Serological techniques are insensitive in detecting cyst carriers. Table 1 is a compilation of data on the reactivity of these tests. Investigators using the IHA test report from 87 to 100% (48, 49, 96) positive in cases of liver abscess and from 85 to 98% positive in acute amebic dysentery. The diagnosis of asymptomatic carriers of *Entamoeba histolytica* cysts is very variable and appears to be dependent on the population from which the sample is drawn. The test was positive for 2 to 6% of the sera from noninfected controls and hospitalized patients sick with bacillary dysentery and other diseases. The percentage of serological reactors was as high as 44% in some endemic areas. IHA titers of 128 and above are reported as positive in our diagnostic laboratory.

Capron et al. (21) reported the sensitivity of the IF and IE tests to be 92 and 99%, respectively. With the advent of axenic cultivation of *E. histolytica* (35), improved soluble antigens have been made, and more reproducible and standardized tests have resulted. Such antigens have been used in the CF, IHA, L, CEP, and IE tests. Commercial kits for CEP and L tests are available; the former are more specific than the latter.

CHAGAS' DISEASE

Chagas' disease can be serologically diagnosed with a high degree of sensitivity and specificity. Three serological tests are commonly employed for diagnosis—CF, IHA, and IF. Cerisola (24) recommended the use of all three tests for maximal sensitivity and specificity. He also reported that 4 to 24 months

Parasitic diseases / Tests	Complement Fixation	Agglutination Tests: Bentonite Flocculation	Agglutination Tests: Indirect Hemagglutination	Agglutination Tests: Latex	Agglutination Tests: Direct Agglutin.	Indirect Immunofluorescence	Immunodiffusion	Immunoelectrophoresis	Countercurrent Electrophoresis	Intradermal
Amebiasis	■	▲	■	▲	○	■	■	■	▲	▲
Chagas'	■		■	▲	▲	■	○	▲	○	○
African Trypanosomiasis	▲		○			▲	▲			
Leishmaniasis	■		■	○	○	▲	○	○		■
Malaria	▲		■	▲		■	■	○	○	
Pneumocystis	■			○		▲				
Toxoplasmosis	■		■	○		■	○			■
Ancylostomiasis	○		■	▲		○		○		▲
Ascariasis	○	■	■			▲	▲	○		▲
Clonorchiasis	■		■					○		■
Cysticercosis	▲		▲	▲		▲	▲	○	○	○
Echinococcosis	■	■	■	▲		■	▲	■	○	■
Fascioliasis	■	○	■	▲		▲	○	○	○	▲
Filariasis	▲	■	■	○		■		○		▲
Paragonimiasis	■	○	○				○	○		■
Schistosomiasis	■	▲	■	○		■	▲	○		■
Toxocariasis	○	■	■			▲	○	○		▲
Trichinellosis	■	■	■	■		■	▲	▲		■

FIG. 1. *Immunodiagnostic tests for parasitic diseases. Symbols:* ■, *evaluated test;* ▲, *experimental test;* ○, *reported in the literature.*

TABLE 1. *Sensitivity and specificity of three serological tests in amebiasis as compiled from reports*

Human serum	Indirect hemagglutination		Double diffusion		Indirect immunofluorescence	
	No. tested	Percent positive	No. tested	Percent positive	No. tested	Percent positive
Amebic abscesses	314	91	622	92	484	98
Amebic dysentery	514	84	595	72	257	58
Asymptomatic cyst carriers	191	9	19	55	74	23
Patients with other diseases[a] and healthy people	658	2	198	10	1,667	1

[a] Including inflammatory bowel disease.

after treatment the tests of 81% of the patients whose tests had been positive became negative. Sensitivity and specificity of the IHA test are shown in Table 2. The L test has been found somewhat less sensitive and specific (74, 108), but it is considered practical for surveys. In addition, the IHA test can also be readily adapted for epidemiological work. Eluates from filter-paper blood samples are adequate for testing by the IHA test (101) and facilitate IHA as a test (47) for surveys. In the CF test, a titer of 8 is positive; in the IHA test, 128; and in the IF test, 64.

A direct agglutination test, introduced recently by Vattuone and Yanovsky (158), is very sensitive with sera from patients with acute infections. This method employs trypsinized, Formalin-fixed epimatigotes obtained from culture. Evaluations indicate high reactivity with sera from patients with acute Chagas' disease and relatively good specificity with regard to cross-reactions with leishmaniasis. The antibody involved in the direct agglutination test is sensitive to 2-mercaptoethanol and may be of the immunoglobulin M (IgM) class. Titers of 512 and above appear to be specific for Chagas' disease.

AFRICAN TRYPANOSOMIASIS

The serological detection of antibody against the African trypanosomes relies mainly on the detection of high levels of nonspecific IgM antibody in the serum by the Mancini test (87). The detection of specific antibody by the IF test (85) is better with homologous antigen than with heterologous antigen, and maximal sensitivity can be achieved when the serum is tested with trypanosomes of the homologous human species (82). Soltys and Woo (135), employing the indirect charcoal-agglutination test for the diagnosis of West African sleeping sickness, found that it was most satisfactory for detecting *Trypanosoma gambiense* infections. Although CF has been used in animal trypanosomiasis (132), it has not been extensively evaluated for human infections.

TABLE 2. *Sensitivity and specificity of the indirect hemagglutination test with six parasitic antigens*[a]

Human antiserum	Antigens: Ascaris	Toxocara	Echinococcus	Filaria	*T. cruzi*[b]	Cysticercus[c]
Ascaris-toxocara	14/21	8/21	1/20	6/22	0/21	0/23
Bacteria-virus	3/39	2/39	0/49	7/84	1/24	0/33
Echinococcus	3/19	0/19	20/20	3/35	0/25	15/21
Filaria	2/23	14/23	2/32	27/37	0/22	4/23
Protozoa	3/18	1/8	1/21	3/38	3/14	1/18
Schistosoma	2/28	1/28	0/24	9/41	1/24	8/29
Trichina	4/33	7/33	1/29	15/43	2/30	1/31
Normal controls	1/24	1/24	0/25	4/84	0/23	1/24

[a] Results show the number positive/number tested.
[b] Sera from Chagas' disease, 11/11.
[c] Sera from cysticercus infections, 10/14.

LEISHMANIASIS

Visceral leishmaniasis can be serologically diagnosed quite adequately by IHA, IF, and CF tests. The diagnosis of cutaneous leishmaniasis, especially in the Americas, is more difficult. For diagnosis the IHA test was employed with antigens of *Leishmania donovani, L. tropica,* and *L. braziliensis.* Since the sensitivity of the IHA test was low, the IF test is being used routinely. Walton et al. (167) reported excellent results from an IF test with amastigote antigen in cutaneous leishmaniasis. Cross-reactions are obtained with sera from patients with Chagas' disease.

The direct agglutination test with trypsinized, Formalin-fixed promastigotes of the three *Leishmania* species, prepared according to the method of Vattuone and Yanovsky (158), has proven to be slightly more sensitive than the IF test with sera from American leishmaniasis (2). Cross-reactions with *T. cruzi* are usually of a lower titer than the specific reaction. In the direct agglutination test for leishmaniasis, a titer of 32 is positive with *L. donovani* antigen, 128 with *L. tropica,* and 64 with *L. braziliensis* antigen.

MALARIA

With the introduction of IF methods, interest in the serological diagnosis of malaria (36, 79, 163) has been renewed. Tobie et al. (156) and Collins et al. (27) have contributed much to the evaluation of this procedure. The test of choice for the serological diagnosis of malaria is the IF test (148, 164). We have adapted for use in the IF test (147) a thick-smear antigen prepared from washed, parasitized blood cells. Evaluation of this antigen indicates a false-positive rate of 1% at a titer of 16. Sensitivity of the test is 95% (149). For high sensitivity and specificity, human homologous malaria antigen should be used, and at present both *Plasmodium falciparum* and *P. vivax* can be maintained in *Aotus trivirgatus,* the South American owl monkey. In the IF test, a titer of 16 is positive.

The IHA test has also been extensively used (32). Stein and Desowitz (141) described an IHA test in which Formalin- and tannic acid-treated sheep red cells sensitized with antigen from *P. cynomolgi* and *P. coatneyi* are used. Mahoney et al. (92) prepared their antigen by disrupting the parasites in a French press and reported good results with the test. Rogers et al. (116), who used *P. knowlesi* antigen prepared by the method of Mahoney et al. (92), reported that the test is both sensitive and relatively specific for malaria. The IHA procedure revealed antibody titers of 16 or greater in 98% of sera from slide-proven cases of malaria and in less than 1% of sera from individuals without a history of malaria. Pyruvic aldehyde-sensitized cells (37), which enhance the usefulness and adaptability of the IHA test for malaria, have been evaluated by Meuwissen and Leeuwenberg (95). We perform the IHA test with double aldehyde-fixed cells (37) sensitized with human malarial antigen for seroepidemiological studies.

PNEUMOCYTOSIS

The tests of choice for pneumocystosis are the CF and the IF tests (104). Serological procedures detect only between 30 and 40% of patients with this infection. The reasons for this may be that many of the patients are immunosuppressed; therefore, antibody may be absent or in exceedingly low concentration, or there is an excess of antigen complexing all available antibody. A direct fluorescent-antibody test has been developed for the detection of parasites in smears of mucus, sputum, and tissue biopsies (83). Use of serological methods is limited drastically by the difficulty in preparing antigens and conjugated antisera for use in the tests. Sensitive techniques, such as radioimmunoassay, are needed to detect antigen in the serum of patients with pneumocystis or to detect very low levels of antibody in the immunosuppressed patient. Before radioimmunoassay can be evaluated, the pneumocystis antigen has to be purified. To this end, methods for cultivating pneumocystis need to be developed.

TOXOPLASMOSIS

The extensive use of the methylene blue dye (MBD) test established a firm basis for the serological diagnosis of toxoplasmosis (121). For technical reasons, laboratory diagnosis is shifting to the use of other tests, especially the IHA and IF tests. Both utilize a killed antigen, are technically simple, pose no threat of infection to the laboratory worker, and are more economical to perform than the MBD test.

Jacobs and Lunde (52) introduced the IHA test for toxoplasmosis, and we are using it in our laboratory for routine diagnosis. Recently, we have also used this test in epidemiological studies (165).

The IF test is as sensitive and specific as the IHA and MBD tests, and its reproducibility is greater than 98% (145). The IF test can also be done with class-specific conjugates of the IgM type. Newborn babies whose sera are positive with an IgM conjugate may have congenital infections. However, such findings must be interpreted with caution.

In our laboratory, IHA titers of 64, 128, and 256 are considered to be of questionable clinical importance. These titers probably represent the low persistent antibody levels detectable in a large percentage of the population. Titers higher than 256 may represent recent experience with the parasite and may be of clinical significance. Titers obtained with the IF test are slightly lower than those obtained with the IHA test, and an IF titer above 64 may be clinically significant. A combination of two tests facilitates interpretation of the reactions. IHA and IF tests are a practical pair which utilize two kinds of antigen. Although high toxoplasmosis serological titers usually correlate strongly with clinical disease, low titers are difficult to interpret. Especially sensitive tests may be useful in uveitis. The detection of antibody in cases of uveitis led Shimada and O'Connor (133) to investigate an immune adherence test, and they reported a relatively high sensitivity with this procedure. Hübner and Uhlíková (50) evaluated a gel diffusion technique and found it to be a more sensitive indicator of cure of toxoplasmosis following treatment than the dye or CF tests.

HELMINTH DISEASES

Ancylostomiasis

Since the comprehensive studies on the serology of ancylostomiasis by Rombert et al. (120) and Vieira and Rombert (159), very little work on the serology of ancylostomiasis has been reported. Ball and Bartlett (8) published a report on the IF, CF, and IHA tests for an experimentally induced human infection. With serum from this person, the CF and IF tests became positive after infection. During the third year after the person had had three exposures to 100 larvae, the IF test indicated relatively high antibody levels, but the CF and IHA tests gave no reaction. The Prausnitz-Küstner tests were positive 4 weeks after infection, indicated the highest titers at 3 months, and became negative after 1 year. There was no observed correlation between concentration of ova in the stools and serological titer. In 1971, Rombert (117) reported on the use of frozen sections in the IF tests. Rombert and Vieira (119) and Vieira and Rombert (160, 161) reported on immunity studies on experimental animals. Sood et al. (136) found the IHA, circumoval precipitin, and DD tests of little value in detecting antibody in infected individuals.

Ascariasis

One normally does not discuss the serology of ascariasis except as it relates to toxocariasis in humans. In a recent publication, Soprunova et al. (137) reported the detection of four- to eight-branched carbon chain volatile fatty acids which correlated with the intensity of infection. This is an important finding because, although it does not deal with serological diagnosis, it does open the door to the biochemical detection of infection. Little work has been done in this area, and the extension of this type of research to the detection of metabolites or antigens in the serum and body fluids is a most intriguing problem for future investigation.

Clonorchiasis

Komiya (77) reviewed the reports on clonorchiasis. The early serology of this disease was based mainly on the precipitin test. Cross-reactions with other trematode antigens and clonorchiasis sera were reported by Nagomoto (99), and the urine precipitin reaction proved to be most specific. CF and intradermal tests have also been used in the diagnosis of clonorchiasis (125, 129, 166, 175). The percentage of positive intradermal reactions increased with the age of the population. With the intradermal test, high levels of cross-reactivity were found with specimens from paragonimiasis patients (125). Melcher-type acid-soluble antigens of adult worms were found to be most sensitive in the intradermal reaction, whereas in the CF test the Melcher acid-insoluble fraction was more satisfactory than the acid-soluble fraction (125, 166). Sawada et al.'s (129) purified antigen for the intradermal test was a defatted adult extract, fractionated by gel filtration and ion-exchange chromatography, and it was found to be specific. Sawada et al. (127) prepared a CF antigen that proved to be a carbohydrate polyglucose antigen. The IHA test proved to be slightly more sensitive than CF or ID tests (107). A gel diffusion test with a metabolic antigen was found to be more sensitive in humans with liver disease (150). Kojima et al. (76) used a passive cutaneous anaphylaxis test in rabbits infected with *Clonorchis sinensis*.

Cysticercosis

The serology of cysticercosis is of interest from both the medical and veterinary points of view. The paucity of sera from proven cases of human cysticercosis in the United States has made these diagnostic tests difficult to evaluate. CF, IHA, and DD reactions have been used. Results obtained with the CF test have been inconsistent. Although comparisons are difficult because of the variations in methods and reagents used, some evidence indicates that the test lacks both sensitivity and specificity. In South Africa, workers (113, 114) have evaluated an IHA test and a DD test with sera from both human and hog cysticercosis. The IHA test yielded 85% positive results with sera from proven cases of cysticercosis in humans, 5% positive results with sera from African hospital patients, and 2% with blood donor sera. The test was more sensitive with serum than with spinal fluid. Of sera from patients with intestinal tapeworm *(Taenia saginata)*, 17% were serologically reactive. The IHA test on hog serum was 100% positive with sera from animals condemned because of heavy infection with cysticerci; only 26% of the sera from animals showing light measles infection were positive. Biagi et al. (12) in Mexico reported the best results with the IHA test. Beltran and Gomez-Priego (9) reported the use of CEP in both human and experimental cysticercosis. Employing four antigens, these workers found excellent correlation between the clinical condition of the cyst in the host and the number of precipitate bands formed. Cross-reactions with sera from patients with *Echinococcus* sp., *T. saginata,* and *Coenurus* sp. infections have been found. In our laboratory, we have tested a small number of sera from patients with proven cases of cysticercosis. Using IHA tests with extracts of whole worms of *T. saginata* and cysticerci of *T. solium,* we observed good sensitivity in most instances. In one case, 3 months after a solitary cyst was removed from a 16-year-old girl, her serum became negative. In three other cases, serology following surgery was positive several months later, but, in each instance, the surgeon was not able to remove all of the cyst. An evaluation of the IHA test with cysticercal antigen is shown in Table 2. Although an IHA titer of 4 may be considered positive with animal infections, higher dilutions may have to be used as a standard with human sera to eliminate false-positive reactions. We have found DD insensitive with both human and animal sera.

Echinococcosis

Many types of tests have been used successfully for the serological diagnosis of hydatid disease (60–62). The IHA, IF, and IE tests are of particular value. Sera producing high IHA titers are usually positive with agglutination and CF tests, and are indicative of infections. However, the significance of low IHA titers is equivocal. They have occurred with sera from patients with collagen diseases and liver cirrhosis (68), with schistosomiasis (16), and with other parasitic infections (Table 3). There are cross-reactions between sera from other cestode infections. Hydatid cysts in the lung and dead or calcified cysts are less frequently detected by serological tests than those in the liver. Antibodies have been measured by IHA, CF, and L tests for many years after surgery (81), but CF and IF tests (3) become negative within 1 year of surgery.

The IF test can best be performed with protoscolices from viable cysts in human or animal organs (3). Ambroise-Thomas and Truong (3) reported that IF showed a sensitivity of 93% with 300 proven infections.

A combination of IHA with one or more of the more specific techniques (BF, L, CF, or gel diffusion tests) can lead to more accurate diagnosis. A combination of IHA and BF tests is routinely performed on all diagnostic sera in our laboratory. The specificity is high only when titers of 256 and above by IHA and 5 and above by BF are considered positive. The L tests of Fischman (40, 41) and Szyfres and Kagan (151) are somewhat simpler to perform. Their specificity is comparable to IHA, but sensitivity is lower. The L test prepared from lyophilized hydatid fluid as used in the IE test is recommended by South American workers (157) as very sensitive.

The IE test has been evaluated in a number of countries (23, 138, 157), and the specificity of band 5 has been confirmed. Although not all sera contain band 5 antibody, the sensitivity of the test is reported as high when performed with carefully standardized reagents in a pre-

TABLE 3. *Sensitivity and specificity of indirect hemagglutination (IHA) and bentonite flocculation (BF) tests for the diagnosis of hydatid disease*

Human antiserum	Serological tests			
	IHA		BF	
	No. positive/no. tested	Percent positive	No. positive/no. tested	Percent positive
Hydatid disease				
Liver	52/59	88	50/58	86
Lung	6/18	33	9/18	50
Controls				
Cysticercus cellulosae	9/9	100	4/8	50
Taenia saginata	0/16	0	2/16	13
Cancer	0/16	0	2/15	13
Other parasitic diseases	5/126	4	8/113	7
Miscellaneous diseases	0/62	0	0/52	0
Normal	0/47	0	0/52	0

scribed manner. Since very large amounts of concentrated reagents are required and the test is time-consuming, it does not lend itself to epidemiological studies. However, since the presence of band 5 is a positive identification, the test has a place in the diagnostic laboratory, but not to the exclusion of other tests.

Fascioliasis

Although fascioliasis in humans is a worldwide problem, both serological and immunological studies have been dwarfed by the work in schistosomiasis. Platzer (111) reviewed the serology of fascioliasis in his chapter on the trematodes of the liver and lung. Stork et al. (143) studied the prevalence of fascioliasis in 1,011 individuals in Peru and reported that 9% of these people were passing eggs of *Fasciola hepatica* in their feces. In a group of 137 children examined for eggs in their stools, intradermal, CF, IF, and IE tests were also performed. The serological tests were made by A. Capron in Lille, France. The results indicate that no one test gives conclusive diagnostic evidence of infection: 61% of the children showed ova in their stools, and 60% of the intradermal tests were positive, as were 14% of the CF tests, 49% of the IF tests, and 48% of the IE tests. Yuthsastr-Kosol et al. (179) prepared an antigen for *F. buski* and showed that antibody could be detected by CF. Cross-reaction with *Opisthorchis viverrini* was high. Fraga de Azevedo and Rombert (42) evaluated the IF test and also reviewed serological work up to 1960. These workers employed miracidia as antigen and obtained good reactivity with animal (74%) and human sera (80%). Benex et al. (10) compared the serological activity of experimental fascioliasis in sheep by L, CF, IHA, IF, IE, and DD tests, and showed that most tests become positive by the second or third week after exposure. Following chemotherapy, antibody titers decreased, and by the 9th week precipitins were lost, but the other type of antibodies persisted longer.

Filariasis

IHA and BF tests, with antigen prepared from *Dirofilaria immitis* adults, are used routinely in our laboratory for the diagnosis of filariasis. The sensitivity of the tests varies with the clinical history of the patient, and the specificity may not be satisfactory (56, 88). In *Loa loa* and *Onchocerca volvulus* infections, titers can be very high. On the other hand, very low titers are the rule with *Acanthocheilonema perstans* infections. Sera from patients with eosinophilic lung may be positive. Because of the many reactions with low titers in sera from people ill with other diseases, interpretation is difficult. The filariasis test cross-reacts with a wide variety of helminth infections and must be interpreted with caution.

In our evaluation, 27 of 37 filariasis sera (73%) were positive by the IHA test (Table 2). Of 152 sera from missionaries with microfilaria in the blood, 64% were positive. In addition, 14% of the approximately 2,877 sera from individuals without microfilaria in the blood were positive.

The filarial infections in humans perhaps epitomize the problems encountered in the nematode group, since broad cross-reactivities are evident. Niel et al. (102) found that antigen of *Ascaris suum* reacted in the DD test for filariasis. Petithory et al. (109) reported that *A. suum, Parascaris equorum,* and *Neoascaris vitulorum* gave 83 to 89% positive reactions in onchocerciasis. Capron et al. (20) reviewed their work in the use of IE with the sera of 172 patients with filariasis. The main antigen used was *Dipetalonema viteae,* a filarial species found in rodents. With this antigen, they detected specific precipitin bands in sera of patients with *O. volvulus, Loa loa,* and *Wuchereria bancrofti.* The sensitivity of the test was 80%.

The IF test has been recently studied by Pinon and Gentilini (110), Ten Eyck (154, 155), and Ambroise-Thomas and Truong (5). Using frozen sections of *D. viteae,* Ambroise-Thomas and Truong (5) found a 90% sensitivity and a group reaction with all species of filaria. Homologous antigen reacted at a higher titer than heterologous antigen. Ten Eyck (154) employed frozen sections of *O. volvulus* and found the IF test to be comparable in sensitivity to skin biopsy for the diagnosis of onchocerciasis. Using both *O. volvulus* and *W. bancrofti* antigens, Ten Eyck (155) found that in bancroftian filariasis the homologous antigen was superior, but for onchocerciasis both antigens were of equal sensitivity. Specimens from patients with microfilaria but with no local or systemic symptoms were nonreactive.

The application of cellular immune techniques is the newest innovation in filariasis diagnosis. Pinon and Gentilini (110) have applied the rosette test and the migration inhibition test employing peripheral leukocytes and have compared these techniques of cellular hypersensitivity with the IF and IHA test by using the sera of 15 patients with filariasis. Sera that were negative by IF and IHA were positive by the other methods. Bloch-Michel and Waltzing (13) have also worked with the rosette technique in the direction of filariasis, but they caution that, until more purified antigens are employed, interpretation of the test's specificity must be guarded.

Paragonimiasis

In his reviews of paragonimiasis, Yokogawa (177, 178) noted the early work on intradermal tests as applied to epidemiological studies. He reviewed the work on the purification of antigens, the evaluation of metabolic product antigen, the evaluation of extracts of adult worms, miracidia, and cercariae, and covered studies on precipitin, flocculation, urine precipitin, and CF tests. Yogore et al. (176) employed agar gel diffusion and IE, and reported specific bands for paragonimiasis in the serum of infected rabbits and humans. Sawada et al. (128), using a variety of gel-filtration and ion-exchange chromatographic methods, isolated a highly purified antigen that did not cross-react with serum from *Schistosoma japonicum,* ascaris, entamoeba, and trichuris infections. Capron et al. (22), employing IE, reported on the antigenic structure and host-parasite relationships for three species of *Paragonimus*. At present, Korean and Japanese workers are actively investigating the immunological aspects of this infection.

Schistosomiasis

A large number of serological tests have been and are still employed for the diagnosis of schistosomiasis. These include intradermal CF, BF, IHA, cholesterol-lecithin (CL), IF, and DD tests as well as certain special reactions, such as the Cercarien Hüllen Reaktion (162) and circumoval precipitation reaction (70). Most tests are sensitive, and many detect antibody in people with old infections and in people living long in endemic areas as well as people with acute disease. Moreover, there are cross-reactions (positive trichina sera are usually also positive with schisto tests) in some populations. In our laboratory, CF and IF tests are performed for routine diagnoses. The CL and BF tests are not being used since too many equivocal results were obtained. Antigens for the CF and IF tests are prepared from adult worms, but cercariae are used as antigens in the CL and BF tests. Results of the CF test correlate closely with active clinical infection, although Buck and Anderson (19) reported that it lacks sensitivity in specimens from children and from persons with chronic infections. The IF test is the most sensitive technique, and, with sections of adult worms used as the antigen, cross-reactions with trichina sera are decreased.

The technique of the IF test has been greatly improved with the introduction of frozen sections of adult worms. Wilson et al. (172) evaluated adult and cercarial antigen of *S. mansoni* for sensitivity and specificity and found the cryostat adult antigen superior in that no cross-reactions with sera from patients with schistosome dermatitis and trichinosis were obtained.

Reis et al. (115) evaluated the DD test with sera from ill patients whose sera were positive by CF. The gel diffusion test was sensitive with sera from patients with acute stages of schistosomiasis but was less sensitive with sera from patients with chronic disease. Colwell et al. (28) evaluated a leukocyte-mediated histamine release technique with platelets from infected rabbits exposed to schistosome antigens. The test was sensitive, and specificity was higher than that obtained with CF or IF. Wolfson et al. (173) demonstrated that, in infected individuals, migration inhibition of peripheral leukocytes could be demonstrated when the leukocytes were incubated with schistosome antigens. Buck and Anderson (19) evaluated both CF and the CL slide flocculation tests in four populations located in Chad and Ethiopia (endemic areas) and Peru and Afghanistan (nonendemic areas). The slide flocculation test exhibited high sensitivity but poor specificity, whereas the CF test exhibited high specificity but poor sensitivity with sera from children, with sera from patients with chronic infections, and in sera from Africans with severe onchocerciasis. Tanaka et al. (152) reported both high sensitivity and specificity for the CF test in cases of *S. japonicum*. CF is probably the test of choice in the serological diagnosis of clinical schistosomiasis. Fiorillo et al. (39) found the IHA test to be more sensitive with sera from persons with acute disease and less sensitive with sera from persons with chronic disease.

Colwell et al. (28) suggested that the histamine release technique will detect nanogram amounts of antigen. Free antigen in the serum of heavily infected mice and hamsters was described by Berggren and Weller (11) in agar gel tests. This antigen was characterized by Nash et al. (100) and found to be a polysaccharide. Antigen could be detected in the sera of 3 of 8 infected patients studied in the United States but was absent in 27 sera collected in Brazil from heavily infected individuals. This antigen, because of its molecular size, must be different from the antigen found in urine. Williams et al. (169) evaluated a radioactive antigen microprecipitin (RAMP) assay for schistosomiasis. The technique is highly reproducible and quantitative, and may indicate the immune response in schistosomiasis.

Toxocariasis

Serological tests for the diagnosis of visceral larva migrans (VLM) have been less than satisfactory. Two antigens, a fraction from a Sephadex column of *Ascaris lumbricoides* perienteric fluid (106) and an extract of *Toxocara canis* adults, are employed in the tests under evaluation. In spite of considerable cross-reactivity, a specific diagnosis may occasionally be reported on the basis of the difference in titers produced by the two antigens. In addition, *Ascaris* antibody can be absorbed with *Ascaris* antigen to reveal specific *Toxocara* antibody. A combination of two tests, IHA and BF, is used in routine diagnosis. Sera reacting in one test are usually reactive in both, but titer differences may contribute some information.

Serological results are often difficult to interpret and evaluate. False-negative reactions are a diagnostic problem, since sera from persons with ascariasis as well as from persons with VLM may be negative serologically. Very few specimens are received from patients with proven VLM. Diagnosis is usually established on the basis of the clinical history. In many strongly presumptive cases of VLM, the serology is negative. A high titer is indicative of present infection or previous experience with the parasite. Serological diagnosis has been discussed by Kagan et al. (59, 64) and Jung and Pacheco (54).

Serological tests for the diagnosis of VLM require much more research and evaluation. Until more specific and sensitive antigens or tests have been prepared and evaluated, the diagnosis of VLM must be based on an interpretation of the combined laboratory and clinical findings in each case.

In our laboratory, the IHA and BF tests are performed. A titer of 32 or greater in the IHA or of 5 or greater in the BF test is considered of diagnostic significance. Sensitivity with these techniques is not over 66%, and specificity is poor (Table 2). Tests with greater sensitivity are required for these infections.

Trichinosis

Many tests are used for the diagnosis of trichinosis. A good test should be sufficiently sensitive and reproducible to measure increase or decrease in serum titer during the acute stage of infection, yet not so sensitive that it reveals residual circulating antibodies from past experience with the parasite. The BF test most nearly meets these prerequisites for a practical diagnostic procedure (58, 78, 103). The BF test, however, is not adequate for testing lightly infected pigs (131). The IF test is the only procedure that demonstrates antibodies in pigs infected with less than one larva per gram of diaphragm muscle tissue (71).

With the BF test, antibodies are detected after the third week of a clinical infection; with the CF test, also a good method, a little earlier. Titers obtained by BF rise rapidly for several weeks until a peak is reached and then drop slowly; specimens from almost all persons are negative 2 to 3 years after infection. The specificity of the BF test is very high (78, 103). The IF test is probably the most reactive diagnostic procedure (80, 123, 144). The other tests available to the diagnostic laboratory, such as the L (14, 98) and CL (7) tests, are good techniques that are particularly suitable for small laboratories because of their simplicity.

In the CDC laboratory, the BF test is the standard test performed for the diagnosis of trichinosis. Sera are titrated in twofold dilutions from 1:5, and a titer of 5 is considered diagnostically significant. Rising titers in a series of serum samples from a patient are particularly important. Since no single test or single antigen will reveal all infections at all stages of the disease, a second test, preferably of a different type, is recommended for confirmation of low titers or to resolve questionable reactions. An evaluation of the BF test is given in Table 4. When 40 sera with BF titers of 5 through 10,240 were tested by L, IHA, DD, and CEP, we found 52% positive by L, 92% by IHA, 77% by DD, and 50% by CEP.

The IF, trichinoscopy, and the digestion method were evaluated by five members of the European Common Market Laboratory for sensitivity and specificity in the detection of lightly infected swine. Serological methods were not as sensitive as the digestion method in the detection of light infections (75). In attempts to overcome the deficiencies of the BF test, Gankavi (46) evaluated the ring precipitin reaction and found it most satisfactory as a screening procedure. Stephanski and Malczewski (142) evaluated a migration inhibition test and reported that cells from animals infected for only 4 days were inhibited. From comparisons of IF, BF, CF, precipitin, and intradermal tests, Gancarz (45) concluded that the intradermal and BF tests were best and the CF test was least valuable. These findings agree with those of other investigators who have compared the tests. BF is the test of choice for the diagnosis of human trichinosis in our laboratory (66). Rombert and

TABLE 4. *Sensitivity and specificity of the bentonite flocculation test for the diagnosis of trichinosis*

Human serum	No. positive/ no. tested	Percent positive
Trichina	38/39	97
Echinococcus	0/28	0
Filaria	0/29	0
Ascaris-toxocara	0/21	0
Schistosoma	0/34	0
Protozoa	0/48	0
Bacteria-virus	0/46	0
Normal controls	0/30	0

Palmeiro (118) employed frozen sections of infected muscle as antigen in the IF test when measuring antibody in experimental infections in rats. Sensitivity of the test was high. A stable cuticular slide antigen was evaluated by Wegesa et al. (168).

Plonka et al. (112) have investigated the IHA test, which has not been used as widely as some of the other tests. They found it to be more sensitive than IF, ring precipitation, and CF tests, and also very specific. Further, interest has been maintained in improving trichinella antigens (33).

Recent advances in the immunology of trichinosis include the introduction of the CEP test. Despommier et al. (34) evaluated this method with a particle-associated antigen from larvae of *T. spiralis* and found it to be very sensitive. In our experience, neither DD nor CEP was as sensitive as BF unless the antibody titers by BF were high. We often found it necessary to concentrate the sera to demonstrate precipitin bands by either diffusion test. A commercial CEP kit for trichinosis is being prepared.

Williams et al. (170) evaluated a radioactive antigen microprecipitin (RAMP) test for trichinosis. With this method, IgE antibodies are measured. Three international congresses on trichinosis have been held, and the proceedings of these meetings reflect a continuing research interest in the serological diagnosis of trichinosis.

SEROLOGICAL TESTS

Complement-fixation test

CF tests for parasitic diseases are the oldest, most widely employed, and most varied of all serological methods. Usually, the CF technique used for syphilis serology is followed, but, without some modifications, it has not been entirely satisfactory with parasitic antigens. Both the quantitative-type test (91) and the modified Kolmer test have been successfully standardized; the results from different laboratories,

however, are often not comparable. All tests employ the 50% hemolysis end point and require precise standardization of reagents and techniques. Since divergent results are caused as much by variation in techniques as by differences in antigens, a single standardized CF test is highly desirable. Such a test, the Laboratory Branch Complement Fixation (LBCF) test, has been devised by the CDC laboratories for viral, bacterial, and parasitic serological diagnosis. It has been used successfully for the diagnosis of Chagas' disease, malaria, amebiasis, pneumocystosis, toxoplasmosis, paragonomiasis, schistosomiasis, cysticercosis, and echinococcosis.

The LBCF test can be performed as a microtitration or a test-tube procedure. A 0.28% sheep cell suspension is prepared in Veronal-buffer-gelatin diluent and standardized (preferably) with a spectrophotometer. Five 50% units of complement are used in each test with optimal concentrations of antigen and sheep cell hemolysin. The first incubation period is 15 to 18 h at 4 to 6 C; the second incubation period (after sensitized cells are added) is 30 min at 37 C. The percentages of hemolysis in the controls and in the tests are read. When controls are satisfactory, reactions showing 0 to 30% hemolysis are recorded as positive and the remainder, as negative. Anticomplementary sera are those reading less than 75% hemolysis in the serum control without antigen.

Directions for the LBCF test are given in detail in *Public Health Monograph No. 74: Standardized Diagnostic Complement Fixation Method and Adaptation to Micro Test*. Single copies are available on request from the Public Inquiries Branch, U.S. Public Health Service, Washington, D.C. 20201.

Inert particle aggregation tests

Tanned red blood cells, bentonite particles, polyvinyl latex particles, and cholesterol crystals have been employed as carriers of antigens in diagnostic tests for parasitic infections. Both test-tube and slide tests have been designed by which antibodies are measured qualitatively or quantitatively. Basic methods for the IHA, BF, and CL tests are fairly well standardized and can be used with several antigens. Latex tests are patterned after the rheumatoid arthritis test of Singer and Plotz (134). Since there is no single method for coating latex particles with parasitic antigens, methods for trichina and echinococcus antigens are described. CL tests require precise proportions of antigens and reagents. Although the CL tests for schistosomiasis and trichinosis are valuable tests, they should be performed with strict adherence to the methods described by their authors (6, 7) and are not included here.

Bentonite flocculation test

The BF test, initially developed with trichina antigen (18), has been adapted for the diagnosis of echinococcosis (40, 105), schistosomiasis (1), VLM (124), and filariasis (67). It is a slide flocculation test in which a small drop of antigen-coated bentonite particles is added to 0.1-ml samples of diluted serum. After 15 min of rotation, the degree of aggregation of the particles is estimated under low-power magnification. In a positive reaction, over 50% of the particles are in small-to-large floccules; less than 50% flocculation is a negative reaction.

Special equipment and reagents.

Antigen solution in 0.85% saline.
Suspension of standard-sized bentonite particles.
Normal serum for negative control and positive serum of known titer. (One serum of low and another of high titer are more satisfactory as positive control sera.)
Saline, 0.85%.
Thionin blue solution in distilled water, 0.1%.
Tween 80. (Keep in refrigerator and do not use after expiration date on bottle.)
Wax ring slides, as for Kline tests.
Glass capillary pipettes calibrated to deliver 60 to 80 drops per ml. (Prepare very fine glass Pasteur pipettes from 3-mm glass tubing and calibrate; syringes with needles are not satisfactory.)
Boerner-type rotating machine for slide flocculation tests.
Dissecting microscope with 1× objective and 12× oculars.
Water bath, 56 C.

Preparation of reagents.

Suspension of standard-sized bentonite particles

All glassware must be scrupulously clean and free from detergents.

1. Suspend 0.5 g of bentonite in 100 ml of glass-distilled water.
2. Homogenize in a Waring Blendor, or equivalent, for 1 min.
3. Transfer suspension to a 500-ml glass-stoppered graduate and add glass-distilled water to make 500 ml. Shake thoroughly.
4. Centrifuge in 50-ml centrifuge tubes for 15 min at $500 \times g$. (When an International Centrifuge, size 1, type SB, with a head radius of 18 cm is used, $500 \times g = 1,550$ rpm.)

5. Pour off and save the supernatant fluid; discard the sediment.
6. Centrifuge the supernatant fluid at $750 \times g$ for 15 min ($750 \times g = 1,990$ rpm).
7. Pour off and discard the supernatant fluid.
8. Resuspend the sediment in 100 ml of distilled water and homogenize in a blender for 1 min. This is the "stock" bentonite, which usually remains stable for at least 4 months without losing its adsorptive properties if stored at 4 C.

Suspensions of antigen-coated particles

Although an excess of antigen is needed to prepare stable stock antigen, some antigens can be too strong to coat the particles properly. Therefore, each fresh lot of antigen is titrated to determine the optimal dilution for the lot. Titration is carried out as described below, except that a series of dilutions of antigen is prepared instead of the "optimal dilution" mentioned.

Stock antigen. Mix 1 volume (10 ml) of optimal dilution of antigen with 2 volumes (20 ml) of bentonite suspension. Incubate at 4 C overnight (or several hours). Add 0.5 volume (5 ml) of a 0.1% thionin blue solution. Let the mixture stand for 1 h to stain the coated particles. This "stock antigen" can be used for at least 3 months after preparation, if kept at 4 C.

Test antigen. Shake stock antigen suspension well and transfer 8 ml to a 15-ml conical centrifuge tube. Wash twice with 0.85% saline by centrifugation at $800 \times g$ for 5 min (this step removes the nonadsorbed antigen).

Resuspend the sedimented particles in 4 ml of saline. At this stage, they will form into loosely aggregated clumps which must be dispersed by carefully adding an anionic detergent.

Prepare a fresh solution of Tween 80 by dissolving 0.5 ml in 99.5 ml of distilled water. Add 0.1 ml or less of the Tween solution to the antigen. Shake well. Test with saline and normal serum (1:100), as described below under Performance of the BF test, steps 3–5. If the particles are still aggregated, add additional small amounts of Tween 80 dilution, and retest until flocculation has entirely disappeared in the negative serum and less than 50% of the particles in the saline are flocculated after 15 min of rotation.

Test two positive control sera, one of high titer and one of low titer. If the titers of the positive control sera are more than one dilution lower than the expected titers, too much Tween 80 has been added. Although the excess can be washed away, it is better to discard the antigen and start with a new 8-ml amount of stock suspension.

The properly adjusted suspension of washed coated particles (test antigen) can be used for from 4 to 6 weeks when stored in the cold. *DO NOT FREEZE.*

Smaller or larger amounts of test antigen can be prepared by washing smaller or larger volumes of stock antigen. The final volume must be half of the original for optimal concentration of particles in each test.

Performance of the BF test.

1. Sera to be tested should be inactivated for 30 min at 56 C.
2. Dilute serially each serum with 0.85% saline 1:5, 1:10, and 1:20. Positive sera are further diluted until flocculation is read as negative.
3. Pipette 0.1 ml of serum dilution into a well of a wax-ringed slide and add 1 drop of standardized test antigen (use a pipette that delivers 60 to 80 drops per ml).
4. Rotate the slide in a horizontal plane on a rotating apparatus for 15 min at 120 rotations per min.
5. Examine with a dissecting microscope for presence of agglutination.

Reading the BF test.

Results are read as follows: 4+ reaction, all particles are agglutinated; 3+ reaction, 75% of the particles are agglutinated; 2+ reaction, 50% of the particles are agglutinated; 1+ reaction, 25% of the particles are agglutinated.

A 3+ or 4+ agglutination is considered positive. A 2+ or 1+ reaction is negative.

In each series of tests, saline control and negative and positive serum controls should be included.

Indirect hemagglutination test (26, 37, 48, 52, 54, 73, 116, 141)

IHA tests in which tanned sheep or human red blood cells are used as the inert carrier of several parasitic antigens have been designed from the technique of Boyden (17). Tests for toxoplasmosis, amebiasis, malaria, hydatid disease, cysticercosis, and VLM are recommended. The technique is relatively simple to perform, and the test is very sensitive. The procedure can be varied and still demonstrate an antigen-antibody reaction. Cells treated with Formalin or glutaraldehyde have been used with slight adjustments in the IHA tests.

Equipment and reagents.

Equipment

Centrifuge, capable of $800 \times g$.
Water baths, 56 and 37 C.
Graduated conical centrifuge tubes, 12 ml.
Glassware: serological pipettes, flasks, graduates, 10×75 mm test tubes, dropping pipettes.
Additional equipment for microtitration test: dropping pipettes of 0.05 and 0.025 ml; loops, 0.05 ml; U plates; vibrator.

Reagents

Alsever's solution or 3.8% sodium citrate.
Buffered saline.
Normal rabbit serum (NRS).
Tannic acid.
Antigen.
Positive serum of known titer and negative control serum.
Erythrocytes: sheep or human "O" (allow cells to age at 4 C for at least 3 days before use).

Preparation of reagents.

Anticoagulating solutions

Sodium citrate, 3.8%:
  Sodium citrate .... 3.8 g
  Distilled water .... 100.0 ml
  (Sterilize at 15 lb of pressure for 15 min and store at 4 C.)

Alsever's solution:
  Dextrose .... 2.05 g
  Sodium citrate .... 0.8 g
  Sodium chloride .... 0.42 g
  Citric acid .... 0.055 g
  Distilled water .... 100.0 ml
  (Sterilize by filtration and store at 4 C.)

Phosphate-buffered saline (PBS)

Stock solutions:
  Na_2HPO_4, 0.15 M ... 21.3 g/liter
  KH_2PO_4, 0.15 M .... 20.4 g/liter
  NaCl, 0.15 M .... 8.8 g/liter

PBS, pH 6.4:
  Na_2HPO_4, 0.15 M ...... 32.3 ml
  KH_2PO_4, 0.15 M .... 67.7 ml
  NaCl, 0.15 M .... 100.0 ml

PBS, pH 7.2:
  Na_2HPO_4, 0.15 M ...... 76.0 ml
  KH_2PO_4, 0.15 M .... 24.0 ml
  NaCl, 0.15 M .... 100.0 ml

Diluent: 1% NRS

Inactive rabbit serum from healthy rabbits at

56 C for 30 min. Inactivated serum can be stored frozen and reinactivated for 10 min immediately before use.

Mix 1 ml of serum with 99 ml of PBS, pH 7.2.

If the diluent reacts with tanned sheep cells or sensitized sheep cells, discard it and replace with serum from nonreactive rabbit.

Preparation of tannic acid dilutions, 1:1,000 and 1:20,000

Immediately before use, prepare a fresh solution of 1:1,000 dilution of tannic acid by dissolving 10 mg of reagent-grade tannic acid in 10 ml of PBS, pH 7.2.

Dilute the 1:1,000 stock solution 1:20 for the 1:20,000 dilution used in the test (2.0 ml of 1:1,000 plus 38.0 ml of PBS, pH 7.2). If the cells show no tanning effect or if spontaneous agglutination occurs, several different concentrations of tannic acid must be tested to determine the optimal dilution for tanning a particular lot of cells.

Performance of the IHA microtiter test.

Preparation of tanned sensitized red cells

1. Wash sheep red cells suspended in Alsever's solution or 3.8% sterile sodium citrate three times with PBS, pH 7.2. Centrifuge at 800 × g for 5 min twice and for 10 min after the third wash. Adjust to a 2.5% suspension by adding 39 ml of buffered saline to each 1 ml of packed cells.

2. Add an equal volume of 1:20,000 tannic acid solution; mix well. Incubate the mixture in a water bath at 37 C for 10 min.

3. Remove the tannic acid-treated cells from the water bath and centrifuge for 5 min at 800 × g. Decant the supernatant fluid. Wash once with PBS, pH 7.2, and resuspend the cells to a 2.5% suspension with PBS, pH 6.4.

4. Sensitize the tanned cells by adding an equal volume of the optimal dilution of antigen in PBS, pH 6.4, to the cell suspension. (Example: add 10 ml of antigen dilution to 10 ml of 2.5% cell suspension.) Incubate the mixture in a 37 C water bath for 15 min. The optimal dilution must be predetermined for each lot of antigen by box titration of dilutions of positive sera of known titer, as shown below.

5. Remove the antigen-treated cells from the water bath and centrifuge for 5 min at 800 × g. Decant the supernatant fluid and wash the cells twice with 1% NRS.

6. Adjust the cells to a 1.5% suspension in 1% NRS after a final pack by centrifugation at 800 × g for 10 min.

Determination of optimal concentration of antigen

1. Prepare four dilutions of antigen in PBS, pH 6.4 (example: 1:25, 1:50, 1:100, 1:150).

2. Sensitize cells with each dilution of antigen as described above in Preparation of tanned sensitized red cells, steps 4, 5, and 6.

3. Check one negative and one positive serum with each dilution by the test procedure given below. The lowest concentration of antigen giving the highest titer with the immune serum and no reaction with the negative serum is considered optimal.

Test procedure

Inactivate the serum specimens for 30 min at 56 C. Prepare serial dilutions of the serum in 1% NRS as follows:

1. Into microtitration U plates, transfer 0.05 ml of 1% NRS with a pipette dropper to all wells in which serum dilutions will be made.

2. With a microtitration loop, transfer 0.05 ml of the test serum to the first well containing 0.05 ml of 1% NRS.

3. Mix thoroughly and prepare 12 twofold serum dilutions by transferring 0.05 ml to each successive well, discarding the final 0.05 ml from the 12th well.

4. Place the plate on a vibrator. With a pipette dropper, add 0.025 ml of 1.5% sensitized cell suspension to each serum dilution while the plate is vibrating.

5. Allow the cells to settle for 2 or 3 h at room temperature.

6. Read the patterns of the cells on the bottom of the wells. A positive reaction (4+) is indicated by a mat or carpet of cells covering the bottom of the well. (In strong reactions the edges can be folded.) A negative test is one in which the cells have settled to form a compact button or ring at the center of the well. Titer is the end-point dilution factor of the highest dilution showing a 3+ or 4+ reaction.

Controls

Diluent control. Transfer 0.05 ml of 1% NRS to several wells in a U plate and add 0.025 ml of the 1.5% suspension of sensitized cells. These reactions should be negative.

Serum control. Prepare a 1.5% suspension of unsensitized tanned cells in 1% NRS. Prepare a duplicate plate of serial dilutions of the sera to be tested, 6 wells for each serum instead of 12. To each well, add 0.025 ml of unsensitized tanned cells. A negative reaction should be obtained with each serum. If the serum is reactive, it must be absorbed with sheep cells and retested.

Performance of the IHA tube test.

Preparation of tanned sensitized red cells

Washing and tanning. Wash sheep red cells in 3.8% sterile sodium citrate three times with PBS, pH 7.2 (centrifuge at 800 × g for 5 min each time). Adjust to a 2.5% suspension by adding 39 ml of PBS, pH 7.2, to each 1 ml of packed cells. Add an equal volume of 1:20,000 tannic acid in PBS, pH 7.2. Mix thoroughly. Incubate the mixture in a water bath at 37 C for 15 min. Remove tannic acid-treated cells from the water bath and centrifuge for 5 min at 800 × g. Decant the supernatant fluid and wash once with PBS, pH 7.2.

Sensitizing. Decant the supernatant fluid. To a measured volume of packed tanned cells, add 5 volumes of the optimal dilution of antigen diluted in PBS, pH 6.4. (Example: to 0.2 ml of packed cells, add 1 ml of antigen dilution.) To a second portion to be used as cell controls, add 5 volumes of PBS, pH 6.4. Mix thoroughly and incubate the antigen-cell mixtures in a water bath at 37 C for 15 min. Add 1 volume of 0.4% NRS diluted with PBS, pH 7.2, and centrifuge for 5 min at 800 × g. Wash one or two times wth 0.4% normal rabbit serum. Resuspend cells to a 2% suspension in 0.4% normal rabbit serum.

Determination of optimal concentration of antigen

1. Prepare four dilutions of antigen in PBS, pH 6.4, (example: 1:10, 1:20, 1:40, 1:80).
2. Sensitize cells with each dilution of antigen.
3. Titrate one negative and one positive serum with each antigen-cell suspension. The highest concentration of antigen yielding the highest specific immune serum titer is considered optimal.

Test procedure

1. Make serial dilutions of the serum to be tested, using 1% NRS in PBS, pH 7.2, as follows. Prepare a rack with 10 × 75 mm test tubes (10 tubes for each serum). Transfer 0.5 ml of 1% NRS to all tubes except the first. In the first tube, put 0.98 ml of 1% NRS and 0.02 ml of the serum. For routine tests, this is the lowest dilution (1:50) tested. Mix well and prepare doubling dilutions by transferring 0.5 ml to each successive tube, discarding 0.5 ml from the last tube.
2. To each tube (0.5 ml of serum dilution), add 0.05 ml of sensitized cells.

3. Shake the rack to mix the cells thoroughly.
4. Allow the cells to settle for 2 to 3 h at room temperature; then read and record the patterns on the bottom of the tubes. (The patterns may be read after overnight settling at 4 C.) The end point of a positive test is indicated by a mat or carpet of cells covering the bottom of the tube; this is equivalent to the 4+ reaction. In a negative test the cells have settled to form a compact button or ring. Diluent and serum controls and sera with known titers are included with each day's test.

Latex agglutination tests (14, 40, 41, 98, 151)

Latex particles are coated with soluble parasitic antigens and then are usually used in rapid slide diagnostic tests which are particularly useful in screen or field testing. They are only moderately sensitive tests. The size and concentration of the latex particles, the suspending buffers, and the concentration of antigens used to coat the particles all influence the preparation of satisfactory antigens. Only the trichina and echinococcus tests are described here.

Special equipment and reagents.

Glycine-buffered saline (GBS).
Suspension of uniform-sized latex particles 0.23 or 0.81 μm in size.
Soluble antigens.
Positive and negative control sera, inactivated at 56 C for 30 min; known titers.
Spectrophotometer: Spectronic-20 or Coleman Junior type.
Glass plates ruled into 2.5-cm squares.
Dropping pipettes delivering 20 to 30 drops per cc.
Wooden applicator sticks or toothpicks.
Lighted viewing box.

Preparation of GBS, pH 8.3

NaCl	9 g
$CaCl_2$	1 g
Glycine	7.51 g
Water	1,000 ml
Adjust to pH 8.2 to 8.4 with 1 N NaOH.	

Preparation of standard latex suspension

Since suspensions of the 0.81-μm latex particle are commercially available, it is used for preparing trichina and echinococcus reagents, although the smaller-sized particle (about 0.23 μm) is better for echinococcus.

1. Prepare an estimated 1% (total solids) latex from the stock latex suspension in GBS, pH 8.3.

2. Measure the optical density of a 1:200 dilution of this 1% suspension (0.1 ml + 19.9 ml of GBS) in a Spectronic-20 colorimeter at a wavelength of 650 nm, or measure a 1:100 dilution in a Coleman Junior spectrophotometer at the same wavelength. An optical density of 0.28 ± 0.02 is optimal when 13 × 100 mm cuvettes are used in a Spectronic-20 colorimeter.

3. Adjust the stock latex suspension with sufficient GBS so that the optical density of a 1:200 dilution is optimal (0.28 ± 0.02). (The standard stock suspension is *not* the 1:200 dilution.)

The adjusted latex suspension can be stored at 4 C as long as it remains uncontaminated. It should not be frozen.

Preparation of sensitized particles

Trichina latex antigens:

Dilute 1 ml of Melcher's acid-soluble fraction (MASF) of trichina larvae (94) with 4 ml of GBS, pH 8.3. Add 5 ml of standard latex suspension. Incubate in a water bath at 37 C for 30 min and overnight at 4 C.

Alternatively, to 3 ml of Witebsky's boiled crude trichina antigen (171), add 2 ml of standard latex suspension. Incubate at 37 C in a water bath for 30 min and overnight at 4 C. Dilute by adding 1 ml of GBS, pH 8.3.

Echinococcus latex antigens:

Dialyze hydatid fluid against running water overnight, then concentrate by pervaporation to $1/10$ or $1/12$ of original volume.

Add 1 ml of concentrated hydatid fluid to 1.5 ml of standard latex suspension. Incubate at 37 C in a water bath for 30 min. Add 2.5 ml of GBS. Refrigerate overnight before use.

Since lots of antigens vary, titrate each new lot. They will be very near the proportions given above, but slightly different amounts or dilutions should be tested. The amounts of latex can also be varied slightly to prepare a suspension of coated particles that will be negative with normal serum, yet give the proper titers with known positive sera. Too little antigen permits flocculation of latex in negative sera. Excess antigen usually is indicated by negative or reduced reactivity with positive sera.

The coated particles will retain their reactivity for several weeks to several months if stored at 4 C (never frozen). Control sera must be tested with each day's run.

Performance of the slide test

1. Inactivate sera at 56 C for 30 min.
2. Prepare serial dilutions of serum in GBS,

1:5, 1:10, 1:20, etc., for a quantitative test. For a qualitative test, do not dilute.

3. Place one drop of undiluted serum (or one drop of each dilution) in separate squares on a marked glass plate.

4. Add one drop of sensitized latex particles to each square and mix with a stick. Spread over an area about the size of a quarter.

5. Rotate the plate for 2 or 3 min by hand or on a mechanical rotator. Rotation by hand for 2 min is adquate for trichina tests; 3 min is required for echinococcus. Rotation by machine at 180 rpm requires 5 min.

6. Read macroscopically for agglutination of particles. Use reflected light or a viewing box.

A negative test shows uniform turbidity and no flocculation, or slight granulation up to 1+ flocculation. A weakly positive reaction shows 2+ (usually fine) aggregation. A positive reaction shows 3+ or 4+ (complete aggregation). Titers are usually very low with these tests.

Indirect immunofluorescence test (15, 38, 53, 79, 122, 126, 145–147, 156, 163, 167)

The IF test has been investigated as a diagnostic technique for several parasitic diseases, including toxoplasmosis, malaria, trichinosis, schistosomiasis, and hydatid disease. The detailed description of the IF test for toxoplasmosis serves as a general model for other antigen-antibody systems.

Special equipment and reagents.

IF binocular microscope equipped with BG-12 exciter and OG-1 ocular filters or the equivalent. For malaria IF, a UG-1 or UG-2 exciter filter and a GG-9 ocular filter or the equivalent are essential.

PBS, pH 7.6.

Buffered glycerol, pH 9.0.

Evans blue dye, 1% in PBS, pH 7.6.

Antigen on slides.

Fluorescein-conjugated anti-human globulins (must be free from specific toxoplasma antibody).

Antisera.

Preparation of reagents.

Stock buffered salt solution

Na$_2$HPO$_4$, anhydrous ...	13.36 g
NaH$_2$PO$_4$·H$_2$O	1.80 g
NaCl	85.00 g
Distilled water to final volume of	1,000 ml

PBS, 0.01 M, pH 7.6

Stock buffered salt solution, 100 ml; distilled water, 900 ml. Check pH and adjust, if necessary.

Buffered glycerol

Prepare a 0.2 M Na_2HPO_4 solution by dissolving 28.4 g of anhydrous Na_2HPO_4 in 1,000 ml of distilled water; pH will be 9.0. Mix 1 volume with 9 volumes of glycerol.

Performance of the IF (slide) test.

The fluorescein-conjugated anti-human globulin should first be assayed with a positive control serum of known titer to determine the best dilution for use. The conjugate is diluted with PBS, pH 7.6, and Evans blue. (For example, for a 1:10 conjugate and 1:500 counterstain dilution, add to 0.1 ml of conjugate 0.2 ml of 1% Evans blue and 0.7 ml of PBS.)

1. Prepare a serial fourfold dilutions of the serum to be tested in PBS, pH 7.6. Dilutions can be started at 1:16, because this is the lowest dilution that is considered significant. Fourfold dilutions of sera are preferred when making comparisons on a test-to-test basis, but twofold dilutions will give more information when sera are to be compared in the same test.

2. Remove antigen slides from freezer and wash in a gentle stream of distilled water.

3. Blot dry (facial tissue is satisfactory).

4. Place the slide on wet paper in a shallow pan with the smears up.

5. Cover each smear with a successive dilution of serum.

6. Cover the pan with a lid or aluminum foil and place in a 37 C incubator for 30 min.

7. Rinse off serum dilutions with a gentle stream of distilled water; then dip several times in a PBS bath.

8. Blot the smears dry and replace the slides in a pan on wet paper.

9. Cover the smears with the optimal dilution of anti-human conjugate diluted in Evans blue in PBS, pH 7.6.

10. Cover the pan and place in the 37 C incubator for 30 min.

11. Repeat washings as in step 7, with a final rinse in water.

12. Blot dry.

13. Place a small drop of buffered glycerol, pH 9, on the smear and cover with a cover slip.

14. Examine with the high-dry objective on fluorescence microscope equipped with a BG-12 exciter and OG-1 ocular filter or the equivalent.

15. Prepare the following controls each time the test is performed: (i) saline, (ii) negative serum, and (iii) positive human serum of known titer. The positive serum is tested at four dilutions: one below, two above, and one at the known titer of the serum. For example, if the control serum has a titer of 1,024, with a fourfold dilution scheme it should be tested at

dilutions of 1:256, 1:1,024, 1:4,096, and 1:16,384. The negative control serum can be tested only at 1:16.

When a large number of diagnostic sera are to be tested, they should be screened at 1:16 and 1:64 dilutions. If a serum is positive at a dilution of 1:64, it should be retested at higher dilutions to determine its titer.

Frozen-sectioned antigens

Tests for schistosomiasis, echinococcosis, and filariasis generally employ cryostat sections of the adult or larval stages as antigen. The test procedure is the same as for toxoplasma except that the slides are not washed with water after being removed from the freezer. Instead, they are allowed to dry and are then immersed in acetone for 10 min.

Reading the toxoplasma IF test.

In the toxoplasmosis test, the reaction is negative when the organisms fluoresce reddish-purple (due to the Evans blue) with no yellow-green fluorescence around the periphery; the reaction is also considered negative when only the anterior ends of organisms fluoresce bright yellow-green with no extension of yellow-green around the posterior end. This "polar staining" will occur only with some sera and at lower dilutions, usually disappearing at a serum dilution between 1:16 and 1:64.

The reaction in toxoplasma serology is positive when yellow-green fluorescence extends around the entire periphery of the organism. This reaction can be intense enough (in lower dilutions of strong positive sera) to mask all internal red counterstain. In higher dilutions, the peripheral staining will become a thin, peripheral halo around an internal, red fluorescence.

The titer is the end-point dilution factor of the highest dilution at which more than half of the organisms exhibit the yellow-green fluorescence around their entire periphery. When fourfold dilutions are tested, the end point is usually sharply defined.

When reading the malaria IF test, both BG-12 and UG-1 or -2 exciter filters are used with the GG-9 ocular filter. Plasmodia are first located, with the BG-12 exciter filter, by refraction of blue light from the pigment; specific fluorescence is then evaluated by using the UG-1 or -2 exciter filter. Presence of at least 10% schizonts in the malaria antigen is recommended for greatest sensitivity.

In the malaria IF test, the reaction is positive when plasmodia can be distinguished against the background by their specific green fluorescence. Titers of reactions with schizonts always equal and often exceed titers observed with other life cycle forms. The reactions with schizonts, therefore, are used in determining titers of diagnostic sera.

Interpretation of the toxoplasma IF test.

Serology serves only as an aid to diagnosis and can rarely be considered diagnostic in itself. The following observations should help the clinician interpret laboratory findings.

A titer of 16 to 64 usually reflects only some past exposure; however, when rising titers appear in later specimens of serum from the same patient, it can signify early stages of disease.

A titer of 1,024 is very significant. The clinician should be advised to consider toxoplasmosis and should attempt to identify the disease by additional tests or isolation of the parasite from biopsied lymph nodes.

Precipitin Tests

Diagnostic precipitin tests for parasitic diseases include the old "ring" test, microprecipitin reactions in which clumps of precipitate form about living larval or other life-cycle stages of parasites when they are incubated in serum containing antibodies, double diffusion in gels, and the newer IE and CEP methods.

Microprecipitin tests (93, 162)

Special equipment and reagents.
Hanging-drop or "well" slides and cover slips.
Sterile physiological saline and solutions of penicillin and streptomycin.
Antisera – not chylous or cloudy. Positive and negative control sera.
Living *Trichinella spiralis* larvae, schistosome cercariae or eggs.

Preparation of parasite antigens for microprecipitin reactions

Trichina larvae. Digest muscle of rats or mice infected for 1 to 2 months with *T. spiralis;* 30 to 50 g of muscle will be digested in 1 liter of artificial digestive fluid (0.7% pepsin, 0.5% HCl in warm water) in a few hours. Collect and wash the larvae several times in warm saline. Finally, wash in 1:10,000 Merthiolate-treated saline for not more than 5 min, and follow by several washes with sterile saline to remove the Merthiolate. Larvae can be used as long as they remain viable. Living larvae are motile or are tightly coiled. Suspend clean, sterile larvae in sufficient sterile saline that a measured number (10 to 100) can be transferred in one drop.
Schistosome cercariae. Transfer several in-

fected snails to a beaker of warm water (37 C) and incubate for 1 h to induce shedding of cercariae. Decant the fluid, and concentrate the cercariae by centrifugation if the yield is low. Wash in fresh water, and resuspend the cercariae so that one drop contains from 30 to 50 organisms. Cercariae can be used after storage at 4 C for as long as 12 h.

Schistosome ova. Collect eggs from infected hamster or mouse livers in 1.75% saline. Separate the eggs and debris by screening through fine mesh screens. The eggs are isolated by sedimentation. Wash eggs in 1.75% saline and suspend so that one drop contains approximately 100 eggs. The egg suspension can be stored in the cold for 12 to 24 h, if necessary.

Performance of microprecipitin tests.

Do not use Merthiolated-treated serum in these tests.

Circumlarval: trichina (93)

1. Transfer a drop of the antigen suspension containing not more than 100 washed, viable larvae (preferably 10 to 50) to the well of a hanging-drop slide.
2. Cover with about 0.5 ml of inactivated antiserum and mix gently with an applicator stick.
3. Place a cover slip over the well, seal with paraffin, and incubate in a moist chamber at 37 C.
4. Examine the slides with low magnification at 2-h intervals for 6 h for the appearance of a granular precipitate attached to the anterior end of the larvae.
5. Return to the incubator overnight. The next day, the precipitates may have loosened and may be floating in the serum.

The percentage of larvae with precipitate and the size of the aggregates of precipitate should be noted and compared with the reactions of positive and negative control sera.

Cercarienhüllenreaktion: schistosomiasis (162)

This test is performed in the same way as the circumlarval test. Use one drop of cercariae containing 30 to 50 organisms and one drop of antiserum that has not been inactivated. To prevent bacterial contamination and to permit longer periods of observation, a small drop of penicillin G (4,000 units per ml) and streptomycin (0.5 mg/ml) can be added to the chamber. Incubate from 4 to 24 h at 22 C. Within this time, if antibodies are present in the serum, the cercariae will be immobilized and surrounded by a "membrane" of precipitate.

Results are read as follows: negative reaction, no envelope in 4 to 24 h; doubtful reaction, appearance of a fine envelope on the tails of a few cercariae; positive reaction, formation of a clearly defined envelope. A thin smooth membrane is a ± reaction. A thin, wrinkled membrane is a + reaction. A discrete thick membrane is a 2+ to 3+ reaction. A heavy loose membrane is a 4+ reaction.

Circumoval precipitin test: schistosomiasis

This test is performed in the same manner as the circumlarval test. Use one drop of a suspension of eggs (about 100) in 1.75% saline and one drop of 0.05 ml of serum which has been inactivated at 56 C for 30 min. Incubate at 37 C for 24 h. Examine after 2 and 24 h, recording the percentage of ova showing precipitates, measuring length, and noting fingerlike shapes of the precipitate. Compare with negative and positive controls.

Weak reaction: precipitates 12.5 μm or less in length. Moderate reaction: precipitates 25 μm in length. Strong reaction: precipitates 37.5 μm and over in length.

The circumoval precipitin reaction is considered more specific for the species of schistosomes than the cercarienhüllenreaktion.

Gel diffusion tests (23, 29, 89, 138, 157)

Diagnostic precipitin tests in gels include the Ouchterlony type of DD, IE, and CEP. They have been evaluated for amebiasis, echinococcosis, trichinosis, and Chagas' disease. Although their usefulness is somewhat limited by the larger quantities of concentrated antigen and the potent or concentrated antisera required, they permit identification of specific and nonspecific components, thus increasing accuracy of the tests. Techniques vary greatly. Described here are basic general methods which should be standardized in each laboratory for each disease.

Special equipment and reagents.

Agar gels: agarose, Difco purified agar, Ionagar, or Noble agar.

Glass slides (5 × 7.5 cm and 2.5 × 7.5 cm) coated with a thin film of dried agar or agarose.

Patterns and cutters. Slides can be cut with small "cork-borer" cutters. Mechanical IE cutters are recommended for IE slides.

Moist chambers and incubators 37 and 25 C.

Power supply and IE apparatus.

Staining solutions.

Veronal buffer solution.

Antigens: Saline or Veronal buffer extracts of parasites; concentrated hydatid fluid. Soluble antigens prepared for other serological tests can often be used after concentration 3- to 10-fold. Crude antigens must produce multiple bands with diagnostic sera and, in the case of hydatid antigen, must include the diagnostic band 5 (23). They can be stored frozen or lyophilized and are usually very stable.

Antisera: Lyophilized or frozen positive and negative control sera of known reactivity which must also show any specific diagnostic bands. Diagnostic sera can be inactivated at 56 C for 30 min.

Preparation of media.

For DD test:

Purified agar (Difco)	10.0 g
NaCl	5.0 g
Glycine	7.5 g
Merthiolate	0.1 g
Distilled water	1,000 ml

1. Dissolve all reagents except the agar in half the water.

2. Adjust the pH to 7.2 to 7.4 with small amounts of 0.1 M NaOH.

3. Dissolve the agar in the remaining water by carefully boiling over direct heat or in a boiling-water bath. (Freely flowing steam in an autoclave can be used to dissolve the agar, but not steam under pressure.)

4. Mix the two solutions, making sure the agar is completely dissolved; if necessary, heat again to make a uniform solution.

5. Dispense in 50- to 100-ml amounts in capped containers. Can be stored in the cold for several weeks without deterioration.

6. For use, melt a container of agar in a boiling-water bath and use the whole amount. Repeated heating can alter gel formation.

For IE and CEP tests

Agarose	9 g
or Special agar-Noble	20 g
Distilled water	500 ml
Veronal buffer, ionic strength 0.075, pH 8.5 ...	500 ml

1. Dissolve agarose or agar in the water with heat.

2. Add Veronal buffer and heat to boiling to insure complete solution.

3. Prepare plates immediately or store as directed for the DD agar medium above.

Stock Veronal buffer, pH 8.5, ionic strength 0.075

Dissolve 5.53 g of barbital in approximately 500 ml of distilled water and 30.90 g of sodium barbital in a second 500 ml of distilled water. Mix and bring up to 2 liters in a volumetric flask. Add 0.4 g of Merthiolate crystals. Dilute with equal parts distilled water for use in the IE bath.

Preparation of other reagents.

Buffered saline (PBS, pH 7.5) for dissolving the nonprecipitated proteins from the agar slides: Mix 200 ml of Sorensen's 0.067 M phosphate buffer, pH 7.5, with 3,800 ml of 0.89% NaCl solution.
Staining solutions:
  0.3% thiazine red R in 1% acetic acid or 0.1% amidoblack in 1% acetic acid.
  1% acetic acid.
  1% acetic acid and 1% glycerol.
  0.4% aqueous solution of bromophenol blue indicator. Dilute to light purple with Veronal buffer for use.

Preparation of slides.

1. Clean 5 × 7.5 cm or 2.5 × 7.5 cm glass slides and coat with a thin layer of agar or agarose by swabbing the entire area with hot, melted 0.1% agar which has been prepared by diluting small amounts of the agar medium with distilled water.
2. Dry in the air or with low heat. Store in dust-free boxes for not less than 16 h before use. They can be stored indefinitely.
3. Place slides, coated side up, on a level surface, and, with a pipette, transfer to each measured amounts of the desired hot, melted agar or agarose: 3 or 4 ml for 2.5 × 7.5 cm slides and 8 ml for 5 × 7.5 cm slides. Cover the whole area of the slide.
4. Allow to solidify at room temperature and store in moist chambers in a refrigerator. Slides should "set" overnight before use to insure maximal gelling. The thickness of the agar can be varied by using different amounts of medium. Slides prepared carefully will be very smooth, uniform, and level.

Cutting slides

1. For DD, it is practical to cut wells in a hexagon about a central well (Fig. 2A). Diameters of the wells and distances between wells must be uniform so that tests can be replicated. Recommended proportions: diameter of well, 8 mm, and space, 10 mm; diameter, 5 mm, and space, 6 mm; diameter, 3 mm, and space, 4 mm.

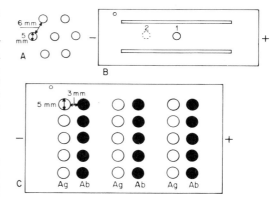

FIG. 2. *Patterns for cutting double diffusion slides.*

2. For IE, cut the antigen well near the center of the Noble agar slide (Fig. 2B-1) and nearer the cathode of the agarose (Fig. 2B-2). Cut a small well for the indicator (bromophenol blue solution).
3. For CEP, cut parallel rows of wells as shown in Fig. 2C. Diameters of wells are 5 mm and the wells are 3 mm apart.

Aspirate the plugs of gel from the wells, but leave the gel in the antiserum slot cut in the IE slide until after electrophoresis. Seal the bottom edge of the wells with a minute drop of hot agar or agarose. Store in moist containers at 4 C or use immediately.

Performance of the DD test.

1. Fill the central well to the top with appropriate dilution of antigen.
2. Fill the six outside wells with unknown sera. Whenever possible, one well should contain a known positive serum. If the supply of reagents permits, run all unknown sera twice. When the sequence of the sera is changed, some weak reactions may be enhanced by being next to a strongly reacting antiserum.
3. Incubate in a moist chamber at 25 C for 3 days or at 37 C for 24 h.
4. Record lines as they appear.
5. Gently flush out remaining reactants from wells with distilled water. Cover the slide with wet filter paper, making certain the wells are filled with fluid. Air-dry overnight.
6. Remove filter paper and soak out excess reactants from the gel in PBS, pH 7.5, for at least 4 h or overnight.
7. To stain: 10 min, distilled water; 10 min, distilled water; 15 min, thiazine red R stain; 10 min, 1% acetic acid; 10 min, 1% acetic acid; 10 min, 1% acetic acid plus 1% glycerol.
8. Air-dry slides and store for reference.

TABLE 5. *Types of antigens recommended for parasitic serology*

Test[a]	Disease	I. Extracts of parasites	II. Partially purified	III. Special
CF	Trichinosis	Saline-larvae	MASF-larvae	
	Echinococcosis			Hydatid cyst fluid
	Schistosomiasis	Saline-adult and saline-cercariae	MASF-adults and delipidized adults (C)[b]	
	Cysticerosis		Delipidized adults and cysticerci	
	Chagas' disease	Maekelt extract-epimastigotes (91)		Exo-antigen (T)[b]
	Toxoplasmosis	Water-*T. gondii*		
	Amebiasis	Saline axenic culture trophozoites (35)		
BF	Trichinosis	Saline-larvae	MASF-larvae	Metabolic products of larvae
	Echinococcosis			Hydatid cyst fluid
	Schistosomiasis		Delipidized cercariae (A)[b]	
	Ascariasis/toxocariasis		Adults	
	Filariasis	Saline-adults *D. immitis*		
	Amebiasis	Saline-axenic culture trophozoites		
Latex	Trichinosis	Saline-larvae, saline-boiled larvae	MASF-larvae	
	Echinococcosis			Concentrated hydatid cyst fluid
CL	Schistosomiasis		Delipidized cercariae (A)[b]	
IHA	Trichinosis		MASF-larvae	
	Echinococcosis			Hydatid cyst fluid
	Ascariasis/toxocariasis		MASF-adults	Fraction of perientric fluid (106)
	Filariasis	Saline-adults *D. immitis*		
	Toxoplasmosis	*T. gondii* from peritoneal exudates		
	Amebiasis	Saline-axenic culture trophozoites		
	Malaria	Saline-*P. knowlesi* in monkey blood sediment		
	Cysticerosis		Delipidized adults and cysticerci	
IF	Trichinosis			Cuticles of larvae
	Schistosomiasis			Whole cercariae
	Toxoplasmosis			Whole organisms
	Malaria			Thick blood smears containing trophozoites and schizonts
	Pneumocytoses			*Pneumocystis carinii* cysts

TABLE 5—*Continued*

Test[a]	Disease	I. Extracts of parasites	II. Partially purified	III. Special
Precipi-tin DD, IE, CEP	Trichinosis	Saline-larval con-centrated 3 to 10×	MASF-larvae con-centrated 5 to 10×	Metabolic concen-trated 3 to 10×
	Echinococcosis			Concentrated hyda-tid fluid (23, 138)
	Amebiasis	Saline-axenic cul-ture trophozoites concentrated 3×		

[a] CF, complement fixation; BF, bentonite flocculation; CL, cholesterol-lecithin; IHA, indirect hemagglu-tination; IF, indirect immunofluorescence; DD, double diffusion; IE, immunoelectrophoresis; CEP, counter-current electrophoresis.

[b] MASF = Melcher's acid-soluble fraction (94); A = Anderson type antigen (6); C = Chaffee type antigen (25); T = Tarrant et al. type antigen (153).

Performance of the IE test.

1. Fill the IE bath with Veronal buffer, ionic strength 0.0375, pH 8.5, to the level recom-mended by the manufacturer.

2. Load the tray with cut agarose or Noble agar slides, and place filter-paper wicks in posi-tion.

3. Carefully fill the antigen well. Place a drop of bromophenol blue solution in the indica-tor well.

4. Turn on the power supply and adjust the current passing through the length of the slide to give a potential difference of about 3 V per cm of agar.

5. When the indicator has reached the previ-ously determined distance (about 3.5 cm) neces-sary for good separation—usually after 1 to 1.5 h—shut off the machine and remove the slides.

6. Remove the agar from the trough and seal the bottom edges with a small amount of hot agar or agarose.

7. Fill the trough with antiserum. Incubate at room temperature in a moist chamber for 3 days, and proceed as in steps 4 through 8 of DD test above.

Performance of the CEP test.

Prepare IE bath and load slides as in steps 1 and 2 for the IE test. Fill wells on the cathodic side (labeled Ag in Fig. 2C) with antigen. Fill anodic wells (Ab in Fig. 2C) with serum sam-ples previously concentrated threefold by ly-ophilization. Turn on the power supply and allow current to pass through the slide until the bromophenol blue indicator has moved the de-sired distance. The optimal separation of reac-tants depends on the type of matrix, concentra-tion of buffers in the matrix and bath, and the size of wells, as well as the type of IE apparatus employed. The machine should be initially standardized with some antigen/antibody sys-tem, and the voltage necessary to produce good bands in 30 to 90 min without overheating the agar should be determined. Most of the para-sitic CEP tests are run 45 min. Remove the slides and examine for bands immediately. Wash out excess reactants and incubate the slides for 1 to 3 h at room temperature. Reex-amine for bands. Dry and stain the slides as in steps 5 through 8 for the DD test.

PARASITIC ANTIGENS FOR SEROLOGICAL TESTS

Most parasitic antigens are complex mix-tures of specific and nonspecific components which have been prepared for use in a single test. Some can be used only in that particular test; others are more adaptable. In Table 5 we have listed the antigens which can be used in the tests described in this chapter. Individual references can be consulted for descriptions of their preparation or you may consult our direc-tions given in the first edition of the *Manual of Clinical Microbiology* (66). Since some idea of the limitations of handling a reagent are desir-able, the general characteristics of the "crude" and the "partially purified" and "special" anti-gens will be given.

In general, the crude extracts are all wet or lyophilized parasites ground in buffered saline. Sonic treatment to rupture the organisms has been limited to the protozoa. The extracting solutions were selected primarily because they were the preferred diluents used in the tests. The pH varied from 6.8 to 8.3 (optimally, 7.4 to 7.6). The period of extraction varied from 3 h to overnight. Longer periods have resulted occa-sionally in less specific antigens. Most prepara-tions were made in the cold because some anti-genic components are labile (schistosomes).

TABLE 6. *Partial list of companies producing commercial parasitic antigens*

Company	Disease	Trade name	Type of reagent[a]
Italdiagnostic, Rome, Italy	Echinococcosis	Agglutinotest	Latex kit
	Toxoplasmosis	Agglutinotest	Latex kit
	Toxoplasmosis		CF antigen
ICN Chemical & Radioisotope Division, Irvine, Calif.	Toxoplasmosis	Para-Tek immunodiagnostics	IF kit
Hyland Laboratories, Los Angeles, Calif.	Amebiasis	Amebogen	Countercurrent electrophoresis kit
	Chagas' disease		Countercurrent electrophoresis kit
	Trichinosis		Latex kit
Behringwerke, Marburg, Germany	Chagas' disease		Latex, CF, IHA kits
	Schistosomiasis		ID antigen
	Echinococcosis		ID antigen
	Toxoplasmosis		CF, latex kits
Wellcome Reagents, Ltd., Beckenham, Kent, England	Amebiasis		IF antigen
	Chagas' disease		IF antigen
	Echinococcosis		IF antigen
	Leishmaniasis		IF antigen
	Schistosomiasis		IF antigen
	Toxoplasmosis		IF antigen
	Trichinosis		IF antigen
	African trypanosomiasis (3 antigens)		IF antigen
Cooke Laboratory Products, Alexandria, Va.	Toxoplasmosis		IF kit
Ames Co., Elkhart, Ind.	Amebiasis	Seramoeba	Latex kit
Electro-Nucleonics Laboratories, Inc., Bethesda, Md.	Toxoplasmosis	Virgo reagents	IF kit
Canalco, Inc., Rockville, Md.	Toxoplasmosis		IHA, microhemagglutination kit
Difco Laboratories, Detroit, Mich.	Trichinosis		Bentonite flocculation test
ICL Scientific, Fountain Valley, Calif.	Trichinosis	Rythrotex reagents	Slide agglutination test
Cordis, Miami, Fla.	Amebiasis		Countercurrent electrophoresis kit
National Veterinary Assay Laboratory, Tokyo, Japan	Toxoplasmosis		IHA sensitized cells

[a] CF, complement fixation; IF, indirect immunofluorescence; IHA, indirect hemagglutination; ID, intradermal; IF, indirect immunofluorescence.

However, some (trichina) can be boiled. Some extracts lose reactivity if lyophilized (toxoplasma, ascaris). All can be stored at -20 C. However, refreezing is not recommended, especially for amoeba and schistosome antigens.

Among those antigens classified as "partially purified" the Melcher's (94) acid-soluble fraction (MASF) is the most stable and can be used in a variety of tests. The method of preparation is harsh, and the resulting MASF can usually be handled with a minimum of care. Some MASF – such as trichina – can be lyophilized, but ascaris and toxocara cannot; generally, however, MASF antigens can be frozen and thawed more than once. MASF is not a "purified" antigen. It still contains all or almost all of the elements demonstrated in the crude extract: the quantities of some, however, including the lipids, are drastically reduced. Delipidization with anhydrous ether, i.e., the Chaffee (25) and Anderson (6) methods, is a much gentler treatment, and usually labile elements are apparently unaffected. The resulting lots of antigen are very uniform. However, most of the antigens should be stored in small amounts and not refrozen. Hydatid cyst fluid and perenteric fluid from ascarids are very rich mixtures and, although they are apparently stable when protected with other elements in the fluid, they may be unstable when purified by fractionation. Hydatid fluid can be dialyzed and lyophilized, but with considerable loss of antigenicity. It is advisable to treat all parasitic antigens as potentially labile.

The number of commercial antigens (Table 6) is increasing, but many parasitic antigens still must be prepared in the laboratory.

LITERATURE CITED

1. Allain, D. S., E. S. Chisholm, and I. G. Kagan. 1972. Use of the bentonite flocculation test for the diagnosis of schistosomiasis. Health Serv. Rep. 87:550–559.

2. Allain, D. S., and I. G. Kagan. 1975. A direct agglutination test for leishmaniasis. Am. J. Trop. Med. Hyg. 24:232–236.

3. Ambroise-Thomas, P., and T. K. Truong. 1970. L'immuno-fluorescence dans le diagnostic serologique et le contrôle post-operataive de l'hydatidose humaine. I. Matériel et methods. Cah. Med. Lyon. 46:2955–2962.

4. Ambroise-Thomas, P., and T. K. Truong. 1972. Fluorescent antibody test in amebiasis. Am. J. Trop. Med. Hyg. 21:907–912.

5. Ambroise-Thomas, P., and T. K. Truong. 1972. Application of the indirect fluorescent antibody test on sections of adult filariae to the serodiagnosis, epidemiology and post therapeutic surveillance of human filariasis. WHO/FIL/72.101, World Health Organization, Geneva.

6. Anderson, R. I. 1960. Serodiagnosis of *Schistosoma mansoni* infections. I. Development of a cercarial antigen slide flocculation test. Am. J. Trop. Med. Hyg. 9:299–303.

7. Anderson, R. I., E. H. Sadun, and M. J. Schoenbechler. 1963. Cholesterol-lecithin slide (TsSF) and charcoal card (TsCC) flocculation tests using an acid soluble fraction of *Trichinella spiralis* larvae. J. Parasitol. 49:642–647.

8. Ball, P. A. J., and A. Bartlett. 1969. Serological reactions to infection with *Necator americanus*. Trans. R. Soc. Trop. Med. Hyg. 63:362–369.

9. Beltran, F., and A. Gomez-Priego. 1973. Evaluacíon de los contrainmunoelectroforesis (CIEF) para la deteccíon de anticuerpos en la cisticercosis experimental y humana. Antioquia Med. 23:472–473.

10. Bénex, J., J. Guilhon, and R. Barnabé. 1973. Étude comparative de diverses méthodes de diagnostic immunologique de la *Faciolose Hépato-biliaire* expérimentale du mouton et influence du traitement sur la persistance des anticorps. Bull. Soc. Pathol. Exot. 66:116–128.

11. Berggren, W. L., and T. H. Weller. 1967. Immunoelectrophoretic demonstration of specific circulating antigen in animals infected with *Schistosoma mansoni*. Am. J. Trop. Med. Hyg. 16:606–612.

12. Biagi, F., F. Navarrete, A. Pina, A. M. Santiago, and L. Tapia. 1961. Estudio de tres reacciones serologicas en el diagnostico de la cisticercosis. Rev. Med. Hosp. Gen. Mexico City 24:501–508.

13. Bloch-Michel, H., and P. Waltzing. 1973. Le phénomène des rosettes appliqué aux filarioses. Étude chez 56 patients. Nouv. Presse Med. 6:382.

14. Bloomfield, N., and G. W. Snook. 1962. Use of slide latex test for detecting trichinosis in hogs. Cornell Vet. 52:569–581.

15. Boonpucknavig, S., and R. C. Nairn. 1967. Serological diagnosis of amoebiasis by immunofluorescence. J. Clin. Pathol. 20:875–878.

16. Botros, B. A. M., R. W. Moch, and I. S. Barsoum. 1973. Echinococcosis in Egypt: evaluation of the indirect hemagglutination and latex agglutination tests for echinococcal serologic surveys. J. Trop. Med. Hyg. 76:243–247.

17. Boyden, S. V. 1951. The adsorption of proteins on erythrocytes treated with tannic acid and subsequent hemagglutination by anti-protein sera. J. Exp. Med. 93:107–120.

18. Bozicevich, J., J. E. Tobie, E. H. Thomas, M. H. Hoyem, and S. B. Ward. 1951. A rapid flocculation test for the diagnosis of trichinosis. Public Health Rep. 66:806–814.

19. Buck, A. A., and R. I. Anderson. 1972. Validation of the complement fixation and slide flocculation tests for schistosomiasis. Geographic variations of test capacities. Am. J. Epidemiol. 96:205–214.

20. Capron, A., M. Gentilini, and A. Vernes. 1968. Le diagnostic immunologique des filarioses. Possibilités nouvelles offertes par l'immuno-électrophorèse. Pathol. Biol. 16:1039–1045.

21. Capron, A., A. Vernes, G. Niel, and M. Bouvry. 1972. Le diagnostic immunonologique de l'amibiase. Med. Chir. Diag. 1:5–13.

22. Capron, A., A. Vernes, M. Tsuji, and D. Afchain. 1969. Human and experimental para-

gonimiasis: antigenic structure and host parasite relationship for species of the genus Paragonimus. Ann. Parasitol. Hum. Comp. 44:709–732.

23. Capron, A., L. A. Yarzabal, A. Vernes, and J. Fruit. 1970. Le diagnostic immunologique de l'echinococcose humaine. Pathol.-Biol. 18:357–365.

24. Cerisola, J. A. 1970. Immunodiagnosis of Chagas' disease: haemagglutination and immunofluorescence tests. J. Parasitol. 56(Sect. II):409–410.

25. Chaffe, E. F., P. M. Bauman, and J. J. Shapilo. 1954. Diagnosis of schistosomiasis by complement fixation. Am. J. Trop. Med. Hyg. 3:905–913.

26. Chordi, A., K. W. Walls, and I. G. Kagan. 1964. Studies on the specificity of the indirect hemagglutination test for toxoplasmosis. J. Immunol. 93:1024–1033.

27. Collins, W. E., G. M. Jeffery, E. Guinn, and J. C. Skinner. 1966. Fluorescent antibody studies in human malaria. IV. Cross reactions between human and simian malaria. Am. J. Trop. Med. 15:11–15.

28. Colwell, E. J., J. R. Ortaldo, M. J. Schoenbechler, J. F. Barbaro, and E. H. Fife, Jr. 1971. Trichinella spiralis and Schistosoma mansoni specificity of in vitro, leucocyte-mediated histamine release from rabbit platelets. Exp. Parasitol. 29:263–270.

29. Crowle, A. J. 1973. Immunodiffusion. Academic Press Inc., New York.

30. Cuadrado, R. R., and I. G. Kagan. 1967. The prevalence of antibodies to parasitic diseases with sera of young army recruits from the United States and Brazil. Am. J. Epidemiol. 86:330–340.

31. de Blasi, R., and L. Magaudda-Borzi. 1958. Revista sintetiche erctiche la sierologia dell' amebiasi. Riv. Parassitol. 19:267–296.

32. Desowitz, R. G., J. J. Saave, and B. Stein. 1966. Application of the indirect hemagglutination test in recent studies on the immunoepidemiology of human malaria and the immune response in experimental malaria. Mil. Med. 131(Suppl.):1157–1166.

33. Despommier, D., and M. Müller. 1970. Functional antigens of Trichinella spiralis. J. Parasitol. 56(Sect. II, Part 1):76.

34. Despommier, D., M. Müller, B. Jenks, and M. Fruitstone. 1974. Immunodiagnosis of human trichinosis using counterelectrophoresis and agar gel diffusion techniques. Am. J. Trop. Med. Hyg. 23:41–45.

35. Diamond, L. S. 1968. Techniques of axenic cultivation of Entamoeba histolytica Schaudinn, 1903 and E. histolytica-like amebae. J. Parasitol. 54:1047–1056.

36. El-Nahal, H. M. S. 1967. Fluorescent antibody studies in the preerythrocytic schizonts of Plasmodium berghei yoelli and Plasmodium cynomolgi (larger strain). Trans. R. Soc. Trop. Med. Hyg. 61:8–9.

37. Farshy, D. C., and I. G. Kagan. 1972. Use of stable sensitized cells in an improved indirect microhemagglutination test for malaria. Infect. Immun. 7:680–682.

38. Fife, E. H., Jr., and L. H. Muschel. 1959. Fluorescent antibody technic for serodiagnosis of Trypanosoma cruzi infection. Proc. Soc. Exp. Biol. Med. 101:540–543.

39. Fiorillo, A. M., J. C. Costa, and J. Passos. 1973. Identification of hemagglutinating antibodies in chronic schistosomiasis. Rev. Inst. Med. Trop. (Sao Paulo) 15:371–376.

40. Fischman, A. 1960. Flocculation tests in hydatid disease. J. Clin. Pathol. 13:72–75.

41. Fischman, A. 1960. A rapid latex test for hydatid disease. N.Z. Med. J. 59:485–487.

42. Fraga de Azevedo, J., and P. C. Rombert. 1965. L'application de l'immunofluorescence au diagnostic de la fasciolase hépatique. Ann. Parasitol. Hum. Comp. 40:529–542.

43. Fulton, J. D. 1962. Diagnosis of protozoal diseases, p. 86–114. In P. P. H. Gell and R. P. A. Coombs (ed.), Clinical aspects of immunology. F. A. Davis Co., Philadelphia.

44. Fulton, J. D. 1963. Serological tests in toxoplasmosis, p. 259–272. In P. C. C. Garnham, A. E. Pierce, and I. Roitt (ed.), Immunity to protozoa. F. A. Davis Co., Philadelphia.

45. Gancarz, Z. 1968. Immunobiological methods in the diagnosis of human and animal trichinosis. Exp. Med. Microbiol. 20:219–225.

46. Gankavi, B. L. 1971. Ring precipitation reactions in trichinellosis in pigs. Veterariya (Moscow) 48:69–70.

47. Goldsmith, R. A., I. G. Kagan, M. A. Reyes-Gonzáles, and J-Cedeño Femeira. 1972. Seroepidemiologic studies in Oaxaca, Mexico. Search for parasitic antibody using the indirect hemagglutination test. Bol. Of. Sanit. Panam. (Engl. Ed.) 6:39–52.

48. Healy, G. R. 1968. The use of and limitations to the indirect hemagglutination test in the diagnosis of intestinal amebiasis. Health Lab. Sci. 5:174–179.

49. Healy, G. R., I. G. Kagan, and N. N. Gleason. 1970. Use of the indirect hemagglutination test in some studies of seroepidemiology of amebiasis in the western hemisphere. Health Lab. Sci. 7:109–116.

50. Hübner, J., and M. Uhlíková. 1973. Use of the microprecipitation method in agar gel (MPA) in the diagnosis of toxoplasmosis. III. Correlation of MPA, complement-fixation reaction (CFT) and Sabin-Feldman dye test (SFT) in serodiagnosis of human toxoplasmosis. J. Hyg. Epidemiol. Microbiol. Immunol. 17:70–84.

51. Jacobs, L. 1967. Toxoplasma and toxoplasmosis. Adv. Parasitol. 5:1–45.

52. Jacobs, L., and M. N. Lunde. 1957. A hemagglutination test for toxoplasmosis. J. Parasitol. 43:308–314.

53. Jeanes, A. L. 1966. Indirect fluorescent antibody test in diagnosis of hepatic amoebiasis.

Br. Med. J. 5501:1464.

54. Jung, R. C., and G. Pacheco. 1960. Use of a hemagglutination test in visceral larva migrans. Am. J. Trop. Med. Hyg. 9:185–191.

55. Kagan, I. G. 1960. Trichinosis: a review of biologic, serologic, and immunologic aspects. J. Infect. Dis. 107:65–93.

56. Kagan, I. G. 1963. A review of immunologic methods for the diagnosis of filariasis. J. Parasitol. 49:773–798.

57. Kagan, I. G. 1963. Seminar on immunity to parasitic helminths. VI. Hydatid disease. Exp. Parasitol. 13:57–71.

58. Kagan, I. G. 1965. Evaluation of routine serologic testing for parasitic diseases. Am. J. Public Health 55:1820–1829.

59. Kagan, I. G. 1968. Serologic diagnosis of visceral larva migrans. Clin. Pediatr. (Philadelphia) 7:508–509.

60. Kagan, I. G. 1968. A review of serologic tests for the diagnosis of hydatid disease. Bull. WHO 39:25–37.

61. Kagan, I. G. 1970. Immunodiagnostico de la enfermedad hidatica humana con limitada referencia a la immunidad en el perro y oveja. Arch. Int. Hid. 24:47–56.

62. Kagan, I. G. 1973. Diagnóstico immunológico de la enfermedad hidática. Torax 23:232–236.

63. Kagan, I. G. 1974. Advances in the immunodiagnosis of parasitic infections. Z. Parasitenkd. 45:163–195.

64. Kagan, I. G., H. A. Fox, K. W. Walls, and G. R. Healy. 1967. The parasitic diseases of childhood with emphasis on the newer diagnostic methods. Clin. Pediatr. (Philadelphia) 6:641–654.

65. Kagan, I. G., and L. Norman. 1969. The serology of trichinosis, p. 222–268. In S. E. Gould (ed.), Trichinosis in man and animals. Charles C Thomas, Publisher, Springfield, Ill.

66. Kagan, I. G., and L. Norman. 1970. Serodiagnosis of parasitic diseases, p. 453–486. In J. E. Blair, E. H. Lennette, and J. P. Truant (ed.), Manual of clinical microbiology, 1st ed. American Society for Microbiology, Bethesda, Md.

67. Kagan, I. G., L. Norman, and D. S. Allain. 1963. An evaluation of the bentonite flocculation and indirect hemagglutination tests for the diagnosis of filariasis. Am. J. Trop. Med. Hyg. 12:548–555.

68. Kagan, I. G., L. Norman, D. S. Allain, and C. G. Goodchild. 1960. Studies on echinococcosis: nonspecific serologic reactions of hydatid-fluid antigen with serum of patients ill with diseases other than echinococcosis. J. Immunol. 84:635–640.

69. Kagan, I. G., J. J. Osimani, J. C. Varela, and D. S. Allain. 1966. Evaluation of intradermal and serologic tests for the diagnosis of hydatid disease. Am. J. Trop. Med. Hyg. 15:172–179.

70. Kagan, I. G., and J. Pellegrino. 1961. A critical review of immunological methods for the diagnosis of bilharziasis. Bull. WHO 25:611–674.

71. Kagan, I. G., and K. D. Quist. 1970. An evaluation of five serologic tests for the diagnosis of trichinosis in lightly infected swine, p. 271–277. In S. K. Singh and B. K. Tandan (ed.), H. D. Srivastava Commemoration Volume. India Veterinary Research Institute Iznatnagan, U.P., India.

72. Kagan, I. G., D. W. Rairigh, and R. L. Kaiser. 1962. A clinical, parasitologic, and immunologic study of schistosomiasis in 103 Puerto Rican males residing in the United States. Ann. Intern. Med. 56:457–470.

73. Kessel, J. F., W. P. Lewis, C. M. Pasquel, and J. A. Turner. 1965. Indirect hemagglutination and complement fixation tests in amebiasis. Am. J. Trop. Med. Hyg. 14:540–550.

74. Knierim, F., G. Eskuche, L. Sandoval, and E. Muñoz. 1971. Reacción de aglutinación con látex para el diagnóstico serológico de enfermedad de Chagas. Bol. Chil. Parasitol. 26:32–35.

75. Kohler, G., and E. J. Ruitenberg. 1974. Evaluation of three diagnostic methods for trichinellosis. Results of a joint EEC project. Bull. WHO 50:413–419.

76. Kojima, S., M. Yokogawa, and T. Tada. 1974. Production and properties of reaginic antibodies in rabbits infected with *Clonorchis senensis* or *Schistosoma japonicum*. Exp. Parasitol. 35:141–149.

77. Komiya, Y. 1966. *Clonorchis* and clonorchiasis. Adv. Parasitol. 4:53–106.

78. Kozar, M., Z. Kozar, and K. Karmanska. 1964. The comparative evaluation of some agglutination tests in the diagnosis of trichinellosis. Wiad. Parazytol. 10:717–737.

79. Kuvin, S. F., J. E. Tobie, C. B. Evans, G. R. Coatney, and P. G. Contacos. 1962. Fluorescent antibody studies on the course of antibody production and serum gamma globulin levels in normal volunteers infected with human and simian malaria. Am. J. Trop. Med. Hyg. 11:429–436.

80. Labzoffsky, N. A., R. K. Baratawidjaja, E. Kuitunen, F. N. Lewis, D. A. Kavelman, and L. P. Morrissey. 1964. Immunofluorescence as an aid in the early diagnosis of trichinosis. Can. Med. Assoc. J. 90:920–921.

81. Lass, N., Z. Laver, and J. Lengy. 1973. The immunodiagnosis of hydatid disease: postoperative evaluation of the skin test and four serological tests. Ann. Allergy 31:430–436.

82. Latif, B. M. A., and K. M. G. Adam. 1973. Differentiation of *Trypanosoma brucei*, *T. rhodesiense* and *T. gambiense* by the indirect fluorescent antibody test. Bull. WHO 48:401–407.

83. Lim, S. K., W. C. Eveland, and R. J. Porter. 1974. Direct fluorescent-antibody method for the diagnosis of *Pneumocystis carinii* pneumonia from sputa or tracheal aspirations

from humans. Appl. Microbiol. 27:144-149.

84. Lobel, H. O., H. M. Mathews, and I. G. Kagan. 1973. Interpretation of IHA titers for study of malaria epidemiology. Bull. WHO 49:485-492.

85. Lucasse, C. 1970. Fluorescent antibody tests applied to serum of patients with gambian sleeping sickness. Trop. Geogr. Med. 22:227-236.

86. Lumsden, W. H. R. 1967. The demonstration of antibodies to protozoa, p. 877-937. In D. M. Weir (ed.), Handbook of experimental immunology, F. A. Davis Co., Philadelphia.

87. Lumsden, W. H. R. 1970. Biological aspects of trypanosomiasis research, 1965; a retrospect, 1969. Adv. Parasitol. 8:227-249.

88. McQuay, R. M. 1967. Parasitologic studies in a group of furloughed missionaries. II. Helminth findings. Am. J. Trop. Med. Hyg. 16:161-166.

89. Maddison, S. E. 1965. Characterization of Entamoeba histolytica antigen-antibody reaction by gel diffusion. Exp. Parasitol. 16:224-235.

90. Maddison, S. E., S. J. Powell, and R. Elsdon-Dew. 1965. Application of serology to the epidemiology of amebiasis. Am. J. Trop. Med. Hyg. 14:554-557.

91. Maekelt, G. A. 1960. Die komplementbindungsreaktion der Chagaskrankheit. Z. Tropenmed. Parasitol. 11:152-186.

92. Mahoney, D. F., B. C. Redington, and M. J. Schoenbechler. 1966. Preparation and serologic activity of plasmodial fractions. Mil. Med. 131(Suppl.):1141-1151.

93. Mauss, E. A. 1940. The in vitro effect of immune serum upon Trichinella spiralis larvae. Am. J. Hyg., Sect. D 32:80-83.

94. Melcher, L. R. 1943. An antigenic analysis of Trichinella spiralis. J. Infect. Dis. 73:31-39.

95. Meuwissen, J. H. E. T., and A. D. E. M. Leeuwenberg. 1972. Indirect haemagglutination test for malaria with lyophilized cells. Trans. R. Soc. Trop. Med. Hyg. 66:666-667.

96. Milgram, E. A., G. R. Healy, and I. G. Kagan. 1966. Studies on the use of the indirect hemagglutination test in the diagnosis of amebiasis. Gastroenterology 50:645-649.

97. Monroe, L. S., E. R. Korn, and S. J. Fitzwilliam. 1972. A comparative study of the latex agglutination and gel diffusion precipitin test in the diagnosis of amebic liver abscess. Am. J. Gastroenterol. 58:52-57.

98. Muraschi, T. F., N. Bloomfield, and R. B. Newman. 1962. A slide latex-particle agglutination test for trichinosis. Am. J. Clin. Pathol. 37:227-231.

99. Nagamoto, T. 1959. Studies on Clonorchis sinensis. II. Immunological studies on clonorchiasis. J. Kurume Med. Assoc. 22:1416-1417.

100. Nash, T. E., B. Prescott, and F. A. Neva. 1974. The characteristics of a circulating antigen in schistosomiasis. J. Immunol. 112:1500-1507.

101. Neal, R. A. and R. A. Miles. 1970. Indirect hemagglutination test for Chagas' disease, with a simple method for survey work. Rev. Inst. Med. Trop. (Sao Paulo) 12:325-332.

102. Niel, G., M. Gentilini, J. Couture, J. M. Pinon, and M. Davis. 1972. Use of antigenic extracts of Ascaris suum for the diagnosis of filariasis by means of double diffusion. Value compared with Onchocera volvulus and Dipetalonema vitae antigens. Bull. Soc. Pathol. Exot. 65:569-580.

103. Norman, L., and I. G. Kagan. 1963. Bentonite, latex, and cholesterol flocculation tests for the diagnosis of trichinosis. Public Health Rep. 78:227-232.

104. Norman, L., and I. G. Kagan. 1973. Some observations on the serology of Pneumocystis carinii infections in the United States. Infect. Immun. 8:317-321.

105. Norman, L., E. H. Sadun, and D. S. Allain. 1959. A bentonite flocculation test for the diagnosis of hydatid disease in man and animals. Am. J. Trop. Med. Hyg. 8:46-50.

106. Oliver-Gonzáles, J., P. Hurlbrink, E. Conde, and I. G. Kagan. 1969. Serologic activity of antigen isolated from the body fluid of Ascaris suum. J. Immunol. 103:15-19.

107. Pacheco, G., D. E. Wykoff, and R. C. Jung. 1960. Trial of an indirect hemagglutination test for the diagnosis of infections with Clonorchis sinensis. Am. J. Trop. Med. Hyg. 9:367-370.

108. Pellegrino, J., and N. Katz. 1971. Comparison of the latex slide agglutination and complement fixation tests for the diagnosis of Chagas' disease. J. Parasitol. 57:771.

109. Petithory, S., L. Brumpt, and M. Bahno. 1973. Études des possibilité diagnostiques serologiques de l'onchocercose par double diffusion aves des antigénes hétérologues. Ann. Parasitol. Hum. Comp. 48:343-350.

110. Pinon, J. M., and M. Gentilini. 1972. Intéret de l'utilisation du teepol dans les réactions d'immunofluorescence indirecte en vue de l'élimination des réactions croisées dans le diagnostic des filarioses. Bull. Soc. Pathol. Exot. 65:306-308.

111. Platzer, E. G. 1970. Trematodes of the liver and lung, p. 1000-1009. In G. J. Jackson et al. (ed.), Immunity to parasitic animals, vol. 2. Appleton-Century-Crofts, Englewood Cliffs, N.J.

112. Plonka, W. S., Z. Gancarz, and B. Zawadzka-Jedrzejewska. 1972. A rapid screening haemagglutination test in the diagnosis of human trichinosis. J. Immunol. Methods 1:309-312.

113. Proctor, E. M., and R. Elsdon-Dew. 1966. Serological tests in porcine cysticercosis. S. Afr. J. Sci. 62:264-267.

114. Proctor, E. M., S. J. Powell, and R. Elsdon-Dew. 1966. The serological diagnosis of cysticercosis. Ann. Trop. Med. Parasitol. 60:146-151.

115. Reis, A. P., N. Katz, and J. Pellegrino. 1970. Immunodiffusion tests in patients with Schistosoma mansoni infections. Rev. Inst.

Med. Trop (Sao Paulo) 12:245–248.

116. Rogers, W. A., Jr., J. A. Fried, and I. G. Kagan. 1968. A modified indirect microhemagglutination test for malaria. Am. J. Trop. Med. Hyg. 17:804–809.

117. Rombert, P. C. 1971. A reaccão de imunofluorescência (RIF) sobre cortes por congelacão no diagnóstico da ancilostomiase. An. Esc. Nac. Saude Publica Med. Trop. (Lisbon) 5:291–295.

118. Rombert, P. C., and J. M. Palmeiro. 1973. Estudo da triquinosé experimental do rato pela técnica de imunofluorèscencia, em cortes de congelacão. Medico 66:88–97.

119. Rombert, P. C., and R. A. Vieira. 1971. Conbribiucão para o estudo da imunidade na ancilostomiase. 1. Estududos serológicos na infeccáo experimental dó cáo. An Esc. Nac. Saude Publica Med. Trop. 5:61–81.

120. Rombert, P. C., R. Viera, and J. Fraga de Azevedo. 1967. O diagnóstico da ancilostomíase pela reaccão do latex. Medico 803:3–32.

121. Sabin, A. B., and H. A. Feldman. 1948. Dyes as microchemical indicators of a new immunity phenomenon affecting a protozoon parasite (Toxoplasma). Science 108:660–663.

122. Sadun, E. H. 1963. Seminar on immunity to parasitic helminths. VII. Fluorescent antibody technique for helminth infections. Exp. Parasitol. 13:72–82.

123. Sadun, E. H., R. I. Anderson, and J. S. Williams. 1962. Fluorescent antibody test for the serological diagnosis of trichinosis. Exp. Parasitol. 12:424–433.

124. Sadun, E. H., L. Norman, and D. S. Allain. 1957. The detection of antibodies to infections with the nematode Toxocara canis, a causative agent of visceral larva migrans. Am. J. Trop. Med. Hyg. 6:562–568.

125. Sadun, E. H., B. C. Walton, A. A. Buck, and B. K. Lee. 1959. The use of purified antigens in the diagnosis of Clonorchiasis sinensis by means of intradermal and complement fixation tests. J. Parasitol. 45:129–134.

126. Sadun, E. H., J. S. Williams, and R. I. Anderson. 1960. A fluorescent antibody technique for the serodiagnosis of schistosomiasis in humans. Proc. Soc. Exp. Biol. Med. 105:289–291.

127. Sawada, T., Y. Nagata, and K. Takei. 1964. Studies on the substance responsible for the skin tests on clonorchiasis. Jpn. J. Exp. Med. 36:315–322.

128. Sawada, T., K. Takei, S. Sato, and G. Matsuyama. 1968. Studies on the immunodiagnosis of paragonimiasis. III. Intradermal skin tests with fractionated antigens. J. Infect. Dis. 118:235–239.

129. Sawada, T., K. Takei, J. E. Williams, and J. W. Moose. 1965. Isolation and purification of antigen from adult Clonorchis sinensis for complement fixation and precipitin tests. Exp. Parasitol. 17:340–349.

130. Schiller, E. L. 1967. Progress and problems in the immunodiagnosis of helminthic infections. Adv. Clin. Chem. 9:43–68.

131. Scholtens, R. G., I. G. Kagan, K. D. Quist, and L. Norman. 1966. An evaluation of tests for the diagnosis of trichinosis in swine and associated quantitative epidemiologic observations. Am. J. Epidemiol. 83:489–500.

132. Seah, S., and P. D. Marsden. 1970. Complement fixation test in Trypanosoma rhodesiense infection with cultured Trypanosoma cruzi as antigen. Trans. R. Soc. Trop. Med. Hyg. 64:279–283.

133. Shimada, K., and G. R. O'Connor. 1973. An immune adherence hemagglutination test for toxoplasmosis. Arch. Ophthalmol. 90:372–375.

134. Singer, J. M., and C. M. Plotz. 1958. Slide latex fixation test. J. Am. Med. Assoc. 168:180–181.

135. Soltys, M. A., and P. T. K. Woo. 1972. Immunological methods in diagnosis of protozoan diseases in man and domestic animals. Z. Tropenmed. Parasitenkd. 23:172–187.

136. Sood, P., O. Prakash, and R. A. Bhujwala. 1972. A trial of hemagglutination, circumoval precipitin and gel diffusion tests in hookworm infection. Indian J. Med. Res. 60:1132–1133.

137. Soprunova, N. J., F. F. Soprunov, and A. A. Lur'e. 1973. Nachweis von Helminthen-metaboliten im Darm des Wirtes als ein neuer diagnostischer Test für Helminthiasen. Angew. Parasitol. 14:11–17.

138. Sorice, F., and L. Castagnari. 1970. Impiego della immuno-precipitazione elettroforetica nella diagnosi immunologica dell'idatidose. G. Mal. Infect. Parassit. 23:1–8.

139. Soulsby, E. J. L. 1962. Antigen-antibody reactions in helminth infections. Adv. Immunol. 2:265–308.

140. Soulsby, E. J. L. 1967. The demonstration of antibodies to helminths, p. 938–966. In D. M. Weir (ed.), Handbook of experimental immunology. F. A. Davis Co., Philadelphia.

141. Stein, B., and R. S. Desowitz. 1964. The measurement of antibody in human malaria by a formalized sheep cell hemagglutination test. Bull. WHO 30:45–49.

142. Stephanski, W., and A. Malczewski. 1972. Specificity of migration inhibition test in parasitic invasion. II. Studies on Trichinella spiralis. Bull. Acad. Pol. Sci. Ser. Sci. Biol. 201:26–28.

143. Stork, M. G., G. S. Venables, S. M. F. Jennings, J. R. Beesley, P. Bendez, and A. Capron. 1973. An investigation of endemic fascioliasis in Perusian village children. J. Trop. Med. Hyg. 76:231–235.

144. Sulzer, A. J., and E. S. Chisholm. 1966. Comparison of the IFA and other tests for Trichinella spiralis antibodies. Public Health Rep. 81:729–734.

145. Sulzer, A. J., and E. C. Hall. 1967. Indirect fluorescent antibody tests for parasitic diseases. IV. Statistical study of variation in

the indirect fluorescent antibody (IFA) test for toxoplasmosis. Am. J. Epidemiol. 86:401–407.

146. Sulzer, A. J., and I. G. Kagan. 1967. Indirect fluorescent antibody tests for parasitic diseases. III. Conjugate-antigen relationships in the tests for trichinosis and schistosomiasis. Am. J. Med. Technol. 33:1–8.

147. Sulzer, A. J., and M. Wilson. 1967. The use of thick-smear antigen slides in the malaria indirect fluorescent antibody test. J. Parasitol. 53:1110–1111.

148. Sulzer, A. J., and M. Wilson. 1971. The fluorescent antibody test for malaria. Crit. Rev. Clin. Lab. Sci. 2:601–619.

149. Sulzer, A. J., M. Wilson, and E. C. Hall. 1969. Indirect fluorescent antibody tests for parasitic diseases. V. An evaluation of a thick-smear antigen in the IFA test for malaria antibodies. Am. J. Trop. Med. Hyg. 18:199–205.

150. Sun, T., and J. B. Gibson. 1969. Antigens of Clonorchis sinensis in experimental and human infections. Am. J. Trop. Med. Hyg. 18:241–252.

151. Szyfres, B., and I. G. Kagan. 1963. A modified slide latex screening test for hydatid disease. J. Parasitol. 49:69–72.

152. Tanaka, H., D. T. Dennis, B. H. Kean, H. Matsuda, and M. Sasa. 1972. Evaluation of a modified complement fixation test for schistosomiasis. Jpn. J. Exp. Med. 42:537–542.

153. Tarrant, C. J., E. H. Fife, Jr., and R. I. Anderson. 1965. Serological characteristics and general chemical nature of the in vitro exoantigens of Trypanosoma cruzi. J. Parasitol. 51:277–285.

154. Ten Eyck, D. R. 1973. Comparison of biopsy and fluorescent antibody staining techniques in the detection and study of onchocerciasis in an Ethiopian population. Am. J. Epidemiol. 98:283–288.

155. Ten Eyck, D. R. 1973. Onchocerca volvulus and Wuchereria bancrofti: fluorescent antibody staining of frozen homologous sections for diagnosis. Exp. Parasitol. 34:154–161.

156. Tobie, J. E., D. C. Abele, G. J. Hill, P. G. Contacos, and C. B. Evans. 1966. Fluorescent antibody studies on the immune response in sporozoite-induced and blood induced vivax malaria and the relationship of antibody production to parasitemia. Am. J. Trop. Med. Hyg. 15:676–683.

157. Varela-Diaz, V. M., and E. A. Coltorti. 1974. Tecnicas para el diagnostico immunologico de la hidatidosis humana. Centro Panamericana Ser. Monogr. 7.

158. Vattuone, N. H., and J. F. Yanovsky. 1971. Trypanosoma cruzi: agglutination activity of enzyme-treated epimastigotes. Exp. Parasitol. 30:349–355.

159. Vieira, R. A., and P. C. Rombert. 1968. Estudos sobre ancilostomideos. 1. Morfologia das larvas filariformes. 2. Taxa de desenvolur-

mento larvae. 3. Immunofluorescencia aplicado ao diagnostica da ancilostomiase. An. Esc. Nac. Saude Publica Med. Trop. (Lisbon) 2:129–161.

160. Vieira, R. A., and P. C. Rombert. 1974. Contribuição para o estudo da immunidade na ancilostomiase 2. Tentativa de imunização do cão pela inoculação de larvas de Ancylostoma caninum atenuadas pelas radiacões ultravioletas. J. Soc. Ciên. Med. Lisbon 138:99–146.

161. Vieira, R. A., and P. C. Rombert. 1974. Contribuição para o estudo da imunidade na ancilostomiase. 3. Nova casvística sobre a imunização do cão com larvas de Ancylostoma caninum atenvadus pelos R.U.V. An. Inst. Hyg. Med. Trop. 2:485–499.

162. Vogel, H., and W. Minning. 1949. Hüllenbildung bei Bilharziacercarien im Serum Bilharzia-infizierter Tiere und Menschen. Zentralbl. Bakteriol. Parasitenk. Infektionskr. Abt. I. Orig. 153:91–105.

163. Voller, A. 1962. Fluorescent antibody studies on malaria parasites. Bull. WHO 27:283–287.

164. Voller, A. 1971. The detection and measurement of malaria antibodies. Trans. R. Soc. Trop. Med. Hyg. 65:111–124.

165. Walls, K. W., I. G. Kagan, and A. Turner. 1967. Studies on the prevalence of antibodies to Toxoplasma gondii. 1. U. S. military recruits. Am. J. Epidemiol. 85:87–92.

166. Walton, B. C., and I. Chyu. 1959. Clonorchiasis and paragonimiasis in the Republic of Korea. Bull. WHO 21:721–726.

167. Walton, B. C., W. H. Brooks, and I. Arjona. 1972. Serodiagnosis of American leishmaniasis by indirect fluorescent antibody test. Am. J. Trop. Med. Hyg. 21:296–299.

168. Wegesa, P., A. J. Sulzer, and A. Van Orden. 1971. A slide antigen in the indirect fluorescent antibody test for Trichinella spiralis. Immunology 21:805–808.

169. Williams, J. S., E. H. Sadun, and R. W. Gore. 1971. A radioactive antigen microprecipitin (RAMP) assay for schistosomiasis. J. Parasitol. 57:220–232.

170. Williams, J. S., R. W. Gore, and E. H. Sadun. 1972. Trichinella spiralis: antigen-antibody interaction assayed by radioactive iodinated antigen. Exp. Parasitol. 31:299–306.

171. Witebsky, F., P. Wels, and A. Heide. 1942. Serodiagnosis of trichinosis by means of complement fixation. N. Y. J. Med. 42:431–435.

172. Wilson, M., A. J. Sulzer, and K. W. Walls. 1974. Modified antigens in the indirect immunofluorescence test for schistosomiasis. Am. J. Trop. Med. Hyg. 23:1072–1076.

173. Wolfson, R. L., S. E. Maddison, and I. G. Kagan. 1972. Migration inhibition of peripheral leucocytes in human schistosomiasis. J. Immunol. 109:123–128.

174. World Health Organization. 1965. Immunology and parasitic diseases. WHO Tech. Rep. Ser. no. 315, p. 64.

175. Wykoff, D. E. 1959. Studies on Clonorchis si-

nensis. II. Development of an antigen for complement fixation and studies on the antibody response in infected rabbits. Exp. Parasitol. 8:51–57.

176. Yogore, M. G., R. M. Lewert, and E. D. Madraso. 1965. Immunodiffusion studies on paragonimiasis. Am. J. Trop. Med. Hyg. 14:586–591.

177. Yokogawa, M. 1966. Paragonimus and paragonimiasis. Adv. Parasitol. 3:99–158.

178. Yokogawa, M. 1969. Paragonimus and paragonimiasis. Adv. Parasitol. 7:375–387.

179. Yuthsastr-Kosol, V., G. Manning, and C. Diggs. 1973. *Fasciolopsis buski*: serum complement-fixing activity in human infection. Exp. Parasitol. 33:100–104.

Section E

VIRAL, RICKETTSIAL, AND CHLAMYDIAL IMMUNOLOGY

Chapter 52

Introduction

PHILIP K. RUSSELL

Immunological tests to evaluate the immune response to viruses, rickettsiae, and chlamydiae are done in clinical laboratories for a variety of purposes. Establishing or confirming an etiological diagnosis of disease is the commonest reason for employing immunological tests in clinical situations; however, immunological testing is also done to evaluate protective immunity, either naturally acquired or vaccine induced, to test for immunological responsiveness of an individual, or to provide information relative to immunopathological processes. The selection of the appropriate test depends on the nature of the information required, the stage of the infectious process, and the nature of the immunological response to the infectious agent in question, as well as technical considerations relating to test systems, such as precision, accuracy, specificity, and the rapidity with which tests can be performed. Cost is often a major consideration for selection of a clinical laboratory test.

Establishing or confirming the etiology of an infectious process due to viruses, rickettsiae, and chlamydiae by immunological tests relies at present almost entirely on serological methods which measure antibody activity against one or more of the antigenic components of the organism in question. Although serological diagnosis is the most commonly used clinical laboratory tool for diagnosis of viral, rickettsial, and chlamydial infection, it must be kept in mind that it is an indirect method and at present cannot supplant viral isolation or direct demonstration of viral antigen in host tissues or secretions for conclusive proof of infection in many instances. Immunological methods have major limitations, most of which relate to the specificity of the reactions. In the case of enteroviruses, because of the large number of serotypes and the high degree of specificity of available tests, serological diagnosis is usually not recommended until an agent has been isolated. The reverse is true for influenza viruses; serological diagnosis can be quite useful since the number of serotypes is limited. Strain-specific diagnosis of influenza does, however, require virus isolation. Chronic viral infections, such

as cutaneous herpes simplex, cytomegalovirus, and hepatitis B, cannot be diagnosed by immunological methods alone; virus isolation or demonstration of viral antigens is essential. The diverse manifestations of viral, rickettsial, and chlamydial infections often require that immunological tests be employed in conjunction with other laboratory methods and evaluated in the context of supporting clinical and epidemiological data.

Immunological tests vary widely in the number and complexity of the antigenic components involved. Complement-fixation (CF) tests which utilize unpurified or partially purified antigens derived from infected cell cultures, mouse brain, embryonated eggs, or similar substrates often contain mixtures of antigens. Viral antigen preparations may contain nonstructural antigens, as well as internal and external components of virions. Use of such antigens may be entirely appropriate for confirming clinical diagnosis if interpreted with knowledge of the limited specificity. It must be kept in mind that antibody activity against nonstructural or internal antigens may be entirely unrelated to protective immunity, although providing reliable evidence for the occurrence of an infection when significant increases in titer are found. Hemagglutination-inhibition (HI) tests measure antibody activity against only viral surface antigens. The hemagglutinin is a capsid or envelope protein or glycoprotein depending on the type of virus, and HI tests measure either antibody specific for the hemagglutinin or antibody directed at other antigens closely associated with the hemagglutinin on the surface of the hemagglutinating particle. In the latter case, steric interference causes inhibition of the HI reaction which causes a positive test; an example is the low-level HI activity of influenza antineuraminidase antibody. The specificity of HI tests depends in large part on the extent of antigenic relatedness of hemagglutinins among viruses of the same group. The HI test for rubella is specific for the rubella virus, since no antigenically related agents are known to exist, whereas cross-reactions among related viruses limit the specificity of myxovirus, paramyxovirus, and togavirus HI tests. Neutralization tests which measure biological activity of antibody against one or more viral surface antigens tend to be more specific than either HI or CF tests and are more closely related to protective immunity, although it is not always the case. Virus neutralization is a complex phenomenon which may proceed through several possible mechanisms depending on the nature of the virus, the type of immunoglobulin (Ig) involved, and whether complement contributes to the in vitro reaction. Some neutralization reactions involve minimal amounts of specific antibody binding to critical surface antigens, which results in nonreversible destruction of infectivity of the virions. In other instances, antibody against one or more surface antigens may inhibit the attachment of virus to susceptible cells by steric effect without irreversibly destroying infectivity of the virion. Complement may enhance the neutralizing activity of some antibody classes either by acting on the lipid envelope of the enveloped viruses or by adding to the steric effect. Since type- or strain-specific antigens are usually external capsid or envelope antigens, neutralization tests have a higher degree of specificity than tests which include reactions with internal viral antigens, such as the nucleocapsid antigen of influenza.

Recent developments in molecular virology and improved biochemical and biophysical techniques have allowed the development of tests for specific viral antigens. A variety of assays utilizing radioimmune precipitation, solid-phase radioimmunoassay, and indirect hemagglutination methods have been devised which allow precise quantitation of antibody to individual nonstructural and subviral antigenic components. The specificity of such tests depends on chemical or physical isolation and purification of the individual antigens. Clinical use of such tests is presently restricted largely to hepatitis B, where a high level of sensitivity is required and conventional tests are inadequate. In diseases where conventional CF, HI, and indirect fluorescent-antibody tests are adequate for diagnostic purposes, radioimmunoassay procedures at present are important tools in research on the immunological response and pathogenesis of viral infections. Increasing use of specific tests for antibody to nonstructural and component antigens may be expected in the future as the utility of the tests becomes better defined and improved methods for antigen preparation are developed.

The following chapters in this section describe tests for antibody to viruses and do not address viral isolation and identification procedures which have been well described in the *Manual of Clinical Microbiology*. There are diseases, however, in which viral isolation has not been done or is not feasible in a clinical laboratory, but detection of viral antigen in blood or stool is possible. These diseases include hepatitis A and B and acute gastroenteritis caused by several parvoviruses (including the Norwalk agent) and reovirus-like agents (also referred to as orbivirus-like agents, duoviruses, or rotaviruses). Hepatitis B antigen can be detected by a variety of immunological methods, including counterimmunoelectrophoresis and radioimmunoassay. Immune electron microscopy (IEM) has been the primary method used to detect hepatitis A virus and the viruses which cause acute nonbacterial gastroenteritis in feces. The IEM technique is described in chapter 67.

Ig-specific tests which measure the antiviral antibody activity of a specific class of antibody have some very useful clinical applications. Detection of IgM antibody in the newborn can be indicative of an intrauterine infection with rubella virus or cytomegalovirus. In some, but not all, virus infections, the presence of IgM antibody reflects a recent infection. Caution is needed in interpretation of tests, since the persistence of IgM antibody is highly variable, and in a small percentage of patients IgM antibody persists for long periods after measles, rubella, and some togavirus infections. Indirect immunofluorescence tests using conjugated class-specific anti-Ig is an efficient method for determining class-specific antibody activity. Separation of Igs by velocity centrifugation and testing of fractions by HI tests is useful for rubella and togaviruses.

There is a rapidly increasing body of evidence which indicates that cell-mediated immunological mechanisms play a major role in the human response to viral and rickettsial infections. The interaction of stimulated lymphocytes and/or macrophages with the infecting agents, their antigens, and with infected cells, are clearly important factors in determining the progression and resolution of infectious processes. Cell-mediated immunological processes acting alone or in conjunction with antibody are recognized as contributors to both protective immunity and pathogenetic processes. The relative importance of cellular versus antibody-mediated mechanisms has not yet been well defined for most viral diseases. Humoral factors are the major, perhaps the most important, mechanisms of protective immunity in many acute viral infections, including respiratory and enteric infections where both local and circulating antibody have a protective action. Cell-mediated mechanisms appear to be of importance in resolution of infection in the previously nonimmune host and in chronic infections. At present, in vitro laboratory tests for cell-mediated immunity to viruses, rickettsiae, and chlamydiae remain mainly research tools. There are potential applications for such tests in clinical medicine, for example, to evaluate specific immunocompetence in patients who are immunologically compromised as a result of disease or therapy. However, recommendations for performing such tests in nonresearch clinical laboratories must await further advancement in technology and understanding of the role of cell-mediated immunity in these diseases.

The usefulness of serological data for diagnosis is highly dependent on the nature of the specimens submitted. For most acute viral, rickettsial, and chlamydial infections, reliable results require demonstration of a rise in antibody titer between acute and convalescent sera. The importance of obtaining a serum specimen early in the course of an illness before an antibody rise occurs plus an appropriately timed convalescent serum cannot be overemphasized.

It is also frequently important that sufficient clinical information be provided to enable laboratory personnel to select the most appropriate tests. Optimal utilization of the diagnostic laboratory requires effective communication with the clinicians who require the test results.

The safety of personnel working in diagnostic laboratories is always a major consideration when infectious agents are used. Many of the CF and HI antigens described in the following chapters contain viable infectious agents which constitute a known hazard; in addition, serum and other specimens from patients are a potential hazard. Antigen preparation and performance of neutralization tests entail the handling of infectious agents. Antigen production may be especially hazardous because of manipulation of large amounts of infected substrates and the potential for generating infectious aerosols. Laboratory personnel should be immunized against those agents for which vaccines are available and thoroughly trained in safe techniques for handling infectious agents. Infectious agents should be restricted to appropriately designed laboratories with the equipment to protect personnel and prevent environmental contamination.

Chapter 53

Herpes Simplex Virus

JOHN A. STEWART AND KENNETH L. HERRMANN

INTRODUCTION

The clinical course of herpes simplex virus (HSV) infection in humans is extremely variable. Primary infection with type 1 (HSV-1) or type 2 (HSV-2) is subclinical or unrecognized a large part of the time. Primary infection, when clinically apparent, may range from minimal stomatitis to severe generalized disease ending fatally. The major clinical conditions associated with HSV infections are gingivostomatitis, keratitis and conjunctivitis, vesicular eruptions of the skin, aseptic meningitis, encephalitis, genital tract infections, neonatal herpes, and generalized primary infection.

Latent infection is established in most seropositive individuals and is associated with recurrent fever blisters in 10 to 15% of the seropositive group. Genital eruptions may recur commonly, but the exact frequency has not been as accurately determined. Primary herpes infection can only be documented by serological methods since individuals having their first clinically apparent infection may have preexisting antibody detected in the early acute serum in response to an earlier unrecognized infection.

Since a majority of individuals in most population groups (15) have been infected by age 20, evidence of serum antibody against HSV by any serological test, except immunoglobulin M (IgM) specific antibody, provides no information as to the time of infection. Diagnosis of current infection depends upon the demonstration of a significant increase in antibody titer. A serum collected as close as possible to the onset of illness and a convalescent serum collected 10 days to 3 weeks later should be tested simultaneously.

Primary infection with either HSV type is easily documented by testing paired sera in any of the common serological tests. Either HSV type may be used as antigen in a given test because of the strong antigenic cross-reaction between the types. However, HSV-1 is recommended when only one antigen is used because it has somewhat broader reactivity.

The immune response to recurrent infection or reinfection is much more complicated and depends upon the HSV type of the initial and of the recurrent infection, the number of previous infections, and the severity of the subsequent infection. After primary infection in children, antibody levels may fall to low or undetectable levels and then be boosted by later clinical or subclinical infections (3). Dascomb et al. (4) showed a significant complement-fixation (CF) or neutralization antibody rise in 5 of 14 adults with recurrent HSV infections. Three of the five patients with antibody rise had systemic symptoms as well. Rises have also been seen with encephalitis in patients with a history of previous herpetic fever blisters. Thus, severe recurrence, whether associated with cutaneous or neurological symptoms, may result in antibody rise. However, most adults after multiple recurrences have moderately high stable titers by CF and neutralization tests that do not fluctuate with subsequent infection (5). The initial infection with HSV-2 is likely to give a significant antibody rise to both herpes group and HSV-2 specific antigens.

The tests which have the widest application for serodiagnosis and serosurveys are CF, indirect immunofluorescence (IIF), neutralization, indirect hemagglutination (IHA), and IHA-inhibition tests.

The CF test is most useful for those laboratories which normally perform this test with multiple antigens for serodiagnosis of other viral diseases. The exact titration required of its multiple components precludes its occasional use for the serodiagnosis of HSV alone. CF detects antibody directed to the intact virion and the soluble antigens produced by infected cells (7). The immune response in humans includes antibody to each of the structural components of the virus, the envelope, capsid, and internal proteins, as well as nonvirion antigens specified by the cell. Nonsedimentable antigen may represent 50% of the total CF antigen (13). In addition, immunization studies with these low-molecular-weight proteins (90,000 and 170,000) must have included some of the envelope glycoproteins since neutralizing antibody was produced. Primary infection is easily detected by crude antigens extracted from infected cell cultures. CF antibodies are stable

416

and long lasting in the adult and are able to give a reliable estimate of the total incidence of HSV infection in serosurveys. However, since HSV-1 and HSV-2 antigens share external, internal, and soluble antigens (7), the CF test using standard crude antigen does not lend itself to epidemiological studies of type-specific infection. Directions for performing the CF test are presented in chapter 58 of this *Manual*. Description of HSV CF reagents and their preparation are given elsewhere (14).

IIF tests with either unfixed or fixed HSV-infected cells will show strong binding of antibody as measured by fluorescein-conjugated anti-human globulin of animal origin. The major advantage of the IIF test is that it can be used to determine the Ig class (IgM, IgA, IgG) of HSV antibody with the use of the appropriate anti-human globulin. Since sera with rheumatoid factor may give a false-positive IgM reaction, they should be absorbed with aggregated IgG and retested for specific IgM. The major disadvantage of the IIF test in survey work is that only a limited number of sera can be processed each day. Measurement of type-specific antibody by the membrane IIF test (8) requires cross-absorption with large quantities of infected cells and is not practical for routine testing.

The delineation of specific type 1 and type 2 antibodies is quite difficult because of the strong cross-reaction between the two viruses. The various tests that have been used to identify specific antibody will be briefly described.

The microneutralization test as developed by Pauls and Dowdle when applied to antibody studies (9) separates sera into three groups, type 1, type 2, and intermediate. Although some sera in the intermediate group have been shown to have specific antibody to both serotypes by inhibition of IHA, this conclusion cannot be made for all intermediate sera. With two other neutralization procedures (11), the plaque-reduction test and kinetic neutralization test, it is also difficult to establish a clear-cut difference between the presence and absence of type 2 antibody. When sera from patients with either recurrent oral lesions or recurrent genital herpes were compared, some overlap in the II/I index was found (1, 11). The neutralization tests are in general more sensitive than CF and also show a better differentiation of HSV-1 and HSV-2 antibody. The major disadvantages of the neutralization tests are their greater complexity, the longer time required to complete the procedures, and the failure to completely differentiate HSV-2 antibody in human sera.

The IHA test for HSV is based on the ability of HSV antibody to agglutinate tanned sheep erythrocytes sensitized with HSV antigens. It is a sensitive and specific procedure for the detection of antibody, and titers are usually 4- to 16-fold higher than by CF. HSV IgM can easily be detected by IHA if the serum is first separated into IgM and IgG fractions. The strong cross-reaction between herpes types 1 and 2 found in other serological procedures is also present in the IHA test. Most patient and animal hyperimmune sera have IHA titers that are either identical or at most twofold higher to one virus type. Thus, the inhibition step is necessary to determine type-specific antibody. However, early convalescent sera from many patients with recent HSV-2 infections and some patients with recent HSV-1 infections (1) have a significant (fourfold greater) response to the homologous antigen. The major advantages of the IHA test are that it can be completed in 1 day and can detect both recently produced antibody in primary infections and stable antibody in latent or chronic infections.

The IHA-inhibition test for type-specific antibody to HSV-1 and HSV-2 is based on the ability of homologous antigen to inhibit completely at least 8 units of antibody while heterologous antigen gives only partial inhibition. The major disadvantages of the IHA-inhibition test are that IHA antigens must largely be produced locally and that relatively few laboratories are experienced with the test. The major advantages of the IHA-inhibition test are that it is relatively simple, requires only standard equipment, can be performed with either fresh or glutaraldehyde-stabilized erythrocytes, yields results much sooner than any of the various neutralization tests, and gives definitive results in typing not only monotype-specific human sera but also human sera containing both HSV-1 and HSV-2 antibodies. Detailed descriptions of the IHA-inhibition test are given by Back and Schmidt (1), Schneweis and Nahmias (12), and Bernstein and Stewart (2).

CLINICAL INDICATIONS

A presumptive clinical diagnosis of infection with HSV can frequently be made in the light of the clinical manifestations. The serological results obtained from testing the convalescent serum collected 10 to 14 days after onset offer little guidance in the clinical management of most patients. When immediate diagnosis is imperative, other procedures such as microscopy for multinucleated giant cells, immunofluorescence for viral antigen, and virus culture should be performed. However, in some patients with encephalitis, and other unusual manifestations, initial diagnostic procedures may provide inconclusive results, and serological procedures could indicate recent infection with herpes. In cases where the specific etiology of viral encephalitis remains undiagnosed, cerebrospinal fluid (6) should be tested for herpes antibody in parallel with serum. Two other groups of patients should be tested for herpes antibody: infants with undiagnosed congenital infection (10) and immunosuppressed patients with prolonged fever of unknown etiology. Procedures to determine type-specific antibody to HSV have their main application in epidemiological studies and are of limited usefulness in the diagnosis of current infection.

INDIRECT HEMAGGLUTINATION-INHIBITION TEST

The IHA part of the IHA-inhibition test is performed essentially as described for cytomegalovirus in chapter 59, with the use of antigens prepared from stable laboratory strains of HSV-1 and HSV-2. The most critical factors in the IHA test are the pH and molarity of buffers, the selection of the optional tannic acid dilution for each batch of sheep erythrocytes, and the use of reasonably potent herpesvirus antigens. Once familiarity is gained with fresh erythrocytes, one can then easily master the use of glutaraldehyde-fixed cells (10). Glutaraldehyde-fixed cells have the advantage that large volumes of sensitized cells can be prepared at one time and are stable for 6 to 12 months at −60 C.

Evaluation of inhibiting antigens

Since inhibition is the key to this test, the inhibiting antigens are checked for their ability to inhibit completely 8 units of IHA antibody with known homologous HSV-1 or HSV-2. To facilitate inhibition, at least an eightfold lower concentration of antigen should be used in sensitization than is used for inhibition, even if this means that the sensitizing antigen is used at slightly less than its optimal dilution. If 8 units of antibody is not completely inhibited under these conditions, the amount of antigen coating the cells must be decreased. To achieve this, the tannic acid concentration is reduced in twofold steps until the desired inhibition occurs.

Serum treatment and antibody titration

Sera to be tested are diluted 1:8 in 1% normal rabbit serum diluent (NRSD), inactivated at 56 C for 30 min, and adsorbed with sheep erythrocytes. Serial twofold dilutions from 1:8 through 1:4,096 in 0.05-ml volumes of NRSD

are then prepared in duplicate flexible polyvinyl chloride microtitration U plates. To each serum dilution on the first plate, 0.025 ml of HSV-1 sensitized cells is added; to each serum dilution on the duplicate plate, 0.025 ml of HSV-2 sensitized cells is added. The plates are sealed with clear tape, placed on a mechanical vibrator for 1 min, and then incubated at room temperature for 2 to 3 h to allow cells to settle.

The IHA titer of the serum to each antigen is judged to be the highest dilution of the serum which causes agglutination of a thin layer of cells over 80% or more of the bottom of the well. At this end-point dilution, the serum contains 1 unit of IHA antibody in 0.05 ml. In the inhibition test an initial dilution of serum is selected that contains 16 units of antibody; this is calculated by dividing the end-point dilution by 16. Since the initial serum dilution is further diluted with an equal volume of control or inhibiting antigen in the first well of the test, the actual starting serum dilution in the test is 8 units of antibody. For example, let us assume that the IHA titer is 512; 512 ÷ 16 = 32 = initial serum dilution which contains 16 units of antibody in 0.05 ml (or 8 units of antibody in 0.05 ml after being mixed with a similar volume of antigen solution in the first well).

Test procedure

Duplicate microtitration U plates are prepared, one for HSV-1 and one for HSV-2 antigen sensitized cells. A 0.05-ml volume containing 16 units of antibody of a known HSV-1 serum is added to the first well of rows 1, 2, and 3 of the duplicate plates. A known HSV-2 serum similarly is added to the first well of rows 4, 5, and 6 of both plates. Unknown serum 1 is added to the first well of rows 7 to 9 of both plates, and unknown serum 2 is added to the first well of rows 10 to 12. Then 0.05-ml volumes of the appropriate initial dilution of any additional unknown sera are added in the same way to other sets of duplicate plates. Now 0.05 ml of the proper dilution of HSV-1 inhibiting antigen is added to the first well of rows 1, 4, 7, and 10 of all plates. HSV-2 inhibiting antigen is added to the first well of rows 2, 5, 8, and 11 of all plates, and the same dilution of uninfected control antigen is added to the first well of rows 3, 6, 9, and 12 of all plates. Gently mix the serum-antigen mixture with a mechanical vibrator and incubate at room temperature for 30 min. After incubation, 0.05 ml of NRSD is added to all test wells except the first of each row, and six serial twofold dilutions of each serum are made by use of 0.05-ml microdiluters. To each serum dilution in one set of plates 0.025 ml of

HSV-1 sensitized cells is added, and to corresponding dilutions in the other set of plates 0.025 ml of HSV-2 sensitized cells is added. The plates are sealed, shaken for 1 min on a mechanical vibrator, and incubated at room temperature for 2 to 3 h or until patterns form. Table 1 shows the patterns of inhibition given by sera containing HSV-1, HSV-2, or both types of antibody. A layer of agglutinated cells covering 80% or more of the bottom of the well is read as lack of inhibition; partial or no agglutination is read as inhibition.

REAGENTS

Indirect hemagglutination and inhibiting antigens

The antigens produced for IHA are used interchangeably as inhibiting antigens. Well-characterized laboratory strains of HSV known to be antigenically stable such as MacIntyre VR_3 (HSV-1) and MS (HSV-2) should be used for antigen production. Antigen is prepared from infected human diploid fibroblasts, HEp-2 cell cultures, or Vero cell cultures showing advanced cytopathic effect in 80% or more of the cells for 12 to 24 h before harvest. The cell monolayers are rinsed once with phosphate-buffered saline (PBS), pH 7.2. Additional PBS is then added to the culture (25 ml/2-liter roller bottle) and frozen as evenly as possible over the cell sheet by rotating the bottle in an alcohol-dry ice bath. The PBS-cell layer can be kept frozen at -60 C for up to 2 weeks before harvest. The fluid overlay obtained after thawing the culture at room temperature is used as IHA antigen. Since HSV cultures typically contain dislodged cells, the antigen is clarified by centrifugation at $500 \times g$ prior to storage in small portions at -60 C without preservative. The antigen titer remains stable for at least 8 to 12 months after preparation. CF antigens from commercial sources (Flow Laboratories, Inc., or Microbiological Associates, Inc.) can also be used in the IHA test. However, CF antigens usually will have a different optimal tannic acid dilution and pH of sensitization than will an IHA antigen prepared as above.

Control antisera

Human antisera should be obtained from patients with recurrent fever blisters and genital herpes infection and evaluated for type-specific antibody. Once characterized, known type 1 and type 2 sera can be used as controls in each test.

INTERPRETATION

Antisera to type 1 and type 2 HSV produce a characteristic inhibition pattern when tested against both types of HSV sensitized cells. In addition, antisera containing both antibody types are distinguished easily. A few sera when tested in the standard inhibition test with 8 units of antibody have been completely inhibited by both HSV-1 and HSV-2 (2). Such "untypable" sera contain primarily IHA antibody activity against the common HSV group antigens and relatively little activity against the type-specific antigens. The serum must then be tested at a greater concentration, 32 to 64 units of antibody, absorbed with enough antigen to remove group-specific antibody, and then tested for residual type-specific antibody.

LITERATURE CITED

1. Back, A. F., and N. J. Schmidt. 1974. Typing *Herpesvirus hominis* antibodies and isolates by inhibition of the indirect hemagglutination reaction. Appl. Microbiol. 28:400–405.
2. Bernstein, M. T., and J. A. Stewart. 1971. Method for typing antisera to *Herpesvirus hominis* by indirect hemagglutination inhibition. Appl. Microbiol. 21:680–684.
3. Buddingh, G. J., D. I. Schrum, J. C. Lanier, and D. J. Guidry. 1953. Studies of the natural history of herpes simplex infections. Pediatrics 11:595–610.
4. Dascomb, H. E., C. V. Adair, and N. Rogers. 1955. Serologic investigations of herpes simplex virus infections. J. Lab. Clin. Med. 46:1–11.
5. Douglas, R. G., Jr., and R. B. Couch. 1970. A prospective study of chronic herpes simplex virus infection and recurrent herpes labialis in humans. J. Immunol. 104:289–295.
6. MacCallum, F. O., I. J. Chinn, and J. V. T. Gostling. 1974. Antibodies to herpes-simplex virus in the cerebrospinal fluid of patients with herpetic encephalitis. J. Med. Microbiol. 7:325–331.
7. Martin, M. L., E. L. Palmer, and R. E. Kissling. 1972. Complement-fixing antigens of herpes

TABLE 1. *Typing of herpes antisera by IHA-inhibition*

IHA results with HSV-1 sensitized cells after absorption of serum with			IHA results with HSV-2 sensitized cells after absorption of serum with			HSV antibody type
HSV-1	HSV-2	Control antigen	HSV-1	HSV-2	Control antigen	
0^a	+	+	0	0	+	1
0	0	+	+	0	+	2
0	+	+	+	0	+	1 and 2
0	0	+	0	0	+	"Untypable"

^{a} Symbols: + = agglutination; 0 = inhibition.

simplex virus types 1 and 2: reactivity of capsid, envelope, and soluble antigens. Infect. Immun. **5**:248-254.

8. Nahmias, A. J., I. Del Buono, K. E. Schneweis, D. S., Gordon, and D. Thies. 1971. Type-specific surface antigens of cells infected with herpes simplex virus (1 and 2). Proc. Soc. Exp. Biol. Med. **138**:21-27.

9. Nahmias, A. J., W. E. Josey, Z. M. Naib, C. F. Luce, and A. Duffey. 1970. Antibodies to *Herpesvirus hominis* types 1 and 2 in humans. I. Patients with genital herpetic infections. Am. J. Epidemiol. **91**:539-546.

10. Palmer, D. F., J. J. Cavallaro, K. L. Herrmann, J. A. Stewart, and K. W. Walls (ed.). 1974. A procedural guide to the serodiagnosis of toxoplasmosis, rubella, cytomegalic inclusion disease, herpes simplex. Immunology Series No. 5, p. 39-41, 46-56, and 89-94. Center for Disease Control, Atlanta, Ga.

11. Plummer, G. 1973. A review of the identification and titration of antibodies to herpes simplex viruses type 1 and 2 in human sera. Cancer Res. **33**:1469-1476.

12. Schneweis, K. E., and A. J. Nahmias. 1971. Antigens of herpes simplex virus type 1 and 2—immunodiffusion and inhibition passive hemagglutination studies. Z. Immunitaetsforsch. Allerg. Klin. Immunol. **141**:471-487.

13. Tokumaru, T. 1965. Studies of herpes simplex virus by the gel diffusion technique. II. The characterization of viral and soluble precipitating antigens. J. Immunol. **95**:189-195.

14. Tokumaru, T. 1969. Herpesviruses, *Herpesvirus hominis, Herpesvirus simiae, Herpesvirus suis,* p. 641-676. *In* E. H. Lennette and N. J. Schmidt (ed.), Diagnostic procedures for viral and rickettsial infection, 4th ed. American Public Health Association, Inc., New York.

15. Wentworth, B. B., and E. R. Alexander. 1971. Seroepidemiology of infections due to members of the herpesvirus group. Am. J. Epidemiol. **91**:496-507.

Chapter 54

Varicella-Zoster Virus

PHILIP A. BRUNELL

INTRODUCTION

The complement-fixation (CF) test is the most commonly employed test for measuring varicella-zoster (V-Z) antibody. The test is applicable to most virology laboratories that are capable of doing CF; antigens are available from commercial sources. The CF test is suitable for confirming the clinical diagnosis of zoster or varicella (2). Heterologous reactions may be observed when sera obtained during convalescence from these illnesses are tested with herpes type 1 antigen (5); reactions with other herpesvirus antigens are rare.

The major disadvantage of the CF technique is its relative insensitivity. Some individuals no longer have detectable antibody within 1 year after onset of varicella (2). The test, for instance, is too insensitive for determining susceptibility to varicella (6). The CF technique is often incapable of detecting antibody responses during the first month of life (1).

The detection by fluorescence microscopy of antibody directed against membrane antigen (FAMA) provides a sensitive and specific method for determining susceptibility to varicella and for confirming the clinical diagnosis of infection (6).

CLINICAL INDICATIONS

The FAMA test for detection of V-Z antibody is most useful for determining susceptibility to varicella. It is invaluable in identification of the immune status of adults whose recollection of previous varicella may be inaccurate. The FAMA technique has also been helpful when hospitalized children develop varicella to identify those at risk.

Zoster and varicella are readily diagnosed clinically in most instances. Some zosteriform lesions, particularly in the facial area, may be caused by herpes simplex virus. Occasionally, disseminated herpes simplex or insect bites may be misdiagnosed as varicella.

Selection of donors for preparation of zoster immune globulin or for immunoprophylaxis with zoster immune plasma necessitates the use of a method for ascertaining that the donor has an acceptable antibody titer factor (4).

Serological methods are preferred to virus isolation techniques for confirming clinical diagnosis, as serological techniques are more rapid. V-Z virus is quite labile, moreover, which makes isolation of virus a less reliable technique. The period that virus can be isolated from skin lesions usually does not exceed more than 4 days following onset of varicelliform rash, which limits the usefulness of isolation as a method of confirming clinical diagnosis.

TEST PROCEDURE

Detection by fluorescence microscopy of antibody directed against membrane antigen (6)

Human embryonic lung fibroblasts (HELF) are infected with V-Z-infected cells. The inoculum should be sufficient to produce nearly complete infection of the monolayer within 48 h. Infected cells are removed by scraping. The cells are sedimented at $1,000 \times g$ for 10 min and washed three times in phosphate-buffered saline (PBS). Volumes of 0.025 ml of V-Z-infected cell suspension, 10^5 cells/ml, are dispensed into wells in a U-shaped microtiter plate. Serum to be tested is diluted in PBS, and 0.025 ml is added to the cells in the microtiter plate. After incubation of the serum and cells in a humidified atmosphere for 30 min at 25 C, the microtiter plates are placed in a holder and centrifuged at $1,000 \times g$ for 10 min. The supernatant fluid is removed by simply inverting the microtiter plate with a brisk flick of the wrist. The pelleted cells are washed three times with PBS. Fluorescein-labeled anti-human globulin (0.025 ml) is then added to each well of the microtiter plate. After incubation, centrifugation, and washing as described above, the pelleted cells are taken up in glycerol-saline, 9:1, and placed on a microscope slide. The cell suspension is covered with a cover slip which is affixed with nail polish. The slide is then examined with a fluorescence microscope fitted with a phase fluorescence condenser. A ring of fluorescence is observed around the V-Z-infected cells if serum contains antibody.

Controls

Uninfected HELF incubated with V-Z antibody containing sera or V-Z-infected cells incubated with sera devoid of V-Z antibody should fail to yield fluorescence.

A dilution of conjugate should be chosen for the test which fails to give positive reactions with a battery of sera obtained from individuals prior to varicella but yields positive results when V-Z-infected cells are tested with sera containing V-Z antibody.

Nuclear fluorescence has been observed with some serum specimens containing antinuclear antibody.

REAGENTS

Fluorescein-labeled antihuman globulin can be purchased from Behring Diagnostics, Somerville, N.J.

Microtiter U plates and the carrier for centrifuging these plates are available from Cooke Engineering, Alexandria, Va.

INTERPRETATION

Individuals who were tested prior to the onset of varicella did not have detectable V-Z FAMA (6). The absence of antibody can be used for evidence of susceptibility to varicella. Only 1 of 70 patients studied soon after the onset of zoster did not have detectable antibody (3). This patient had been receiving intensive immunosuppressive therapy. It is possible, therefore, that patients who are immunosuppressed may be immune and yet be devoid of antibody.

Antibody can be detected in normal patients with varicella or zoster within 2 days after the onset of rash in almost all instances (3). In immunosuppressed patients, e.g., patients receiving anticancer therapy, the appearance of antibody may be delayed until the 2nd week of varicella. Antibody will usually be detectable in patients with zoster, but a rise may not occur until 2 to 3 weeks after onset in immunosuppressed patients. The magnitude of the peak antibody response is as great in the immunocompromised patient even though the peak response may be later than in the normal group. Delayed peak responses occur in both disseminated and localized zoster (3).

Heterologous responses following other herpesvirus infections have not been observed thus far (6).

LITERATURE CITED

1. Brunell, P. A. 1966. Placental transfer of varicella-zoster antibody. Pediatrics **38**:1034–1038.
2. Brunell, P. A., and H. L. Casey. 1964. A crude tissue culture antigen for the detection of varicella-zoster. Complement fixing antibody. Public Health Rep. **70**:839–842.
3. Brunell, P. A., A. A. Gershon, S. A. Uduman, and S. Steinberg. 1975. Varicella-zoster immunoglobulins during varicella, latency, and zoster. J. Infect. Dis. **132**:49–54.
4. Brunell, P. A., A. Ross, L. Miller, and B. Kuo. 1969. Prevention of varicella with zoster immune globulin. N. Engl. J. Med. **280**:1191–1194.
5. Ross, C. A. C., J. H. S. Sharpe, and P. Terry. 1965. Antigenic relationships of varicella-zoster and herpes simplex. Lancet **2**:708–711.
6. Williams, V., A. A. Gershon, and P. A. Brunell. Varicella-zoster antibody directed against surface antigens on infected cells. J. Infect. Dis. **130**:1034–1038.

Chapter 55

Cytomegalovirus

J. L. WANER, T. H. WELLER, AND J. A. STEWART

INTRODUCTION

Human cytomegaloviruses (CMV) are members of the herpesvirus group that are ubiquitous in humans. The host, after the primary infection, characteristically becomes latently infected. An infection during pregnancy may be transmitted to the fetus or to the infant during birth. The congenitally infected infant usually is viruric for a prolonged period, and the pathological consequences range from no overt illness to severe central nervous system damage. Infection in the adult may be asymptomatic, or various syndromes including CMV mononucleosis, hepatitis, or pneumonitis may result. In the immunocompromised patient the clinical consequences of infection are more overt.

The presence of active infection with CMV can only be inferred from serological data and must be confirmed by viral isolation. Preferred sources are urine and saliva, although virus may be isolated from various body secretions and tissues. CMV exhibits a strict species-specific growth requirement, and in vitro replication is best in fibroblasts; therefore, cultures of diploid human fibroblasts are routinely used for isolation attempts. Human CMV are identified by the characteristic cytopathic effect (enlarged, rounded cells with prominent intranuclear inclusions), species-specific requirement for growth in vitro, the absence of significant amounts of cell-free virus during the initial passages in cell cultures, and by application of immunological procedures. CMV antigens can be detected in infected cells by the indirect fluorescent-antibody (IFA) test with the use of human immune sera devoid of antibodies to the other herpesviruses. A direct fluorescent-antibody test has also been applied in rapid screening of urine samples for CMV (1). Animal antisera to several strains of CMV have been prepared but are not yet available for routine use.

A degree of antigenic heterogeneity has been demonstrated between human strains of CMV with human and animal-prepared immune sera. The significance of these findings is not yet established, but immunological data based on use of an antigen prepared from a single strain of CMV may be misleading.

TEST PROCEDURES

Complement-fixation test

The complement-fixation (CF) test is the method commonly used for determining levels of CMV antibody and is conveniently performed by the microtiter technique. Reagents from commercial sources should be tested for potency before use; antigen preparations are "block"-titered with arbitrarily selected reference sera of known reactivity.

CF antigens are usually prepared from a broadly reactive strain such as AD169. If cell culture facilities are available, potent antigens can be prepared from locally isolated CMV strains. A degree of strain specificity has been reported with the CF test (2, 19). The following protocol is recommended for antigen preparation. Only small amounts of CF antigen are present in the fluid phase of infected cultures, and antigen must be extracted from infected cells (3). Infected cultures showing maximal cytopathic effect should be held an additional 24 h before the antigen is extracted. The cells are dislodged with a rubber policeman into glycine-buffered saline (0.05 M glycine, pH 9.0) and centrifuged for 15 min at $250 \times g$. The supernatant fluid is discarded, fresh buffer is added and discarded after a second centrifugation, and the cell pellet is then resuspended in glycine buffer to make a 10% suspension. The infected cells may be disrupted mechanically by the use of tissue grinders, sonic treatment, or three cycles of freeze-thawing. The supernatant fluid obtained after centrifugation of the disrupted cell suspension at $250 \times g$ for 15 min constitutes the CF antigen. A useful modification entails extraction of the disrupted cell suspension in buffer overnight at 4 C with two or three episodes of vigorous shaking before centrifugation. The antigen preparation is distributed in convenient volumes and stored at -70 C. Thereafter, when thawed, antigen is not refrozen for subsequent use. The potency of the antigen is determined by block titration with a reference serum of known titer.

In performance of the CF test, Veronal-buffered saline (pH 7.2) is the recommended diluent, although Kolmer's saline is adequate. Twofold dilutions of sera, inactivated at 56 C for 30 min, are reacted with 2 units of antigen and 2 units of complement overnight at 4 C. A control antigen prepared from uninfected cells is included in each test in addition to the usual controls. The serum titer is the reciprocal of the highest dilution showing 75% fixation as judged by the degree of hemolysis. Sera reactive at a minimal dilution of 1:8 are indicative of prior exposure to the virus.

Indirect fluorescent-antibody test

The IFA test is a sensitive and broadly reactive immunological method for determining antibody levels to CMV. The procedure is rapid and permits measurement of antibody belonging to specific immunoglobulin (Ig) classes. Additional details may be found in comprehensive texts on fluorescent-antibody methods (5, 16). Fluorescein isothiocyanate-conjugated anti-gamma globulins are available from commercial sources or may be prepared locally (22). Commercial reagents vary in quality and should be checked for potency and specificity before use.

Infected cells serve as antigens and may be prepared by either of two procedures, with similarly prepared uninfected cells serving as antigen controls. Cultured cells infected for at least 3 days and exhibiting approximately 70% cytopathic effect are dislodged with 0.25% trypsin, washed twice with phosphate-buffered saline (PBS; 0.15 M, pH 7.2), and adjusted to a final concentration of approximately 10^7 cells/ml. One drop of cell suspension is placed in a circumscribed area on a glass slide and air-dried (4). Several such areas may be prepared per slide. An alternate and preferred method is to use intact infected (40 to 50%) cell monolayers grown on cover glasses, or eight-chambered slides (Lab-Tek Products, Naperville, Ill.). Intact monolayers are washed with buffered saline and air-dried. In both methods the air-dried cells are fixed with cold acetone for 15 min at 4 C and may then be used directly or stored at -20 C. Sera for testing are diluted initially 1:4 in PBS. Then serial twofold dilutions of sera are prepared, and each dilution is individually applied dropwise to a batch of dried cells in a moist chamber for 30 min at 37 C. The preparations are washed twice with PBS and overlaid with a drop of fluorescein-conjugated anti-human IgG for 30 min at 37 C. (Conjugates are first block-titrated with a known reactive serum to determine optimal dilution for use.) The conjugate is removed, the cells are washed twice with PBS, and the preparation is covered

with PBS-buffered glycerol solution (9 parts glycerol, 1 part PBS, pH 8.0). A counterstain such as Evan's blue (0.05 to 0.001% in PBS) may be included to improve contrast. It is applied for 5 min as a wash either before or after addition of conjugate. Positive and negative serum controls are included in each test. Reactivity is assessed by specific nuclear fluorescence observed by microscopic examination with ultraviolet illumination. The serum titer is expressed as the reciprocal of the highest serum dilution showing fluorescence.

IFA may be used to measure CMV antibody in the IgM class of Ig's by using an anti-IgM conjugate. This is useful in the investigation of immune response in newborns when cord sera are available (6).

The detection by IFA of antibody reacting with antigens (early antigens) that are not dependent on viral deoxyribonucleic acid synthesis may be helpful in defining recently acquired infections (15). The IFA test is modified in that cell cultures are fed with medium containing 20 μg of cytosine arabinoside hydrochloride/ml at the time of infection and are washed and fixed 3 days later. Antibody to early antigen appears as a speckled fluorescence distributed over the nucleus.

Neutralization test

Neutralizing antibody in human sera may show a degree of CMV strain specificity. The choice of strain of virus is therefore important. Virus isolated from the patient would be preferable, but usually is not practicable. Even if the homologous virus is on hand, serial cultivation for months may be required before sufficient quantities of cell-free infectious virus become available. Therefore, culture-adapted CMV strains, such as AD169 and Davis, are usually used. These strains show some antigenic differences in neutralization tests (7, 20).

Neutralizing antibody titers are best determined by the plaque reduction method (12), which is more accurate than the cell-culture tube neutralization technique. The diluent needs to be chosen with caution because some strains of CMV are relatively labile in the presence of $NaHCO_3$ (17). Eagle's minimal essential medium (MEM) with 6.6 mM $NaHCO_3$ or tris(hydroxyethyl)aminomethane-buffered saline, both containing added heat-inactivated calf serum in a concentration of 4%, is used as diluent in different laboratories. Although human sera contain complement-independent neutralizing antibody, the incorporation of 4% fresh guinea pig serum usually enhances neutralizing activity and allows detection of antibody at greater dilutions. Sera are inactivated at 56 C for 30 min before testing. Serial twofold serum dilutions then are mixed with equal volumes of virus suspension containing 200 plaque-forming units/0.2 ml. Virus controls prepared with diluent without serum are processed in parallel. The mixtures are incubated at 37 C for 30 min. Each serum dilution-virus mixture is then inoculated in 0.2-ml amounts onto duplicate cultures of actively growing confluent human fibroblast cells contained in 60-mm tissue culture dishes. Cell cultures are maintained with MEM and 5% fetal calf serum. After an absorption period of 1 h at 37 C, the inoculated cultures are washed once with diluent and overlaid with maintenance medium containing 2% methyl cellulose (12) or 0.3% agarose (21), and then they are incubated at 37 C in a humidified 5% CO_2 atmosphere. One to two weeks later, the overlay medium is removed, and the cultures are fixed with 10% formalin for 10 min at room temperature and stained with 0.03% methylene blue. Plaques are counted with the aid of a microscope. The CMV antibody titer is expressed as the highest serum dilution which neutralizes 60% of the virus (compared with plaque counts of the control virus plates).

A rapid IFA method of assaying infectious virus has been applied to neutralization tests (18). The test is conducted as above except that cell cultures on cover glasses or, preferably, chamber slides are inoculated and no semisolid overlay is added. Between 72 and 96 h after infection, the cultures are fixed in acetone as for the IFA test and are allowed to react with pooled human anti-CMV sera and anti-human IgG conjugate. The number of fluorescing cells is determined, and the antibody titer is expressed as in the plaque reduction method.

Indirect hemagglutination test

The indirect hemagglutination (IHA) test detects IgM and IgG antibodies and can be completed in 1 day. Reagents designated for use in the IHA test are not commercially available, but CMV CF antigens from commercial sources can be used. The procedure (10) as used at the Center for Disease Control follows. Antigen for IHA can be prepared from infected cell cultures showing maximal cytopathic effect for at least 24 h. The cell sheets are rinsed once with PBS (pH 7.2). PBS is then added to the culture (25 ml/2-liter roller bottle; 5 ml/1-liter prescription bottle) and frozen as evenly as possible over the cell sheet by rotating the bottle in an alcohol-dry ice bath. The PBS-cell layer can be kept frozen for up to 2 weeks before harvest. The

fluid overlay recovered after the culture is thawed at room temperature is used as IHA antigen. If the fluid contains dislodged cells, the antigen is clarified by centrifugation at 500 × g, prior to storage in small portions without preservative at −60 C.

All reagents used in the IHA test should be at room temperature since refrigeration of sheep cells during tanning and sensitization causes fuzzy agglutination and less sensitivity in detecting antibody. This protocol describes the use of fresh sheep cells, which are easier to use than fixed cells because they show less spontaneous agglutination and the tannic acid optimal dilution can be determined more precisely. Once familiar with the IHA method, one can then master the use of glutaraldehyde-fixed cells (10) so that, at one time, large volumes of sensitized cells can be prepared which are stable upon storage at −60 C. Most of the problems that have occurred in first applying the IHA test have involved errors in the pH or molarity of buffers. To avoid such problems, the formulas for the two PBS solutions provided here should be followed exactly.

PBS (pH 6.7) is prepared by mixing 100 ml of 0.15 M NaCl with 100 ml of a buffer composed of 32.3 ml of 0.15 M Na_2HPO_4 and 67.7 ml of 0.15 M KH_2PO_4. PBS (pH 7.2) is prepared by mixing 175 ml of 0.15 M NaCl with 9.5 ml of 0.15 M Na_2HPO_4 and 3.0 ml of 0.15 M NaH_2PO_4. The pH should be ±0.05 the expected pH. If the pH is outside these limits, adjust with 1 N NaOH or 1 N HCl.

Tanned erythrocytes are prepared from sheep blood collected in sterile 3.8% sodium citrate or Alsever's solution. Blood is aged 1 to 6 weeks at 4 C and then washed three times with PBS (pH 7.2). The buffy coat layer is removed by aspiration, and the packed cells are resuspended to make a 2.5% concentration. The optimal tannic acid (reagent grade) dilution may vary from 1:20,000 to 1:160,000 and should be determined for each fresh batch of cells. The tannic acid is diluted in PBS (pH 7.2) within 1 h of use. Equal volumes of the 2.5% erythrocyte suspension and the tannic acid solution are mixed and incubated in a 37 C water bath for 10 min. The cells are centrifuged at 500 × g for 10 min and washed once with PBS (pH 7.2). They are then resuspended to a 2.5% concentration in PBS (pH 6.7).

To *sensitize the cells* with CMV, the antigen is diluted in PBS (pH 6.7), and 1 volume of the optimal antigen dilution and 1 volume of 2.5% tanned cells are mixed and incubated for 30 min at room temperature. The cells are centrifuged at 500 × g for 10 min, washed twice with a 1% normal rabbit serum diluent (NRSD), and then adjusted to a 1% suspension in the same diluent. To prepare the NRSD, rabbit serum is heat-inactivated (56 C for 30 min), pretested for absence of sheep cell agglutinins, and diluted with 99 parts of PBS (pH 7.2).

Sera to be tested are diluted 1:8 in NRSD, inactivated at 56 C for 30 min, and adsorbed at 4 C for 30 min by using 0.1 ml of 50% washed sheep erythrocytes per ml of diluted serum. Twofold dilutions in 0.05-ml volumes are then prepared in flexible polyvinyl chloride microtitration U plates. To each serum dilution, 0.025 ml of sensitized cells is added. The plates are sealed with clear tape, shaken, incubated at room temperature for 2 to 3 h, and then refrigerated until read. Settling patterns are read as positive when the cells are completely and uniformly agglutinated or when a large circle of partially agglutinated cells nearly coats the bottom of the cup. Small rings of agglutinated cells are read as plus-minus, and buttons are read as negative. The highest serum dilution which produces complete or almost complete agglutination is the end-point dilution. Controls consist of (i) a 1:8 dilution of the test serum plus tanned erythrocytes treated with PBS only, (ii) a 1:8 dilution of the test serum plus erythrocytes sensitized with uninfected fibroblast tissue culture antigen, and (iii) a positive control consisting of a complete titration of a known CMV-positive serum.

Immunoprecipitin and platelet agglutination techniques

Antibody to CMV in human sera also may be assayed by the immunoprecipitin and platelet agglutination techniques (9, 11). The immunoprecipitin test is less sensitive than the CF test, and the platelet agglutination test is more sensitive. Neither method is commonly used.

DISCUSSION

The presence in the infant of transplacentally acquired CMV antibody of the IgG class complicates the interpretation of serological results during the first 6 months of life. Detection of specific IgM antibody to CMV in the serum of a newborn, however, usually indicates congenital infection since maternal IgM cannot cross the intact placenta; additionally, the prenatally infected child will usually be excreting virus. Excretion of virus does not begin until 3 to 12 weeks after birth in the perinatally infected child (14). The IgM antibody response is similar to that of the prenatally infected infant. CMV IgM antibody may persist for months after primary infection, and therefore its detection in a single serum specimen is of limited value in the timing of a primary infection.

CMV IgM antibody is commonly demonstrated by the IFA test but can also be detected by IHA if the serum is first separated into IgM and IgG fractions. The CF reaction primarily reflects IgG antibodies. All results require careful interpretation since false-positive IgM reactions may be otained with sera from patients with heterophile-positive mononucleosis, varicella, or rheumatoid factor (8). Sera with rheumatoid factor may be absorbed with aggregated IgG and retested for specific IgM. Indeed, the usefulness of the IgM response is questioned by the report that fetal IgM antibody is produced to maternal IgG and may yield a false-positive IFA test (13).

Serial serum specimens derived from individuals over 6 months of age that exhibit a fourfold or greater rise in CF antibody titer suggest a recent infection. However, some asymptomatic latently infected individuals may exhibit labile CF titers (19). The IFA and IHA tests appear to be more sensitive than the CF method in detecting IgG antibody. Thus, a seroconversion may be detected earlier.

Postnatal CMV disease may be due to reactivation of a latent infection, reinfection with a similar or different antigenic strain, or a primary infection. Depending on socioeconomic factors, geographical locality, and the test employed, CMV seroreactivity of a population over 30 years of age may range between 40 and 100%. Even when a base-line serum is available, a serum unreactive by CF may not be indicative of the absence of previous CMV infection. It is to be emphasized that antibody rises of fourfold or greater indicate recent antigenic stimulation but per se are not confirmatory either of a recent primary infection or of reactivation of a preexisting latent process with active viral excretion. Parallel studies on viral excretion are indicated.

LITERATURE CITED

1. Anderson, C. H., and R. H. Michaels. 1972. Cytomegalovirus infection: detection by direct fluorescent antibody technique. Lancet 2:308–309.
2. Baron, J., L. Youngblood, C. M. F. Siewers, and D. N. Medearis. 1969. The incidence of cytomegalovirus, herpes simplex, rubella, and toxoplasma antibodies in microencephalic, mentally retarded, and normocephalic children. Pediatrics 44:932–939.
3. Benyesh-Melnick, M., V. Vonka, F. Probstmeyer, and J. Wimberly. 1966. Human cytomegalovirus: properties of the complement-fixing antigen. J. Immunol. 96:261–267.
4. Chiang, W., B. B. Wentworth, and E. R. Alex-

ander. 1970. The use of an immunofluorescence technique for the determination of antibodies to cytomegalovirus strains in human sera. J. Immunol. 104:992–999.

5. Goldman, M. 1968. Fluorescent antibody methods. Academic Press Inc., New York.

6. Hanshaw, J. B. 1969. Congenital cytomegalovirus infection: laboratory methods of detection. J. Pediatr. 75:1179–1185.

7. Hanshaw, J. B., R. F. Betts, G. Simon, and R. C. Boynton. 1965. Acquired cytomegalovirus infection: association with hepatomegaly and abnormal liver function tests. N. Engl. J. Med. 272:602–609.

8. Hanshaw, J. B., J. C. Neiderman, and L. N. Chessin. 1972. Cytomegalovirus macroglobulin in cell-associated herpesvirus infections. J. Infect. Dis. 125:304–306.

9. Jung, M., P. C. Price, G. S. Kistler, and U. Krech. 1973. Immunoprecipitation studies with antigens of human cytomegalovirus. Z. Immunitaetsforsch. 145:S.191–198.

10. Palmer, D. F., J. J. Cavallaro, K. Herrmann, J. A. Stewart, and K. W. Walls (ed.). 1974. A procedural guide to the serodiagnosis of toxoplasmosis, rubella, cytomegalic inclusion disease, herpes simplex. Immunology Series No. 5, p. 23–56. Center for Disease Control, Atlanta, Ga.

11. Penttinen, K., L. Kääriainen, and G. Myllyla. 1970. Cytomegalovirus antibody assay by platelet aggregation. Arch. Gesamte Virusforsch. 29:189–194.

12. Plummer, G., and M. Benyesh-Melnick. 1964. A plaque reduction neturalization test for human cytomegalovirus. Proc. Soc. Exp. Biol. Med. 117:145–150.

13. Reimer, C. B., C. M. Black, D. J. Phillips, L. C. Logan, E. F. Hunter, B. J. Pender, and B. E. McGrew. 1975. The specificity of fetal IgM; antibody or anti-antibody. Ann. N.Y. Acad. Sci. 254:77–93.

14. Reynolds, D. W., S. Stagno, T. S. Hostly, M. Tiller, and C. A. Alford, Jr. 1973. Maternal cytomegalovirus excretion and perinatal infection. N. Engl. J. Med. 289:1–5.

15. The, T. H., G. Klein, and M. M. A. C. Langenhuysen. 1974. Antibody reactions to virus specific early antigens (EA) in patients with cytomegalovirus (CMV) infection. Clin. Exp. Immunol. 16:1–12.

16. Vogt, P. K. 1969. Immunofluorescent detection of viral antigens, p. 316–326. In K. Habel and N. P. Salzman (ed.), Fundamental techniques in virology. Academic Press Inc., New York.

17. Vonka, V., and M. Benyesh-Melnick. 1966. Thermoinactivation of human cytomegalovirus. J. Bacteriol. 91:221–226.

18. Waner, J. L., and J. E. Budnick. 1973. Threeday assay for human cytomegalovirus applicable to serum neutralization tests. Appl. Microbiol. 25:37–39.

19. Waner, J. L., T. H. Weller, and S. V. Kevy. 1973. Patterns of cytomegaloviral complement-fixing antibody activity: a longitudinal study of blood donors. J. Infect. Dis. 127:538–543.

20. Weller, T. H., J. B. Hanshaw, and D. E. Scott. 1960. Serologic differentiation of viruses responsible for cytomegalic inclusion disease. Virology 12:130–132.

21. Wentworth, B. B., and L. French. 1970. Plaque assay of cytomegalovirus strains of human origin. Proc. Soc. Exp. Biol. Med. 135:253–258.

22. Wood, B. T., S. H. Thompson, and G. Goldstein. 1965. Fluorescent antibody staining. III. Preparation of fluorescein-isothiocyanate-labeled antibodies. J. Immunol. 95:225–229.

Chapter 56

Epstein-Barr Virus

WARREN A. ANDIMAN AND GEORGE MILLER

INTRODUCTION

The Epstein-Barr (EB) virus is an infectious agent ubiquitous throughout the world. Primary infection in young children is generally asymptomatic or accompanied by nonspecific minor illness. In developing countries and in socioeconomically deprived areas of the United States, about 80% of 5-year-old children are seropositive; in economically privileged areas, about 40 to 50% of children aged 5 years have antibodies. In persons who remain uninfected into adolescence, primary infection is often manifest as a self-limited, symptomatic disease in the form of infectious mononucleosis. Certain populations develop EB virus-associated neoplastic disease in the form of Burkitt's lymphoma (BL) and nasopharyngeal carcinoma (NPC); however, these diseases are not thought to be the result of primary infection. There are firm lines of evidence suggesting a causal relationship between EB virus and these two human cancers. Undoubtedly, there are strong genetic and environmental factors which influence the expression of these diseases.

EB virus was discovered by Epstein, Barr, and Achong in 1964 in lymphoblasts cultured from Burkitt's lymphoma. On the basis of morphology and the structure of its genome, the agent is a herpesvirus. Mature, enveloped particles measure 150 to 200 nm in diameter. The virus genome contains double-stranded deoxyribonucleic acid (DNA) of molecular weight $\sim 90 \times 10^6$ to 100×10^6. Intracellular circular forms of the viral genome occur, and the virus is thought to behave as an episome.

TESTS AVAILABLE: COMMON USES AND THEIR RELATIONSHIP TO CLINICAL DISEASES

Within the past 10 years, several distinct EB virus-related cell-associated antigens have been characterized by immunofluorescence and other serological procedures (Table 1). These include EB viral capsid antigens (VCA; 2), EB virus membrane antigens, EB nuclear antigen (EBNA) (8), EB virus-induced early antigens (5), which are subdivided into restricted and diffuse components, and various soluble anti-gens. The first four classes can be demonstrated by immunofluorescence techniques and the last by complement fixation and immunodiffusion. There are also several techniques now available which can display the presence of neutralizing antibodies to EB virus.

Serological procedures are utilized most often for the following reasons: (i) to determine susceptibility or immunity to infectious mononucleosis; (ii) to determine whether a heterophile antibody-negative mononucleosis syndrome in an individual patient is etiologically related to EB virus (since all heterophile-positive mononucleosis is due to EB virus, it is rarely necessary to measure specific EB virus antibodies as a diagnostic procedure in mononucleosis); (iii) to determine whether the EB virus can be implicated as the etiological agent in a variety of atypical clinical syndromes, such as transverse myelitis and infectious polyneuritis, which have occasionally been associated with EB virus infection; (iv) to determine susceptibility or immunity to infection in primates used in experimental EB virus inoculation experiments; (v) to determine whether a lymphoblastoid cell line contains antigenic markers of EB virus expression; and (vi) as epidemiological tools in specific populations; in particular, seroepidemiological methods have been used to distinguish patients with EB virus-associated tumors from individuals with inapparent infection.

During primary infection, recognizable as infectious mononucleosis, antibodies develop to the diverse EB virus-associated antigens. Whereas nearly all acute-phase sera of infectious mononucleosis patients contain VCA antibodies, it has been shown by prospective study that these antibodies are absent before infectious mononucleosis. The titer of this antibody peaks around the second week of illness, and about 20% of acutely infected individuals have a fourfold or greater increase in antibodies to VCA in the interval between collection of the first and subsequent acute-phase sera. Anti-VCA titers gradually decline to levels seen in 18- to 30-year-old control blood donors, persist for life, and appear to be associated with permanent immunity. Sera from about 80% of newly infected persons reveal antibodies to the diffuse

TABLE 1. *EB virus-associated antigen systems and tests for EB virus-antibody*

Antigen system	Source of antigen	Usual negative antigen control	Test used to demonstrate antigen[a]	Usual method used to demonstrate antibody in human serum
1. "Viral capsid"	Acetone-fixed cell smears of "producer" lymphoblastoid cell lines	Nonproducer lymphoblastoid cell lines	Immunofluorescence	Indirect immunofluorescence with fluorescein-conjugated antihuman IgG or antihuman IgM
2. "Early"	Acetone- or methanol-fixed cell smears of nonproducer lymphoblastoid cell lines treated with virus concentrates of the P_3J-HR1 line ("superinfection") or with halogenated pyrimidines ("induction")	Nonproducer lymphoblastoid cell line, not induced or superinfected	Immunofluorescence	Indirect immunofluorescence with fluorescein-conjugated antihuman IgG
3. "Membrane"	Living cells from Burkitt lymphoma biopsies and some producer lymphoblastoid cell lines	EB virus genome free cell line; autologous bone marrow	Immunofluorescence	Ability of unknown human serum to block immunofluorescence caused by fluorescein-conjugated reference human serum
4. "Nuclear"	Acetone-fixed cells of Burkitt lymphoma biopsies or of any EB virus genome containing lymphoblastoid cell line	EBV genome free cell line	Anticomplement immunofluorescence	Ability of unknown human serum to fix human complement in the presence of the antigen; complement fixation detected by indirect immunofluorescence with fluorescein-conjugated antihuman B1c globulin
5. Complement fixing	Crude extracts of EB virus genome containing lymphoblastoid cell lines, e.g., Raji	Extracts of EB virus genome free lymphoblastoid cell lines, e.g., MOLT-4, CEM	Complement fixation	Complement fixation
6. Immunoprecipitating	Crude extracts of EB virus genome containing lymphoblastoid cell lines, e.g., Raji	Extracts of EBV genome free lymphoblastoid cell lines, e.g., MOLT-4, CEM	Immunodiffusion	Immunodiffusion
7. Neutralization of abortive infection (viral envelope antigens)	Concentrated extracellular fluid from the P_3J-HR1 Burkitt lymphoma cell line	Concentrated extracellular fluid from a nonproducer cell line	Early antigen production following superinfection of nonproducer cells or inhibition of colony formation by nonproducer (Raji) cells	Serum neutralizaton

Table 1 —cont.

Antigen system	Source of antigen	Usual negative antigen control	Test used to demonstrate antigen[a]	Usual method used to demonstrate antibody in human serum
8. Neutralization of transformation (viral envelope antigens)	Concentrated extracellular fluid from the B95-8 line (transformed producer marmoset) or from the Kaplan (mononucleosis line); directly from oropharyngeal secretions	Concentrated extracellular fluid from a nonproducer cell line or from the P₃J-HR-1 line	Transformation of primary human leukocytes into continuous lines or stimulation of cellular DNA synthesis in primary human leukocytes	Serum neutralization

[a] In all instances, the antigen is demonstrated by the use of reference human antisera empirically determined to be with or without reactivity to the antigen system under study. Reprinted with permission from G. Miller, 1975, "Epstein-Barr herpesvirus and infectious mononucleosis," in *Progress in Medical Virology–1976*, S. Karger, Basel.

component of early antigen. This class of antibodies reflects extensive, current, or very recent disease and is also commonly found in those patients with Burkitt's lymphoma or nasopharyngeal carcinoma who also have very high anti-VCA titers. Antibodies to EB nuclear antigen begin to appear in a minority of patients in the third or fourth week after onset of infectious mononucleosis (3). By 6 months, however, all convalescent infectious mononucleosis patients carry this antibody, which thereafter persists for life. Thus, anti-EB nuclear antigen responses may be used to diagnose primary EB virus infections. Neither the height of the antibody titer to VCA and EB nuclear antigen nor the time required for their development correlates with severity or duration of illness in infectious mononucleosis.

In the following section two of these tests will be described in detail, those for measuring antibodies to VCA and for demonstrating the presence of antibodies to the EB nuclear antigen. Although a variety of other tests will be described briefly, it is assumed that for the foreseeable future they will remain specialized research tools.

FLUORESCENT-ANTIBODY TESTS

Indirect fluorescent-antibody test for antibodies to viral capsid antigen

This indirect fluorescent-antibody test is the most widely used test for determining the presence of antibody to the virus and was the test used in the massive epidemiological investigations that have implicated EB virus as the etiological agent of infectious mononucleosis. Capsid antigens are found only in those human or nonhuman primate lymphoid cell lines which are producers of virus. A maximum of 5 to 10% of the cells in those lines are activated to express the capsid antigen, though all the cells contain the viral genome. Antigen smears are prepared by removing 3 ml of cells from a suspension of virus-productive cell stock (EB3, B95-8, HR1K) at a concentration of 10⁶ cells/ml. To control for anticellular antibodies which might be present in the serum under test, antigen should also be prepared from a nonproducer (VCA-negative) cell line, such as Raji or transformed umbilical cord leukocytes. The cells are pelleted, the supernatant fluid is removed, and the cells are resuspended in 0.1 ml of phosphate-buffered saline (PBS). The cell suspension is dropped from a capillary pipette onto a microscope slide (5 or 6 drops per slide) and allowed to air-dry. Slides are fixed in acetone at 20 C. Store at −20 C.

Test proper

1. Sera are serially diluted in a microtiter tray with PBS (usually from 1:10 to 1:160).

2. Fixed cell smears are circled with a Martex pen (Martex Corp., Englewood, N.J.).

3. Add 1 drop of serum dilution per smear.

4. Incubate for 45 min at 37 C in a moist chamber.

5. Rinse slides with cold PBS and wash twice for 5 min.

6. Dry slides (hairblower may be used).

7. Fluorescein isothiocyanate-conjugated rabbit antihuman IgG (Antibodies, Inc., Davis, Calif.) is diluted 1:10 with PBS.

8. Add 1 drop of conjugate per smear.

9. Incubate for 45 min at 37 C and repeat step 5.

10. Wash with distilled water for 2 min and dry.

11. Mount long cover slips (22 × 50 mm) with buffered glycerol, pH 9.0.

12. Read slides with a Leitz-Wetzlar indirect illuminating fluorescence microscope.

Note: A test for the presence of VCA in a cell line of unknown producer status can be performed by using sera known to be positive or negative for anti-VCA antibodies.

Test for presence of antibodies to EBNA

EB nuclear antigen was discovered in the course of attempts to localize the intracellular site of production of soluble complement-fixing antigens. The test utilizes an anticomplement immunofluorescence technique. The antigen is present in all EB virus genome carrying lymphoblast cell lines and in biopsies of Burkitt's lymphoma, nasopharyngeal carcinoma, and experimental lymphoma induced by EB virus. The EB nuclear antigen seems to be an early expression of information contained in the genome.

Antigen smears are prepared from 3 ml of actively growing cell suspensions with a density of 10^6 cells/ml; the fraction of viable cells must be high, because degenerating cells do not contain EB nuclear antigen. To control for antinuclear antibodies in the serum under test, a control antigen should be prepared from a lymphoblast cell line (e.g., MOLT-4, CCRF-CEM) which lacks EB nuclear antigen. One drop from a capillary pipette is drawn between two 22 × 22 mm cover slips. The smears are permitted to air-dry; they are then fixed in acetone for 10 min at room temperature and stored at −70 C until use.

Hanks buffered saline solution (HBSS), which is used for all washes and for all dilution of sera, is adjusted to an exact pH of 6.9 before use and is kept on ice.

All tests for anti-EB nuclear antigen must be run with a known positive and a known negative serum as controls. Each serum under test is mixed with 0.8 ml of HBSS and inactivated in a 56 C water bath for 30 min. A 0.1-ml amount of fresh human serum lacking EB virus antibodies is added as the complement source to each serum dilution, bringing the final dilution of sera to 1:10. From this point, all sera must be kept on ice.

Test proper

1. Cover slips are dipped in HBSS and gently blotted.

2. Cover slips are placed in a box lined with moist absorbent cotton.

3. Three drops of diluted serum is put on each cover slip and spread out with capillary.

4. Incubate for 30 min at 37 C.

5. Cover slips are blotted and washed in stirred HBSS for 30 min. The wash is changed every 10 min, and dishes are kept covered.

6. Three drops of a 1:10 dilution of fluorescein-conjugated goat antiserum to human complement $\beta iC/\beta iA$ (Hyland Laboratories, Costa Mesa, Calif.) is put on each cover slip.

7. Incubate for 30 min at 37 C.

8. Blot and wash as in step 5.

9. Blot and wash in distilled water for 2 min. Blot again.

10. Air-dry and mount face down with buffered glycerol, pH 9.0.

Note: In performing this test, we have found the following items indispensable to successful completion: the pH of the HBSS, keeping all reagents on ice, and ensuring that the cell smears *not* be allowed to dry until the final step.

Indirect immunofluorescence test for immunoglobulin M antibodies to EB virus

In 1972, Schmitz and Scherer (10) described a test which demonstrates, by immunofluorescence, the presence of IgM antibodies in the sera of all patients acutely ill with heterophile-positive infectious mononucleosis. These antibodies were found to persist for only a 2- to 3-month period after onset of symptoms, and their presence indicated recent infection. The test appears to hold promise as a useful diagnostic tool in those cases of infectious mononucleosis which are heterophile negative.

Test for "early antigens"

The so-called "early antigens" can be made to appear in normally nonproductive lymphoblastoid cell lines (e.g., Raji, 64-10) either by superinfection with virus concentrates of the P_3J-HR1 Burkitt line (5) or by "induction" (1) with various halogenated pyrimidines, e.g., 5-iododeoxyuridine (IUdr) or bromodeoxyuridine. The antigen consists of at least two components, D and R, which can be distinguished on the basis of their distribution through the cell and by their stability to methanol (4).

Antibodies to early antigens are found in selected human sera and reflect current or recent disease processes that are associated with the virus, including BL and NPC. Antibodies to early antigens disappear rapidly following recovery from infectious mononucleosis.

In our laboratory superinfection is accomplished by adding 3 ml of the supernatant fluid of the HR1K virus subline to each 3 ml of Raji growing at a concentration of 10^6 cells/ml. Cell smears are prepared from washed, pelleted cells 4 days after superinfection.

"Induction" of early antigen is accomplished by adding IUdR (Calbiochem, San Diego, Calif.) to stock suspensions in a concentration of 60 μg/ml, removing the IUdR through several wash and pelleting procedures 48 h later, and then allowing further growth of the leukocytes for an additional 5 to 7 days before cell smears are prepared.

NEUTRALIZATION TESTS

Two types of neutralization tests have been described based on the two main biological properties of EB virus. The first assesses the ability of antibody-positive human sera to neutralize the capacity of EB virus to transform human leukocytes in vitro into continuous lymphoblastoid cell lines (6) or to inhibit the stimulation of DNA synthesis which follows addition of EB virus to human umbilical cord lymphocytes (8a). The second measures the ability of immune sera to neutralize the induction of early antigen in a nonproductive cell line (Raji) by the P_3J-HR1 Burkitt tumor virus (7). Induction of early antigen is accompanied by inhibition of cell growth and inhibition of colony formation. A microtiter neutralization test is based on the ability of antibody-positive sera to prevent colony inhibition after addition of the HR1K virus (9). These assays are different from tests measuring antibody to cell-associated antigens. They detect reactivity between immune sera and antigens present at or near the surface of biologically active infectious virus. The presence of EB virus-neutralizing activity correlates with the presence of antibody to EB virus capsids but not with the heterophile antibody.

ACKNOWLEDGMENTS

This work was supported by Public Health Service grants CA-12055, CA-16038, and HD-00177, by American Cancer Society grant VC-107, and by the Damon Runyon-Walter Winchell Cancer Fund. G.M. is an Investigator of the Howard Hughes Medical Institute.

LITERATURE CITED

1. Gerber, P., and S. Lucas. 1972. Epstein-Barr virus-associated antigens activated in human cells by 5-bromodeoxyuridine. Proc. Soc. Exp. Biol. Med. 141:431–435.
2. Henle, G., and W. Henle. 1966. Immunofluorescence in cells derived from Burkitt's lymphoma. J. Bacteriol. 91:1248–1256.
3. Henle, G., W. Henle, and C. A. Horwitz. 1974. Antibodies to Epstein-Barr virus-associated nuclear antigen in infectious mononucleosis. J. Infect. Dis. 130:231–239.
4. Henle, G., W. Henle, and G. Klein. 1971. Demonstration of two distinct components in the early antigen complex of Epstein-Barr virus-infected cells. Int. J. Cancer 8:272–282.
5. Henle, W., G. Henle, B. Zajac, G. Pearson, R. Waubke, and M. Scriba. 1970. Differential reactivity of human serums with early antigens induced by Epstein-Barr virus. Science 169:188–190.
6. Miller, G., J. C. Niederman, and D. Stitt. 1972. Infectious mononucleosis: appearance of neutralizing antibody to Epstein-Barr virus measured by inhibition of formation of lymphoblastoid cell lines. J. Infect. Dis. 125:413–416.
7. Pearson, G., F. Dewey, G. Klein, G. Henle, and W. Henle. 1970. Relation between neutralization of Epstein-Barr virus and antibodies to cell membrane antigens induced by the virus. J. Natl. Cancer Inst. 45:989–995.
8. Reedman, B. M., and G. Klein. 1973. Cellular localization of an Epstein-Barr virus-associated complement-fixing antigen in producer and non-producer lymphoblastoid cell lines. Int. J. Cancer 11:499–520.
8a. Robinson, J., and G. Miller. 1975. Assay for Epstein-Barr virus based on stimulation of DNA synthesis in mixed leukocytes from human umbilical cord blood. J. Virol. 15:1065–1072.
9. Rocchi, G., and J. Hewetson. 1973. A practical and quantitative microtest for determination of neutralizing antibodies against Epstein-Barr virus. J. Gen. Virol. 18:385–391.
10. Schmitz, H., and M. Scherer. 1972. IgM antibodies to Epstein-Barr virus in infectious mononucleosis. Arch. Gesamte Virusforsch. 37:332–339.

Chapter 57

Influenza Virus

WALTER R. DOWDLE

INTRODUCTION

The typical clinical course of influenza begins abruptly with fever and chills followed by fatigue, headache, myalgia, and, often, a slight nonproductive cough. Recovery from uncomplicated influenza begins 3 to 4 days after onset, although weakness and fatigue may persist for several weeks. Pulmonary complications of viral or bacterial origin sometimes develop, but fatal complications are most frequent among the aged and among those with underlying chronic debilitating illnesses. Influenza is most often recognized by its characteristic epidemic pattern. Epidemics, or outbreaks, of influenza type A may occur every 1 to 2 years, and epidemics of type B, every 4 to 6 years. Influenza does not always appear in epidemics or the classic clinical form. Sporadic cases frequently occur in nonepidemic years. The diagnosis of influenza on clinical grounds may be difficult or impossible against a background of other respiratory diseases in the community, and for this reason a laboratory diagnosis of influenza is required.

Influenza virus type C is associated with mild, often subclinical, disease and is rarely considered in the differential diagnosis of acute febrile respiratory infections. Techniques for diagnosis of type C infections differ slightly from those used for the other influenza viruses (2, 7).

Evidence of serum antibody against influenza type A or B viruses by any serological test is indicative of infection, but it provides no information as to when the infection occurred. Since most individuals by school age have been infected with influenza virus at least once, diagnosis of current disease depends upon the demonstration of a significant increase in antibody titer. An increase in titer is determined by simultaneous testing of serum collected at the onset of illness and convalescent serum collected 2 to 3 weeks later. The only exceptions to this requirement for paired sera are the presence of specific antibody in convalescent sera after an epidemic of a totally new antigenic subtype or antibody titers proven to be statistically higher than expected.

In theory, a serodiagnosis of influenza can be made upon demonstration of a significant rise in antibody titer to any of the four major virus antigens (matrix [M] protein, nucleoprotein [NP], neuraminidase [NA], and hemagglutinin [HA]). In practice, it is far more complex. Antibody titer rises to each antigenic component do not occur at the same rate or with equal frequency, and various tests have different degrees of sensitivity. The primary advantage of using the influenza virus internal M and NP antigens is that these proteins do not undergo variation, and few tests antigens are required. The major disadvantage of tests for M antibody is that antibody rises to this antigen usually are associated only with the most severe disease (6). Tests for NP antibody are far more sensitive. Since the surface HA and NA structures undergo antigenic drift and, less often, antigenic shift (11), antibody to these proteins may indicate, within broad limits, the probable infecting strain. A significant rise in antibody titer following infection occurs less frequently with the NA antigen than with the HA antigen. Also, the enzyme inhibition test (1) for NA antibody is complex and is not a practical procedure for routine diagnostic use. Tests for antibody to the HA antigen are most sensitive and most practical, and these are usually used for serodiagnosis. Antibodies to the HA antigen are also most closely associated with virus neutralization and protection against disease.

The three tests which have the widest application for serodiagnosis and serosurveys are single radial immunodiffusion (SRD), complement fixation (CF), and hemagglutination inhibition (HI).

The SRD test is a simple two-component system for detection of influenza virus antibodies. In this test the influenza virus antigen is incorporated in an agar or agarose gel, and antisera are allowed to diffuse radially from their points of application. The formation of antigen-antibody complexes changes the optical characteristics of the gel and results in zones of opalescence which can be easily seen. This test can be designed to assay antibody to each of the four major virus antigens. Antibody is quantitated by the size of the opalescent zone formed after diffusion of serum. The SRD has been reported to be more sensitive than the CF test for detection of NP antibody rises and as sensitive as the HY test for HA antibody rises (6). The advantages of the test are numerous: simplicity of application, absence of nonspecific inhibitors, the requirement for minimal amounts of sera, and more precise quantitation than is possible by conventional tests. The major disadvantage of the SRD test is the large amount of antigen required for incorporation into agar. The test is impractical for small laboratories unless the antigen can be provided by a central source or unless the test becomes commercially available. Methods for preparing reagents and performing the SRD test have been given elsewhere (7, 9).

CF is most useful for those laboratories which routinely perform the test with a battery of antigens for serodiagnosis of other viral diseases. Its complexity precludes occasional use for serodiagnosis of influenza. The test may be performed with whole virion (HA and NA) or NP antigens. Results with the former antigen parallel those obtained by the HI test, but CF has the added advantage of not being affected by nonspecific inhibitors which interfere in the HI test. Results with the type-specific NP antigen may not always parallel results with the HA antigen. Antibody rises to the NP antigen are often poor in early childhood but respond rapidly to infection in later years. In older adults titers tend to persist longer and are less likely to show significant increases after infection. Directions for performing the CF test are presented in chapter 58 of this *Manual*. Descriptions of influenza virus CF reagents and their preparation have been given elsewhere (5).

The HI test for antibody to the HA antigen is based on the ability of influenza viruses to agglutinate erythrocytes and the ability of specific HA antibody to inhibit this agglutination. The major disadvantage of the HI test is that nonspecific inhibitors can be found in a wide variety of animal sera, and treatment of sera is required to prevent false-positive reactions. The major advantages of the HI test are that it is simple, requires only standard equipment, and can be performed with a variety of erythrocytes over a wide range of hydrogen ion concentrations and temperatures. Because of its sensitivity, simplicity, and versatility, the HI test is probably the most frequently used test for influenza serodiagnosis and serosurveys.

Detailed reviews of the techniques for influenza virus identification and serodiagnosis were given by Schild and Dowdle (8), Dowdle and Coleman (2), and Hoyle (4).

CLINICAL INDICATIONS

Because of the requirement for simultaneous testing of acute and convalescent paired sera for diagnosis, serological procedures provide little or no guidance for clinical management of the patient with acute influenza. Retrospective diagnosis of influenza, however, can be important in establishing the presence of influenza in the community and in the management of clinically similar cases. In many instances, outbreaks of influenza may be diagnosed in less than 24 h by testing 10 or more acute and an equal number of convalescent sera collected from different individuals matched with respect to age. The basis for this test is the observation that, by the time the presence of an outbreak in the community is recognized, a number of persons usually are already convalescing from the illness and a number of other persons are in the early acute stages. The use of unpaired sera for rapid diagnosis of influenza outbreaks has been previously described in detail (7).

HEMAGGLUTINATION-INHIBITION TEST (MICROTITER)

Hemagglutination titration

Titrate influenza virus suspensions representing contemporary type A and B strains with washed erythrocytes suspended in 0.01 M phosphate-buffered physiological saline (PBS), pH 7.2. Use guinea pig (0.4%), human type O (0.4%), or chicken (0.5%) erythrocyte suspensions. Dilute the virus suspensions 1:10 in PBS. Prepare twofold serial dilutions from 1:10 through 1:2,560 in 0.05-ml volumes in microtiter plates. Add 0.05 ml of erythrocyte control (diluent plus erythrocytes). Mix and incubate at room temperature until erythrocytes settle. Hemagglutination is determined by tilting the plates and noting the absence of "tear-shaped" streaming of erythrocytes which flow at the same rate as erythrocyte controls (Fig. 1). The highest dilution of virus which causes agglutination is considered the titration end point; that dilution contains 1 hemagglutination unit (HA unit) per 0.05 ml.

Preparation of test antigen

Perform the HI test with a test antigen preparation containing 4 HA units in 0.025 ml. Since 0.025 ml of the HA end point dilution would contain only 0.5 HA unit, determine the proper dilution of virus to be used in the HI test by dividing the HA titer by 8. For example, if

PATTERNS OF COMPLETELY AGGLUTINATED CELLS

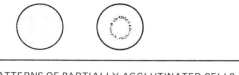

PATTERNS OF PARTIALLY AGGLUTINATED CELLS

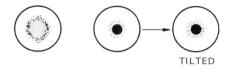

TILTED

PATTERNS OF NON AGGLUTINATED CELLS

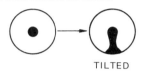

TILTED

FIG. 1. *Examples of settled erythrocyte patterns in the HI test. From Palmer et al. (7).*

the HA titer is 160 with titration volumes of 0.05 ml (by definition 0.05 ml of the end point dilution contains 1 unit), then a 1:20 dilution contains 8 HA units in 0.05 ml or 4 HA in 0.025 ml.

To control possible errors in dilution and to confirm the HA titer, retitrate the test or working virus dilution. Prepare a row of six wells, each containing 0.05 ml of diluent. Add 0.05 ml of the working dilution of virus (8 HA units) to the first well, and make the twofold dilution series through five wells. To the sixth well add 0.05 ml of diluent in place of virus. This will serve as the cell control. Add 0.05 ml of the erythrocyte suspension to all wells and mix; allow the contents to settle. The cell control and the last two wells should show compact buttons of normal settling. Agglutination in the first three wells of the series indicates that the working dilution contains 8 HA units of virus per 0.05-ml volume or 4 HA units per 0.025-ml volume to be used in the HI test. Adjust the virus concentration of the working dilution, if necessary, by adding PBS (if more than three wells show agglutination) or by adding virus (if fewer than three wells show agglutination). If adjustment of working antigen dilution is required, confirm its HA titer by retitration as just described.

Serum treatment. Many influenza viruses are highly sensitive to serum factors which may nonspecifically inhibit agglutination. Such inhibitors, which are usually sialic acid-containing mucoproteins, can successfully be removed

from human sera with the receptor-destroying enzyme (RDE) of *Vibrio cholerae* or with potassium periodate (KIO$_4$).

For RDE treatment, add 4 volumes of RDE (100 units per ml) to each volume of serum. Incubate the mixture overnight in a water bath at 37 C. Add 3 volumes of 2.5% sodium citrate and incubate the mixture at 56 C for 30 min. Add 2 volumes of PBS to yield a final 1:10 dilution of treated serum.

For KIO$_4$ treatment, add 0.3 ml of 0.011 M KIO$_4$ to 0.1 ml of serum. Incubate the serum-KIO$_4$ mixtures for 15 min at room temperature. Add 0.3 ml of 1% glycerol-saline solution to neutralize excess KIO$_4$. Add 0.3 ml of PBS to bring the serum dilution to a final 1:10.

Nonspecific agglutination of human O or chicken erythrocytes by human sera occurs infrequently. However, if serum control wells (PBS substituted for virus) indicate nonspecific agglutination, absorb the serum by adding 0.1 ml of 50% erythrocytes to 1 ml of the 1:10 dilution of treated serum. Allow absorption to proceed for 1 h at 4 C and remove erythrocytes by centrifugation.

Test procedures

Test paired human sera for influenza diagnosis with one or more contemporary type A and B strains. Include reference antisera to confirm the identity of each strain used in the test. Prepare twofold dilutions of treated antiserum from 1:10 through 1:2,560 in 0.025-ml volumes. The number of rows depends upon the number of antigens to be used. Add 0.025 ml of the test virus suspension containing 4 HA units to each well. To test for agglutinins in the serum, add diluent instead of antigen to a well containing the lowest dilution of serum. Also prepare cell controls (PBS only) and antigen controls (PBS and antigen) for each test. Shake and incubate the plates for 30 min at room temperature.

Add 0.05 ml of erythrocytes to each well, and then shake and incubate the plates at room temperature until the cell control shows the button of normal settling. The HI titer is defined as the dilution factor of the highest dilution of serum which completely inhibits hemagglutination. Determine complete inhibition by tilting the plates and observing the "tear-shaped" streaming of cells which flow at the same rate as control cells.

REAGENTS

Hemagglutination antigen

Prepare influenza virus antigens for use in the HI test in 10- or 11-day-old embryonated hen eggs. Swab eggs directly over the air sac with 70% alcohol, and punch a small hole in the shell. Place the egg on a candler with air sac up to note position and confirm viability of the embryo. Inject 0.1 ml of seed virus into the allantoic cavity, and seal the hole in the shell with "model airplane cement" or wax. Incubate the eggs at 33 C for 72 h. Chill eggs overnight to minimize bleeding during harvesting. Swab the area over the air sac with 70% alcohol, and break the shell away to the level of the allantoic membrane. Pull the membrane away with sterile forceps, and harvest the fluid with pipette or syringe. Infected allantoic fluid may be stored for several months at 4 C. Sodium azide may be added to a final concentration of 0.1% as a preservative. Contemporary type A and B virus antigen for the HI test may also be obtained commercially (Flow Laboratories, Inc.; Microbiological Associates, Inc.).

Erythrocyte suspension

Add 1 volume of whole blood to 4 volumes of Alsever's solution. Erythrocytes suspended in Alsever's solution may be kept under refrigeration for as long as 1 week. Before suspensions are used, wash them three times with PBS, centrifuge at $250 \times g$ for 10 min, and resuspend to a concentration of 0.4% for guinea pig and human O erythrocytes and 0.5% for chicken erythrocytes.

Potassium periodate (KIO₄) for serum treatment

Prepare 0.011 M KIO_4 by adding 129 mg to 50 ml of distilled water, and dissolve with the aid of a magnetic stirrer. Prepare 1% glycerol-saline solution by adding 0.5 ml of glycerol to 49.5 ml of 0.85% NaCl solution in distilled water.

Reference antisera

Dilute infected allantoic harvests to contain approximately 160 HA units/ml. Obtain a preliminary 2-ml blood sample from the wing vein of each chicken to be injected, and examine by HI test for absence of preexisting antibody. Using a 5-ml hypodermic syring fitted with a 25-gauge hypodermic needle, slowly inject 5 ml of virus suspension into a wing vein. Nine or 10 days after injection, exsanguinate the chicken by cardiac puncture with a 50-ml hypodermic syringe fitted with an 18-gauge, 9-cm hypodermic needle.

Antiserum produced by infection of susceptible animals or injection with inactivated whole virus suspensions may contain antibodies to the NA as well as the HA antigen. Under some conditions in the HI test, the NA antibody may cause low-level inhibition of some strains and suggest false antigenic relationships (10). This is not a problem when sera are used as controls in a diagnostic test. Reference antisera may also be obtained from commercial sources (Flow Laboratories, Inc.; Microbiological Associates, Inc.).

INTERPRETATION

Evaluation of the microtiter HI test for all myxoviruses has shown within-test reproducibility to be 80 to 90% for exact titers and 100% for titers differing by no more than one dilution (3). In a still larger evaluation of the test for serodiagnosis of influenza, the World Health Organization Collaborating Center for Influenza in Atlanta, Ga., found within-test reproducibility to be 95% for titers differing by no more than one dilution. A fourfold or greater change in antibody titer under these standard test conditions is highly significant. A fourfold or greater increase in antibody titer between acute and convalescent sera can therefore be interpreted as compatible with recent influenza virus infection or vaccination.

To achieve maximal HI test results, all possible sources of error must be eliminated. For example, sera must be treated adequately to remove nonspecific inhibitors. The reference virus strain should be known to be sensitive to HA antibody in the HI test. Erythrocytes should be fresh and have normal settling patterns. Errors which are frequently made by misinterpretation of erythrocyte settling patterns should be avoided by reading the test for "streaming" of erythrocytes. Finally, in interpreting HI test results from an HA antibody serosurvey, it should be recognized that low HI titers under some conditions may result from NA antigen-antibody interaction (10). NA antibody is unlikely to interfere when the HI test is used for serodiagnosis of recent infections.

Fourfold or greater antibody rises to the type A or B virus used in the test indicate an infection or vaccination with that virus type but not necessarily with that strain. Anamnestic responses frequently occur, depending upon the previous immunological experiences of the individual. In many instances, antibody titers to an older strain may increase at a faster rate and exceed the titer to the infecting strain. For this reason, diagnostic efficiency can often be increased by including recently prevalent as well as currently prevalent strains.

The sensitivity of the HI test for serodiagnosis of infection is difficult to assess. Studies which have compared the HI test with the type-specific (NP) CF test have shown HI to be superior in some instances and CF in others. The superiority of either one of these tests depends upon the age and previous antigenic experience of the individual, the strain used in the test, and the interval between acute and convalescent sera. Some laboratories use both tests for maximal diagnostic efficacy. Even then, diagnosis cannot always be assured. Reports vary, but it is clear that a small percentage of patients may be ill, shed virus, and still fail to respond with significant increases in antibody titer.

LITERATURE CITED

1. Aymard-Henry, M., M. T. Coleman, W. R. Dowdle, W. G. Laver, G. C. Schild, and R. G. Webster. 1973. Influenza virus neuraminidase and neuraminidase-inhibition test procedures. Bull. WHO 48:199–202.
2. Dowdle, W. R., and M. T. Coleman. 1974. Influenza virus, p. 678–685. In E. H. Lennette, E. H. Spaulding, and J. P. Truant (ed.), Manual of clinical microbiology, 2nd ed. American Society for Microbiology, Washington, D.C.
3. Hierholzer, J. C., M. T. Suggs, and E. C. Hall. 1969. Standardized viral hemagglutination and hemagglutination-inhibition test. II. Description and statistical evaluation. Appl. Microbiol. 18:824–833.
4. Hoyle, L. 1968. The influenza viruses. Virol. Monogr. No. 4.
5. Lief, F. S. 1963. Antigenic analysis of influenza viruses by complement fixation. VII. Further studies on production of pure anti-S serum and on specificity of type A S antigens. J. Immunol. 90:172–177.
6. Mostow, S. R., G. C. Schild, W. R. Dowdle, and R. J. Wood. 1975. Application of the single radial immunodiffusion test for assay of antibody to influenza type A virus. J. Clin. Microbiol. 2:351–540.
7. Palmer, D. F., W. R. Dowdle, M. T. Coleman, and G. C. Schild. 1975. Advanced laboratory techniques for influenza diagnosis. Center for Disease Control, Atlanta, Ga.
8. Schild, G. C., and W. R. Dowdle. 1975. Influenza virus characterization and diagnostic serology, p. 315–372. In E. D. Kilbourne (ed.), The influenza viruses. Academic Press Inc., New York.
9. Schild, G. C., M. Henry-Aymard, and H. G. Pereira. 1972. A quantitative single-radial-immunodiffusion test for immunological studies with influenza virus. J. Gen. Virol. 16:231–236.
10. Schulman, J. L., and E. D. Kilbourne. 1969. Independent variation in nature of influenza virus: distinctiveness of the hemagglutinin. Proc. Natl. Acad. Sci. U.S.A. 63:326–333.
11. WHO Expert Committee. 1971. A revised system of nomenclature for influenza viruses. Bull. WHO 45:119–124.

Chapter 58

Respiratory Syncytial Virus and the Parainfluenza Viruses

MAURICE A. MUFSON

INTRODUCTION

Respiratory syncytial virus and parainfluenza viruses types 1, 2, 3, and 4 commonly cause acute lower respiratory tract diseases, mainly bronchiolitis and pneumonia, in infants and children and upper respiratory tract illness in adults (6, 9, 10). Infrequently do these agents cause pneumonia in adults. Serological evidence of infection with respiratory syncytial virus and the parainfluenza viruses can be determined by several methods, including complement-fixation and neutralization procedures, and, additionally, for the parainfluenza viruses, hemagglutination inhibition.

As routine diagnostic antibody tests, complement-fixation procedures for respiratory syncytial and parainfluenza viruses and hemagglutination-inhibition tests for the parainfluenza viruses are easy methods for measuring circulating antibody responses during infection. For the survey of antibody status among groups of individuals to respiratory syncytial and the parainfluenza viruses, virus neutralization tests detect protective antibody and indicate the level of immunity in individuals in the group. Neutralization tests can be conducted in roller tube tissue cultures, petri dishes, or microtiter plates (3, 7, 12). Since antibody measured by hemagglutination inhibition correlates well with the level of protective antibody assayed by neutralization, such tests for the parainfluenza viruses provide a reliable and more rapid method for survey of type-specific antibody.

CLINICAL INDICATIONS

The choice of test to assay antibody to the parainfluenza and respiratory syncytial viruses depends on the information needed concerning the immunological status of the individual, on the one hand, and the rapidity and ease of its performance, on the other. Both complement-fixation and hemagglution-inhibition procedures provide specific and reliable assays for measurement of antibody in acute- and convalescent-phase paired sera and can be performed in hospital laboratories as routine tests. These tests are usually done by use of microtiter procedures (13). By contrast, virus neutralization procedures seem too laborious for the measurement of antibody responses during the course of an individual patient's illness. The neutralization test should be reserved for special surveys and research purposes rather than the routine measurement of parainfluenza or respiratory syncytial virus antibody responses as would be usually undertaken by hospital laboratories.

Unfortunately, serological tests for the measurement of antibody responses during acute virus infections require paired sera for simultaneous testing to detect rising levels of antibody. Of necessity, the test cannot be performed until a convalescent serum has been obtained late in the course of illness. Usually the patient has recovered by this time. Nonetheless, the measurement of antibody responses of individual patients can provide retrospective evidence of infection with respiratory syncytial and the parainfluenza viruses, especially in the absence of virus isolation, and signal the presence of an outbreak of these viruses in the community.

TEST PROCEDURES

Complement fixation

The measurement of antibody by complement fixation is performed with microtiter procedures, because it conserves antigen, provides ease of operation, and allows the simultaneous testing of many sera quickly and accurately. The characteristics of this system have been described in detail (8).

For the measurement of antibody to the parainfluenza viruses and respiratory syncytial virus in sera from infants and children, it is important that 8 units of the viral antigen be used; 4 units of antigen suffices for testing of sera from adults (1). Tissue culture-grown antigens can be purchased from commercial sources. Respiratory syncytial virus antigen can be produced by a low multiplicity infection of HEp-2 cells (supplemented with inactivated chicken serum), and parainfluenza virus antigen can be produced by infection of rhesus monkey kidney cells and harvest of the cultures when maximal cytopathic effect (CPE) develops.

The guinea pig complement should be tested to assure that it lacks antibody to the parainfluenza viruses, and other myxoviruses, because guinea pigs can readily acquire these infections. Test each lot of guinea pig complement for parainfluenza, influenza, and mump virus antibodies before use; purchase additional complement from a negative lot.

Initially, test each serum for anticomplementary activity. Any serum found to be anticomplementary can be treated with mouse liver powder and then retested to determine whether or not the anticomplementary activity has been eliminated (11). Briefly, the procedure is as follows:

1. Mix 200 mg of mouse liver powder with 1.0 ml of serum and shake continuously for 1 h at room temperature.

2. Centrifuge the mixture at 2,000 to 2,500 rpm for 20 min.

3. Remove the serum with a fine-pointed pipette and inactivate at 56 C for 30 min.

The use of four dilutions, 1:8, 1:16, 1:32, and 1:64, for testing acute and convalescent sera provides an efficient scheme for the detection of antibody responses, and at the same time conserves antigen. Occasionally, however, no end point is reached with this dilution series, and the test must be repeated with higher dilutions of sera, e.g., 1:8, 1:16, 1:32, 1:64, 1:128, 1:256, and 1:512. Low-level rises in paired sera from infants and children may only be detected with serum dilutions starting at 1:2. Acute- and convalescent-phase sera from a single patient must be tested in the same test.

Briefly, the procedure for the complement-fixation test is as follows:

1. Dispense 0.025 ml of 0.85% saline containing magnesium and calcium (diluent), in appropriate wells of a disposable "U" well plastic disposable microtiter plate. Prepare diluent by adding 1 ml of magnesium-calcium saline ($MgCl_2 \cdot 6H_2O$, 10 g, and $CaCl_2 \cdot 2H_2O$, 4 g, in 100 ml of distilled water) to 1,000 ml of 0.85% saline. Use this diluent throughout the test.

2. Inactivate serum at 56 C for 30 min. Make twofold dilutions of serum with a 0.025-ml microdilutor (or "loop").

3. Add by pipette dropper 0.025 ml of antigen to each dilution of serum.

4. Prepare serial twofold dilutions of a positive serum control from 1:2 to 1:64 with a 0.025-ml microdilutor.

5. To the positive serum control, add with a pipette-dropper 0.025 ml of diluent to each well; for an antigen control, add 0.025 ml of diluent to each of six wells; for the erythrocyte control, add 0.075 ml of diluent to each of four wells; and, for the complement control, add 0.05 ml of

diluent to each of eight wells.

6. Add 0.025 ml of antigen diluted to contain 4 or 8 units (as required) to each well containing dilutions of the positive serum control.

7. Make successive twofold dilutions, usually 1:2 to 1:64, of antigen, using 0.025 ml, and add 0.25 ml of diluent to each antigen control well.

8. Dilute complement in cold diluent to contain 2 exact units. Further twofold dilutions of complement are made to contain 1, 0.5, and 0.25 units of complement.

9. Add 0.025 ml of each dilution of complement to the appropriate control wells.

10. Add 0.025 ml of the initial complement dilution containing 2 units to the remainder of the test, except for the erythrocyte control wells.

11. Tap the plates gently on all four sides to mix, cover with transparent adhesive cellophane tape, and incubate overnight at 4 C.

12. The next morning, warm the plates to room temperature for approximately 20 min, and add 0.05 ml of sensitized sheep erythrocytes to each well (prepared by mixing equal volumes of the erythrocyte suspension and hemolysin diluted to contain 2 units).

13. Tap the plate gently on all four sides to mix the erythrocytes, and incubate at 37 C for 30 to 45 min or until the complement controls show cell lysis. When the complement controls show the appropriate degree of hemolysis, transfer the plates from the 37 C incubator to a refrigerator at 4 C. The complement control wells containing 2 units should show complete hemolysis, and the 1-unit wells should show nearly complete or complete hemolysis; the erythrocytes in the 0.5- and 0.25-unit wells should not be hemolyzed. Remove the plates from 4 C after 1 h, warm to room temperature for 20 min, and read the test. Dilutions of test serum showing hemolysis of 75% or more of the erythrocytes are considered antibody positive.

Hemagglutination inhibition for parainfluenza virus antibody

Hemagglutination-inhibition procedures easily provide data on serological responses in parainfluenza virus infection, especially when microtiter techniques are used. Antigen consisting of tissue culture harvests of untreated virus can be prepared by low-multiplicity infection of rhesus monkey kidney cells and harvest of virus at maximal hemagglutination activity. Test a sample of culture media daily and harvest on the day of high-titer antigen, usually after the fifth day of incubation. Freeze the untreated harvest in small portions at -70 C, incorporating 0.5% bovine serum albumin at final concentration for antigen stabilization. Add 0.1 ml of a 10% suspension of sterile bovine serum albumin to each 1.9 ml of virus antigen, and adjust to pH 7 with one or two drops of 1 N sodium hydroxide.

Treatment of tissue culture harvests with Tween 80 and ether increases the hemagglutinin titer (5). Briefly, add Tween 80 to the tissue culture harvest at a final concentration of 0.1%. Mix and add ether to increase the total volume by one-third. Mix vigorously for 5 to 15 min at 4 C. Centrifuge and pipette the lower aqueous phase into a flask gently. Bubble nitrogen through the antigen to remove residual ether. Hemagglutination antigens can also be purchased from commercial sources.

For the microtiter procedure, "U" well plastic disposable plates are preferred. The hemagglutination patterns in "U" wells are easily interpreted. Initially, antigen lots must be titrated and a dilution of antigen containing 1 hemagglutinin unit per unit of volume must be determined. Use 4 units of antigen per unit of volume in the hemagglutination-inhibition test.

The procedure for determining the hemagglutinin content of the antigen preparation is as follows:

1. Dispense 0.05 ml of 0.85% phosphate-buffered saline (PBS) into duplicate columns of 10 wells each, and 5 additional wells for erythrocyte controls.

2. Make twofold dilutions of antigen with a 0.05-ml microdilutor in duplicate, starting in the first well and proceeding to the tenth well.

3. Dispense 0.05 ml of a 1% solution of guinea pig erythrocytes in PBS into each virus-containing well and into the erythrocyte control wells. Prepare erythrocyte dilutions fresh daily; the stock erythrocytes should be between 1 and 4 days old.

4. Tap gently on all four sides of the plate to mix.

5. Incubate at room temperature for 1 h and read the test.

6. The end point is the last dilution showing hemagglutination of about 50% of the cells. This represents 1 hemagglutinin unit per 0.05 ml, and in the hemagglutination-inhibition test use 4 hemagglutinin units in a 0.025-ml volume (or eight times the concentration of the dilution containing 1 hemagglutinin unit as measured in the hemagglutination test in which 0.05-ml volumes are employed).

The procedure for the hemagglutination-inhibition test is as follows:

1. Treat serum to remove nonspecific inhibitors of hemagglutination, by using receptor-destroying enzyme (RDE), which can be purchased from commercial sources. Add 0.1 ml of RDE to 0.1 ml of sera and incubate overnight at 37 C. The next morning, add 0.3 ml of PBS to the mixture and inactivate at 56 C for 30 min. This is a 1:5 dilution of serum, which can be used immediately or stored at −20 C for testing later.

2. Test each serum in duplicate, and acute and convalescent sera in the same test.

3. Serum should be tested starting at a dilution of 1:10, twofold dilutions are carried out to 1:1,280 or 1:2,560.

4. Dispense 0.025 ml of PBS in the appropriate number of wells.

5. Dip a 0.025-ml microdilutor into the 1:5 dilution of treated serum and loop it into the first well PBS; mix and continue the dilution process. The initial serum dilution of the first well is now 1:10.

6. Add 0.025 ml of antigen containing 4 units per 0.025 ml to each serum dilution.

7. Tap gently on all four sides of the plate to mix, and incubate at room temperature for 1 h.

8. For the serum control, mix 0.025 ml of the 1:5 dilution of treated serum in a well with 0.025 ml of the PBS and then add 0.025 ml of PBS with a dropper pipette.

9. For the virus control titration (virus "back titration"), drop 0.05 ml of PBS in five wells, and in the first well loop 0.05 ml of the dilution of virus antigen used in the test; continue the dilution process through the five wells. For interpretation, the first well (or highest concentration) is designated 4 units, and the succeeding dilutions, 2, 1, 0.5, and 0 units.

10. After 1 h of incubation at room temperature, add 0.05 ml of 1% guinea pig erythrocytes in PBS to each well, tap the plate gently on all four sides to mix, incubate at room temperature for 1 h, and read. Note that the erythrocytes in wells with serum will settle more quickly and may be read at 30 to 45 min, but the cell control and virus titration usually require the full 60 min of incubation.

11. The pattern of the virus control titration should show complete hemagglutination in the wells estimated to contain 4, 2, and 1 units of hemagglutination, and no hemagglutination in the remaining two wells. Slight variations from this pattern are acceptable.

12. The serum hemagglutination-inhibition end point is the last dilution showing complete inhibition of hemagglutination.

Neutralization test for respiratory syncytial virus antibody

The measurement of neutralizing antibody to respiratory syncytial virus can be performed by plaque reduction, tube neutralization procedures, or in microtiter plates (1, 3, 7). Plaque assay provides an especially sensitive measure of neutralizing antibody. Its use and interpretation are facilitated by techniques which produce large clear plaques (1 to 2 mm in diameter) in susceptible cell monolayers (usually HEp-2 cells). The sensitivity of HEp-2 cells for replication of respiratory syncytial virus varies with the source of the cells, and several lines may have to be tested to find a sensitive one. Several plaque procedures for respiratory syncytial virus antibody measurement have been described, each with slight but not major variations in the conduct of the test (3, 7). The plaque procedure used in our laboratory provides end points in 5 to 6 days.

The *plaque reduction test* for respiratory syncytial virus antibody is performed as follows:

1. HEp-2 cells grown in plastic (or glass) flat-sided bottles are treated with 0.25% trypsin for 15 to 20 min, and the dispersed cells are washed and suspended in growth media consisting of Eagle's minimal essential medium (EMEM) supplemented with 10% calf serum and appropriate antibiotics.

2. Seed the cell suspension into plastic 60-mm tissue culture petri dishes and incubate in a 5% carbon dioxide atmosphere at 37 C.

3. Wash the confluent cell sheets twice with Hanks balanced salt solution (HBSS).

4. Inactivate test sera at 56 C for 30 min and make dilutions of virus in growth media. Use 1:10, 1:40, 1:160, and 1:320 dilutions of sera in the initial test, but if no end point is reached adjust dilutions in the repeat test.

5. Mix 0.2 ml of respiratory syncytial virus diluted to contain approximately 20 to 50 plaque-forming units (PFU) with an equal volume of each serum dilution and incubate at room temperature for 1 h.

6. Inoculate duplicate dishes with 0.2 ml of virus-serum mixture.

7. Add 0.2 ml of HBSS solution to each dish to prevent drying during virus absorption.

8. Gently agitate the plates every 15 min during the 2-h absorption period to allow equal distribution of the inoculum.

9. After absorption, rinse the plates with HBSS and overlay the cells with 10 ml of a fresh 2% methylcellulose (viscosity, 15 counts/s) solution in EMEM.

10. Incubate the plates for 5 to 6 days in a 5% carbon dioxide atmosphere at 37 C.

11. At the end of the incubation period, decant the overlay and add 5 ml of 10% formalin to each dish to preserve the cells.

12. The following day, rinse the cells in tap water and air-dry.

13. Plaques appear as 1- to 2-mm diameter defects in the confluent cell monolayer. Microscopically, the defects are respiratory syncytial virus syncytia, some of which have become detached in part from the dish. Optionally, the cells can be stained with Giemsa stain.

14. Control plates include virus alone and diluent alone.

15. Express the plaque reduction neutralizing antibody titer as a reciprocal of the serum dilution producing a 50% reduction in plaque count from the virus control.

Alternatively, a *tube neutralization procedure* can be used for the measurement of neutralizing antibody to respiratory syncytial virus. The test can be performed as follows:

1. Inactivate serum specimens at 56 C for 30 min, and dilute in EMEM supplemented with 5% inactivated chicken serum and appropriate antibiotics.

2. Serum dilutions used are 1:4, 1:8, 1:16, 1:32, 1:64, and 1:128.

3. Mix each serum dilution with an equal volume of virus diluted to contain approximately 100 TCD_{50} per ml.

4. Inoculate 0.2 ml of each serum virus mixture into duplicate roller tube cultures containing a light growth of HEp-2 cells.

5. At daily intervals after the third day, the virus control tubes are examined for CPE.

6. Read the test when the virus control tubes exhibit CPE involving all or nearly all of the cell sheet (75 to 100% CPE).

7. Add neutral red at a final concentration of 1:80,000 to each tube and incubate the tubes for 1 h at 37 C. Neutral red stains respiratory syncytial virus syncytium red and facilitates their visual identification with a scanning objective. After neutral red has been added to the roller tube cultures, they must be protected from light, usually by wrapping the entire rack of tubes in aluminum foil; once ready for reading, the tubes should be examined quickly and protected as much as possible from stray light.

8. The end point is the dilution of serum which inhibits the formation of CPE so that no more than one-fourth of the cell sheet shows involvement by respiratory syncytial virus syncytia.

Measurement of neutralization antibody for the parainfluenza viruses

For the measurement of antibody to the four parainfluenza viruses, individual tests must be carried out with the specific virus type as the challenge virus in the neutralization test. Since the parainfluenza viruses do not usually produce CPE in tissue culture, but do exhibit hemadsorption, the end point of the neutralization procedure is the demonstration of hemadsorption inhibition.

The procedure is as follows:

1. Inactivate serum specimens as 56 C for 30 min and prepare serial twofold dilutions in EMEM without serum, but containing the appropriate antibiotics. Usually, the dilutions tested include 1:4, 1:8, 1:16, 1:32, and 1:128.

2. Mix equal volumes of each serum dilution and virus containing approximately 100 TCD_{50} per 0.1 ml and incubate at room temperature for 1 h.

3. Inoculate duplicate roller tube cultures of rhesus monkey kidney cells with 0.2 ml of each virus-serum mixture.

4. Include a virus (back titration) and serum controls.

5. Incubate cell cultures on a stationary rack at 37 C.

6. After the third day, all virus control tubes are tested for hemadsorption by the addition of 0.25 ml of a 0.4% solution of sterile guinea pig erythrocytes in saline. Once the erythrocytes have been added to the roller tube cultures, refrigerate the tubes for 20 min and then examine them for hemadsorption. On the day the virus titration shows a titer between 32 and 100 TCD_{50} of virus, add erythrocytes to all tubes, refrigerate for 20 min, and read the test.

7. The end point is the dilution of serum showing complete inhibition of hemadsorption.

REAGENTS

Small amounts of certified antigens for complement-fixation and hemagglutination-inhibition tests can be obtained from the Center for Disease Control, Atlanta, Ga. These antigens should be used to evaluate and standardize commercial reagents. Seed virus for producing complement-fixation and hemagglutination-inhibition or virus neutralization tests is available from the American Type Culture Collection, Rockville, Md., and the Infectious Diseases Branch, National Institute of Allergy and Infectious Diseases, Bethesda, Md.

Commercial sources

Complement-fixation and hemagglutination-inhibition antigens: Microbiological Associates, Bethesda, Md.; Flow Laboratories, Bethesda, Md.; and BioQuest, Cockeysville, Md.

Complement: Texas Biological Laboratories, Inc., Fort Worth, Tex.

Tissue culture media: Microbiological Associates; Flow Laboratories; BioQuest; Grand Island Biological Co., Grand Island, N.Y.; and International Scientific Industries, Cary, Ill.

Methylcellulose: Dow Chemical Co., Midland, Mich.

These reagents are also available from other sources. It behooves each user to evaluate the quality of purchased reagents.

INTERPRETATION

The serological diagnosis of respiratory syncytial and parainfluenza virus infections, or an acute virus infection in general, requires the detection of a fourfold or greater increase in antibody during convalescence compared with the acute-phase antibody level. The detection of at least this magnitude of increase in antibodies confirms the occurrence of infection. Usually one-half or more of infants and children and adults develop diagnostic antibody rises for respiratory syncytial and the parainfluenza viruses by complement fixation. Hemagglutination-inhibition tests provide similar sensitivity for parainfluenza virus infection.

Heterotypic antibody responses detected by complement fixation and hemagglutination inhibition frequently occur with parainfluenza virus infections. Parainfluenza virus antibody rises also occur following mumps virus infections (2). Consequently, it is difficult to establish the type of the infecting virus based on serological procedures alone. Virus isolation procedures must be performed to do this.

With respiratory syncytial virus infection of infants and children, usually only approximately one-half of them develop fourfold or greater rises in complement-fixation antibody (1, 9, 10). Slightly less than one-half of these individuals also develop rises in neutralization antibody. By contrast, most adults who develop diagnostic respiratory syncytial virus antibody rises also develop neutralization antibody rises (4).

Unchanging high levels of antibody in acute- and convalescent-phase sera suggest recent virus infection. Possibly the high level of antibody in the acute-phase serum reflects the development of antibody as a consequence of recent infection, but the collection of the serum occurred after the onset of infection and antibody had appeared. Unchanging high levels of antibody also can represent past virus infection with persistence of high antibody levels. Consequently, considering unchanging high levels of antibody as diagnostic of a recent virus infection entails a value judgement. Similar arguments preclude definitely considering the detection of a fourfold or greater declining titer of antibody between acute- and convalescent-phase sera as evidence of a recent virus infection, especially if the acute-phase serum was not collected as early as possible after the onset of infection or the convalescent-phase serum was obtained late, or both.

LITERATURE CITED

1. Chanock, R. M., H. W. Kim, A. J. Vargosko, A. Deleva, K. Johnson, C. Cumming, and R. H. Parrott. 1961. Respiratory syncytial virus. I. Virus recovery and other observations during 1960 outbreak of bronchiolitis, pneumonia and minor respiratory diseases in children. J. Am. Med. Assoc. 176:647–653.

2. Chanock, R. M., D. Wong, R. J. Huebner, and J. A. Bell. 1960. Serologic response of individuals infected with parainfluenza viruses. Am. J. Public Health 50:1858–1865.

3. Coates, H. V., D. W. Alling, and R. M. Chanock. 1966. An antigenic analysis of respiratory syncytial virus isolates by plaque reduction neutralization test. Am. J. Epidemiol. 83:299–313.

4. Johnson, K. M., H. H. Bloom, M. A. Mufson, and R. M. Chanock. 1962. Natural reinfection of adults by respiratory syncytial virus: possible relation to mild upper respiratory illness. N. Engl. J. Med. 267:68–72.

5. Killgore, G. E., and W. R. Dowdle. 1970. Antigenic characterization of parainfluenza 4A and 4B by the hemagglutination-inhibition test and distribution of HI antibody in human sera. Am. J. Epidemiol. 93:308–316.

6. Kim, H. W., J. O. Arrobio, C. D. Brandt, B. C. Jeffries, G. Pyles, J. L. Reid, R. M. Chanock, and R. H. Parrott. 1973. Epidemiology of respiratory syncytial virus infection in Washington, D.C. I. Importance of the virus in different respiratory tract disease syndromes and temporal distribution of infection. Am. J. Epidemiol. 98:216–225.

7. Kisch, A. L., and K. M. Johnson. 1963. A plaque assay for respiratory syncytial virus. Proc. Soc. Exp. Biol. Med. 112:583–589.

8. Lennette, E. H. 1969. General principles underlying laboratory diagnosis of viral and rickettsial infections, p. 1–65. In E. H. Lennette and N. J. Schmidt (ed.), Diagnostic procedures for viral and rickettsial infections, 4th ed. American Public Health Association, Inc., New York.

9. Mufson, M. A., H. D. Levine, R. E. Wasil, H. E. Mocega-Gonzalez, and H. E. Krause. 1973. Epidemiology of respiratory syncytial virus infection among infants and children in Chicago. Am. J. Epidemiol. 98:88–95.

10. Parrott, R. H., H. W. Kim, J. O. Arrobio, D. S. Hodes, B. R. Murphy, C. D. Brandt, E. Camargo, and R. M. Chanock. 1973. Epidemiology of respiratory syncytial virus infection in Washington, D.C. II. Infection and disease with respect to age, immunologic status, race and sex. Am. J. Epidemiol. 98:289–300.

11. Rapp, F., G. M. Gnesh, and I. Gordon. 1955. A practical method for removal of anticomplementary properties from human serum. Proc. Soc. Exp. Biol. Med. 90:335–339.

12. Schmidt, M. J., E. H. Lennette, and M. F. Hanahoe. 1966. A micromethod for performing parainfluenza virus neutralization tests. Proc. Soc. Exp. Biol. Med. 122:1062–1067.

13. Sever, J. L. 1962. Application of a microtechnique to viral serological investigations. J. Immunol. 88:320–329.

Chapter 59

Measles and Mumps

FRANCIS L. BLACK

INTRODUCTION

The infectious agents of both measles and mumps are paramyxoviruses, and both carry several distinct polypeptides capable of stimulating an immune response. Measles virus antigens, however, are unique for agents infecting humans, and the immune response is, to all effects, specific (3). Infection with measles virus results in primary reactions in each aspect of the immune response. Mumps antigens are related to those of the parainfluenzas and Newcastle disease. Mumps antibodies may rise in response to infection with other agents, and differential degrees of relatedness between the several antigens of mumps and parainfluenza means that in mumps virus infection some components of the immune response will usually be primary in nature and some secondary. Both viruses possess hemagglutinins, but red cell specificity differs, and only mumps virus possesses a neuraminidase which may release hemagglutination.

The choice of a serological test for measles can be made purely on the basis of sensitivity and convenience, because the several manifestations of the immune reaction move in synchrony, and all are measles virus specific. On both scores, the hemagglutination-inhibition (HI) test is usually preferred.

A serological test for current mumps infection must be capable of demonstrating qualitative as well as quantitative changes if specific reactions are to be distinguished from anamnestic rises in response to other infections. On the other hand, a test for mumps immunity must be chosen primarily on the basis of specificity. For diagnosis, the change in relative complement-fixation (CF) titer with released virus (V) and cell-associated (S) antigens has long been used (7). Antibody to the S antigen usually rises before V antibody, presumably because the S antigens are less specific and more influenced by prior sensitization. Recently, fluorescent-antibody binding (4) and radioimmune adherence (6) techniques have been proposed. With either of these newer techniques, distinguishing immunoglobulin M (IgM) from IgG is relatively easy, and they will probably provide a more reliable index of current infection than the CF test. Both methods, however, require special reagents or cell cultures that are not readily available, and experience with the tests has been limited to date. For determination of mumps immunity, there is general agreement that the neutralization reaction gives the most specific indication of immunity (5), but the HI test may offer a satisfactory alternative, and it does not require a stock of titrated live virus or living cell cultures.

Cell-mediated immunity plays a very important role in the protection of the host from measles and mumps. The techniques for studying cell-mediated immunity (9, 10), however, have been little used because of their newness and technical demands. At the time of writing, the special values of these tests have been too sketchily delineated to permit evaluation of usefulness.

CLINICAL INDICATIONS

Immunological tests should be used to confirm measles or mumps infection when the clinical symptomatology is atypical or when the risk of secondary cases is an important consideration. Clinical criteria may be adequate for diagnosis of both diseases in typical cases, but atypical infections, especially (meningo-)encephalitis are not clinically distinguishable from similar disease caused by other agents. Identification of recent measles or mumps infection in these patients may be essential to making the differential diagnosis.

Measles serological tests may be useful in making a positive distinction between possible etiologies in rash disease in pregnant women. When rubella serology is negative, a positive test for measles, which rarely causes teratological effects, may provide confidence in a benign outcome.

Measles serology is an important element in diagnosing subacute sclerosing panencephalitis (SSPE).

There are highly effective vaccines available for both measles and mumps. In neither instance are untoward effects noted when these vaccines have been administered to previously immune individuals, but neither is any good done. Common practice condones vaccination of young children who have a negative history without serological confirmation of need. In older age groups, unrecognized infections and poor memory account for a large proportion of negative histories, and conservative practice would call for serological confirmation of need, before vaccine is administered to these persons.

TEST PROCEDURES

Hemagglutination inhibition

Measles antigen. Tissue culture-grown measles virus provides a convenient source of antigen. Any of a variety of human or old-world primate cell tissue culture lines may be used to grow the virus. The Vero green monkey kidney line is highly appropriate. When the measles virus-infected culture shows extensive cytopathic effect, it should be frozen and thawed, and the cell debris is then removed by low-speed centrifugation. It may be necessary to test several pools to obtain a good hemagglutination titer (1:8 or more). Commercially sold antigens are also generally satisfactory. The antigen should be treated either with Tween-ether or ultrasound, to increase antigen titer and test sensitivity. In the first procedure, 0.1 volume of 1% Tween 80 solution is slowly stirred into the antigen preparation. Then 0.5 volume of anesthetic-grade ether is added and the mixture is stirred for 5 h at room temperature. The phases are then allowed to separate, the ether phase is removed, and dissolved ether is taken off by bubbling nitrogen through the preparation. Alternatively, a 10-min treatment in an ice bath with a Bronwill Biosonic sonic oscillator at 25% power, or equivalent instrument, may be used. Treatment of the antigen will increase its titer at least fourfold without increasing its antibody-binding capacity. Treated preparations may be held for several days at 4 C.

Mumps antigen. Mumps hemagglutinating antigen preparations may be the same as mumps V CF antigen (see below) or may be any high-titer virus preparation. They should be treated as above with either Tween 80-ether or ultrasound. Not only does this treatment increase the specific hemagglutinating activity, but it also reduces neuraminidase activity and results in more stable agglutination patterns.

Red blood cells. Cells from the measles test must be derived from an old-world monkey. The genus *Cercopithecus* (e.g., African green monkey) has generally proved most useful, but *Macaca* or *Erythrocebus* may also be satisfactory.

For the mumps test, chicken or goose cells may be used and have the advantage of more rapid settling. Monkey or human O cells are also satisfactory, and these make possible the integration of tests for mumps with tests for other viruses.

The donor animal will commonly have antibody to the disease in question, and it is important that this be removed by thorough washing. Sedimenting at least three times from 10 or more volumes of phosphate-buffered saline (PBS) is required.

Sera. Sera are treated to remove nonspecific inhibitors of agglutination by mixing with 9 volumes of 14% kaolin in PBS. The kaolin is removed after 20 min by low-speed centrifugation and one-fourth the serum volume of packed red blood cells is added. After 1 h at 4 C, sedimentation of the red blood cells removes cell-directed agglutinins. The supernatant fluid is considered a 1:10 serum dilution. Cerebrospinal fluid (CSF) may be used without kaolin extraction and without dilution. Kaolin extraction should not be used if sera are fractionated for differential determination of IgM and IgG.

The test. Either microtiter technique or 10 × 75 mm test tubes with 0.1-ml samples may be used. Serial twofold serum or CSF dilutions are made in PBS. An equal volume of antigen, diluted to contain 3 to 4 hemagglutinating units, is added. If test tubes are used, they are shaken. The test is held for 1 h at room temperature, and 1 volume of 0.5% red blood cells in PBS is then added. The test is shaken again, if in tubes, and the cells are allowed to settle.

With measles agglutinin, settling at 37 C gives a small increase in sensitivity over room temperature. If the test is reshaken and settles a second time, the patterns are usually clearer, but there will be a fractional loss in sensitivity.

With mumps agglutinin settling should take place at 4 C to minimize elution, and reshaking is no help.

Controls should include known positive and negative sera and the unknown sera at a 1:10 dilution with diluent replacing antigen. Fifty percent agglutination is usually taken as the end point.

Mumps complement-fixation test

Good mumps V and S CF antigens and controls are commercially available, or they may be prepared from embryonated eggs (8). The V antigen is composed of released virions, whereas the S antigen includes cell-associated material and unassembled virus components.

Serum should be heated at 56 C for 30 min and adsorbed with an equal volume of 10% sheep red blood cells. The test itself is then carried out by any standard procedure (see chapter 58). If reactions are obtained with the control antigen, preadsorption of the serum with this reagent may be called for. The two antigens should be run in parallel with paired specimens collected as early as possible and after an interval of 1 to 2 weeks.

REAGENTS

Measles and mumps hemagglutinating antigens: Flow Laboratories, Rockville, Md.; Microbiological Associates, Inc., Bethesda, Md.

Mumps V and S CF antigens: Microbiological Associates, Inc.

Kaolin, acid-washed: Fisher Chemicals.

Tween 80: ICN Life Sciences Group, Cleveland, Ohio.

PBS (quantities in grams unless otherwise designated):

Solution A — NaCl, 8.0; KCl, 0.2; $CaCl \cdot 2H_2O$, 0.132; $MgCl \cdot 6H_2O$, 0.1; water, 800 ml.

Solution B — Na_2HPO_4, 1.15; KH_2PO_4, 0.2; water, 200 ml. Dissolve ingredients of solutions A and B separately and then combine.

INTERPRETATION

Measles

The development of measles HI antibody is closely synchronized with symptomatology, and maximal values are approached 2 weeks after rash. Demonstration of an increasing titer must be done on paired specimens collected within this period, but a significant (fourfold) increase may be demonstrable in specimens taken as little as 2 or 3 days apart during the first week after rash. If the initial specimen is collected after the first week but within the first month, HI activity in IgM can be demonstrated. The proportion of activity in the IgM fraction is usually too small to be demonstrated convincingly by inactivation of IgM and determination of titer loss, but, if the IgM is separated by sucrose in gradient centrifugation, a positive finding is indicative of recent infection (1). An exception occurs in the presence of multiple sclerosis where activity persists in the IgM.

A positive measles HI titer at a 1:10 serum dilution is indicative of immunity. Less than 5% of naturally immunized persons will have titers lower than 10, and the proportion of these very low titers does not usually exceed 10% after vaccination. Nonspecific positive reac-

tions are not a common problem.

A serum HI titer of 1,280 or greater in the absence of recent infection is suggestive of SSPE. However, this cannot be considered diagnostic because the titers in SSPE patients overlap extensively with the upper portion of the normal range. An HI titer in the CSF that is more than $1/80$ of the serum titer is useful confirmation of SSPE. This may also be found in multiple sclerosis.

Mumps

An increasing mumps V CF titer with increasing ratio of V to S titer in the paired sera is indicative of recent (less than 30 days) mumps infection. Increasing titers without the appropriate change in ratio are equivocal. Negative or stable titers are indicative of no recent mumps infection.

An HI titer of 40 or more is indicative of mumps immunity (2). Titers of 10 or 20 are equivocal. Normal range extends to about 160 in long-term immunity.

LITERATURE CITED

1. Black, F. L. 1974. Measles virus, p. 709–715. *In* E. H. Lennette, E. H. Spaulding, and J. P. Truant (ed.), Manual of clinical microbiology, 2nd ed. American Society for Microbiology, Washington, D.C.

2. Black, F. L., and W. J. Houghton. 1967. The significance of mumps hemagglutinin inhibition titers in normal populations. Am. J. Epidemiol. 85:101–107.

3. Black, F. L., and L. Rosen. 1962. Patterns of measles antibodies in residents of Tahiti and their stability in the absence of re-exposure. J. Immunol. 88:725–731.

4. Brown, G., J. V. Baublis, and T. P. O'Leary. 1970. Development and duration of mumps fluorescent antibodies in various immunoglobulin fraction of human serum. J. Immunol. 104:86–94.

5. Buynak, E. B., J. E. Whitman, Jr., R. R. Roehm, E. H. Morton, G. P. Lampson, and M. R. Hilleman. 1967. Comparison of neutralization and hemagglutination-inhibition techniques for measuring mumps antibody. Proc. Soc. Exp. Biol. Med. 125:1068–1071.

6. Daugharty, H., D. T. Warfield, W. D. Hemingway, and H. L. Casey. 1973. Mumps class-specific immunoglobulins in radioimmunoassay and conventional serology. Infect. Immun. 7:380–385.

7. Henle, G., S. Harris, and W. Henle. 1948. The reactivity of various human sera with mumps complement fixation antigens. J. Exp. Med. 88:133–147.

8. Henle, W. 1969. Mumps virus, p. 457–482. *In* E. H. Lennette and N. J. Schmidt (ed.), Diagnos-

tic procedures for viral and rickettsial infections, 4th ed. American Public Health Association, Inc., New York.

9. Labowskie, R. J., R. Edelman, R. Rustigian, and J. A. Belanti. 1974. Studies of cell-mediated immunity to measles virus by *in vitro* lymphocyte-mediated cytotoxicity. J. Infect. Dis. **129:**233–239.

10. Utermohlen, V., and J. B. Zabriskie. 1973. A suppression of cellular immunity in patients with multiple sclerosis. J. Exp. Med. **138:**1591–1595.

Chapter 60

Adenoviruses

FRANKLIN H. TOP, JR.

INTRODUCTION

Diseases caused by adenoviruses include upper and lower respiratory tract infections (1), acute gastroenteritis of children (5, 7), conjunctivitis (11), and hemorrhagic cystitis (6). Although adenoviruses may be associated with a large proportion of the last two syndromes, they cause less than 10% of respiratory tract infections except in military trainees, in whom they cause epidemics of acute respiratory disease (12). Currently, 33 types of human adenovirus are recognized; however, most disease has been associated with a limited number of serotypes, types 1–8, 11, 14, 19, and 21.

Serological diagnosis of adenovirus infection is based upon a rise in antibody titer between the acute and convalescent phase of the illness. Serum should be collected during the acute illness and 2 to 3 weeks after the onset of illness. Three serological tests have been used commonly for serodiagnosis: the complement fixation (CF) test, the hemagglutination-inhibition (HI) test, and the neutralization test.

Undoubtedly the most useful single antibody assay is the CF test which measures group-specific antibody. In this test a single adenovirus antigen can be used to detect infection with any of the adenovirus serotypes. A second advantage is that, with the exception of the antigen, reagents and procedures for the adenovirus CF test are identical to those used for CF tests for other viruses. The CF test is less sensitive than the HI or neutralization test (10), especially in young children and in military trainees immunized with adenovirus vaccines.

Both the neutralization test and the HI test detect type-specific antibodies. Since the presence of neutralizing antibody has been shown to correlate with protection against disease caused by a specific adenovirus type (13), the neutralization test is especially valuable in surveys of a population's immunity to a specific adenovirus and in studies of adenovirus vaccine immunogenicity. When many serotypes need be included in serological tests, the lesser expense and greater simplicity of the HI test may afford advantages over the neutralization test.

CLINICAL INDICATIONS

Serological diagnosis of adenovirus infection should be considered in patients with any of the diseases mentioned previously—febrile upper and lower respiratory tract infections, acute gastroenteritis, keratoconjunctivitis, and hemorrhagic cystitis. Generally, specimens for virus isolation should be obtained together with the acute serum. In syndromes in which limited numbers of adenovirus types cause disease and in which a large proportion of cases are associated with adenoviruses (for example, keratoconjunctivitis or hemorrhagic cystitis), serological diagnosis without resort to viral isolation may be practical. Unfortunately, the vast majority of recognized human adenovirus illnesses occur as acute respiratory tract disease, a syndrome caused by many viruses other than adenoviruses. Since the many types of adenovirus cause but a small proportion of all respiratory tract infections, type-specific diagnosis by serology alone is impractical unless the involved adenovirus is identified.

TEST PROCEDURES

Complement fixation

Adenovirus CF tests are performed by standard microtiter procedures detailed in chapter 58 of this *Manual* and elsewhere (8). A CF antigen prepared from one adenovirus type serves to detect the group-reactive antibody raised by infection with other adenovirus types. Satisfactory adenovirus CF antigen is available from commercial sources, or the antigen can be easily prepared by propagation of type 2, 4, 5, or 7 in bottle cultures of human embryonic kidney (HEK), HeLa, or KB cells maintained with Eagle's minimal essential medium (MEM) with 2% fetal bovine serum (FBS) by a method similar to that described by Rose (8). An inoculum of virus which produces complete cytopathic effect (CPE) within 5 to 7 days is used. Medium is not changed after 3 days regardless of acidity. The culture is held for an additional 2 days after nearly all cells are detached, and then the mixture is centrifuged.

The supernatant fluid is saved, and the cellular pellet is resuspended in several milliliters of the supernatant fluid, rapidly frozen and thawed five times, and centrifuged. The supernatant fluid is added to that originally saved. This pool serves as the CF antigen without further treatment. An antigen control is made from an uninfected bottle culture harvested with a rubber policeman and treated similarly. Four units of antigen are used in the CF test.

Neutralization

Neutralization tests are performed with tube cultures of HEK cells, which can be purchased from all major companies supplying cell cultures. HEK cells are maintained in L-15 medium with 2% FBS. Prepare virus seeds titering approximately 7 to 8 $\log_{10}$ $TCID_{50}$/0.1 ml by harvesting infected HEK cell cultures at complete CPE, rapidly freezing and thawing the cultures three times, and harvesting the supernatant fluid after centrifugation at $1,200 \times g$ for 10 min. Since the slow and inconsistent development of CPE at high dilutions of adenovirus seed virus tends to obscure end points, use a dilution of virus which titers 100 $TCID_{50}$ between 3 and 5 days after inoculation. Generally, this is a 1:100 dilution of virus seed and titers approximately 5 to 6 $\log_{10}$ $TCID_{50}$/0.1 ml.

After incubation of acute and convalescent serum specimens at 56 C for 30 min, dilute the specimens 1:4 through 1:256 in sterile tubes, leaving 0.2 ml of each dilution remaining. To each tube add 0.2 ml of the dilution of seed virus. Shake the tubes and incubate them at room temperature for 1 h. Then pipette 0.1 ml of each virus-serum dilution into each of two HEK tube cultures. Make a 1:2 dilution of the virus seed in Hanks balanced salt solution, and then make four subsequent 10-fold dilutions. Inoculate 0.1 ml of each dilution into each of two (or six) HEK tubes. Uninoculated HEK tubes serve as cell controls. Known positive and negative sera should be included in each test. Since cell toxicity is induced uncommonly by serum and is easily differentiated from adenovirus CPE, serum controls generally are not necessary.

Examine the cultures daily, and score the test when 32 to 320 $TCID_{50}$ are apparent in the virus titration, using the Reed-Muench method. (Generally, the tubes inoculated with the 1:2 dilution of virus seen show 3 to 4+ CPE at this time.) A slightly greater sensitivity (which is required for evaluation of vaccine immunogenicity) is obtained if the test is read at 10 $TCID_{50}$. The highest serum dilution in which both tubes show no adenovirus CPE is considered the end point.

Hemagglutination inhibition

A method used at the Center for Disease Control by Hierholzer et al. (3, 4) is useful for adenovirus HI tests. As in other HI tests, erythrocyte suspensions are best standardized by spectrophotometric procedures (3). A 0.4% erythrocyte concentration is employed in adenovirus HI tests. Rhesus monkey erythrocytes are used for adenovirus types of Rosen's group I (types 3, 7, 11, 14, 16, 20, 21, 25, and 28), whereas rat erythrocytes are used for adenovirus group II (types 8, 9, 10, 13, 15, 17, 19, 22, 23, 24, 26, 27, 29, and 30) and group III (types 1, 2, 4, 5, and 6). Many members of group III agglutinate rat erythrocytes completely only in the presence of antisera of a heterologous type in that group; therefore, a 1:100 dilution of a type 6 immune serum (previously adsorbed with rat erythrocytes) in buffer is used in HI tests with adenoviruses of group III. Rats should be preselected for erythrocytes sensitive to viral hemagglutination, and rat erythrocytes should be used within 2 days after collection. Adenovirus types 12, 18, and 31 do not hemagglutinate simian or rodent erythrocytes.

Diluent used in HI tests is 0.01 M phosphate-buffered saline which contains 0.00772 M Na_2HPO_4, anhydrous, 0.00228 M $NaH_2PO_4 \cdot H_2O$, and 0.146 M NaCl at pH 7.2. In the Center for Disease Control laboratory, rigid styrene U plates are preferred over V plates for adenovirus HI tests (4).

Adenovirus hemagglutinating (HA) antigens for types 1 to 7 are obtainable commercially. HA antigens for these or other types can be made by inoculation of susceptible cell lines (HEK, HeLa, or KB cells) maintained in Eagle's MEM containing 2% FBS with a virus dose causing complete CPE between 3 and 5 days after inoculation. The antigen is harvested when cellular degeneration is complete. The supernatant fluid of a low-speed centrifugation ($1,500 \times g$ for 10 min) serves as antigen which is stable indefinitely at -20 C.

Although kaolin was used to remove nonspecific serum inhibitors in the original adenovirus HI test (9), more recent experience in two independent laboratories has been that kaolin adsorption may result in a less sensitive test (4, 10). Hierholzer et al. (4) suggest that routine removal of nonspecific inhibitors of hemagglutination is not necessary and recommends that human sera be heated at 56 C for 30 min, diluted 1:5, and adsorbed appropriately with

50% rhesus or rat erythrocytes prior to use in HI tests. Sera are diluted from 1:10 to 1:10,240 with standard loops, leaving 0.025 ml of each serum dilution in a well. Then 0.025 ml containing a predetermined 4 units of antigen is added to each well, and the plates are gently agitated and incubated at room temperature for 1 h. To each well 0.05 ml of the appropriate 0.4% erythrocyte suspension is added. After gentle shaking, the plates are incubated for 1 h at 37 C. The end point is the last tube that shows no evidence of hemagglutination.

Necessary controls include erythrocytes alone and the initial (1:10) dilution of serum plus erythrocytes. In addition, the amount of antigen used in the test should be established by titration.

REAGENTS

Adenovirus CF antigen and HA antigen (types 1–7) can be prepared in the laboratory as described above in the section on test procedures, or they can be obtained commercially (CF antigen from Microbiological Associates, Inc., Bethesda, Md., Flow Laboratories, Inc., Bethesda, Md., or BioQuest, Cockeysville, Md.; HA antigen from Microbiological Associates, Inc.).

INTERPRETATION

Serological tests for the diagnosis of adenovirus infections require both acute and convalescent serum specimens obtained 2 to 3 weeks apart. With each test, a significant rise in antibody titer ($\geq$fourfold) between acute and convalescent sera is required for serological diagnosis. Consequently, the test cannot be performed until late in the convalescent period when results are of lesser clinical importance than in the acute illness. Nevertheless, the results may be of epidemiological importance or of clinical interest in establishing an association of an unusual or severe illness with adenovirus infection.

Whether a patient's illness is due to the adenovirus infection is a more difficult question which cannot be answered by serological means alone. Many adenovirus infections are asymptomatic and persistent (2). Particularly in infants, antibody may not develop until months after the onset of infection. Serological evidence of adenovirus infection (and even isolation of an adenovirus) thus may be coincidental to a disease caused by infection with a different agent. Isolation of an adenovirus (especially in high titer) from a diseased organ or its secretions, or previous epidemiological association of the patient's syndrome with adenovirus infection, is evidence that adenovirus may be the etiological agent of the illness.

As mentioned previously, the CF test detects antibody stimulated by infection with any human adenovirus. Although it is a valuable screening test for adenovirus infection, it will not yield information as to the type of infecting adenovirus. Also, it is less sensitive than the neutralization and HI tests, especially in younger children. The neutralization and HI tests are more sensitive provided that the infecting adenovirus type is included as an antigen in these tests. Rises in antibody titers to heterotypic adenoviruses may occur with both HI and neutralization tests in as high as 25% of adult infections, generally between types included within an adenovirus group (9). For these reasons, serological tests on individual patients cannot be considered to establish firmly the infecting adenovirus type in the absence of virus isolation.

LITERATURE CITED

1. Brandt, C. D., H. W. Kim, A. J. Vargosko, B. C. Jeffries, J. O. Arrobio, B. Rindge, R. H. Parrott, and R. M. Chanock. 1969. Infections in 18,000 infants and children in a controlled study of respiratory tract diseases. I. Adenovirus pathogenicity in relationship to serologic type and illness syndrome. Am. J. Epidemiol. **90:**484–500.

2. Fox, J. P., C. D. Brandt, F. E. Wasserman, C. E. Hall, I. Spigland, A. Kogon, and L. R. Elveback. 1969. The virus watch program: a continuing surveillance of viral infections in metropolitan New York families. VI. Observations of adenovirus infections. Am. J. Epidemiol. **89:**25–50.

3. Hierholzer, J. C., and M. T. Suggs. 1969. Standardized viral hemagglutination and hemagglutination-inhibition tests. I. Standardization of erythrocyte suspensions. Appl. Microbiol. **18:**816–823.

4. Hierholzer, J. C., M. T. Suggs, and E. C. Hall. 1969. Standardized viral hemagglutination and hemagglutination-inhibition tests. II. Description and statistical evaluation. Appl. Microbiol. **18:**824–833.

5. Moffet, H. L., H. K. Shulenberger, and E. R. Burkholder. 1968. Epidemiology and etiology of severe infantile diarrhea. J. Pediat. **72:**1–14.

6. Numazaki, Y., S. Shigeta, T. Kumasaka, T. Miyazawa, M. Yamanaka, N. Yano, S. Takai, and N. Ishida. 1968. Acute hemorrhagic cystitis in children. Isolation of adenovirus type 11. N. Engl. J. Med. **278:**700–704.

7. Ramos-Alvarez, M., and J. Olarte. 1964. Diarrheal diseases of children. Am. J. Dis. Child. **107:**218–231.

8. Rose, H. M. 1969. Adenoviruses, p. 205-226. In E.

H. Lennette and N. J. Schmidt (ed.), Diagnostic procedures for viral and rickettsial diseases. American Public Health Association, Inc., New York.

9. Rosen, L. 1961. Hemagglutination-inhibition antibody responses in human adenovirus infections. Proc. Soc. Exp. Biol. Med. **108**:474–479.

10. Schmidt, N. J., E. H. Lennette, and C. J. King. 1966. Neutralizing, hemagglutination-inhibiting and group complement-fixing antibody responses in human adenovirus infections. J. Immunol. **97**:64–74.

11. Sprague, J. B., J. C. Hierholzer, R. W. Currier II, M. A. W. Hattwick, and M. D. Smith. 1973. Epidemic keratoconjunctivitis: a severe industrial outbreak due to adenovirus type 8. N. Engl. J. Med. **289**:1341–1346.

12. Top, F. H., Jr. 1975. Control of adenovirus acute respiratory disease in U. S. Army trainees. Yale J. Biol. Med. **48**:185–195.

13. Van der Veen, J., M. F. W. Abarbanel, and K. G. Oei. 1968. Vaccination with live type 4 adenovirus; evaluation of antibody response and protective efficacy. J. Hyg. **66**:499–511.

Chapter 61

Rubella Virus

WILLIAM E. RAWLS AND MAX A. CHERNESKY

INTRODUCTION

Two clinical entities are caused by rubella virus. Infection acquired postnatally usually results in a benign, self-limiting illness; however, in utero infections may be severe, and death or life-long disability is a not infrequent outcome. There are three circumstances in which laboratory support may be of value. These include the diagnosis of congenital rubella, the diagnosis of postnatal rubella, and the determination of the immune status of women during their reproductive years of life. Isolation of rubella virus in tissue culture is laborious and requires several weeks. In contrast, serological techniques are easily performed, rapid, and reliable. Except for the diagnosis of congenital rubella in the newborn period, serological techniques are the method of choice. In addition, the presence of detectable antibodies to rubella virus indicates that the patient is immune and, if exposed, will not develop clinical rubella.

The basis for serological diagnosis of rubella rests upon the rapid rise in antibody titers to the virus in the convalescent phase of the illness. The initial serum sample should be collected while the patient has the rash, and a second serum sample should be collected approximately 1 week later. A fourfold or greater rise in antibody titers to rubella virus between the acute and convalescent sera is diagnostic of a recent infection when both sera are tested together in one of the following serological tests: hemagglutination inhibition (HI), complement fixation (CF), neutralization, or indirect immunofluorescence. In addition, antibodies can be detected by precipitation in agar gel. Of the techniques described, the HI test has been found to be sensitive, rapid, and reliable. Thus, the HI test is the technique of choice both for diagnosing rubella and for surveys of populations in which immunity to the virus is being assessed.

Of special interest is the relatively late rise of antibodies which are detected in the CF test when compared with the HI test. This is of practical importance in that it is sometimes possible to demonstrate a fourfold rise in antibodies by the CF test after the antibody titers detected in the HI test are no longer increasing. HI antibodies rise rapidly as the rash fades, and peak titers are reached by 10 to 14 days, whereas CF antibodies become detectable about 1 week after the rash and reach maximal levels 1 to 2 weeks later. CF antibodies do not persist as long as HI antibodies, and the absence of CF antibodies does not imply susceptibility to infection by rubella virus.

Since the original description of the HI test for rubella (10), several modifications have been introduced. These include the choice of indicator erythrocyte (2), optimal pH of reagents (3), methods for removal of nonspecific inhibitors from sera (5), methods for preparation of the antigen (9), and duration of incubation of antigen with the sera (1, 6). Two more detailed accounts of the subject (7, 8) are recommended to the interested reader.

CLINICAL INDICATIONS

Rubella is a benign, self-limiting disease, usually of childhood, which is characterized by mild upper respiratory symptoms, suboccipital lymphadenopathy, and an erythematous rash. Mild complications of arthralgias and arthritis may occur following the disappearance of rash in young adults. The prime indication for laboratory diagnosis of rubella resides in the potential risk of this disease to the fetus of women in the early stages of pregnancy. Susceptibility to rubella virus can be altered by administering live virus vaccine. Women of child-bearing age should be assessed by antibody analysis for susceptibility to rubella; those found susceptible should be vaccinated with due regard taken for the potential dangers of vaccination during pregnancy. Some physicians determine the rubella antibody status of pregnant women at the patient's first prenatal visit. Those without antibodies are monitored through early pregnancy for seroconversion. Finally, pregnant women who develop symptoms suggestive of rubella or who are exposed to a suspected case of rubella should be investigated for antibodies to the virus. Analysis of acute and convalescent sera from women with a rubella-like illness will show a rise in antibody titers if the disease is rubella. A serum sample is collected soon after exposure, and a second sample is collected 4 to 5 weeks later. Analysis will reveal a rise in antibody titers if infection occurred. Serological examination of the supposed contact also can be helpful in this situation (4).

A special problem arises when a woman in the first trimester seeks medical attention after the rash has faded. Serological confirmation of recent rubella can sometimes be accomplished by demonstrating IgM antibodies to rubella virus. With the usual HI test, IgM antibodies can be detected for 4 to 8 weeks after the illness; however, recent reports (1, 6) indicate a much longer persistence of IgM which can be detected when the IgM antibodies are incubated overnight at 4 C before indicator erythrocytes are added. Antibodies of the IgM class are demonstrable by a number of techniques including indirect immunofluorescence with the use of fluoroisothiocyanate-conjugated antihuman IgM, degradation of HI activity in the serum sample by 2-mercaptoethanol, adsorption of IgG activity from the sample with staphylococcal protein-A, or physical separation of IgM from IgG by chromatography or by density gradient centrifugation. In our laboratory, we have found physical separation of IgM by density gradient centrifugation to be the most reliable method.

TEST PROCEDURES

Although different laboratories use modifications of the standard rubella HI test, the following is a description of the test which we have found consistently to give good results. The test is conveniently performed in disposable plastic or vinyl V-bottom microtiter plates. The rubella hemagglutinating (HA) antigen is titrated each time the test is performed. Serial twofold dilutions of the antigen are made in 0.025 ml of dextrose-gelatin-Veronal (DGV) buffer to which 0.025 ml of the same diluent is subsequently added before the addition of each cup of 0.025 ml of a 0.25% washed suspension of pigeon erythrocytes. Control cups containing no antigen are included. The plates are sealed and placed at 4 C for 1 h, after which time they are placed at room temperature for 15 min before being read. The highest dilution that produces a pattern of complete hemagglutination is considered 1 HA unit. Four units are used in the HI test.

To perform the HI test, first remove the nonspecific inhibitors of hemagglutination and nonspecific agglutinins from the serum. To 0.1 ml of test serum add 0.1 ml of DGV and 0.6 ml of a 25% suspension of kaolin. Mix the suspension well by shaking, and allow it to sit at room temperature for 20 min with frequent agitation. Sediment the kaolin in a clinical centrifuge, and after transferring the supernatant fluid to a clean tube add 0.05 ml of a 50% suspension of pigeon erythrocytes. After 60 min of incubation at 4 C, sediment the erythrocytes by centrifugation, and remove the supernatant fluid and heat it at 56 C for 30 min. This final sample, which represents a dilution of 1:8, is now ready to be incorporated into the test.

Alternatively, the nonspecific inhibitor may be removed by precipitation with heparin and manganous choride. The serum sample is diluted 1:4 with 0.15 M NaCl. To each 0.8 ml of diluted serum are added 0.03 ml of sodium heparin (200 units) and 0.04 ml of 1 M manganous chloride. The sample is held at 4 C for 20 min, and the precipitate which forms is pelleted by centrifugation. The supernatant fluid is then adsorbed with pigeon erythrocytes as described above.

Known positive and negative control sera are treated similarly. Further serial twofold dilutions of each serum are made in 0.025-ml amounts of DGV. An area of the plate is reserved for duplication of the first three dilutions of each serum. These received DGV in place of antigen and serve as serum controls. To the other dilutions of serum are added 4 HA units of antigen in a volume of 0.025 ml, and the antigen is back-titrated in a separate part of the plate by doubling dilutions in 0.025 ml of DGV to represent 4, 2, 1, and 0.5 HA units. The plates are incubated for 1 h at room temperature, after which 0.025 ml of a 0.25% suspension of pigeon erythrocytes is added to each well. The hemagglutination pattern is read after 1 h at 4 C, and that dilution of serum which completely inhibits hemagglutination is taken as the end point.

The CF test is performed by a standard technique (9). Detection of IgM antibodies by density gradient centrifugation entails diluting the test serum 1:5 in phosphate-buffered saline (PBS) and adsorbing with pigeon erythrocytes. After removal of the erythrocytes, layer the diluted serum onto a gradient which is constructed by layering 1.5 ml of 40, 25, and 10% (wt/vol) solution of sucrose in PBS into a 5-ml Lusteroid tube. Prior to layering the test serum, equilibrate the gradient by overnight diffusion in a refrigerator. Centrifuge the specimen at 157,000 × g for 18 h. Puncture the bottom of the tube with a needle, and collect six fractions of 0.8 ml each. Perform HI tests on the fractions without further treatment or after dialysis against PBS to remove excess sucrose. The bottom two fractions contain IgM; IgG is located primarily in the middle two fractions, and the nonspecific inhibitor of agglutination is located at the top of the gradient.

REAGENTS

To prepare HA antigen, infect monolayers of BHK-21 cells grown in 32-oz bottles with 5 to 10 ml of rubella stock containing 10^4 or more $TCID_{50}$ per ml. After the virus has adsorbed for 2 h at 37 C, cover the monolayers with Eagle's medium containing 2% fetal calf serum that has previously been adsorbed with kaolin. Change the medium after 24 h and then harvest for HA antigen after the 5th and 7th days of incubation. High-titered antigen can be extracted from the monolayers by extracting the cell-associated antigen with alkaline buffers (9). The cell-associated antigen preparations have CF activity and can be used as the antigen source in the CF test. We have found that good quality CF and HI antigens in lyophilized form can be purchased from commercial sources such as Flow Laboratories, Inc., Microbiological Associates, Inc., or Connaught Laboratories.

Whole blood is collected by drawing from the pigeon's wing vein into Alsever's solution. The erythrocytes are washed three times in DGV buffer, and the packed cells are resuspended in an equal volume of DGV to make a 50% suspension; part of this suspension is used to adsorb nonspecific agglutinins from the test sera. A 10% working suspension is made in DGV from which the 0.25% suspension to be used in the test is made.

Acid-washed kaolin powder can be purchased from most scientific supply companies. A 25-g amount of kaolin is washed with tris(hydroxymethyl)aminomethane (Tris) buffer until a pH of 7.0 or greater is achieved. The Tris buffer is made by mixing 12.1 g of Trisma base (Sigma Chemical Co.), 80 ml of 1 N HCl, and 0.85 g of NaCl, and bringing the volume to 1 liter. This solution is then further diluted 1:10 for washing the kaolin. After the final wash in Tris buffer, the kaolin pellet is resuspended in 100 ml of Tris-bovine albumin (TBA) buffer. TBA is made by adding to 96.67 ml of Tris buffer the following ingredients: 0.33 ml of a 35% sterile solution of bovine albumen (Nutritional Biochemicals Corp.), 1 ml of 0.5% $MgCl_2 \cdot 6H_2O$

solution, 1 ml of an 8% NaN_3 solution, and 1 ml of 0.5% $CaCl_2$ solution.

DGV buffer is made by dissolving 0.60 g of gelatin in 250 ml of distilled water which is held in a stoppered 1-liter flask in a boiling-water bath. To this flask, 0.58 g of barbital (Veronal) is added. In a separate container 0.02 g of $CaCl_2$ is dissolved in 50 ml of distilled water before being added to the barbital-gelatin mixture. The following solution dissolved in 500 ml of water is then added: 0.38 g of sodium barbital, 0.12 g of $MgSO_4 \cdot 7H_2O$, 8.5 g of NaCl, and 10 g of dextrose. The volume is then brought to 1 liter. This solution is filtered and then is dispensed into 100-ml volumes and frozen at −20 C. On the day of the test, the DGV is thawed and supplemented with bovine albumin fraction V to a concentration of 0.4%, and the pH is adjusted to 6.2 with HCl.

INTERPRETATION

The presence of HI antibody in a patient's serum at titers of 1:8 or greater indicates that the patient has been infected with the virus and is immune to rubella. Patients without detectable antibodies at a serum dilution of 1:8 are usually susceptible to infection by rubella virus; however, a small percentage of adults may not have detectable HI antibodies at this dilution and yet are immune. Neutralizing antibodies at low dilutions can usually be detected in the sera of these patients. The lack of a serological response to rubella virus vaccine in women who do not have detectable HI antibodies is often due to low levels of neutralizing antibodies.

Confirmation of rubella requires the demonstration of a fourfold rise in antibody titers between paired sera. There is considerable variability in the antibody titers maintained during life, and a firm diagnosis cannot be made on the absolute titer of a single serum sample. Because of day to day variations in the results of HI tests, paired sera should be tested in parallel. Fourfold differences in titers of paired sera tested on different days may reflect test to test variation and not a true change in antibody concentration. This is especially important when paired sera are collected from pregnant women who have not experienced clinical illness. Judgments regarding therapy should be withheld until the sera have been reexamined in parallel.

Often an acute serum is not collected, and the laboratory is asked to make a diagnosis on later convalescent sera which have been collected but show no difference in titer because an apparent plateau of HI antibody has been achieved.

These sera require special consideration. CF antibodies appear later and rise more slowly than antibodies detected by HI. Paired sera collected later in convalescence and tested for antibodies by the CF test may be diagnostic. It is also possible to analyze the serum for IgM antibodies to rubella virus. Special techniques are required for assaying IgM antibodies, and studies of this nature require consultation between the laboratory and the physician.

LITERATURE CITED

1. Al-Nakib, W., J. M. Best, and J. E. Banatvala. 1975. Rubella-specific serum and nasopharyngeal immunologic responses following naturally acquired and vaccine induced infection-prolonged persistence of virus-specific IgM. Lancet 1:182–185.
2. Gupta, J. D., and J. D. Harley. 1970. Use of formalinized sheep erythrocytes in the rubella hemagglutination-inhibition test. Appl. Microbiol. 20:843–844.
3. Gupta, J. D., and V. J. Peterson. 1971. Use of a new buffer system with formalinized sheep erythrocytes in the rubella hemagglutination-inhibition test. Appl. Microbiol. 21:749–750.
4. Larke, R. P. B., and M. A. Chernesky. 1975. Rubella testing and the pregnant patient. Canadian Family Physician 21:83.
5. Liebhaber, H. 1970. Measurement of rubella antibody by hemagglutination inhibition. II. Characteristics of an improved HAI test employing a new method for removal of non-immunoglobulin HA inhibitors from serum. J. Immunol. 104:826–834.
6. Pattison, J. R., D. S. Dane, and J. E. Mace. 1975. Persistence of specific IgM after natural infection with rubella virus. Lancet 1:185–187.
7. Person, D. A., and E. C. Herrmann, Jr. 1971. Laboratory diagnosis of rubella virus infections and antibody determinations in routine medical practice. Mayo Clin. Proc. 46:477–483.
8. Rawls, W. E., and D. A. Person. 1974. Rubella virus, p. 716–722. In E. H. Lennette, E. H. Spaulding, and J. P. Truant (ed.), Manual of clinical microbiology, 2nd ed. American Society for Microbiology, Washington, D.C.
9. Schmidt, N. J., and E. H. Lennette. 1966. Rubella complement fixing antigens derived from the fluid and cellular phases of infected BHK-21 cells: extraction of cell-associated antigen with alkaline buffers. J. Immunol. 97:815–821.
10. Stewart, G. L., P. D. Parkman, H. E. Hopps, R. D. Douglas, J. P. Hamilton, and H. M. Meyer, Jr. 1967. Rubella-virus hemagglutination-inhibition test. N. Engl. J. Med. 276:554–557.

Chapter 62

Togaviruses, Bunyaviruses, and Colorado Tick Fever Virus

THOMAS P. MONATH

INTRODUCTION

Of the viruses transmitted to vertebrates by hematophagous arthropods (arboviruses), those of major clinical importance belong to three families (Togaviridae, Bunyaviridae, and Reoviridae) and to four genera of ribonucleic acid-containing viruses differentiated by their physicochemical properties, electron microscopic features, and serological reactivities (Table 1).

The serological diagnosis of clinical Toga- and Bunyavirus infection depends upon the demonstration of a significant change in the titer of specific antibodies in paired serum samples by means of one or more serological methods: hemagglutination-inhibition (HI), complement-fixation (CF), or neutralization tests. The fluorescent-antibody, indirect-hemagglutination, and precipitation tests have not been widely employed for routine serology, but the solid-phase radioimmunoassay with the use of purified antigens and immunoglobulin-specific indicators shows promise for the future. Each of the serological methods may also be used in retrospective surveys to define remote infections by detection of antibody in single serum samples.

Unlike the Toga- and Bunyaviruses, the diagnosis of Colorado tick fever (CTF) is most reliably established by the isolation of virus from the red cell fraction of whole blood or by demonstration of viral antigen in the patient's erythrocytes by direct fluorescent-antibody staining. Serological findings following CTF infection are often complicated because CF antibodies appear inconsistently and usually are of low titer. The plaque reduction neutralization test (PRNT) is more useful, but the indirect fluorescent-antibody technique (for details, see chapter 55) performed with infected BHK-21 or Vero cells as a substrate is the most sensitive test for early serological diagnosis (9).

Hemagglutination-inhibition test

Certain Toga- and Bunyaviruses reproducibly agglutinate goose erythrocytes; inhibition of hemagglutination (HA) by specific antibody forms the basis for the HI test (5, 10). The test is relatively simple, and results are rapidly obtained. Serological cross-reactivities between members of some virus groups are great; thus, inclusion of an antigen in the HI test may provide a useful screening procedure for diagnosis of infection with heterologous members of the same virus group. The marked cross-reactivity of HI antibodies to many Togaviruses is, however, also a limitation of the technique, since virus-specific diagnosis may be impossible. Other limitations of the technique include: (i) the presence of nonspecific inhibitors of HA in serum phospholipid fractions (12); (ii) the difficulty of preparing HA antigens for some viruses; and (iii) the specificity of the reaction with certain Bunyaviruses, such that infection with a closely related serotype may be missed.

HI antibodies appear during the first 3 to 10 days after primary infection. Peak antibody titers are attained approximately 1 month after infection and often decline over the next month. Thereafter, HI titers decline very slowly and antibody may persist for many years.

Complement-fixation test

A technique for the CF test is described in chapter 58 of this *Manual*. CF antibodies to Toga- and Bunyaviruses appear during the 2nd or 3rd week after primary infection and reach peak titer at 1 or 2 months. Antibody may decline to undetectable levels 1 to 2 years after infection; therefore, the test is most useful for the diagnosis of infection within a definite period prior to collection of the serum sample. In contrast to the general rule, primary dengue virus infection is often followed by high CF antibody titers which may persist for many years. The CF test is more specific than the HI test for the diagnosis of Togavirus infections and can be carried out with viral antigens which fail to hemagglutinate. The failure of some individuals to produce CF antibodies to some viruses limits the diagnostic usefulness of the test.

TABLE 1. *Classification of arthropod-borne viruses (arboviruses) of public health importance in the Western Hemisphere*

Virus	Classification			Arthropod vector
	Physicochemical		Serological	
	Family	Genus		
Eastern equine encephalomyelitis	Togaviridae	Alphavirus	Group A	Mosquito
Western equine encephalomyelitis	Togaviridae	Alphavirus	Group A	Mosquito
Venezuelan equine encephalomyelitis	Togaviridae	Alphavirus	Group A	Mosquito
Yellow fever	Togaviridae	Flavivirus	Group B	Mosquito
St. Louis encephalitis	Togaviridae	Flavivirus	Group B	Mosquito
Dengue	Togaviridae	Flavivirus	Group B	Mosquito
Powassan	Togaviridae	Flavivirus	Group B	Tick
Oriboca	Bunyaviridae	Bunyavirus	Group C	Mosquito
Caraparu[a]	Bunyaviridae	Bunyavirus	Group C	Mosquito
Guaroa[a]	Bunyaviridae	Bunyavirus	Bunyamwera	Mosquito
Oropouche	Bunyaviridae	Bunyavirus	Simbu	Not known
LaCrosse[a]	Bunyaviridae	Bunyavirus	California	Mosquito
Chagres[a]	Bunyaviridae	Bunyavirus	Phlebotomus fever	Phlebotomine fly
Catu[a]	Bunyaviridae	Bunyavirus	Guama	Mosquito

[a] Other members of serogroup are known to cause human disease.

Neutralization test

The basis of the neutralization test is the ability of an immune serum to render a suspension of virus nonpathogenic for a susceptible host, either laboratory animal or cell culture (7). A widely employed test performed with monolayer cell cultures measures the reduction in viral plaque infectivity of a constant amount of virus afforded by serial dilutions of the test serum. As opposed to the neutralization test in mice, the PRNT offers many advantages including sensitivity, quantitative precision, specificity, and simplicity of the titration of antibody (2, 8). Because the test is essential to specific diagnosis, its advantages far outweigh its disadvantages, which include the expense of maintaining cells and the relatively long time required to obtain results.

Neutralizing antibody may appear within the first few days after infection. Peak titers are reached at 1 to 2 months; antibody persists for a prolonged period, probably lifetime.

Choice and sequence of tests

For serological diagnosis of arbovirus infections, an acute serum collected 0 to 7 days after onset and an early convalescent serum collected 10 to 21 days after the first serum specimen are needed. A late convalescent serum collected 6 to 8 weeks after onset may also be useful for detection of a decline in HI or CF antibody titers. The CF test may be used as the primary diagnostic procedure; however, because of the earlier appearance of HI antibody and the greater sensitivity of the test, it is preferable initially to screen sera by HI against an appropriate battery of antigens. If a serum is positive to one or more antigens used in the HI test, the acute and convalescent sera should then be tested by the CF and/or neutralization test for extension and confirmation of results. To assure comparable serological results, paired acute and convalescent sera must be examined in the same test.

CLINICAL INDICATIONS

The clinical and epidemiological features of the case are important in the decision to employ serological tests and in the choice of antigens. Meningoencephalitis, aseptic meningitis, and fever with headache are manifestations of infection with eastern equine encephalitis (EEE), western equine encephalitis (WEE), St. Louis encephalitis (SLE), Powassan, and California group viruses. SLE infection with central nervous system signs occurs most frequently in older individuals and may be clinically confused with cerebrovascular accident. Toga- and Bunyaviruses cause acute fatal or self-limited infections; other etiologies should be sought in persons with prolonged or recurrent febrile or neurological disease.

The neotropical viruses associated with human disease (e.g., members of serogroups C, Bunyamwera, Simbu, Guama, and Phlebotomus fever) cause nonspecific febrile syndromes with headache, myalgia, and arthralgia. With the exception of dengue and Guaroa viruses, rash is not a feature. Yellow fever virus infection is suspected when jaundice and hemorrhage appear, but atypical, mild infections are frequent.

A history of tick bite introduces the possibility of CTF or Powassan infection in North America. CTF, which occurs in the western United States, is characterized by fever, headache, myalgia, gastrointestinal symptoms, and occasional rash.

TEST PROCEDURES

Hemagglutination inhibition

Materials.

1. Patient's sera to be tested.
2. Hemagglutinating viral antigens, homologous viral antisera, and normal serum (see below, Reagents).
3. Borate-saline solution, pH 9.0 (0.05 M borate-0.12 M NaCl).
4. Bovine albumin (Armour fraction V), 0.4%, in borate-saline, pH 9.0 (BABS).
5. Acid-washed kaolin, 25% (wt/vol), in BABS.
6. A series of phosphate-buffered saline solutions (virus-adjusting diluents [VADs]; see below, Reagents) which provide optimal pH for hemagglutination when combined in equal quantities with BABS.
7. Male domestic goose erythrocytes, washed three times and suspended at 8% (optical density 0.45 at 490 nm) in dextrose-gelatin-Veronal (0.60 g of gelatin, 0.38 g of sodium Veronal, 0.029 g of $CaCl_2$, 0.125 g of $MgSO_4 \cdot 7H_2O$, 8.5 g of NaCl, 10.0 g of dextrose; suspended in 1 liter of water and autoclaved).
8. Plastic microtiter plates with 8 rows of 12 U-shaped wells (Cooke Laboratory Products, Alexandria, Va.), 0.025- and 0.05-ml loop diluters, 0.025- and 0.05-ml droppers, 1.0-ml serological pipettes, and sealing tape.
9. Mechanical shaking device (optional) and reflecting stage for reading plates.

Treatment of sera to remove nonspecific inhibitors of HA and nonspecific erythrocyte agglutinins. Dispense 0.2 ml of each test serum into a tube, and add 0.8 ml of borate-saline and 1.0 ml of 25% kaolin suspension. Shake at 5-min intervals for 20 min at room temperature, and then centrifuge (2,000 rpm for 10 min). Removal of erythrocyte agglutinins is accomplished by adding 0.1 ml of washed packed goose erythrocytes to the decanted supernatant fluid. Tubes are held at 4 C, shaken occasionally, and after 30 min are centrifuged (4 C, 1,500 rpm for 5 min). Decant sera, which are now at a dilution of 1:10.

Preliminary HA titrations. Prepare serial twofold dilutions of antigen in microtiter plates by adding 0.1 ml of antigen to the first and 0.05 ml of BABS to the remaining wells of each row; dilute with 0.05-ml loops through well 11.

Select VAD buffers over a range to give final pH values from 5.75 to 7.2 that will permit determination of the optimal value for each antigen. Prepare 1:24 dilutions of standardized goose erythrocytes in each of the selected VADs. Add 0.05 ml of cell suspension prepared in the appropriate VAD to each well, including the 12th well, which serves as an erythrocyte control. Plates are shaken either during the addition of cells (by use of a mechanical shaker) or afterwards by tapping the corners with a ruler, and results are read after 30 min of incubation. Optimal incubation temperature to achieve highest HA titers varies from 4 to 37 C, but room temperature may be used as an acceptable standard for most antigens. Record HA patterns as complete agglutination (+), partial agglutination ($\oplus$, a ring of agglutinated cells surrounding a partial button), trace agglutination ($\pm$), or no agglutination (0). One HA unit is contained in 0.05 ml of the highest dilution of antigen causing complete or partial agglutination. For the HI test, 4 to 8 units *contained in 0.025 ml* are required. *Example:* If the HA titer at the optimal pH is 1,280 (1 HA unit in 0.05 ml of antigen diluted 1:1,280), an antigen suspension diluted 1:160 would contain 8 HA units in 0.05 ml, and a suspension diluted 1:80 would contain 8 units in 0.025 ml.

HI test. Add 0.05 ml of kaolin-erythrocyte adsorbed serum to the first and last of a row of wells in the microtiter plate and 0.025 ml of BABS to the remaining wells. Make twofold dilutions of the serum through the next to the last well using 0.025-ml loops. Add antigen containing 4 to 8 HA units in 0.025 ml to each well except the last, which serves as the serum control. Include antisera known to contain antibodies to each of the antigens used in the test as a control. Prepare a back titration of the antigen suspension used in the test.

Incubate plates overnight at 4 C or at room temperature for 2 h. Dilute the back titration of antigen using 0.05-ml loops, and then add to each well 0.05 ml of erythrocyte suspension diluted in the VAD giving optimal viral HA. Shake the plates, and incubate them for 30 min.

The HI titer is recorded as the highest serum dilution completely inhibiting HA. Agglutination of goose erythrocytes should be absent in the serum control. Specific controls to test for removal of serum nonspecific inhibitors of HA are not done; therefore, inclusion of several serologically unrelated antigens in the test may help interpretation. Nonspecific inhibition is suspected if a serum is "positive" to several serologically unrelated viruses or to a virus unlikely to have caused infection on epidemiological grounds. The back titration of antigen indicates any change in HA units after test incubation.

Complement-fixation test. A CF test is described in chapter 58 of this *Manual.*

Neutralization test: constant virus-varying serum dilution plaque reduction test in cell culture. Primary Pekin duck embryo cells are recommended for tests with the alphaviruses and SLE, and the Vero cell line is recommended for tests with many Bunyaviruses and CTF virus. Cell lines useful for work with flaviviruses include porcine kidney (6), LLC-MK2 for dengue viruses, and rabbit embryonic kidney (MA-111) for yellow fever.

For the preparation of primary duck embryo cultures, harvest 1-day-old embryos; remove the heads, feet, and wings, and wash the remaining tissue three times in Hanks balanced salt solution (BSS). Mince the embryos into small pieces (3 mm), and disperse the cells by addition of 0.25% trypsin in Hanks BSS. After trypsinization, decant the cell suspension through four layers of sterile gauze and centrifuge it. Wash the cell sediment, and suspend the cells in growth medium (see below, Reagents). Count the cells using a hemacytometer, and seed 1-oz prescription bottles with 3.5 ml of a suspension containing 700,000 cells/ml. Incubate the bottles at 37 C for approximately 3 days or until monolayers are confluent. Monolayer cultures may also be prepared in plastic plates (Linbro Scientific Co., New Haven, Conn.), which must be incubated in a 5% CO_2 atmosphere or buffered by addition to the growth medium of N-2-hydroxylethyl piperazine-N'-2-ethanesulfonic acid (HEPES), 6.0 g/ liter.

Continuous cell lines such as Vero (available at the 121st passage level from the American Type Culture Collection, Rockville, Md.) are maintained by weekly passage in stationary or roller bottles. After 25 to 30 passages in the laboratory, it is advisable to return to cells near the original passage level. Cells in stock cultures are dispersed with trypsin-ethylenediaminetetraacetic acid solution (Microbiological Associates, Inc., Bethesda, Md.), suspended in growth medium, and counted. One-ounce bottles are seeded with 3.5 ml of a suspension containing 150,000 cells/ml.

To assay virus seeds for plaque infectivity titer, prepare serial 10-fold dilutions in growth medium. Add 0.1 ml of each dilution to duplicate cell cultures. Cultures are incubated at 37 C for 45 min to facilitate virus adsorption and are then overlaid with 1% Noble agar in Earle's BSS. Neutral red is incorporated into this primary overlay at a final concentration of 1:40,000 for viruses such as EEE, WEE, and SLE, which cause rapidly developing plaques, or into a second overlay (at a final concentration of 1:25,000) applied after several days of incubation for viruses which form plaques more slowly. Plaques appear as clear areas surrounded by normal cells vitally stained by neutral red.

For the PRNT, prepare serial twofold dilutions of the sera to be tested in growth medium, and dispense in 0.1-ml volumes into sterile tubes. A virus suspension diluted to contain approximately 200 plaque-forming units (PFU) in 0.1 ml is added in equal volumes (0.1 ml) to each test serum dilution and to six control tubes containing normal human serum. Normal human serum (containing "labile serum factor" [4]) obtained fresh and stored in portions at −70 C is incorporated into the virus suspension at a dilution not to exceed 1:8. This restores neutralizing capacity of sera lost during storage and improves the precision of test results by reducing the appearance of partially inhibited plaques.

Virus-serum mixtures, held until this point in an ice bath, are incubated in a water bath at 37 C, and 0.1 ml of each mixture is inoculated onto cell monolayers. Procedures for adsorption of virus, agar overlay, and staining are as described for virus assays above. The neutralization titer is expressed as the highest dilution of serum causing a 90% or greater reduction in PFU over the average number of PFU in normal serum controls.

REAGENTS

Antigens

Antigens for use in the HI and CF tests are prepared by extraction of infected tissue with sucrose-acetone (5). In a biological safety cabinet, prepare a 20% (wt/vol) suspension of infected brains (livers for some group C Bunyaviruses) in chilled 8.5% sucrose. Homogenize for 1 min (Omni-Mixer; Ivan Sorvall, Inc., Norwalk,

Conn.), and add 1 volume of homogenate to 20 volumes of chilled acetone by rapid injection from a syringe and needle. Avoid splashing by placing the needle point beneath the surface of the acetone. Stopper, shake vigorously, allow settling for 15 min in an ice bath, and siphon off the supernatant fluid. Add 20 volumes of chilled acetone, shake, and allow settling at 4 C for 1 h; then decant the acetone, and dry the particulate material to a powder by vacuum (2 to 2.5 h), keeping the flask cold while drying. Reconstitute with 0.1 M tris(hydroxymethyl)-aminomethane (Tris) in borate saline, pH 9.0, to twice the volume of the original brain. Centrifuge at 10,000 rpm for 1 h, and decant the supernatant fluid containing the antigen.

If an inactivated antigen is desired, β-propiolactone (BPL) in cold 0.85% NaCl is added to a final concentration of 0.3%. The mixture is held at 4 C with gentle mechanical stirring for 72 h. Portions of the antigen may then be lyophilized or stored frozen.

Satisfactory inactivated HA and CF antigens for alphaviruses and CF antigens for many other viruses can also be prepared as crude 10% suspensions of infected suckling mouse brain in 0.1 M Tris in borate-saline, pH 9.0, and treated with BPL as previously described.

Sonic treatment and treatment with trypsin may be necessary to prepare HA antigens for some Bunyaviruses (1). LaCrosse virus HA antigens can be prepared from infected BHK-21 cells grown in suspension and then extracted with Tween 80-ether (3).

Viral antigens are not commercially available; however, small quantities for reference purposes may be obtained from the Biological Reagents Branch, Scientific Resources Division, Center for Disease Control, Atlanta, Ga.

Antisera

Antisera for use as homologous controls in serological tests may be prepared by a series of intraperitoneal (i.p.) inoculations of adult mice with 0.5 ml of 10% suspension (in phosphate-buffered saline) of infected mouse brain. Antigens inactivated with BPL should be used for the first two immunizing inoculations if the live virus will kill adult mice. Mice immunized by inoculations on days 1, 3, 21, and 24 are then bled on day 34. Complete Freund's adjuvant may be added to the inocula if desired. Hyperimmune mouse ascitic fluids may be prepared by the i.p. inoculation of sarcoma-180 cells prior to the final immunizing dose of virus. Guinea pigs, rabbits, monkeys, goats, or horses may be used as alternative hosts to mice for preparation of antisera.

Virus-adjusting diluents

Phosphate buffers for adjusting the pH of goose erythrocyte suspensions are prepared by mixing stock solutions of 0.15 M NaCl-0.2 M Na_2HPO_4 and 0.15 M NaCl-0.2 M NaH_2PO_4, as shown in Table 2.

Growth medium for cell cultures

Medium 199 (10×) with Hanks BSS containing L-glutamine (this and other reagents available from Microbiological Associates, Inc.) .... 100 ml
Fetal calf serum, heated at 56 C for 30 min .... 50 ml
$NaHCO_3$ (sterilized by filtration), 7.5% .... 16.5 ml
Gentamicin solution, 50 mg/ml ... 0.5 ml
Sodium penicillin G, 1,000,00 units, and streptomycin, 1.0 g, dissolved in 10 ml of sterile distilled water and brought to 1 liter with doubly distilled sterile water .... 1.0 ml

INTERPRETATION

A positive result is indicated by an HI antibody titer of $\geq 1:10$ or a CF titer of $\geq 1:8$. In the serum dilution neutralization test in cell culture, $\geq 90\%$ plaque reduction by an undiluted serum may be considered positive, and 70 to 89% plaque reduction is equivocal. Lack of correlation between HI or CF and PRNT results may indicate a technical error or infection with an antigenically related virus which induces antibody that is cross-reactive by HI or CF but not by the more specific viral neutralization.

For serological confirmation, it is necessary to interpret comparative titrations of paired sera collected at appropriate intervals in relation to

TABLE 2. *Virus adjusting diluents for addition to goose erythrocyte suspensions*

Final pH[a]	0.15 M NaCl-0.2 M Na_2HPO_4 (%)	0.15 M NaCl-0.2 M NaH_2PO_4 (%)
5.75	3.0	97.0
5.9	7.7	92.3
6.0	12.5	87.5
6.1	17.3	82.7
6.2	22.0	78.0
6.4	32.0	68.0
6.6	45.0	55.0
6.8	55.0	45.0
7.0	64.0	36.0
7.2	72.0	28.0

[a] The final pH is that measured after mixing equal volumes of virus-adjusting diluent and BABS, pH 9.0.

the onset of clinical symptoms. A fourfold or greater rise or fall in antibody titer confirms recent infection with the virus used in the test and indicates that the illness was etiologically related to it. Twofold changes in antibody titers are regarded as inconsequential and may be found if the paired serum samples are taken within too short an interval. Stable HI and/or neutralization antibody titers in both an early acute and a convalescent serum and absence of CF antibody in the latter suggest remote infection unrelated to the current illness. The absence of detectable HI antibody in a serum obtained 2 weeks or more after onset of clinical symptoms is presumptive evidence against a Togavirus infection, but absence of neutralization antibody is more conclusive.

Primary infection is usually followed by the development of antibodies which are immunologically monotypic. With time, antibodies which are more cross-reactive with heterologous antigens may develop. Advantage can be made of the cross-reactivity of Togavirus HI antibodies, since infection with a member of a serological group may be detected despite omission from the test of the specific antigen responsible for infection. Because of the antigenic sharing between members of the alpha- and flavivirus groups and the different specificities of the available tests, serological interpretation is' most reliable when HI and CF antibody titers are compared with a variety of antigens within the serogroup and when confirmation by the PRNT tests has been achieved. A fourfold or higher titer to one virus antigen than to other members of a serogroup generally indicates infection with that agent, although heterotypic reactions may occur (see below). Results should be reviewed with regard to their compatibility with the known seasonal activity of arthropod-borne virus infection and with the geographical distribution of the viruses in question.

Definitive diagnosis is most difficult when infection occurs in an individual previously naturally infected or vaccinated with an antigenically related virus. This problem is particularly evident in tropical regions where two or more related viruses are endemic, although in the United States past yellow fever vaccinations and remote infection with dengue virus have complicated interpretation of serological results in patients with SLE infection. Superinfection usually results in the development of a rapid and broad anamnestic response that may preclude the demonstration of a rise in titer or prevent specific diagnosis. In some instances, the antibody response may be heterotypic with a higher titer to the original antigen than to the agent responsible for the current illness. The spectrum of serological responses in persons with flavivirus superinfections has been described in detail by several authors (11, 13).

Review of the technical laboratory procedures is essential to diagnostic interpretation. Because of unavoidable variability between tests, titers of paired sera may be reliably compared only if the sera were tested together at the same time. When titers to serologically related antigens are compared, moreover, it is important to assure that differences are not related to quantitative variations in the amount of HA or CF antigen employed.

LITERATURE CITED

1. Ardoin, P., D. H. Clarke, and C. Hannoun. 1969. The preparation of arbovirus hemagglutinations by sonication and trypsin treatment. Am. J. Trop. Med. Hyg. 18:592–598.
2. Bergold, G. H., and R. Mazzali. 1968. Plaque formation by arboviruses. J. Gen. Virol. 2:273–284.
3. Chappell, W. A., P. E. Halonen, R. F. Toole, C. H. Calisher, and L. Chester. 1969. Preparation of La Crosse virus hemagglutinating antigen in BHK-21 suspension cell cultures. Appl. Microbiol. 18:433–437.
4. Chappell, W. A., D. R. Sasso, R. F. Toole, and T. P. Monath. 1971. Labile serum factor and its effect on arbovirus neutralization. Appl. Microbiol. 21:79–83.
5. Clarke, D. H., and J. Casals. 1958. Techniques for hemagglutination and hemagglutination-inhibition with arthropod-borne viruses. Am. J. Trop. Med. Hyg. 7:561–573.
6. DeMadrid, A. T., and J. S. Porterfield. 1969. A simple micro-culture method for the study of group B arboviruses. Bull. WHO 40:113–121.
7. Dulbecco, R., M. Vogt, and A. G. R. Strickland. 1956. A study of the basic aspects of neutralization of two animal viruses, Western equine encephalitis virus and poliomyelitis virus. Virology 2:162–205.
8. Earley, E., P. H. Peralta, and K. M. Johnson. 1967. A plaque neutralization method for arboviruses. Proc. Soc. Exp. Biol. Med. 125:741–747.
9. Emmons, R. W., D. V. Dondero, V. Devlin, and E. H. Lennette. 1969. Serologic diagnosis of Colorado tick fever. Am. J. Trop. Med. Hyg. 18:796–802.
10. Hammon, W. McD., and G. E. Sather. 1969. Arboviruses, p. 227–280. In E. H. Lennette and N. J. Schmidt (ed.), Diagnostic procedures for viral and rickettsial infections, 4th ed. American Public Health Association, Inc., New York.
11. Monath, T. P., D. C. Wilson, and J. Casals. 1973. The 1970 yellow epidemic in Okwoga District, Benue Plateau State, Nigeria. 3. Serological

responses in persons with and without preexisting heterologous group B immunity. Bull. WHO **49:**235–244.

12. Porterfield, J. S., and C. E. Rowe. 1960. Hemagglutination with arthropod-borne viruses and its inhibition by certain phospholipids. Virology **11:**765–770.

13. Theiler, M., and J. Casals. 1958. The serological reactions in yellow fever. Am. J. Trop. Med. Hyg. **7:**585–594.

Chapter 63

Arenaviruses

FREDERICK A. MURPHY

INTRODUCTION

The arenaviruses are a taxon established on the basis of common details of virion structure, and reinforced on the basis of distant, varying serological cross-reactivities (20, 21, 27). This taxon contains several viruses which are significant human pathogens: lymphocytic choriomeningitis (LCM) virus, Lassa virus (the etiological agent of Lassa fever), Machupo virus (Bolivian hemorrhagic fever), and Junin virus (Argentinian hemorrhagic fever). In addition, there are six other member viruses which have not been associated with human disease (Amapari, Latino, Parana, Pichinde, Tacaribe, and Tamiami viruses; 22). Arenaviruses have rather similar natural histories, each being perpetuated in nature by a single or limited number of rodent species (12). The viruses usually are not pathogenic in their natural rodent hosts, but infection patterns include slow clearance or persistence and chronic shedding (11, 13, 14). These characteristics, and the limited geographical location of each virus-rodent pairing (except LCM virus in *Mus musculus*), relate to human exposure and, therefore, to the risk of natural human disease.

Pathogenic arenaviruses become an extreme biohazard in conventional viral diagnostic and serology laboratories; in clinical settings (e.g., when drawing specimens) and in clinical chemistry and hematology laboratories, the biohazard is similar. This is obvious with viruses such as Lassa, Machupo, and Junin, but it should also be remembered that LCM virus may cause severe meningoencephalitis, or in rare instances may be lethal. Procedures in which Lassa, Machupo, or Junin virus is used must be limited to laboratories with "class 3" containment, such as the Maximum Security Laboratory at the Center for Disease Control (CDC). Procedures that require the use of field isolates of LCM virus should be limited to laboratories meeting the containment and staff competence standards defined by the U.S. Public Health Service (24).

Three general serological methods have been used for clinical, epidemiological, and reference assays of human experience with pathogenic arenaviruses, or of human immune status. These methods are complement fixation (CF), indirect immunofluorescence (IIF), and neutralization. Preference has most often reflected the kind of containment facilities available rather than the real merits of different tests. For example, Machupo virus serology has primarily been done by plaque reduction neutralization at the Middle America Research Unit, where the staff is immune by virtue of previous field infection. In contrast, Lassa virus serology has primarily been done by CF and IIF at the CDC, where the staff must work in glove-port cabinets.

CLINICAL INDICATIONS

Indications for serological testing for particular arenavirus antibodies usually come from clinico-epidemiological judgments relating to serious febrile illness, febrile illness with prostration and shock, aseptic meningitis, or illness with an unusually high case fatality rate. Clinical signs and symptoms of each arenavirus disease may vary somewhat in character and severity, but differential diagnoses should include arenaviruses which are prevalent in those geographical areas where infections have occurred and/or areas known to harbor reservoir rodent species. Clinical indications regarding Lassa fever have been published by Monath (19), and those for Bolivian hemorrhagic fever, by Johnson and colleagues (11). LCM infection must be considered in relation to exposure to wild mice and pet rodents (16); clinical indications have been reported by Lehmann-Grube (14). These are "emerging" diseases, and increased demand for clinical laboratory testing must be anticipated; in such instances, speed of serological methods will determine clinical value. Likewise, demands for more epidemiological survey data are to be anticipated, and in such instances the capacity for handling large numbers of specimens must be considered along with the specificity and sensitivity of methods. In all cases, serology should be complemented by virus isolation attempts from appropriate specimens.

TEST PROCEDURES

Complement-fixation testing

CF testing is carried out in microtiter systems according to a standardized technique (3). Antigens may be prepared from infected Vero cells harvested late in infection (5 to 7 days; 26); supernatant fluids plus cells may be frozen and thawed several times, clarified, and used without further treatment. LCM antigen is often made from infected suckling mouse brain by extraction with sucrose-acetone (5, 7, 28) or with a fluorocarbon such as Genetron or Freon 113 (4). Antigens may be inactivated with β-propiolactone (1), but they must then be tested rigorously for residual infectivity. CF testing has been used successfully with all arenaviruses (see also chapter 58).

Indirect immunofluorescence

IIF methods vary only in the substrate used (6). Vero cells (25), or BHK-21 or L cells for LCM, may be grown in culture chambers (Lab-Tek, 8 chambers/slide; Miles Laboratories, Westmont, Ill.) or in Leighton tubes on cover slips. Cultures are inoculated, and when at least 30% of the cells are infected (via immunofluorescence assay, 3 to 11 days postinfection) they are processed as substrates (H. Wulff, personal communication). Alternatively, cells may be grown and infected in bottles as monolayers (23) or as spinner cultures (17; V. J. Lewis, P. D. Walter, W. L. Thacker, and W. G. Winkler, in preparation), and samples of detached cells are dried as spots in the uncoated circles on epoxy-coated slides (Cel-Line Associates, Minotola, N.J.). In both cases, the infected cells are air-dried, fixed in acetone for 10 min at room temperature (or for 24 h at -20 to -70 C), dried, and stored at -70 C, where they are stable indefinitely. When needed, substrates are thawed, air-dried, and flooded with human serum (at 1:2 or 1:4 dilution for screening or in serial twofold dilutions for titration). After 30 min at room temperature in a moist chamber, serum is washed off with phosphate-buffered saline (PBS; one short wash followed by two 10-min immersions with agitation), and fluorescein isothiocyanate (FITC)-conjugated anti-human immunoglobulin (or anti-human IgG and IgM for class-specific testing) at a predetermined working dilution is added for 30 min. FITC conjugates are available from many commercial sources. The same washing procedure is followed by air drying and mounting under a cover slip in PBS-buffered glycerol (1:9). Conventional immunofluorescence microscopy equipment is used, and dilution end points are chosen where brightness of immunofluorescence just begins to diminish. This judgment may be made with double-blind coded specimens for added objectivity. Because of the possibility of prozone effects, full titrations of human sera may be indicated in some circumstances. The substrates for IIF testing are infectious, and attempts to avoid this biohazard by using immunologically related nonpathogenic viruses have failed; however, Machupo virus substrates have been shown to be inactivated by the drying and acetone fixation steps (23). One major advantage of the cell monolayer substrates from chambers or Leighton tubes (relative to infected cells deposited as spots on slides) is that viral antigen is maintained in its normal aggregate or granular form in infected cell cytoplasm. This acts as an additional control; all positive sera must yield the same pattern. Standard positive and negative serum controls are always included, and specificity controls must be included when more than one arenavirus is suspected (23). IIF testing has been successfully used with nearly all of the arenaviruses.

Neutralization

Neutralization methods vary greatly, and no single method has overall superiority. For many years, LCM neutralization was done by intracerebral inoculation of 3-week-old Swiss mice with mixtures of undiluted serum and 10-fold dilutions of virus. More recently, LCM neutralizing antibody was measured by its inhibition of mouse footpad swelling evoked by the virus (8, 9, 18). These in vivo neutralization methods have not been shown to be suitable for other arenaviruses; cell culture methods now predominate, but methods vary widely. An LCM neutralization may be carried out in tubes with cells which support virus growth but do not exhibit cytopathic changes (e.g., L cells); end points are determined by CF on supernatant fluids (14). Similarly, neutralization on LCM and other arenaviruses may be done in Lab-Tek chambers with immunofluorescent-focus inhibition used to determine serum end points (31). For this test, virus is diluted to yield 30 to 50 focus-forming units per chamber sample; after incubation for 1 h at 37 C with serum dilutions, the mixture is adsorbed to Vero or other susceptible cells in the slide chambers. At about 48 h, when each focus of residual infectivity contains 4 to 10 cells, conventional immunofluorescence staining (direct or indirect) is done. Serum end points are determined from dilutions which inhibit 80% of the foci present with normal serum controls. Arenaviruses other than LCM plaque in Vero and several other cell lines, so neutralization methods based upon plaque reduction in monolayers are widely used. The Machupo virus neutralization (29, 30) is done with Vero cells grown in disposable plastic trays containing 96 flat wells (#96CF clear; Linbro Chemical Co., Inc., New Haven, Conn.). After adsorption of serum-virus mixtures (80 to 100 plaque-forming units of virus) for 1 h at 36 C in a 4% CO_2 atmosphere, agar is overlaid and incubation is continued. An indicator overlay is added, and plaques are counted at 5 to 8 days; 80% plaque reduction end points are calculated. The failure of LCM virus to plaque in this kind of system has been offset by the recent demonstration of microplaques in an agarose cell suspension technique (10). In this case, dispersed BHK-21 cells in agarose are added to microtiter plates already containing serum-virus mixtures (6 to 10 microplaque-forming units per well) in a solid agar layer. An indicator overlay is added at 4 days, and microplaques are counted with a hand lens.

Other assays for arenavirus antibodies have been used occasionally. Immunodiffusion has merit because massive amounts of soluble antigen are characteristically formed in infected cells in vivo (e.g., LCM-infected mouse brain) or in cell culture (all arenaviruses in Vero cells). A bold precipitin line is formed with antisera from many kinds of experimental animals, but human convalescent sera have not been tested comparatively.

INTERPRETATION

Choice of particular serological methods and the clinical or epidemiological interpretation of serological results will, of course, vary according to laboratory settings. The three general methods, CF, IIF, and neutralization, may be compared in typical settings. CF for LCM has advantages (i) when integrated into an antigen battery used for all aseptic meningitis specimens, (ii) when used on large numbers of specimens, or (iii) when required of a laboratory without competence for handling the virus. On the other hand, CF antibody is (i) the least specific, (ii) relatively low in titer and subject to insensitivity problems, (iii) subject to anticomplementary problems, (iv) slow to arise after infection (often remaining undetectable from 3 to 4 weeks after infection), and (v) the first assay to return to negative after infection. These factors limit CF usefulness from both clinical and epidemiological standpoints.

IIF is becoming the single most useful assay for arenavirus antibodies by virtue of its (i) extreme sensitivity, which allows easy detection of fourfold rises between acute and convalescent sera, (ii) usefulness with improperly handled sera, (iii) rapid seroconversion after infection (often becoming positive within a few days to a week after the beginning of illness), (iv) safety when carried out with inactivated substrates (allowing field assays without biohazard), and (v) storability of substrates for immediate use. The real shortcoming of IIF lies in the difficulty in handling large numbers of specimens. Another shortcoming is the lack of IIF specificity, but the geographical isolation of arenaviruses (LCM excepted) reduces this diagnostic problem.

Neutralization methods will continue to be used only in specialty laboratories because of biohazard, cost, and complexity. However, because of the extreme sensitivity combined with specificity of several of the newer in vitro methods, neutralization retains its value for confirmation of the presumptive data obtained with other tests. Of all the serological methods, only neutralization is indicative of protection against reinfection. These characteristics and the fact that response occurs late after infection and persists indefinitely make neutralization of the most value to the epidemiologist and of the least to the clinician.

In most instances in which arenavirus antibodies are found in human sera, meaningful interpretations follow. The severity of several of the arenavirus diseases and the high case fatality rates often mean that public health measures to limit human risk are of immediate concern when antibody and/or other evidences of infection are found in a population group (2, 15). Clinical judgments also improve when serological evidence of arenavirus activity contributes to differential diagnosis considerations. Finally, rodent control measures are often warranted when antibody patterns indicate particular population risks.

LITERATURE CITED

1. Buckley, S. M., and J. Casals. 1970. Lassa fever, a new virus disease of man from West Africa. III. Isolation and characterization of the virus. Am. J. Trop. Med. Hyg. 19:680–691.
2. Casals, J., and S. M. Buckley. 1973. Lassa fever virus, p. 325–339. In F. Lehmann-Grube (ed.), Lymphocytic choriomeningitis virus and other arenaviruses. Springer-Verlag, Berlin.
3. Casey, H. 1965. Standardized diagnostic complement fixation method and adaptation to microtest. In Public Health Monogr. no. 74, Public Health Service Publ. no. 1228. U.S. Government Printing Office, Washington, D.C.

4. Chastel, C., and P. LeNoc. 1968. Antigène fixateur du complément de titre élevé et de préparation simple pour le virus de la chiorome méningite lymphocytaire. Ann. Inst. Pasteur Paris 114:698–704.

5. Clarke, D. H., and J. Casals. 1958. Techniques for hemagglutination and hemagglutination-inhibition with arthropod-borne viruses. Am. J. Trop. Med. Hyg. 7:561–573.

6. Cohen, S. M., I. E. Triandaphilli, J. L. Barlow, and J. Hotchin. 1968. Immunofluorescent detection of antibody to lymphocytic choriomeningitis virus in man. J. Immunol. 96:777–784.

7. Gresikova, M., and J. Casals. 1963. A simple method of preparing a complement-fixing antigen for lymphocytic choriomeningitis virus. Acta Virol. (Prague) 7:380–388.

8. Hotchin, J. 1962. The footpad reaction of mice to lymphocytic choriomeningitis virus. Virology 17:214–216.

9. Hotchin, J., L. Benson, and E. Sikora. 1969. The detection of neutralizing antibody to lymphocytic choriomeningitis virus in mice. J. Immunol. 102:1128–1135.

10. Hotchin, J., and W. Kinch. 1975. Microplaque reduction: a new assay for neutralizing antibody to lymphocytic choriomeningitis virus. J. Infect. Dis. 131:186–188.

11. Johnson, K. M., S. B. Halstead, and S. N. Cohen. 1967. Hemorrhagic fevers of Southeast Asia and South America: a comparative appraisal. Prog. Med. Virol. 9:105–158.

12. Johnson, K. M., P. A. Webb, and G. Justines. 1973. Biology of Tacaribe-complex viruses, p. 241–258. In F. Lehmann-Grube (ed.), Lymphocytic choriomeningitis virus and other arenaviruses. Springer-Verlag, Berlin.

13. Justines, G., and K. M. Johnson. 1969. Immune Machupo virus. Nature (London) 222:1090–1091.

14. Lehmann-Grube, F. 1971. Lymphocytic choriomeningitis. Virol. Monogr. 10:1–173.

15. Lehmann-Grube, F. 1973. Lymphocytic choriomeningitis virus and other arenaviruses. Springer-Verlag, Berlin.

16. Lewis, A. M., W. P. Rowe, H. C. Turner, and R. J. Huebner. 1965. Lymphocytic choriomeningitis virus in hamster tumor: spread to hamsters and humans. Science 150:363–364.

17. Lewis, V., and D. Clayton. 1969. Detection of lymphocytic choriomeningitis virus antibody in murine sera by immunofluorescence. Appl. Microbiol. 18:289–290.

18. Mims, C. A., and R. V. Blanden. 1972. Antiviral action of immune lymphocytes in mice infected with lymphocytic choriomeningitis virus. Infect. Immun. 6:695–698.

19. Monath, T. P. 1973. Lassa fever. Tropical Doctor 4:155–161.

20. Murphy, F. A., P. A. Webb, K. M. Johnson, and S. G. Whitfield. 1969. Morphological comparison of Machupo with lymphocytic choriomeningitis virus: basis for a new taxonomic group. J. Virol. 4:535–541.

21. Murphy, F. A., P. A. Webb, K. M. Johnson, S. G. Whitfield, and W. A. Chappell. 1970. Arenoviruses in Vero cells: ultrastructural studies. J. Virol. 6:507–518.

22. Murphy, F. A., S. G. Whitfield, P. A. Webb, and K. M. Johnson. 1973. Ultrastructural studies of arenaviruses, p. 273–285. In F. Lehmann-Grube (ed.), Lymphocytic choriomeningitis and other arenaviruses. Springer-Verlag, Berlin.

23. Peters, C. J., P. A. Webb, and K. M. Johnson. 1973. Measurement of antibodies to Machupo virus by the indirect fluorescent technique. Proc. Soc. Exp. Biol. Med. 142:526–531.

24. Public Health Service Committee on the Safe Shipment and Handling of Etiologic Agents. 1974. Classification of etiologic agents on the basis of hazard, 4th ed. Center for Disease Control, Atlanta, Ga.

25. Rhim, J. S., K. Schell, B. Creasy, and W. Case. 1969. Biological characteristics and viral susceptibility of an African green monkey kidney cell line (Vero). Proc. Soc. Exp. Biol. Med. 132:670–678.

26. Rhim, J. S., B. Simizu, and N. H. Wiebenga. 1967. Growth of Junin virus, the etiologic agent of Argentinian hemorrhagic fever, in cell cultures. Arch. Gesamte Virusforsch. 21:243–252.

27. Rowe, W. P., W. E. Pugh, P. A. Webb, and C. J. Peters. 1970. Serological relationship of the Tacaribe complex of viruses to lymphocytic choriomeningitis virus. J. Virol. 5:289–292.

28. Shope, R. E. 1974. Arboviruses, p. 740–745. In E. H. Lennette, E. H. Spaulding, and J. P. Truant (ed.), Manual of clinical microbiology, 2nd ed. American Society for Microbiology, Washington, D.C.

29. Webb, P. A., K. M. Johnson, J. B. Hibbs, and M. L. Kuns. 1970. Parana, a new Tacaribe complex virus from Paraguay. Arch. Gesamte Virusforsch. 32:379–388.

30. Webb, P. A., K. M. Johnson, and R. B. Mackenzie. 1969. The measurement of specific antibodies in Bolivian hemorrhagic fever by neutralization of virus plaques. Proc. Soc. Exp. Biol. Med. 130:1013–1019.

31. Winn, W. C., Jr., F. A. Murphy, and M. R. Flemister. 1973. The pathogenesis of Tamiami virus meningoencephalitis in newborn mice, p. 299–311. In F. Lehmann-Grube (ed.), Lymphocytic choriomeningitis virus and other arenaviruses. Springer-Verlag, Berlin.

Chapter 64

Immune Electron Microscopy as a Method for the Detection, Identification, and Characterization of Agents Not Cultivable in an In Vitro System

ALBERT Z. KAPIKIAN, JULES L. DIENSTAG, AND ROBERT H. PURCELL

INTRODUCTION

Recently, there has been a renewed interest in the technique of immune (or immuno-) electron microscopy (IEM), a method which can be defined as the direct observation of antigen-antibody interaction by electron microscopy (2, 30). It is indeed surprising that this method had not been utilized to its fullest potential until recently, for it was first described as long ago as 1941 in the United States and in Germany (4, 5). Workers in both countries independently observed by electron microscopy that a mixture of tobacco mosaic virus (TMV) and a specific antiserum resulted in aggregation of the virus particles, whereas, in contrast, when TMV virus was mixed with a control serum, aggregation was not observed. In addition, the United States workers showed the specificity of this reaction by demonstrating that TMV did not aggregate in the presence of anti-tomato bush stunt virus serum and that the latter virus did not react with anti-TMV serum. With the introduction of the technique of negative staining, which greatly enhanced contrast, antigen-antibody reactions were demonstrated with great clarity (9, 32, 33; T. F. Anderson, N. Yamamoto, and K. J. Hummeler, J. Appl. Phys. 32:1639, 1961). However, until recently, studies utilizing the technique were performed predominantly with purified antigens which were known to be of high titer. This chapter will deal exclusively with the use of IEM (i) as a means of detecting fastidious viral agents which do not grow in vitro and for which other practical methods of detection do not exist or are limited and (ii) as a serological technique for demonstrating evidence of infection with such fastidious agents. The technique has also been utilized for demonstrating immunological and other properties of different viruses and for typing viruses, but these procedures will not be described in detail. The technique of IEM has been reviewed by Almeida and Waterson (2), Doane (13), and Kapikian et al. (25).

CLINICAL INDICATIONS

IEM is still essentially a research tool since electron microscopes are not generally available, and even when microscopes are accessible individuals adequately trained in the method of IEM are found only infrequently. However, as microscopes become more generally available, the technique has the potential of being utilized as a routine laboratory test (1a, 35). The technique itself is quite simple, but its interpretation may pose problems to inexperienced individuals.

In dealing with certain diseases such as nonbacterial epidemic gastroenteritis, IEM is the only in vitro method available for detection and identification of etiological agents from clinical specimens. For hepatitis type A, IEM was the first in vitro method available for the detection and identification of the etiological agent of this disease and remains a mainstay in the study of this virus from clinical specimens. Thus, study of specimens by IEM from patients with these illnesses will be described. IEM has also been used effectively in the study of hepatitis type B, but other more practical methods have been developed for the study of this disease (50).

Studies of agents of acute infectious nonbacterial gastroenteritis by immune electron microscopy

It appears that viral gastroenteritis is comprised of at least two entities with distinct epidemiological characteristics (21, 22). The first tends to occur in family or community-wide outbreaks and affects adults, school-age children, family contacts, and most probably young children as well. The clinical features usually last 24 to 48 h, and the illness is usually mild with combinations of nausea, vomiting, diarrhea, abdominal cramping, malaise, and low-grade fever. In spite of intensive efforts, the etiological agents of this form of viral gastroenteritis have not been definitely propagated in any in vitro or animal system, nor had they been recognized by conventional electron microscopy (6, 14, 15). However, utilizing the technique of IEM, we (29) were able to visualize a 27-nm particle in an infectious human stool filtrate derived from an outbreak in Norwalk, Ohio (1). The particles which were heavily coated with antibody were not randomly distributed but were present as aggregates that could easily be differentiated from other round structures which lacked antibody (Fig. 1). In this technique, a stool filtrate was allowed to react with convalescent serum

from a volunteer who had developed the disease. This approach was taken so that virus particles, if present, would appear in the form of aggregates, thereby enabling the visualization and identification of a viral agent present in low titer and of such small size that it would not be recognized by conventional electron microscopy (23, 25, 27, 29). In further studies in which a stool filtrate containing the 27-nm particle was used as antigen in tests with patients' paired sera, it was found that most individuals who developed illness due to this agent

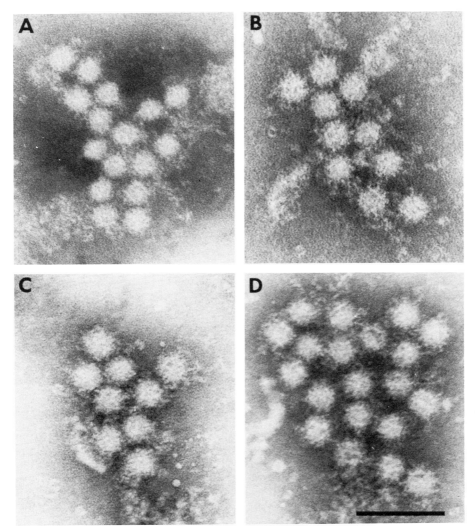

FIG. 1. *Aggregates observed after (i) incubation of 0.4 ml of the 8FIIa stool filtrate with 0.1 ml of a 1:10 dilution of convalescent serum from a volunteer who developed gastroenteritis after challenge with the Norwalk filtrate and (ii) further preparation for electron microscopy. (A) An aggregate observed in the initial experiment (incubation of serum-stool filtrate for 1 h). (B, C, and D) Aggregates observed in the second experiment (incubation of serum-stool filtrate for 1.75 h). The particles are coated with antibody. Bar = 100 nm and applies to A–E. (B) From Kapikian et al. (29). (A, C, and D) From Kapikian et al. (25).*

also developed serological evidence of infection by IEM. From this and other evidence, the 27-nm particle was implicated as the etiological agent of Norwalk gastroenteritis (29). Additional IEM studies later revealed a close temporal association of illness with the presence of the 27-nm particles in stools during experimental infection (46). More recently, particles which resemble the Norwalk agent morphologically have also been observed by IEM in stool filtrates derived from two family outbreaks of gastroenteritis, one in Hawaii and the other in Montgomery County, Md. (T. S. Thornhill et al., in preparation). By IEM, antibody responses to these agents were found in most individuals with naturally occurring or experimentally induced illness, and reciprocal IEM studies demonstrated that the Norwalk and Hawaii agents were distinct. By IEM also, the density of these three particles was found to be about 1.37 to 1.41 g/cm^3 in cesium chloride (26; Thornhill et al., in preparation). Thus, numerous studies could be carried out by IEM on as yet uncultivable agents found in the stools of patients with gastroenteritis, and such uncultivable agents were implicated as etiological agents of epidemic gastroenteritis.

IEM has also been utilized for the detection of agents in a second form of gastroenteritis which could be designated sporadic infantile gastroenteritis (28, 36). This form of gastroenteritis has been associated with a severe form of diarrhea which is often accompanied by vomiting and occurs predominantly in infants and young children. The etiological agent is a reovirus-like agent which cannot yet be propagated efficiently in any in vitro system but has been shown to produce illness in several animal models (47, 51). Although IEM may be used for the detection of this agent in stools, conventional electron microscopy is quite adequate for its detection because, in contrast to the Norwalk agent, the reovirus-like particle is relatively large (70 nm) and has a quite distinct morphological appearance; thus, it may be recognized readily even when appearing as a single particle without an antibody covering (28). Serological evidence of infection with the reovirus-like agent has been demonstrated by IEM, but this method is not routinely used at present since a complement-fixation (CF) test for the human reovirus-like agent has been developed (24, 28).

Immune electron microscopy studies with viral hepatitis type A

As with epidemic nonbacterial gastroenteritis, the etiological agent of type A hepatitis has not been cultivated in any in vitro system. However, it has been transmitted serially in nonhuman primates (38).

Prompted by the success in visualizing the Norwalk agent by IEM, Feinstone, Kapikian, and Purcell (17) examined stool filtrates made from stools of volunteers who had developed experimental type A hepatitis illness (7). Filtrates were allowed to react either with a convalescent serum from a volunteer who had developed the disease or with immune human serum globulin (since we assumed that antibody would be present in the latter also), and 27-nm particles coated with antibody were readily visualized (Fig. 2). These particles would not have been recognized without the addition of the antibody-containing serum or gamma globulin. As with the Norwalk agent, the 27-nm particles stood out clearly from the surrounding matter and were easily differentiated from other spherical objects devoid of antibody, which are usually seen in stool filtrates. The hepatitis A particles appeared as single particles heavily coated with antibody or as particles in groups aggregated by antibody. In addition, individuals with both naturally occurring and experimentally induced hepatitis A were found to develop serological evidence of infection in IEM studies in which a stool filtrate which contained the 27-nm-particle was used as antigen in tests with paired sera. From this and other evidence, the 27-nm particle was implicated as the etiological agent of viral hepatitis type A (17). Since these studies, the 27-nm particle has been visualized by IEM in stools of hepatitis A patients in Arizona (19), in Melbourne, Australia (37), and in a recent outbreak in California (12; Fig. 3). In each study, serological responses to the hepatitis A particles were also demonstrated by IEM. IEM has thus provided the first in vitro method for demonstrating serological evidence of infection with hepatitis A antigen.

IEM was also utilized to study the buoyant density of the hepatitis A particle in cesium chloride (8, 16). In addition the shedding patterns of hepatitis A antigen in stools from both experimentally and naturally infected individuals were examined by IEM (10, 12). Such studies revealed that (i) shedding approximates the time of acute illness, (ii) shedding tends to occur before illness is clinically apparent, and (iii) by the time transaminases peak and jaundice develops, it is usually too late to detect the hepatitis A antigen in stools. The technique of IEM has also been used to determine the shedding pattern of the hepatitis A particle in experimentally infected nonhuman primates and to study their serological responses to it (11). In such studies, the technique enabled the selec-

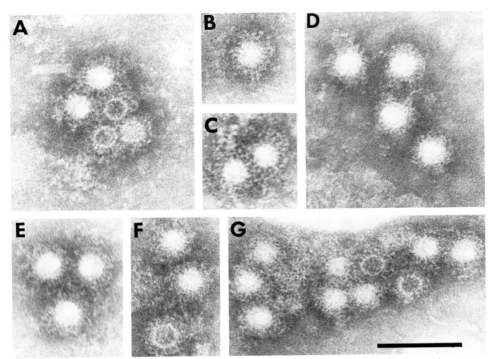

FIG. 2. *Hepatitis A virus-like particles observed after 1 ml of the 2% stool filtrate was incubated with 0.1 ml of a 1:10 dilution of a convalescent serum or a 1:20 dilution of immune serum globulin (human) followed by further preparation for electron microscopy. An aggregate (A), a single particle (B), and a doublet (C) observed after incubation of the stool filtrate with a convalescent serum from a patient from the Joliet, Ill., study. The particles are heavily coated with antibody. The quantity of antibody in this serum to the hepatitis A particle was rated 3 to 4+. (D, E, F, and G) Hepatitis A virus-like particles observed after incubation of 1 ml of the stool filtrate with immune serum globulin. The particles are heavily coated with antibody also. The quantity of antibody in this lot of immune serum globulin to the hepatitis A particle was scored 3 to 4+ also. Bar = 100 nm and applies to A–G. (A, B, F, G) From Feinstone, Kapikian, and Purcell (17). (C, D, and E) From Kapikian et al. (25).*

tion not only of particle-containing inocula but of seronegative animals as well. It also enabled a comparison of the immunological and biophysical properties of animal- and human-derived hepatitis A antigens. In addition, the technique was utilized to study the role of the hepatitis "A" particle in non-hepatitis B post-transfusion hepatitis; such studies revealed a lack of association between hepatitis A infection and post-transfusion hepatitis (18, 30a, 34). Thus, as with the Norwalk agent, such studies were carried out on an agent that had not been cultivated in any in vitro system, and sufficient evidence was obtained from such IEM studies to implicate the 27-nm particle as the etiological agent of viral hepatitis type A (17, 43, 44).

Recently CF (41) and immune adherence hemagglutination (IAHA) tests (39) have been developed for detecting serological responses to the 27-nm hepatitis A particle by use of antigen prepared from livers of marmosets (*Saguinus*

mystax) infected with hepatitis A virus (42). It appears that for hepatitis A the IAHA test is more specific, more sensitive, and simpler to carry out than the CF test (31). The IAHA test should provide a valuable tool for both diagnosis and large-scale epidemiological investigations of type A hepatitis infection. The CF and IAHA tests are without doubt much simpler to perform than the IEM test and thus more practical for the detection of hepatitis A infection. However, a limiting factor in these more practical tests is that the source of antigen for them is also quite limited, since infected marmoset livers are not readily available. However, in recent studies, purified hepatitis A antigen for the IAHA test has been prepared from stools containing hepatitis A antigen particles (39a).

Although the IAHA test is to be used in preference to the IEM method for detecting type A hepatitis infection, IEM will have to be utilized in special circumstances. Recently, the

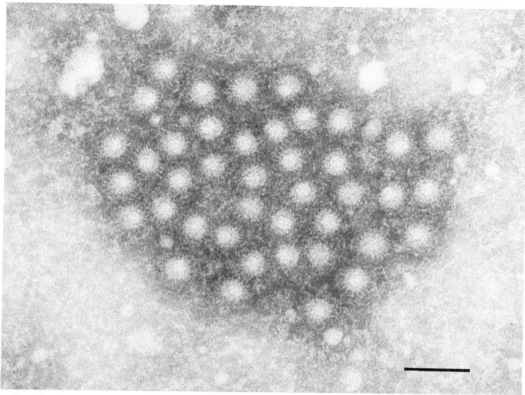

FIG. 3. *Aggregate of hepatitis A antigen particles, heavily coated with antibody in a 2% stool filtrate from a patient in California with naturally occurring hepatitis A virus infection (12). The filtrate was incubated with convalescent serum obtained from a volunteer experimentally infected with the MS-1 strain of hepatitis A virus (7). Phosphotungstic acid (3%) used as negative stain. Bar = 100 nm. From Purcell et al. (43) with permission, Charles B. Slack, Inc., publisher.*

temporal relationship between the development of IEM and IAHA antibody was assessed in serially collected serum samples from a chimpanzee experimentally infected with hepatitis A virus (Fig. 4; 9a). Antibody to hepatitis A antigen was detected about 4 weeks earlier by IEM than by IAHA. Thus, the IEM test may be necessary for early diagnosis of hepatitis A. It was noteworthy that by both methods antibody to hepatitis A antigen was still detectable at quite high levels almost 2 years after the development of hepatitis. In addition, since IEM is the only method for direct observation of antigen-antibody interaction, it may be necessary to test by IEM those occasional sera which by IAHA and CF have anticomplementary activity or give nonspecific reactions (9a). In further studies, to be described in greater detail later in the chapter, comparing antibody quantitation by IEM and IAHA, excellent agreement was found between the two tests (9a). It was noteworthy that the IEM and IAHA results

were found to have a higher correlation coefficient than the IAHA and CF tests. Thus, although the IAHA test is the more practical test and represents a major contribution to the study of hepatitis type A, IEM will remain a valuable technique which specialized laboratories should be able to perform. One advantage of the IEM test under present conditions is that antigen in the IEM test consists of a relatively crude low-titered stool filtrate, whereas for the IAHA and CF tests the antigen must be purified by biophysical methods from materials containing high titers of virus. Indeed, only approximately 10 to 20% of stools or of marmoset livers positive for hepatitis A antigen by IEM are suitable for antigen in the IAHA test (J. L. Dienstag and R. H. Purcell, unpublished data).

REAGENTS

Antigen

For initial screening tests, prepare about 10

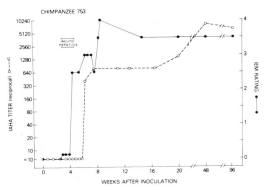

FIG. 4. *Antibody to hepatitis A°antigen rated in a single 1:10 serum dilution by immune electron microscopy (IEM) and titered in serial twofold dilutions by immune adherence hemagglutination (IAHA) in longitudinally collected serum samples from a chimpanzee with experimental hepatitis A virus infection. From Dienstag, Alling, and Purcell (9a).*

ml of a 2% stool filtrate as follows (46). Weigh 200 mg of a stool and mix it with 10 ml of veal infusion broth (VIB) containing 0.5% bovine serum albumin (BSA). Shake the diluted stool with glass beads for about 10 min to homogenize the stool. After the stool has been thoroughly mixed with the VIB containing BSA, clarify it in a refrigerated centrifuge for 2 h at 3,000 rpm to remove debris. Collect the supernatant fluid and filter it in a Swinnex 47-mm filter apparatus containing a prefilter, a 1,200-nm filter, a Dacron mesh, and a 450-nm filter (Millipore Corp.). The filtrate is the material to be examined. Appropriate containment facilities should be available for the various steps involved in the preparation of stool filtrates, especially if the presence of a hepatitis agent is suspected.

(When using cell culture harvests of viruses as an antigen for typing, etc, simply harvest the culture fluid and use it as antigen; clarification by low-speed centrifugation is usually not necessary.)

Sera

Acute- and convalescent-phase sera or immune serum globulin are used. Inactivation of sera is not necessary with unenveloped viruses such as the gastroenteritis and hepatitis A particles. However, when dealing with enveloped viruses, sera should be inactivated at 56 C for 30 min to inactivate complement. Reaction of an enveloped agent with uninactivated serum containing specific antibody may result in the formation of "complement holes" in the envelope (2). Clarification of sera is not usually

necessary. If sera have too much background material by electron microscopy, centrifuge at 40,000 rpm for 1.0 h and harvest the supernatant fluid (2). This is usually an unnecessary step and is not routinely practiced in our laboratory.

TEST PROCEDURE

Detection of virus-like particles in stool filtrates

Add 0.2 ml of a 1:5 dilution of convalescent serum (or, if not available, immune serum globulin) to an appropriate tube. As a control to this procedure, add 0.2 ml of phosphate-buffered saline (PBS) to another tube. To each tube, add 0.8 ml of the stool filtrate antigen, cover, and mix by inverting 15 to 20 times. (For hepatitis A studies we routinely use 0.9 ml of antigen and 0.1 ml of a 1:10 dilution of serum [10, 17].) Allow the mixture to incubate at room temperature for 1 h. Occasionally, it may be advantageous to incubate overnight at 4 C. The mixtures are then centrifuged at 17,000 rpm for 90 min in a Sorvall (RC2B) centrifuge with an SS-34 fixed angle rotor or at 23,000 rpm for 90 min in a Beckman L2-65B ultracentrifuge with a 40.2 fixed angle rotor or an equivalent centrifuge or rotor. The supernatant fluid is carefully discarded, and the tubes are inverted in a beaker to allow the remaining fluid to drain. The pellet or sediment is resuspended with a few drops of distilled water, stained with 2% phosphotungstic acid (pH 7.2), and placed on a 400 mesh Formvar carbon-coated grid; the excess fluid is removed with the edge of a filter-paper disk. The grid is examined at a magnification of about 40,000 in an electron microscope. Appropriate containment facilities should be available for these steps also, especially if the presence of a hepatitis agent is suspected.

Detection of serological responses

If particles are seen with a convalescent serum, the significance of these particles must be determined. This is done by taking the same stool filtrate and allowing it to react in the same test with an acute-phase or pre-illness serum and with the convalescent-phase serum (used previously) from the patient in an attempt to show that a serological response occurred to that antigen. In addition, the filtrate should ideally be reacted with PBS as a control, especially if only one serum pair is being examined. In studies with paired sera, each is diluted 1:5 or 1:10 and the same procedure outlined in the preceding paragraph is repeated with each serum and with PBS in the same test. Paired sera and the PBS control should be examined under code to eliminate the possibility of biased interpretation.

INTERPRETATION

In order to quantitate the amount of antibody in each preparation, five squares of each grid are routinely examined, and the relative concentration of antibody in each serum specimen is estimated by judging the amount of antibody coating aggregated or single particles on a 0 to 4+ scale. Three or more particles in a group are considered to constitute an aggregate. A rating of 0, i.e., no antibody, is assigned when single particles or doublets or groups of particles are observed without antibody. A 4+ rating indicates that particles are so heavily coated with antibody that they are almost obscured. Ratings of 1+, 2+, and 3+ indicate the presence of antibody in lesser amounts than those rated 4+. A 1+ change in antibody rating between

paired sera is considered significant. In convalescent sera, the antibody coating the particles appears to be of the immunoglobulin G class morphologically (2).

Examples of aggregates of the Norwalk agent scored as 1+ and 4+ are shown in Fig. 5. The pre-illness serum of volunteer A was scored as 1+ since the particles were well defined and appeared to be covered with very little antibody, whereas the convalescent serum of volunteer B was scored as 4+ because the particles were so heavily coated with antibody that they were almost obscured. Heavily coated particles were usually found in small aggregates or as single particles or as doublets, whereas those with less antibody usually formed larger aggregates. An example of a significant seroresponse as shown in a gastroenteritis volunteer's paired sera is shown in Fig. 6.

With the hepatitis A antigen, particles are not usually seen following incubation with pre-challenge or pre-illness sera, whereas when such sera or PBS are incubated with a Norwalk

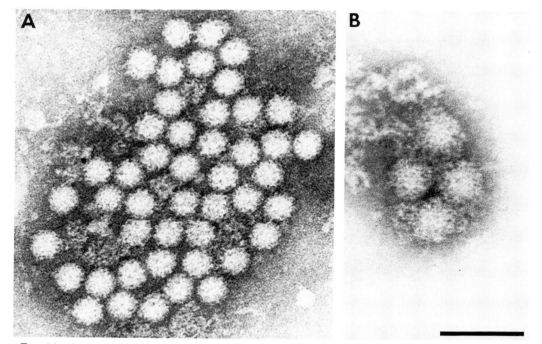

FIG. 5A. *Aggregate observed after incubation of 0.8 ml of the Norwalk stool filtrate with 0.2 ml of a 1:5 dilution of prechallenge serum of volunteer "A" and further preparation for electron microscopy. The quantity of antibody on these glistening particles was rated as 1+. From Kapikian et al. (29).*

FIG. 5B. *Aggregate observed after incubation of 0.8 ml of the Norwalk stool filtrate with a 1:5 dilution of postchallenge serum of volunteer "B" and further preparation for electron microscopy. The particles were very heavily coated with antibody. Heavily coated particles were usually found to be in small aggregates, whereas those with less antibody were usually in larger aggregates. The quantity of antibody on these particles was rated as 4+. Bar = 100 nm and applies to A also. From Kapikian et al. (29).*

particle-containing filtrate, aggregation of particles is occasionally observed. Therefore, with the Norwalk agent nonspecific aggregation may occur and ratings of less than 3+ cannot be considered significant when examining only a single serum such as in a prevalence study. Antibody ratings of 3+ and 4+ have not been observed nonspecifically. Thus, one of the pitfalls in an IEM study of a single specimen is the presence of nonspecific aggregation, as aggregation of particles per se does not signify the presence of antibody. To establish the specificity of aggregation, one may vary the dilution of antigen or antibody and examine the size of aggregates and the amount of antibody coating the particles as the reaction goes from antigen

excess to antibody excess. In antibody excess particles occur as predominantly single particles or doublets heavily coated with antibody, whereas at approximate antigen-antibody equivalence large aggregates lightly coated with antibody are observed; in antigen excess particles may occur singly without aggregation. When one examines paired sera by IEM, nonspecific aggregation is usually not a problem, since the same conditions exist for each serum. Since spontaneous aggregation of particles is not observed with hepatitis A antigen, the antibody determination for this agent is usually simple, even with a single serum specimen. Since, however, patients often already have developed low-level antibody (up to IEM

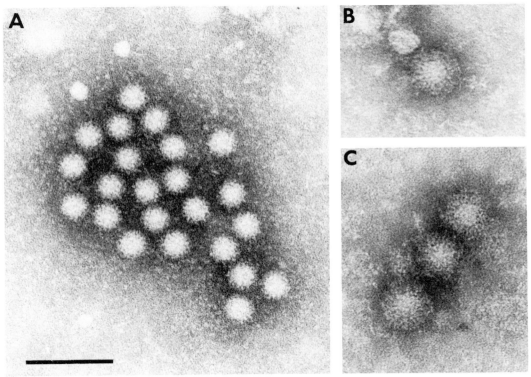

Fig. 6A. *Aggregate observed after incubation of 0.8 ml of the Norwalk stool filtrate with 0.2 ml of a 1:5 dilution of a volunteer's prechallenge serum and further preparation for electron microscopy. This volunteer developed gastroenteritis after challenge with a second passage Norwalk filtrate which had been heated for 30 min at 60 C (14). The quantity of antibody on the particles in this aggregate was rated 1-2-2 +, and this prechallenge serum was given an overall rating of 1 to 2 +. Bar = 100 nm and applies to B and C also. From Kapikian et al. (25).*

Fig. 6B and C. *A single particle (B) and three single particles (C) observed after incubating 0.8 ml of the Norwalk stool filtrate with 0.2 ml of a dilution of the same volunteer's convalescent serum and further preparation for electron microscopy. These particles are very heavily coated with antibody. The quantity of antibody on these particles was rated 4 +, and the serum was given an overall rating of 4 + also. The difference in the quantity of antibody coating the particles in the prechallenge and postchallenge sera is clearly evident. From Kapikian et al. (25).*

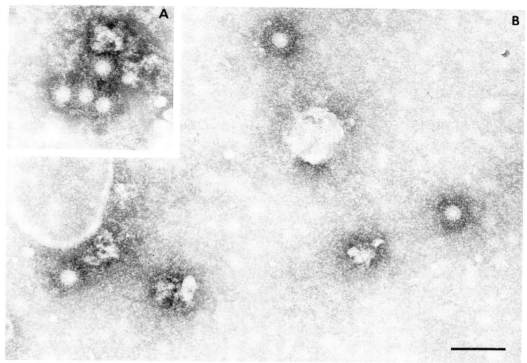

Fig. 7. A small aggregate of three particles plus a single particle (A) and three single particles (B) observed after (i) incubation of 0.9 ml of the stool filtrate with 0.1 ml of a 1:10 dilution of convalescent serum from a patient who developed hepatitis during the naturally occurring outbreak in American Samoa and (ii) further preparation for electron microscopy. The particles are clearly covered with antibody. The ready recognition of both the antibody-coated particles in the aggregate and the antibody-coated single particles illustrates clearly the use of the technique of immune electron microscopy in these studies. Bar = 100 nm and applies to A also. From Kapikian et al. (25).

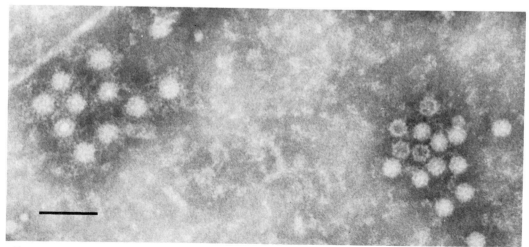

Fig. 8. Aggregate of hepatitis A antigen particles heavily coated with antibody appears on the left. On the right is a group of 22-nm (approx.) particles commonly found in stool with little, if any, antibody. Phospho-tungstic acid (3%) used as negative stain. Bar = 100 nm. From Purcell et al. (43) with permission, Charles B. Slack, Inc., publisher.

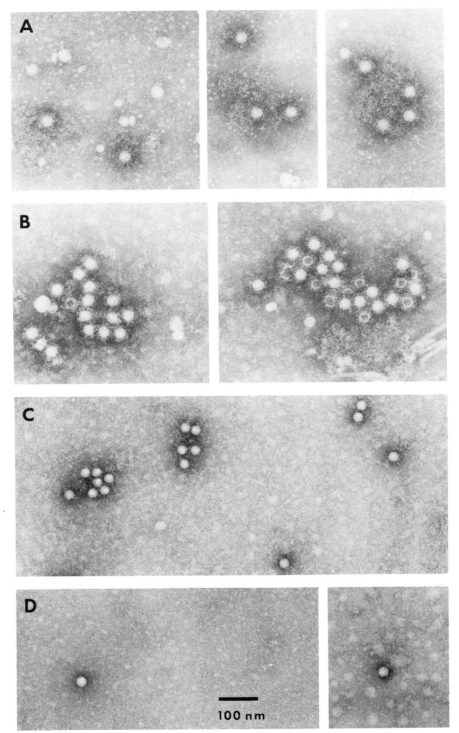

FIG. 9. *Hepatitis A antigen particles incubated with serially diluted antibody concentrations (1:64, 1:640, 1:6,400, and 1:64,000 for A, B, C, and D, respectively). (A) Extreme antibody excess; immune electron microscopy (IEM) antibody rating 3 to 4+. (B) Approximate antigen-antibody equivalence; IEM antibody rating 2 to 3+. (C) Relative antigen excess; IEM antibody rating 1+. (D) Extreme antigen excess with trace IEM antibody. Note the decrease in interparticle distance and in antibody halo density with successive antibody dilution. All particles measure 27 nm, but those with more antibody appear deceptively larger. Phosphotungstic acid (2%) with bacitracin (20) used as negative stain. Bar applies to A–D. From Dienstag, Alling, and Purcell (9a).*

ratings of 1 to 2+) during the acute phase of illness, if the convalescent serum sample is obtained too early, an increase in antibody may not be discerned. In this system, therefore, the ideal interval between paired acute and convalescent sera is at least 4 to 6 weeks (12). An example of hepatitis A particles in a stool filtrate following preparation for IEM is shown in Fig. 7. The particles may appear as single particles or aggregates coated with antibody. These particles would not be recognized without the addition of the antibody-containing serum.

Not infrequently, stool preparations containing occasional aggregates of approximately 22-nm particles with little or no antibody may be seen. These particles have been observed in both Norwalk and hepatitis A particle positive stool filtrates. The size of the aggregates and the amount of antibody on them does not change significantly in tests with paired sera. Thus, they appear to be present nonspecifically. An example of approximately 22-nm particles observed in a stool filtrate containing hepatitis A particles is shown in Fig. 8.

The IEM test is quite reproducible, and in recent studies it has been shown that for a serially diluted serum sample 1+ differences in ratings represent approximate 10-fold differences in antibody titer (9a). For hepatitis A antigen it was found that a 1:64 dilution of a convalescent serum from a patient naturally infected with hepatitis A virus had an IEM rating of 3 to 4+; a 1:640 dilution, a rating of 2 to 3+; a 1:6,400 dilution, a rating of 1+; and a 1:64,000 dilution, only a trace of antibody. Examples of such ratings as the reaction proceeded from extreme antibody excess to extreme antigen excess are shown in Fig. 9. In addition, as noted previously, the IEM ratings of a single serum dilution were compared with the IAHA titers determined on serial (twofold) dilutions on 92 serum samples from patients with hepatitis or other illnesses (9a). As can be seen in Fig. 10, there was excellent agreement in antibody quantitation by the two methods. It would be optimal, of course, to do titrations of sera by IEM. However, because of the time-consuming nature of the IEM test, we have found that a single dilution of serum gives satisfactory, reproducible results which agree with quite conventional test systems. For example, we have examined paired sera of diarrhea patients who shed the human reovirus-like (HRVL) agent and have demonstrated serological (IEM) responses to the HRVL agent which were later confirmed by the CF technique (28) (Table 1). An example of an IEM study with the HRVL agent and paired sera from an infant

who developed HRVL agent illness is shown in Fig. 11. Figure 11 also shows the HRVL agent from another patient but without the addition of serum prior to examination by electron microscopy.

Finally, another use of this technique, mentioned earlier, is the typing of viruses. This method has been used for the typing of enteroviruses (3, 13), rhinoviruses (25), and adenoviruses (49). In such typing experiments, the virus preparation is mixed with specific antiserum and the presence or absence of specific aggregation by antibody is determined. These tests are rather easy to interpret since the antigen is prepared from tissue culture prepara-

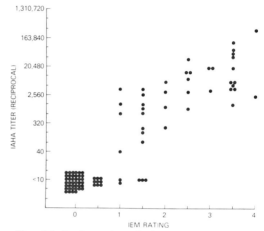

FIG. 10. *Reciprocal antibody titer, determined by immune adherence hemagglutination (IAHA), plotted as a function of antibody rating, determined on a 1:10 dilution of the same serum sample, by immune electron microscopy (IEM). From Dienstag, Alling, and Purcell (9a).*

TABLE 1. *Serological response of patients with diarrhea to the human reovirus-like (HRVL) agent by immune electron microscopy (IEM) and complement fixation (CF)[a]*

Age (mo)	HRVL agent in stool	Antibody measured by IEM[b]		Antibody measured by CF[c]	
		Acute	Convalescent	Acute	Convalescent
8	+	0–1	4	<4	≥64
10	+	0	3–4	<4	32
11	+	0	2–3	<4	≥64
13	+	0	2–3	<4	32
20	No stool	0	3–4	<4	≥64

[a] From Kapikian et al. (22); adapted from Kapikian et al. (28).

[b] On a 0 to 4+ scale.

[c] The reciprocal antibody titer is shown.

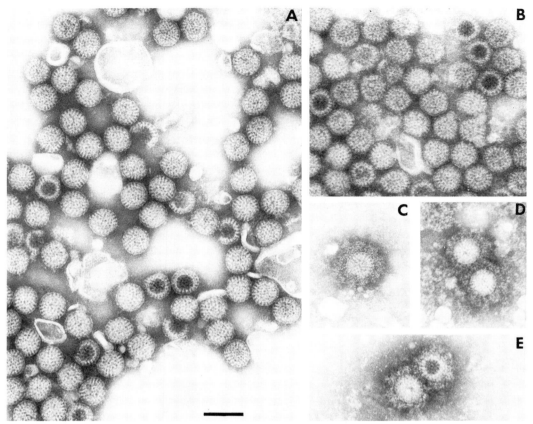

FIG. 11. *(A) Reovirus-like particles observed in a stool filtrate of patient F after incubation of the stool filtrate with phosphate-buffered saline and further preparation for electron microscopy. The particles had a definite capsomere structure and appeared to have a double-shelled capsid. Occasional "empty" particles were seen. (B) Reovirus-like particles observed after the stool filtrate of patient Ru was incubated with a 1:5 dilution of acute-phase serum from this same patient and then prepared for electron microscopy. No definite antibody was seen on these particles. This serum was given an overall rating of 1 + for antibody to the reovirus-like agent (Table 1). (C, D, and E) Reovirus-like particles observed after incubation of the stool filtrate of patient Ru with a 1:5 dilution of convalescent serum from this same patient and further preparation for electron microscopy from the same experiment as B above. The particles appear to be heavily coated with antibody. The quantity of antibody on these particles was scored as 4 +. This convalescent serum was given an overall rating of 4 + for antibody to the reovirus-like agent (Table 1). Bar represents 100 nm and applies to A–E. From Kapikian et al. (28).*

tions and they contain relatively little debris. Modifications and variations in the application and performance of the technique of IEM have been described (2, 13, 40, 45, 48, 52; Hughes et al., Abstr. Annu. Meet. Am. Soc. Microbiol. 1975, S170, p. 242).

IEM is a simple tool which has had and will have many other practical and basic research applications in the future. However, its most exciting application is in its use as a tool for detection of heretofore unrecognized etiological agents of human disease.

LITERATURE CITED

1. Adler, J., and R. Zickl. 1969. Winter vomiting disease. J. Infect. Dis. **119**:668–673.
1a. Almeida, J. D. 1975. Visualization of fecal viruses (editorial). N. Engl. J. Med. **292**:1403–1404.
2. Almeida, J. D., and A. P. Waterson. 1969. The morphology of virus antibody interaction. Adv. Virus Res. **15**:307–338.
3. Anderson, N., and F. W. Doane. 1973. Specific identification of enteroviruses by immuno-electron microscopy using a serum-in-agar

diffusion method. Can. J. Microbiol. 19:585–589.

4. Anderson, T. F., and W. M. Stanley. 1941. A study by means of the electron microscope of the reaction between tobacco mosaic virus and its antiserum. J. Biol. Chem. 139:339–344.

5. Ardenne, M. von, H. Friedrich-Freksa, and G. Schramm. 1941. Elektronenmikroskopischen Untersuchung der Pracipitinreaktion von tabakmosaik Virus mit kaninchen Antiserum. Arch. Gesamte Virusforsch. 2:80–86.

6. Blacklow, N. R., R. Dolin, D. S. Fedson, H. DuPont, R. S. Northrup, R. B. Hornick, and R. M. Chanock. 1972. Acute infectious non-bacterial gastroenteritis: etiology and pathogenesis. A combined clinical staff conference at the Clinical Center of the National Institutes of Health. Ann. Intern. Med. 76:993–1008.

7. Boggs, J. D., J. L. Melnick, M. E. Conrad, and B. F. Felsher. 1970. Viral hepatitis: clinical and tissue culture studies. J. Am. Med. Assoc. 214:1041–1046.

8. Bradley, D. W., C. L. Hornbeck, C. R. Gravelle, E. H. Cook, and J. E. Maynard. 1975. CsCl banding of hepatitis A associated virus-like particles. J. Infect. Dis. 131:304–306.

9. Brenner, S., and R. W. Horne. 1959. A negative staining method for high resolution electron microscopy of viruses. Biochim. Biophys. Acta 34:103–110.

9a. Dienstag, J. L., D. W. Alling, and R. H. Purcell. 1976. Quantitation of antibody to hepatitis A antigen by immune electron microscopy. Infect. Immun. 13:1209–1213.

10. Dienstag, J. L., S. M. Feinstone, A. Z. Kapikian, R. H. Purcell, J. D. Boggs, and M. E. Conrad. 1975. Fecal shedding of hepatitis A antigen. Lancet 1:765–767.

11. Dienstag, J. L., S. M. Feinstone, R. H. Purcell, J. H. Hoofnagle, L. F. Barker, W. T. London, H. Popper, J. M. Peterson, and A. Z. Kapikian. 1975. Experimental infection of chimpanzees with hepatitis A virus. J. Infect. Dis. 132:532–545.

12. Dienstag, J. L., J. A. Routenberg, R. H. Purcell, R. R. Hooper, and W. O. Harrison. 1975. Food-handler-associated outbreak of hepatitis type A: an immune electron microscopic study. Ann. Intern. Med. 83:647–650.

13. Doane, F. W. 1974. Identification of viruses by immunoelectron microscopy, p. 237–255. In E. Kurstak and R. Morrisset (ed.), Viral immunodiagnosis. Academic Press Inc., New York.

14. Dolin, R., N. R. Blacklow, H. DuPont, R. F. Buscho, R. G. Wyatt, J. A. Kasel, R. Hornick, and R. M. Chanock. 1972. Biological properties of Norwalk agent of acute infectious non-bacterial gastroenteritis. Proc. Soc. Exp. Biol. Med. 140:578–583.

15. Dolin, R., N. R. Blacklow, H. DuPont, S. Formal, R. F. Buscho, J. A. Kasel, R. P. Chames, R. Hornick, and R. M. Chanock. 1971. Transmission of acute infectious nonbacterial gastroenteritis to volunteers by oral administration of stool filtrates. J. Infect. Dis. 123:307–312.

16. Feinstone, S. M., A. Z. Kapikian, J. L. Gerin, and R. H. Purcell. 1974. Buoyant density of the hepatitis A virus-like particle in cesium chloride. J. Virol. 13:1412–1414.

17. Feinstone, S. M., A. Z. Kapikian, and R. H. Purcell. 1973. Hepatitis A: detection by immune electron microscopy of a virus-like antigen associated with acute illness. Science 182:1026–1028.

18. Feinstone, S. M., A. Z. Kapikian, R. H. Purcell, H. J. Alter, and P. V. Holland. 1975. Transfusion-associated hepatitis not due to viral hepatitis type A or B. N. Engl. J. Med. 292:767–770.

19. Gravelle, G. R., C. L. Hornbeck, J. E. Maynard, C. A. Schable, E. H. Cook, and D. W. Bradley. 1975. Hepatitis A: report of a common-source outbreak with recovery of a possible etiologic agent. II. Laboratory studies. J. Infect. Dis. 131:167–171.

20. Gregory, D. W., and B. J. S. Pirie. 1973. Wetting agents for biological microscopy. I. General considerations and negative staining. J. Microsc. (Oxford) 99:251–265.

21. Kapikian, A. Z. 1974. Acute viral gastroenteritis. Prev. Med. 3:535–542.

22. Kapikian, A. Z., et al. 1976. Recent advances in the etiology of viral gastroenteritis. Ciba Symp., Diarrhoea in Childhood, in press.

23. Kapikian, A. Z., J. D. Almeida, and E. J. Scott. 1972. Immune electron microscopy of rhinoviruses. J. Virol. 10:142–146.

24. Kapikian, A. Z., W. L. Cline, C. A. Mebus, R. G. Wyatt, A. R. Kalica, H. D. James, Jr., D. VanKirk, and R. M. Chanock. 1975. New complement-fixation test for the human reovirus-like agent of infantile gastroenteritis. Lancet 1:1056–1081.

25. Kapikian, A. Z., S. M. Feinstone, R. H. Purcell, R. G. Wyatt, T. S. Thornhill, A. R. Kalica, and R. M. Chanock. 1975. Detection and identification by immune electron microscopy of fastidious agents associated with respiratory illness, acute non-bacterial gastroenteritis, and hepatitis A. Perspect. Virol. 9:9–45.

26. Kapikian, A. Z., J. L. Gerin, R. G. Wyatt, T. S. Thornhill, and R. M. Chanock. 1974. Density in cesium chloride of the 27-nm "8FIIa" particle associated with acute infectious nonbacterial gastroenteritis: determination by ultracentrifugation and immune electron microscopy. J. Infect. Dis. 129:709–714.

27. Kapikian, A. Z., H. D. James, Jr., S. J. Kelly, and A. L. Vaughn. 1973. Detection of coronavirus strain 692 by immune electron microscopy. Infect. Immun. 7:111–116.

28. Kapikian, A. Z., H. W. Kim, R. G. Wyatt, W. J. Rodriguez, S. Ross, W. L. Cline, R. H. Parrot, and R. M. Chanock. 1974. Reovirus-like agent in stools: association with infantile diarrhea and development of serologic tests. Science 185:1049–1053.

29. Kapikian, A. Z., R. G. Wyatt, T. S. Thornhill, A. R. Kalica, and R. M. Chanock. 1972. Visualization by immune electron microscopy of a 27-nm particle associated with acute infectious nonbacterial gastroenteritis. J. Virol. 10:1075–1081.

30. Kelen, A. E., A. E. Hathaway, and D. A. McLeod. 1971. Rapid detection of Australian/SH antigen and antibody by a simple and sensitive technique of immuno electron microscopy. Can. J. Microbiol. 17:993–1000.

30a. Knodell, R. G., M. E. Conrad, J. L. Dienstag, and C. J. Bell. 1975. Etiologic spectrum of post-transfusion hepatitis. Gastroenterology 69:1278–1285.

31. Krugman, S., H. Friedman, and C. Lattimer. 1975. Viral hepatitis, type A. Identification by specific complement fixation and immune adherence tests. N. Engl. J. Med. 292:1141–1143.

32. Lafferty, K. J., and S. J. Oertelis. 1961. Attachment of antibody to influenza virus. Nature (London) 102:764–765.

33. Lafferty, K. J., and S. J. Oertelis. 1963. The interaction between virus and antibody III. Examination of virus-antibody complexes with the electron microscope. Virology 21:91–99.

34. Lancet. 1975. Non-A, non-B. Lancet 2:64–65.

35. Lancet. 1975. Rapid diagnosis of virus diseases. Lancet 1:1411.

36. Lancet. 1975. Rotaviruses of man and animals. Lancet 1:257–259.

37. Locarnini, S. A., A. A. Ferris, A. C. Stott, and I. D. Gust. 1974. The relationship between a 27-nm virus-like particle and hepatitis A as demonstrated by immune electron microscopy. Intervirology 4:110–118.

38. Maynard, J. E., D. Lorenz, D. W. Bradley, S. M. Feinstone, D. H. Krushak, L. F. Barker, and R. H. Purcell. 1975. Review of infectivity studies in non-human primates with virus-like particles associated with MS-1 hepatitis. Am. J. Med. Sci. 270:81–85.

39. Miller, W. J., P. J. Provost, W. J. McAleer, O. L. Ittensohn, V. M. Villarejos, and M. R. Hilleman. 1975. Specific immune adherence assay for human hepatitis A antibody, application to diagnostic and epidemiologic investigations. Proc. Soc. Exp. Biol. Med. 149:254–261.

39a. Moritsugu, Y., J. L. Dienstag, J. Valdesuso, D. C. Wong, J. Wagner, J. A. Routenberg, and R. H. Purcell. 1976. Purification of hepatitis A antigen from feces and detection of antigen and antibody by immune adherence hemagglutination. Infect. Immun. 13:898–908.

40. Patterson, S. 1975. Detection of antibody in virus-antibody complexes by immunoferritin labelling and subsequent negative staining. J.

Immunol. Methods 9:115–122.

41. Provost, P. J., O. L. Ittensohn, V. M. Villarejos, and M. R. Hilleman. 1975. A specific complement-fixation test for human hepatitis A employing CR326 virus antigen. Diagnosis and epidemiology. Proc. Soc. Exp. Biol. Med. 148:962–969.

42. Provost, P. J., B. S. Wolanski, W. J. Miller, O. L. Ittensohn, W. J. McAleer, and M. R. Hilleman. 1975. Physical, chemical and morphologic dimensions of human hepatitis A virus strain CR326. Proc. Soc. Exp. Biol. Med. 148:532–539.

43. Purcell, R. H., J. L. Dienstag, S. M. Feinstone, and A. Z. Kapikian. 1975. Relationship of hepatitis A antigen to viral hepatitis. Am. J. Med. Sci. 270:61–71.

44. Purcell, R. H., S. M. Feinstone, and A. Z. Kapikian. 1975. Recent advances in hepatitis A research, p. 11–26. In T. J. Greenwalt and G. A. Jamieson (ed.), Transmissible disease and blood transfusion. Grune & Stratton, New York.

45. Rigby, C., and C. M. Johnson. 1972. Immunoelectron microscopy of herpes simplex virus. Can. J. Microbiol. 18:1337–1341.

46. Thornhill, T. S., A. R. Kalica, R. G. Wyatt, A. Z. Kapikian, and R. M. Chanock. 1975. Pattern of shedding of the Norwalk particle in stools during experimentally induced gastroenteritis in volunteers as determined by immune electron microscopy. J. Infect. Dis. 132:28–34.

47. Torres-Medina, A., R. G. Wyatt, C. A. Mebus, N. R. Underdahl, and A. Z. Kapikian. 1975. Diarrhea in gnotobiotic piglets caused by reovirus-like agent of human nonbacterial gastroenteritis. J. Infect. Dis., in press.

48. Valters, W. A., L. G. Boehm, E. A. Edwards, and M. J. Rosenbaum. 1975. Detection of adenovirus in patient specimens by indirect immune electron microscopy. J. Clin. Microbiol. 1:472–475.

49. Vassall, J. H., II, and C. G. Ray. 1974. Serotyping of adenovirus using immune electron microscopy. Appl. Microbiol. 28:623–627.

50. WHO Study Group. 1970. Viral hepatitis and tests for the Australia (hepatitis-associated) antigen and antibody. Bull. WHO 42:957–992.

51. Wyatt, R. G., D. L. Sly, W. T. London, A. E. Palmer, A. R. Kalica, D. H. VanKirk, R. M. Chanock, and A. Z. Kapikian. 1976. Induction of diarrhea in colostrum-deprived newborn rhesus monkeys with the human reovirus-like agent of infantile gastroenteritis. Arch. Virol. 50:17–27.

52. Zuckerman, A. J. 1970. Viral hepatitis and tests for the Australia (hepatitis-associated) antigen and antibody. VI. Electron microscopy and immune electron microscopy. Bull. WHO 42:975–978.

Chapter 65

Hepatitis B Virus

LEWELLYS F. BARKER AND ROBERT H. PURCELL

INTRODUCTION

Hepatitis B virus (HBV) is a deoxyribonucleic acid (DNA)-containing virus which consists of a 27-nm nucleocapsid core surrounded by an outer lipoprotein coat. The intact virion is approximately 40 to 42 nm in diameter. Virus infectivity in serum or plasma resists heating for up to 4 h at 60 C and treatment with lipid solvents and proteolytic enzymes. The virus is probably less stable after purification and suspension in aqueous solutions. The outer coat, originally described as Australia antigen, is now termed hepatitis B surface antigen (HB$_s$ Ag); HB$_s$ Ag is immunologically distinct from the nucleocapsid core, which is called hepatitis B core antigen (HB$_c$ Ag). The core particles replicate in hepatocyte nuclei, and HB$_s$ Ag is produced in the cytoplasm of infected hepatocytes. Production of excess HB$_s$ Ag results in release into the bloodstream of quantities of this material sufficient for direct immunological detection by a variety of methods. The number of HB$_s$ Ag particles in serum usually exceeds the number of intact virions by several orders of magnitude.

HBV infection produces a broad spectrum of clinical manifestations, ranging from the absence of overt disease and minimal aberrations of liver function tests to acute fulminant disease which is usually fatal. Symptoms and signs of overt disease commonly include malaise, anorexia, weight loss, hepatomegaly, and jaundice. Infected individuals may become chronic HB$_s$ Ag carriers as a result of HBV persistence in the liver; chronic HBV infections frequently follow mild or subclinical acute illnesses.

Support of HBV replication has not yet been achieved in any in vitro system, but the production of massive amounts of HB$_s$ Ag in infected individuals and the antibody responses to HB$_s$ Ag and HB$_c$ Ag have made possible the development of a number of serological tests for diagnosis and epidemiological studies. In view of the problem of HBV transmission by blood and blood products, HB$_s$ Ag detection has come into widespread use to avoid transfusion of material collected from infected blood donors. Since different methods may be suitable for various applications, a number of laboratory techniques will be discussed. Inoculation of susceptible animals, particularly chimpanzees, is the only available method for detection of infectious HBV; although there are several valuable applications of infectivity determinations in experimental animals, this approach is obviously not practical for routine diagnostic and epidemiological studies.

The course of serological events in type B hepatitis is illustrated in Fig. 1. Since HB$_s$ Ag is generally evanescent in acute infections and is often present in highest titer at the onset of clinical illness, samples obtained early in acute disease are preferred for diagnosis by HB$_s$ Ag detection. Subsequent diagnosis and epidemiological data can be obtained by detection of antibody to HB$_s$ Ag (anti-HB$_s$) and to HB$_c$ Ag (anti-HB$_c$). Anti-HB$_c$ often appears while HB$_s$ Ag is still present, whereas anti-HB$_s$ may lag several months behind HB$_s$ Ag disappearance. Anti-HB$_s$ may not be detected during convalescence in a small proportion of individuals with self-limited infections.

SEROLOGICAL DIAGNOSIS

Detection of hepatitis B surface antigen and antibody to hepatitis B surface antigen

Serum or plasma, stored either refrigerated or frozen, is suitable for essentially all diagnostic procedures. The most frequently used serological procedures for HB$_s$ Ag detection are listed in Table 1. They are grouped as first, second, and third generation methods according to sensitivity. Since the third generation methods (radioimmunoassay and reversed passive hemagglutination) are the most sensitive, they are the preferred methods in most clinical situations, but there are valuable special applications of the other methods which merit their inclusion in this chapter. All commercially available reagents for HB$_s$ Ag and anti-HB$_s$ detection are subject to federal licensure and control and are accompanied by detailed directions for use (Table 2). Reference reagents may be obtained from the Reference Resources Branch, National

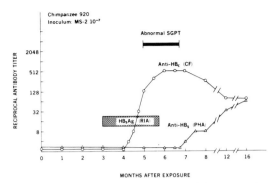

MONTHS AFTER EXPOSURE

FIG. 1. *Serological events in a chimpanzee infected with a 1-ml intravenous inoculation of a 10^{-7} dilution of human plasma containing the ayw subtype of HBV. HB_s Ag appears several weeks before liver damage, manifested by enzyme elevations. Anti-HB_c appears while HB_s Ag and elevated enzymes are present, and anti-HB_s appears during convalescence. SGPT = serum glutamic pyruvic transaminase; CF = complement fixation; RIA = radioimmunoassay; PHA = passive hemagglutination.*

TABLE 1. *Methods for detection of hepatitis B surface antigens[a]*

Classification	Test
First generation $(1\times)$[b]	Agar gel diffusion
Second generation $(5\text{-}10\times)$	Counterelectrophoresis Rheophoresis Complement fixation Reversed passive latex agglutination
Third generation $(100\times)$	Radioimmunoassay Reversed passive hemagglutination

[a] Licensed reagents are commercially available for all of these methods.

[b] Relative sensitivity.

Institute of Allergy and Infectious Diseases, Bethesda, Md. 20014.

Agar gel diffusion. The original studies of the relationship of HB_s Ag to type B hepatitis were carried out with the agar gel diffusion or Ouchterlony method (7, 23, 27). Although less sensitive than other methods, agar gel diffusion has the advantages of demonstrating specificity by the formation of lines of identity between HB_s Ag in test samples and in postive control sera and of distinguishing among subtypes of HB_s Ag by lines of partial identity or spur formation (3, 21). The method is relatively slow, requiring 24 to 72 h for optimal results, but it is the simplest available method for HB_s

Ag and anti-HB_s detection, as no special equipment is required. A number of different well configurations and agar and buffer combinations have given satisfactory results. Optimal test conditions are somewhat dependent on the antiserum used. There are many potential sources of satisfactory antisera (Table 3). Since agar gel diffusion is a relatively insensitive method for detecting anti-HB_s as well as HB_s Ag, it provides a convenient method for identifying very potent antisera.

Counterelectrophoresis. Counterelectrophoresis (CEP) is 5 to 10 times as sensitive as agar gel diffusion for HB_s Ag detection and provides results in 1 to 2 h (2, 8). There are a number of commercially available CEP reagents and kits (Table 2, footnote). Alternatively, the test may be set up by coating lantern slides, $3^1/4$ by 4 inches (8.3 by 10.2 cm), with 16 ml of agarose (L'Industrie Biologique Francaise SA), at a 1%

TABLE 2. *Commerical sources of third generation[a] reagents*

Test	Source of reagents
Radioimmunoassay (solid phase)	
For HB_s Ag	Abbott Laboratories Curtis Nuclear Electro-Nucleonics, Inc.
For anti-HB_s	Abbott Laboratories
Reversed passive hemagglutination for HB_s Ag	Abbott Laboratories
Passive hemagglutination for anti-HB_s	Electro-Nucleonics, Inc.

[a] A complete list of licensed manufacturers for other test methods can be obtained by writing to the Director, Bureau of Biologics, Food and Drug Administration, Bethesda, Md. 20014.

TABLE 3. *Sources of antisera for detection of hepatitis B surface antigen (HB$_s$Ag)*

Human

Multiply transfused patients, e.g., hemophiliacs, thalassemics

Anamnestic response after transfusions of blood and blood products

Stimulation with noninfectious HB_s Ag positive material, e.g., plasma protein fraction

Sporadic, not associated with blood and blood products

Animal hyperimmunization with purified HB_s Ag

Laboratory animals: guinea pigs, rabbits, mice, monkeys, chimpanzees

Domestic animals: horses, sheep, goats

concentration in barbital buffer (0.05 M, pH 8.6). Two double parallel rows of 15 wells, 3 mm in diameter and 7 mm apart, edge-to-edge, are cut after the agar has cooled. Wells in one of each of the double set of rows are filled with test samples, and in the other rows, with anti-HB$_s$ of adequate potency to form a precipitin reaction in agar gel diffusion. The slides are connected to the same barbital buffer in an electrophoresis cell by wicks of chromatographic paper (Schleicher and Schuell, no. 470C), with the anti-HB$_s$-containing wells proximal to the anode and the test samples proximal to the cathode. Electrophoresis is carried out for 2 h at 15 mA constant current per slide. Slides may be examined for immunoprecipitin reactions from 1 to 24 h after completion of electrophoresis. An HB$_s$ Ag positive control serum should be included on each slide. Many variations of this technique have been described in the literature. Careful selection of the anti-HB$_s$ reagent is essential to obtain optimal sensitivity with CEP.

Rheophoresis. Rheophoresis is a simple method which uses the same principle as agar gel diffusion but provides increased sensitivity, roughly equivalent to CEP (15). The increased sensitivity is obtained by using an agar gel diffusion dish with an outer moat filled with tris(hydroxymethyl)aminomethane (Tris) buffer, 0.01 M, pH 7.6. After filling the wells with test sera and reagents and the moat with buffer, a cover with a small central hole over the well containing anti-HB$_s$ is placed over the dish, and it is incubated at 30 to 37 C. In this manner the buffer in the moat and the antigens in the outer wells are encouraged to migrate centrally by evaporation through the central hole. This method is particularly convenient for determining HB$_s$ Ag subtypes with appropriate subtype-specific antisera.

Complement fixation. The microtiter complement-fixation (CF) technique provides two- to fourfold greater sensitivity than CEP for HB$_s$ Ag detection, with a prerequisite being a potent and specific complement-fixing antiserum (30). Test samples are heated for 30 min at 56 C and diluted in microtiter plates starting at 1:4. Four to eight units of antibody and 1.7 to 2 exact units of complement are added to each well in the microtiter plates. All test components are diluted in Veronal-buffered saline supplemented with calcium and magnesium. After overnight incubation of the plates at 4 C, a 1% suspension of sheep red blood cells sensitized with hemolysin is added; the plates are incubated at 35 C for 30 min with shaking at 10-min intervals to keep the red blood cells in suspen-

sion. The end point is the highest serum dilution at which 3 to 4+ fixation of complement occurs.

Reversed passive latex agglutination. The most rapid and simple second generation test for HB$_s$ Ag is reversed passive latex agglutination (20). The test is based on agglutination of latex particles coated with anti-HB$_s$ by HB$_s$ Ag in test samples. The samples and latex reagent are mixed on a plastic plate; after gentle mixing for 5 min at room temperature, the test sample reactions are compared with positive and negative controls for evidence of agglutination. Since false-positive results are rather common, confirmation of all agglutination reactions by another method of equal or greater sensitivity is essential.

Passive hemagglutination. Agglutination of human erythrocytes coated with HB$_s$ Ag (passive hemagglutination) or with anti-HB$_s$ (reversed passive hemagglutination) is the basis of very sensitive, rapid, and simple methods for detecting anti-HB$_s$ and HB$_s$ Ag, respectively (25, 33). As is the case for all of the methods heretofore described, standardized coated-cell reagents are available commercially for both of these methods. The tests are performed in microtiter plates in which dilutions of the test samples are mixed with the coated cells. Since both of these methods give nonspecific false-positive results with some sera, confirmation by specific inhibition of the agglutination reactions with HB$_s$ Ag or anti-HB$_s$ or by testing the samples with another method of at least equivalent sensitivity is necessary before interpreting the results as positive or negative.

Radioimmonoassay. The most sensitive methods for detecting HB$_s$ Ag and anti-HB$_s$ are radioimmunoassays (11, 19, 22, 26, 34). The two most widely used methods are the solid-phase radioimmunoassay and the double antibody or radioimmunoprecipitation (RIP) tests. The solid-phase radioimmunoassay system for HB$_s$ Ag detection utilizes the sandwich principle in which test samples are added to plastic tubes or beads coated with anti-HB$_s$ (22, 26). After an initial incubation step, the sample is removed and the tubes or beads are washed prior to the addition of ^{125}I-labeled anti-HB$_s$. Following a second incubation and a second washing step, the tubes or beads are counted in a gamma counter. The counts are compared with counts produced by negative control serum which is used to establish a cut-off point above which the samples are considered to contain HB$_s$ Ag. Confirmation of positive results by showing that they are repeatable and are specifically inhibited by unlabeled anti-HB$_s$ is essential because of the occurrence of occasional nonspecific false-positive results.

In the RIP method for HB_s Ag, known quantities of anti-HB_s and ^{125}I-labeled HB_s Ag are incubated with test samples and then reacted with antibody against gamma globulin which precipitates antigen-antibody complexes (11). The presence of HB_s Ag in the test sample competitively inhibits the reaction between anti-HB_s and radiolabeled HB_s Ag, resulting in a high ratio of free ^{125}I-HB_s Ag to bound and precipitated ^{125}I-HB_s Ag. By mixing test samples with ^{125}I-HB_s Ag alone, the RIP method can be used for detection of anti-HB_s in the samples (11, 19). Radioimmunoassay methods are approximately 10-fold more sensitive than hemagglutination methods and 1,000 or more times more sensitive than second generation methods such as CEP for HB_s Ag and anti-HB_s detection.

Determination of antigen and antibody subtype specificities

There are four major subtypes of HB_s Ag, termed *adw, ayw, adr,* and *ayr* (3, 21). The *adw* and *ayw* subtypes predominate in most parts of the world, but the *adr* subtype is common in Southeast Asia; *ayr* appears to be the least common of the four subtypes. Subtype-specific antisera are prepared by hyperimmunization of guinea pigs or rabbits with purified HB_s Ag. They may then be used in any of several methods, particularly agar gel diffusion, CEP, rheophoresis, and radioimmunoassay, for determining HB_s Ag subtypes (10). The subtype specificities of antibodies may be determined with the passive hemagglutination or radioimmunoassay techniques for anti-HB_s detection by studying inhibition of the antibody reactions with different known HB_s Ag subtypes.

Detection of hepatitis B core antigen and antibody to hepatitis B core antigen

Several procedures for detecting HB_c Ag and anti-HB_c have been developed (Table 4); although most of these are research tools at present, some are adaptable to clinical testing (1, 4, 9, 12, 14, 24, 32). Tests for HB_c Ag are seldom used in the diagnosis of type B hepatitis, but tests for anti-HB_c have proven valuable for diagnostic and seroepidemiological studies of HBV infection (13, 18). At present, there are no commercially available tests or reagents for HB_c Ag or anti-HB_c detection, and lack of availability of HB_c Ag reagent has limited the use of tests for anti-HB_c to research laboratories. Reference anti-HB_c may be obtained from the Reference Resources Branch, National Institute of

TABLE 4. *Methods for detection of antibody to hepatitis B core antigen (HB_c Ag)*

Method	Sensitivity	Source of HB_c Ag
Complement fixation	1×	Liver
Counterelectrophoresis	1×	Liver
Immune adherence hemagglutination	10×	Plasma, liver
Radioimmunoprecipitation	300×	Plasma

Allergy and Infectious Diseases, Bethesda, Md. 20014.

HB_c Ag suitable for use in serological tests has been purified from HB_s Ag-positive liver or plasma. Extensive serological studies have been carried out with HB_c Ag purified by differential centrifugation and isopycnic banding in cesium chloride from the liver of an immunosuppressed chimpanzee experimentally infected with HBV. HB_c Ag has also been purified from plasma of chronic carriers of HB_s Ag which contains large numbers of Dane particles. The Dane particles are purified by isopycnic and rate zonal centrifugation procedures. The HB_s Ag coat is removed by treatment of the plasma-derived Dane particles with a nonionic detergent. The free cores are then purified by isopycnic banding in cesium chloride. Two populations of cores have been detected by such means: "heavy" cores with a density of approximately 1.37 g/cm^3 and a high specific DNA polymerase activity, and "light" cores deficient in DNA polymerase activity, with a density of approximately 1.30 to 1.32 g/cm^3. Heavy cores have served as a source of antigen for RIP tests of anti-HB_c, and light cores have been used successfully as a source of antigen for CF and immune adherence hemagglutination tests (IAHA) for anti-HB_c.

Complement fixation. CF has been the most widely used and best characterized serological technique for detecting anti-HB_c (12). The CF test will detect anti-HB_c following most clinical acute hepatitis B virus infections, but is insufficiently sensitive to diagnose many subclinical and inapparent infections. Almost all patients with chronic infection, whether clinical or subclinical, have anti-HB_c detectable by CF. The CF test for anti-HB_c is performed as described above for anti-HB_s. Antigen for the CF test has been purified from chimpanzee liver. A disadvantage of the CF test is the relatively large quantity of antigen required when compared with other serological tests for anti-HB_c.

Counterelectrophoresis. CEP is approximately as sensitive as CF for detecting anti-HB$_c$ but provides results within 2 h (14). The CEP test is performed as described above for HB$_s$ Ag and anti-HB$_s$, with the use of antigen purified from chimpanzee liver. As with CF, the test requires relatively large quantities of HB$_c$ Ag.

Immune adherence hemagglutination. IAHA is approximately 10 times as sensitive as CF and CEP for detecting anti-HB$_c$ (32). It uses relatively small quantities of antigen and, therefore, can be performed with HB$_c$ Ag purified from Dane particle-rich plasma as well as with antigen derived from liver. Test sera are heated at 56 C for 30 min and diluted in Veronal-buffered saline (pH 7.6) containing 0.1% (wt/vol) gelatin or bovine serum albumin, 1.5 × 10^{-4} M calcium, and 5 × 10^{-4} M magnesium (GVB). Duplicate twofold dilutions are prepared in U-bottom microtiter plates. To one set of dilutions is added 25 μliters of HB$_c$ Ag in GVB, and to the other, 25 μliters of GVB. The microtiter plate is briskly agitated and incubated at 37 C for 60 min or at 4 C overnight. Four 50% hemolytic units of guinea pig complement in 25 μliters of GVB are added to each well, and the plate is briskly shaken and incubated at 37 C for exactly 40 min. A 25-μliter amount of a solution of dithiothreitol (3 mg per ml) in GVB containing 4 × 10^{-2} M ethylenediaminetetraacetate (EDTA-GVB) and 25 μliters of a human type O erythrocyte suspension (1%, vol/vol) in EDTA-GVB are added. The plate is briskly agitated and allowed to stand at room temperature for 60 min. The IAHA titer is expressed as the highest serum dilution which produces at least 2+ hemagglutination on a scale of 0 to 4. The serum is considered positive for anti-HB$_c$ if the titer is at least fourfold greater than the titer obtained with the GVB diluent control. The IAHA test is very sensitive to slight variations in the quality of the reagents, and, therefore, it is necessary to preselect human erythrocytes for their sensitivity as indicators of hemagglutination in the test.

Radioimmunoassay. The most sensitive methods for detecting HB$_c$ Ag and anti-HB$_c$ are radioimmunoassays. The solid-phase radioimmunoassay for detection of HB$_c$ Ag is similar to one of the methods used for detecting HB$_s$ Ag (29). Samples to be tested are incubated with the solid phase (in this case, the wells of microtiter plates) coated with anti-HB$_c$. After washing, the microtiter wells are inoculated with ^{125}I-labeled anti-HB$_c$ and reincubated. Following an additonal wash, the solid phase is evaluated for residual radioactivity in a gamma spectrometer. Samples with residual counts significantly greater than counts remaining in nega-

tive control samples are considered positive for HB$_c$ Ag.

Anti-HB$_c$ may also be measured by a double antibody RIP test utilizing tritium-labeled HB$_c$ Ag (9, 24). High-density Dane particle cores purified from HB$_s$ Ag-positive plasma are intrinsically labeled with [^{3}H]thymidine triphosphate ([^{3}H]TTP) via the DNA polymerase of the core (see below). Newly synthesized [^{3}H]DNA is retained within the core, and radiolabeled cores are purified from unreacted [^{3}H]TTP by density gradient centrifugation in cesium chloride. The radiolabeled HB$_c$ Ag is mixed with the serum sample to be tested for antibody and incubated at 4 C for 3 or more days. Sufficient antihuman gamma globulin is added to precipitate all of the immunoglobulin G (including that bound to labeled HB$_c$ Ag), and the mixture is incubated at 37 C for 1 h and at 4 C overnight. After centrifugation to pellet the precipitated globulins, a measured sample of the supernatant fluid is removed and mixed with scintillation fluid, and the radioactivity is measured in a beta particle spectrometer. The percentage of radioactive HB$_c$ Ag precipitated and, therefore, bound to anti-HB$_c$ is calculated. Serum samples that precipitate 50% or more of the radiolabeled HB$_c$ Ag are considered positive for anti-HB$_c$. Low levels of anti-HB$_c$, perhaps consisting of antibodies cross-reactive with other unidentified antigens, are sometimes encountered. It is therefore important to test paired serum samples to establish the diagnosis of HBV infection by this means.

Deoxyribonucleic acid polymerase

DNA-dependent DNA polymerase activity has been detected in a high-density subpopulation of Dane particle cores (17, 24, 31). A low-density subpopulation of plasma-derived Dane particle cores, as well as cores purified from chimpanzee liver, appear to be deficient in such polymerase activity. DNA polymerase-positive Dane particles probably represent fully infectious hepatitis B virions; low density polymerase-deficient Dane particles probably represent incomplete virions which are deficient in or lack genetic material.

DNA polymerase activity can sometimes be detected in the sera of individuals acutely infected with HBV. In addition, a proportion of patients with chronic type B hepatitis exhibit serum DNA polymerase activity. Although useful as an ancillary diagnostic criterion, serum DNA polymerase activity is a less sensitive indicator of HBV infection than serum HB$_s$ Ag. Furthermore, serum DNA polymerase activity is usually more transient than HB$_s$ Ag (6, 16, 18).

Serum DNA polymerase activity is measured by incubating the serum sample with a reaction mixture consisting of deoxyadenosine-5'-triphosphate, deoxycytidine-5'-triphosphate, deoxyguanosine-5'-triphosphate, and thymidine [³H]methyl-5'-triphosphate in Tris buffer (pH 8.0) with $MgCl_2$, KCl, 2-mercaptoethanol, and Nonidet P-40. After incubation of the reaction mixture at 37 C for 3 h, reacted radioactive substrate is separated from the unreacted reagent on diethylaminoethyl cellulose paper, washed in phosphate-buffered saline, and counted in a beta particle spectrometer. Several variations on this procedure have been described (6, 16, 17, 24, 31); the original papers should be consulted for details.

The specificity of DNA polymerase activity is confirmed by demonstrating specific immune precipitation of polymerase activity, and, hence, of Dane particles, by anti-HB$_s$ prior to detergent treatment (9, 17, 31). This confirmatory test is necessary because contamination of serum with bacteria can result in false-positive DNA polymerase results.

Virus isolation: animal models

Since HBV has not been successfully isolated in tissue culture, presence of the virus can be directly demonstrated only by inoculation of susceptible animals. Although chimpanzees, gibbons, and rhesus monkeys have been experimentally infected with HBV, only the chimpanzee has been fully evaluated and demonstrated to be a sensitive indicator of HBV infectivity (5, 6). HBV infection in the chimpanzee resembles HBV infection in humans but is generally less severe. All of the serological markers of type B hepatitis, including HB$_s$ Ag, anti-HB$_s$, anti-HB$_c$, and serum DNA polymerase activity have been detected in association with HBV infection in chimpanzees.

Applications of test methods

The availability of a wide variety of laboratory techniques for detecting HBV infection makes it necessary to select the optimal method for various practical and research applications. The major practical uses of these tests are to identify blood donors who are infected with HBV and to establish the etiology of clinical cases of hepatitis. For both of these applications, the demonstration of HB$_s$ Ag in serum or plasma provides the most direct, unequivocal evidence of active HBV infection. The third generation methods (reversed passive hemagglutination and radioimmunoassay) are the methods of choice for these applications because of their high sensitivity, and, in fact, blood banks in the United States are now required to

test each unit collected by one of these methods. For diagnosis of clinical hepatitis cases when HB$_s$ Ag is not detected, sensitive methods for detecting the development of anti-HB$_s$ (passive hemagglutination or radioimmunoassay) or anti-HB$_c$ (CF, IAHA, radioimmunoassay) in paired sera obtained during the acute phase of the illness and during convalescence should be employed.

Serological tests for anti-HB$_c$ have found limited usefulness for routine serodiagnosis and seroepidemiology, in large part because of the limited quantities of reagents available for testing and the complex nature of some of the techniques. From the standpoint of balance between practicality and sensitivity, IAHA is an attractive technique for serological studies of anti-HB$_c$.

The same methods are also optimal for studying the epidemiology of type B hepatitis, although HB$_s$ Ag prevalence may be established with somewhat less accuracy, albeit at much lower cost, by using first or second generation methods for HB$_s$ Ag detection. Anti-HB$_s$ detection by the less sensitive methods is particularly useful for identifying donors whose plasma contains high anti-HB$_s$ titers and is therefore suitable for the manufacture of hepatitis B immune globulin (HBIG) and potent antisera for in vitro diagnostic methods (28). In evaluating the safety and effectiveness of passive and active immunization with experimental HBIG preparations and vaccines, the highly sensitive third generation methods are preferred. Determination of HB$_s$ Ag subtypes by any of a number of methods is of great value as an epidemiological tool and also for answering basic questions regarding the importance of subtypes in protection against reinfection with HBV and in vaccine effectiveness.

LITERATURE CITED

1. Almeida, J. D., D. Rubenstein, and E. J. Stott. 1971. New antigen-antibody system in Australia antigen positive hepatitis. Lancet 2:1224–1227.
2. Alter, H. J., P. V. Holland, and R. H. Purcell. 1971. Counterelectrophoresis for detection of hepatitis-associated antigen: methodology and comparison with gel diffusion and complement fixation. J. Lab. Clin. Med. 77:1000–1010.
3. Bancroft, W. H., F. K. Mundon, and P. K. Russell. 1972. Detection of additional determinants of hepatitis B antigen. J. Immunol. 109:842–848.
4. Barker, L. F., J. D. Almeida, J. H. Hoofnagle, R. J. Gerety, D. R. Jackson, and P. P. McGrath. 1974. Hepatitis B core antigen: immunology and electron microscopy. J. Virol.

14:1552–1558.

5. Barker, L. F., F. V. Chisari, P. P. McGrath, D. W. Dalgard, R. L. Kirschstein, J. D. Almeida, T. S. Edgington, D. G. Sharp, and M. R. Peterson. 1973. Transmission of type B viral hepatitis to chimpanzees. J. Infect. Dis. 127:648–662.

6. Bradley, D. W., J. E. Maynard, K. R. Berquist, and D. H. Krushak. 1974. Hepatitis B and serum DNA polymerase activities in chimpanzees. Nature (London) 251:356–357.

7. Gocke, D. J., H. B. Greenberg, and N. B. Kavey. 1969. Hepatitis antigen. Detection of infectious blood donors. Lancet 2:248–249.

8. Gocke, D. J., and C. Howe 1970. Rapid detection of Australia antigen by counterelectrophoresis. J. Immunol. 104:1031–1034.

9. Greenman, R. L., W. S. Robinson, and G. N. Vyas. 1975. A sensitive test for antibody against the hepatitis B core antigen (anti-HB$_c$). Vox Sang. 29:77–80.

10. Holland, P. V., R. H. Purcell, H. Smith, and H. J. Alter. 1972. Subtyping of hepatitis-associated antigen (HB$_s$ Ag); simplified technique with counterelectrophoresis. J. Immunol. 109:420–425.

11. Hollinger, F. B., V. Vorndam, and G. R. Dreesman. 1971. Assay of Australia antigen and antibody employing double-antibody and solid-phase radioimmunoassay techniques and comparison with the passive hemagglutination methods. J. Immunol. 107:1099–1111.

12. Hoofnagle, J. H., R. J. Gerety, and L. F. Barker. 1973. Antibody to hepatitis B virus core in man. Lancet 2:869–873.

13. Hoofnagle, J. H., R. J. Gerety, L. Y. Ni, and L. F. Barker. 1974. Antibody to hepatitits B core antigen. A sensitive indicator of hepatitis B virus replication. N. Engl. J. Med. 290:1336–1340.

14. Huang, S. N., and V. Grah. 1973. A study on antibodies produced with liver tissue containing Australia antigen and virus-like particles. Lab. Invest. 29:743–750.

15. Jambazian, A., and J. C. Holper. 1972. Rheophoresis: a sensitive immuno-diffusion method for detection of hepatitis associated antigen. Proc. Soc. Exp. Biol. Med. 140:560–564.

16. Kaplan, P. M., J. L. Gerin, and H. J. Alter. 1974. Hepatitis B-specific DNA polymerase activity during post-transfusion hepatitis. Nature (London) 249:762–764.

17. Kaplan, P. M., R. L. Greenman, J. L. Gerin, R. H. Purcell, and W. S. Robinson. 1973. DNA polymerase associated with human hepatitis B antigen. J. Virol. 12:995–1005.

18. Krugman, S., J. H. Hoofnagle, R. J. Gerety, P. M. Kaplan, and J. L. Gerin. 1974. Viral hepatitis, type B. DNA polymerase activity and antibody to hepatitis B core antigen. N. Engl. J. Med. 290:1331–1335.

19. Lander, J. J., H. J. Alter, and R. H. Purcell. 1971. Frequency of antibody to hepatitis-associated antigen as measured by a new radioimmunoassay technique. J. Immunol. 106:1166–1171.

20. Leach, J. M., and B. J. Ruck. 1971. Detection of hepatitis associated antigen by the latex agglutination test. Br. Med. J. 4:597–598.

21. LeBouvier, G. L. 1971. The heterogeneity of Australia antigen. J. Infect. Dis. 123:671–675.

22. Ling, C. M., and L. R. Overby. 1972. Prevalence of hepatitis B virus antigen as revealed by direct radioimmunoassay with ^{125}I-antibody. J. Immunol. 109:834–841.

23. London, W. T., A. I. Sutnick, and B. S. Blumberg. 1969. Australia antigen and acute viral hepatitis. Ann. Intern. Med. 70:55–59.

24. Moritsugu, Y., J. W. M. Gold, J. Wagner, R. Y. Dodd, and R. H. Purcell. 1975. Hepatitis B core antigen: detection of antibody by radioimmunoprecipitation. J. Immunol. 114:1792–1798.

25. Peterson, D. A., G. G. Froesner, and F. W. Deinhardt. 1973. Evaluation of passive hemagglutination, solid-phase radioimmunoassay, and immunoelectroosmophoresis for the detection of hepatitis B antigen. Appl. Microbiol. 26:376–380.

26. Peterson, M. R., L. F. Barker, and D. S. Schade. 1973. Detection of antibody to hepatitis-associated antigen in hemophilia patients and in voluntary blood donors. Vox. Sang. 24:66–75.

27. Prince, A. M. 1968. An antigen detected in the blood during the incubation period of serum hepatitis. Proc. Natl. Acad. Sci. U.S.A. 60:814–821.

28. Prince, A. M., W. Szmuness, K. R. Woods, and G. F. Grady. 1971. Antibody against serum hepatitis antigen. Prevalence and potential use as immune serum globulin in prevention of serum hepatitis infections. N. Engl. J. Med. 285:933–938.

29. Purcell, R. H., J. L. Gerin, J. D. Almeida, and P. V. Holland. 1973/74. Radioimmunoassay for the core of the Dane particle and antibody to it. Intervirology 2:231–243.

30. Purcell, R. H., P. V. Holland, J. H. Walsh, D. C. Wong, A. G. Morrow, and R. M. Chanock. 1969. A complement-fixation test for measuring Australia antigen and antibody. J. Infect. Dis. 120:383–386.

31. Robinson, W. S., and R. L. Greenman. 1974. DNA polymerase in the core of the human hepatitis B virus candidate. J. Virol. 13:1231–1236.

32. Tsuda, F., T. Takahasi, K. Takahashi, Y. Miyakawa, and M. Mayumi. 1975. Determination of antibody to hepatitis B core antigen by means of immune adherence hemagglutination. J. Immunol. 115:834–838.

33. Vyas, G. N., and N. R. Shulman. 1970. Hemagglutination assay for antigen and antibody associated with viral hepatitis. Science 170:332–333.

34. Walsh, J. H., R. Yalow, and S. A. Berson. 1970. Detection of Australia antigen and antibody by means of radioimmunoassay techniques. J. Infect. Dis. 130:383–386.

Chapter 66

Antibody Assays for Enteroviruses and Reoviruses

Enteroviruses

INTRODUCTION

The human enterovirus group is comprised of 67 distinct antigenic types, including 3 polioviruses, 29 coxsackieviruses, 31 echoviruses, and 4 newly recognized types which are classified simply as enteroviruses without being assigned to any of the three subgroups. Although heterotypic antibody responses commonly occur in human enterovirus infections, they are not consistent enough or sufficiently well-defined to permit the use of one, or a few, antigens for group-specific serological diagnosis.

The neutralization test is generally considered to be the most sensitive and specific of the conventional serological procedures for detection of enterovirus antibodies. Hemagglutination-inhibiting (HI) antibodies appear to parallel neutralizing antibodies, but the test is severely limited by the fact that only about one-third of the currently recognized enterovirus immunotypes agglutinate erythrocytes. The complement-fixation (CF) test is useful for serodiagnosis of poliovirus infections, but not for other enterovirus infections. In coxsackievirus infections, the presence of heterotypic CF antibody generally prevents type-specific diagnosis, and, further, high levels of CF antibody are usually present in acute-phase sera, making it impossible to demonstrate diagnostically significant increases in antibody titer between acute- and convalescent-phase specimens. In echovirus infections the problem of heterotypic CF antibody also obtains, and, in addition, many infected individuals fail to produce CF antibody. The heterotypic reactivity of human sera with the coreless capsid antigens of coxsackieviruses and echoviruses in immunodiffusion and immunofluorescent staining tests limits the value of these procedures for serodiagnosis of infection (4, 8).

CLINICAL INDICATIONS

Although serological methods alone are not generally used for laboratory diagnosis of enterovirus infections, neutralization tests may be employed in outbreak situations where the predominating enterovirus type(s) is known, and tests can be limited to one or a few virus types. Tests against selected virus types may also be used in certain clinical syndromes such as hand-foot-and-mouth disease, pleurodynia, or paralytic illness, in which only certain immunotypes have been implicated. Neutralizing antibody assays are sometimes performed against the homologous virus type on patients from whom an enterovirus has been isolated, in an effort to strengthen the etiological role of the isolate in the patient's illness; the demonstration of a significant rise in antibody titer establishes a temporal association of the enterovirus infection with the current illness. Neutralizing antibody assays for polioviruses are the only reliable means for determining immunity status, since CF antibodies are of shorter duration than neutralizing antibodies, and often are not produced in response to vaccination.

Although the neutralization test is the most satisfactory method for serological diagnosis of enterovirus infections, its value is limited to some extent by the rapid development of neutralizing antibodies in response to infection, which may preclude the detection of a diagnostically significant increase in antibody titer. Thus, early collection of the acute-phase serum specimen is particularly important.

Virus isolation is the most suitable method for laboratory diagnosis of enterovirus infections, but paired sera should also be submitted to the laboratory to provide serological support on the etiological role of an enterovirus isolate, and also to rule out other viral infections which produce similar syndromes, and for which satisfactory in vitro serological tests are available, e.g., herpes simplex virus, mumps virus, and certain arboviruses.

TEST PROCEDURE

Enterovirus neutralization tests in which inhibition of the viral cytopathic effect (CPE) is read microscopically are the most generally adaptable to antibody assays and identification of viral isolates. These can be performed in cell cultures in tubes, or in micro cell cultures in wells in plastic plates. The cells most frequently employed are primary rhesus or grivet monkey kidney, human fetal diploid fibroblast strains, or continuous monkey kidney cell lines such as the BS-C-1 line of grivet monkey kidney cells. Tube and bottle cultures or suspensions of these cell types are available from commercial sources (Flow Laboratories, Rockville, Md.; Grand Island Biological Co., Grand Island, N.Y.; Microbiological Associates, Bethesda, Md.). Detailed methods for initiating and subpassaging various types of cells are given elsewhere (7). A satisfactory cell culture maintenance medium for enterovirus neutralization tests consists of Eagle's minimal essential medium (MEM) supplemented with 2% inactivated fetal bovine serum.

Seed enterovirus preparations are available from the American Type Culture Collection, Rockville, Md., and from the Research Resources Branch (RRB), National Institutes of Health, Bethesda, Md., and these can be used to prepare working stocks. Before they are employed in neutralization tests, the identity of stock virus preparations should be confirmed by testing against homotypic immune serum prepared in another, reliable laboratory. Well-characterized enterovirus antisera may be obtained from the RRB, National Institutes of Health, and enterovirus antisera are also available commercially (Microbiological Associates).

Certain enterovirus strains, or virus in certain preparations, may have a strong tendency to aggregate, and thus be insusceptible to neutralization by homologous antisera. If it is necessary to use such a preparation for neutralization tests, virus can be disaggregated by treatment with sodium deoxycholate (1). One part of a 1% solution of sodium deoxycholate (prepared in distilled water) is mixed with nine parts of the virus preparation, which is then stirred on a vortex mixer for 1 min and incubated at 37 C for 15 min.

1. Infectivity titers of enterovirus preparations to be used as challenge virus are determined in the same cell type and culture vessels to be used for neutralization tests. Log$_{10}$ dilutions of the virus are prepared in maintenance medium, and each dilution is inoculated into four tube cultures in a volume of 0.1 ml (0.05 ml for micro cell cultures). Tests incubated at 36 to 37 C for 7 days, and examined microscopically for viral CPE. The TCD$_{50}$ end point is calculated by the method of Karber or Reed and Muench (3). The dilution of virus preparation containing a challenge dose of 100 TCD$_{50}$ is

determined by adding 2 to the negative log of the titer.

Example: TCD$_{50}$ titer = $10^{-6.0}$ per 0.1 ml

$$\begin{array}{r} -6.0 \\ +2.0 \\ \hline -4.0 \end{array}$$ = log of dilution of virus preparation containing 100 TCD$_{50}$ in 0.1 ml

2. Test sera are heated at 56 C for 30 min to inactivate heat-labile, nonspecific viral inhibitory substances, and twofold dilutions are prepared in maintenance medium.

3. Equal volumes of the serum dilutions and test virus diluted to contain 100 TCD$_{50}$ per 0.1 ml are mixed and incubated at room temperature or 37 C for 1 h.

4. As a control on the test dose of virus, the working dilution and successive 10-fold dilutions prepared from this dilution are mixed with equal volumes of maintenance medium and incubated under the same conditions as the serum-virus mixtures. This control indicates the infectious dose of virus actually present in the test. A test dose below 32 TCD$_{50}$ may give falsely high antibody titers, and one above 320 TCD$_{50}$ may result in an insensitive test, as low levels of antibody may fail to neutralize the large challenge virus dose.

5. The serum-virus mixtures and virus-diluent mixtures are inoculated into tube cultures in a volume of 0.2 ml. Generally, two cell cultures are inoculated with each serum-virus mixture, and four with each virus dilution.

6. Known high- and low-titered positive sera and a negative serum should be included as controls in each run. The titers of the positive sera should vary by no more than twofold from the median, and the negative serum should show no neutralization.

7. Tests are incubated at 36 to 37 C and observed at 2- to 3-day intervals; final readings are made when the virus control shows that 100 TCD$_{50}$ are present in the test. The antibody end point is the highest initial dilution of serum which inhibits CPE of the test virus dose.

Modifications for micro cell cultures

Cell cultures are prepared in microtiter plates (with flat-bottom wells) which have been processed for tissue culture (Falcon Plastics, Oxnard, Calif.; Linbro Chemical Co., New Haven, Conn.). BS-C-1 or human fetal diploid lung (HFDL) cells are suspended in growth medium (90% Eagle's MEM and 10% fetal bovine serum) at a concentration of 50,000 BS-C-1 cells per ml or 100,000 HFDL cells per ml, and are planted in a volume of 0.15 ml per well. The plates are incubated in a CO_2 incubator for 2 to 3 days until the cells become confluent. Growth medium is then removed from each cup and replaced with 0.1 ml of maintenance medium.

Virus is diluted to contain 100 TCD_{50} in a volume of 0.05 ml, and serum-virus mixtures or virus-diluent mixtures are added in a volume of 0.1 ml per well.

Plates are incubated at 36 to 37 C in a CO_2 incubator, or they may be incubated in a regular incubator after adding 0.1 ml of sterile mineral oil (350 Seyboldt units viscosity) to each well and sealing the plate with Paklon tape (Minnesota Mining and Manufacturing Co., St. Paul, Minn.).

Tests are read with an inverted microscope.

Metabolic inhibition tests have been developed for large-scale enterovirus neutralizing antibody assays, e.g., surveys to determine immunity status to polioviruses. The tests are based upon differences in the color of the phenol red indicator in cell cultures degenerated by virus and in those protected by neutralizing antibody, and the chief advantage is that the tests can be read colorimetrically and do not require microscopic observation. The methods are described in detail elsewhere (7).

A few of the group A coxsackieviruses can be propagated only in suckling mice, and neutralization tests must be performed in this host system (5). However, these virus types appear to be of minor clinical importance, and serological diagnosis is rarely attempted.

INTERPRETATION

A fourfold or greater increase in neutralizing antibody titer to an enterovirus usually indicates a current infection with that virus type. Occasionally, however, there is recall of neutralizing antibody to closely related enteroviruses with which the patient has been previously infected, and this may confuse type-specific diagnosis, particularly in group B coxsackievirus infections. When neutralizing antibody titer rises occur to more than one enterovirus type, it is sometimes possible to identify the current infecting type by the fact that antibody is absent or at a low level in the acute-phase serum, while elevated antibody titers may be present to previous infecting virus types.

Reoviruses

INTRODUCTION

Each of the three reovirus serotypes has been isolated from individuals with a wide variety of clinical illnesses, but their role in the etiology of human disease has not been well established. Most infections are inapparent and are acquired early in life. Antibody assays are rarely done for serodiagnosis of reovirus infections, but, as in the case of enteroviruses, they may be performed on individuals from whom virus is isolated in order to strengthen the association of the isolate with the patient's illness.

Methods available for assay of reovirus antibodies include HI, neutralization, and CF tests. The HI test is the method of choice because of its relative simplicity and its sensitivity. Sera with low levels of reovirus antibody may fail to neutralize the large test doses of virus which are required to produce CPE in neutralization tests, and many infected individuals fail to produce detectable levels of reovirus CF antibody. However, most reovirus infections elicit the production of HI antibodies. The HI test is based upon the fact that reoviruses have sites on their surfaces (hemagglutinins) which attach to human erythrocytes (and also bovine erythrocytes in the case of reovirus type 3) and agglutinate them, and that this hemagglutination reaction is inhibited when specific antibody combines with the virus.

TEST PROCEDURE

The following procedure is conducted by the microtiter method in "V" plates. A macro method performed in tubes (6) may also be employed. For the test described below, 0.01 M phosphate-buffered saline (PBS) containing 0.2% bovine albumin (Fraction V, Armour Pharmaceutical Co.) is used as a diluent for erythrocytes, serum, and antigen.

Standardization of indicator (human group O) erythrocyte suspension

Erythrocyte suspensions standardized by the cyanmethemoglobin (CMG) method (2) give the most accurate and reliable results, and the method is applicable for use with a variety of spectrophotometers. An alternative, but less satisfactory, method is to prepare a 0.5% suspension of erythrocytes based upon packed cell volume. The CMG method is based upon lysing the erythrocytes, converting the hemoglobin released to CMG with a reagent containing potassium cyanide and potassium ferricyanide (Cyanmethemoglobin Reagent, Hycel, Inc.), and then reading the concentration of CMG against a standard on a spectrophotometer.

Construction of a standard CMG curve. CMG is diluted in CMG reagent to contain 80, 60, 40, 20, and 0 (blank) mg of CMG/100 ml. The optical density of each dilution is read on a spectrophotometer at a wavelength of 540 nm. These readings should fall on a straight line when plotted on regular graph paper against the milligrams of CMG per 100 ml.

Calculation of the factor to be used in determining the target OD. For each spectrophotometer the factor to be used in determining the target optical density (OD) must be calculated from the OD readings obtained for the standards.

Factor = sum of concentrations (mg of CMG/100 ml) of standards (80 + 60 + 40 + 20 + 0) divided by the sum of the OD readings of the standards.

Calculation of the target OD for the 0.5% erythrocyte suspension.

Target OD = target mg of CMG/100 ml divided by the factor. In the case of a 0.5% suspenson of mammalian erythrocytes, the target mg of CMG/100 ml is 6.255.

The factor and target OD can be used for subsequent standardizations with the spectrophotometer if the instrument is not moved or unduly jarred. The reliability of the instrument should be checked before each use by reading the OD of the 40 mg/100 ml CMG standard; this standard will remain stable for several months if kept refrigerated and free from contamination.

Washing erythrocytes. Human group O red cells collected in Alsever's solution should be stored at 4 C for 18 to 24 h prior to use. The blood is then filtered through gauze and the cells are washed three times in physiological saline by centrifugation at 700 × g for 7 min; the buffy coat is carefully removed after each washing. The erythrocytes are then packed in a graduated centrifuge tube by centrifugation at 700 × g for 10 min, and the volume of packed cells is noted. The supernatant fluid is removed and a stock 4% suspension of erythrocytes is prepared in dextrose-gelatin-Veronal (DGV) solution.

Standardization of the 0.5% working dilution of human group O red cells.

1. A 1-ml amount of the 4% suspension of erythrocytes is transferred to a 25-ml volumetric flask, and 0.1 ml of 5% aqueous saponin solution is added to enhance lysis of the cells. The flask is then filled to the mark with CMG reagent, and the contents are mixed well.

2. After standing at room temperature for 5 to 10 min, the OD of the solution is read at 540 nm against the reagent blank.

3. The dilution necessary to adjust the 4% erythrocyte suspension to the desired OD for the 0.5% suspension is calculated:

$$\frac{\text{OD of 4\% suspenson} \times \text{volume of 4\% suspension (1 ml)}}{\text{target OD}} = \text{dilution factor}$$

The 4% erythrocyte suspension is diluted appropriately to prepare the working suspension, which is stored at 4 C until added to the test. A working suspension of erythrocytes should be used only for a single day's tests.

Antigen titration

Reovirus hemagglutinating antigens are generally prepared from infected rhesus monkey kidney cell cultures. The cells and fluids are harvested 72 h after the cultures show maximal viral CPE, frozen and thawed three times, and stored at −70 C. Only reovirus type 3 hemagglutinating antigen is available commercially (Microbiological Associates). Antigens are clarified by low-speed centrifugation (700 × g for 10 min) prior to use in the test.

1. Duplicate twofold dilutions of each antigen (starting with undiluted) are prepared in a volume of 0.025 ml by use of microdiluters.

2. To each antigen dilution is added 0.025 ml of diluent. Three wells in the plate receive only 0.05 ml of diluent. These are "cell controls" to indicate whether the erythrocytes settle properly under the conditions of the test.

3. To each antigen and cell control well is added 0.025 ml of the standardized 0.5% human group O red cell suspension, and the reagents are mixed by shaking the plates or agitating them on a vibrating platform.

4. Tests are incubated at 37 C for 1 h, or until the erythrocytes in the cell control wells settle into a tight button. Tests may also be incubated at room temperature, but settling of the erythrocytes may require a longer time.

5. The end point of the antigen titration is the highest dilution producing complete agglutination of the erythrocytes. This represents 1 hemagglutinating (HA) unit, and antigen is diluted to contain 4 HA units in a volume of 0.025 ml for the test proper.

Example: Final titer = 1:32

$$\frac{1}{32} \times 4 = \frac{1}{8}$$

or 1:8 dilution of antigen contains 4 HA units.

6. The antigen concentration of the working dilution is checked before it is used in the test proper. Five dilutions are prepared in duplicate from the working dilution. To the first wells in each set is added 0.05 ml of antigen. With microdiluters, four serial twofold dilutions are prepared from this in 0.025-ml volumes. The

wells thus contain 4, 2, 1, 0.5, and 0.25 units of antigen. To each antigen well is added 0.025 ml of diluent, and wells containing 0.05 ml of diluent are prepared for cell controls. Each well then receives 0.025 ml of the 0.5% suspension of erythrocytes, and the tests are mixed and incubated as described above. The first three antigen dilutions (containing 4, 2, and 1 HA units) should show complete agglutination, the fourth partial or no agglutination, and the fifth no agglutination. The antigen concentration of the working dilution is adjusted upward or downward as necessary.

Hemagglutination-inhibition test

For serodiagnosis of reovirus infection, acute- and convalescent-phase sera are tested in parallel in the same run against antigens to each of the three reovirus types.

1. To remove nonspecific (nonantibody) inhibitors of reovirus hemagglutination, sera diluted 1:4 are absorbed with an equal volume of a 25% suspension of acid-washed kaolin (25 g of kaolin in 100 ml of PBS, pH 7.4) for 20 min at room temperature with occasional shaking. After centrifugation at $700 \times g$ for 15 min to sediment the kaolin, the supernatant fluid, representing approximately a 1:8 dilution of absorbed serum, is removed.

2. Human sera do not require absorption with human group O red cells, but animal sera must be absorbed to remove natural agglutinins. To each 1 ml of kaolin-treated serum is added 0.1 ml of a 50% suspension of human group O red cells. After incubation at 4 C for 1 to 2 h, the erythrocytes are sedimented by centrifugation at $700 \times g$ for 15 min at 4 C, and the supernatant fluid (absorbed serum) is removed. Sera are not heat-inactivated for testing.

3. Twofold dilutions of serum (from 1:8 through 1:2,048) are prepared in 0.025-ml volumes for tests against each of the three reovirus antigen types, and dilutions of 1:8 through 1:32 are prepared in the same volumes for a "serum control." This set of dilutions receives diluent rather than antigen, and indicates whether the test serum itself agglutinates the indicator erythrocytes.

4. The working dilution (containing 4 HA units) of each reovirus antigen is added to the appropriate set of serum dilutions in a volume of 0.025 ml, and 0.025 ml of diluent is added to each of the serum control dilutions.

5. Again, controls on the working dilution of antigen are prepared as indicated above in step 6 under Antigen titration.

6. Cell control wells containing 0.05 ml of diluent are prepared.

7. Tests are incubated for 1 h at room temperature.

8. To each well is added 0.025 ml of the 0.5% human group O erythrocyte suspension, and the contents of the wells are mixed.

9. Tests are incubated at 37 C for 1 h, or at room temperature until the erythrocytes in the cell control wells show proper settling.

10. The HI antibody titer of a serum is the highest dilution which completely inhibits hemagglutination by the 4 units of test antigen.

The controls in the test should show the following results. Agglutination should not occur in the serum control dilutions; if it does, the test on that serum cannot be considered valid unless the inhibition titer of the serum is fourfold higher than the titer of natural agglutinins. The "back titration" of the working dilution of antigen should show the results indicated above in step 6 under Antigen titration; if less than 2 or more than 8 units of antigen were used in the test, it cannot be considered valid. Known positive and negative sera for each antigen should be included as controls in each run; these should be treated to remove inhibitors and agglutinins together with the test sera, rather than being pretreated. The titers of the positive control sera should vary by no more than twofold from the median titer, and the negative serum should show no inhibition. The erythrocyte controls should show no agglutination.

INTERPRETATION

A fourfold or greater increase in HI antibody titer to a reovirus antigen is considered evidence of a current reovirus infection, but it may not be possible to determine the infecting virus type. Infections with type 3 virus generally produce only a homotypic HI antibody response, but type 1 and type 2 infections usually elicit heterotypic HI antibody titer increases. The demonstration of reovirus HI antibody in a single serum specimen from a survey indicates a past reovirus infection but, again, the specific type(s) may be uncertain.

LITERATURE CITED

1. Gwaltney, J. M., Jr., and A. M. Calhoun. 1970. Viral aggregation resulting in the failure to correctly identify an unknown rhinovirus. Appl. Microbiol. 20:390–392.
2. Hierholzer, J. C., and M. T. Suggs. 1969. Standardized viral hemagglutination and hemagglutination-inhibition tests. I. Standardization of erythrocyte suspensions. Appl. Microbiol. 18:816–823.
3. Lennette, E. H. 1969. General principles under-

lying laboratory diagnosis of viral and rickettsial infections, p. 1-65. *In* E. H. Lennette and N. J. Schmidt (ed.), Diagnostic procedures for viral and rickettsial infections, 4th ed. American Public Health Association, Inc., New York.

4. MacWilliam, K. M., and M. A. Cooper. 1974. Antibody levels in human sera measured by the fluorescent antibody technique against the coxsackie B virus types 1-5 grown in HEp2 cells compared with results obtained by neutralization. J. Clin. Pathol. 27:825-827.

5. Melnick, J. L., and H. A. Wenner. 1969. Enteroviruses, p. 529-602. *In* E. H. Lennette and N. J. Schmidt (ed.), Diagnostic procedures for viral and rickettsial infections, 4th ed. Ameri-can Public Health Association, Inc., New York.

6. Rosen, L. 1974. Reoviruses, p. 735-739. *In* E. H. Lennette, E. H. Spaulding, and J. P. Truant (ed.), Manual of clinical microbiology, 2nd ed. American Society for Microbiology, Washington, D.C.

7. Schmidt, N. J. 1969. Tissue culture technics for diagnostic virology, p. 79-178. *In* E. H. Lennette and N. J. Schmidt (ed.), Diagnostic procedures for viral and rickettsial infections, 4th ed. American Public Health Association, Inc., New York.

8. Schmidt, N. J., and E. H. Lennette. 1973. Advances in the serodiagnosis of viral infections. Prog. Med. Virol. 15:244-308.

Chapter 67

Chlamydiae

JULIUS SCHACHTER

INTRODUCTION

The human chlamydial infections include psittacosis, lymphogranuloma venereum (LGV), trachoma-inclusion conjunctivitis (TRIC), and the genital tract infections associated with agents capable of producing eye diseases. There are no wholly satisfactory serological methods for diagnosing these infections. The tests that are useful for diagnosing one of the diseases may be totally useless in attempting to diagnose some of the others. Problems stem from inadequate antibody response for certain tests, inability to obtain appropriately paired sera because of long incubation periods or inapparent infections, and high background reactor rates in high-risk populations.

For practical purposes, only two serological methods can be recommended. These are the complement-fixation (CF) test (8) and Wang's microimmunofluorescence (micro-IF) technique (17). The CF test (reviewed by Meyer and Eddie, 8) is most useful in the diagnosis of psittacosis and LGV (systemic infections), considerably less helpful in diagnosing TRIC agent oculogenital infections, and virtually useless in the diagnosis of trachoma (superficial infections). The recently developed micro-IF test has not been used in the routine diagnosis of psittacosis, although it may be adapted to this use in the future (5), but it is most useful in the diagnosis of chlamydial oculogenital infections and trachoma. Both tests are useful in serological surveys, perhaps more so than for diagnosing individual infections.

A variety of other serological techniques have been used, largely in research projects. Some of these tests are untried in the routine diagnosis of human infections, and others have been tried and found wanting. For example, the microagglutination tests once used in diagnosing avian chlamydial infections were successful only with sera from certain avian species. Despite the fact that agglutination tests are standard in some laboratories, my experience specifically recommends against their use with human sera. The radioisotope immune precipitation test has been applied in specialized serological surveys

and appears to be considerably more sensitive, although of similar specificity to the CF test (2, 11). The long-range usefulness of this test has not been determined, but it will probably be limited because the test is expensive and group reactive.

The CF test is a group-specific test. It measures antibodies to an antigenic determinant common to all chlamydiae (the active moiety is apparently an eight-carbon sugar, 2-keto-3 deoxyoctanoic acid [1]). This includes the species designated as *Chlamydia trachomatis* and *C. psittaci* (10). In contrast, the micro-IF test measures specific antibodies that are not detected by the CF test. Wang and Grayston introduced the micro-IF test in 1970 (17), initially for the serotyping of *C. trachomatis*, but further studies from the same and other laboratories found it to be a highly sensitive and specific indicator of antichlamydial antibodies (3, 9, 11, 18).

The CF and micro-IF tests when applied to individual sera are generally carried through an appropriate dilution range to allow determination of end points against the antigens. In survey work to determine the prevalence of antichlamydial antibodies, it may be possible to simplify testing by screening sera at the specific dilutions which are considered to be indicative of significant titers. The micro-IF test may involve many antigens (up to 13 serotypes may be used [6, 19]), but many studies could focus on antigenic types prevalent in the specific geographical area and associated with the disease conditions under consideration. This is particularly applicable in studies on childhood trachoma. Even in other studies it may be possible, in fact, to use only one or two types in the micro-IF test. For instance, our studies on genital tract infections in San Francisco, Calif., revealed that at least 75% of reactive sera had detectable antibodies to either type E or LGV II. Similar results have been obtained in Washington (9). Wang and Grayston (18) have found type-specific patterns in 79% of their sera from isolate-positive patients. Even in this study it is apparent that approximately 75% of these patients' sera react with type E or LGV II, although much higher titers were observed with homologous serotypes.

CLINICAL INDICATIONS

The CF test should be used routinely whenever LGV is considered in the differential diagnosis, such as in the case of young men being examined for inguinal lymphadenopathy, with or without systemic complications. In untreated cases, if a laboratory is available, efforts should be made to isolate chlamydiae from aspirates of fluctuant nodes. The bubonic form of LGV is less often seen in women. Women usually present with what are considered to be the later sequelae of LGV (vaginal-rectal syndrome involving rectal strictures and proctolitis or proctitis).

The disadvantage of the CF test is not its lack of specificity (for there are no known defined cross-reactions), but the ubiquitous nature of some of the chlamydial parasites and the group specificity of the test. Thus, the positive serological result may support a diagnosis of LGV but cannot prove it. Serological proof of the diagnosis would be based on demonstration of rising titers (a greater than fourfold difference in paired acute and convalescent sera), but in most cases the patient has had the chlamydial infection for too long a period of time before the test is performed. Even in acute lymphadenopathy in the male, there is usually a 3- to 4-week period from infection to presentation. Since there may have to be reliance on a static titer, with LGV one will feel much more comfortable in accepting a serological diagnosis when the CF titers are high (1:64 or greater), although any titer above the 1:8 or 1:16 range is considered significant. The titers in men take on greater meaning than those in women, because the common chlamydial infections causing nongonococcal urethritis in the male tend not to produce either as high a rate or as high a titer as do the genital tract infections in women (cervicitis). It is very rare to find a man with chlamydial urethritis having a CF titer above the 1:16 level (Table 1). Any patient tested for LGV should also have a serological test for syphilis. Some patients will have both, and Venereal Disease Research Laboratory reactive sera may react with both LGV and normal yolk sac antigens.

The CF test should be performed whenever a diagnosis of psittacosis is considered. Any acute or chronic febrile disease following exposure to birds, a pneumonitis, or a persistent influenzal disease would be clinical indications for considering psittacosis in the differential diagnosis. Here the CF test is much more satisfactory for

TABLE 1. *Distribution of chlamydial CF titers in patients with proven infections*

Disease	No. tested	No. with CF titer				
		<1:16	1	1:32	1:64	≥1:128
Lymphogranuloma venereum	15	0	1	2	0	12
Psittacosis	30	0	2	5	5	18
Adult inclusion conjunctivitis	93	46	28	11	6	2
Cervicitis, females ..	55	30	9	6	4	6
Urethritis, males ...	60	51	8	1	0	0

diagnosis, since acute and convalescent sera can be obtained and often demonstrate rising titers. In fact, in my experience, the great majority of psittacosis cases may be diagnosed in this manner. The diagnosis may have to be based upon a single high titer if the patient has a persistent or relapsing disease, but such a titer would clearly support the clinical impression. The problems of cross-reactions and previous exposure to other chlamydiae are clearly the same. In general, psittacosis infections produce high CF antibody levels (1:64 or greater). If a patient has had early and persistent treatment with tetracyclines, the antibody levels may be suppressed. There have been a number of human infections (proven by agent isolation) where no serological response was obtained because of early therapy.

The CF test is useless in the diagnosis of trachoma and not particularly useful in the diagnosis of oculogenital infections (14). At best, only 50% of individuals with eye and genital tract infections will have significant (greater than 1:16) CF titers (12). In the uncomplicated genital tract infections such as urethritis or cervicitis, the CF reactor rates are even less. The CF test is almost useless in the diagnosis of urethritis as only 15% of men with proven urethritis caused by chlamydiae have shown significant CF levels. However, approximately 40% of the women with chlamydial cervicitis have significant CF levels (12). CF titers in the background populations, i.e., sexually active men or sexually active women, will show a similar distribution in reactor rates. Women will have a higher background rate of CF reactors than men. Cytological or chlamydial isolation methods are the alternatives for diagnosing oculogenital infections, with tissue culture isolation being the method of choice.

The clinician may choose to utilize the delayed hypersensitivity test (Frei test), which is only applied in diagnosing LGV but is actually group reactive and positive at varying rates among patients with psittacosis or the TRIC agent infections. However, Frei test antigens currently available are not particularly potent, and routine use of this test is not recommended. In my experience the CF test is virtually always positive in LGV patients who have positive Frei tests, and is positive in LGV patients (agent recovered) who have negative skin tests (15). CF antibody levels tend to be persistent, but rapid declines in CF titers have been noted both spontaneously and after effective chemotherapy. One should not interpret falling titers in convalescence as supporting the diagnosis.

The micro-IF test measures specific antibodies to antigenic determinants present in the cell walls of the elementary body particles. It is much more sensitive than the CF test (9). For example, in one series of 55 isolate-positive patients, we found 29 with significant CF reactions whereas all 55 were positive in the micro-IF test. The respective geometric mean titers were 1:12 and 1:164. The micro-IF test can be applied to patients with LGV or to the TRIC agent ocular or oculogenital infections (3, 9, 11, 18). The presence of a reaction in a single serum specimen simply reflects present or past exposure. Changing titers may be seen in patients who are examined relatively early in the course of an infection, but this is usually not the case. One advantage of the micro-IF test is that information on the specific serotype responsible for the infection may be obtained. The micro-IF test offers the added advantage of determining the immunoglobulin class of the reactive antibodies since the presence of IgM antibodies may lend further support to diagnosis of active infections. Unfortunately, many of these infections tend to be chronic, and the best assessment is that the IgM antibody response may last for approximately 1 month following infection (18). In one study only 33% of patients with active infections had IgM antibodies (9). The major disadvantage of this test is that its results reflect the high prevalence of chlamydial infection in certain groups (13). In other words, in appropriate populations there may be very high reactor rates from previous exposure to the chlamydiae, and these antibody levels may persist for life, although in some patients they disappear spontaneously (18), possibly reflecting brief antigenic exposure. The significant level in the micro-IF test has been chosen as 1:8.

TEST PROCEDURES

Complement fixation

The CF test (8) may be performed in either the tube system or the microsystem. I strongly prefer the standardization of reagents in the tube system, regardless of which system is being used for test. The microtiter systems are most useful in screening large numbers of sera, but it is preferable to retest all positive results in the tube system. Occasionally, sera giving titers in the 1:4 to 1:8 range in the microsystem are positive at 1:16 (which I consider the significant level) in the tube system. The micro-system uses standard plates and volumes one-tenth those used in the tube test. The CF test is performed on serum specimens heated at 56 C for 30 min (preferably acute and convalescent paired sera tested together). In each test a positive control serum of high titer is included together with known negative serum. The reagents for the CF test are standardized by the Kolmer technique and include special buffered saline, group antigen, antigen (normal yolk sac) control, the positive serum, the negative serum, guinea pig complement, rabbit anti-sheep hemolysin, and sheep red cells. The hemolytic system is titrated and the complement unitage is determined. The standard units used in the test are 4 units of antigen and 2 exact units of complement. The test may be performed by either the water bath technique or the overnight (icebox) technique, the former being preferable. Doubling dilutions of the serum (from 1:2) are made in a 0.25-ml volume of saline. The antigen is added at 4 units (0.25 ml), and 2 exact units of complement (0.5 ml) are added. Standard reagent controls are always included. The normal yolk sac control is used at the same dilution as the group antigen. The tubes are shaken well and incubated in a water bath at 37 C for 2 h. Then 0.5 ml of sensitized sheep red cells is added, and the tubes are placed in the water bath for another hour. The tubes are read for hemolysis on a 1+ to 4+ scale roughly equivalent to 25 to 100% inhibition of red cell lysis. The end point of the serum is considered the highest dilution producing at least 50% (2+) hemolysis after a complete inhibition of hemolysis has been observed. It is general practice in my laboratory to shake the tubes to resuspend the settled cells, then refrigerate them overnight, and recheck the results the following morning.

Microimmunofluorescence

The micro-IF test is performed against chlamydial organisms grown in yolk sac (18). The individual yolk sacs are selected for elementary body richness and are pretitrated to give an even distribution of particles. It is generally found that a 1 to 3% yolk sac suspension (phosphate-buffered saline, pH 7.0) is satisfactory. The antigens may be stored as frozen portions, and after thawing they are well mixed in a Vortex mixer before use. Antigen dots are placed on a slide in a specific pattern with separate pen points used for each antigen. Each cluster of dots includes all the antigenic types to be tested. The antigen dots are air-dried and fixed on slides with acetone (15 min at room temperature). Slides may be stored frozen. When thawed for use they may sweat, but they can be conveniently dried (as can the original antigen dots) with a hair dryer. The slides have serial dilutions of serum (or tears or exudate) placed on different clusters. The clusters of dots are placed sufficiently separated to avoid the running of the serum from cluster to cluster. After addition of the serum dilutions, the slides are incubated for 0.5 to 1 h in a moist chamber at 37 C. They are then placed in a buffered saline wash of 5 min, followed by a second 5-min wash. The slides are then dried and stained with fluorescein-conjugated anti-human globulin. These conjugates are pretitrated in a known positive system to determine appropriate working dilutions. This reagent may be prepared against any class of globulin being considered (IgA or secretory piece for secretions, IgG or IgM). Counter-stains such as bovine serum albumin conjugated with rhodamine may be included. The slides are then washed twice again, dried, and examined by standard fluorescence microscopy. Use of a monocular tube is recommended to allow greater precision in determining fluorescence for individual elementary body particles. The end points are read as the dilution giving bright fluorescence clearly associated with the well-distributed elementary bodies throughout the antigen dot. Identification of the type-specific response is based upon dilution differences reflected in the end points for different prototype antigens (5, 18).

For each run of either CF or micro-IF, known positive and negative sera should always be included. These sera should always duplicate their titers as previously observed within the experimental (one dilution) error of the system.

REAGENTS

The commercially available antigens have occasionally presented sizable problems. In the CF test an antigen with the highest possible titer should be used to allow greatest dilution of the crude preparations being used and for reasons of economy. Several commercial preparations are available, but none can be recommended. Commercial preparations often have titers in the 1:8 or 1:16 range; the working dilution would be 1:2 to 1:4, which is unsatisfactory. In the CF system a major problem has been

obtaining complement free from antibodies to chlamydiae. Guinea pig inclusion conjunctivitis is a very common chlamydial infection in guinea pig colonies. The antigens appear to be anticomplementary, whereas they are simply reacting with the antibody present in the complement. This can often be shown when the complement does not react with the normal yolk sac control. One should always attempt to purchase complement certified to be nonreactive with chlamydial antigens. Unfortunately, the certification is not always accurate, and testing for antichlamydial antibodies prior to use is essential.

The CF hemolytic system reagents may be readily obtained commercially. There is, however, no commercial source of antigen which is highly potent. Therefore, the antigens must be prepared in the laboratory. There are several methods available that produce suitable antigens. The deoxycholate-extracted group antigen or the ether-extracted 16 (and acetone-precipitated if preferred) group antigens are perfectly satisfactory. Virtually any chlamydial strain can be used to prepare a group antigen, as it appears to be the major antigenic component for all strains. Comparative tests have shown that some strains or isolates are to be preferred over others; for instance, the psittacosis antigens have been superior to the LGV antigens even with LGV serum. The 6BC strain which has been used at the Hooper Foundation for many years is available from the American Type Culture Collection or the World Health Organization (WHO) Reference Centre at the Hooper Foundation. The technique of preparation involves inoculation of 7-day-old embryonated hen eggs via the yolk sac route with a standardized inoculum (0.25 ml containing approximately 10^5 egg LD_{50}) which kills most of the embryos in approximately 96 h. Embryos dying before 72 h are discarded. When approximately 50% of the embryos are dead, all the eggs are refrigerated for 3 to 24 h. The yolk sacs are harvested and examined microscopically (Giminez or Macchiavello stain; 4) for elementary bodies. If rich in particles, they are pooled and weighed. Yolk sacs are then ground thoroughly with sterile sand, and a 20% suspension in nutrient broth (pH 7.0) is prepared. Sterility tests are performed, and the material is held in a refrigerator for 6 weeks. During this period, the antigen preparation is occasionally shaken. The suspension is then centrifuged lightly (200 $\times$ g for 30 min) to remove coarse tissue debris and is steamed at 100 C for 30 min. After cooling, phenol is added to a final concentration of 0.5%. This antigen is divided into portions and stored in a refrigerator for use. It should titer at least 1:256. If stored properly and protected from contamination by using aseptic technique, the antigens will be stable for years. Small quantities of antigen are available from the WHO Reference Centre for reference purposes. The normal yolk sac control is prepared in a similar manner from uninfected embryos.

The routine immunofluorescent reagents used in the micro-IF test are available from Antibodies Inc., Hyland Laboratories, or Microbiological Associates, Inc., among others. The yolk sac antigens, however, are not available commercially and must be prepared in the laboratory. For a complete battery of test antigen, types A, B, Ba, C, D, E, F, G, H, I, J, and K, and LGV antigens L I, L II, and L III must be included. For routine screening of human sera, a simplified antigen pattern involving fewer antigen dots is useful. Closely related antigens may be pooled, for example, D and E, L I and L II, G and F, C and J (S. P. Wang, personal communication). The antigens are generally prepared from infected yolk sac suspensions. Tissue culture preparations may be used although they tend not to be as rich in particles. The yolk sacs are inoculated with suspensions of chlamydiae titrated to kill the embryos in approximately 7 days. In some instances, a greater time period may be required. When 50% of the eggs are dead, the rest are chilled, the yolk sacs are harvested, and individual yolk sacs are examined microscopically; those rich in elementary bodies are selected for use. They are homogenized to approximately 5% with sterile phosphate-buffered saline, and final antigen dilution is selected on the basis of morphological screening in a fluorescence system. The working dilution (usually 1 to 3%) may be frozen in portions at −60 C and stored until needed for making slides. The antigen suspensions when frozen and the slides when frozen are stable, but thawed suspensions should be used within 1 to 2 weeks.

INTERPRETATION

The normal backgrounds of the test (which reflect diseases prevalent in the community) will vary depending upon the geographical area where they are performed and the specific population group to be tested. (Table 2 presents the results obtained at the Hooper Foundation when the CF and micro-IF tests were used in parallel in different population studies.) In the CF test, for example, at a 1:16 level the general population in the San Francisco area tests 2 to 3% positivity. However, if one were testing veterinarians, one would find between 10 and

TABLE 2. *Antichlamydial antibodies in selected populations tested at the Hooper Foundation*

Group	CF $\geq 1:16$ (%)	Micro-IF $\geq 1:8$ (%)
Screening studies		
Normal adults, all ages	2–3	25–45
Pediatric sera	<1	10
Trachoma endemic population	5–15	>80
Males, venereal disease study, young adults	5–10	20–25
Females, venereal disease study, young adults	15–20	50–70
Prostitutes	30–60	Up to 85
Proven chlamydial infections (isolation)		
Lymphogranuloma venereum	100	100
Psittacosis	100	ND[a]
Adult inclusion conjunctivitis	50	100
Male, urethritis	15	90
Female, cervical infection	45	99

[a] Not determined.

20%, with significant CF levels depending on the type of practice. Further, if one were testing sexually active individuals, one would find the background to be approximately 5% for men and 15 to 20% for women. In patients with Reiter's syndrome, there is approximately a 25% seropositivity rate, and approximately 10% of the patients with Reiter's syndrome have very high antibody levels such as those often seen in psittacosis or LGV. CF titers of 1:64 or higher are rarely seen in the normal population or in sexually active males, although they do occur in sexually active females. This is the level which would be highly supportive of a diagnosis of psittacosis or lymphogranuloma venereum. There has not been similar broad experience with the micro-IF test, but the published results together with unpublished data from the Hooper Foundation indicate no problem with the group-specific cross-reactions. For example, we have tested psittacosis convalescent sera with CF titers of 1:512 and found them completely nonreactive in the micro-IF test. But there is a problem of background reactor rates. For example, asymptomatic sexually active men have a background reactor rate of approximately 25%. Sexually active young women may have reactor rates of 60 to 70%. Thus, a single positive titer could again only be used to determine previous exposure (the proviso here being that these tests are being done for diagnostic and not epidemiological purposes). In epidemiological studies, type-specific reactions could be of considerable interest in detecting predominant serotypes, transmission chains, patterns of clustering, etc. IgM antibodies in the micro-IF test may give greater support for active infection, but the experience indicates that only 28 to 33% of patients with active infections have these antibodies, and some patients who have IgM antibodies do not have demonstrable chlamydial infection (9, 11). There is an increasing reactor rate with age, but the background is approximately 10% in the pediatric population. The stimulus for this antibody response is not known (neonatal asymptomatic infections?). Patients with LGV tend to have high CF titers and very high and broadly reactive micro-IF antibody responses (18). Often, LGV patients have CF titers of 1:128 or 1:256 and micro-IF titers of 1:4,000 or higher. Specific antichlamydial IgA or IgG in tears may indicate active chlamydial infection of the conjunctiva (7).

In either CF or micro-IF, it is clear that a fourfold or greater rise in titer will support the diagnosis of chlamydial infection in the clinical syndrome being considered. Unfortunately, this is usually not observed, and often the clinician must simply use the titer observed in the point study and determine where it falls in the scheme of known background patterns to determine whether it supports his clinical diagnosis.

LITERATURE CITED

1. Dhir, S. P., S. Hakomori, G. E. Kenny, and J. T. Grayston. 1972. Immunochemical studies on chlamydial group antigen (presence of a 2-keto-3-deoxycarbohydrate as immunodominant group). J. Immunol. 109:116–122.
2. Gerloff, R. K., and R. O. Watson. 1967. The radioisotope precipitation test for psittacosis group antibody. Am. J. Ophthalmol. 63:1492–1498.
3. Hanna, L., E. Jawetz, B. Nabli, I. Hoshiwara, B. Ostler, and C. Dawson. 1972. Titration and typing of serum antibodies in TRIC infections by immunofluorescence. J. Immunol. 108:102–107.
4. Hanna, L., J. Schachter, and E. Jawetz. 1974. Chlamydiae (psittacosis-lymphogranuloma venereum-trachoma group), p. 795–804. In E. H. Lennette, E. H. Spaulding, and J. P. Truant (ed.), Manual of clinical microbiology, 2nd ed. American Society for Microbiology, Washington, D.C.
5. Jones, B. R. 1974. Laboratory tests for chlamydial infection: their role in epidemiological studies of trachoma and its control. Br. J. Ophthalmol. 58:438–454.
6. Kuo, C. C., S. P. Wang, J. T. Grayston, and E. R. Alexander. 1974. TRIC Type K, a new immunological type of Chlamydia trachomatis. J. Immunol. 113:1–20.

7. McComb, D. E., and R. L. Nichols. 1969. Antibodies to trachoma in eye secretions of Saudi Arab children. Am. J. Epidemiol. 90:278–284.
8. Meyer, K. F., and B. Eddie. 1956. Psittacosis, p. 399–430. In E. H. Lennette and N. J. Schmidt (ed.), Diagnostic procedures for virus and rickettsial diseases, 2nd ed. American Public Health Association, Inc., New York.
9. Philip, R. N., E. A. Casper, F. B. Gordon, and A. L. Quan. 1974. Fluorescent antibody responses to chlamydial infection in patients with lymphogranuloma venereum and urethritis. J. Immunol. 112:2126–2134.
10. Page, L. A. 1974. Order II. Chlamydiales Storz and Page 1971, 334, p. 914–928. In R. E. Buchanan and N. E. Gibbons (ed.), Bergey's manual of determinative bacteriology, 8th ed. The Williams & Wilkins Co., Baltimore.
11. Reeve, P., R. K. Gerloff, E. Casper, R. N. Philip, J. D. Oriel, and P. A. Powis. 1974. Serological studies on the role of Chlamydia in the aetiology of non-specific urethritis. Br. J. Vener. Dis. 50:136–139.
12. Schachter, J., C. R. Dawson, S. Balas, and P. Jones. 1970. Evaluation of laboratory methods for detecting acute TRIC agent infection. Am. J. Ophthalmol. 70:375–380.
13. Schachter, J., L. Hanna, E. C. Hill, S. Massad, C. W. Sheppard, J. E. Conte, S. N. Cohen, and K. F. Meyer. 1975. Are chlamydial infections the most prevalent venereal disease? J. Am. Med. Assoc. 231:1252–1255.
14. Schachter, J., C. H. Mordhorst, B. W. Moore, and M. L. Tarizzo. 1973. Laboratory diagnosis of trachoma: a collaborative study. Bull. WHO 48:509–515.
15. Schachter, J., D. E. Smith, C. R. Dawson, W. R. Anderson, J. J. Deller, Jr., A. W. Hoke, W. H. Smartt, and K. F. Meyer. 1969. Lymphogranuloma venereum. I. Comparison of the Frei test, complement fixation test, and isolation of the agent. J. Infect. Dis. 120:372–375.
16. Volkert, M., and P. M. Christensen. 1955. Two ornithosis complement-fixing antigens from infected yolk sacs. I. The phosphatide antigen, the virus antigen and methods for their preparation. Acta Pathol. Microbiol. Scand. 38:211–218.
17. Wang, S. P., and J. T. Grayston. 1970. Immunologic relationship between genital TRIC, lymphogranuloma venereum, and related organisms in a new microtiter indirect immunofluorescence test. Am. J. Ophthalmol. 70:367–374.
18. Wang, S. P., and J. T. Grayston. 1974. Human serology in Chlamydia trachomatis infection with microimmunofluorescence. J. Infect. Dis. 130:388–397.
19. Wang, S. P., J. T. Grayston, and J. L. Gale. 1973. Three new immunologic types of trachoma-inclusion conjunctivitis organisms. J. Immunol. 110:873–879.

Chapter 68

Rickettsiae

J. WILLIAM VINSON

INTRODUCTION

The rickettsial diseases of humans are listed in Table 1 together with their etiological agents, geographical distribution, and mode of transmission to humans. The five rickettsial diseases indigenous to the United States are Rocky Mountain spotted fever (RMSF), Q fever, murine (flea-borne) typhus, Brill-Zinsser (BZ) disease, and rickettsialpox. In terms of reported numbers of cases, RMSF has the highest incidence, followed by Q fever and murine typhus. BZ disease, or recrudescent typhus, occurs in persons who contracted primary epidemic typhus, generally in middle Europe or Russia, before immigrating to the United States. Rickettsialpox is seldom reported. In addition to the rickettsial diseases indigenous to the United States, both epidemic typhus and scrub typhus have been diagnosed in persons who were infected in endemic areas and came to the United States by fast air travel during the incubation period of their disease.

The Weil-Felix (WF) reaction was the first serological procedure developed for a rickettsial infection, and despite its limitations it is still almost universally employed. This is probably due to accessibility of antigens and simplicity of performance. The WF reaction (11) is based on the fact that certain antibodies elicited during the course of several rickettsial infections react with the polysaccharide O antigens of the so-called OX strains of two *Proteus* species, the OX-19 and OX-2 strains of *P. vulgaris* and the OX-K strain of *P. mirabilis*. The patterns of reactions of these antigens with antibodies to the typhus group, to the spotted fever group (except for rickettsialpox), and to scrub typhus are shown in Table 2. Sera from patients with rickettsialpox, Q fever, and trench fever do not give a WF reaction, and this reaction is usually negative in BZ disease.

A wide variety of procedures more satisfactory than the WF reaction have been devised to detect specific antibodies to all rickettsial agents. Antigens are prepared from rickettsiae propagated in the yolk sacs of chick embryos, in cell cultures, or, in the case of *Rochalimaea*

quintana, on cell-free media. Q fever and trench fever rickettsiae have antigens unique to themselves. Both epidemic and murine typhus share a common antigen, and members of the spotted fever group share a common antigen. In addition, there are minor antigenic crossovers between the typhus and the spotted fever groups. Most of the serological procedures detect only the common group antigen, but some have been modified to allow distinctions to be made between the species within the groups.

Serological procedures include complement fixation (CF), agglutination (4) and microagglutination (5), hemagglutination (2), and immunofluorescence (IF; 3, 6), all of which have been amply summarized (4, 9). Many state public health laboratories perform the CF test for rickettsial diseases, and they can obtain antigens from the Center for Disease Control (CDC). At present, rickettsial CF antigens are not consistently available directly from commercial sources. Performance of the remaining specific serological tests is confined to laboratories involved in rickettsial research.

During about the first 3 weeks after onset of disease, the predominant antibody produced is immunoglobulin M (IgM), whereas IgG predominates in later convalescence. Treatment of sera with ethanethiol inhibits IgM antibody but not IgG antibody. This fact is exploited for the serological diagnosis of BZ disease, in which IgG appears early in the disease (8). Pretreatment of the sera with ethanethiol before performance of the test does not reduce the CF antibody titer as compared with the titer of the matched untreated sera.

Serological diagnosis of scrub typhus by rickettsial antigens presents particular difficulties because of the diversity of antigenic strains of *R. tsutsugamushi*. To date, the preferred serological test for scrub typhus is the IF technique (1), but it generally is restricted to research laboratories.

In short, serological diagnosis of rickettsial infections in clinical laboratories by necessity is generally restricted to the less than satisfactory WF reaction, which can give at best only a presumptive diagnosis. No matter what the

TABLE 1. *Rickettsial diseases of humans*

Antigenic classification	Etiological agent	Disease	Geographical distribution	Transmission to humans
Typhus group	*Rickettsia prowazeki*	Epidemic typhus	Worldwide	Infected louse feces
	R. prowazeki	Brill-Zinsser disease	Worldwide	Recrudesence of latent infection
	R. mooseri	Murine typhus	Worldwide	Infected flea feces
Spotted fever group	*R. rickettsii*	Rocky Mountain spotted fever	Western hemisphere	Tick bite
	R. conorii	Fièvre boutonneuse	Mediterranean littoral, Africa, India	Tick bite
	R. sibirica	Siberian tick typhus	Siberia, Mongolia	Tick bite
	R. australis	Queensland tick typhus	Australia	Tick bite
	R. akari	Rickettsialpox	United States, USSR	Mite bite
Scrub typhus	*R. tsutsugamushi*	Scrub typhus	Asia, Australia, Pacific Islands	Mite bite
Trench fever	*Rochalimaea quintana*	Trench fever	Mexico, Central and South America, Middle East, Europe	Infected louse feces
Q fever	*Coxiella burnetii*	Q fever	Worldwide	Infectious aerosol from livestock

TABLE 2. *Usual Weil-Felix reactions in rickettsioses*

Disease	OX-19	OX-2	OX-K	Day after onset positive[a]	Cases with positive reactions[a] (%)
Murine typhus . .	+ + + +	+	0	8–15	95
Epidemic typhus	+ + + +	+	0	8–15	95
Brill-Zinsser disease	—[b]	—[b]	0	8–15	20
Spotted fever . . .	+ + + +	+	0	8–15	80
	+	+ + + +	0	8–15	
Scrub typhus . . .	0	0	+ +	10–14	40–60
Rickettsialpox . .	0	0	0	—	—
Q fever	0	0	0	—	—
Trench fever	0	0	0	—	—

[a] If treatment is begun early in the disease, the Weil-Felix reaction may not become significantly positive.

[b] Usually negative.

outcome of the WF reaction, the sera should be sent to the state public health laboratory for confirmation with specific rickettsial agents.

CLINICAL INDICATIONS

Diagnosis of rickettsial infections depends almost solely on clinical recognition and is aided by such epidemiological features as recent exposure to relevant arthropods, residence or recent travel in endemic areas both at home and abroad, or, in the case of Q fever, exposure to infected livestock. Present serological tests for detection of rickettsial diseases are mainly useful in confirming an initial clinical diagnosis or in establishing a retrospective diagnosis. The tests depend on demonstration of a rise in antibody titer during the course of the disease. By the time the results of serological tests become available to the physician, the patient is dead, under treatment, or recovering. All rickettsial infections can be successfully treated with broad-spectrum antibiotics, such as tetracycline, provided therapy is begun early in the disease. Early clinical diagnosis and treatment are therefore crucial to the prevention of severe disease and death. The importance of this point is emphasized when it is recalled that the case fatality rate for undiagnosed and untreated RMSF hovers around 25%.

Blood serum specimens should be obtained during the early acute and convalescent stages of the disease and tested simultaneously. WF tests on a single serum specimen rarely furnish information of significant value. If an early serum specimen is not available, a specimen should be obtained 2 months after infection and tested simultaneously with the convalescent serum against *rickettsial* antigens. A drop in titer can be helpful in establishing a retrospective diagnosis. The sera can be tested in the clinical laboratory for the typhus and spotted fever groups and for scrub typhus by means of the WF reaction. Only a presumptive serological diagnosis can be made from the WF reaction. Results should always be confirmed by submitting the sequentially obtained sera to the state public health laboratory for examination with specific rickettsial antigens. If the latter laboratory is not equipped for performing the procedures, it will forward the sera to the CDC. The CDC does not accept specimens submitted privately. If Q fever, rickettsialpox, or BZ disease is suspected, sequentially obtained serum specimens are sent directly to a state public health laboratory for testing by the CF or other methods. When submitting sera, the dates the specimens were obtained as well as the date of *onset of disease* should *always* be stated. This information is of vital importance for interpreting results of the serological tests.

TEST PROCEDURES

The WF and CF tests are described, as well as the procedure for distinguishing between IgM and IgG antibodies.

Weil-Felix reaction

Two types of WF test are available, the rapid slide test and the tube test. Antigens for the agglutination reaction can be prepared in the laboratory or purchased commercially. Directions for performance of both types accompany the commercially obtained *Proteus* antigens. Sera should be tested concurrently against OX-19, OX-2, and OX-K antigens, since the pattern of reaction with them aids in the interpretation of results.

Rapid slide test. Instructions for performing the rapid slide agglutination test accompany the commercial antigens. The antigens should be standardized with human convalescent sera. Positive control sera of known titer, preferably human convalescent sera, as well as a known negative serum should be included as controls with each test. The value of the slide test is the rapidity with which results can be obtained. Positive results may be confirmed with the tube test.

Tube method. For each serum to be tested, place in a holder 10 Wassermann or Kahn tubes in each of three rows. Pipette 0.5 ml of saline into the three tubes in row 10 for an antigen control. In other tubes make nine serial 10-fold dilutions of the test serum in saline from 1:10 through 1:2,560. Starting with the highest dilution, transfer 0.5 ml to each of the three tubes in row 9, and continue this procedure downward through the remaining eight dilutions. To one series of dilutions, plus the saline blank in row

10, add 0.5 ml of OX-19 antigen, to another add the OX-2 antigen, and to the third add OX-K antigen. If antigens are bought commercially, dilute them according to instructions. If prepared as detailed in the Reagents section, use without further dilution. Include titrations of both positive and negative control sera. The antigen plus saline acts as an antigen control. Agitate to mix; incubate for 2 h at 37 C and then overnight at 4 C. Tubes are held up to shielded light for reading. The antigen control should show an even turbidity. In a positive reaction, antigen will settle to the bottom of the tube and the supernatant fluid will be clear. On gentle shaking, the agglutinated bacilli will be dislodged with some difficulty but will finally swirl upward to show a fine granular type of agglutination. Results are read from 4 (complete agglutination) through 1 to ± to 0 (no agglutination) and are reported in terms of the final serum dilution.

Complement fixation

The CF test can be performed either in tubes or in the microtiter system as described in chapter 58 of this *Manual*. Before testing unknown sera, the antigen should be standardized against the corresponding human convalescent serum. Twofold falling dilutions of antigen are titrated in checkerboard fashion against twofold falling dilutions of known positive serum. The highest dilution of antigen completely fixing complement in the presence of the highest serum dilution is considered to be 1 unit of antigen. This titration is generally made with immune serum having a high concentration of IgG antibody. Sera obtained early in infection should be tested against 4 to 6 units of antigen, since the IgM CF antibodies which predominate during the first 3 weeks of disease are more readily detected by the higher antigen concentration (7). Two units of antigen are used when making sero-epidemiological studies, since the antibodies detected are generally residual IgG immunoglobulins. An antigen titration should be included in all subsequent tests. As usual, tests of known positive and negative sera should be included. Results are graded 0, ±, 1^+, 2^+, 3^+, or 4^+, according to the amount of complement fixed, with 0 representing no fixation and 4^+ complete fixation of complement.

Differentiation between immunoglobulin M and G antibodies

IgM antibodies are selectively inhibited by ethanethiol, leaving IgG antibodies intact. The ethanethiol is removed by the heat of serum inactivation before performance of the CF or other tests. The test serum is diluted 1:5 in Veronal buffer, and portions are placed in each of two tubes. The specimen in the first tube is brought to a dilution of 1:10. To the second tube is added an equal volume of 0.06 M ethanethiol. Both specimens are allowed to stand at 26 C for 3 h, after which they are both inactivated at 56 C for 30 min. The two specimens are immediately titrated in the CF test as usual. A lowering of CF titer in the treated serum, as compared with the untreated control, indicates that the serum contains largely IgM antibody. If the two titers are similar, the immunoglobulins are IgG.

REAGENTS

Weil-Felix antigens

WF antigens consist of whole unflagellated bacilli of the OX-19, OX-2, and OX-K strains of *Proteus* species. They can be either viable or killed. Antigens can be prepared in the laboratory or purchased commercially as kits from several sources, including Sylvana, Lederle Laboratories, and Beckman Instruments, Inc. (Diagnostic Operations). These companies also sell antisera produced in rabbits against the homologous *Proteus* strains. Although the antigens agglutinate in the presence of homologous antisera, they may not invariably react with rickettsial antibodies. Ideally, therefore, WF antigens should be standardized with the appropriate human convalescent sera. Such sera should also be used as positive controls in performing the test.

Proteus antigens can also be prepared in the laboratory. A modification of the method of Plotz (10) is given here. Cultures can be purchased from the American Type Culture Collection. As suggested in the Introduction, only O or nonmotile variants can be used. This is crucial to the performance of the test since agglutination of the bacilli by antibody cannot occur if the somatic O antigens are obscured by the H antigens of flagellated bacilli. Stock cultures are maintained by streaking smooth, or nonspreading, colonies on dry agar slants and incubating them at 37 C for 18 to 24 h.

To prepare the antigen, streak the stock *Proteus* strain on a nutrient agar plate. After incubation at 37 C for 18 to 24 h, inoculate smooth nonspreading O-type colonies into broth. After incubation for 18 h, examine a drop of the broth in a hanging drop slide to test for motility of the microorganisms. If the bacilli are nonmotile, inoculate the broth culture into Roux bottles containing nutrient agar; use 4 to 5 ml per bottle. After 18 h of incubation at 37 C, wash the growth off with 0.5% Formal saline,

using approximately 20 ml per bottle. Pool the bacterial suspensions and wash them free from medium by three cycles of centrifugation at 1,000 × g. Suspend sedimented cells from the final centrifugation in sufficient 0.5% Formol saline to give a turbidity reading equal to 3 on the McFarland nephelometer scale or a reading of 179 with a no. 42 filter in a Klett-Summerson colorimeter. Store the antigen at 4 C.

Complement-fixing antigens

Rickettsial antigens, including the group antigens for the typhus and spotted fever groups as well as Q fever antigen, are available to state public health laboratories on request to the Biologic Products Division, Bureau of Laboratories, CDC, Atlanta, Ga. Guinea pig and human convalescent sera for standardization of antigens and for use as positive controls can be obtained from the same source.

Ethanethiol can be purchased from Eastman Organic Chemicals, Rochester, N.Y.

INTERPRETATION

Weil-Felix test

The patterns of the WF reactions in rickettsial infections are presented in Table 2. Also given are the times of appearance of agglutinins in relation to onset of disease and the expected proportion of cases which will conform to this pattern. These are idealized generalizations, and the results of the WF reactions must be interpreted with caution. Because of the ubiquity of *Proteus* species and the occurrence of antibodies to them in low titer in a high percentage of the population, serum titers of less than 1:160 cannot be considered significant. Occasionally, serum from a normal person may contain agglutinins reaching a titer of 1:160. Interpretation of results of testing a single serum specimen is therefore especially hazardous. It is essential to show at least a fourfold rise in titer between acute and convalescent sera. When WF agglutinins develop, they may appear as early as the 6th day after onset of disease, but they are generally present by the 12th day. Titers peak early in convalescence and then decline fairly rapidly over the next several months.

Proteus infections, especially of the urinary bladder, may also elicit agglutinins. Antibiotic therapy started early in rickettsial disease may suppress the development of *Proteus* agglutinins.

The WF reaction does not distinguish between epidemic and murine typhus. Sometimes epidemiological considerations may allow a distinction to be made. In addition, there are usually agglutinins to OX-2 in low titer. Exact serological differentiation may be possible by the use of tests involving specific rickettsial agents in a state or research laboratory. The WF reaction may remain negative in some cases of the typhus group, and it is usually negative in BZ disease, especially when the span between primary and recrudescent disease is less than 15 years.

In the tick-borne members of the spotted fever group, agglutinins appear to OX-19 or to OX-2, sometimes in approximately equal titer to both and occasionally to neither. These reactions do not distinguish between members of the group and do not invariably distinguish the typhus from the spotted fever groups.

The WF reaction in scrub typhus presents several difficulties. Ideally, agglutinins appear to OX-K antigen. In fact, only 40 to 60% of cases develop OX-K agglutinins. Frequently, titers do not rise to 1:160, and a tentative diagnosis may have to rely on a fourfold rise in titer, e.g., from 1:20 to 1:80, during the course of the disease. Further increasing the nonspecificity of the reaction is the fact that most cases of relapsing fever elicit a rise in agglutinins to the OX-K antigen.

A negative WF reaction does not necessarily exclude rickettsial disease. The reaction is invariably negative in rickettsialpox, Q fever, and trench fever, and it is usually negative in BZ disease. The WF reaction therefore provides a presumptive serological diagnosis. Additional tests with specific rickettsial antigens should always be performed.

Complement fixation

The CF test is valuable in diagnosing all rickettsioses except scrub typhus, in which, as suggested earlier, IF is the preferred procedure. A fourfold rise in titer between early and convalescent sera must be demonstrated. A titer of 1:8 or greater is considered significant. CF antibodies generally appear in detectable concentrations during the 2nd week of the disease, peak from the 15th to the 20th day, and gradually decline. Residual antibody can frequently be detected years after infection.

Both epidemic and murine typhus rickettsiae share a common antigen, and each possesses a species-specific antigen. In addition, there is some crossover with the antigens of the spotted fever groups. The usual CF antigens do not distinguish between murine and epidemic typhus. Differentiation may be possible on epidemiological grounds or by use of species-specific antigens, in which case the antibody titer will be higher to the homologous than to the heterologous antigen. A modification of the IF test (6) in which antibody to the common antigen is removed from the test serum can also be used to identify the disease.

A similar problem arises with members of the spotted fever group, which share a common CF antigen. Differentiation among them may sometimes be made on epidemiological grounds.

Several million males in the United States were inoculated with epidemic typhus vaccine during their military sevice. As a consequence, they may have low residual antibody titers to both group and specific antigens of R. prowazeki. If they contract murine typhus, the resulting antibody pattern may be difficult to interpret. There will be an anamnestic antibody response to the group antigen, a primary response to specific R. mooseri antigen, and the presence of residual antibody to specific R. prowazeki antigen. A person previously immunized with epidemic typhus vaccine who contracts RMSP may also show an antibody pattern difficult to interpret because of the cross-reactions between the typhus and spotted fever groups.

In BZ disease an early anamnestic antibody response of the IgG class occurs. This serves to differentiate it from primary epidemic and murine typhus, in which IgM antibody predominates for the first 3 weeks of the disease. The rapid rise of CF antibody within 4 to 5 days of onset and peak titers on the 9th or 10th day are suggestive of BZ. Differentiation can also be made by treatment of the sera with ethanethiol, which selectively lowers the titer of IgM CF antibody but does not interfere with the IgG CF reaction with CF typhus antigen (7).

In human Q fever CF antibodies are elicited both to phase I and II antigens of Coxiella burnetii. Those against phase II appear first, and those against phase I appear erratically in low titer weeks or months after the onset of disease. In cases of Q fever with subacute endocarditis, however, both CF phase I and phase II antibodies appear in high titer, e.g., up to 1:2,048 (9).

Early treatment with broad-spectrum antibiotics may delay the appearance of CF antibody but rarely prevents the production of antibodies.

LITERATURE CITED

1. Bozeman, F. M., and B. L. Elisberg. 1963. Serological diagnosis of scrub typhus by indirect immunofluorescence. Proc. Soc. Exp. Biol. Med. 112:568–573.
2. Chang, R. S.-M., E. S. Murray, and J. C. Snyder.

1954. Erythrocyte-sensitizing substances from the rickettsiae of the Rocky Mountain spotted fever group. J. Immunol. **73**:8–15.

3. Elisberg, B. L., and F. M. Bozeman. 1966. Serological diagnosis of rickettsial diseases by indirect immunofluorescence. Arch. Inst. Pasteur Tunis **43**:193–204.

4. Elisberg, B. L., and F. M. Bozeman. 1969. Rickettsiae, p. 826–868. *In* E. H. Lennette and N. J. Schmidt (ed.), Diagnostic procedures for viral and rickettsial infections, 4th ed. American Public Health Association, Inc., New York.

5. Fiset, P., R. A. Ormsbee, R. Silberman, M. Peacock, and S. H. Spielman. 1969. A microagglutination technique for the detection and measurement of rickettsial antibodies. Acta Virol. **13**:60–66.

6. Goldwasser, R. A., and C. C. Shepard. 1959. Fluorescent antibody methods in the differentiation of murine and epidemic typhus sera; specificity changes resulting from previous immunization. J. Immunol. **82**:373–380.

7. Murray, E. S., J. A. Goan, J. M. O'Connor, and M. Mulahasanovic. 1965. Serologic studies of primary epidemic typhus and recrudescent typhus (Brill-Zinsser disease). I. Differences in complement-fixing antibodies: high antigen requirement and heat lability. J. Immunol. **94**:723–733.

8. Murray, E. S., J. M. O'Connor, and J. A. Gaon. 1965. Differentiation of 19s and 7s complement fixing antibodies in primary versus recrudescent typhus by ethanethiol or heat. Proc. Soc. Exp. Biol. Med. **119**:291–297.

9. Ormsbee, R. A. 1974. Rickettsiae, p. 805–815. *In* E. H. Lennette, E. H. Spaulding, and J. P. Truant (ed.), Manual of clinical microbiology, 2nd ed. American Society for Microbiology, Washington, D.C.

10. Plotz, H. 1944. The rickettsiae, p. 559–578. *In* Laboratory Methods of the United States Army, 5th ed. Lea & Febiger, Philadelphia.

11. Weil, E., and A. Felix. 1916. Zur serologischen Diagnose des Fleckfiebers. Wien. Klin. Wochenschr. **29**:no. 2.

Chapter 69

Microplate Enzyme Immunoassays for the Immunodiagnosis of Virus Infections

ALISTER VOLLER, DENNIS BIDWELL, AND ANN BARTLETT

INTRODUCTION

Antibodies and antigens labeled with fluorescent dyes or isotopes have been used extensively for immunodiagnosis over the past two decades, and their applications to various areas of clinical immunology are discussed at length elsewhere in this volume. However, they do have some disadvantages. Immunofluorescence usually depends upon subjective assessment of the end result, and this technique is often laborious. Radioimmunoassay, although subjective, is expensive, carries some risks and, because it requires expensive equipment, is restricted to central facilities. The use of enzyme-labeled reactants overcomes some of the above-listed disadvantages. These are safe, have long shelf life, and yield objective results with the same sensitivity as radioimmunoassay yet can be used with relatively cheap, simple equipment. This chapter deals with enzyme-linked immunosorbent assays (ELISA) (1, 2) for immunoserology of virus infections and some practicable versions used in our laboratory (3). The basic ELISA test depends on two assumptions: (i) that antigen or antibody can be attached to a solid-phase support yet retain immunological activity and (ii) that either antigen or antibody can be linked to an enzyme and the complex retain both immunological and enzymatic activity. Experience has shown that these assumptions are true for many antigen-antibody systems. Antibodies and many antigens can be readily attached to paper disks or to plastic surfaces, such as polyvinyl or polystyrene, either chemically or by passive adsorption, and still retain their activity. Antibodies and antigens have been linked to a variety of enzymes including peroxidase, glucose oxidase, β-galactosidase, and alkaline phosphatase, yielding stable, highly reactive reagents.

Competitive assays utilizing a "known" enzyme-labeled reagent, as in most radioimmunoassays, can be used. However, we have found that the noncompetitive methods — the "double antibody sandwich" for detection of antigen and the indirect method for detection of antibody — are the most useful in practice.

Double antibody sandwich method for detection and measurement of antigen (Fig. 1)

1. The wells in polystyrene plates are coated with immunoglobulin containing specific antibody to the antigen. Plates are washed.
2. The test solutions thought to contain antigen are incubated in the sensitized wells. Washing removes unreacted material, and any antigen remains attached to the immobilized antibody on the plastic surface.
3. The conjugate consisting of enzyme-labeled specific antibody is then incubated in each well. This will react with any antigen already "captured" by the antibody on the well surface. A further washing removes excess conjugate.
4. Finally, the enzyme substrate is added. Its rate of degradation depends on the amount of enzyme-labeled antibody present and that, in turn, depends on the amount of antigen in the test sample. The enzyme substrate is chosen to give a color change upon degradation, and this can be assessed visually or measured in a spectrophotometer. Additional sensitivity may be imparted by using unlabeled specific antibody followed by enzyme-labeled anti-species immunoglobulin (Ig) as the indicator.

Applications of double antibody sandwich method

This method has been used by us to assay plant viruses and is the basis of the "microelisa" test for hepatitis B antigen which has been introduced by Organon Inc. Preliminary trials show that this enzyme immunoassay for hepatitis B antigen, even when read visually, has the same range of sensitivity as radioimmunoassay.

Indirect microplate ELISA method for detection and measurement of antibody (Fig. 2)

1. Wells of polystyrene microhemagglutination plates are sensitized by passive adsorption with the relevant antigen; the plates are then washed.
2. The test samples are incubated in the sen-

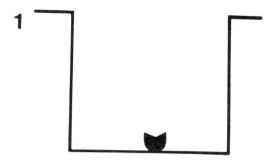

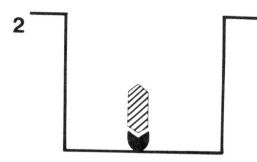

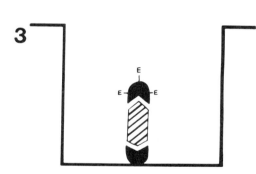

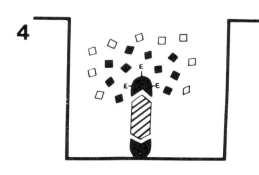

sitized well and the plates are again washed; antibody present reacts with the immobilized antigen on the well surfaces.

3. Enzyme-labeled anti-human Ig conjugate is incubated in the wells; this reacts with any "captured" antibody in step 2. Excess reagent is washed away.

4. Enzyme substrate is added and the plates are incubated; the rate of degradation is indicated by a color change, which is proportional to the antibody concentration in the test samples in step 2.

5. The reaction is stopped, and the color change is assessed visually or in a spectrophotometer.

Applications of the indirect microplate ELISA method for virus infections

This method can be used for the assay of antibodies to any infectious agent if the relevant antigen can be adsorbed satisfactorily to the solid-phase surface. To date for immunodiagnosis of infections, antibodies to viruses, parasites, and fungi have been measured in a microplate system; applications to virus infections are described below, and examples are given in Table 1.

The first reported work on virus infections was on rubella (3); in this study, the microplate ELISA values correlated with the traditional hemagglutination inhibition (HI) titers. Later work showed that by means of Ig-specific conjugates it is possible to detect rubella IgM antibody; this is, of course, of particular importance in clinical diagnosis. In these studies some commercially available rubella HI antigen preparations (Microbiological Associates) were found to be quite suitable for the microplate ELISA tests (3). Similar methods were used for detection of antibody to cytomegalovirus (4), and the CFT antigen available from Microbiological Associates was used as antigen. A detailed description of the method for the assay of antibody to cytomegalovirus is given in the appendices. The same method has been found to be appropriate for the measurement of antibodies to herpesviruses, adenoviruses, coxsackie B vi-

FIG. 1. *Double antibody sandwich method for microplate ELISA for the detection and measurement of antigen. (1) Antibody is adsorbed to the plate. The plate is then washed. (2) Test solution containing antigen is added. The plate is washed. (3) Enzyme-labeled specific antibody is added. The plate is washed. (4) Enzyme substrate is added. The amount of hydrolysis is proportional to the amount of antigen present. (Reproduced by kind permission of the Editor, Bulletin of the World Health Organization.)*

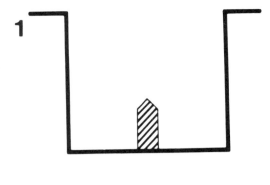

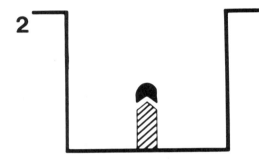

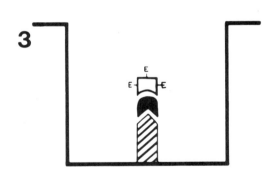

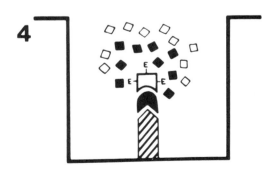

ruses, and measles virus. In all instances, commercially available antigens were used.

The microplate ELISA is particularly suitable for epidemiological studies because the same basic method can be used to measure antibody to various antigens. The feasibility of such surveys is illustrated in Table 2, which shows the results of microplate ELISA tests carried out simultaneously for antibodies to rubella and measles antigen. Tests were on blood samples obtained by finger prick, and different plates were sensitized with the relevant antigen.

In a recent collaborative study (de Thé et al.), it was shown that antibodies to Epstein-Barr virus can be detected by microplate ELISA. The antigen was an extract of P3HR1 cells, and the results (Table 3) show a correlation with immunofluorescent titers to the viral capsid antigen.

The virtues of enzyme immunoassays include low cost for supplies and materials, reagent stability, safety, sensitivity, reproducibility, and ease of procedure. An obvious application is for the screening of pregnant women simultaneously for rubella virus, cytomegalovirus, toxoplasmosis, and herpesvirus. The procedures are simple enough to be performed in even poorly equipped laboratories. There is an inherent danger that such assays may not be adequately standardized and controlled, with consequent misleading results. All tests, therefore, should be related to positive and negative reference samples. Interlaboratory standardization will be necessary for enzyme immunoassays, and this can only be achieved by means of stable reference reactants that can be exchanged.

APPENDIX I

Preparation of Enzyme-Labeled Anti-Human Globulin Conjugates

(Comparable conjugates are obtainable from Microbiological Associates, Bethesda, Md.)

Typical sources of antisera

Rabbit antiserum to human IgG

FIG. 2. *Indirect method for microplate ELISA for the detection and measurement of antibodies. (1) Antigen is adsorbed to the plate. The plate is then washed. (2) Serum is added (any specific antibody attaches to the antigen). The plate is washed. (3) Enzyme-labeled antiglobulin, which attaches to the antibody, is added. The plate is washed. (4) Substrate is added. The amount hydrolyzed is proportional to the amount of antibody present. (Reproduced by kind permission of the Editor, Bulletin of the World Health Organization.)*

TABLE 1. *Reagents and conditions suitable for viral microplate ELISA tests*

Antigen	Source	Antigen dilution for use	Test serum dilution for use
Cytomegalovirus	Microbiological Associates, Bethesda, Md.	1:100	1:200
Measles	Microbiological Associates, Bethesda, Md.	1:100	1:100
Herpes	Microbiological Associates, Bethesda, Md.	1:400	1:400
Rubella	Microbiological Associates, Bethesda, Md.	1:200	1:100
Adenovirus	Institute of Medical Microbiology, CH9000, St. Gallen, Switzerland	1:100	1:200
Mumps	Institute of Medical Microbiology, CH9000, St. Gallen, Switzerland	1:50	1:400
Picornavirus antigen	Institute of Medical Microbiology, CH9000, St. Gallen, Switzerland	1:100	1:100
Epstein-Barr P3HR1	International Agency for Cancer Research, Lyon, France	1:1,600	1:200
Arbovirus	Laboratory prepared	1:250	1:250
Mycoplasma pneumoniae	Laboratory prepared	1:400	1:200

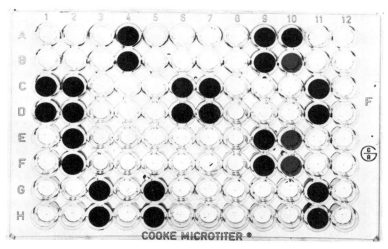

FIG. 3. *Results of microplate ELISA tests for measles; dense wells represent positive results.*

Sheep antiserum to human Ig
Goat antiserum to human IgM

Immunoglobulin preparation

1. To a mixture of 1.0 ml of antiserum plus 1.0 ml of phosphate-buffered saline (PBS; pH 7.4) add 2.0 ml of 36% Na_2SO_4. Mix; stir gently for 30 min at room temperature.

2. Centrifuge at $3,000 \times g$ for 10 min. Discard supernatant. Wash precipitate twice in 18% Na_2SO_4 solution. Centrifuge; discard supernatant.

3. Dissolve precipitate in 0.8 ml of PBS. Add an equal quantity of 24% Na_2SO_4 solution. Centrifuge at $3,000 \times g$ for 10 min. Wash precipi- tate with 12% Na_2SO_4.

4. Redissolve precipitate in 1.0 ml of PBS. Transfer to dialysis sac. Dialyze extensively at +4 C against PBS.

5. Determine protein concentration by absorption at 280 nm.

Alkaline phosphatase labeling

Source: Calf mucosa; Sigma type VII; specific activity, 300 to 1,100 units.

1. Centrifuge enzyme suspension; discard supernatant. Add 2 mg of Ig in 1.0 ml of PBS to 5 mg of enzyme. Mix at room temperature. Dialyze extensively at +4 C with several changes of PBS.

TABLE 2. Results of microplate ELISA tests for rubella and measles on sera from a population resident in New Guinea (Takia)[a]

Age group (years)	No. tested	Rubella[b]		Measles[b]	
		% +ve	Mean ELISA value	% +ve	Mean ELISA value
0–4	32	43	0.252	25	0.204
5–9	48	77	0.495	87	0.505
10–16	37	89	0.557	100	0.563
17–30	27	93	0.595	100	0.525
Over 30	22	100	0.603	100	0.508

[a] Positive readings = E400 greater than 0.2. Alkaline phosphatase-labeled sheep anti-human IgG used as indicator.

[b] Antigens: Microbiological Associates, Bethesda, Md.

TABLE 3. Results of microplate ELISA tests for antibody to Epstein-Barr virus (EBV) in various groups of subjects[a]

Group	No. in group	ELISA results[b]	
		% Patients +ve (>0.2)	Mean value
Controls			
EBV-IFA − ve	31	10	0.14
EBV-IFA + ve	30	50	0.23
Infectious mononucleosis	10	80	0.29
Nasopharyngeal cancer	20	100	0.59
Burkitt's lymphoma	10	100	0.76

[a] Antigen used: Sonic extract of P3HR1 cells. Sera diluted 1:200. Indicator: Sheep anti-human IgG labeled with alkaline phosphatase. (Results, reproduced with permission, from a collaborative study with the International Agency for Cancer Research, coordinated by Dr. de Thé.)

[b] Results expressed as E400.

2. Add 25% glutaraldehyde to give a final concentration of 0.2%. Mix, incubate for 1 to 2 h at room temperature, and then dialyze again at 14 C against several changes of PBS.

3. Transfer dialysis tube to 0.05 M tris-(hydroxymethyl)aminomethane (Tris) buffer (pH 8.0); continue to dialyze extensively at +4 C with several buffer changes.

4. Dilute conjugate to 4.0 ml with Tris buffer containing 1.0% bovine serum albumin and 0.02% sodium azide. Store in the dark at +4 C.

Determination of working strength of the conjugate

1. The assessment of a preparation of alkaline phosphatase-labeled anti-human IgG is given as an example. Cooke M29AR disposable polystyrene hemagglutination plates (Dynatech Laboratories) are used as carrier surface.

Human gamma globulin (KABI) is diluted to 100 ng/ml in coating buffer (see Appendix 2). A 0.2-ml volume of this solution is added to each well in the first four rows of the plate (48 wells). The plate is covered, placed in a humid chamber, and incubated overnight at +4 C. Contents of the plate are shaken out; wells are refilled with PBS-Tween and are left for 3 min. This washing procedure is repeated twice more.

Dilutions of the stock conjugate are made in PBS-Tween. These dilutions are 1:200, 1:400, 1:600, 1:800, 1:1,200, 1:1,400, 1:1,600, 1:1,800, 1:2,000, 1:2,200, and 1:2,400.

Volumes (0.2 ml) of each of the dilutions of the conjugate are added to duplicate coated wells and also to duplicate uncoated wells. PBS-Tween is added to two coated and two uncoated wells. Plates are incubated for 3 h at room temperature (about +23 C) in a humid chamber. The washing procedure is then repeated.

Two-tenths-milliliter volume of p-nitrophenyl phosphate substrate solution (see Appendix 2) is added to each well. The time of addition is noted. The color development is observed in the plates visually, and after 30 min at room temperature (about 23 C) the reaction in all wells is stopped by the addition of 0.05 ml of 3 M NaOH. The absorbance of the contents of each well is then read at 400 nm in a microcuvette in a spectrophotometer (E400).

The conjugate dilution giving an absorbance value of about 1.0 with the IgG solution at 100 ng/ml is then further assessed as described below.

2. An indirect microplate ELISA (see Appendix 2) is then carried out using the three conjugate dilutions close to that determined as described above. The antigen will be that which is to be used in subsequent clinical assays. For general purposes, rubella antigen is suitable for assessing conjugates. A positive reference serum and a negative reference serum are tested with a series of dilutions. The conjugate dilution that yields a high positive value (e.g., 1.0) and a low negative value (e.g., <0.1) in about 30 min of substrate incubation time is used for all subsequent tests.

APPENDIX 2

Materials Used

Carrier surface

Disposable polystyrene microhemagglutination plates. Cooke M29AR (Dynatech Laboratories).

Coating buffer

Carbonate-bicarbonate (pH 9.6): 1.59 g of Na$_2$CO$_3$, 2.93 g of NaHCO$_3$, and 0.2 g of NaN$_3$ made up to 1 liter with distilled water. Store at +4 C for not more than 2 weeks.

PBS-Tween

Consists of: 8.0 g of NaCl, 0.2 g of KH$_2$PO$_4$, 2.9 g of Na$_2$HPO$_4 \cdot 12H_2O$, 0.2 g of KCl, 0.5 ml of Tween 20, and 0.2 g of NaN$_3$ in 1 liter of distilled water. pH is 7.4. Store at +4 C.

Diethanolamine buffer (10%)

Consists of: 97 ml of diethanolamine, 800 ml of water, 0.2 g of NaN$_3$, 100 mg of MgCl$_2 \cdot 6H_2O$; 1 M HCl is added until the pH is 9.8. The total volume is made up to 1 liter with water. Store at +4 C in the dark.

Remove a sufficient amount (1 ml = three tests) 1 to 2 h before the substrate solution is to be used and allow to warm to room temperature.

Substrate solution

Substrate solution is p-nitrophenyl phosphate (1 mg/ml). Sigma 104 phosphate substrate is used. Tablets (5 mg) are stored at -20 C in the dark until used. Immediately before use, one (5 mg) tablet is dissolved in each 5 ml of 10% diethanolamine buffer, which has been warmed to room temperature. It must be used the same day.

Sodium hydroxide

NaOH (3 M) is used.

Enzyme-antibody conjugates

(See Appendix 1.) These are stored at +4 C as a concentrated stock solution and are diluted in PBS-Tween at room temperature immediately before use.

APPENDIX 3

Determination of Optimum Conditions for Indirect Microplate ELISA for Viral Systems

The estimation of cytomegalovirus antibody is presented as an example (Table 4).

Preparations for test

1. Stock virus antigen (Microbiological Associates CFT antigen no. 30-101 prepared from infected, cultured W138 human embryonic living cells) is diluted 1:50, 1:100, 1:200, and 1:400 in carbonate buffer, and 200-μliter amounts of each dilution are used to coat 12 wells, horizontally, of a polystyrene microtiter plate and kept at 4 C overnight.

2. The plates are washed as described previously.

3. Positive and negative reference sera are diluted 1:100, 1:200, 1:400, 1:800, and 1:1,600 in PBS-Tween, and 200-μliter amounts of each dilution are added to each vertical row of wells of the plate. Two blank wells (no serum) are included in each antigen row. The plate is incubated at room temperature for 2 h.

4. The plate is washed as described previously.

5. Alkaline phosphatase-labeled anti-human globulin conjugate is diluted 1:1,000 in PBS-Tween; 200-μliter amounts are added to each well and incubated at room temperature for 2 h.

6. The plate is washed as before.

7. Equal amounts (200 μliter) of substrate solution are added to each well and incubated at room tempeature for 30 min.

8. The reaction is stopped by the addition of 50 μliters of 3 M NaOH.

TABLE 4. *Sample test for cytomegalovirus (CMV) infection by ELISA*[a]

Antigen dilution	Dilution of positive reference serum					Dilution of negative reference serum				
	100	200	400	800	1,600	100	200	400	800	1,600
CMV										
1:50	1.5	1.1	1.0	0.93	0.7	0.13	0.1	0.05	0.02	0.04
100	1.3	1.05	0.94	0.87	0.65	0.1	0.08	0.05	0.02	0.03
200	1.05	0.93	0.85	0.59	0.46	0.1	0.09	0.05	0.03	0.02
400	0.85	0.72	0.63	0.48	0.3	0.11	0.08	0.06	0.02	0.01
Control										
1:50	0.14	0.05	0.02	0.02	0.01	0.05	0.02	0.02	0.05	0
100	0.09	0.07	0.09	0.01	0.03	0.04	0.03	0.1	0.03	0.01
200	0.07	0.05	0.04	0.05	0.03	0.04	0.05	0.03	0.02	0.03
400	0.03	0.02	0.06	0.02	0.02	0.02	0.02	0.06	0.02	0

[a] The highest dilution of CMV antigen and of positive antiserum giving a value of about 1.0 after 30 min of substrate incubation was used in all subsequent tests. In the example shown, the antigen was used at 1:100 and the sera were diluted 1:200 in subsequent tests. (Two blanks were run for each antigen dilution.) Results are expressed as E400.

9. The color change in each well is estimated spectrophotometrically at 400 nm (E400).

This checker board estimation is carried out simultaneously on a control antigen prepared for uninfected W138 cell cultures (Microbiological Associates control CFT antigen no. 30-102F). The results of a typical experiment are shown in Table 4.

Indirect microplate ELISA method

Test. The example given is for cytomegalovirus. Antigen used: Cytomegalovirus CFT antigen (Microbiological Associates catalog no. 30-101) used at a dilution of 1:100. Antigen is made up in coating buffer immediately before plates are coated.

1. A 200-μliter volume of cytomegalovirus antigen solution is added to each well of plate and incubated in a humid chamber at +4 C overnight.

Plates are then washed.

2. Test sera are diluted 1:200 in PBS-Tween. A 200-μliter volume of each of the diluted sera is added to each plate well. Each serum is tested in duplicate. Six wells contain positive reference samples and four wells contain negative reference samples. Plates are incubated for 2 h at room temperature.

Plates are washed as before.

3. A 200-μliter amount of freshly diluted conjugate is added to each well. Plates are incubated for 2 h at room temperature.

Plates are washed as before.

4. A 200-μliter amount of substrate solution is added to each well, and incubation is carried out at room temperature. The time of addition of substrate is noted.

Samples are taken from the wells containing the positive reference samples, and the absorbance is quickly read at 400 nm in a spectrophotometer. When the reference samples reach a predetermined absorbance value, the reaction is stopped by the addition of 50 μliters of 3 M NaOH. The absorbance of the contents of each well is then read at 400 nm in a spectrophotometer. The test is duplicated using control CFT antigen (Microbiological Associates catalog no. 30-102F) diluted 1:100 and test sera diluted 1:200. The substrate reaction is stopped after an incubation time comparable to that of the test antigen plate.

Interpretation of results. The results of microplate ELISA tests can only be interpreted if (i) a positive reference serum is available, (ii) a negative reference serum is available, and (iii) a group of normal (uninfected individuals) sera is available.

The test is set up, as described earlier, with the positive and negative reference samples. Dilutions of the positive sample can be made, and the unknown samples values can be expressed as a dilution titer of the known reference sample. Samples are only considered to be positive when they yield values above that of the normal (uninfected) individuals, which provide the base-line level. This must be determined for each system.

LITERATURE CITED

1. Engvall, E., and P. Perlmann. 1971. Enzyme-linked immunosorbent assay (ELISA). Quantitative assay of IgG. Immunochemistry 8:871.
2. Engvall, E., and P. Perlmann. 1972. ELISA III. Quantitation of specific antibodies by enzyme-linked anti-immunoglobulin in antigen coated tubes. J. Immunol. 109:129.
3. Voller, A., and D. E. Bidwell. 1975. A simple method for detecting antibodies to Rubella. Br. J. Exp. Pathol. 56:338.
4. Voller, A., and D. E. Bidwell. 1976. Enzyme immunoassays for antibodies in measles, cytomegalovirus infections and after Rubella vaccination. Br. J. Exp. Pathol., in press.

Section F

IMMUNOHEMATOLOGY

Chapter 70

Introduction

H. HUGH FUDENBERG

The immunohematological laboratory procedures described in this section were selected as being the techniques most useful in a modern clinical setting. Blood grouping, compatibility testing, and associated immunohematological test procedures (Rosenfield) are clearly the most frequently used techniques. Their importance has increased as blood bank operations have expanded to meet hospital requirements. About 300 blood group antigens have been discovered to date, and approximately 50 unrelated antigens are present in a high frequency of the population. In most hospitals, the technical needs of the blood transfusion service are limited to obtaining compatible blood for patients, and when problems arise, blood bank laboratories or commercial laboratories are consulted. However, there are now many sophisticated panels of red cell antigens commercially available to clinical laboratories, and use of the techniques described here is becoming increasingly widespread. In addition to their use for safe transfusion therapy, blood typing and compatibility testing are necessary for management of pregnancy, i.e., for typing and screening sera from pregnant women for antibodies, and for evaluation of the newborn.

Although there is as yet no convincing hypothesis to explain fully the immunosuppressive action of Rh immunoglobulin, which was first applied in 1964, the technique for Rh immune suppression has provided great fiscal benefits in terms of prevention of mental retardation and other birth defects that would otherwise require long-term medical care and/or institutionalization. The question of its mode of action is interesting also in terms of understanding the control of antibody formation. Reiss and Pollack have proposed a model to explain both suppression and augmentation (by anti-D) of the Rh immune response, based on a "suppressor mode" of the Rh immune mechanism involving a "helper" subpopulation of thymocytes. Further basic studies should answer these intriguing questions, which in turn may lead to improvements and additions to the clinical and laboratory techniques described here.

Inhibitors of clotting factors and their immunology (Blatt and Roberts) are most important in inherited and acquired hematological disorders. Hemorrhagic diseases, most notably hemophilia, are now better understood as a result of new and important discoveries in this area. Detection of the relevant antibodies by clotting assays and immunological techniques has enabled us to classify genetic variants of these disorders, and, using specific human antibodies to purify antigens by affinity chromatography, it is now possible to detect the carrier state of one such variant, hemophilia A. The field is expanding rapidly, and further discoveries should be forthcoming.

In autoimmune and drug-immune hemolytic anemias (Petz), the importance of precise diagnosis is emphasized, since prognosis and appropriate management vary considerably in the various disorders. Techniques for laboratory diagnosis of these disorders and characterization of antibodies in eluates of patient sera are valuable clinical tools. In this respect an area that is receiving increased attention, as a consequence of recent advances in research on alloantibodies in blood, is the occurrence of hemolytic transfusion reactions. Successful prevention of such reactions by allotyping of donors and recipients should provide a considerable increase in patient safety and protection.

Antigen detection and quantitation by inhibition of hemagglutination using the chromic chloride method (Koistinen and Fudenberg) is especially useful for detection of human antibodies to human IgA and allotypes thereof. This is important since administration of as little as 55 ml of IgA- or Am-incompatible plasma during transfusion therapy can cause severe or even fatal anaphylactic reactions in recipients who have anti-IgA or anti-Am. Anti-IgA is probably significant in transplantation as well, and maternal anti-IgA apparently resistant to IgG is often detected in cord serum, suggesting a possible role in the production of selective IgA deficiency.

Chapter 71

Blood Typing and Associated Immunohematological Test Procedures

RICHARD E. ROSENFIELD

INTRODUCTION

Blood typing (grouping) data are needed for safe transfusion therapy, management of pregnancy, and evaluation of the newborn. Routine blood typing consists of three groups of tests: (i) tests of red cells to determine the presence or absence of the membrane antigens, A, B, and Rh1 (Rh$_0$ or D), (ii) tests of serum to determine the presence or absence of expected anti-A and anti-B hemagglutinating activity, and (iii) other tests of serum to detect unexpected hemagglutinating activity.

ABO blood types (groups)

The relation between the presence of A and B erythrocytic antigens and the occurrence of expected serum hemagglutinins is shown in Table 1.

Type O red cells lack both A and B erythrocytic membrane antigens and, consequently, are not agglutinated by serum of any ABO type. Type AB red cells carry both A and B, and are agglutinated by the serum of any ABO type other than that of type AB. Type A blood has A but not B on its red cells, and the serum of type A agglutinates any red cells that carry B. Finally, type B blood has B but not A on its red cells, and type B serum agglutinates any red cells that carry A. In summary, anti-A in serum occurs whenever the red cells lack A, whereas anti-B in serum occurs whenever the red cells lack B.

The chemical structures of the A and B sub-

TABLE 1. *Relation between occurrence of erythrocytic A and B antigens and the presence of serum anti-A and anti-B activity*

Erythrocytic membrane antigens	Serum anti-A and anti-B activity				Actual ABO type
	O	A	B	AB	
None	−[a]	+	+	+	O
A	−	−	+	+	A
B	−	+	−	+	B
A and B ...	−	−	−	−	AB

[a] Agglutination observed (+) or not observed (−) in tests with red cells of differing ABO types.

stances are well known (6). They are similar oligosaccharides, but each possesses a unique terminal immunodominant sugar unit, namely, N-acetyl-D-galactosamine (GalNac) for A substance and D-galactose (Gal) for B substance. These two sugars are also very similar, differing only at their carbon-2 position where GalNac carries N-acetyl instead of the hydroxyl of Gal. Oligosaccharide structures like these are also found on the cell membranes of many other species including bacteria. Exposure to such foreign structures accounts for the very regular appearance of naturally occurring anti-A and anti-B in humans whenever the respective A and/or B antigen is not synthesized.

A and B are heritable co-dominant traits, but they are secondary rather than primary gene products. The primary gene products of A and B genes are transferase enzymes which place the terminal immunodominant sugar unit in $\alpha 1 \rightarrow 3$ glycosidic bond with the galactose unit of a trisaccharide, L-fucose-$\alpha 1 \rightarrow$ 2-D-galactose-$\beta 1 \rightarrow$ 4-N-acetyl-D-glucosamine. This trisaccharide carries an antigen, H, until either GalNac or Gal is attached. Furthermore, the amount of A or B that can be formed (and also the amount of H which is abolished) is a function of transferase efficiency: strong enzymes produce strong type A or type B cells with little H, whereas weaker enzymes produce weaker A (or B) with considerable residual H (22). Strength of expression of A and B is thus a function of A and B genes. Ordinary strong type A cells (called A$_1$) carry about 10^6 sites per cell, ordinary type B carries about 7.5×10^5 sites, and moderately weak type A (called A$_2$) carries about 2.5×10^5 sites per cell (4).

Humans respond to A and B antigens by making three classes of serum antibodies: immunoglobulin M, G, and A (IgM, IgG, IgA). In addition, secretory dimer IgA occurs in saliva and breast milk. All of these antibodies are excellent agglutinins: IgM and secretory IgA by virtue of their size and multiple specific combining sites, and IgG and serum IgA because of very large numbers of A and B antigen sites on tested cells. With IgG anti-A, agglutination is observed when the reaction system contains at least 20,000 antibody molecules per red cell; with IgM anti-A, only 50 antibody molecules per cell are needed (5). Although secretory IgA does not interact with complement and is not lytic, serum antibodies are all lytic (Rosenfield, unpublished data). IgM and the IgG subtypes 1 and 3 activate the classical complement pathway, and IgA and IgG subtypes 2 and 4 activate the alternate or properdin complement pathway (H. L. Spiegelberg, O. Götze, and H. J. Müller-Eberhard, Fed. Proc. 31:655, 1972). A-anti-A and B-anti-B hemolysis, however, is not very efficient, presumably because the A and B antigens are not presented optimally at the cell surface. For example, lytic anti-A often partly lyses strong A_1 cells but not weaker A_2 cells even though the same A_2 cells are readily agglutinated. Immune hemolysis, therefore, is not a very reliable blood typing method.

In summary, ABO blood types are defined by hemagglutination tests that (i) identify A and/or B antigen on red cells and (ii) detect expected anti-A and/or anti-B activity in serum. The tests themselves are relatively simple to perform and interpret, but a small number of blood samples (<1%) present three kinds of problems:

1. Unusually weak expression of A or B. Either A or B in an occasional blood sample may present as antigen that will not support hemagglutination with specific blood typing reagent (18). The problem is usually recognized as absence of expected anti-A or anti-B serum activity. Such red cells must be evaluated by tests for adsorption and elution, as discussed below (Preparation of eluates). These blood types, known as A_x and B_x, although not directly agglutinable, can bind anti-A or anti-B and, after washing, release their bound antibodies in appropriate eluates which can then be tested for capacity to agglutinate other red cells that have normal expressions of A or B. Rarely, A_x and B_x may present *with* anti-A or anti-B serum agglutinating activity; these specimens may be very difficult to identify. Absence of expected anti-A and/or anti-B serum activity may, however, reflect low serum gamma globulin levels (e.g., agammaglobulinemia) or non-response to A and B antigens (i.e., children up to the age of 6 to 12 months; 18).

2. Partial, or mixed field, agglutination. ABO types slightly stronger than A_x and B_x are called A_3 and B_3 (18). When tested with anti-A and anti-B, only some of the tested red cells are agglutinated. This is called partial, or mixed field, agglutination. Partial agglutination also occurs with blood samples from type A or type B patients who have been given transfusions with type O red cells. But there is a difference: the A (or B) agglutinates can be separated from type O red cells in the transfused patients whereas no efficient separation can be achieved with either type A_3 or B_3.

3. Unexpected serum anti-A or anti-B. The regular occurrence of natural anti-A and anti-B is due to the fact that everyone is immunologically challenged repeatedly with A-like and B-like bacterial polysaccharides. Sometimes this results in a type A person making demonstrable anti-A, or a type B person making demonstrable anti-B. This phenomenon is rarely seen in persons with "strong" A or B blood types, but is not uncommon in persons with "weaker" types. Such types include A_2 and A_2B; B_2 exists only in some A_1B blood types where "very strong" A creates an unusually weak B (i.e., "A_1B_2"). These antibodies tend to be cold-reactive (i.e., more readily seen at lower temperatures); they also distinguish "strong" from "weak" blood types more readily than do ordinary blood typing reagents.

Rh blood type (20)

Rh differs considerably from ABO. Firstly, its chemical structure has not as yet been determined, but Rh does not appear to be carbohydrate. Secondly, it is not associated with naturally occurring serum antibody and, thus, cannot be evaluated by an independent test of serum. Finally, there are far fewer Rh sites on red cells than sites for A or B, so that a different form of testing is required to determine the presence or absence of Rh antigen on red cells and of Rh antibody in the serum of a person who may have been immunized.

Rh antibodies are human allogeneic responses to parenteral foreign red cells. This may occur as a consequence of either pregnancy or blood transfusion, and the immune response is almost always IgG. As stated in the preceding section, binding of about 20,000 IgG antibody molecules per red cell is needed before agglutination can be observed. The average Rh-positive red cell has only 10^4 to 4×10^4 sites per cell (19), and this creates a situation in which Rh-positive erythrocytes suspended in physiological salt solution (0.85% NaCl) cannot be effectively cross-linked by specific IgG antibodies as can type A or type B red cells. In contrast to Rh, type A and type B cells have so many sites that, when enough IgG anti-A or anti-B is present, the occurrence of sufficient weak intercellular molecular bridges will sustain visible agglutination.

To achieve hemagglutination by Rh-anti-Rh, steps must be taken to overcome a counterion cloud barrier around all normal red cells. Normal erythrocytes carry a very significant net negative electrical charge. This creates a counterion cloud around each cell (17). For cells in saline, this cloud is about 15 nm thick, and tends to prohibit firm cross-linking by IgG antibody molecules that can extend only 15 nm. IgM antibody molecules can extend 30 nm; they are effective hemagglutinins, but they are uncommon immune responses to Rh.

Several measures are available for Rh tests to reduce the effects of the counterion cloud surrounding normal erythrocytes:

1. Reduction of electrical conductance with high concentrations of symmetrical hydrophilic colloid. This involves the use of albumin (either human or bovine, but usually the latter). At a final concentration in the reaction mixture of >15%, IgG Rh antibody will softly agglutinate Rh-positive red cells. The test can be performed on a glass slide or tile, where the cell concentration should be >20%, or it can be performed in test tubes with far fewer cells by using centrifugation to bring the antibody-coated cells into contact with one another. With enough antibody, these tests are quite effective and, accordingly, they are used for Rh blood typing. They are not very sensitive, however, and are not of great value for detecting weak Rh antibodies.

2. Protease treatment of red cells. The bulk of the net negative charge of erythrocytes arises from sialic acid residues. In theory, therefore, Rh-positive red cells treated with neuraminidase should become agglutinable by IgG anti-Rh. They do, but the effect is not nearly as good as that produced by treating such cells with a protease. Proteases cleave membrane glycopeptides that carry sialic residues, thereby removing some of the negativity, and exert an additional potentiating effect on IgG Rh antibody cross-linking, mostly, perhaps, in the form of antigen site clustering (S. P. Masouredis, personal communication; 15a). Fairly strong and reasonably sensitive agglutination by IgG anti-Rh can be seen with protease-treated red cells. All proteases active at pH 7 are effective, and the ones used most commonly are ficin, papain, trypsin, and bromelin.

3. The IgG antiglobulin test. Although IgG Rh antibody fails to agglutinate Rh-positive erythrocytes suspended in saline, it does coat these cells. If such coated cells are washed sufficiently to reduce soluble IgG protein $10^{-4} \times$ below its original serum concentration, addition of appropriately diluted animal (usually rabbit) antihuman IgG will agglutinate these cells. The phenomenon is dependent on several factors: (i) Enough IgG Rh antibody must remain bound through the preparatory washing process so that at least 100 to 150 bound antibody molecules are on each washed red cell (2). (ii) Animal IgG-antihuman IgG is also an anti-gen-antibody reaction that follows mass law. Therefore, the antihuman IgG must be used at an appropriate dilution because either too much (prozone) or too little results in failure to agglutinate weakly coated red cells. In general, animal antihuman IgG serum, as a manual reagent for the antiglobulin test, should contain 7 μg of N IgG antibody per ml (16).

4. Other test procedures require costly and complicated instrumentation in the form of AutoAnalyzers or the Groupamatic. All are based on the use of rouleaux formation to augment sensitivity. They include assymmetrical hydrophilic colloids such as polyvinylpyrrolidone (K-90, average molecular weight ~ 3 × 10^5), lowered ionic and pH test conditions, addition of positively charged macromolecules (protamine sulfate, polybrene), use of a protease, and various combinations of these maneuvers (1).

Rh, like A or B, may present as a very weak antigen. This is called Rh:w1, Rh_0, or D^u. Some examples are recognized by weak agglutination on direct blood typing, but others are so weak that even weak direct agglutination will not be seen unless the cells are optimally treated beforehand with a protease. Such cells will, however, be IgG coated. After washing, such coated cells can be agglutinated by antiglobulin serum. They can also release their bound antibody in eluates where the antibody can be identified by its specific capacity to agglutinate more normal Rh-positive erythrocytes. Rh:w1 is usually not very immunogenic (23) and, therefore, does not create a serious problem in the Rh typing of blood donors.

The Rh1 (Rh_0 or D) antigen is commonly associated with Rh2 (rh′ or C) and/or Rh3 (rh″ or E) in white and oriental people (20). For this reason, Rh:-1 blood samples have, customarily, been retested with anti-Rh1,2 (Rh_0′ or DC) and anti-Rh1,3 (Rh_0″ or DE) reagents, and only Rh:-1,-2,-3 (rh or dce) donor blood has been called Rh-negative. Rh:-1,2,-3 (rh′ or dCe), Rh:-1,-2,3 (rh″ or dcE), and Rh:-1,2,3 (rh_y or dCE) blood samples together rarely exceed 1% of all tested samples, and the cost of the extra reagents is considerable. In addition, the Rh3 immune response does not cross-react with Rh1, and the Rh2 antigen is very poorly immunogenic except perhaps for one variant, Rh:-1,w2 (rh^{Gu} or G^u), encountered infrequently in blacks. In consequence, major blood centers are now attempting to eliminate the additional tests of Rh-negative blood donors.

The problem with patients is somewhat different. Rh:w1 patients should be considered to be Rh-positive, but Rh:-1 is always Rh-negative regardless of status in regard to Rh2 and Rh3.

Patients present another problem: they may be "partly" Rh-positive. Rh1 does not appear to be a single antigen (20) but, rather, to consist of at least four antigens, Rh13 (Rh^A), Rh14 (Rh^B), Rh15 (Rh^C), and Rh16 (Rh^D). Absence of one or more of these can allow the patient to be immunized, but this blood type will not necessarily present as Rh:w1; indeed, it may seem to be normally Rh-positive. Fortunately, these people are quite rare.

Unexpected serum agglutinins

About 0.5 to 1% of unselected blood specimens have unexpected serum agglutinating activity. For this reason, all blood typing should include a search for such antibodies so that they may be identified as soon as possible. These antibodies can be naturally occurring like, but not as regular as, anti-A and anti-B. Anti-I, anti-A$_1$, anti-P1, anti-H, anti-Le^a, anti-Le^b, anti-M, anti-N, and anti-S are in this category. Some, especially anti-Le^a, can cause serious reaction to blood transfusion with incompatible red cells.

Allogeneic immunization is an even more dangerous cause of unexpected serum antibodies. Here, one encounters antibodies to antigens in the Rh, Kell, Kidd, and Duffy systems, and these usually cause very serious blood transfusion reactions. What must be remembered is that these immune responses may result from pregnancy as well as from previous blood transfusion. Kidd antibodies are particularly dangerous because, while they do not seem to cause clinically apparent erythroblastosis, they do cause particularly violent transfusion reactions.

Screening for unexpected antibodies is also associated with problems. Firstly, the serum or plasma being tested may contain unusually high concentrations of assymmetrical proteins such as fibrinogen or gamma globulin. These can cause erythrocytes to aggregate in rouleaux, flat surface to flat surface, which resemble hemagglutination. When suspected, such aggregated cells should be washed once with saline to reduce the concentration of the rouleaux-inducing protein. This maneuver will not significantly reduce unpotentiated true hemagglutination. Secondly, the serum may contain a relatively innocuous cold agglutinin. Although the effect of such an antibody can be abolished by warming to 37 C, it should be characterized for specificity, titer, and perhaps both thermal amplitude and capacity to fix complement. Indeed, the patient may require all blood transfusions to pass through an appropriate warming device.

Cold agglutinins are just one form of autolo-gous serum antibody activity that trouble blood typing laboratories. Patients with "warm" acquired hemolytic anemia may appear to be incompatible with all blood, and yet transfusion may be needed to counteract life-threatening anemia. There is no way for the blood typing laboratory to avoid the problem of acquired hemolytic anemia and, for this reason, diagnostic tests are included in this chapter.

ROUTINE BLOOD TYPING

Reagents and equipment

The usual reagents used for routine blood typing are anti-A, anti-B, anti-Rh1, diluent used in manufacture of the anti-Rh1 (e.g., 22% bovine albumin), antiglobulin serum (usually antihuman IgG), and 2% red cell suspensions in saline of A$_1$ cells, pooled O cells, and pooled protease-treated O cells. Anti-A,B may also be used for the typing of red cells, and A$_2$ cells may be used additionally to test serum for expected anti-A and anti-B hemagglutinating activity. The use of pooled O cells should be restricted to technicians who can detect partial, or mixed field, agglutination; less experienced personnel should use single sources of type O red cells in separate tests.

Anti-A. Anti-A is obtained from type B human volunteers after one to three subcutaneous booster immunizations with 1 mg of porcine A substance. Postimmunization antibody levels should exceed 1:256 with A$_1$ cells, 1:128 with A$_2$ cells, and 1:64 with A$_2$B cells. Avidity can be improved by adding NaCl to a final concentration of 2%. Anti-A is colored with methylene blue.

Anti-B. Anti-B is obtained from type A volunteers after immunization by 1 to 3 mg of equine B substance. The titer should exceed 1:256. Avidity can be improved with 2% NaCl. Anti-B is colored with acriflavine.

Anti-A,B. Anti-A,B is obtained from O volunteers who responded to both porcine A and equine B. Its titer should exceed that of both anti-A and anti-B. It is uncolored.

Anti-Rh1. Anti-Rh1 (Rh$_0$ or D) is serum from immunized Rh:-1 persons. This serum must be made free from other antihuman red cell antibodies such as anti-A, anti-B, anti-Rh12 (rh^G or G), anti-K1 (Kell), etc. It is diluted in bovine albumin solution (~22%) to have a titer, after dilution, of 1:32 when tested with Rh-positive red cells suspended in albumin. This reagent must be specific under all conditions of testing, including use of protease-treated red cells and use of the antiglobulin test.

Antiglobulin serum. Antiglobulin serum comes from animals (usually rabbits) that have been immunized with human IgG. The serum must be diluted 1:40 or more in 0.5% bovine albumin so that the final product will contain 7 μg of N IgG antibody per ml. This will maximally agglutinate red cells that have been minimally coated with IgG Rh antibody. The reagent must not have other antibodies. Other animal antiglobulin reagents include anti-C3 (anti-β1C globulin) and anti-C4 (anti-β1E globulin). These are made from specifically immunized animals. For ordinary manual tests, they rarely can be diluted beyond 1:10 or 1:20 and often must be adsorbed with washed normal human red cells to be made specific. Polyvalent antiglobulin reagents are also available; they are mostly anti-IgG but contain some anti-C3, anti-IgM, and anti-IgA. Their usefulness is restricted by our lack of knowledge of their actual antibody content.

Red cell suspensions. Red cells, as 2% suspensions (vol/vol) in saline, are used to test sera for agglutinin activity. Type A_1 cells (also if desired type A_2) are used to detect anti-A, and type B cells are used to detect anti-B. Type O cells are used both to control tests for anti-A and anti-B and to detect other antibodies. For the latter purpose, type O cells are selected to carry Rh2 (rh' or C), Rh3 (rh'' or E), K1 (Kell), homozygous expression of both Rh4 (hr' or c) and Rh5 (hr'' or e), Fy^a, Fy^b, JK^a, JK^b, S, and s. Rh8 (rh^{w1} or C^w), Rh10 (hr^v or V), and K3 (Penney) are convenient to have but are not as important. When used as a pool, at least one-third should be Rh:3 and K:1, otherwise, weak antibodies with these specificities may be overlooked.

Protease-treated O cells. A sample of the type O cells can be treated with any protease active at pH 7 (15). Ficin (from fig), extremely simple to use and one of the most effective, can be obtained from Enzyme Development Corp., New York, N.Y. A stock solution consists of 250 mg of ficin powder dissolved in 25 ml of 0.85% NaCl. This should be well mixed and stored at -20 C in 1- to 2-ml amounts. For use, 1 ml of stock solution is mixed with 9 ml of 0.1 M phosphate buffer, pH 7.4 $\pm$ 0.3. After 1 volume of this working solution is added to 1 volume of three times washed packed red cells, the cell suspension should be incubated at 37 C for 15 min. These treated red cells, washed twice in saline and resuspended at 2% concentration (vol/vol) for use, are stable at 4 C for 12 to 24 h.

Equipment. In addition to test tubes and racks for their support, a suitable small centrifuge (e.g., Serafuge, Clay-Adams, New York, N.Y.) is needed.

Magnification facilitates inspection of tested red cells to detect agglutination. This can be a 6$\times$ or 7$\times$ hand lens. Alternatively, gently transfer a tiny sample to a glass slide and examine at 50$\times$ or 100$\times$ under a microscope.

Typing of blood specimens from patients other than infants

For each blood specimen arrange eight small test tubes (8 mm [inner diameter] $\times$ 75 mm) into two groups of four each. One set of four test tubes will be used for serum tests to be described in Step 3. The other set of four test tubes is used for red cell tests now to be described.

Step 1: Red cell typing. Add 1 drop of specific reagent to each of these four test tubes as follows:

> Tube 1 – 1 drop of anti-A
> Tube 2 – 1 drop of anti-B
> Tube 3 – 1 drop of anti-Rh1
> Tube 4 – 1 drop of bovine albumin

With four wooden applicator sticks, transfer red cells from the specimen to be typed into each of the four test tubes containing reagent. Slightly redden 5 to 10 mm of the end of each applicator stick in the blood specimen, drain off excess blood, and introduce this reddened tip into one reagent. Avoid clots. Twist and shake so as to resuspend a small number (10^7) of red cells in the reagent, and then discard the applicator stick. Use a fresh applicator for each reagent.

An alternative method consists of preparing a washed 2% (vol/vol) cell suspension from the blood specimen to be tested. One drop of this suspension can then be added to each of four empty test tubes. Two of these test tubes should now be centrifuged to sediment the red cells and allow removal, with a fine glass pipette, of the supernatant fluid. One of these latter test tubes now receives 1 drop of anti-Rh1; the other receives 1 drop of bovine albumin. The other two test tubes receive 1 drop of anti-A and 1 drop of anti-B, respectively.

After mixing, tests with anti-A and anti-B should either be allowed to stand at room temperature for 5 to 10 min or be centrifuged at 1,000 $\times$ g for 10 s. Tests with anti-Rh1 and bovine albumin should be centrifuged at 1,000 $\times$ g for 1 min, and then 2 drops of saline should be added to each to reduce the viscosity of the albumin. Finally, all four test tubes should be shaken *very gently*, just to dislodge the sedimented red cells so that they can be inspected for evidence of agglutination. Results and their significance are given in Table 2.

Step 2: Additional tests for presumptively Rh-negative specimens.

1. Repeat the test with another source of anti-Rh1 reagent.

TABLE 2. *Results of presumptive tests for ABO and Rh, and their significance*

Agglutination of red cells with		Presumptive meaning in regard to ABO type	Agglutination of red cells with		Meaning
Anti-A	Anti-B		Anti-Rh1	Bovine albumin	
Neg	Neg	Type O	Neg	Neg	Presumptively Rh-negative
Pos	Neg	Type A	Pos	Neg	Definitely Rh-positive
Neg	Pos	Type B	Pos	Pos	Other tests needed
Pos	Pos	Type AB	Neg	Pos	Impossible[a]

[a] Anti-Rh1 diluted in albumin. When possible, the actual diluent used in the manufacture of the anti-Rh1 should be available for use in the "bovine albumin test."

2. Incubate both the first and the second test for Rh1, and the control test with bovine albumin, for 1 h at 37 C.

3. Wash the red cells of all three tests four times. Fill the test tube with saline for each wash, centrifuge at $1,000 \times g$ for 1 min and pour off all of the supernatant saline. Shake the sedimented red cells in the residual saline from the wet walls of the test tube, and refill the test tube with fresh saline.

4. After the fourth wash, shake the sedimented red cells, add 1 drop of antiglobulin serum (antihuman IgG), mix, and centrifuge at $1,000 \times g$ for 10 s. Shake very gently, just to dislodge the sedimented red cells, and inspect for evidence of agglutination.

5. Results of these tests and their significance are given in Table 3.

Step 3: Tests for expected and unexpected hemagglutinins. We now return to the second set of four test tubes mentioned above. Each of these test tubes receives 1 drop of a specific red cell suspension, as follows:

> Tube 1 – 1 drop of type A suspension
> Tube 2 – 1 drop of type B suspension
> Tube 3 – 1 drop of type O suspension
> Tube 4 – 1 drop of ficin-treated type O suspension

Centrifuge the patient's blood specimen so that supernatant serum or plasma is available. Transfer 1 drop of serum or plasma to each of these four test tubes. Mix and immediately centrifuge at $1,000 \times g$ for 10 s the test tubes with A, B, and O cells. Shake very gently, just to dislodge the sedimented cells, and inspect for evidence of agglutination. The results and their significance may be inferred from Table 1. When these results imply the same ABO type as do the results of cell typing (Step 1), they are confirmatory and final.

Note that O cells will not normally be agglutinated. Such agglutination implies unexpected antibody activity. This, as well as any discrepancy between the results of cell (Step 1) and serum (Step 3) tests, must be explained without delay.

To complete tests for unexpected antibodies, incubate both the test tube with type O cells and the test tube with ficin-treated O cells at 37 C for 1 h. At the end of this period, the sedimented cells in both tubes are inspected very gently for evidence of agglutination. Finally, the red cells in the test with O cells are washed four times, 1 drop of antiglobulin serum is added to the washed cells, the test tube is centrifuged at $1,000 \times g$ for 10 s, and the sedimented red cells are again inspected very gently for evidence of agglutination.

These tests with pooled O cells can only be performed by technicians who are competent to detect partial, or mixed field, agglutination. Less experienced technicians must use single sources of O cells, and this can mean three to five separate tests rather than one test with pooled cells. To learn how to discern partial agglutination tests, technicians should prepare known mixtures of washed A and O cells, and of Rh-positive and Rh-negative cells, and use the

TABLE 3. *Results of antiglobulin tests for Rh, and their significance*

Anti-Rh1		Bovine albumin	Meaning
Test 1	Test 2		
Neg	Neg	Neg	Rh-negative (Rh:1)
Pos	Pos	Neg	Rh:w1 (Rh$_0$ or D^u)
Pos	Pos	Pos	Positive direct antiglobulin test, method invalid[a]
Neg	Pos	Neg	Invalid[b]

[a] For positive result in albumin test, adsorption and elution with anti-Rh1 will allow eluates to be tested for anti-Rh1 activity. If positive, the specimen is Rh-positive; if negative, or if weakly agglutinated Rh-positive cells cannot be distinguished from weakly agglutinated Rh-negative cells, the specimen is Rh-negative. Saline agglutinating (IgM) anti-Rh1 can also be used, but these reagents are not usually as sensitive as adsorption and elution.

[b] Either anti-Rh1 test 2 contains an unwanted non-anti-Rh1 antibody, anti-Rh1 test 1 is deficient in respect to a component of Rh1, or someone forgot to add serum to test 1.

different test methods described until they can invariably detect from 5 to 95% agglutinated cells in artificial mixtures. It is not too difficult to discern 2 to 98%.

Typing of cord blood specimens

In these tests, only the red cells are evaluated because, with rare exception, serum hemagglutinins are IgG antibodies derived from the mother.

For these tests, five rather than four test tubes are used. Four of the test tubes are handled in exactly the same fashion as in Steps 1 and 2 above: one test is used for A-anti-A, another for B-anti-B, another for Rh1-anti-Rh1, and the last for albumin control. The results of these tests and their significance are also the same except that the result of ABO typing is final instead of presumptive. Only Step 3 has been omitted.

The fifth test tube in cord blood typing is used for a direct antiglobulin test, an important diagnostic procedure for recognition of erythroblastosis. This test begins with a test tube filled with saline. Erythrocytes (10^7) are introduced by applicator stick (as in Step 1), the test tube is centrifuged at $1,000 \times g$ for 1 min, and the supernatant saline is poured off. This is repeated three more times. Finally, 1 drop of antiglobulin serum is added to the washed red cells and, after mixing, the test tube is centrifuged at $1,000 \times g$ for 10 s. The sedimented red cells are gently inspected for evidence of agglutination. A positive result is characteristic of erythroblastosis. Strong agglutination is typical of Rh disease. Very weak agglutination may signify ABO disease (e.g., O mother with A or B baby). A complement antiglobulin test is rarely positive and does not imply clinical erythroblastosis.

OTHER PROCEDURES RELATED TO BLOOD TYPING

Preparation of eluates

Eluates are necessary to (i) study the specificity of cell-bound autologous antibodies, (ii) resolve doubts as to the presence or absence of a possible weakly expressed red cell antigen, and (iii) separate a mixture of antibodies on the basis of their specificity.

Beginning with antibody-sensitized red cells, these cells are washed, usually six times with 0.85% NaCl. The washing process should be achieved rapidly, and preferably at 4 C, to reduce antibody loss by spontaneous elution.

Of three methods to recover cell-bound antibodies (pH 3.0 from stroma [11], ether [21], and heat [12]), heat is readily available and is a reasonably efficient procedure. Add 2 to 3 volumes of saline to each volume of washed, packed erythrocytes and incubate with constant mixing at 56 C for 15 min. Centrifuge for 60 s at $1,000 \times g$ and quickly remove the supernatant fluid. This eluate may be tested immediately for its antibody activity, or it may be stored for several weeks at either 4 C or lower temperatures.

Inherent inefficiency of the heat method of elution is observed when comparing eluates from "strong" and "weak" blood types: a better eluate is usually obtained from the "weaker" cells. Thus, anti-A bound to type A cells is recovered better when the red cells used for adsorption are type A_2 (or A_3) rather than type A_1. A similar pattern is seen for Rh where better eluates are obtained from Rh:w1 (Rh or D^u) than from Rh:1 (normal Rh or D). For Rh antibodies, and also for Kell, much more efficient recovery of bound antibody is observed with the ether and pH 3.0 from stroma methods; both methods give better eluates from "strong" red cells.

Eluates, especially those prepared from cells known to be strongly agglutinated by anti-IgG, are expected to have agglutinating activity. If an eluate does not, suspect penicillin sensitivity and test with penicillin-treated erythrocytes (13).

Determination of the specificity of unexpected agglutinins

The specificity of an unexpected agglutinin is determined by tests with a series of blood specimens that have been selected on the basis of the membrane antigens carried by the red cells of each one. There are generally 6 or 12 type O specimens in such a "panel." All important red cell antigens should be present in at least one panel specimen and absent in at least one other. Used additionally are A_1, A_2, and B cells, cells from the patient, and type O cord blood cells. Two sets of washed cell suspensions, 2% (vol/vol) in strength, are prepared from each cell. One set is treated with protease; the other set is not. One drop of patient's serum is tested with 1 drop of each reagent cell suspension, and evidence for agglutination is sought, with both normal and protease-treated cells, and by antiglobulin testing, as in screening tests for unexpected hemagglutination. The pattern of negative and positive results obtained with the patient's serum is compared with the known distribution of each antigen in the "panel" cells.

More than one specificity within a single serum may be recognized by dissimilar reactions (e.g., strong versus weak, protease test versus antiglobulin test), but trial adsorptions are often necessary.

If a red cell blood group alloantibody is in the patient's serum, the patient's red cells should lack that alloantigen.

Serological evidence of incompatibility ("compatibility tests" or "cross-matches")

There is no method of testing that will guarantee the compatibility of donor blood. All that can be done is to perform a series of tests that are more likely than not to disclose some evidence in the event that serious incompatibility does exist between patient and donor. A simple method for doing this is to take two test tubes, 8 mm (inner diameter) × 75 mm, fill each one with 0.85% NaCl, introduce donor red blood cells into each (e.g., approximately 10^7 cells by applicator stick), centrifuge at 1,000 × g for 1 min, and remove the saline. Introduce 1 drop (0.05 ml) of 0.5% bromelin solution (see below) into only one of the tubes and then 1 drop of patient's serum into each of the two tubes. Mix and centrifuge the tube *without bromelin* at 1,000 × g for 10 s. Inspect cells for evidence of agglutination. Now incubate *both tubes* at 37 C for 10 min. Centrifuge the tube *with bromelin* and inspect cells for evidence of agglutination. Wash the cells in the other tube *(without bromelin)* four times, remove saline, add antiglobulin serum (anti-IgG), centrifuge, and inspect cells gently for evidence of agglutination. If all three tests fail to disclose agglutination, the donor blood is considered acceptable.

This method has a number of advantages. It is fast, and all tests for agglutination are made with cells suspended in saline so that interpretations require no weighting for viscosity. The three tests are designed to detect a wide variety of blood type reactions, including all known to cause serious reactions. The method also has some deficiencies because, rarely, some antigen-antibody reactions can be observed better by an alternative, albeit more time-consuming, technique. Bromelin-treated cells are unduly sensitive to agglutination by relatively weak and clinically unimportant cold agglutinins.

Alternative methods include:

1. Addition of a high concentration (~22%) of bovine albumin to a test. Although first incubated at 37 C for 1 h, this kind of test is thereafter handled like Rh typing (see above, Step 1 under Typing of blood specimens from patients other than infants).

2. Use of special equipment (e.g., Auto-Analyzer) that permits tests of direct agglutination under either low or normal ionic conditions (1). The low ionic automated test incorporates positively charged macromolecules, like protamine sulfate; the normal ionic automated test incorporates both bromelin and a rouleaux-inducing agent such as K-90 polyvinylpyrrolidone. Sensitive antiglobulin tests can also be performed by AutoAnalyzer (2).

There are emergency situations in which blood must be used before laboratory tests, even rapid ones, can be completed. Under such conditions, the attending physician assumes full responsibility for this life-threatening state of affairs and administers type O red cells. An obstetrician, knowing that his patient is Rh-negative, will use type O, Rh-negative red cells. In either event, the blood bank must be promptly notified, given appropriate specimens and requests, and asked to inform the attending physician as soon as adequate tests have been completed. If slightly more time is available, the blood bank may be requested to provide ABO type-specific blood on the basis of incomplete tests for evidence of serological incompatibility. In this situation, the results of completed tests will often be available before the transfusion has even been started.

Bromelin solution. Bromelin, a proteolytic enzyme derived from pineapple, can be obtained from Mann Research Laboratories, Division Becton-Dickinson, Rutherford, N.J. Suspend 150 mg of bromelin (1,200 activity) in 3.0 ml of 0.15 M phosphate buffer, pH 5.5. Add 27.0 ml of 0.85% NaCl, mix, and centrifuge at 1,000 × g for 20 min. Store the supernatant fluid in small portions at −20 C.

Measurement of agglutinins by titration

For some, but not all, erythrocyte antigen-antibody reactions, this is an easy way to roughly estimate antibody concentration; a simple method follows:

Arrange a row of 10 test tubes for each test (not specimen) to be evaluated. For cold agglutinins this would be minimally two tests: one for cells from a normal adult and one for cells from cord blood. For Rh this would also be minimally two tests: one for ficin-treated Rh-positive cells and one for normal cells using the antiglobulin test.

In parallel, arrange five larger master tubes (10 mm [inner diameter] × 75 mm). Alternate the position of these so that they are opposite test tubes 1, 3, 5, 7, and 9.

To construct a 2-drop, twofold dilution titration in duplicate, one adds 9 drops of 0.9% NaCl to each of the last four master tubes. Also add 1 drop of 0.9% NaCl to test tubes 2, 4, 6, 8, and 10 of each row. Tube 1 of the master tubes should contain the serum for titration. From this tube, add 2 drops to test tube 1 of each row, 1 drop to tube 2 of each row, and 3 drops to the next master tube. One now has, in each row, 2 drops of undiluted serum in tube 1, 2 drops of a 1:2 dilution of serum in tube 2, and 12 drops of 1:4 diluted serum in the next master tube. Rinse the pipette well, mix the master tube well, and then dispense 2 drops of the 1:4 dilution to tube 3 of each row, 1 drop of this dilution to tube 4 of each row, and 3 drops of this dilution to the next master tube. Here, 3 drops + 9 drops = 12 drops but $\frac{1}{4} \times \frac{1}{4}$ = 1:16, and the dilution is now 1:16. continue to the end of the titration. Add appropriate cells in 2-drop amounts to each test tube of each row. After incubation, centrifugation, antiglobulin test, etc., the last tube in each row that contains distinctly agglutinated erythrocytes is indicative of the titration value for that test.

When drops are delivered accurately from a uniformly positioned Pasteur pipette the reproducibility of this method for a 10-tube, twofold dilution titration is excellent. A flow diagram is given in Fig. 1.

The technique is the same when three or four rows are used instead of two. For three rows, add 12 drops of saline to the master tubes and transfer 4 drops. For four rows, add 15 drops of saline to the master tubes and transfer 5 drops.

Tests for acquired hemolytic anemia

Direct antiglobulin tests. Take two small test tubes (8 mm × 75 mm) for each specimen. Label one tube IgG and the other C3. Transfer 10^7 red cells to each of these two test tubes. Wash both test tubes four times and remove the saline. Add 1 drop of anti-IgG to the tube labeled IgG, and add 1 drop of anti-C3 to the tube labeled C3. Mix and centrifuge both tubes at $1,000 \times g$ for 10 s. Inspect for agglutination.

If polyvalent antiglobulin serum is used, add 1 drop of IgG solution (10 mg/ml of saline) to one tube of washed red cells and 1 drop of saline to the other. Mix and then add 1 drop of the polyvalent antiglobulin serum to each tube. Mix, centrifuge, and inspect for evidence of agglutination. The tube *without added IgG* solution gives the result for all antibodies, but anti-IgG is the strongest antibody in the reagent. The tube *with added IgG* gives the result for all non-anti-IgG antibodies, of which anti-C3 is the strongest.

Absence of agglutination generally, but not invariably, indicates absence of disease. Strongly positive C3 and negative IgG (or no stronger IgG + C3) usually indicates cold agglutinin disease. Strongly positive IgG and more weakly positive C3 usually indicates active warm acquired hemolytic anemia. Strongly positive IgG with negative C3 may or may not indicate active warm acquired hemolytic anemia.

These manual tests are neither very sensitive nor very revealing of adherent proteins at the red cell surface. With more sensitive tests using K-90 polyvinylpyrrolidone to augment agglutination and an AutoAnalyzer to perform tests and record results, sera against all five immunoglobulins and both C3 and C4 can be used (10). Under these conditions, the following

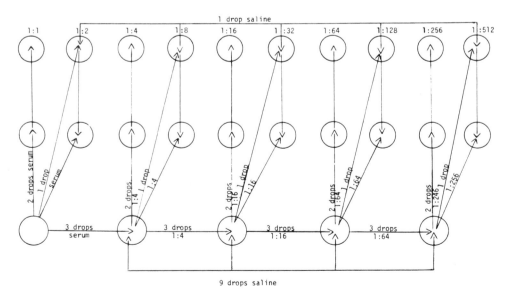

Fig. 1. Flow diagram for twofold titration to be used with either two different cells or two different test conditions.

disease states are usually characterized by positive specific antiglobulin tests as shown below.

Paroxysmal cold hemoglobinuria
1. Very acute, postviral: Negative, all involved red cells are quickly and completely lysed in vivo.
2. Late acute: C3 + C4.

Cold agglutinin disease
1. Monoclonal IgM cold agglutinins: C3 + C4. Weak IgG and, less commonly, weak IgA, IgD, and IgE may be seen.
2. Mixed cryoglobulin cold agglutinins: IgM + IgG (sometimes + IgA) + C3 + C4.

Warm acquired hemolytic anemia (AHA)
1. Monoclonal IgG: Very strong IgG carrying either κ or λ light chains but not both. Sometimes weak C4.
2. IgM (warm agglutinins): Spontaneous agglutination in polyvinylpyrrolidone, sometimes disruption by anti-IgM, IgG usually present, and sometimes IgA. There are always C4 and C3.
3. Mild AHA (sometimes partial remission): IgA and C3, but not C4 (properdin pathway). IgG may be seen.
4. Clinically inactive AHA: Polyclonal IgG carrying both κ and λ light chains. Sometimes IgA also. No complement components.

Sugar-water test for paroxysmal nocturnal hemoglobinuria (8). Mix 1 volume of patient's defibrinated whole blood with 9 volumes of 10% sucrose in water. Incubate at 37 C for 30 min and observe for lysis. Do the same with normal blood as a control.

Lysis of paroxysmal nocturnal hemoglobinuria (PNH) cells will be observed within 30 min because, under these lowered ionic conditions, large amounts of immunoglobulin and complement will interact at the cell surface. These will not lyse normal cells because decay of complement components will be more rapid than the immune lytic process, but PNH cells are more sensitive to lysis and they will be destroyed.

Ham test for PNH (7). To 1 part of washed 20% suspension of red cells add 9 parts of fresh, normal, ABO-compatible human serum that previously has been acidified to pH 6.7 by addition of 10% (vol/vol) 0.2 N HCl. Addition of 0.005 M Mg^{2+} potentiates the reaction (14). Incubate at 37 C for 60 min and observe for partial lysis. Two controls are essential: (i) inactivated acidified serum, and (ii) normal red cells instead of those of the patient being tested. Serum of the patient is usually not as strongly hemolytic.

Red cells in a rare disease, hereditary erythroblastic multinuclearity with positive acid

serum test (HEMPAS; 3), will also give a positive Ham test. This disease, also known as congenital dyserythropoietic anemia (CDA), can be recognized by performing the Ham test with two incubation stages, 30 min at 4 C and then 30 min at 37 C. PNH cells show no change, whereas HEMPAS (CDA) cells display much more lysis.

Cold-warm lysins of paroxysmal cold hemoglobinuria (9). Inactivate serum of the patient at 56 C for 10 min, cool, and dilute with an equal volume of fresh normal human serum. To 9 parts of this serum mixture, add 1 part of a washed 50% suspension of normal type O red cells. Mix at room temperature. Incubate in an ice bath (4 C) for 30 min and then at 37 C for an additional 30 min. Observe for lysis. As controls, (i) reverse the incubation temperatures, and (ii) substitute heat-inactivated for fresh human serum.

LITERATURE CITED

1. Berkman, E. M., J. Nusbacher, S. Kochwa, and R. E. Rosenfield. 1971. Quantitative blood typing profiles of human erythrocytes. Transfusion (Philadelphia) 11:317–332.
2. Burkart, P., R. E. Rosenfield, T. C. S. Hsu, K. Y. Wong, J. Nusbacher, S. H. Shaikh, and S. Kochwa. 1974. Instrumented PVP-augmented antiglobulin tests. I. Detection of allongeneic antibodies coating otherwise normal erythrocytes. Vox Sang. 26:289–304.
3. Crookston, J. H., M. C. Crookston, K. L. Burnie, W. H. Francombe, J. V. Dacie, J. A. Davis, and S. M. Lewis. 1969. Hereditary erythroblastic multinuclearity associated with a positive acidified-serum test: a type of congenital dyserythropoietic anemia. Br. J. Haematol. 17:11–26.
4. Economidou, J., N. C. Hughes-Jones, and B. Gardner. 1967. Quantitative measurements concerning A and B antigen sites. Vox Sang. 12:321–328.
5. Greenbury, C. L., D. H. Moore, and L. A. C. Nunn. 1963. Immunology 6:421–433.
6. Hakomori, S., and A. Kobata. 1973. Blood group antigens, p. 79–140. In M. Sela (ed.), The antigens, vol. 2. Academic Press Inc., New York.
7. Ham, T. H. 1937. Chronic hemolytic anemia with paroxysmal nocturnal hemoglobinuria. N. Engl. J. Med. 217:915–917.
8. Hartmann, R. C., and D. E. Jenkins, Jr. 1966. The "sugar-water" test for paroxysmal nocturnal hemoglobinuria. N. Engl. J. Med. 275:155–157.
9. Hinz, C. F., Jr., and A. M. Mollner. 1962. Initiation of the action of complement in a human auto-immune hemolytic system, the Donath-Landsteiner reaction. J. Clin. Invest. 41:1365–1366.
10. Hsu, T. C. S., R. E. Rosenfield, P. Burkart, K. Y. Wong, and S. Kochwa. 1974. Instrumented PVP-augmented antiglobulin tests. II. Evalu-

ation of acquired hemolytic anemia. Vox Sang. 26:305–325.

11. Kochwa, S., and R. E. Rosenfield. 1964. Immunochemical studies of the Rh system. I. Isolation and characterization of antibodies. J. Immunol. 92:682–692.

12. Landsteiner, K., and C. P. Miller, Jr., 1925. Serological studies on the blood of the primates. II. The blood groups in anthropoid apes. J. Exp. Med. 42:853–862.

13. Ley, A. B., J. P. Harris, M. Brinkley, B. Liles, J. A. Jack, and H. Cahan. 1958. Circulating antibody directed against penicillin. Science 127:1118–1119.

14. May, J. E., W. Rosse, and M. M. Frank. 1973. Paroxysmal nocurnal hemoglobinuria. Alternate-complement-pathway-mediated lysis induced by magnesium. N. Engl. J. Med. 289:705–709.

15. Miller, W. V., et al. (ed.). 1974. Technical methods and procedures of the American Association of Blood Banks, 6th ed., p.326–330.

15a. Nicholson, G. L. 1972. Topography of membrane concanavalin A sites modified by proteolysis. Nature (London) New Biol. 239:193–197.

16. Pollack, W., H. J. Hager, and L. L. Hollenbeck, Jr. 1962. The specificity of antihuman gamma globulin reagents. Transfusion (Philadelphia) 2:17–30.

17. Pollack, W., H. J. Hager, R. Reckel, D. A. Toren, and H. O. Singher. 1965. A study of the forces involved in the second stage of hemagglutination. Transfusion (Philadelphia) 5: 158–183.

18. Race, R. R., and R. Sanger. 1968. Blood groups in man, p. 19–33, 44–47. F. A. Davis Co., Philadelphia.

19. Rochna, E., and N. C. Hughes-Jones. 1965. The use of purified ^{125}I-labelled anti-γ globulin in the determination of the number of D antigen sites on red cells of different phenotypes. Vox Sang. 10:675–686.

20. Rosenfield, R. E., F. H. Allen, Jr., and P. Rubinstein. 1974. Genetic model for the Rh blood group system. Proc. Natl. Acad. Sci. U.S.A. 70:1303–1307.

21. Rubin, H. 1963. Antibody elution from red blood cells. J. Clin. Pathol. 16:70–73.

22. Schacter, H., M. A. Michaels, M. C. Crookston, C. A. Tilley, and J. H. Crookston. 1971. A quantitative difference in the activity of blood group A-specific N-acetylgalactosaminyl transferase in serum of A_1 and A_2 human subjects. Biochem. Biophys. Res. Commun. 45:1011–1018.

23. Schmidt, P. J., E. G. Morrison, and J. Shohl. 1962. The antigenicity of the Rh_0 (D^u) blood factor. Blood 20:196–202.

Chapter 72

Autoimmune and Drug-Immune Hemolytic Anemias

LAWRENCE D. PETZ

INTRODUCTION

This chapter describes the means of definitively diagnosing the autoimmune and drug-immune hemolytic anemias on the basis of their distinctive serological characteristics. A classification of immune hemolytic anemias is listed in Table 1.

It is essential that a precise diagnosis be made in each case since prognosis and management differ strikingly among the various hemolytic anemias. For example, successful therapeutic regimens for warm antibody autoimmune hemolytic anemia (AIHA) consists of corticosteroids, splenectomy, and, to a lesser extent, immunosuppressive drugs. In contrast, cold agglutinin disease is best managed by keeping the patient strictly warm. If further therapy is necessary, chlorambucil may produce significant improvement, but corticosteroids and splenectomy are rarely effective and thus generally contraindicated. (If either warm or cold AIHA is associated with an underlying disorder such as a lymphoma, treatment of the underlying disease may cause improvement in the hemolysis.) Finally, patients with drug-immune hemolytic anemias are effectively treated merely by discontinuing the offending drug, with other supportive measures (transfusions, corticosteroids) at times being necessary temporarily.

CHARACTERISTIC SEROLOGICAL FINDINGS IN IMMUNE HEMOLYTIC ANEMIAS

The serological tests described below are utilized to characterize the antibodies present on the patient's red cells and in his serum. The results of such studies may be diagnostic of warm antibody AIHA (Table 2), cold agglutinin disease (Table 3), or paroxysmal cold hemoglobinuria (Table 4).

In addition, a history of drug administration must be sought. Aldomet (and, rarely, L-dopa and mefenamic acid) causes development of hemolytic anemia with serological characteristics similar to warm antibody AIHA. Penicillin (and, rarely, cephalothin) when administered in high doses (greater than 10×10^6 units per day) may cause hemolytic anemia characterized by a strongly positive direct antiglobulin (Coombs) test (DAT) but with no antibody detectable in the patient's serum or red cell eluate unless antibiotic-treated red cells are used for antibody detection. Other drug-induced immune hemolytic anemias are usually characterized clinically by acute intravascular hemolysis, hemoglobinemia, hemoglobinuria, and renal failure, often after ingestion of only a small quantity of the offending drug. Serologically, such patients have weakly or moderately positive DATs, and drug-related serum antibody is detectable only when the patient's serum, the drug, and normal red cells are all incubated together.

LABORATORY DIAGNOSIS OF IMMUNE HEMOLYTIC ANEMIAS

The diagnosis of immune hemolytic anemias is based on the finding of characteristic serological abnormalities in a patient with clinical evidence of hemolysis. In order to distinguish among the diagnostic possibilities listed in Table 1, a detailed laboratory evaluation is required. The serological tests to be performed determine whether the patient's red cells are coated with immunoglobulin G (IgG), complement components, or both; and whether the red cells are weakly or strongly sensitized. The performance of the DAT supplies such information. Further, tests must be performed to determine the characteristics of the antibodies in the patient's serum and in an eluate from his red cells. Screening tests followed by steps required for a more detailed characterization of the antibodies are described below.

DIRECT ANTIGLOBULIN (COOMBS) TEST

Collection of specimens

Blood for the DAT should be collected in ethylenediaminetetraacetate (EDTA) anticoagulant (0.01 M) to inactivate complement and thus prevent in vitro sensitization of red cells by clinically insignificant cold antibodies (e.g., normal incomplete cold antibody), which

TABLE 1. *Immune hemolytic anemias*

I. Autoimmune hemolytic anemias (AIHA)
   A. Warm antibody AIHA
      1. Idiopathic (unassociated with another disease)
      2. Secondary (associated with chronic lymphocytic leukemia, lymphomas, systemic lupus erythematosus, etc.)
   B. Cold antibody AIHA
      1. Idiopathic cold hemagglutinin syndrome
      2. Secondary cold hemagglutinin syndrome
         a. Associated with *Mycoplasma pneumoniae* infection
         b. Associated with chronic lymphocytic leukemia, lymphomas, etc.
      3. Paroxysmal cold hemoglobinuria
         a. Idiopathic
         b. Secondary to syphilis or acute viral infections

II. Immune drug-induced hemolytic anemia
   A. Aldomet-induced hemolytic anemia
   B. Penicillin-induced hemolytic anemia
   C. Other drug-induced hemolytic anemias

III. Alloantibody-induced immune hemolytic anemia
   A. Hemolytic transfusion reactions
   B. Hemolytic disease of the newborn

TABLE 2. *Warm antibody autoimmune hemolytic anemia*

1. Direct antiglobulin (Coombs) test
   A. Usually IgG-strongly positive
   B. Frequently complement
   C. Occasionally IgM, IgA

2. Serum antibody
   A. Incomplete antibody
   B. Moderate titer
   C. Maximal activity at 37 C
   D. Frequent Rh "specificity"
   E. Rarely lytic in vitro

3. Eluates
   A. Antibody activity demonstrable

would result in a false-positive reaction. Vacutainer tubes (Becton-Dickinson, Parsippany, N.J.) containing EDTA are adequate for this purpose. If positive reactions are obtained with red cells that have been separated from a clotted specimen or in another anticoagulant and have been allowed to cool to room temperature or lower, the DAT should be repeated on a freshly drawn specimen anticoagulated with EDTA.

Performance of test with broad-spectrum antiglobulin serum

A licensed "broad-spectrum" antihuman globulin serum containing anti-IgG and anti-C3d antibodies should be used for initial tests. The manufacturer's instructions should be followed carefully, and the reactivity of the serum should be checked against appropriate controls (see below). In general, the technique is as follows:

1. Place 1 drop of a 2 to 5% saline suspension of red cells in a labeled 10 × 75 mm tube. Wash three or four times with saline. After the last wash, decant completely, add 1 or 2 drops of antihuman globulin serum, and mix.

2. Centrifuge for approximately 15 s at 900 to 1,000 RCF (equivalent to centrifugation in a Serofuge [Clay-Adams, Inc., Parsippany, N.J.] at 3,400 rpm). Examine for agglutination macroscopically and, if negative, microscopically. The manner in which the red cells are dislodged from the bottom of the tube is critical. The tube should be held at an angle and shaken gently until all cells are dislodged. Then it should be tilted back and forth gently until an even suspension of cells or agglutinates is observed. If the tube containing antiglobulin serum is negative, add 1 drop of IgG sensitized red cells (commercially available), and recentrifuge. If the patient's cells were washed adequately in the first stage of the test, then the control cells should be agglutinated and the negative result on the patient is valid.

Agglutination is graded as follows:
   4+   One solid aggregate. No free cells.
   3+   Several large aggregates. Very few free cells.

TABLE 3. *Cold agglutinin disease*

1. Direct antiglobulin (Coombs) test
   A. Moderately positive with broad-spectrum or anticomplement antiglobulin sera
   B. Negative with anti-IgG antiglobulin serum

2. Serum antibody
   A. IgM agglutinin maximally reactive at 4 C
   B. Very high titer (usually >1:1,000)
   C. Upper thermal limit of activity: usually about 30 C
   D. Usually anti-I specificity
   E. Idiopathic cases have monoclonal antibody
   F. Causes in vitro lysis
      1) Complement dependent
      2) Accentuated by acidification
      3) Especially enzyme-treated red cells

TABLE 4. *Paroxysmal cold hemoglobinuria*

1. "Cold" antibody—Thermal range usually up to 10–15 C
2. Acts mainly as a hemolysin (biphasic)
3. Lysin titer greater than agglutinin titer
4. IgG antibody
5. Specificity of anti-P

2+ Medium-sized aggregates. Free cells in background.

1+ Small aggregates with turbid reddish background.

w+ Tiny aggregates with turbid reddish background, or microscopic aggregates.

0 No agglutination.

Monospecific antiglobulin sera

A simple extension of the routinely performed DAT gives valuable information regarding the differential diagnosis of immune hemolytic anemias (16). The DAT should be performed with monospecific antisera against IgG and C3d. (Other immune globulins [e.g., IgM, IgA] sensitize red cells infrequently and usually in association with IgG. Other complement components [especially C4] may be detected on erythrocytes but always in association with C3d in patients with AIHA.) Such antisera are available as precipitating reagents from commercial manufacturers, but no licensing standards exist regarding hemagglutinating reactions; thus, quality control procedures must be performed to verify appropriate reactivity (3). Such sera must first be tested by agglutination against normal group A, B, and O erythrocytes, and, if necessary, absorbed at 4 C for 2 h with an equal volume of washed packed red cells. (The following procedures should also be applied in checking the adequacy of a broad-spectrum antiserum).

Anti-IgG. For determination of anti-IgG activity of an antiglobulin serum, a serum containing an IgG alloantibody should be selected that reacts 1+ to 2+ by the indirect antiglobulin test (IAT), but is negative in saline or albumin media. (See below for details of the IAT and agglutination in saline or albumin media.) If the reaction is stronger than this, the antibody should be diluted in normal human serum. Especially for initial evaluation, it is advisable to test more than one IgG antibody, e.g., anti-Rh$_0$(D), anti-K, or anti-Fy^a. Thereafter, periodic quality control of that batch of antiglobulin serum may be performed with just one antibody, usually anti-Rh$_0$(D).

Procedure

1. Label tubes: test sample and negative control. Identify the antibody used.

2. Add 1 drop of antibody-containing serum to each.

3. Prepare 2 to 5% saline suspensions of red cells positive for the antigenic determinant [e.g., Rh$_0$(D)] and negative for the antigenic determinant.

4. Add 1 drop of the appropriate suspension to each tube.

5. Incubate at 37 C for 15 to 30 min.

6. Wash all tubes three times with saline.

7. Add antiglobulin reagent to each tube and mix.

8. Centrifuge.

9. Observe for agglutination.

A monospecific anti-IgG antiserum should give the appropriate positive and negative results and should also give negative results when tested against cells strongly sensitized with complement (see below).

Anticomplement. Red cells sensitized with complement in vivo are coated with C3d, a fragment of the third component of complement. They may also have other components of complement (e.g., C4, C5, C6, C8) but always with the concomitant presence of C3d in patients with hemolytic anemias.

Commercially available antisera to C3 that are marketed for use in immunodiffusion may be adequate as antiglobulin sera. They must give negative reactions against normal erythrocytes and against erythrocytes strongly sensitized with IgG [as can readily be prepared by reacting Rh$_0$(D) positive red cells with commercially available anti-Rh$_0$(D)]. To test for C$_3$ reactivity, complement-sensitized red cells may be prepared by adding 1 ml of whole blood anticoagulated in ACD or CPD to 10 ml of 10% sucrose. The mixture is incubated at 37 C for 15 min, and the cells are then washed in saline four times. Such red cells are sensitized with C3 and C4.

To prepare cells coated with C3d, 1 volume of the above sensitized packed erythrocytes is added to an equal volume of 0.1% trypsin. The mixture is incubated at 37 C for 30 min. As a negative control, normal red cells without complement sensitization are incubated with trypsin simultaneously. After incubation, the red cells are washed three times. The complement-sensitized red cells will now react with anti-C3d (α_2D), but not anti-C3d (β_{1A}/β_{1C}) or anti-C4.

Antiglobulin test titrations and scores

It is useful to perform titrations of the monospecific antiglobulin reagents against antiglobulin test positive red cells in order to assess the relative strength of the reactions. For anti-IgG antisera, the use of fourfold dilutions from 1:1 to 1:4,096 is usually adequate. For anti-C3, doubling dilutions from 1:1 to 1:128 are usually optimal, although other dilutions may be chosen depending on the potency of the individual antiserum.

Semiquantitative direct antiglobulin test.

1. Prepare a 2 to 5% suspension of patient's red cells in saline.

2. Place 1 drop into tubes labeled 1:1 to 1:4,096 (for anti-IgG).

3. Wash the cells four times in isotonic saline.

4. Prepare serial dilutions from 1:1 to 1:4,096 of the antiglobulin serum (e.g., 0.1-ml amounts) in saline; starting from the highest dilution, transfer 2 drops of each dilution to the appropriate tube containing a button of washed red cells; resuspend the cells completely.

5. Centrifuge and check for agglutination in each tube.

By grading the strength of the antiglobulin test reactions at each dilution for both anti-IgG and anti-C3, one achieves a better understanding of the strength of the reactions. A numerical score may also be assigned to specific degrees of agglutination so that an antiglobulin test titration score may be developed for each antiglobulin test. One such method assigns a value of 10 for 4+ agglutination, 8 for 3+, 6 for 2+, 4 for 1+, 2 for w+ reactions, and 0 for negative. (See Table 5.)

Interpretation and precautions

In patients with warm antibody AIHA, the DAT will reveal IgG and C3d in about 50% of patients, IgG only in 30%, and C3d only in 20%. The red cells of patients with cold antibody AIHA are sensitized with C3d but not with IgG. Patients with drug-induced immune hemolytic anemia caused by penicillin and Aldomet typically have red cells strongly sensitized by IgG but without fixation of complement. Other drug-immune hemolytic anemias are usually characterized by weak to moderate sensitization of red cells by complement components without detectable immune globulins. However, some such patients do have IgG on their red cells, more often in association with complement.

Table 6 summarizes the characteristic antiglobulin test results in various hemolytic anemias.

One point that must be emphasized is that about 30% of patients with immune hemolytic anemias will appear to have a negative DAT unless the antiglobulin serum used contains antibodies against complement components (18).

Although the results of the DAT provide valuable information if performed as above, they must be interpreted in conjunction with clinical and other laboratory data to avoid erroneous conclusions. A positive DAT occurs in situations other than immune hemolytic anemias. A positive DAT does not necessarily indicate the presence of autoantibody; furthermore, even if

TABLE 5. *Direct antiglobulin (Coombs) test titers*

Anti-IgG		Anti-C3	
Dilution	Aggluti-nation	Dilution	Aggluti-nation
1:4	4+	1:4	4+
1:16	4+	1:8	3+
1:64	4+	1:16	3+
1:256	3+	1:32	2+
1:1,024	2+	1:64	1+
1:4,096	1+	1:128	0
Saline	0	Saline	0
Anti-IgG titration score: 48[a]		Anti-C3 titration score: 36[a]	

[a] Titration score is derived by assigning a value of 10 for complete agglutination (4+), 6 for a strong reaction with a number of large agglutinates (2+), etc. The score is the sum of the values obtained at each dilution of antiglobulin serum. The examples illustrate reactions obtained when potent monospecific antiglobulin sera were allowed to react against red cells strongly sensitized with IgG and moderately strongly sensitized with C3. Such reactions are frequently found in patients with warm antibody autoimmune hemolytic anemia.

TABLE 6. *Antiglobulin tests in immune hemolytic anemias*

Anemia	IgG	C3[a]
Warm antibody		
AIHA (50%)	+	+
(30%)	+	0
(20%)	0	+
Cold agglutinin disease	0	+
Paroxysmal cold hemoglobinuria	0	+
Penicillin- or Aldomet-induced	+	0
Other drug-induced immune hemolytic anemias[b]	0	+
Warm antibody AIHA associated with systemic lupus erythematosus	±	+

[a] Such cells are primarily sensitized with the $\alpha_2 D$ component of C3.

[b] The most common pattern of red cell sensitization is indicated, but occasionally IgG may be detected with or without C3.

autoantibody is present, the patient may or may not have a hemolytic anemia. Thus, an independent clinical assessment must be made to determine the presence or absence of hemolytic anemia, and the role of the DAT is to aid in the evaluation of the etiology of hemolysis when present.

A positive DAT may result from any of the following:

1. Formation of autoantibodies against red cells.
2. Antibody formation against drugs rather than against intrinsic red cell antigens, e.g., penicillin, cephalothin, stibophen, quinidine, phenacetin.
3. Abnormalities of the red cell membrane
   a. T antigen activation (a rare phenomenon characteristically associated with sepsis). Normal rabbit serum contains anti-T and therefore antiglobulin serum may agglutinate T-activated red cells.
   b. Associated with weak M or N antigens. Rare cases of weak M and N antigens associated with a positive DAT have been described. It has been postulated that the abnormal red cell membrane may absorb proteins in a nonimmunological fashion.
   c. Following exposure to drugs. The cephalosporins can alter the red cell membrane so that it takes up proteins nonimmunologically.
4. The attachment of transferrin to reticulocytes reacting with antitransferrin in the antiglobulin sera. This is rarely a problem since commercial broad-spectrum antiglobulin sera do not have antitransferrin, or, if they do, the antitransferrin is attenuated beyond its range of reactivity by the dilution at which the sera are marketed.
5. Unknown mechanisms: A small percentage of hospitalized patients will have a positive DAT if potent antiglobulin reagents are used. Such patients do not have a hemolytic anemia and have no abnormal red cell antibodies; the cause of the positive antiglobulin test is uncertain. It is typically only weakly positive, and red cell sensitization is usually by complement components only.
6. Refrigerated clotted samples may give a positive DAT due to in vitro complement sensitization by normal incomplete cold antibody.
7. Delayed transfusion reactions: A careful transfusion history is very important in the investigation of AIHA, as a patient presenting with a positive DAT and perhaps hemolysis, due to a delayed transfusion reaction, can mimic the reactions seen in AIHA.

CHARACTERIZATION OF ANTIBODIES IN SERUM AND ELUATE

The patient's serum is examined to determine whether it contains antibodies. If so, one must determine the characteristics of the antibodies, particularly their thermal range and specificity. Also of significance is whether they are agglutinins or "incomplete" antibodies, and whether they have hemolytic activity. In addition, a red cell eluate is tested for reactivity by IAT and by agglutination of enzyme-treated red cells, and, if reactive, the specificity of the antibody should be determined.

Screening tests should first be performed utilizing several different temperatures and techniques. Information derived from such screening tests with the patient's fresh uninactivated serum and with a red cell eluate are useful in planning the best procedures for definitive evaluation.

Preparation of eluate from patient's red cells

I prefer to use a modification of Rubin's method. Landsteiner and Miller's method is equally easy, but eluates may be less potent. Kochwa and Rosenfield's method is technically more difficult, and, in limited comparative studies, I have not found eluates to be more potent than those prepared by the modification of Rubin's method.

Rubin's method (20).

1. Allow patient's EDTA whole blood sample to incubate at 37 C for 10 min to allow any cold autoantibodies present to dissociate.
2. Wash as many cells as possible four times in large volumes of saline; keep approximately 1 ml of the last saline wash. (The last saline wash should always be tested in parallel with the eluate. This ensures that one has washed the red cells free from serum, and thus the eluate has only red cell sensitizing antibody present and is not contaminated with diluted serum antibody.)
3. Add twice the volume of ether and half the volume of saline to washed packed red cells; mix thoroughly for 1 min.
4. Incubate at 37 C for 15 to 30 min (see below).
5. Centrifuge at 900 to 1,000 RCF for 10 min.
6. Separate off the red bottom layer into a labeled, unstoppered test tube and incubate at 37 C for 30 min to allow excess ether to evaporate.

Hughes-Jones, Gardner, and Telford (9) have estimated that, if elution was carried out for 1 min in the manner described above, about 50% of the original antibody would be eluted, and, if the elution process was continued for a further 30 min at 37 C, about 70% of the antibody would be recovered. Landsteiner and Miller's method would yield only about one-third as much antibody from the same volume of sensitized cells.

Landsteiner and Miller's method (11). A volume of 0.9% NaCl equal to the volume of saline which will be used for the eluate is added to washed packed red cells and mixed thor-

oughly. The mixture is centrifuged at 900 to 1,000 RCF for 10 min, and the supernatant fluid is taken off and kept as a control. The same volume of saline is then added to the packed red cells, and the mixture is placed in a water bath at 56 C for 5 to 10 min, with repeated shaking. At the end of this time, the mixture is centrifuged rapidly while still hot, and the cherry-red supernatant fluid is removed; this is the eluate.

Since antibodies may deteriorate rapidly in saline, there is a possible advantage in substituting group AB serum or 6% albumin for saline in the elution process. The actual volume of either medium added to the washed packed cells depends on the strength of the antiglobulin test: if this is very strong, a volume equal to twice that of the red cells should be used; if moderately strong, a volume equal to that of the red cells; and, if weak, a volume equal to half the volume of the red cells.

Kochwa and Rosenfield's method (10). Washed red cells are made up to a 10% suspension in 0.9% NaCl and lysed at 4 C by adding 0.5 ml of a 0.5 g/100 ml solution of digitonin to every 10 ml of the red cell suspension. If a large volume (e.g., 100 ml or more) of red cell suspension is to be dealt with, it may be centrifuged at 1,000 × g at 4 C to achieve preliminary packing of the stroma. After the supernatant fluid has been removed, the lightly packed stroma is pipetted into one or more small centrifuge tubes, e.g., of 10-ml capacity, which can be centrifuged at high speed, i.e., at 10,000 to 30,000 × g. The tightly packed stroma is then washed three to five times in a large volume of saline for 20 min at 20,000 to 30,000 × g and at 4 C until the supernatant fluid is free from hemoglobulin. Finally, glycine buffer, pH 3.0, is added to the washed packed stroma in a volume equal to that of the original packed red cells; the contents of the tubes are well mixed and left at 37 C for about 5 min, and they are then recentrifuged at 20,000 to 30,000 × g for 20 min. The elution process is repeated twice more, and all three eluates are then dialyzed for 12 to 24 h at 4 C against a large volume of buffered saline, pH 7.0 (100 to 200 times the volume of the eluates). The eluates are concentrated, if necessary, by vacuum dialysis.

Preparation of enzyme-treated red cells

Enzymes enhance the reactivity of red cells with certain alloantibodies such as those of the Kidd, Lewis, Rh-Hr, and P systems. In warm antibody AIHA, autoantibody is detectable in the patient's serum in over 80% of cases by use of enzyme-treated erythrocytes, whereas the IAT will detect antibody in only 35%.

Enzymes commonly used are bromelin, trypsin, papain, ficin, and multienzyme preparations. Enzymes may be employed in a simple one-stage (direct) technique, where the enzyme is mixed directly with the test cells and serum to be tested, or in a two-stage (indirect) technique, where the test cells are pretreated before use. I prefer the two-stage technique utilizing papain since it is more sensitive than the one-stage technique.

One-stage papain technique.

1. Place in a tube 2 volumes of the patient's serum, 1 volume of 5% suspension of red cells, and 1 volume of activated papain solution, pH 5.4 (see below).
2. Incubate at 37 C for 15 to 30 min.
3. Centrifuge; examine for hemolysis and agglutination.
4. Record results.

Two-stage papain technique.

1. Place in a small tube 2 volumes of the patient's serum and 1 volume of premodified cells (see below).
2. Incubate at 37 C for 15 to 60 min.
3. Centrifuge; examine for hemolysis and agglutination.
4. Record results.

Preparation of premodified cells.

1. To 1 volume of washed packed reagent O cells, add 1 volume of 0.1% papain solution, pH 7.3.
2. Incubate at 37 C for 15 to 30 min. This time will vary from batch to batch of the papain solution.
3. Wash twice with saline and resuspend to 2 to 5% suspension in saline.

The enzyme-treated cells must always be set up against inert serum as a negative control and a weak incomplete Rh antiserum as a positive control.

Preparation of 1% activated papain solution.

1. In a mortar grind 1.0 g of papain with 50 ml of 0.067 M phosphate buffer at pH 5.4.
2. Centrifuge at 3,000 rpm for 10 min or filter.
3. To the clear supernatant fluid, add 5.0 ml of 0.5 M cysteine hydrochloride.
4. Dilute the solution to 100 ml with more buffer, pH 5.4.
5. Incubate at 37 C for 1 h.
6. Store at −20 C in small portions which are discarded after use. Do not freeze.

For the two-stage method the same solution can be used diluted 1:10 in phosphate buffer, pH 7.3. Some workers add sodium hydroxide to the cysteine hydrochloride solution to bring it to a neutral pH before adding it to the papain.

Ficin test. A stock ficin solution is made by dissolving 1.0 mg of ficin in 100 ml of pH 7.3 buffered saline. Once made, the stock solution should be stored frozen (-20 C or below) to retain activity of the enzyme. Some people may have dangerous hypersensitivity to raw ficin; they should work with it under a hood and wear gloves.

1. Prepare a 0.1% solution of ficin by mixing 1 volume of the 1% ficin stock solution with 9 volumes of pH 7.3 buffered saline.

2. To 1 volume of washed packed red cells, add 1 volume of working 0.1% ficin solution.

3. Incubate at 37 C for 15 min.

4. Wash cells three times in 0.85% saline.

5. Cells at this time are ready for use and should be used according to methods in use in the laboratory.

Notes: Different workers use different strength ficin solutions. Concentrations from 0.05 to 1% are recommended in the literature. Generally, 0.1% ficin is recommended for pretreatment of cells for use in antibody screening and identification procedures, and 1% ficin is recommended for pretreatment of cells to be used for absorption procedures, i.e., autoabsorption for removal of cold autoagglutinins.

It must be stressed that enzymes considerably enhance the reactivity of cold autoagglutinins. Therefore, the great majority of normal sera will react with enzyme-pretreated cells at room temperature and in some instances demonstrate carry-over reactivity at 37 C due to the presence of cold autoagglutinins in these sera. On these occasions, it is frequently helpful to warm the enzyme-pretreated cells and serum under test separately to 37 C before mixing. This technique prevents the cold autoagglutinins from reacting with their antigen at temperatures below 37 C.

It should also be noted that, if enzyme-pretreated cells are used with antiglobulin serum, the reagent must be shown to be free from unwanted antibody activity (i.e., anti-A, anti-B, anti-H, antispecies) that might demonstrate increased reactivity with enzyme-pretreated cells.

Screening tests for serum antibodies

Room temperature tests. The patient's serum is tested against reagent red cells suitable for antibody detection (i.e., either a single sample of group 0 cells or a pool of two containing all the Rh antigens and as many other antigens as possible). The cells are used untreated and enzyme-treated (e.g., papain-treated). The patient's serum is tested with and without the addition of fresh normal serum at pH 6.5 (0.1 volume of 0.2 N HCl added to serum). The tests are incubated at room temperature (20 C if possible) and 37 C.

As a screening procedure it is suggested that the following be set up:

Room temperature tests

1. Add 2 drops of patient's serum to four test tubes.

2. Add 2 drops of fresh normal serum acidified to pH 6.5, as a source of complement, to tubes 2 and 4.

3. Add 1 drop of 5% screening ("reagent") red cells to the first two tubes.

4. Add 1 drop of 5% enzyme-treated red cells to tubes 3 and 4.

5. The tests are left at room temperature for 15 to 60 min before centrifugation.

6. They are examined for hemolysis and then are agitated gently and inspected for agglutination.

37 C tests

1. Add 2 drops of patient's serum to four test tubes.

2. Add 2 drops of fresh normal serum acidified to pH 6.5, as a source of complement, to tubes 2 and 4.

3. Add 2 drops of 30% bovine albumin to the first tube.

4. Allow to warm to 37 C (5 to 10 min).

5. Add 1 drop of 5% screening cells to tubes 1 and 2. (It is preferable that these cells also be warmed to 37 C before being added to the serum.)

6. Add 1 drop of 5% enzyme-treated red cells to tubes 3 and 4. (It is preferable that these cells also be warmed to 37 C before being added to the serum.)

7. The tests are left at 37 C for 15 to 60 min before centrifugation (preferably at 37 C).

8. They are then examined for hemolysis and are agitated gently and inspected for agglutination.

9. The cells are then washed four times, and antiglobulin serum is added to the button of cells and read.

Specificity antibody in serum and eluate (warm antibodies)

1. Prepare serial doubling dilutions of patient's serum and red cell eluate, in saline, from 1:1 to 1:512 (e.g., 0.1-ml amounts).

2. Starting from the highest dilution, transfer 2 drops from each tube to small tubes (10 × 75 mm) labeled 1, 2, 4, 8, etc.

3. Add 2 drops of 30% albumin to each tube.

4. Add 1 drop of 5% screening (reagent) red cells to each tube; mix. (It is preferable that these cells be warmed to 37 C before being added to the serum.)

5. Incubate tubes at 37 C for 15 to 60 min.

6. Wash four times in isotonic saline.

7. Add antiglobulin serum to the button of washed cells.

8. Examine for agglutination.

9. Select a dilution that reacts 1 to 2+ with reagent screening cells.

10. Dilute the patient's serum and eluate accordingly; test this and the undiluted materials against a panel of red cells (should include cord cells and Rh_{null}, -D-, LW negative, and U negative if possible), proceeding as from steps 3–8 above.

If the antibody detected on screening only reacted with enzyme-treated erythrocytes, then enzyme-treated erythrocytes should be substituted for untreated erythrocytes in step 4. It is not necessary to add albumin in this case.

The specificity of the autoantibodies associated with warm antibody AIHA is very complex (18). The main specificity is directed against the Rh complex but may only be obvious if very rare cells such as -D- or Rh_{null} are available (23). If these cells are available, then one can demonstrate Rh specificity, in the broadest sense, in approximately 70% of warm antibody AIHA. Clear-cut specificity such as anti-$Rh_0(D)$, rh'(C), rh''(E), hr'(c), and hr''(e) is present only very rarely, anti-hr''(e) being the most common. Usually, the undiluted eluate or serum will react with all cells of common genotypes tested, but variations in strength of reaction may be seen. If dilutions of the serum (or eluate) are tested against erythrocytes of various genotypes, the serum may react to higher titer with cells of some Rh genotypes than others. For example, the titer may be 1:32 against cells having the hr''(e) antigen and 1:8 against cells lacking that antigen. In reference to AIHA, this is frequently referred to as Rh "specificity." Cross-absorptions and -elutions with the use of erythrocytes of various genotypes will yield even more information (24). Apart from the Rh specificity, there have been reports of anti-U, anti-LW, and anti-I^T being associated with warm antibody AIHA (18, 25).

Cold agglutinins

IgM cold agglutinins in cold agglutinin disease are usually present to a titer of greater than 1,000 at 4 C. Thus, a useful screening test is as follows. Prepare a 1:64 dilution of serum in 0.9% NaCl, add 1 drop of the diluted serum to a 10 × 75 mm tube, add 1 drop of a 2% saline suspension of pooled group O red cells, and incubate at 4 C for 1 to 2 h. If there is no agglutination at this dilution, cold agglutinin disease is excluded. If strong agglutination occurs, a cold agglutinin titer, thermal amplitude tests, and specificity tests should be performed. In addition, characterization of the antibody's ability to lyse red cells in vitro in the presence of complement is of interest.

Special technical considerations. It is preferable that the blood be collected and the serum be separated *strictly* at 37 C. To do this properly, blood should be collected into a warmed syringe or Vacutainer tube and immediately immersed in a 37 C water bath or thermos flask. If blood cannot be collected at 37 C, then the sample should be put at 37 C as soon as possible. The dangers of letting the blood cool are that the auto-antibody will combine with the cells causing:

1. Agglutination of the cells; leading to difficulties in typing.

2. Loss of antibody from the serum, therefore giving a false low cold agglutinin titer, etc.

3. Binding of more complement as more antibody combines at the lower temperature (e.g., 20 C), leading to a stronger positive DAT than the patient really has.

4. Possible direct hemolysis of the cells utilizing antibody and complement, again leading to false, low laboratory values and possible misinterpretation of in vitro hemoglobinemia as being an in vivo occurrence.

If the samples have inadvertently cooled, warming to 37 C for at least 10 min will cause the cold antibody to elute back from the cells into the serum and the auto-agglutination will disperse completely in most cases. It should be noted that complement bound to the cells in the cooling will remain on the cells. Therefore, the DAT should be carried out on a sample of blood collected into EDTA, as this will prevent any complement being bound in vitro, even if cooling occurs.

The serum should be separated from the cells strictly at 37 C. Ideally, this means working completely in a 37 C warm room or using a heated, jacketed centrifuge. We have found that samples transferred from a 37 C water bath and centrifuged immediately in a Serofuge at room temperature drop approximately 7 to 8 C after only 1 min of centrifugation. Therefore, we keep a Serofuge in an incubator at 45 C; at this temperature, the samples spin at 37 C. It is important to remove samples immediately after centrifugation. The same principle applies to washing cells. We use saline at 40 to 45 C, which we find drops a few degrees as soon as it enters a test tube and a few more degrees when centrifuging is in progress. A few experiments on each apparatus are essential before selecting a routine procedure.

Cold agglutinin titration, thermal amplitude, and specificity. A master series of doubling dilutions of serum is made in 0.9% NaCl, starting with undiluted serum and ending at a dilution of 1:2,000 or 1:4,000. One drop of each serum dilution is then pipetted into three rows of 10×75 mm tubes so that three replicate titrations are made. The tubes are placed in a 37 C water bath until the contents reach 37 C (e.g., 10 min), and 1 drop of a 2% suspension of saline-washed red cells that have been warmed to 37 C is added to each tube: normal pooled group O adult red cells are added to the first row; normal pooled group O cord red cells are added to the second row; and, if available, the rare adult i cells are added to the third row. The contents of the tubes are mixed, and the tubes are incubated for 1 to 2 h. Agglutination is read macroscopically, reading each tube directly from the water bath to prevent cooling. The tubes are then incubated at 30 C for 60 min, and agglutination is again read macroscopically. The procedure is repeated at 20 C and at 4 C. If centrifugation is employed, it must be carried out strictly at the required temperature (e.g., 4 C).

In a patient with hemolytic anemia who has a moderately or strongly positive DAT caused by complement sensitization of his red cells, the finding of a cold agglutinin in the above tests to a titer of 1:1,000 at 4 C with reactivity up to at least 30 C satisfies the criteria of cold agglutinin disease. In patients with hemolytic anemia but with borderline cold agglutinin activity, the above tests should be repeated with the use of a 30% albumin medium instead of saline. This causes enhanced agglutination of many cold agglutinins, and it is very rare for a patient to have hemolytic anemia caused by a cold agglutinin if it does not react to at least 30 C in 30% albumin (6).

The specificity of such antibodies, whether in the idiopathic disease or secondary to mycoplasma pneumonia infections or lymphoma, is usually anti-I. Other antibodies, including those from some of the patients with infectious mononucleosis, have anti-i specificity. Rarely, the antibody is anti-Pr (anti-SP$_1$); see below.

For practical purposes, one usually uses the cord cell as an "I negative." When investigating antibodies of the I system, one must keep in mind that a truly I negative red cell has not been described. Some cells have less I than others; i.e., normal homozygote I adults, normal heterozygote adults [i (cord)], i$_2$ adults (usually Negro), and i$_1$ (usually Caucasian), the foregoing in decreasing order of I strength.

When dealing with high-titer anti-I, it is very difficult to determine specificity unless titrations are performed. As one raises the temperature, the specificity becomes more apparent. For instance, at 4 C an anti-I may react to a titer of 2,000 with adult I cells and 256 with i (cord) cells, but at 25 C it may still react to a titer of 128 with adult cells and give no reaction with cord cells. If adult i cells are available, specificity is more obvious. Anti-i reacts with adult i cells more strongly than i (cord) cells and much more weakly with adult cells. If all cells are equally agglutinated, then a mixture of anti-I and -i, or anti-Pr should be suspected. Anti-Pr is easily distinguished, as the antigen seems to be destroyed by enzyme treatment. Both anti-I and anti-i give much higher titers against enzyme-treated cells. Therefore, if both adult and cord cells give much weaker reactions after enzyme treatment, then anti-Pr should be strongly suspected (5).

Some rarities to watch for in the Ii system are reactions against joint antigens as IA, IB, IH, iH, and IP$_1$. An unusual antibody that reacts more strongly with i (cord) than adult i and more weakly with adult I has been termed anti-I^T (7). Some authors have described rare examples of anti-H and "anti-O."

Hemolysis tests

If the screening test reveals that the antibody causes lysis in vitro, semiquantitative tests may then be performed as follows.

A master series of dilutions of the patient's acidified serum (pH 6.8) is made in acidified fresh normal serum (pH 6.8). (For acidification it is convenient to add to the sera 0.1 volume of 0.2 N HCl.) Relatively large volumes should be used so that lysis may be readily visible, and it is convenient to add 1 drop of a 50% suspension of the test red cells in buffered saline to 10 drops of each dilution. It is essential that the serum dilutions and red cells be warmed to the appropriate temperature before they are mixed (20 to 25 C for cold hemolysins and 37 C for warm). Care should be taken to deliver the cell suspension directly into the serum because, if the concentrated cell suspension comes into contact with the side of the tube, this by itself may lead to lysis.

Either untreated or enzyme-treated red cells

or both are tested depending on the results of the serum screening test.

The contents of the tubes are gently remixed after incubation for 1 h, and the tubes are then centrifuged at the temperature at which they were incubated. Lysis is read visually by comparing each supernatant fluid with that in a tube containing the same serum dilution but to which no red cells have been added. For warm hemolysins, if a 37 C centrifuge is not available, lysis must be read after the cells have spontaneously sedimented. The suspensions must not be allowed to cool even momentarily, as this may be sufficient for a high-thermal-range cold antibody to bring about lysis.

Control tests comprising acidified fresh normal serum and all the test red cell samples should be set up and must show no lysis.

Antibodies capable of bringing about lysis in vitro of normal red cells at 37 C ("warm hemolysins") have seldom been detected in the sera of AIHA patients. Nevertheless, they are not unknown, and patients forming them have usually been acutely ill. In contrast to the rarity with which normal cells are lysed, enzyme-treated red cells are lysed much more frequently. It is significant that patients whose sera cause lysis of these modified cells, but not normal cells, do not necessarily suffer from a serious degree of hemolysis.

In the cold hemagglutinin disease the patient's serum is not infrequently deficient in complement and causes lysis of normal red cells only when fresh serum is added. The titration should be carried out at 20 to 25 C, and the serum and cells must be allowed to reach this temperature separately before they are mixed.

A temperature of 25 C is about optimal for the demonstration of lysis by high-titer cold antibodies. Below 15 C lysis will not take place because some complement components will not bind at these temperatures; above 28 C—depending on the thermal range of the antibody—lysis is prevented because the antibody is not adsorbed.

Serological tests in paroxysmal cold hemoglobinuria

Paroxysmal cold hemoglobinuria is the rarest form at AIHA. It can be transitory or of long standing. It is historically associated with long-standing syphilis (usually congenital) but more often accompanies other (usually viral) diseases or is "idiopathic."

Direct antiglobulin test. The same principles apply here as in cold agglutinin disease, in that the autoantibody, even though IgG, is a "cold" antibody and sensitizes in the peripheral circulation. It binds complement to the cell membrane and then elutes from the cell into the serum at 37 C. Thus, the DAT, if positive, is due to sensitization with complement components only.

Eluate. As in cold agglutinin disease, there is usually no point in making eluates from these complement-coated cells.

Serum. The autoantibody is known as the Donath-Landsteiner (DL) antibody and is classically described as biphasic in that it will sensitize cells in the cold and then hemolyze them when they are moved to 37 C in the presence of complement. This is the basis of the diagnostic test for this disease, the DL test. The antibody is of the IgG immunoglobulin class, usually agglutinating normal cells at 4 C only to low titers (e.g., less than 1:64), and usually does not sensitize cells above 15 C. We have, however, seen one exceptional case in which the antibody sensitized cells up to 32 C and caused lysis up to this temperature (19).

Specificity. The antibody has been shown almost always to have specificity within the P blood group system (i.e., anti-P). That is to say, it will react with all cells except the rare pp or P^k cells.

Donath-Landsteiner test. Serum from the patient is obtained from blood allowed to clot undisturbed at 37 C. One volume of a 50% suspension of washed normal group O, P-positive red cells is added to 9 volumes of patient's unacidified serum. The suspension is chilled in crushed ice at 0 C for 1 h and then placed in the water bath at 37 C. The tube is centrifuged after 30 min at 37 C.

Lysis visible to the naked eye indicates a positive test. In some cases this occurs within 1 min or so of warming. An additional tube containing patient's serum diluted with an equal volume of normal serum should be subjected to the same procedure to allow for the possibility that the patient's serum is deficient in complement, as it may be soon after a hemolytic attack. A further control tube, kept strictly at 37 C throughout, should show no hemolysis.

DRUG-INDUCED IMMUNE HEMOLYTIC ANEMIAS

Approximately 16% of immune hemolytic anemias are related to drug administration, and by far the most common causes are Aldomet and penicillin (4, 17). Other drug-induced hemolytic anemias occur very rarely but must be kept in mind, particularly in patients with hemolytic anemia and a positive DAT but with no detectable antibody in the serum or eluate that is reactive against normal erythrocytes (unless the appropriate drug is added to the in vitro test system).

Aldomet-induced immune hemolytic anemia

In 1966, Carstairs, Worlledge, and co-workers (2, 26) described the first positive DATs and AIHA due to the drug α-methyldopa (Aldomet). This reaction is different from any of the others described below because patients receiving this drug produce antibodies which react directly with normal red cells, even in the absence of the drug. Indeed, the antibody seems to be directed mainly against the rhesus blood group antigens. In contrast, the antibodies made by patients receiving the drugs mentioned below (except L-dopa and mefenamic acid) are directed against the drug itself and not the red cell. In such instances, the red cells are only innocent bystanders in the reaction, but nevertheless are affected as if antibody has been directed against them directly.

Two other drugs recently have been described as acting in a fashion similar to α-methyldopa. One is a closely related drug, L-dopa, which was described as causing positive DATs in about 6% of patients receiving the drug. Recently, hemolytic anemia associated with L-dopa also have been described. The other drug, mefenamic acid, is unrelated to methyldopa and has been described as causing positive DATs and AIHA.

Characteristics of methyldopa-induced abnormalities

1. The serological findings are indistinguishable in the laboratory from "idiopathic" warm-type autoimmune anemia.

2. A positive DAT is found in 15% of patients receiving methyldopa (reports vary from 10 to 36%). The incidence seems to vary between racial groups, being highest in Caucasians, lower in Chinese, and almost absent in Blacks.

3. The positive IAT is due to sensitization with IgG. One of the most distinctive aspects of the serological results in patients with Aldomet-induced hemolytic anemia is the fact that the DAT titration score (see above, section on antiglobulin test titrations and scores) is extraordinarily high with anti-IgG antiglobulin serum and negative with anti-complement serum. This combination of results occurs very uncommonly in AIHA not associated with Aldomet administration.

4. The DAT usually becomes positive after 3 to 6 months of treatment. (It is interesting to note that this delay is not shortened when a patient who previously exhibited a positive test is restarted on the drug.)

5. The development of the positive DAT appears to be dose-dependent. About three times as many patients (36%) have positive tests when taking more than 2 g of the drug daily compared with 11% of patients taking less than 1 g daily; 19% become positive on 1 to 2 g daily.

6. Various reports indicate that from 0 to 5% of patients receiving methyldopa have hemolytic anemia. The cumulative incidence is 0.8%.

7. The positive direct antiglobulin reaction gradually becomes negative once methyldopa is stopped. This may take from 1 month to 2 years. Fortunately, the clinical and hematological values improve much more rapidly, usually within 1 to 3 weeks.

In conclusion, α-methyldopa is one of the most common causes of a positive DAT due to drugs. The total of methyldopa-induced AIHA exceeds the total of all other drug-induced immune hemolytic anemias so far described. Thus, the laboratory evaluation of Aldomet-induced hemolytic anemia is identical to that for warm antibody AIHA described above. Final proof that Aldomet is responsible for causing hemolytic anemia can only be obtained clinically by stopping Aldomet administration and observing resolution of the hemolysis.

Penicillin-induced hemolytic anemia

In 1958, Ley et al. (14) first reported the presence of circulating penicillin antibody. In the course of routine blood bank testing, a serum was encountered which agglutinated the red cells of 25 group O members of an antibody identification panel. This panel had been stored in a preservative solution containing penicillin. The same panel, with no penicillin present, did not react with the serum. In the paper, a patient was described who had developed a positive DAT and hemolytic anemia after receiving penicillin. In 1966, Petz and Fudenberg (15) defined the role of penicillin in causing immune hemolytic anemia.

Penicillin is one of the few drugs which binds firmly to proteins. Penicillin will combine with the protein on normal red cell membranes both in vivo and in vitro. The drug cannot be removed even by multiple washes in saline. This means that one very easily can "sensitize" cells with penicillin in the laboratory and then use these treated cells for the detection of penicillin antibodies. This is in contrast to most other drugs, where it is not possible to prepare drug-coated cells for antibody detection.

Considerable experimental work has demonstrated that the immunogenicity of penicillin is due to its ability to react chemically with tissue proteins to form several different heptenic groups. The major haptenic determinant is the benzylpenicilloyl (BPO) group. It is not yet clear whether the BPO group is formed by the direct reaction of penicillin with amino groups of protein, or through the intermediate formation of benzylpenicillenic acid.

Penicillin can be detected on the red cell membranes of all patients receiving high doses of penicillin.

If a sensitive technique is used, about 90% of unselected sera can be shown to contain penicillin (BPO) antibodies (1, 13). Most sera contain IgM antibodies alone (approximately 80%); approximately 13% contain IgG antibodies as well. The high percentage of penicillin antibodies in the normal population is probably due to continual exposure to penicillin in our modern environment. The titer of such normal antibodies is usually less than 1:50, whereas titers greater than 1:1,000 are usually found in patients with penicillin-induced hemolytic anemia.

Approximately 3% of patients receiving massive doses of intravenous penicillin will develop a positive DAT. A small percentage of these will develop hemolytic anemia. The mechanism of the positive DAT and hemolytic anemia seems clear. The drug is adsorbed to the red cells, and an immune antibody, i.e., anti-penicillin, is produced by the patient and will react with the penicillin on the red cells. The end product, therefore, is a red cell sensitized with IgG.

Complement is not usually involved in this reaction, and no intravascular hemolysis occurs. The red cells are destroyed extravascularly by the reticuloendothelial system, probably in the same way as rhesus (IgG) sensitized cells.

The essentials for penicillin-induced immune hemolytic anemia are

1. Administration of large doses of penicillin (in the order of more than 20×10^6 units per day).
2. High-titer IgG penicillin antibody present in serum.
3. Strongly positive DAT, due to sensitization with IgG.
4. Antibody eluted from patient's red cells will react against penicillin-treated normal red cells.

The last point is very important. If investigations are being performed to elucidate the cause of a positive DAT, then eluates from the red cells should always be prepared. If an eluate prepared from cells strongly sensitized with IgG does not react against normal red cells, then a drug-induced phenomenon should be strongly suspected. This is particularly true if no antibody activity against normal red cells is present in the serum. If the patient is found to be receiving penicillin, then it is a simple matter to treat some cells with penicillin and test the eluate with these cells. If a reaction is obtained with the penicillin-treated cells, but no reaction occurs with the same cells untreated with the drug, then the answer is clear; the positive DAT is due to sensitization with a penicillin antibody.

The only other drugs which will attach firmly to red cells and cause a positive DAT by the same mechanism as penicillin are cephalothin and possibly carbromal. Cephalothin has been described as a rare cause of immune hemolytic anemia but, so far, carbromal has not.

Detection of antibodies to penicillin (and cephalosporins)

Preparation of penicillin-sensitized cells (22).

1. Wash group O cells (preferably fresh) three times in saline.
2. Add 10^6 units (approximately 600 mg) of potassium benzyl penicillin G dissolved in 15 ml of pH 9.6 barbital buffer to 1 ml of packed washed cells. (In the original publication, T.M.A. buffer was used, but this has rather an obnoxious smell; barbital buffer [pH 9.6] has been found to be satisfactory for routine use. Sodium barbital, 0.1 M [20.6 g/liter], is adjusted to pH 9.6 with 0.1 N HCl [approximately 15 ml].)
3. Incubate for 1 h at room temperature with gentle mixing.
4. Wash cells three times in saline.

Slight lysis may occur during incubation, and a small "clot" may form in the red cells which can be removed with applicator sticks before washing cells. Once prepared, the cells may be kept in ACD at 4 C for up to 1 week, but they do deteriorate slowly during this time.

Preparation of cephalothin (Keflin)-coated cells (22).

1. Wash group O cells (preferably fresh) three times in saline.
2. Add 40 mg of Keflin dissolved in 10 ml of pH 9.6 barbital buffer to 1 ml of washed packed cells.
3. Incubate at 37 C for 2 h with gentle mixing.
4. Wash cells three times in saline.

Detection of antibodies to penicillin and Keflin. For titrations of large numbers of sera, the following method of Levine and co-workers (12) is convenient:

1. Prepare serial dilutions of patient's sera in a special diluent [50 ml of pH 8.2 tris(hydroxymethyl)aminomethane buffer + 25 ml of 6% dextran + 1 ml of normal rabbit serum, which has been absorbed with penicillin and Keflin-treated cells].

2. Add to 0.2 ml of each dilution 1 drop (approximately 0.03 ml) of 2% antibiotic-"coated" cells suspended in the same diluent.

3. Mix and incubate at room temperature for 1 h.

4. Centrifuge in a Serofuge for 1 min and read macroscopically for agglutination. This method detects both IgM and IgG antibodies.

The Levine method is a sensitive method but rather impractical for those who only occasionally investigate a penicillin- or Keflin-induced positive DAT. It is recommended that, in such cases, standard saline agglutination and IATs be employed on the patient's serum and eluate as follows:

1. If the patient has a positive DAT and penicillin is suspected as the cause, then an eluate should be prepared by a standard method (see above, section on preparation of eluate from patient's red cells).

2. The eluate and the patient's serum should be tested against normal group O cells and the same cells treated with penicillin. Usually, serial dilutions of the patient's serum are tested.

3. Two volumes of eluate or serum dilutions should be incubated in saline with 1 volume of a 2% suspension of penicillin-treated and untreated group O cells.

4. Incubate at room temperature for 15 min; centrifuge and inspect for agglutination.

5. Move tubes to 37 C for 30 min; centrifuge and inspect for agglutination.

6. Wash cells four times in saline.

7. Add antiglobulin serum to the button of washed cells; centrifuge; inspect for agglutination.

IgM penicillin antibodies will agglutinate saline-suspended penicillin-treated cells but not the same cells untreated. (It should be noted that Levine's method is more sensitive for the detection of IgM antibodies.) IgG penicillin antibodies will react by the IAT against penicillin-treated cells but not against the same cells untreated. The IAT is equal in sensitivity to Levine's method in the detection of serum IgG antibodies, and is superior when testing eluates from red cells of patients with positive DATs.

If IATs are used to detect Keflin antibodies, it must be remembered that Keflin-treated red cells can absorb proteins nonimmunologically. Therefore, all normal sera will give a positive IAT if incubated with Keflin-treated cells for a long enough period. The reaction does not usu-

ally occur once the normal serum is diluted to more than 1:20. The amount of protein present in red cell eluates does not seem to be enough to give nonspecific results, so a positive result usually indicates the presence of antibody to Keflin or a cross-reacting penicillin antibody.

Other drug-induced immune hemolytic anemias

Table 7 lists most of the drugs known to cause a positive DAT.

Shulman (21) proposed a mechanism which is accepted by most investigators as the most probable explanation for the reactions seen with all of the drugs mentioned in Table 7, except penicillin, cephalosporin, α-methyldopa, L-dopa, and possibly carbromal. He showed that drugs such as quinine, quinidine, and stibophen have a far stronger affinity for their respective antibodies than for cell membranes. Such drugs when present together with antibody in the patient's plasma will combine to form an immune complex which may be absorbed to the cell membrane, often activating complement in the process. It is unknown why this immune complex, once formed, sometimes causes red cell destruction only and other times platelet destruction only.

The patient usually presents with acute intravascular hemolysis, with hemoglobinemia and hemoglobinuria. Renal failure is frequent. The patient need only take a small quantity of the drug to precipitate these reactions.

The serum antidrug antibody is often IgM and capable of activating complement. The DAT is positive often due to the presence of complement components on the red cell surface, usually without detectable immunoglobulins. This may be explained by the fact that the immune complex does not bind very firmly to the red cells and may dissociate from the cells and be free to react with other cells. This in turn may explain why such a small amount of drug complex can cause so much red cell destruction. Furthermore, red cell sensitization by IgM antibodies is not readily detectable by the antiglobulin test (3). Some reports of negative DATs, particularly in the earlier literature, may be due to inadequate anticomplement properties of the antiglobulin serum. In vitro reactions (agglutination, lysis, and/or sensitization to antiglobulin sera) are usually only observed when the patient's serum, drug, and red cells are all incubated together.

Detection of other drug-related antibodies. In a patient with immune hemolytic anemia whose serum and red cell eluate does not react with normal red cells, and who is receiving drugs, antibodies reactive with red cells in the

Table 7. *Drugs that have been reported to cause positive direct antiglobulin tests and hemolytic anemia*

Stibophen (Fuadin)
Quinidine
p-Aminosalicylic acid
Quinine
Phenacetin
Penicillins (penicillin G, ampicillin, methicillin)
Chlorinated hydrocarbon-containing insecticides (toxaphene, heptachlor, dieldrin)[a]
Antihistamine (antistin, antazoline)[a]
Sulfonamides (sulfapyridine, sulfamethazine, sulfasomidine, sulfisoxazole)
Isonicotinic acid hydrazine (isoniazid, INH)
Chlorpromazine (Thorazine)[a]
Aminopyrine (Pyramidon)[a]
Dipyrone[a]
α-Methyldopa (Aldomet)
Melphalan (Alkeran)[a]
Cephalosporins (cephalothin, cephaloridine,[b] cephalexin,[b] cefazolin[b])
Mefenamic acid (Ponstel, Ponstan)
Carbromal (Carbrital)[a,b]
Sulphonylureas (chlorpropamide, tolbutamide)
Insulin[a]
Levodopa
Rifampin
Tetracycline

[a] Single report in literature.
[b] Drugs having been reported to cause direct antiglobulin tests but not hemolytic anemia.

presence of the drug should be sought. Methods used vary widely, and for drugs in Table 7 the original method should be utilized. (References to original descriptions of these methods are in reviews [4, 17].)

In addition, the following should be done in instances in which the originally described method gives negative results or for drugs not previously shown to cause hemolytic anemia.

A trial and error approach is recommended. The patient's serum and eluate should be tested against normal untreated and enzyme-treated red cells in the presence of dilutions of the drugs which the patient is receiving. Dilutions should be made starting with a saturated solution and progressing to a physiological dilution of the drug (i.e., average dose of drug circulating per millimeter of blood). The mixtures are usually incubated at 37 C for 1 to 2 h, but one should consider extending these incubation times if negative results are obtained. A duplicate set of tubes with the addition of fresh normal serum (i.e., complement) is also recommended. The tubes are then inspected for agglutination, hemolysis, and sensitization to antiglobulin sera. If no reactions are obtained, an attempt should be made to pretreat the red cells with the drug as in the penicillin techniques.

LITERATURE CITED

1. Abraham, G. N., L. D. Petz, and H. H. Fudenberg. 1968. Immunohaematological cross-allergenicity between penicillin and cephalothin in humans. Clin. Exp. Immunol. 3:343–357.
2. Carstairs, K. C., A. Breckenridge, C. T. Dollery, and S. M. Worlledge. 1966. Incidence of a positive direct Coombs' test in patients on α-methyldopa. Lancet 2:133–135.
3. Garratty, G., and L. D. Petz. 1971. An evaluation of commercial antiglobulin sera with particular reference to their anticomplement properties. Transfusion (Philadelphia) 11:79–88.
4. Garratty, G., and L. D. Petz. 1975. Drug-induced immune hemolytic anemia. Am. J. Med. 58:398–407.
5. Garratty, G., L. D. Petz, I. Brodsky, and H. H. Fudenberg. 1973. An IgA high-titer cold agglutinin with an unusual blood group specificity within the Pr complex. Vox Sang. 25:32–38.
6. Garratty, G., L. D. Petz, and J. K. Hoops. 1973. The correlation of cold agglutinin titrations in saline and albumin with hemolytic anemia. Transfusion (Philadelphia) 13:363.
7. Garratty, G., L. D. Petz, R. O. Wallerstein, and H. H. Fudenberg. 1974. Autoimmune hemolytic anemia in Hodgkin's disease associated with anti-I[T]. Transfusion (Philadelphia) 14:226–231.
8. Gilliland, B. C., E. Baxter, and R. S. Evans. 1971. Red-cell antibodies in acquired hemolytic anemia with negative antiglobulin serum tests. N. Engl. J. Med. 285:252–256.
9. Hughes-Jones, N. C., B. Gardner, and R. Telford. 1963. Comparison of various methods of dissociation of anti-D, using ¹³¹I-labelled antibody. 1963. Vox Sang. 8:531–536.
10. Kochwa, S., and R. E. Rosenfield. 1964. Immunochemical studies of the Rh system. I. Isolation and characterization of antibodies. J. Immunol. 92:682–692.
11. Landsteiner, K., and C. P. Miller. 1925. Serological studies on the blood of primates. II. The blood groups in antropoid apes. J. Exp. Med. 42:853–862.
12. Levine, B. B., M. J. Fellner, and V. Levytska. 1966. Benzylpenicilloyl-specific serum antibodies to penicillin in man. I. Development of a sensitive hemagglutination assay method and haptenic specificities of antibodies. J. Immunol. 96:707–718.
13. Levine, B. B., M. J. Fellner, V. Levytska, E. D. Franklin, and N. Alisberg. 1966. Benzylpenicilloyl-specific serum antibodies to penicillin in man. II. Sensitivity of the hemagglutination assay method, molecular classes of the antibodies detected, and antibody titers of randomly selected patients. J. Immunol. 96:719–726.
14. Ley, A. B., J. P. Harris, M. Brinkley, B. Liles, J. A. Jack, and A. Cahan. 1958. Circulating antibody directed against penicillin. Science 127:1118–1119.

15. Petz, L. D., and H. H. Fudenberg. 1966. Coombs-positive hemolytic anemia caused by penicillin administration. N. Engl. J. Med. **274:**171–178.

16. Petz, L. D., and G. Garratty. 1974. Complement in immunohematology. Prog. Clin. Immunol. **2:**175–190.

17. Petz, L. D., and G. Garratty. 1975. Drug-induced haemolytic anaemia. Clin. Haematol. **4:**181–197.

18. Petz, L. D., and G. Garratty. 1975. Laboratory correlations in immune hemolytic anemias, p. 139–153. *In* G. Vyas, D. P. Stites, and G. Brecker (ed.), Laboratory diagnosis of immunologic disorders. Grune & Stratton, New York.

19. Ries, C. A., G. Garratty, L. D. Petz, and H. H. Fudenberg. 1971. Paroxysmal cold hemoglobinuria: report of a case with an exceptionally high thermal range Donath-Landsteiner antibody. Blood **38:**491–499.

20. Rubin, H. 1963. Antibody elution from red cells. J. Clin. Pathol. **16:**70–73.

21. Shulman, N. R. 1964. A mechanism of cell destruction in individuals sensitized to foreign antigens and its implications in autoimmunity. Ann. Intern. Med. **60:**506–521.

22. Spath, P., G. Garratty, and L. D. Petz. 1971. Studies on the immune responses to penicillin and cephalothin in humans. I. Optimal conditions for titration of hemagglutinating penicillin and cephalothin antibodies. J. Immunol. **107:**854–859.

23. Vos, G. H., L. D. Petz, and H. H. Fudenberg. 1970. Specificity of acquired haemolytic anaemia autoantibodies and their serological characteristics. Br. J. Haematol. **19:**57–66.

24. Vos, G. H., L. D. Petz, and H. H. Fudenberg. 1971. Specificity and immunoglobulin characteristics of autoantibodies in acquired hemolytic anemia. J. Immunol. **106:**1172–1176.

25. Vos, G. H., L. D. Petz, G. Garratty, and H. H. Fudenberg. 1973. Autoantibodies in acquired hemolytic anemia with special reference to the LW system. Blood **42:**445–453.

26. Worlledge, S. M., K. C. Carstairs, and J. V. Dacie. 1966. Autoimmune haemolytic anaemia associated with alphamethyldopa therapy. Lancet **2:**135–139.

Chapter 73

Immunology of Inhibitors to Clotting Factors

PHILIP M. BLATT AND HAROLD R. ROBERTS

INTRODUCTION

The mechanism of blood coagulation is still not completely understood. Nevertheless, many of the blood clotting factors have been purified and chemically characterized. In addition, the general interactions of the various clotting components have been elucidated. To introduce the reader to the general concept of blood coagulation, a list of the blood clotting factors, their synonyms, in vivo half life, molecular weight, and associated diseases are shown in Table 1. A simplified version of the blood clotting reactions is shown in Fig. 1.

The purpose of this report is to review the presently available information concerning the immunology of acquired circulating inhibitors that are directed against plasma procoagulants. Reviews of this subject have been published recently by Feinstein and Rapaport (35), Roberts et al. (103), Bidwell (9), and Shapiro and Hultin (115).

Recent advances in technology have permitted immunochemical characterization of many of the inhibitors. Whereas the pathogenesis of these inhibitors has not been completely worked out, there are some hints that might be exploited in the future. Furthermore, the human inhibitors have been used to study some of the properties of certain procoagulants, and the results of such studies will be covered in this review where appropriate.

ACQUIRED INHIBITORS TO FACTOR I (FIBRINOGEN)

Acquired inhibitors specific for fibrinogen are rare but have been reported in patients with congenital afibrinogenemia (9, 18, 30, 87) and in otherwise normal persons (85, 108). As yet there is no unequivocal evidence that antifibrinogen inhibitors have occurred in patients with abnormal fibrinogens. With one exception, the antibody nature of the fibrinogen inhibitors has not been well established, but the evidence is suggestive that such is so. In one case (18) the patient's plasma reacted with red cells coated with fibrinogen, and in another the life span of transfused fibrinogen was short (30).

Rosenberg et al. (108) have described an antibody directed against the cross-linking sites on the fibrinogen-fibrin molecule. This patient had been taking isoniazid when the inhibitor was discovered, and it was shown that the inhibitor could be neutralized in vitro by heterologous antisera raised against human immunoglobulin G (IgG). This case is particularly interesting since the antibody had no inhibitory effect on factor XIII and did not inhibit the rate of fibrin monomer formation.

Shainoff and Braun (111) reported that, by injecting relatively pure fibrinogen in rabbits, antifibrinogen antibodies could be raised. These antibodies could then be highly purified by precipitating them in combination with fibrinogen. By redissolving the complex and salting out at pH 2.4, relatively pure antifibrinogen antibodies were obtained. The ground work is thus available for characterization and purification of the human antifibrinogen inhibitors by use of immunochemical techniques.

Infusion of fibrinogen into patients with antifibrinogen inhibitors has been associated with severe anaphylaxis, and caution is indicated when and if fibrinogen therapy is necessary for such patients. The occurrence of anaphylaxis in some afibrinogenemic patients with inhibitors suggests that such inhibitors are indeed antibodies.

Laboratory diagnosis

In the case of Rosenberg et al. (108), the inhibitor was found to block cross-linking sites on the fibrin molecule. The detection of this inhibitor required demonstration of clot dissolution in 1% monochloroacetic acid, and delayed γ and α chain cross-linking, required for stabilization of the fibrin clot. The inhibitor was shown to be of the IgG class since antisera against IgG neutralized the inhibitor.

ACQUIRED INHIBITORS TO FACTOR II (PROTHROMBIN)

Hereditary prothrombin "deficiency" is the rarest of the inherited coagulation disorders (110). In fact, it is likely that prothrombin is not actually "deficient" but rather present in a

TABLE 1. *Nomenclature and properties of the blood clotting factors*

Factor	Synonym	Half-life	Mol wt	Disease
I	Fibrinogen	3.3–5.6 days	340,000	Afibrinogenemia Dysfibrinogenemia
II	Prothrombin	55–80 h	68,000	Dysprothrombinemia
III	Tissue thromboplastin			None
IV	Calcium			None
V	Accelerator-globulin, AC globulin, Labile factor Proaccelerin	36 h	≈400,000	Parahemophilia Factor V deficiency
VII	Stable factor Proconvertin Autoprothrombin I Serum prothrombin converting accelera- tor	3–5.5 h	63,000	Factor VII deficiency
VIII	Antihemophilic factor (AHF) Antihemophilic globu- lin (AHG) Thromboplastinogen	10–12 h	1.2×10^6	Classic hemophilia Von Willebrand's disease[a]
IX	Plasma thromboplastin component (PTC) Christmas factor Autoprothrombin II	24–31 h	72,000	Christmas disease PTC deficiency
X	Stuart factor	42 h	55,000	Factor X deficiency Stuart's disease
XI	Plasma thromboplastin antecedent (PTA)	40–84 h	160,000	PTA deficiency Factor XI deficiency
XII	Hageman factor	54 h	140,000	Factor XII deficiency
XIII	Fibrin stabilizing factor (FSF)	4–6 days (estimated)	320,000	Factor XIII deficiency

[a] Associated with long bleeding time, decreased platelet adhesiveness, and autosomal dominant inheritance.

structurally altered form. Affected patients have minimal bleeding problems and consequently require infrequent transfusions. It is not surprising, therefore, that specific inhibitors to prothrombin have not been described in patients afflicted with congenital hypoprothrombinemia. Specific decreases in prothrombin activity have been well documented in systemic lupus erythematosus, as will be described in a later section.

ACQUIRED INHIBITORS TO FACTOR V

In 1972, Fratantoni et al. (43) reported a patient who was congenitally deficient in factor V

and developed an antifactor V antibody. This is the only such case reported to date. The antibody was of the IgG class. Its activity increased over 20 min with incubation at 37 C. When the patient's antifactor V antibody decreased to undetectable levels in vivo, the patient's plasma was allowed to react with the specific antifactor V antibody which had been partially purified. Under these circumstances it was noted that the patient's plasma did not neutralize the antibody. Thus, the patient's plasma had no detectable material capable of cross-reacting with the antibody. On this basis, the authors classified the patient's plasma as being cross-reacting

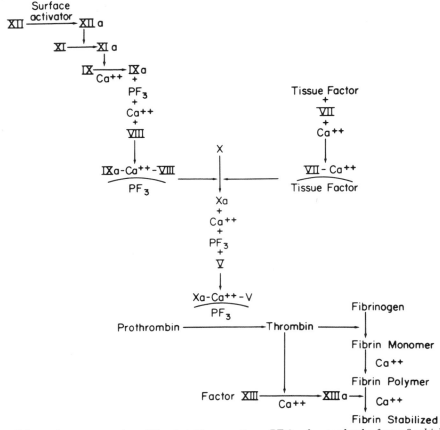

FIG. 1. *Schematic representation of blood clotting reactions. PF-3 refers to platelet factor 3 which presumably provides a phospholipid surface for the reactions to take place.*

material-negative, i.e., CRM−, suggesting that the factor V deficiency was due to absence of factor V molecules or to the presence of molecules structurally altered to the extent that they did not cross-react with the antifactor V antibody. Feinstein et al. (39) and Crowell (26), using a human antifactor V antibody from a patient *without* congenital factor V deficiency, had previously found three factor V deficient patients to be CRM−.

Approximately 10 antifactor V antibodies have apparently arisen spontaneously in patients without known prior coagulation abnormalities (26, 38, 39, 40, 56, 77, 91, 120). Most of the inhibitors arose in the postoperative period in patients who had received blood products and antibiotics. The antibiotic most commonly associated with the inhibitor was streptomycin, with Keflin, penicillin, and chloramphenicol being less frequent. The antifactor V inhibitor associated with Keflin administration (91) was an IgG. This case is interesting in view of re-

cent data presented by Raccuglia and Waterman (97). These authors were attempting to document that the powder form of Keflin would prevent wound infections. While carrying out their study, they noted unexpected hemorrhage from the wound surface. They subsequently showed in vitro that a blood concentration of Keflin greater than 11 mg/ml inhibited factor V. The factor V inhibitors which have been immunologically studied were all of the Ig class (26, 38, 39, 40, 56, 91, 120). Three of these antibodies were heterogeneous as to light chain types; i.e., both kappa and lambda light chains were detected by immunological techniques (26, 38, 39).

The degree of bleeding associated with antifactor V inhibitors is variable, but usually has not resulted in life-threatening hemorrhage. All of the inhibitors occurring in patients without previous clotting abnormalities have been transient, lasting no longer than a few months. Some investigators have advocated treatment with immunosuppressive therapy, but it appears that appropriate treatment entails cessation of all possible offending agents and the use cf general supportive measures.

Laboratory diagnosis

The inhibitor can be detected by clotting tests. In factor V deficiency both the prothrombin and partial thromboplastin times are prolonged. However, these tests can be corrected by the addition of normal plasma. When an inhibitor is present in the patient's plasma, however, the inhibitor will neutralize factor V in normal plasma such that the correcting effect of normal plasma on the prothrombin and partial thromboplastin times will not be observed (Table 2). Similarly, when patients' plasma (diluted appropriately) is added to normal plasma, the factor V content of normal plasma will be decreased whereas other procoagulant levels will be normal. This type of test, shown in Table 3, is used to show the specificity of an inhibitor.

To show that the factor V inhibitor is an Ig, heterologous antisera to human Ig can be raised. If the inhibitor is human Ig, specific heterologous antisera, when mixed with plasma containing the inhibitor, should precipitate the human inhibitor, permitting removal by centrifugation. Thus the supernatant plasma should be free from inhibitor. An example is given in Table 4.

FACTOR VII INHIBITORS

Specific antibodies to factor VII have not been shown to exist.

FACTOR VIII INHIBITORS

Factor VIII inhibitors arise in 5 to 10% of patients with severe classic hemophilia (11, 17, 64), rarely in patients with mild to moderate hemophilia A (7, 25, 71, 123), and in patients with a number of other conditions including (35, 47, 53, 70, 86, 101, 106, 112): middle and older aged people with no other associated illness; postpartum females; allergic reactions to drugs (especially penicillin and sulfa); collagen vascular diseases (especially systemic lupus erythematosus and rheumatoid arthritis); exfoliative skin disease; inflammatory bowel disease; neoplasms; and patients with paraproteins.

It has been established that antifactor VIII inhibitors are antibodies (2, 5, 10, 13, 37, 73, 75, 81, 96, 106, 114, 117). The interaction of factor VIII with the factor VIII antibody is time, temperature, and pH dependent (73). With the exceptions of the antifactor V antibodies de-

TABLE 2. *Clotting tests for detection of an inhibitor to factor V*

Sample	Pro-thrombin time (s)	Partial thromboplastin time (s)
Normal plasma	12.0	40
Factor V deficient plasma without inhibitor[a]	40	180
Factor V deficient plasma with inhibitor[b]	54.2	180
Mixture of inhibitor plasma with normal plasma	25	60
Mixture of factor V deficient plasma without inhibitor with normal plasma	13.0	45

[a] Notice that clotting studies on factor V deficient plasma with and without inhibitor are similar. Only on mixing inhibitor plasma with normal plasma can the inhibitor be detected.

[b] Assume an inhibitor titer as determined by dilution tests to be about 1:16 to 1:32.

TABLE 3. *Specificity of inhibitor to factor V[a]*

Factor	Percentage of normal control
II	100
V	<1
VII	100
X	100

[a] Inhibitor: inhibitor plasma plus normal plasma.

scribed by Fratantoni et al. (43), Feinstein et al. (39), and Crowell (26), no other antibodies to coagulation factors possess these characteristics. Practically speaking, to detect low to moderate levels of antibodies, incubation of the antibody with factor VIII at 37 C for at least 2 h (112) is required before activity of the antibody can be appreciated in vitro.

Early studies which supported the assumption that factor VIII inhibitors were antibodies included those of Leitner et al. (73), who showed that the factor VIII inhibitors could be completely saturated by a sufficient quantity of factor VIII. Roberts et al. (106), using hemagglutination and hemagglutination-inhibition techniques, obtained data suggesting the factor VIII inhibitor was an antibody. Bidwell et al. (10) conclusively showed that rabbit antihuman IgG neutralized the antifactor VIII inhibitor and therefore definitely established the immune nature of such inhibitors.

In 1967, Shapiro (112) demonstrated that the factor VIII inhibitors in his patients were highly restricted in immunochemical composition. By studying three patients (patients with

TABLE 4. *Immunochemical characterization of a factor V inhibitor*[a]

Heterologous antiserum	Expected residual factor V (%)	Presence of inhibitor
Antihuman IgG	100	−
Antihuman IgA	<1	+
Antihuman IgM	<1	+
Control (heated adsorbed normal rabbit serum)[b]	101	

[a] In this experiment, the following conditions obtained:

1. Inhibitor plasma is mixed with specific heterologous antisera and incubated in the cold at 4 C for 18 h. The precipitate is centrifuged and the supernatant fluid is used in step 2 below.

2. Supernatant plasma is mixed 1:1 with normal plasma and the percent residual factor V is measured. The amount of factor V remaining is directly proportioned to the amount of inhibitor neutralized.

3. In this experiment, it is apparent that heterologous IgG antisera neutralized the factor V inhibitor. Hence, the factor V inhibitor is of the IgG class.

[b] When using normal rabbit serum as a control, it must be heated at 56 C for 1 h and adsorbed with $Al(OH)_3$ or $BaSO_4$ to remove clotting factors and nonspecific inhibitors (93).

factor VIII inhibitors associated with hemophilia A, the postpartum state, and ulcerative colitis, respectively), he found the antibodies to consist of IgG heavy chains and only kappa light chains. The antigen-antibody interaction was felt to be a first-order reaction consistent with one to one stoichiometry.

As recently summarized by Barrow and Graham (6), Shapiro (113), and Shapiro and Hultin (115), the human factor VIII antibodies which have been characterized have been of the class IgG (5, 37, 96, 101, 112–114) with rare exceptions. Lusher et al. (81) described a child with classical hemophilia with a low-molecular-weight IgM antibody and, in addition, an IgG antibody. McKelvey and Kwaan (83) described a 63-year-old man with a 2-year history of arthralgia and Raynaud's phenomenon whose factor VIII antibody consisted of IgM globulins. Castaldi and Penny (19) described a 49-year-old female with Waldenstrom's macroglobulinemia with a monoclonal IgM protein with specific activity against factor VIII. Finally, Glueck and Hong (47) described a patient with IgA myeloma and a factor VIII inhibitor consisting of IgA heavy chains. This inhibitor could be adsorbed from the patient's plasma with heterologous IgA antiserum.

Most of the IgG factor VIII antibodies are restricted to the IgG_4 sublcass (5, 6, 101, 113,

116). Light chain subtyping has revealed both kappa and lambda light chains or only one of the two (5, 6, 81, 101, 116, 119). When only one type of light chain was present, the kappa type was found more often than the lambda light chain, as would be expected if the light chains occurred at random. As is true of other antigen-antibody reactions, it has been clearly shown that the factor VIII antibody binding sites reside on the Fab fragment (37, 116).

In addition to their obvious clinical importance, homologous and heterologous antifactor VIII antibodies have become important tools in helping to further the understanding of the molecular defect in hemophilia A. Early reports implied that the defect of hemophilia A was due to the lack of production of the factor VIII molecule, since severely affected patients showed no in vitro procoagulant activity. This concept was first challenged by a report that the plasma of a hemophilia A patient neutralized the capacity of rabbit antiserum to inhibit factor VIII activity (J. N. Shanberge and I. Gore, J. Lab. Clin. Invest. 50:954, 1957). As reviewed by Barrow and Graham (6), Ratnoff and Bennett (98), Hoyer (62), and Hershgold (58), this report has been repeatedly confirmed. The percentage of hemophilia A plasmas containing material that cross-reacts with specific *human* antibody (which neutralizes factor VIII coagulant activity but does not precipitate) has been reported to be about 10%. Conversely, when *animal* antibodies, specifically rabbit (which precipitate factor VIII antigen), are raised to human factor VIII, it has been shown that virtually all hemophilia A plasmas contain cross-reacting material. The nature of the antigenic material in hemophilia A patients detected by the animal antibody is unclear, but Ratnoff and Bennett (98) and Stites et al. (121) suggested that hemophilia A patients synthesize an abnormal factor VIII molecule which is devoid of functional clotting activity but maintains recognizable antigenic sites.

In addition to enhancing our understanding of the disease, the discovery of Shanberge and Gore (J. Lab. Clin. Invest. 50:954, 1957) is now being applied to carrier detection studies. It is recognized that only 25 to 35% of female carriers will have a subnormal level of factor VIII procoagulant activity. Since female carriers of hemophilia A carry only one abnormal X chromosome, one would expect, on the basis of the Lyon hypothesis, that such carriers would have about 50% factor VIII activity as measured by clotting tests. On the other hand, immunological assays using heteroantisera should reveal normal levels of factor VIII. In fact, Zimmerman et al. (127), Bennett and Ratnoff (8), Hoyer

(62), and Denson (28) have found this to be the case and believe that they can predict the carrier state in 75 to 90% of females—a striking increase from the 25 to 35% figure previously possible.

The kinetics of the interaction of the factor VIII molecule with the human antifactor VIII antibody is variable and complex. As previously noted, the reaction of factor VIII antigen with its factor VIII antibody is time, temperature, and pH dependent (112) as measured by neutralization of factor VIII clotting activity. The kinetics of this reaction appear to follow one of two different patterns (3). The first pattern has the characteristics of a second-order reaction (3, 4, 13, 94). In this reaction there is initial rapid loss of activity followed by a plateau of factor VIII activity occurring in 2 to 4 h. Many authors believe that these second-order reactions are attributable to the formation of stable antigen-antibody complexes (12, 53, 112). This type of reaction generally occurs with antibodies incubated with the human factor VIII molecule, although Allain and Frommel (3) also noted second-order kinetics when they caused human factor VIII antibodies to react with porcine factor VIII.

The second type of reaction is more complex (65). It, too, demonstrates an initial rapid destruction of factor VIII, but this is followed by a continuing slow decline of factor VIII activity rather than by a plateau effect. Allain and Frommel (3) found that the antigen-antibody complexes which demonstrated this kinetic reaction were easily dissociable, probably because of weaker antigen-antibody interaction. To complicate matters further, these same authors found that, upon treatment, hemophiliacs may develop a heterogeneous population of antibodies which possess dissimilar kinetic properties.

After initial sensitization, repeated stimulation by factor VIII can produce an anamnestic rise in the factor VIII antibody titer. The increase in antibody titer begins 3 to 7 days after the antigenic stimulus, peaks in 10 to 20 days, and then declines or stabilizes over the ensuing months. Those patients whose antibodies react in this manner are said to be high responders, whereas those who demonstrate little or no anamnestic response are low responders. Allain and Frommel (in preparation) studied 10 older hemophiliac patients who developed antibodies after a long cumulative exposure to factor VIII; all were initially low responders and have remained low responders. Kasper (64), Strauss (123), and we have had a somewhat different experience, since some patients who were initially low responders have become high

responders, and a long cumulative exposure and initial low response to factor VIII is not always correlated with a continuing low responder state.

Although most nonhemophiliacs with spontaneous factor VIII antibodies are low responders, it is unclear which patients with hemophilia A will fall into this category.

Finally, brief comment is warranted concerning inhibitors developing in patients with von Willebrand's disease. Sarji et al. (109), with a modification of the ristocetin assay (54, 55, 109) initially described by Howard and Firkin (61), found an inhibitor directed against the putative *von Willebrand factor* in a severely affected patient who had received multiple transfusions. Evidence that the inhibitor is directed against the von Willebrand factor included the observation that, as the amount of inhibitor was increased in the test system, the level of ristocetin-induced platelet aggregation decreased. In the presence of even higher titers of inhibitor, the ristocetin-induced aggregation could be totally inhibited. Moreover, the inhibitor did not inhibit adenosine diphosphate, epinephrine, or collagen induced platelet aggregation. Finally, when the patients' platelets were exposed to the inhibitor and then washed, they remained fully susceptible to aggregation by ristocetin. Additionally, platelet "adsorption" did not reduce the titer of the inhibitor. These latter two bits of information suggest that the inhibitor is not directed against the platelet membrane.

The inhibitor is heat stable at 56 C for 30 min and is stable to freezing and thawing. Recent data from our institution and from others (R. I. Handin and W. C. Moloney, Blood 44:933, 1975) suggest that the inhibitor to the von Willebrand factor is an IgG.

Laboratory diagnosis

In a patient with classical hemophilia with a high-titer inhibitor, inhibitory activity can be detected by mixing the patient's plasma and normal plasma and performing a partial thromboplastin time on the mixture. Instead of correcting the hemophilic defect as normal plasma usually does, the inhibitor in the patient's plasma will result in a prolonged partial thromboplastin time, usually at least 30 s longer than the control. This is illustrated in Table 5. Since specific inhibitors to factor VIII are time and temperature dependent, the *immediate* mix may not detect the inhibitor, especially if the inhibitor is present in low titer. Rather, the mixture of normal plasma and hemophilic plasma may have to be incubated for 1 to 2 h at 37 C before the inhibitor can be detected. The

TABLE 5. *Detection of a circulating inhibitor in plasma from a classical hemophiliac*

Sample	PTT[a] (s)
Normal plasma	60
Hemophilic plasma	250
Normal plasma plus hemophilic plasma (without inhibitor), 1:1 mix .	68
Normal plasma and hemophilic plasma (with inhibitor), 1:1 mix	160

[a] Partial thromboplastin time. Unactivated.

inhibitor to factor VIII can be specifically assayed in units. These assays are all based on the ability of the inhibitor to neutralize factor VIII, and the units vary according to the method used. This is illustrated in Fig. 2. The specificity of the inhibitor in classical hemophilia is shown in Table 6. It can be seen that the inhibitor significantly neutralizes only factor VIII. More recent experiments have shown that the human inhibitor to factor VIII inhibits factor VIII clotting activity, but may have a slight effect on the von Willebrand factor, as measured by the ristocetin cofactor activity (109).

An example of the immunochemical characterization of a factor VIII antibody is shown in Table 7. Note that the inhibitor shown in Table 7 consists of IgG heavy chains or kappa light chains. Not all inhibitors are so restricted in Ig composition, but the case presented suffices for illustrative purposes.

Inhibitors to the von Willebrand factor can be detected by an assay for this factor as described by Sarji et al. (109). The principle of this test is that the von Willebrand factor in the presence of ristocetin will induce platelet aggregation. In the absence of von Willebrand factor or in the presence of a specific inhibitor to it, platelet aggregation is retarded or absent and can be measured as a percentage of a normal control. Table 8 shows the effect of various dilutions of a von Willebrand factor inhibitor on von Willebrand factor neutralization. Note that at low dilutions of inhibitor little or no von Willebrand activity is detected, whereas at high dilutions the effect of the inhibitor is obscured.

The immunological nature of at least one von Willebrand inhibitor is shown in Table 9. Notice that, in this particular patient, the inhibitor could be neutralized by heterologous antisera to IgG heavy chains and kappa light chains.

FACTOR IX INHIBITORS

Approximately 2 to 10% of patients with hemophilia B will develop inhibitors (11, 102). Additionally, spontaneous factor IX inhibitors in

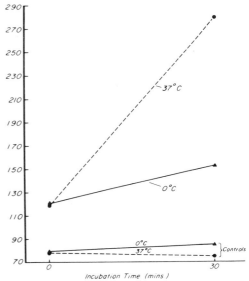

FIG. 2. *Effect of temperature on the reaction between inhibitor and normal plasma. Hemophilic plasma containing an inhibitor was mixed with normal plasma in a 1:1 ratio. A partial thromboplastin time (PTT) was performed immediately. Part of the mix was then incubated for 30 min at 0 C, and part was incubated for 30 min at 37 C. After incubation, a PTT was performed on both samples. Notice that after 30 min of incubation the mixture which had been incubated at 37 C had a much longer PTT than the mixture incubated at 0 C. Controls are shown at the bottom of the graph and consisted of normal plasma mixed 1:1 with hemophilic plasma without an inhibitor.*

TABLE 6. *Specificity of inhibitor in classical hemophilia for factor VIII[a]*

Factor	Percentage of normal control
V	106
VII	80
VIII	<1
IX	71
X	91
XII	151

[a] Inhibitor: 0.2 ml of a 1:50 dilution of inhibitor added to 0.8 ml of normal human plasma.

nonhemophilic patients have been described (20, 67, 69), but their occurrence is considerably rarer than the spontaneous factor VIII antibodies arising in nonhemophilic patients.

As demonstrated by Roberts et al. (105) and George et al. (45), the factor IX inhibitors are stable over a wide range of pH and temperature and are found in the IgG fraction of plasma. Unlike factor VIII antibodies, however, the interaction of factor IX with its inhibitor is vir-

TABLE 7. *Immunochemical characterization of an inhibitor to factor VIII*[a]

Heterologous antiserum	Human factor VIII inhibitor concn (units)
Saline control	2.1
Anti-IgG	0
Anti-IgA	2.1
Anti-IgM	2.1
Anti-kappa	0
Anti-lambda	1.5

[a] The antiserum or saline control was added to the inhibitor plasma in a ratio of 1:1. Residual inhibitor was measured in units described by Shapiro in the article from which the above data were taken (112).

TABLE 8. *Effect of various dilutions of inhibitor plasma on the von Willebrand factor (VWF)*[a]

Inhibitor	Dilution	Residual VWF activity (%)
VWF inhibitor	1:1	0
	1:2	20
	1:4	40
	1:8	100
Buffer control		100

[a] Data from Sarji et al. (109).

TABLE 9. *Neutralization of bovine von Willebrand factor (VWF) by inhibitor plasma adsorbed with heterologous antisera*[a]

Antiserum	Ristocetin assay for VWF macroscopic aggregation (s)	
	Inhibitor plasma	VWD control plasma[b]
Buffer (control) ...	>60	31
Anti-IgG	28	24
Anti-IgA	>60	28
Anti-kappa	24	32
Anti-lambda	>60	35

[a] Data taken from Stratton et al. (122).
[b] VWD, von Willebrand's disease.

tually immediate rather than time dependent.

Colombani and Terrier (21) first suggested that the factor IX inhibitor was an antibody, based on the results of hemagglutination techniques. McLester et al. (84), using an immunosorbent technique, showed that the factor IX inhibitor could be completely exhausted by adding sufficient amounts of factor IX. George et al. (45) described a family in which three or four members with factor IX deficiency developed antibodies which were IgG in nature. Two human factor IX antibodies have been fully characterized by immunochemical techniques (93; W. J. Yount et al., Clin. Res. 23:25A, 1975). Both of these antibodies arose in patients with hemophilia B. The first antibody (93) appeared to be a monoclonal IgG which contains IgG_4 heavy chains and lambda light chains. The second antibody (Yount et al., Clin. Res. 23:25A, 1975), however, was polyclonal and contained a mixture of IgG subclasses and both types of light chains in a kappa to lambda ratio of 6:1.

When the antibody to factor IX is used to detect cross-reacting material in the plasma of hemophilia B patients, it is apparent that there are several molecular variants of hemophilia B. Fantl et al. (34) first showed this when they found that the plasma of one of three patients with hemophilia B neutralized a human anti-factor IX antibody whereas that of the two other patients did not. Many subsequent authors (27, 32, 33, 60, 88, 104, 124) have demonstrated the presence of various amounts of cross-reacting material in patients affected with hemophilia B. The results vary from patient to patient and are also affected by the technique and type of antibody used, but it appears that about 10% of hemophilia B patients are CRM+. Other patients have a reduced amount of CRM roughly proportional to clotting activity, and some severely affected patients have no detectable CRM.

The vast number of variants may well make immunological determinations relatively unrewarding as an aid in the diagnosis of hemophilia B carriers. Elödi (31, 32) has shown that most female carriers contain equal amounts of immunological and procoagulant IX when a rabbit factor IX antibody is used to detect CRM. Roberts et al. (105), with a human antibody, found that carriers from CRM+ kindred have normal immunological material, whereas carriers from CRM− kindred have lower amounts of CRM. Neal et al. (90) have shown that rabbit antibody to factor IX can detect CRM in only about 10% of affected hemophilia B patients. Thus Neals' data conflict with the data of Elödi but appear to be in agreement with recent data (K. Z. Ørstavik and B. Østerud, Congr. Int. Soc. Thromb. Homeostasis, 5th, Paris, 1975). Thus, at present, repeated assays of factor IX activity are the preferred way of screening for the hemophilia B carrier state.

Laboratory studies

The homologous factor IX inhibitor acts almost immediately and can be detected by a prolonged partial thromboplastin time on a mixture of the patients' plasma and normal plasma, as shown in Table 10.

When the inhibitor is diluted to 1:64, its activity can no longer be detected, whether it is incubated for 60 min at 37 C or not incubated at

TABLE 10. *Detection of inhibitor in the plasma of patients with factor IX deficiency[a]*

Dilution of inhibitor plasma	Partial thromboplastin time (s)[b]	
	0-min incubation	60-min incubation
1:1	280	210
1:2	185	148
1:4	188	145
1:8	184	140
1:16	190	145
1:32	188	145
1:64	90	90
Control	90–95	90–95

[a] The tests were performed with 1 part normal plasma plus 1 part dilution of patient plasma. The control was 1 part normal plasma and 1 part buffer

[b] Unactivated.

all. The longer times observed for the unincubated samples in Table 10 can be abolished by activating the partial thromboplastin time with kaolin. The meaning of this unusual observation is unclear. However, the longer clotting times at 0 min of incubation do not reflect a higher concentration of the inhibitor since the inhibitor titer at 0 and 60 min is the same.

The specificity of the inhibitor for factor IX can be easily shown, as demonstrated in Table 11. Notice that when the inhibitor is not in excess only factor IX activity is neutralized.

The antibody nature of the inhibitor in factor IX deficient patients can be demonstrated by adding specific heterologous antibodies to inhibitor plasma, as shown in Table 12. By using the test outlined in Table 12, the results obtained in Table 13 were obtained. These data indicate that this particular inhibitor was an Ig consisting almost, if not entirely, of γG heavy chains. To determine γG subclass, the procedure outlined in Table 12 was repeated with heterologous antisera to γG1, γG2, γG3, and γG4. The data are shown in Table 14. As can be seen, the inhibitor contained only γG4 heavy chains. Further experiments with this particular antifactor IX antibody showed that only lambda light chains could be detected (Table 15). Not all human antifactor IX antibodies are so restricted in Ig composition, but by using the techniques described, the composition of the antifactor IX antibodies can be determined.

FACTOR X INHIBITORS

In 1967, Robinson et al. (107) described a family with a congenital deficiency caused by an "inactivator" of factor Xa, and in 1971 Lechner (69) described a nonhemophilic patient with an inhibitor to factor X. There were no data presented in either report supporting the view

TABLE 11. *Specificity of an inhibitor from a hemophilia B patient for factor IX[a]*

Factor	Percentage of normal
V	103
VII	106
VIII	113·
IX	5
X	100
XII	100

[a] Inhibitor: 0.1 ml of a 1:5 dilution of inhibitor plasma with 0.9 ml of normal plasma. Inhibitor must be diluted to the extent that it will not inhibit the IX in the substrates used in assaying factors other than IX. Thus, the inhibitor is diluted such that detectable IX is left in the test plasma. See Roberts et al. (105).

TABLE 12. *Neutralization of factor IX inhibitor with specific heterologous antibodies[a]*

Mixture 1. Neutralization phase
  a. Inhibitor plasma and specific heterologous antisera to human immunoglobulin → precipitate → centrifuge
  b. Assay supernatant fluid for residual antigen and antibody to insure that mixture is in zone of antibody excess
Mixture 2.
  a. 1 part supernatant from Mixture 1 and 1 part normal plasma
  b. Assay residual factor IX
  c. Residual factor IX is directly proportional to amount of inhibitor neutralized

[a] Modified from Pike et al. (93).

TABLE 13. *Immunochemical characterization of factor IX inhibitor[a]*

Heterologous antisera to	Residual factor IX (% of control)	Residual inhibitor
Anti-IgA	<1	Present
Anti-IgD	<1	Present
Anti-IgE	<1	Present
Anti-IgG	123, 104	Absent
Anti-IgG (absorbed with purified IgG) .	<1	Present
Anti-IgM	<1	Present

[a] Modified from Pike et al. (93).

that either inhibitor was an antibody. There are no other reports in the literature of inhibitors to factor X. This is not surprising in view of the rarity of this disorder. It has been recognized (29, 46), by using various techniques, that many variants of factor X deficiency exist. There is no reason to presume that antibodies to factor X will not be discovered in the future.

TABLE 14. *IgG subclass of the human factor IX antibody[a]*

Anti-Ig	Residual factor IX (% of control)	Residual inhibitor
Anti-IgG1	<1	Present
Anti-IgG2	<1	Present
Anti-IgG3	<1	Present
Anti-IgG4	84, 90	Absent
Anti-IgG4 (absorbed with purified G4) ..	<1	Present

[a] Modified from Pike et al. (93).

TABLE 15. *Light chain type of factor IX inhibitor[a]*

Heterologous antisera to	Residual factor IX (% of control)	Residual inhibitor
Anti-kappa	<1	Present
Anti-lambda	107, 99	Absent
Anti-lambda (adsorbed with purified lambda light chains)	<1	Present

[a] Modified from Pike et al. (93).

ACQUIRED ANTIBODIES TO FACTORS XI AND XII

Factor XI deficiency is an uncommon disorder associated with a mild bleeding tendency. Factor XII deficiency is also uncommon and is rarely associated with hemorrhage. It is not surprising, therefore, that inhibitors against these factors have only rarely been described.

In 1972, Castro et al. (20) described four patients with systemic lupus erythematosus and circulating inhibitors. These patients had normal prothrombin times and prolonged partial thromboplastin times. The first patient appeared to have a specific factor IX inhibitor. The next two had normal levels of factors V, X, VII, IX, and XII but low levels of factor XI, indicating that the inhibitor was specific for factor XI. The fourth patient in this series had an inhibitor which lowered the activity of both factors XI and XII. No studies were performed in these four patients to determine whether the inhibitors were antibodies. Interestingly, the two patients with inhibitors directed against factor XI had hemorrhagic problems. The first had a subarachnoid hemorrhage at a time when factor XI was low. The second patient bled massively in the gastrointestinal tract and lower extremities, but, since the partial thromboplastin time was normal and the patient was thrombocytopenic, the anticoagulant probably had no relationship to the hemorrhage.

In 1975, Krieger et al. (66) reported a patient with systemic lupus erythematosus with an inhibitor which appeared to interfere with the ability of activated factor XI to convert factor IX to its activated form. With gel filtration techniques, more of the inhibitor was found in fractions containing IgM, although smaller amounts of inhibitor were found in fractions containing IgG proteins.

In 1972, Åberg and Nilsson (1) described an inhibitor directed against factors XI and XII in an otherwise healthy 16-year-old white female with discoid lupus erythematosus. This inhibitor migrated in the gamma globulin region on agarose gels. No other immunological characterization was performed. It is of interest that this patient had no undue bleeding but instead had two episodes of lower extremity thrombosis. The first episode occurred 18 months prior to the discovery of the anticoagulant while the patient was taking birth control pills. The second occurred when the anticoagulant was present, but at a time when the patient aborted a 7-month-old fetus.

In 1973, Cronberg and Nilsson (24) reported a third patient with systemic lupus erythematosus with an inhibitor directed against factors XI and XII. In addition, this patient, who had neither hemorrhage nor thrombosis, had platelets which showed intense spontaneous aggregation. No immunological data concerning the inhibitor was presented in this paper.

Forbes and Ratnoff (42), using a heterologous rabbit antibody to factor XI, tested 10 patients with hereditary factor XI deficiency and found that their plasma lacked detectable factor XI antigen. Smink et al. (119), using a similar technique in patients with hereditary factor XII deficiency, likewise found that their plasma lacked detectable factor XII antigen.

FACTOR XIII INHIBITORS

Inhibitors directed against factor XIII have been found in patients with and without congenital factor XIII deficiency. At least two of the former have been described (50, 80). Lorand et al. (80) described a patient who developed a neutralizing antibody following replacement therapy. This antibody was not further characterized. Godal's patient (50) was a 24-year-old female with a life-long history of oozing following minor trauma, profuse menses, and significant bleeding following childbirth. Despite this history, it is not entirely clear that the patient had congenital factor XIII deficiency, since the family history was negative and the patient was not tested prior to discovery of the inhibitor. The factor XIII inhibitor in this patient appeared to be a gamma globulin which acted against activated factor XIII.

Factor XIII inhibitors more commonly arise in patients without a congenital factor XIII deficiency. In many patients a definite relationship exists between the development of the inhibitor and therapy with isoniazid (41, 74, 76, 78, 79, 92, 108). Lewis et al. (76) first reported this relationship in a 78-year-old man on isoniazid therapy. The factor XIII inhibitor was nondialyzable, heat stable to 70 C, and present in the globulin fraction as tested by continuous-flow electrophoresis. When Lorand et al. (78) studied this same inhibitor, their data suggested that the inhibitor was not an antibody, but rather an unusual isoniazid metabolic product which somehow interfered with fibrin cross-linking in the presence of activated factor XIII.

The inhibitor reported by Fiore et al. (41) occurred in a patient who had taken isoniazid and p-aminosalicylic acid for 8 years. The inhibitor to factor XIII acted rapidly, was stable at 56 C but not 75 C, and was found in the gamma to beta globulin areas on continuous-flow electrophoresis. The inhibitor inactivated factor XIII preactivated with thrombin.

In 1972, Lewis (74) summarized data on eight patients with spontaneous inhibitors to factor XIII. Six patients were on isoniazid, one was taking Dilantin, and the medication of one patient was uncertain. Lewis suggested that factor XIII inhibitors might be directed against the factor XIII zymogen, activated factor XIII, factor XIII activators, or cross-linking sites on the fibrin molecule.

Lorand et al. (79) described a patient with a factor XIII inhibitor who had been treated with isoniazid "in the past." This inhibitor appeared in the IgG fractions. In 1974, Rosenberg et al. (108) reported a 57-year-old female with sarcoidosis who had been taking isoniazid for 8 years when spontaneous ecchymoses arose. This patient's inhibitor blocked the cross-linking sites on fibrinogen and fibrin but had no direct effect upon factor XIII or XIIIa. This inhibitor was shown to be an IgG. The most recent report (92) involved an inhibitor which was present predominantly in the beta area on starch zone electrophoresis and in the second peak on Sephadex G-200 gel filtration. The inhibitor's activity persisted after heating to 90 C. This heated material did not react with Ig antisera. The last two pieces of information indicate that this inhibitor is probably not an Ig.

In most of the above-reported cases, the inhibitors disappeared within weeks to months of stopping the isoniazid. Thus, the question of whether all isoniazid-induced inhibitors to factor XIII are indeed Igs remains undecided.

At least one inhibitor specific for factor XIII arose in a patient who had never received isoniazid (52, 82). This inhibitor developed in a man with a left femoral artery thrombosis and was characterized as an IgG antibody consisting of IgG_1 heavy chains and lambda light chains. This antibody did not block fibrin receptor sites for XIIIa but acted against factor XIII itself. Subsequent work (S. Lopaciuk, R. P. McDonagh, and J. McDonagh, Congr. Int. Soc. Thromb. Hemostasis, 5th, Paris, 1975) with two human factor XIII antibodies has revealed that they react only with the a subunit of human, horse, cat, goat, sheep, pig, rat, chicken, goose, and turtle factor XIII.

Laboratory studies

A factor XIII inhibitor can be detected when inhibitor-containing plasma is mixed with normal plasma and clotted. If the clot dissolves in a solution of 1% monochloroacetic acid or 5 M urea, an inhibitor to factor XIII should be suspected. Normal clots, covalently cross-linked in a reaction catalyzed by activated factor XIII, are stable in such solutions. If factor XIII is inhibited or the fibrin cross-linking sites are obstructed, lysis of the clot will usually occur in a few minutes.

A more specific inhibitor assay is based on the observation that activated factor XIII catalyzes the incorporation of monodansyl cadaverine into casein. This reaction can be monitored fluorometrically, and factor XIII activity can be expressed in arbitrary units as described by Lorand and colleagues (80).

If dilutions of plasma containing a factor XIII inhibitor are mixed with normal plasma and residual factor XIII is determined by Lorands' assay, values similar to those shown in Table 16 might be expected.

Immunological techniques similar to those described for factor IX can then be used to show the antibody nature of a factor XIII inhibitor. One inhibitor, characterized immunochemically by Graham and colleagues (52), was a γG1 λ antibody that reacted with the α chain of factor XIII (52; Lopaciuk et al., Congr. Int. Soc. Thromb. Hemostasis, 5th, Paris, 1975).

LUPUS ANTICOAGULANT

Circulating anticoagulants directed against factors VIII (48, 49, 53, 86, 101), IX (20), XI (20), and XII (1, 24), the action of activated factor XI on factor IX (66), and the von Willebrand factor (63, 95, 118) have been reported in patients with collagen vascular diseases—especially in those with systemic lupus erythemato-

TABLE 16. *Factor XIII inhibitor titer*

Inhibitor plasma dilution[a]	Residual factor XIII (units/ml)	
	Observed	Expected[b]
1:2	1	8
1:4	1.5	8
1:8	2	8
1:16	2.5	8
1:32	4	8
1:64	5.5	8
1:128	8	8
Buffer control	8	8

[a] Each dilution was mixed 1:1 with normal plasma.

[b] Undiluted normal plasma contains 16 to 21 units of factor XIII activity by the monodansyl incorporation assay. When diluted 1:1, the expected activity in the absence of inhibitor is about 8 units/ml.

sus (SLE). Such inhibitors, directed against specific clotting factors, have been described elsewhere in this chapter and will not be further discussed. The more common coagulation abnormality associated with SLE, however, is the "lupus anticoagulant" first described by Conley and Hartmann (22).

This inhibitor occurs in 5 to 10% of patients with SLE (35). The precise mode of action of the inhibitor has not been defined. Breckenridge and Ratnoff (16) suggested that the inhibitor blocked the interaction of activated factor X with factor V, whereas Biggs and Denson (14) suggested that the inhibitor delayed the interaction between factors VIII and IX in a noncompetitive manner. Many authors (35, 36, 125) presently favor the concept that the inhibitor interferes with the interaction of prothrombin activator and prothrombin. Yin and Gaston (126) provided strong evidence that the inhibitor interfered with the formation of the prothrombin activator, for in their work they demonstrated that additional prothrombin activator overcame the effect of the lupus inhibitor.

Many authors (14, 72, 86, 89, 125, 126) have demonstrated that the inhibitory effects were clearly potentiated by reducing the phospholipid content of clotting mixtures. Bowie et al. (15) showed that the addition of phospholipid in vitro could correct the abnormal prothrombin consumption tests found in some patients with the lupus inhibitor. Approximately 50% of patients with the lupus inhibitor have thrombocytopenia (22, 86). In 1970, Hemker et al. (57) suggested that factors VIII and IX and factors V and X are adsorbed onto a phospholipid surface during the course of blood clotting. It may well be, therefore, that the lupus inhibitor covers up sites on the lipid surfaces and therefore interferes with normal interaction of various

blood clotting factors. This may provide an explanation as to why a decrease in phospholipid (blood platelets serve as the phospholipid source for the intrinsic system) potentiates the lupus inhibitor.

The immunological data presently available suggest that the lupus inhibitor is an autoantibody which is IgG in some cases (72, 126; S. Schiffman et al., in preparation), IgM in some cases (68, 69), and mixed IgG-IgM in other cases (51, 68, 69).

The activity of the lupus inhibitor requires the presence of a cofactor which has been felt to be either prothrombin (15) or a gamma globulin (126). The cofactor is present in the plasma of normal subjects and patients with SLE. Recent work by Rivard et al. (100) has added immensely to our knowledge of the cofactor for the lupus inhibitor. Their data indicate that the cofactor is neither prothrombin nor an Ig but rather is unique and shares some properties of both. Specifically, the cofactor resembles prothrombin in that it is precipitated from plasma at 50 to 75% ammonium sulfate saturation, it is reduced in activity in a patient with hereditary prothrombin deficiency, and it is reduced in serum. On the other hand, the cofactor differs from prothrombin in that its activity is normal or even increased in some patients with hereditary prothrombin deficiency, it is present in normal amounts in patients receiving vitamin K antagonists, and its activity is not removed from citrated plasma by adsorption with $Al(OH)_3$. Rivard et al. (100) also found that the cofactor is sparingly adsorbed to $BaSO_4$ and elutes in the IgG region from Sephadex G-200 columns. However, commercial gamma globulin lacks cofactor, and anti-Ig antiserum does not reduce cofactor activity.

A third aspect of the lupus inhibitor is hypoprothrombinemia which is sometimes associated with it (23, 35, 44, 59). The cause of the specific decrease in prothrombin activity is unclear.

The most sensitive screening test for the lupus inhibitor is the partial thromboplastin time. The prothrombin time may or may not be abnormal depending on the strength and dilution of the thromboplastin used. The thrombin time is generally normal. When mixing experiments are carried out with equal parts of the patient's and pooled plasma, the prolonged partial thromboplastin time is not further prolonged with incubation at 37 C for 1 h. Prothrombin consumption tests may be normal or abnormal. As pointed out by Feinstein and Rapaport (36), the lupus anticoagulant delays but does not totally inhibit the conversion of prothrombin to thrombin. Thromboplastin generation tests are generally abnormal when the patient's plasma is used as substrate, but normal when normal plasma is used as substrate. One-stage clotting assays for factors VIII, IX, XI, and XII usually yield low results but may be normal provided that the patient's plasma is sufficiently diluted. One-stage assays for factors V, VII, and X are usually normal.

Perhaps the most interesting aspect of the lupus inhibitor is that it is very rarely if ever associated with bleeding (even following major stress such as surgery) unless a concomitant abnormality of platelets (99) and/or a decrease in prothrombin is present. Veltkamp et al. (125) have suggested that vast amounts of phospholipid are formed in vivo during platelet plug formation. This extra phospholipid serves to adsorb clotting factors not complexed to the inhibitor. If, however, the patient has abnormal platelets, platelet phospholipid liberation does not occur.

In our experience, the course of the inhibitor is unpredictable. Since it is not associated with clinical bleeding, therapy is usually not necessary. If hypoprothrombinemia and/or platelet abnormalities are present, therapy with corticosteroids may be of benefit.

CONCLUSIONS

In this chapter, we have reviewed the immunology of acquired inhibitors to clotting factors and have given examples of how these antibodies might be detected by clotting assays and immunological techniques. The results to date have led to new and important discoveries related to the hemorrhagic disorders. The most notable have been the immunological classification of genetic variants, the use of specific human antibodies for purification of the respective antigens by affinity chromatography, the detection of the carrier state for hemophilia A, and interesting explorations into the causes and nature of these specific antibodies. The field is expanding rapidly, and it can be expected that studies of the clotting mechanism, by use of immunological techniques, will continue to lead to new and important data.

ACKNOWLEDGMENTS

This work was supported by Public Health Service grants HL 06350 and AM 05345 and by Clinical Research Unit grant FR 66.

We thank Gloria Stutts for excellent technical assistance.

LITERATURE CITED

1. Åberg, H., and I. M. Nilsson. 1972. Recurrent thrombosis in a young woman with a circulating anticoagulant directed against factors XI and XII. Acta Med. Scand. 192:419–425.

2. Allain, J. P., and D. Frommel. 1973. Antibodies to factor VIII. I. Variations in stability of antigen-antibody complexes in hemophilia A. Blood 42:437–444.

3. Allain, J. P., and D. Frommel. 1974. Antibodies to factor VIII: specificity and kinetics of iso- and hetero-antibodies in hemophilia A. Blood 44:313–322.

4. Allain, J. P., and H. R. Roberts. 1975. Treatment of acute bleeding episodes in hemophilic patients with specific factor VIII antibodies, p. 659–671. In K. M. Brinkhous and H. C. Hemker (ed.), Handbook of hemophilia. Excerpta Medica, Amsterdam.

5. Andersen, B. R., and W. D. Terry. 1968. Gamma G₄-globulin antibody causing inhibition of clotting factor VIII. Nature (London) 217:174–175.

6. Barrow, E. M., and J. B. Graham. 1974. Blood coagulation factor VIII (antihemophilic factor): with comments on von Willebrand's disease and Christmas disease. Physiol. Rev. 54:23–74.

7. Beck, P., J. E. Giddings, and A. L. Bloom. 1969. Inhibitor of factor VIII in mild haemophilia. Br. J. Haematol. 17:283–288.

8. Bennett, B., and O. D. Ratnoff. 1973. Detection of the carrier state for classic hemophilia. N. Engl. J. Med. 288:342–345.

9. Bidwell, E. 1969. Acquired inhibitors of coagulants. Annu. Rev. Med. 20:63–74.

10. Bidwell, E., K. W. E. Denson, G. W. R. Dike, R. Augustin, and G. M. Lloyd. 1966. Antibody nature of the inhibition to antihaemophilic globulin (factor VIII). Nature (London) 210:746–747.

11. Biggs R. 1974. Jaundice and antibodies directed against factors VIII and IX in patients treated for haemophilia or Christmas disease in the United Kingdom. Br. J. Haematol. 26:313–329.

12. Biggs, R., D. E. G. Austen, K. W. E. Denson, R. Borrett, and C. R. Rizza. 1972. The mode of action of antibodies which destroy factor VIII. II. Antibodies which give complex concentration graphs. Br. J. Haematol. 23:137–155.

13. Biggs, R., D. E. G. Austen, K. W. E. Denson, C. R. Rizza, and R. Borrett. 1972. The mode of action of antibodies which destroy factor VIII. I. Antibodies which have second-order concentration graphs. Br. J. Haematol. 23:125–135.

14. Biggs, R., and K. W. E. Denson. 1964. The mode of action of a coagulation inhibitor in the blood of two patients with disseminated lupus erythematosus (DLE). Br. J. Haematol. 10:198–216.

15. Bowie, E. J. W., J. H. Thompson, C. A. Pascuzzi, and C. A. Owen. 1963. Thrombosis in systemic lupus erythematosus despite circulating anticoagulants. J. Lab. Clin. Med. 62:416–430.

16. Breckenridge, R. T., and O. D. Ratnoff. 1963.

Studies on the site of action of a circulating anticoagulant in disseminated lupus erythematosus. Am. J. Med. 35:813–819.

17. Brinkhous, K. M., H. R. Roberts, and A. E. Weiss. 1972. Prevalence of inhibitors in hemophilia A and B. Thromb. Diath. Haemorrh. 51:315–320.

18. Brönnimann, V. R. 1954. Kongenitale Afibrinogenämie. Mitteilung eines Falles mit multiplen Knochencysten und Bildung eines spezifischen Antikörpers (Antifibrinogen) nach Bluttransfusionen. Acta Haemat. 11:40–51.

19. Castaldi, P. A., and R. Penny. 1970. A macroglobulin with inhibitory activity against coagulation factor VIII. Blood 35:370–376.

20. Castro, O., I. R. Farber, and L. P. Clyne. 1972. Circulating anticoagulants against factors IX and XI in systemic lupus erythematosus. Ann. Intern. Med. 77:543–548.

21. Colombani, J., and E. Terrier. 1962. Immunological investigation of a Christmas factor inhibitor by means of Boyden's technique. Nature (London) 196:1111–1112.

22. Conley, C. L., and R. C. Hartmann. 1952. A hemorrhagic disorder caused by circulating anticoagulant in patients with disseminated lupus erythematosus. J. Clin. Invest. 31:621–622.

23. Corrigan, J. J., J. H. Patterson, and N. E. May. 1970. Incoagulability of the blood in systemic lupus erythematosus. A case due to hypoprothrombinemia and a circulating anticoagulant. Am. J. Dis. Child. 119:365–369.

24. Cronberg, S., and I. M. Nilsson. 1973. Circulating anticoagulant against factors XI and XII together with massive spontaneous platelet aggregation. Scand. J. Haematol. 10:309–314.

25. Crowell, E. B. 1970. A factor VIII inhibitor in a mild hemophiliac. Am. J. Med. Sci. 260:261–263.

26. Crowell, E. B. 1975. Observations on a factor V inhibitor. Br. J. Haematol. 29:397–404.

27. Denson, K. W. E. 1973. Molecular variants of haemophilia B (ed.). Thromb. Diath. Haemorrh. 29:217–219.

28. Denson, K. W. E. 1973. The detection of factor VIII-like antigen in haemophilia carriers and in patients with raised levels of biologically active factor VIII. Br. J. Haematol. 24:451–461.

29. Denson, K. W. E., A. Lurie, F. De Cataldo, and P. M. Mannucci. 1970. The factor X defect: recognition of abnormal forms of factor X. Br. J. Haematol. 18:317–327.

30. De Vries, A., T. Rosenberg, S. Kochwa, and J. H. Boss. 1961. Precipitating antifibrinogen antibody appearing after fibrinogen infusions in a patient with congenital afibrinogenemia. Am. J. Med. 30:486–494.

31. Elödi, S. 1974. Hemophilia -B carriers (letter). Lancet 2:1273.

32. Elödi, S. 1975. Factor IX activity and factor IX antigen in haemophilia B carriers. Thromb. Res. 6:39–51.

33. Elödi, S., and E. Puskas. 1972. Variants of haemophilia B. Thromb. Diath. Haemorrh. 28:489–495.

34. Fantl, P., R. J. Sawers, and A. G. Marr. 1956. Investigation of a haemorrhagic disease due to beta-prothromboplastin deficiency complicated by a specific inhibitor of thromboplastin formation. Australas. Ann. Med. 5:163–176.

35. Feinstein, D. I., and S. I. Rapaport. 1972. Acquired inhibitors of blood coagulation. Prog. Hemostasis Thromb. 1:75–95.

36. Feinstein, D. I., and S. I. Rapaport. 1974. Anticoagulants in systemic lupus erythematosus, p. 438–444. In E. L. Dubois (ed.), Lupus erythematosus: a review of the current status of discoid and systemic lupus erythematosus and their variants. Univ. of Southern California Press, Los Angeles.

37. Feinstein, D., S. I. Rapaport, and M. N. Y. Chong. 1969. Immunologic characterization of 12 factor VIII inhibitors. Blood 34:85–90.

38. Feinstein, D. I., S. I. Rapaport, and M. M. Y. Chong. 1973. Factor V inhibitor: report of a case, with comments on a possible effect of streptomycin. Ann. Intern. Med. 78:385–388.

39. Feinstein, D. I., S. I. Rapaport, W. G. McGehee, and M. I. Patch. 1970. Factor V anticoagulants: clinical, biochemical, and immunological observations. J. Clin. Invest. 49:1578–1588.

40. Ferguson, J. H., C. L. Johnston, and D. L. Howell. 1958. A circulating inhibitor (anti-AcG) specific for the labile factor-V of the blood-clotting mechanism. Blood 13:382–397.

41. Fiore, P. A., L. D. Ellis, H. L. Dameshek, and J. H. Lewis. 1971. Factor XIII inhibitor and antituberculous therapy. Clin. Res. 19:418.

42. Forbes, C. D., and O. D. Ratnoff. 1972. Studies on plasma thromboplastin antecedent (factor XI) PTA deficiency and inhibition of PTA by plasma: pharmacologic inhibitors and specific antiserum. J. Lab. Clin. Med. 79:113–127.

43. Fratantoni, J. C., M. Hilgartner, and R. L. Nachman. 1972. Nature of the defect in congenital factor V deficiency: study in a patient with an acquired circulating anticoagulant. Blood 39:751–758.

44. Frick, P. G. 1955. Acquired circulating anticoagulants in systemic "collagen disease"—auto-immune thromboplastin deficiency. Blood 10:691–706.

45. George, J. N., G. M. Miller, and R. T. Breckenridge. 1971. Studies on Christmas disease: investigation and treatment of a familial acquired inhibitor of factor IX. Br. J. Haematol. 21:333–342.

46. Girolami, A., M. Lazzarin, R. Scarpa, and A. Brunetti. 1971. Further studies on abnormal factor X (factor X Friuli) coagulation disorder: a report of another family. Blood 37:534–541.

47. Glueck, H. I., and R. Hong. 1965. A circulating anticoagulant in γ1A multiple myeloma: its

modification by penicillin. J. Clin. Invest. 44:1866–1881.

48. Gobbi, F., and M. Stefanini. 1962. Circulating anti-AHF anticoagulant in a patient with lupus erythematosus disseminatus. Effect on a cephalin complex in vivo. Acta Haematol. 28:155–162.

49. Gobbi, F., and M. Stefanini. 1962. SLE and VIII inhibitor. Acta Hematol. 28:155–162.

50. Godal, H. C. 1970. An inhibitor to fibrin stabilizing factor (FSF, factor XIII). Scand. J. Haematol. 7:43–48.

51. Gonyea, L., R. Herdman, and R. A. Bridges. 1968. The coagulation abnormalities in systemic lupus erythematosus. Thromb. Diath. Haemorrh. 20:457–464.

52. Graham, J. E., W. J. Yount, and H. R. Roberts. 1973. Immunochemical characterization of a human antibody to factor XIII. Blood 41:661–669.

53. Green, D. 1968. Spontaneous inhibitors of factor VIII. Br. J. Haematol. 15:57–75.

54. Griggs, T. R., H. A. Cooper, W. P. Webster, R. Wagner, and K. M. Brinkhous. 1973. Plasma aggregating factor (bovine) for human platelets: a marker for study of antihemophilic and von Willebrand factors. Proc. Natl. Acad. Sci. U.S.A. 70:2814–2818.

55. Griggs, T. R., W. P. Webster, H. A. Cooper, R. H. Wagner, and K. M. Brinkhous. 1974. Von Willebrand factor: gene dosage relationship and transfusion response in bleeder swine — a new bioassay. Proc. Natl. Acad. Sci. U.S.A. 71:2087–2090.

56. Handley, D. A., and B. M. Duncan. 1969. A circulating anticoagulant specific for factor V. Pathology 1:265–272.

57. Hemker, H. C., M. J. P. Kahn, and P. P. Devilee. 1970. The adsorption of coagulation factors onto phospholipids. Thromb. Diath. Haemorrh. 24:214–223.

58. Hershgold, E. J. 1974. Properties of factor VIII (antihemophilic factor). Prog. Hemostasis Thromb. 2:99–139.

59. Hougie, C. 1964. Naturally occurring species specific inhibitor of human prothrombin in lupus erythematosus. Proc. Soc. Exp. Biol. Med. 116:359–361.

60. Hougie, C., and J. J. Twomey. 1967. Haemophilia B_m: a new type of factor IX deficiency. Lancet 1:698–700.

61. Howard, M. A., and B. G. Firkin. 1971. Ristocetin — a new tool in the investigation of platelet aggregation. Thromb. Diath. Haemorrh. 26:362–369.

62. Hoyer, L. W. 1973. Immunologic properties of antihemophilic factor, p. 191–221. In E. B. Brown (ed.), Progress in hematology, vol. 8. Grune and Stratton, New York.

63. Ingram, G. I. C., P. J. Kingston, J. Leslie, and E. J. W. Bowie. 1971. Four cases of acquired von Willebrand's syndrome. Br. J. Haematol. 21:189–199.

64. Kasper, C. K. 1973. Incidence and course of inhibitors among patients with classic hemo-

philia. Thromb. Diath. Haemorrh. 30:263–271.

65. Kernoff, P. B. A. 1972. The relevance of factor VIII inactivation characteristics in the treatment of patients with antibodies directed against factor VIII. Br. J. Haematol. 22:735–742.

66. Krieger, H., J. P. Leddy, and R. T. Breckenridge. 1975. Studies on a circulating anticoagulant in systemic lupus erythematosus: evidence for inhibition of the function of activated plasma thromboplastin antecedent (factor XIa). Blood 46:189–197.

67. Largo, R., P. Sigg, A. von Felten, and P. W. Straub. 1974. Acquired factor-IX inhibitor in a nonhaemophilic patient with autoimmune disease. Br. J. Haematol. 26:129–140.

68. Lechner, K. 1969. A new type of coagulation inhibitor. Thromb. Diath. Haemorrh. 21:482–499.

69. Lechner, K. 1971. Acquired inhibitors in auto and isoimmune disease. Thromb. Diath. Haemorrh. 45:227–241.

70. Lechner, K. 1974. Acquired inhibitors in non-hemophilic patients. Haemostasis 3:65–93.

71. Lechner, K., E. Ludwig, H. Niessner, and E. Thaler. 1972–1973. Factor VIII inhibitor in a patient with mild hemophilia A. Haemostasis 1:261–270.

72. Lee, S. L., and M. Sanders. 1955. A disorder of blood coagulation in systemic lupus erythematosus. J. Clin. Invest. 34:1814–1822.

73. Leitner, A., E. Bidwell, and G. W. R. Dike. 1963. An antihemophilic globulin (factor VIII) inhibitor: purification, characterization and reaction kinetics. Br. J. Haematol. 9:245–258.

74. Lewis, J. H. 1972. Hemorrhagic disease associated with inhibitors of fibrin cross linkage. Ann. N.Y. Acad. Sci. 202:213–219.

75. Lewis, J. H., J. H. Ferguson, and T. Arends. 1956. Hemorrhagic disease with circulating inhibitors of blood clotting: anti-AHF and anti-PTC in eight cases. Blood 11:846–855.

76. Lewis, J. H., I. L. F. Szeto, L. D. Ellis, and W. L. Bayer. 1967. An acquired inhibitor to coagulation factor XIII. Johns Hopkins Med. J. 120:401–407.

77. Lopez, V., R. Pflugshaupt, and R. Butler. 1968. A specific inhibitor of human clotting factor V. Acta Haematol. 40:275–285.

78. Lorand, L., A. Jacobsen, and J. Bruner-Lorand. 1968. A pathological inhibitor of fibrin cross-linking. J. Clin. Invest. 47:268–273.

79. Lorand, L., N. Maldonado, J. Fradera, A. C. Atencio, B. Robertson, and T. Urayama. 1972. Haemorrhagic syndrome of autoimmune origin with a specific inhibitor against fibrin stabilizing factor (factor XIII). Br. J. Haematol. 23:17–27.

80. Lorand, L., T. Urayama, J. W. C. de Kiewiet, and H. L. Nossel. 1969. Diagnostic and genetic studies on fibrin-stabilizing factor with a new assay based on amine incorporation. J. Clin. Invest. 48:1054–1064.

81. Lusher, J. M., J. Shuster, R. K. Evans, and M. D. Poulik. 1968. Antibody nature of AHG (factor VIII) inhibitor. J. Pediatr. 72:325–331.

82. McDevitt, N. B., J. McDonagh, H. L. Taylor, and H. R. Roberts. 1972. An acquired inhibitor to factor XIII. Arch. Intern. Med. 130:772–777.

83. McKelvey, E. M., and H. C. Kwaan. 1972. An IgM circulating anticoagulant with factor VIII inhibitory activity. Ann. Intern. Med. 77:571–575.

84. McLester, W. D., H. R. Roberts, and R. H. Wagner. 1965. Use of an immunosorbent technique in a study of a PTC inhibitor: a new method for the investigation of blood coagulation. J. Lab. Clin. Med. 66:682–687.

85. Mammen, E. F., K. P. Schmidt, and M. I. Barnhart. 1967. Thrombophlebitis migrans associated with circulating antibodies against fibrinogen. Thromb. Diath. Haemorrh. 18:605–611.

86. Margolius, A., D. P. Jackson, and O. D. Ratnoff. 1961. Circulating anticoagulants: a study of 40 cases and a review of the literature. Medicine (Baltimore) 40:145–202.

87. Ménaché, D. 1973. Abnormal fibrinogens: a review. Thromb. Diath. Haemorrh. 29:525–535.

88. Meyer, D., E. Bidwell, and M. J. Larrieu. 1972. Cross-reacting material in genetic variants of hemophilia B. J. Clin. Pathol. 25:433–436.

89. Mueller, J. F., O. D. Ratnoff, and A. W. Heinle. 1951. Observations on the characteristics of an unusual circulating anticoagulant. J. Lab. Clin. Med. 38:254–261.

90. Neal, W. R., D. T. Tayloe, A. I. Cederbaum, and H. R. Roberts. 1973. Detection of genetic variants of hemophilia B with an immunosorbent technique. Br. J. Hematol. 25:63–68.

91. Nilsson, I. M., U. Hedner, M. Ekberg, and T. Denneberg. 1974. A circulating anticoagulant against factor V. Acta Med. Scand. 195:73–77.

92. Otis, P. T., D. I. Feinstein, S. I. Rapaport, and M. J. Patch. 1974. An acquired inhibitor of fibrin stabilization associated with isoniazid therapy: clinical and biochemical observations. Blood 44:771–781.

93. Pike, I. M., W. J. Yount, E. M. Puritz, and H. R. Roberts. 1972. Immunochemical characterization of monoclonal γ G4, λ human antibody to factor IX. Blood 40:1–10.

94. Pool, J. G., and R. G. Miller. 1972. Assay of the immune inhibitor in classic haemophilia: application of virus-antibody reaction kinetics. Br. J. Haematol. 22:517–528.

95. Poole-Wilson, P. A. 1972. Acquired von Willebrand's syndrome and systemic lupus erythematosus. Proc. Soc. Exp. Biol. Med. 65:561–582.

96. Poon, M. C., A. C. Wine, O. D. Ratnoff, and B. S. Bernier. 1975. Heterogenecity of human circulating anticoagulants against antihemophilic factor (factor VIII). Blood 46:409–416.

97. Raccuglia, G., and N. G. Waterman. 1969. Anticoagulant effect of sodium cephalothin (Keflin). Am. J. Clin. Pathol. 52:245–247.

98. Ratnoff, O. D., and B. Bennett. 1973. The genetics of hereditary disorders of blood coagulation. Functional and immunological studies provide evidence for the heterogeneity of many familial clotting disorders. Science 179:1291–1298.

99. Regan, M. G., H. Lackner, and S. Karpatkin. 1974. Platelet function and coagulation profile in L. E. (studies in 50 patients) Ann. Intern. Med. 81:462–468.

100. Rivard, G. E., S. Schiffman, and S. I. Rapaport. 1974. Cofactor of the "lupus anticoagulant." Thromb. Diath. Haemorrh. 32:554–563.

101. Robboy, S. J., E. J. Lewis, P. H. Schur, and R. W. Colman. 1970. Circulating anticoagulants to factor VIII. Immunochemical studies and clinical response to factor VIII concentrates. Am. J. Med. 49:742–752.

102. Roberts, H. R. 1971. Acquired inhibitors in hemophilia B. Thromb. Diath. Haemorrh. 45:217–225.

103. Roberts, H. R., A. I. Cederbaum, and C. W. McMillan. 1975. Immunology of acquired inhibitors to coagulation factors, p. 647–658. In K. M. Brinkhous and H. C. Hemker (ed.), Handbook of hemophilia. Excerpta Medica, Amsterdam.

104. Roberts, H. R., J. E. Grizzle, W. D. McLester, and G. D. Penick. 1968. Genetic variants of hemophilia B: detection by means of a specific PTC inhibitor. J. Clin. Invest. 47:360–365.

105. Roberts, H. R., G. P. Gross, W. P. Webster, I. I. Dejanov, and G. D. Penick. 1966. Acquired inhibitors of plasma factor IX: a study of their induction, properties and neutralization. Am. J. Med. Sci. 251:43–50.

106. Roberts, H. R., M. B. Scales, J. T. Madison, W. P. Webster, and G. D. Penick. 1965. A clinical and experimental study of acquired inhibitors to factor VIII. Blood 26:805–818.

107. Robinson, A. J., P. M. Aggeler, G. P. McNicol, and A. S. Douglas. 1967. An atypical genetic haemorrhagic disease with increased concentration of a natural inhibitor of prothrombin consumption. Br. J. Haematol. 13:510–527.

108. Rosenberg, R. D., R. W. Colman, and L. Lorand. 1974. A new hemorrhagic disorder with defective fibrin stabilization and cryofibrinogenaemia. Br. J. Haematol. 26:269–284.

109. Sarji, K. E., R. D. Stratton, R. H. Wagner, and K. M. Brinkhous. 1974. Nature of Von Willebrand factor: a new assay and a specific inhibitor. Proc. Natl. Acad. Sci. U.S.A. 71:2937–2941.

110. Seeler, R. A. 1972. Congenital "hypoprothrombinemias." Med. Clin. North Am. 56:127–132.

111. Shainoff, J. R., and N. E. Braun. 1973. Purification of antifibrinogen antibodies. Anal. Biochem. 55:206–212.

112. Shapiro, S. 1967. The immunologic character of acquired inhibitors of antihemophilic globulin (factor VIII) and the kinetics of their interaction with factor VIII. J. Clin. Invest. 46:147–156.

113. Shapiro, S. S. 1975. Characterization of factor VIII antibodies. Ann N.Y. Acad. Sci. 240:350–361.

114. Shapiro, S. S., and K. S. Carroll. 1968. Acquired factor VIII antibodies: further immunologic and electrophoretic studies. Science 160:786–787.

115. Shapiro, S. S., and M. Hultin. 1975. Acquired inhibitors to the blood coagulation factors. Seminars in thrombosis and hemostasis, vol. 1, p. 336–385.

116. Shulman, N. R., and R. J. Hirschman. 1969. Acquired hemophilia. Trans. Assoc. Am. Physicians 82:388–397.

117. Shulman, N. R., and R. J. Hirschman. 1969. Acquired hemophilia. Clin. Res. 17:466.

118. Simone, J. V., J. A. Cornet, and C. A. Abildgaard. 1968. Acquired von Willebrand's syndrome in systemic lupus erythematosus. Blood 31:806–812.

119. Smink, M. M., T. M. Daniel, O. D. Ratnoff, and A. B. Stavitsky. 1967. Immunologic demonstration of a deficiency of Hageman factor-like material in Hageman trait. J. Lab. Clin. Med. 69:819–832.

120. Stenbjerg, S., S. Husted, and K. Mygind. 1975. A circulating factor V inhibitor: possible side effect of treatment with streptomycin. Scand. J. Haematol. 14:280–285.

121. Stites, D. P., E. J. Hershgold, J. D. Perlman, and H. H. Fudenberg. 1971. Factor VIII detection by hemagglutination inhibition: hemophilia A and von Willebrand's disease. Science 171:196–197.

122. Stratton, R. D., R. H. Wagner, W. P. Webster, and K. M. Brinkhous. 1975. Antibody nature of circulating inhibitor of plasma Von Willebrand's factor. Proc. Natl. Acad. Sci. U.S.A. 72:4167–4171.

123. Strauss, H. S. 1969. Acquired circulating anticoagulants in hemophilia A. N. Engl. J. Med. 281:866–873.

124. Twomey, J. J., J. Corless, L. Thornton, and C. Hougie. 1969. Studies on the inheritance and nature of hemophilia B_M. Am. J. Med. 46:372–379.

125. Veltkamp, J. J., P. Kerkhoven, and E. A. Loeliger. 1973–1974. Circulating anticoagulant in disseminated lupus erythematosus. Haemostasis 2:253–259.

126. Yin, E. T., and L. W. Gaston. 1965. Purification and kinetic studies on a circulating anticoagulant in a suspected case of lupus erythematosus. Thromb. Diath. Haemorrh. 14:88–115.

127. Zimmerman, T. S., O. D. Ratnoff, and A. S. Littell. 1971. Detection of carriers of classic hemophilia using an immunologic assay for antihemophilic factor (factor VIII). J. Clin. Invest. 50:255–258.

Chapter 74

Detection and Semiquantitation of Fetal Cells (Fetal Hemoglobin) in the Maternal Circulation

ALICE M. REISS AND WILLIAM POLLACK

INTRODUCTION

It is generally acknowledged that transplacental hemorrhages are a frequent occurrence in full-term pregnancies. Usually, the transplacental hemorrhage is less than 15 ml in total red cell volume, and the Rh-negative woman delivered of her Rh-positive infant is specifically and effectively immunosuppressed by a single 300-μg dose of $Rh_0(D)$ immune globulin. There remain, however, a small percentage (approximately 0.3%) of women who experience transplacental hemorrhages that represent volumes above 15 ml. This obstetrical complication can cause immunization in the Rh-negative woman unless the 300-μg doses of the specific immune globulin are commensurate with the volume of Rh-positive fetal red cells that have entered her circulation.

It is rare that the transplacental hemorrhage is of such magnitude that clinical signs of anemia are apparent in the infant at delivery. Most such hemorrhages are silent occurrences, and a test of the infant's hemoglobin value is not usually informative. However, when the cord or venous hemoglobin is below 13.5/100 ml or the capillary hemoglobin is below 14.5/100 ml, it can be surmised that the infant has lost as much as 25 ml of its red cell volume (5).

Extensive efforts have been made to modify the cross-match and the D^u procedures in order to detect and quantitate minor populations of fetal Rh-positive blood in maternal Rh-negative blood. The data obtained have shown lack of sensitivity and reproducibility in the qualitative detection procedures and have proved to be completely inadequate when attempts were made to relate the number of microagglutinates counted to the percentage of fetal Rh-positive cells in the blood mixtures.

The only procedure that has met the screening and semiquantitation needs of the laboratory has been the chemical acid-elution test of Kleihauer et al. (1, 3) or one of its many modifications. However, the great care required to prepare these reagents has relegated their use primarily to the large, research-oriented centers who have the time and the staff available for this purpose.

Reagents (such as FETALDEX, supplied by Ortho) have now been developed for a simplified acid-elution procedure that can be performed by all laboratories with little or no previous experience in such techniques. The reagents can be rigidly controlled during the manufacturing process and are stable in the form in which they are supplied. One considerable advantage of the method is that the adult cells are not fragmented and retain a lightly stained quality in contrast to the brightly stained, highly visible fetal cells. Thus, the ratio of fetal to adult red cells is quite simple to determine.

DESCRIPTION OF REAGENTS

The reagents are supplied in disposable containers, each set consisting of fixing reagent (83% methanol), eluting reagent (malate buffer, pH 4.1), and staining reagent (erythrosin B, 0.5%). Both the eluting and staining reagents are reconstituted with 40 ml of distilled water prior to use.

Each set of reagents should be used once only for one unknown and one control blood smear run simultaneously through the entire procedure.

SPECIMEN COLLECTION AND HANDLING

The maternal blood is drawn into ethylenediaminetetraacetic acid (EDTA), 1.5 mg of EDTA per ml of whole blood. The specimen should be collected as soon as possible after delivery of the baby. This is particularly important in Rh-negative mothers with ABO incompatible pregnancies, i.e., presence of maternal antibodies reactive with fetal A and/or B red cell antigens. In these situations the overall incidence of finding fetal cells is much lower, and the number of fetal cells is generally much smaller.

The anticoagulated whole blood can be stored at 2 to 8 C until used for testing, but storage should not extend beyond 24 h.

MATERIALS

Microscope: Although 250 magnification is recommended, magnifications varying from 200 to 450 may be used as long as a minimum of 4,000 adult red blood cells are counted.

Ocular grid (reticle): Although not essential for screening maternal blood smears that have no or very few fetal cells, it is virtually impossible to achieve meaningful ratios when the decision for more than 300 μg of Rh$_0$ immune globulin must be made unless an ocular grid is used.

Water bath, at 37 C: Accuracy of the water bath temperature is requisite for proper conduct of the test.

Stopwatch.

Thermometer.

Cool air blower or Rh typing box.

Glass microscope slides.

Pasteur pipettes.

Test tubes.

Graduate, to measure 40 ml of distilled water.

Distilled water.

Aqueous sodium chloride solution, 0.85%.

EDTA.

PROCEDURE

Explicit directions accompany the reagents. Briefly, the procedure is as follows.

1. The maternal blood is anticoagulated with EDTA.

2. The maternal blood sample is diluted 1:3 in 0.85% aqueous sodium chloride solution and mixed completely.

3. A thin smear of the diluted blood is prepared and examined at 250 magnification to insure that a one-cell thick monolayer has been achieved.

4. The smear is placed in the fixing reagent at room temperature for 6 min.

5. After rinsing and drying, the smear is placed in the eluting reagent, at 37 C, for 20 s.

6. The smear is transferred to the staining reagent at room temperature for 1 min.

7. After rinsing and drying, the smear is scanned at 250 magnification.

8. Eight fields are randomly selected, and the fetal erythrocytes and the adult erythrocytes in each field are counted and recorded.

9. The ratio of fetal red blood cells to adult red blood cells is determined by dividing the total number of fetal red cells counted by the total number of adult red cells counted, and the result is expressed as a decimal.

The preparation of a thin smear of the diluted blood is extremely important and should be practiced prior to using the reagents. One-half drop (0.025 ml) of diluted blood on a clean glass microscope slide is spread across the entire slide to achieve a monolayer of red cells. To determine whether this has been achieved, the air-dried slide can be scanned under a micro-

scope and the process can be repeated until a smear has been made that shows an even, one-cell thick monolayer, with no crowding of the red cells. If this is not achieved, optimal elution of the adult hemoglobin cannot occur.

The control slide can be made by mixing ABO compatible adult and cord blood in a 2:1 ratio prior to dilution with 0.85% aqueous sodium chloride. The control slide eluted and stained simultaneously with the unknown slide establishes the necessary laboratory proof that fetal red cells, if present in the unknown, will be properly stained in contrast to the adult red cells (Fig. 1).

RESULTS AND INTERPRETATION

In calculating the volume of fetal red cells in the maternal circulation from the fetal-adult red cell ratio, the following considerations must be taken into account:

1. The red cell volume of the mother.

2. The larger mean corpuscular volume (MCV) of fetal and red cells compared with adult red cells.

3. The percentage of fetal red cells containing fetal hemoglobin as compared with those containing adult hemoglobin.

4. The average overall accuracy of the test procedure as determined by clinical experience.

These considerations, which are further elaborated below, result in a factor (3,268) that can

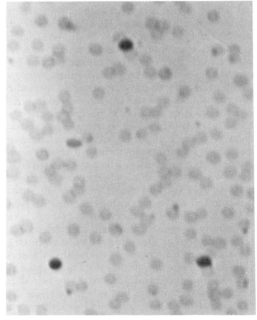

FIG. 1. *Blood smear of adult-fetal blood mixture.*

be used for calculation of the transplacental hemorrhage. Thus, if one counts a total of 4,000 adult red cells among which are distributed 30 fetal red cells, the calculations are

$$30 \div 4,000 \times 3,268 = 24.5 \text{ ml of fetal red cells}$$

Since each 300-μg single dose vial of $Rh_0(D)$ immune globulin will only "neutralize" 15 ml of red cells, the 24.5 ml requires two vials to be effective in suppressing an immune response to Rh.

When no fetal cells are counted in 4,000 adult cells, one 300-μg dose of Rh_0 immune globulin must still be administered, since it is impossible to be sure that fetal red cells did not gain access to the maternal circulation several weeks before delivery. Also, as little as 0.1-ml volumes of Rh-positive blood have been shown to result in sensitization of Rh-negative individuals (2, 7) while being below the level of certain detectability.

Considerations for derivation of the factor (3,268)

1. The average red cell volume of a recently delivered woman is generally accepted to be 1,800 ml (8). However, if the woman is greater than 240 pounds in weight and greater than 5 ft 5 inches in height, then the use of a blood volume of 2,600 ml is more reasonable and the factor increases from 3,268 to 4,718 (4).

2. The MCV of fetal red cells is approximately 22% greater than adult red cells so that the volume present is greater by a factor of 1.22 than indicated by the fetal red cells counted (6).

3. The fetus synthesizes a variable quantity of adult hemoglobin prior to birth. Thus, some fetal cells will stain the same as the maternal cells. To compensate for this under estimation of fetal cells, the factor of 1.25 was used based on the fact that about 80% of fetal cells do contain fetal hemoglobin and will retain the bright red stain (8).

4. The average overall accuracy was derived from four independent laboratories, each of which prepared, stained, and counted eight microscopic fields on 104 coded samples. The data were in good agreement with our own experience when evaluated by analysis of variance and linear regression methods. The average accuracy was found to be about 94%.

The procedure given appears to parallel the accuracy of the Kleihauer procedure when the latter is performed by technicians experienced in the technique. The test described was found to maintain this accuracy even with inexperienced personnel.

Of interest in this study was the finding that the results obtained by technicians with different concentrations of adult and fetal red cells tended to parallel the expected results. In other words, if their tendency was to overestimate the number of fetal red cells at low levels, then this tendency persisted at all higher concentrations. The same was found to be true with underestimation. To avoid undercounting, the accuracy was reduced to 84%, or a factor of 1.19. In the example cited earlier, the transplacental hemorrhage would have been calculated at 21.9 ml rather than the 24.5 ml shown if the experimentally obtained level of accuracy had not been reduced from 94 to 84%. The small increase in volume, which errs on the side of safety, seems reasonable when differences in technical abilities and practices of laboratories in general are taken into consideration.

LITERATURE CITED

1. Betke, K., and E. Kleihauer. 1958. Fetaler und bleibender Blutfarbstoff in Erythrozyten und Erythroblasten von menschlichen Feten und Neugeborenen. Blut 4:241–242.
2. Jennings, E. R., H. H. Dibbern, F. H. Hodel, C. H. Monroe, N. H. Peckham, J. F. Sullivan, and W. Pollack. 1968. Long Beach (California) experience with Rh immunoglobulin. Transfusion (Philadelphia) 8:146.
3. Kleihauer, E., H. Braun, and K. Betke. 1957. Demonstration von fetalem Hämoglobin in den erythrocyten eines blautausstrichs. Klin. Wochenschr. 35:637–638.
4. Nadler, S. B., J. U. Hidalgo, and T. Bloch. 1962. Prediction of blood volumes in normal human adults. Surgery 51:224–230.
5. Oski, F. A., and J. L. Naiman. 1966. Hematologic problems in the newborn, vol. 4: Major problems in clinical pediatrics. W. B. Saunders Co., Philadelphia.
6. Wintrobe, M. M. 1967. Clinical hematology, ed., p. 86. Lea and Febiger, Philadelphia.
7. Woodrow, J. C., and R. Finn. 1966. Transplacental hemorrhage. Br. J. Haematol. 12:297–309.
8. World Health Organization. 1971. Prevention of Rh sensitization. WHO Tech. Rep. Ser. No. 468.

Chapter 75

Antibodies to Allotypes, with Special Reference to the Allotypes of Immunoglobulin A

JUKKA KOISTINEN AND H. HUGH FUDENBERG

INTRODUCTION

History

Hemagglutination became widely used in clinical laboratories when it was discovered that serum from patients with rheumatoid arthritis usually reacted with gamma globulin (2). However, subsequent developments revealed the existence of a whole host of anti-gamma globulins in serum from various individuals (4):

1. Rheumatoid factor
2. Anti-Gm, -Am, and -Mm
3. Anti-antibody
4. Agglutinators to proteolytic fragments
   (a) Pepsin agglutinator
   (b) Papain agglutinator
   (c) Cyanogen bromide agglutinator
   (d) Trypsin agglutinator
   (e) Plasmin agglutinator

It soon became apparent that inhibition of agglutination systems could discriminate among many of these antiglobulin factors. Thus, true rheumatoid factor is inhibited by immunoglobulin G (IgG) from any normal serum, and by rabbit IgG to a better extent than human IgG (aggregated human IgG inhibits far better than nonaggregated).

Anti-gamma globulins directed towards various genetic markers of IgG (the so-called Gm factors) were inhibited by some sera (those possessing the Gm antigen in question) but not by others. Thus, cells coated nonspecifically with pooled IgG and agglutinated by a serum containing, e.g., anti-Gm(a) are easily inhibited by Gm(a+) serum or the IgG thereof, but are not inhibited by Gm(a−) serum or the IgG thereof (7). Further, another sort of antiglobulin, termed anti-antibodies, are not inhibited by any normal serum or the IgG thereof, but only by antigen-antibody complexes (4), and may indeed directly agglutinate IgG-coated cells without addition of anti-IgG's. Thus, inhibition of agglutination tests are necessary to discriminate among the various forms of antiglobulins. The situation is rendered even more complicated by the fact that plasmin, papain, trypsin,

and other enzymes, some found naturally in human blood, cleave IgG to reveal "buried determinants" (10). Most, if not all, normal sera contain IgG which will react with such determinants (termed pepsin, papain, and trypsin agglutinators in humans—"homo reactant" in rabbits). Thus, if the IgG coat has been fragmented during storage (pooled IgG often contains plasmin), inhibition tests with known intact IgG and IgG fragments prepared by proteolysis are mandatory for discrimination.

Passive hemagglutination in localization of antigenic determinants

If an antigen on a molecule inhibits a passive hemagglutination-inhibition system, it is possible to cleave the molecule into smaller fragments and determine the antigenic site; from this, one can sometimes draw conclusions as to the structure of the molecule. For example, use of papain to split IgG into Fab and Fc fragments and demonstration that the Gm factors were on the Fc fragment of IgG, but not present on IgA or IgM, and demonstration that the Inv genetic factors were present on the Fab fragments of IgG, IgA, and IgM led to the conclusions that the immunoglobulins probably contained two separate and distinct types of chains, one common to IgG, A, and M, and the other restricted to each class of immunoglobulin molecules, and that probably two sets of each chain appeared in each immunoglobulin molecule (two Fab fragments; 6). This prediction was shortly confirmed by the finding that there are two light chains present in each IgG, A, and M molecule, and two heavy chains distinctive for each molecule, namely, γ, α, and μ, or its subunit (IgM is a polymer of five such four-chain subunits; 1, 3).

Quantitation of an antigen within a given molecular species

Inhibition of passive hemagglutination can also be utilized to determine what percentage of molecules of a given type bear a genetic or another antigen. Thus in Gm(n+) Caucasians, about 2 to 4% of the IgG molecules contain the

Gm(n) factor. This can be demonstrated by setting up an inhibition of agglutination system and measuring the inhibitory capacity therein of a normal Gm(n+) myeloma (myelomas are not only electrophoretically homogenous, but never contain more than one major Gm factor). The 2 to 4% figure given above is based on the fact that a Gm(n/a+) serum containing 1,200 mg of IgG/100 ml inhibited the Gm(n) system by four to five less twofold dilutions than did a Gm(n+) myeloma, isolated and concentrated to 1,200 mg/100 ml of saline, and suspended in agammaglobulinemic serum (Fudenberg, unpublished data).

CLINICAL IMPLICATIONS OF HUMAN ANTIBODIES TO HUMAN IMMUNO-GLOBULIN A

The chromic chloride method is especially useful for detection of human antibodies to human IgA and subclasses or allotypes (Am markers) thereof (5, 21). This is important since administration of as little as 25 ml of IgA or Am incompatible plasma can cause severe (14, 23) and indeed sometimes fatal (Fundenberg, unpublished data) anaphylactic reactions in recipients who have anti-IgA or anti-Am; therefore, anti-IgA is a clinically significant antiglobulin in transfusion (16, 23) and probably in transplantation as well. One group of patients with or without symptoms of immunological deficiency disease characterized by selective absence of IgA (IgA deficiency is present in about 0.2% of normal Caucasians [12]) can produce very potent anti-IgA with titers higher than 1:1,000, most often in response to IgA received parenterally with blood or its components. Such antibodies react with almost all IgA coats (usually purified IgA myeloma proteins) and are, therefore, termed "class-specific." Class-specific anti-IgA has caused serious anaphylactic reactions upon administration of whole blood, plasma, or gamma globulins (14, 16). Some patients with anti-IgA of "limited specificity" (antibody reacts with only some of the IgA paraprotein coats), and usually with very low titers, have been reported to get mild transfusion reactions. These reactions have been characterized by urticarial, diffuse erythema, or anaphylactoid symptoms, namely, a feeling of flush and respiratory distress. In several patients with anti-IgA of limited specificity, evidence has been obtained implicating anti-IgA-IgA interaction as a cause of the transfusion reaction (25), but the question is still somewhat controversial (13). The significance of anti-IgA in clinical practice is indicated in Table 1. Most often the anti-IgA antibodies are of the IgG class and bind complement (14). Hence, clinical reactions

are presumably kinin-mediated.

The role and mode of production of anti-IgA of limited specificity in about 15% of the sera of recently delivered mothers is yet unclear (24) and can be evaluated only by a clinical and laboratory study. Since maternal anti-IgA resistant to treatment with β-mercaptoethanol, and therefore presumably IgG, is often detected in cord serum, the biological effect of such antiglobulins in the production of selective deficiency of IgA merits investigation.

Immunological subclasses of human immunoglobulin A

The antigenic differentiation of IgA myeloma proteins into two generally accepted subclasses of IgA globulins (IgA₁ and IgA₂) has been based on the reactivity with specific antisera made against IgA₁ and IgA₂ in Ouchterlony analysis. These classes do not represent genetic variants of IgA. Most IgA₂ proteins have a unique structure, in that the two L chains are bound to the two alphachains by noncovalent bonds, detectable by acid urea starch-gel electrophoresis (9). IgA₂ protein is always present in human serum (25). It has been estimated that the IgA₂ levels are about 7% of total IgA in human serum (18).

TABLE 1. *Incidence of human anti-IgA antibodies in various clinical conditions*

Subject classification	No. tested	Anti-IgA antibodies			
		No. negative	Positive		
			Class specific	Limited specificity	Percent
Normal adults	255	251	0	4[a]	2
Antiglobulin positive for Ripley	216	214	0	2	1
Absence of IgA and ataxia telangiectasia	34[b]	19	15	0	44
Kidney transplants	18	17	0	1[a]	5
Post-open-heart surgery and transfusion	55	46	0	9	16
Anaphylactoid transfusion reactions with rash and hives	29	4	3	22[a]	86
Total			18	38	

[a] Failed to agglutinate IgA anti-Rh (Avga)-coated cells.

[b] With total absence of IgA; 3 cases of reaction to transfusion are included in 18 of the series with absence of IgA. Six of these sera agglutinated IgA anti-Rh (Avga)-coated cells.

Genetic variations in IgA

Anti-IgA antibody of *limited specificity* has proved useful in clearly defining the two genetic markers of IgA$_2$. In keeping with the established Gm nomenclature for γ chains, these have been named A$_2$m(1) and A$_2$m(2), A$_2$ denoting the α_2 subclass, and m denoting the genetically determined marker. Thus far, no allotypic markers have been found on IgA$_1$ proteins, but an antigenic determinant occurring as allotype in IgA$_2$ subclass and as isotype in the IgA$_1$ subclass has been reported (19).

The first serum which contained anti-IgA defining the genetically determined marker was obtained from a Caucasian woman (W.F.) who had a severe anaphylactoid reaction to a blood transfusion during and after hysterectomy. She had no history of previous transfusions or injections of gamma globulin; she had had one abortion and two normal pregnancies; her IgA$_1$ and IgA$_2$ levels were normal. A pretransfusion specimen of this serum agglutinated some but not all IgA coats from a panel of 20 different proteins (Table 2). A postreaction specimen showed a marked drop in titer of anti-IgA, but 3 weeks later the titer had risen to pretransfusion level, where it remained for the next 15 weeks. IgA (5) was selected for use in further characterization of the anti-IgA antibody of W.F. and was shown to define Am(1) [A$_2$m(1); see below] by family and population studies.

Immunogenetic studies

The results of A$_2$m(1) typing on the phenotype frequencies in Caucasians, Negroes, Japanese, and Chinese are listed in Table 3.

To establish the inheritance of A$_2$m(1), serum samples from 264 members of 51 Japanese families were typed for A$_2$m(1) (Table 4). The parental combinations and the frequencies of A$_2$m(1) and A$_2$m(−1) offspring are shown in Table 4. The inheritance of A$_2$m(1) was established by genetic analysis of family and population data.

Gene frequencies from Table 4:

    A$_2$m(1) = 0.5130

    A$_2$m(−1) = 0.4870

The expected genotype frequencies of various matings and their offspring were calculated from these data. The calculated values were then used for deriving the expected phenotype frequencies of matings and the proportion of A$_2$m(1) and A$_2$m(−1) offspring from each mat-

TABLE 2. *Purified proteins used in characterizing specificity of anti-Am(1) agglutinator and the limits for the detection of Am(1) in relation to protein concentration*

Protein	Source	Paraprotein typing of		Am(1)	Detection limit
		γA subclass	L chains		
IgA (1)	Br myeloma	γA$_1$	λ	−	0.004 mg/ml
IgA (2)	Lo myeloma	γA$_2$	κ	+	
IgA (3)	Wo myeloma	γA$_1$	κ	−	
IgA (4)	Jo myeloma	γA$_1$	λ	−	
IgA (5)	Ch myeloma	γA$_1$	λ	−	
IgA (6)	He myeloma	γA$_2$	λ	+	0.002 mg/ml
IgA (7)	Cr myeloma	γA$_1$	κ	−	
IgA (8)	Ha myeloma	γA$_1$	λ	−	
IgA (9)	Dij myeloma	−	−	−	
IgA (10)	Rij myeloma	−	−	−	
IgA (11)	Ja myeloma	−	−	−	
IgA (12)	Za myeloma	λA$_2$	κ	+	0.003 mg/ml
IgA (13)	Zeph myeloma	λA$_1$	κ	−	
IgA (14)	Fo myeloma	λA$_1$	λ	−	
IgA (GNV)	Normal adult	−	−	+	0.062 mg/ml
IgA (pool)	120 normal	−	−	+	0.062 mg/ml
IgG	Cohn fraction II	−	−	−	
IgM	Pool of 4 IgM para-proteins	−	−	−	
L. ch.	Pooled L chains	−	−	−	
B.J. κ	Bence Jones pro-tein	−	κ	−	
B.J. λ	Bence Jones pro-tein	−	λ	−	
aIgA serum	L.G., absent IgA	−	−	−	At 1:4 dilution
Am(1) serum	J.M., Caucasian	−	−	+	At 1:256 dilution
Am(−1)	G.S., Negro	−	−	−	At 1:2 dilution

TABLE 3. *Frequency of allotype of human IgA [Am(1)] in various races*

| Race | No. tested | Am(1) phenotype | | | | Gene frequency | |
| | | Positive | | Negative | | Am(1) | Hypothetical allele |
		No.	Percent	No.	Percent		
Caucasian ...	351	344	98.00	7	2.00	0.9858	0.0142
Negro	103	56	51.85	52	48.15	0.3061	0.6939
Japanese	116	85	76.28	31	25.72	0.5130	0.4870
Chinese	50	28	56.00	22	44.00	0.3367	0.6633

TABLE 4. *Inheritance of $A_2m(1)$ studied in 51 Japanese families*

| Matings | No. of families | | No. of offspring | | | |
| | Obs.[a] | Exp. | $A_2m(1)$ | | $A_2m(-1)$ | |
			Obs.	Exp.	Obs.	Exp.
$A_2m(1) \times A_2m(1)$	29	30	84	83	9	10
$A_2m(1) \times A_2m(-1)$	19	18	44	43	20	21
$A_2m(-1) \times A_2m(-1)$	3	3	0	0	5	5
Total	51		128		34	

[a] Obs., observed; Exp., expected.

ing. The observed and expected frequencies of $A_2m(1)$ and $A_2m(-1)$ offspring are compared in Table 4. These data provide convincing evidence of the inheritance of $A_2m(1)$. The distribution of $A_2m(1)$ and $A_2m(2)$ (see below) in family trees indicates an autosomal co-dominant mode of inheritance.

Other examples of anti-$A_2m(1)$ have subsequently been detected, usually as a result of unexplained transfusion reactions. Another serum from a patient with unexplained transfusion reaction agglutinated other IgA-coated cells, all $A_2m(-1)$. Further investigations of this serum similar to those described for $A_2m(1)$ led to delineation of its allele, $A_2m(2)$ (20).

Genotype frequencies in Japanese:

$A_2m(1) A_2m(1) = 0.2632$
$A_2m(1) A_2m(2) = 0.4996$
$A_2m(2) A_2m(2) = 0.2372$

$A_2m(1)$ in saliva and cord blood

Since IgA is the major immunoglobulin of exocrine secretions (17), it is possible to test samples of saliva in the $A_2m(1)$ system. The results of $A_2m(1)$ typing of saliva and serum from the same subject are concordant and independent of one's ABH secretor status.

The cord serum is not usually inhibitory in the $A_2m(1)$ system. The $A_2m(1)$ antigen is fully developed, with inhibitory titers of 1:40 and higher, in infants at the age of 1 year.

TEST PROCEDURE

Methods of absorption of heterophile antibodies

To avoid false-positive agglutination, any antibody reacting with the indicator red cells must be removed by absorption of the test serum. If sheep erythrocytes are used in passive hemagglutination assay, the naturally occurring heterophile antibodies to the indicator red cells in the antisera in passive hemagglutination systems and in test sera in inhibition of agglutination systems must be removed by absorption before these systems can be utilized for passive hemagglutination or inhibition thereof. If the test serum is freshly drawn or kept frozen after collection, complement should be inactivated by heating the serum at 56 C for 30 min before absorption.

One easy absorption method merely involves exposure of 0.5 volume of washed packed cells to the inactivated test serum and centrifugation. More than one such absorption may be necessary before the heterophile antibody is completely removed.

Red blood cells

In addition to conventionally used human group O or sheep erythrocytes, the red cells of the other animals such as rabbit, mouse, chicken, pig, horse, monkey, and guinea pig have also been used. Originally, sheep cells were most extensively used. However, because a consistent supply of group O blood is easy to obtain, it has recently become customary to use group O human red blood cells in passive hemagglutination reactions. Such blood may be collected in any one of the commonly used anticoagulants, e.g., Alsever's solution, acid-citrate-dextrose, and trisodium ethylenediaminetetraacetate, or others, and the blood can be stored at 3 to 5 C for no more than 2 weeks before being used for the coating procedure. Defibrinated sheep blood can be kept at 4 C for 3 to 4 days. Indeed, better reactions are obtained (for unknown reasons) with 3- to 4-day-old blood than with fresh samples. Sheep blood collected aseptically in Alsever's solution containing antibiotics can be stored at 4 C for at least 2 weeks. Heparinized blood should not be stored for more than 2 days at 4 C.

Chromic chloride method

Trivalent cations have been used for labeling albumin employed in an obsolete method for estimating blood volumes. Jandl and Simmons (11) demonstrated the ability of $CrCl_3$ to bind proteins to erythrocytes. This method has been used for the detection of antigens and antibodies by us and our associates (5, 8, 12, 15, 21, 22). The following list shows some of the various antigen-antibody systems for which the assay has been successfully employed:

Human albumin
Alpha globulins
Beta globulins
Gamma globulins
IgG pooled
Ovalbumin
γ_2-Macroglobulin
Hemocyanin (KLH)
Transferrin
Bence Jones proteins
IgG (including IgG of various subclasses and allotypes)
IgA (including IgA of various subclasses and allotypes)
IgM
Complement $C'3$
Bovine serum albumin
Antibody fragments
Rhinovirus
Insulin
Achinostoma antigens
Antihemophilic factor (factor VIII)
Australia antigen
Pneumococcal polysaccharide

Although various physical and chemical parameters such as temperature, ionic strength, pH, inhibitors, and certain kinetics of the protein binding to red cells have been studied (11), little is known of the mechanisms of the underlying chemical reaction, mode of binding, stability of the bonds, or other factors which appear to be significant in the binding process.

It appears that any protein in isolated form can be coupled to red blood cells by use of the chromic chloride technique. The same is true of at least some and perhaps all polysaccharide antigens.

Reagents.

Human group O erythrocytes.
The isolated protein to be coupled on the red blood cells.
Chromic chloride, $CrCl_3 \cdot 6H_2O$, can be stored in

4 C as 1% (0.0375 M) stock solution in a dark bottle.
Polyvinylpyrrolidone (PVP).
Bovine serum albumin (BSA).
Tween 80.
Phosphate-buffered saline, pH 7.2 (PBS).

TVP solution, containing Tween 80 (1:20,000) and PVP (0.0025%) in PBS, can be used as the stock solution to which BSA (0.5 to 1%) is added daily to obtain the TAP solution, into which the red cell suspension and antiserum dilutions are made.

Coating of red blood cells.

1. Red blood cells (stored in 4 C for 1 to 14 days) are washed four times in physiological saline.

2. One volume of washed packed red cells is mixed with one volume of the protein to be coated on the erythrocytes and with one volume of the appropriate dilution of $CrCl_3$. The mixture is incubated in room temperature for 5 min, after which the coated cells are washed three times with saline. The centrifuging of the coated erythrocytes has to be done carefully to avoid spontaneous clumping of the erythrocytes. Usually, 30 s of spinning with an Adams Serofuge is enough to bring the cells down without causing spontaneous agglutination.

3. A 0.1 to 0.2% solution of erythrocytes is made in TAP to be used in the V-bottom plates. U-bottom plates require 0.5 to 1% erythrocyte suspension.

The coating can be checked immediately after washing by the direct Coombs test. The right concentrations for the proteins and chromic chloride can be found by the "checkerboard method" in which erythrocytes are coated with the use of different concentrations of both (for $CrCl_3$ usually varying from 0.025 to 0.1%, and for the antigen protein usually 0.25 to 4.0 mg/ml; Table 5).

When the optimal dilutions are found, the same concentrations can usually be used with success thereafter. The chromic chloride solution should always be freshly made from the 1% stock solution.

It should be emphasized that only saline is used in washing the cells, and as a diluent for $CrCl_3$ and as a solvent for protein solution. Any protein antigen solution in phosphate buffer or tris(hydroxymethyl)aminomethane buffer must be dialyzed against saline to render it suitable for the coating procedure.

Microtiter method

The method of Wegman and Smithies (26) has been found very useful for serial twofold titration of antiserum for use against antigen-

TABLE 5. *Checkerboard method of determining optimal conditions of coating protein with the use of specific antiserum*

Protein concn (mg/ml)	Dilutions of 1% CrCl$_3$					Saline control
	1:5	1:10	1:15	1:20	1:25	
4.0	N.S.[a]	32[b]	32	16	0	0
3.5	N.S.	N.S.	32	8	0	0
3.0	N.S.	16	16	8	0	0
2.5	N.S.	32	32	16	0	0
2.0	Agg.[c]	8	32[d]	8	0	0
1.5	Agg.	8	16	4	0	0
1.0	Agg.	N.S.	8	2	0	0
0.5	Agg.	Agg.	4	0	0	0
Saline	Agg.	Agg.	Agg.	Agg.	Weak Agg.	0

[a] Nonspecific agglutination caused by normal human serum.

[b] Reciprocal of the highest dilution of antiserum showing distinct agglutination.

[c] Visible agglutination of cells caused by CrCl$_3$ as a result of low protein concentration in the absence of antibody.

[d] Protein concentration of 2 mg/ml and 1:15 dilution of CrCl$_3$ is selected in such a case.

coated cells. The interpretation of agglutination in microtiter plates is objective, and the results are highly reproducible. The microtiter technique can be automated for mass screening (e.g., Cook Engineering Co., Alexandria, Va., and Canalco, Rockville, Md.).

Microtiter plates with either V- or U-shaped wells can be used. The method for plates with V-bottom wells:

1. A double dilution series is made in TAP of the serum to be tested for the antibody; 0.025 ml of each dilution is dropped to each well.

2. One drop (0.025 ml) of antigen-coated cell suspension (0.1 to 0.2%) is added to each well.

3. In one well, one drop (0.025 ml) of coated cells and one drop of TAP is dropped to control for the spontaneous agglutination of the coated cells. Antiserum with noncoated cells in another well tests the ability of the serum to agglutinate cells without the antigen.

4. The plates are agitated for good mixing of the reagents and incubated for 1 h at room temperature followed by centrifugation at 1,200 rpm for 30 s in a special holder (Microtiter).

5. After centrifugation, the microtiter plates are placed on an illustrated platform inclined at an angle of 60° to the horizontal.

6. After 15 to 20 min, visual discrimination of agglutination is performed. The unagglutinated cells stream down the vertex of the V-shaped well, whereas the agglutinated cells remain as a single button (Fig. 1).

Hemagglutination tests in U-bottom wells

can be performed in the same manner with few exceptions:

1. The red cell suspension should be stronger, about 1%.

2. After gentle agitation of the mixture, the plates are allowed to stand at room temperature for 2 h before the results are read. No centrifugation is needed. The unagglutinated cells float down to the bottom of the well, forming a small button. The agglutinated cells cover the well as an even surface, and sometimes even very coarse agglutination can be seen.

For determining the titer of antiserum, the highest dilution showing a definite button of agglutinated cells in the V-bottom wells is reckoned as the end point, ignoring one or two dilutions showing intermediate reactions before the reaction is completely negative.

The specificity of antibody reacting with coated cells must always be established by inhibition of agglutination with isolated purified antigens.

Antigen detection and quantitation by inhibition of hemagglutination using the chromic chloride technique

Usually, a dilution of antibody (the agglutinator) two- to fourfold lower than the end point of titration is used as the standard dilution in an agglutination-inhibition system, but lower doses are used if the antigen sought is present in very low concentration in the test fluid (e.g., IgM in serum).

1. Twofold serial dilution of the test material is made in the microtiter plates, 0.025 ml in each well.

2. Into the wells containing the test material, 0.025 ml of appropriate dilution of the agglutinator is added.

3. The plates are agitated and incubated for 10 min at room temperature to allow the antigen-antibody reaction to take place.

4. Then 0.025 ml of the appropriate suspension of coated cells is added to each well.

5. The incubation, centrifugation, and reading of the results is done as described above for both V- and U-bottom plates.

6. Mandatory controls are agglutinator plus buffer plus coated cells (cell control) and test sample plus coated cells (sample control).

In testing for serum IgA by inhibition of hemagglutination with the chromic chloride method, inhibitory titers of 1:2,000 to 1:10,000 can be expected by normal human serum, which should always be used as the control having IgA. Samples in which no IgA can be detected by double diffusion may give inhibitory titers of the order of 1:16 to 1:64 in this system.

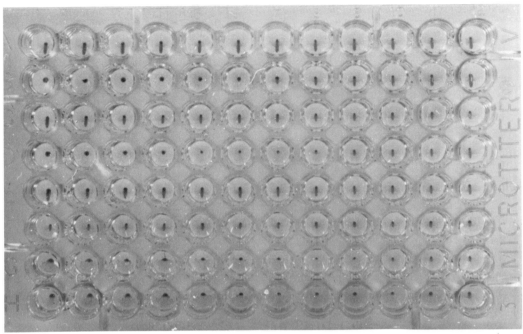

FIG. 1. *Hemagglutination patterns in a microtiter plate with V-shaped wells.*

ACKNOWLEDGMENTS

This work was supported by Public Health Service grants AI-09145 and HD-09938.

LITERATURE CITED

1. Edelman, G. M., and M. D. Poulik. 1961. Studies on structural units of γ-globulins. J. Exp. Med. 113:861–867.
2. Epstein, W., A. Johnson, and C. Ragan. 1956. Observations on a precipitin reaction between serum of patients with rheumatoid arthritis and a preparation (Cohn Fr II) of human γ-globulin. Proc. Soc. Exp. Biol. Med. 91:235–239.
3. Fleishman, J. B., R. H. Pain, and R. H. Porter. 1962. Reproduction of 7S globulins. Arch. Biochem. Biophys. Suppl. 1:174–182.
4. Fudenberg, H. H. 1967. Compleat immunology: science or septophrenia? Clin. Exp. Immunol. 2:1–18.
5. Fudenberg, H. H., E. R. Gold, G. N. Vyas, and M. R. MacKenzie. 1968. Human antibodies to human IgA globulins. Immunochemistry 5:203–212.
6. Fudenberg, H. H., J. F. Heremans, and E. C. Franklin. 1963. A hypothesis for the genetic control of synthesis of the gamma-globulins. Ann. Inst. Pasteur (Paris) 104:155–168.
7. Fudenberg, H. H., and N. L. Warner. 1970. Genetics of immunoglobulins, p. 131–209. *In* H. Harris and K. Hirschhorn (ed.), Human genetics review, vol. 2. Plenum Press, New York.
8. Gold, E. R., and H. H. Fudenberg. 1967. Chromic chloride: a coupling reagent for passive hemagglutination reactions. J. Immunol. 99:859–866.
9. Grey, H. M., C. A. Abel, W. J. Yount, and H. G. Kunkel. 1968. A subclass of human gamma-A-globulins (gamma A₂) which lacks the disulfide bonds linking heavy and light chains. J. Exp. Med. 128:1223–1228.
10. Henney, C. S., and E. F. Ellis. 1968. Antibody production to aggregated human γ-G globulin in acquired hypogammaglobulinemia. N. Engl. J. Med. 278:1144–1146.
11. Jandl, J. H., and R. L. Simmons. 1957. The agglutination and sensitization of red cells by metallic cations: interactions between multivalent metals and the red-cell membrane. Br. J. Haematol. 3:19–38.
12. Koistinen, J. 1975. Selective IgA deficiency in blood donors. Vox Sang. 29:192–202.
13. Koistinen, J., and J. Leikola. 1976. Weak anti-IgA antibodies with limited specificity and nonhemolytic transfusion reactions. Vox. Sang., in press.
14. Leikola, J., J. Koistinen, M. Lehtinen, and M. Virolainen. 1973. IgA-induced anaphylactic transfusion reactions: a report of four cases. Blood 42:111–119.
15. MacKenzie, M. R., G. Mackey, and H. H. Fudenbeg. 1967. Antibodies to IgM in normal human sera. Nature (London) 216:691–693.
16. Miller, W. V., and P. V. Holland, E. Sugarbaker, W. Strober, and T. A. Waldman. 1970. Anaphylactic reactions to IgA: a difficult transfusion problem. Am. J. Clin. Pathol. 54:618–621.

17. Tomasi, T. B., and J. Bienenstock. 1968. Secretory immunoglobulins. Adv. Immunol. **9:**1–96.

18. Vaerman, J. P., J. F. Heremans, and C. B. Laurell. 1968. Distribution of alpha-chain subclasses in normal and pathological IgA-globulins. Immunology **14:**425–429.

19. van Loghem, E., G. de Lange, and J. Koistinen. 1976. The first isoallotype of human IgA proteins: an antigenic determinant occurring as allotype in the IgA$_2$ subclass and as isotype in the IgA$_1$ subclass. Scand. J. Immunol. **5:**161–164.

20. van Loghem, E., A.-C. Wang, and J. Shuster. 1973. A new genetic marker of human immunoglobulins determined by an allele at the alpha-2 locus. Vox Sang. **24:**481–488.

21. Vyas, G. N., and H. H. Fudenberg. 1969. Am(1), the first genetic marker of human immunoglobulin A. Proc. Natl. Acad. Sci. U.S.A. **64:**1211–1216.

22. Vyas, G. N., H. H. Fudenberg, H. M. Pretty, and E. R. Gold. 1968. A new rapid method for genetic typing of human immunoglobulins. J. Immunol. **100:**274–279.

23. Vyas, G. N., L. Holmdahl, H. A. Perkins, and H. H. Fudenberg. 1969. Serologic specificity of human anti-IgA and its significance in transfusion. Blood **34:**573–581.

24. Vyas, G. N., A. S. Levin, and H. H. Fudenberg. 1970. Intrauterine isoimmunization caused by maternal IgA crossing the placenta. Nature (London) **225:**275–276.

25. Vyas, G. N., H. A. Perkins, and H. H. Fudenberg. 1968. Anaphylactoid transfusion reactions associated with anti-IgA. Lancet **2:**312–315.

26. Wegman, T. G., and O. Smithies. 1966. A simple hemagglutination system repairing small amounts of red cells and antibodies. Transfusion (Philadelphia) **6:**67–73.

Section G

LABORATORY EXAMINATION OF PATIENTS WITH ALLERGIC AND IMMUNODEFICIENCY DISEASES

Chapter 76

Introduction: Diagnostic Tests in Allergic Diseases

LAWRENCE M. LICHTENSTEIN

This section of the *Manual* describes a number of tests which are among those most widely utilized in the practice of medicine. Human illness due to allergic disease, and I here use the term in a limited sense to refer to immediate hypersensitivity reactions, affects almost 20% of the population at one time or another and is one of the major causes of morbidity in this country. The laboratory aids to diagnosis in these disorders have progressed vigorously in the past decade as a result of the elucidation of the nature of the responsible immunoglobulin, IgE, by the Ishizakas. This progress was materially advanced by the discovery of several IgE myelomas and by the diagnostic technology which was largely developed by Johannson, Bennich, and Wide in Sweden. In spite of this progress, the use of these techniques in clinical practice is only beginning, and confusion abounds. This section includes all of the currently used techniques for diagnoses in this disease process.

The chapter by Gleich and Yunginger provides technology in the most critical area which remains to be settled in a definitive fashion. This is the lack of federally or professionally approved standardization of allergens; until this is corrected, a comparison of diagnostic procedures from one center to another is impossible. As Gleich outlines, there is no cogent reason for this lack, since the techniques for standardization are readily available to any minimally established diagnostic laboratory. It is incumbent upon any group which chooses to carry out allergy diagnostic tests to establish their own standards which can be used in a seriatim way in their own work and, eventually, will be used to bring their results in line with those of others.

Standardization can be carried out by any of the three techniques in fairly common usage, which are outlined in the next several chapters. Skin testing, which has been used for the diagnosis of allergic disorders for over four decades, is a powerful tool. It is, however, almost universally misused in that standardized antigens are not employed and little effort is made to quantitate the results. We have shown in detailed clinical studies that positive skin test reactions to common inhalant allergens may occur in patients who have no clinical disease when high concentrations are used. It is, therefore, necessary, in order for these tests to be useful, to use either end-point or mid-point titrations. Norman's chapter (see also the chapter by Gleich and Yunginger) spells out in great detail the techniques which are necessary. One critical point, which again is almost universally ignored, is that the dilute solutions of allergens which are commonly used for testing are readily denatured or absorbed in glass in the absence of a protective material such as Tween or protein.

The techniques involved in histamine release are described by Siraganian. This procedure is an in vitro counterpart of the skin test but is approximately 100-fold more precise. The correlation between results obtained by skin test and histamine release is quite excellent (0.8 to 0.9), although not complete. The histamine release technique can be used to measure patient sensitivity, to characterize and standardize antigens, and for the measurement of blocking (IgG) antibodies (see below). To date, it has largely been a tool for investigators rather than a routine diagnostic tool. As a result, however, of the work of Siraganian, automated technology has been introduced which makes this procedure as feasible, both economically and with regard to time, as either skin testing or the radioallergosorbent test (RAST). The choice between these techniques depends upon the capability of the diagnostic laboratories.

RAST technology and total IgE antibody determinations are important new procedures. The total IgE antibody level, although not of great diagnostic significance, provides useful information in the variety of disease processes outlined by Adkinson. The RAST technique is a powerful tool for diagnosis, and in routine clinical practice could replace either skin testing or histamine release. Although this appears likely and has, in fact, occurred in Sweden, the exact parallel between this test, other diagnostic tests, and clinical symptomatology needs to be resolved with respect to multiple allergens and disease processes. When a large volume of samples is to be handled, the standardization and economy which accrues to this technique will likely make it the technique of choice for large centers.

No chapter had been included which describes the technology for measuring blocking or IgG antibodies in allergic disease processes. This is, first, because the utility of measurements of these antibodies in ascertaining the efficacy of immunotherapy has not been established and, second, because the study of such responses is generally beyond the interest of a general diagnostic laboratory. Those interested in this technology I refer to a recent article by Sobotka et al. (2).

The remaining two chapters in this section also concern problems which are frequently seen in the clinical immunology laboratory, although the volume of work devoted to these techniques is considerably less. Hypersensitivity pneumonitis or allergic alveolitis is being recognized with increasing frequency, leading investigators to question how much these processes contribute to idiopathic, chronic lung diseases. The pathogenesis of this type(s) of disease has not been established, but it is necessary for most modern clinical immunology laboratories to have the ability to investigate the various immunological correlates of this type of hypersensitivity phenomenon. Fink has dealt with these techniques in detail.

Finally, immune deficiency diseases remain one of the most difficult diagnostic problems for the clinical immunologist. Unfortunately, these syndromes encompass many and diverse defects, and the workup cannot be codified. There are many ways of approaching this problem and Hong, who has long experience with the diagnostic difficulties, has outlined these and provided a general approach to handling the patient in whom immune deficiency is suspected. He rightly points out that these tests must be interpreted with a great deal of caution and that clinical experience remains perhaps more important here than in any of the disease processes considered above.

In closing this introduction, I would like to attempt to clarify some terminology which may cause confusion. A number of chapters refer to allergic disorders as being type I, II, III, and IV. This is based on what has become a widely accepted classification of allergic reactions by Gell and Coombs (1). Type I reactions are caused by the interaction of an allergen with target cells (basophils and mast cells) which have been sensitized by IgE antibody; disease results from the release of pharmacologically active mediators. Type II reactions involve direct cell or tissue damage caused by an antibody which is directed either against the cell body or against haptens or proteins which have become absorbed in the cell membrane. These are usually complement-dependent reactions. Type III reactions are defined as resulting from immune complexes, when antigen and antibody precipitate in tissue spaces or in the blood, and cause direct damage or damage by the involvement of complement factors or granulocytic cells which are attracted to the site of deposition. Type IV reactions involve classical delayed hypersensitivity. That is, the disease process is caused by sensitized T lymphocytes which produce tissue lesions by mechanisms that are still incompletely understood, but presumably involve the release of a number of lymphokines which are destructive themselves or which attract other cell types to the lesion.

In my opinion, this classification of allergic reactions has little utility. In fact, with the possible exception of anaphylactic reactions, it is highly unlikely that any human disease process involves, even primarily, only one of these categories. The long duration of allergic rhinitis, for example, and the utility of corticosteroids (which have no effect on mediator release) in treating this disease is one example. Another is the demonstration that immune complex disease of the kidney does not occur unless there is first the release of mediators following the IgE-antigen interaction. Even in cellular immunity, the involvement of immediate hypersensitivity reactions is being increasingly appreciated. Numerous other examples of human allergic disorders which clearly involve many or all of the four categories of allergic reactions and which cannot clearly be assigned to any one category could be listed. Therefore, although this classification is defined here because of its wide usage, I cannot recommend it as a guide on which to base one's analysis of human allergic disorders.

ACKNOWLEDGMENTS

This work was supported by Public Health Service grants AI07290 and AI08270 from the National Institute of Allergy and Infectious Diseases.

Publication no. 219 from the O'Neill Research Laboratories, The Good Samaritan Hospital.

LITERATURE CITED

1. Gell, P. G. H., and R. R. A. Coombs. 1968. Clinical aspects of immunology, 2nd ed. F. A. David, Philadelphia.
2. Sobotka, A. K., M. D. Valentine, K. Ishizaka, and L. M. Lichtenstein. 1976. Measurement of IgG blocking antibodies: development and application of a radioimmunoassay[1,2,3]. J. Immunol., in press.

Chapter 77

Standardization of Allergens

GERALD J. GLEICH AND JOHN W. YUNGINGER

INTRODUCTION

Allergens are a special class of antigens which cause hypersensitivity reactions. In the broadest sense, antigens causing any of the four types of allergic reactions (8) may be classified as allergens, e.g., horse serum in a type III reaction and tuberculin in a type IV reaction. However, for the purposes of this presentation, we shall restrict the definition to materials causing type I reactions in humans, such as allergic rhinitis and allergic asthma. These reactions are mediated by homocytotropic antibodies of the immunoglobulin E (IgE) class (13) and probably of the IgG class (22). Because IgE antibodies are responsible for the vast majority of type I allergic reactions and because IgE antibodies can be used to measure allergens, we shall further restrict our discussion to homocytotropic antibodies of this class.

At the present time, a large number of materials are implicated in the causation of IgE-mediated allergic reactions. Ideally, all of these materials should be standardized in terms of their content of allergen. The magnitude of this task can be illustrated by inspection of one manufacturer's catalogs; over 400 different allergenic extracts are listed, ranging from those commonly recognized, such as extracts of ragweed and grass pollens, to extracts of tobacco smoke, cotton, and Seven-Up. It seems unlikely that all of these materials actually function as allergens, although one must keep in mind the remarkable capability of the atopic individual to become sensitized to various substances. Even when materials of questionable allergenicity are not considered, the manufacturer's lists still contain a large number of extracts which appear capable of triggering allergic reactions.

The simplest procedure for determination of the potency of allergy extracts is the measurement of their ability to produce a wheal-and-flare skin reaction. In this way the potencies of various extracts can be compared in terms of their content of arbitrary skin test end-point titration units. These measurements can be useful for estimation of potency, but they suffer from two drawbacks: (i) they require sensitive

patients who are available for the procedure, and (ii) they are imprecise (± fivefold, at best).

The early efforts at in vitro standardization of allergy extracts were directed toward evaluation of the procedures in use at that time (7). The most widely accepted procedure, at least in the United States, for measurement of potency in vitro was described by Stull and his associates (24), who determined the quantity of nitrogen precipitable by phosphotungstic acid and expressed the potency of the extract in terms of "protein nitrogen units" (PNU). Because allergens may constitute only a small proportion of the total protein in a crude pollen extract, it is not surprising that the PNU content frequently is a poor correlate of in vivo potency. In several recent studies of ragweed (1, 12), grass (2; G. J. Gleich et al., J. Allergy Clin. Immunol., in press), and Alternaria extracts (J. W. Yunginger, R. T. Jones, and G. J. Gleich, J. Allergy Clin. Immunol., in press), the PNU measurement of potency correlated with measurement of potency by skin testing or leukocyte histamine release in three of the five studies. Surprisingly, the manufacturer's measurements of PNU are often quite different from those of reference laboratories, in spite of the apparent simplicity of this procedure (1, 2). Thus, the PNU is at best a crude measure of extract potency, and in view of the development of in vitro methods for measurement of the interaction of IgE antibody and allergen, in the future it will probably not be commonly performed.

Another in vitro procedure which can be used to determine allergen potency is histamine release from washed human leukocytes (19, 21). Washed leukocytes from sensitive subjects are exposed to various concentrations of different extracts, and the quantity of extract required for release of 50% of the total histamine is measured. This method could be applied to the general problem of allergen standardization, and in two studies it has been used for measurement of the potency of ragweed extracts (1) and to compare the reactivity of various allergens derived from stinging insects (23). The procedure is comparable to the skin test end-point titration in that suspensions of peripheral blood leukocytes from sensitive subjects are exposed to various concentrations of allergen, but it is considerably more precise than skin testing because the released histamine can be accurately measured. However, for standardization of allergenic extracts, one requires fresh leukocytes from sensitive patients, and, because the leukocytes cannot be stored, the patients must be readily available. Clearly it would prove difficult to identify and procure a large number of patients with a variety of sensitivities as would be needed if leukocyte histamine release were used as a general method for allergen standardization.

Another approach to the problem of allergen extract standardization has been through the isolation of the principal allergens of the extracts. Initially, this was accomplished for antigen E (AgE) from short ragweed (16), and subsequently the AgE content of the extract was used as a measure of the potency of the extract (1, 12). Because the AgE molecule is rather labile (17), it should be a good indicator of changes in the potency of the extract. The assay procedure used for AgE is radial immunodiffusion, and a monospecific antiserum and standard are needed. Comparison of AgE content and biological activity of short ragweed extracts as determined by leukocyte histamine release revealed that these were related (1). One assumes that the other antigens in ragweed extract, AgK, Ra3, and Ra5, would be present in relatively constant proportions to AgE, although this has not been tested to date. Surprisingly, the precipitating antibody to short ragweed AgE is poorly cross-reactive with the AgE-like material from giant ragweed (26). Therefore, this assay system is limited to extracts of short ragweed. In the case of grass extracts, three major allergens have been purified from rye grass, termed group I, group II, and group III (20). Animal antisera to the group I allergen have been used to measure the quantity of this allergen in various grass pollen extracts by radial immunodiffusion. In contrast to AgE from short ragweed, antiserum to rye group I recognizes a similar material in related species of grasses, including fescue, sweet vernal, red top, June, and velvet, and the content of the group I allergen correlated with the biological activity of the grass extracts as determined by skin test end-point titrations (2). Thus, this assay can be used to standardize a variety of related grasses, although group I from certain grasses such as timothy and Bermuda does not cross-react sufficiently with the rye group I antiserum to permit its use for standardization of these extracts.

The measurement of the content of individual allergens by radial immunodiffusion appears to be the ideal at the moment because it requires only a precipitating antibody and a standard. In practice, however, this approach to standardization is limited by the small number of extracts from which allergens have been purified. Following the discovery of IgE (3, 13) and the identification of patients with IgE myeloma proteins, reagents for measurement of allergenic activity by the radioallergosorbent test (RAST) became available (25). The RAST is discussed in detail in chapter 79 of this *Manual*. Briefly, the RAST is a two-step procedure similar in principle to the indirect Coombs test. In the first step allergens covalently bound to solid-phase supports, such as cellulose disks or particles, are allowed to react with allergic serum containing IgE antibodies. IgE antibodies, as well as antibodies of the other immunoglobulin classes, react with the allergens present on the solid-phase supports and form allergen-antibody complexes. IgE antibodies directed against allergens, other than those on the solid-phase support, as well as other serum components, are washed away at the end of the first step of the reaction. In the second step of the RAST, the washed solid-phase allergen-antibody complexes are allowed to react with radio-iodinated affinity chromatography-purified antibody to human IgE. The purified antibodies to IgE react with the IgE on the surface of the cellulose-allergen complex. After another washing step to remove unbound anti-IgE, the radioactivity associated with the complex is measured in a gamma scintillation counter. The quantity of radioactivity is related to the quantity of IgE antibody present in the allergic serum. The RAST has been used for the diagnosis of allergy to various allergens (3, 25), for the measurement of the changes in IgE antibodies to specific allergens (18, 27), and also for the measurement of the potency of allergy extracts (6, 9, 10, 12). For the measurement of the potency of allergy extracts by RAST, two approaches have been employed: (i) various quantities of extracts have been coupled to solid-phase supports and the quantity of coupled extract needed to achieve a given degree of reactivity in the RAST has been determined, and (ii) soluble extracts have been tested to determine their inhibitory capacities in the first step of the RAST as shown in Fig. 1. The former procedure is often referred to as the direct RAST measurement of potency, and the latter procedure is referred to as RAST inhibition. In both of these methods, IgE antibodies in the allergic sera define the specificities associated with the various allergens. The advantages of these procedures for standardization of allergenic extracts are numerous: (i) the solid-phase

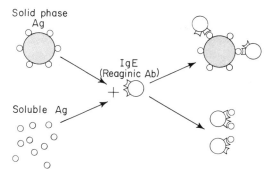

FIG. 1. *Diagrammatic representation of the first stage of RAST inhibition procedure. There is competitive binding between soluble and solid-phase allergens for the available IgE antibodies (12).*

allergens are remarkably stable, and we have found that solid-phase short ragweed has a shelf-life of over 4 years (G. J. Gleich and J. W. Yunginger, unpublished data); (ii) the IgE antibodies could be stored indefinitely after lyophilization; and (iii) it appears that virtually any allergen can be standardized providing that it can be covalently bound to a solid-phase support. However, before the RAST can be used for standardization of a given extract, the investigator must verify that the relevant allergens have been bound to the solid-phase support. In practice, this means that he must demonstrate that the solid-phase allergen is able to bind and thus remove from the allergic serum all of the IgE antibodies reactive with the crude extracts. In our laboratory we have exposed serum to solid-phase allergen and have tested the supernatant fluids by the Prausnitz-Kustner (P-K) passive transfer testing using the crude allergen mixture to challenge the sensitized skin sites. In the case of solid-phase Alternaria (J. W. Yunginger, G. D. Roberts and G. J. Gleich, J. Allergy Clin. Immunol., in press) and ragweed, we found that essentially all of the P-K reactivity was removed by such absorption. These experiments indicated that all of the major allergens recognized by the IgE antibodies were bound to the solid-phase support. Ideally, one should show that all of the allergens are represented on the solid-phase support in the same proportions as in the original allergen mixture. To date, this has not been shown for any complex allergen mixture. If it were possible to bind *all* of the available allergen to the solid-phase support, the investigator could be confident that all major and minor allergens were present on the solid-phase support in essentially the same proportion as in the original mixture. Future work needs to be directed toward developing solid-phase supports of such

high binding capacity that all or virtually all of the allergen can be bound to the support.

CLINICAL INDICATIONS

At the present time there is no United States standard of potency for allergy extracts marketed for diagnosis and treatment of allergic patients. Extracts are labeled with the number of PNU per milliliter or simply in terms of the weight per volume of solid to solvent used to prepare the extract. Certain companies will provide the content of short ragweed AgE per milliliter of extract, but this is the only purified allergen presently used commercially for standardization. Several producers are in the process of applying the RAST procedures for standardization, but it seems likely that routine labeling of extracts in terms of their RAST potency is years away. Thus, at the present time, individual users of allergy extracts are presented with a dilemma. Even though the labels of different extracts indicate the same potency, in terms of weight per volume or PNU per milliliter, it is clear that the true biological potencies of the extracts may differ by 10- to 1,000-fold. One solution is to purchase a large quantity of a given extract, especially those more commonly used, so that the supply will be adequate for 1 year or longer. Then, when a new lot is purchased, it can be compared with the old lot to determine its relative potency. Unfortunately, this approach is limited to fairly large practices and to fairly commonly used extracts. For the remaining extracts, the physician must always exercise caution by using limiting quantities of any new lot until he has had sufficient experience to estimate its biological potency. One hopes that this situation will be changed in the near future because it is evident that standardization of extracts can be accomplished in terms of their content of purified allergens or in terms of their potency in the RAST.

TEST PROCEDURES

From the discussion above, it is apparent that only a few of the various methods available are of practical value for standardization of allergenic activity. For example, measurement of the number of PNU per milliliter of extract bears at best an inconstant relationship to allergenic potency. Nonetheless, because in some situations it may be desirable to determine PNU for a given extract, this procedure will be described. Some of the other procedures, such as leukocyte histamine release and radial immunodiffusion, are described in detail elsewhere in this *Manual*. Consequently, only a brief general description of these procedures is included.

Measurement of the protein nitrogen unit

In this procedure, the soluble proteins of the allergy extract are precipitated with phosphotungstic acid (PTA), and the quantity of nitrogen in the precipitate is determined. The procedure listed below is that utilized by the Bureau of Biologics of the Food and Drug Administration of the United States Government. (This procedure represents that presently utilized by the Food and Drug Administration and may be modified as a result of continuing study of the variables in the method.)

1. Concentrated HCl, 1.3 ml, is added to 2.0 ml of the allergenic extract in a 12-ml conical centrifuge tube. The 2-ml amount of extract is used when the approximate PNU is not known. When the approximate PNU is known, the volume of extract should be altered as described in Table 1.

2. A 1.0-ml amount of 10% PTA in 10% HCl is added and thoroughly mixed with the extract.

3. The precipitate is allowed to stand for 1 h at room temperature.

4. The samples are centrifuged at room temperature at 2,700 rpm for 10 to 15 min.

5. The completeness of precipitation is tested by adding five drops of 10% PTA in 10% HCl to the supernatant fluid. If cloudiness develops, an additional 0.5 ml of 10% PTA in 10% HCl is added, and the mixtures are left for another 1 h at room temperature. Step 4 is then repeated.

6. The supernatant solution is decanted, and the residual fluid in the tube is drained by inversion. The precipitate forms a pellet in the bottom of the conical centrifuge tube, and inversion should not dislodge it.

7. The precipitate is dissolved in 10 ml of 2% NaOH; it is *not* washed. Two milliliters of 2% NaOH is added with a volumetric pipette, and a vortex mixer is used to dislodge the precipitate from the apex of the tube. After the precipitate has dissolved, an additional 8.0 ml of 2% NaOH is added with a volumetric pipette.

8. After the solutions above have been thoroughly mixed, a nitrogen determination is performed on the solubilized precipitate. This can be accomplished by the micro-Kjeldahl procedure (15), by the Nessler procedure (5), or by the use of an ammonia electrode (4). In all of these procedures, the precipitate must first be digested (15).

Skin test end-point titration

The general description of skin testing is presented in chapter 78 of this *Manual*. For determination of allergen potency, the skin tests must be performed on patients with definite sensitivity to the extract in question. These patients should have a typical history of allergic rhinitis or allergic asthma with worsening of their symptoms on exposure to the allergen and a positive skin test or provocation test. They should not be ingesting drugs, such as antihistamines, which interfere with the development of the wheal and flare reactions, and they should not have been treated by injection of pollen extracts (hyposensitization). For assaying the potency of extracts, the dilution of the extract producing a standard end point, e.g., a 6 × 6 mm wheal and flare (2+), is determined. Fivefold dilutions of the extracts are prepared in pH 7.4 phosphate-buffered saline containing approximately 0.5% human serum albumin, and a series of intradermal skin tests are performed to determine the reactivity of the individual patients. The volume of extract injected should be just sufficient to raise an initial 3 × 3 mm wheal; with practice, this wheal size can be readily reproduced. The total volume of extract injected is approximately 0.004 ml. In a preliminary test the extracts are titrated on the forearm at three sites with the use of dilutions differing by 25-fold, and that dilution best approximating the 6 × 6 mm wheal is identified. The tests are then repeated in duplicate on the upper arm, and the dilution best approximating the 6 × 6 mm wheal is bracketed by dilutions fivefold more and fivefold less concentrated. When the resultant wheal sizes are not exactly 6 × 6 mm, the end point can be extrapolated. For example, if the ninth fivefold dilution yields reactions of 7 × 6 and 6.5 × 6 mm for the duplicate determinations, then the mean for the two dilutions is obtained by averaging the product of the wheal diameters. In this case the mean equals $\frac{(7 \times 6) + (6.5 \times 6)}{2} = 40.5$. If the tenth fivefold dilution yields reactions of 5 × 5 and 5 × 5 mm, the mean is $\frac{(5 \times 5) + (5 \times 5)}{2} =$ 25. The extrapolated score for the extract is obtained by determining the difference between the score for the ninth extract and 36 (the score for the hypothetical 6 × 6) and dividing this by the difference between the scores for the ninth and tenth extracts. The extrapolated value in

TABLE 1. *Determination of PNU*

PNU per ml	Amt of allergenic extract used (ml)
>60,000	1
30,000–60,000	1
20,000–30,000	2
10,000–20,000	3
5,000–10,000	4
<5,000	5

this case is $\dfrac{40.5 - 36}{40.5 - 25} = \dfrac{4.5}{15.5} = 0.29$, and the final score for the extract is 9.29. The potency of the extract is expressed in terms of skin test units, i.e., the number of dilutions necessary to achieve that concentration yielding a 6×6 mm wheal. In the example above, the potency of the extract is $5^{9.29}$ or 3.11×10^6 skin test units. We have noted considerable difference in reactivity between the upper and lower arms so that we believe it important to make the final comparisons on the same regions of the skin. In our experiments, up to 12 extracts were tested. Usually, half of the skin tests were performed at one session, and the remaining skin tests were performed a day later. In some cases, the entire battery of skin tests was performed at one sitting. In all cases, the skin test titrations were performed in a double-blind manner. Finally, nonsensitive subjects should be tested with the extract to ensure that extracts are not provoking nonspecific irritant reactions.

Measurement of the potency of allergy extracts by leukocyte histamine release

Histamine release from leukocytes is described in detail in chapter 80 of this *Manual*. For measurement of allergen potency, various quantities of extract are added to the same number of sensitive leukocytes, and the amount of extract needed for release of 50% of total leukocyte histamine is determined from the dose response curves. The potencies of the extracts are then compared in terms of the quantities needed for 50% histamine release.

Measurement of purified allergens by radial immunodiffusion

The detailed description of radial immunodiffusion is presented in chapter 2 of this *Manual*. For measurement of AgE from ragweed pollen or group I from grass pollen, monospecific antiserum to the allergen is incorporated into the gel, and standards containing known quantities of the allergen are analyzed with the unknown. The quantity of allergen in the unknown is determined by reference to the calibration curve yielded by the standards.

Measurement of the potency of allergy extracts by the radioallergosorbent test

As described in the Introduction, allergenic extracts can be standardized by the RAST either by a direct procedure in which various quantities of the extract are coupled to a solid-phase support and then carried through the usual RAST procedure, or by an indirect or inhibition method in which the fluid-phase and solid-phase allergens compete for IgE antibodies. The principles of these procedures have been described in the Introduction.

Use of the direct RAST. Various quantities of allergen extract are covalently bound to either microcrystalline cellulose particles or paper disks (6). In the latter case, the disks are washed with distilled water and then added to a 2.5% aqueous solution of cyanogen bromide (CNBr). Usually, 1 g of disks is activated with 2 g of CNBr. The pH is maintained at 11 for 5 min at room temperature by addition of NaOH with an automatic titrator. The molarity of the NaOH can be varied from 2 to 10, depending on the quantity of disks being activated. The suspension of activated disks is repeatedly washed with ice-cold 0.1 M $NaHCO_3$, water, and finally acetone. The disks are dried for 2 h at 4 C and stored in a disiccator at 4 C. The test extracts are dialyzed with the use of casing with a cutoff at 3,500 daltons to remove preservatives, such as phenol and glycerol. Single activated disks are placed in test tubes, and various quantities of extract are added to the tubes. The volume is brought to a convenient level, e.g., 1.0 to 1.8 ml, by addition of 0.2 M H_3BO_3–0.04 M NaOH–0.16 M NaCl, pH 8.0 (borate-saline), and the disks are tumbled overnight at 4 C. The disks are repeatedly washed with borate-saline, water, and finally RAST diluent. After the last wash, the RAST diluent is completely aspirated, and 0.05 ml of human serum rich in IgE antibodies to the allergen in question is added to the tube. This volume should just cover the disk. After overnight incubation at room temperature, the disks are washed thrice with 2.5 ml of 0.15 M NaCl, and radiolabeled affinity chromatography-purified antibody to IgE, 20 ng in a volume of 0.1 ml, is added to the disk. We have also used 10 ng of antibody to IgE with little difference in results. After another overnight incubation at room temperature, the disk is washed thrice with saline, and the quantity of radioactivity associated with the disk is measured in a gamma scintillation counter. The number of counts in tubes containing only the radiolabeled antibody to IgE is determined, and the results are expressed as counts bound divided by counts added $\times$ 100. These percentages are plotted on semilog paper against the volume of extract used in the coupling procedure. The results of a direct RAST assay for allergen potency are shown in Fig. 2. As controls in the assay, normal human serum and buffer, respectively, are added to disks to determine the degree of nonspecific binding of radiolabeled antibody to IgE. These should not contain greater than 1 to 2% of counts.

Use of RAST inhibition. For the measure-

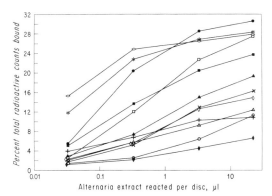

FIG. 2. *Measurement of the potency of Alternaria extracts by direct RAST. Various quantities of dialyzed extracts were reacted with CNBr-activated filter-paper disks. These were washed, and their reactivity with IgE antibodies in a serum pool from 10 subjects allergic to Alternaria was determined. The symbols used in this figure and Fig. 3 indicate the behavior of the same Alternaria extracts in the two RAST assays.*

ment of allergen potency by this procedure, one needs to prepare a sufficient quantity of solid-phase allergen, either disks or particles, to analyze in many assays. The allergen extract coupled to the solid-phase support must be potent, and we usually prepare fresh extracts of pollens or other allergens by extraction of 10 parts by weight of allergen with 90 parts by weight of distilled water with magnetic stirring overnight at room temperature. A drop of toluene is added to the extracting vessel to inhibit bacterial growth. The pH is maintained at near neutrality by addition of 1 N NH_4OH. The dry weight of the extract may be estimated by drying the extract overnight in an oven.

For covalently attaching allergens to microcrystalline cellulose, the following procedure is used. A 1-g amount of microcrystalline cellulose suspended in 10 to 15 ml of 0.1 M $NaHCO_3$ is activated by reaction with 2 g of CNBr dissolved in 2 ml of N,N-dimethylformamide, and the pH is maintained at 11 by addition of 4 N NaOH. The activation procedure is carried out in a chemical hood at 4 C in an ice bath for 45 min. The activated cellulose is washed twice with borate-saline and suspended in a volume of approximately 10 ml of extract containing from 1 to 500 mg of dissolved solids; the pH is adjusted to 8.5. The suspension is tumbled in a 40-ml tube at 4 C for 72 h. The cellulose is repeatedly washed with borate-saline until the absorbance of the washings at 280 nm is less than 0.05. Usually, less than 50% of the absorbance units (absorbance at 280 nm × ml) contained in the extract are bound to the solid-

phase support. Finally, the solid-phase allergen is suspended in RAST diluent.

The RAST inhibition procedure is carried out in the following manner. First, a pool of sera from individuals highly allergic to the allergen in question is obtained. This pool should be obtained from at least 5 and preferably 10 individuals sensitive to the allergen and should possess sufficient reactivity in the RAST so that the positive control tubes in the absence of inhibition yield 10 to 20% binding and the negative controls yield no greater than 1 to 2%. In the experiments with standardization of ragweed extracts, 0.1 ml of a 1:5 dilution of the serum pool yielded 19 to 22% binding, whereas the controls, either normal human serum or fetal calf serum (FCS) yielded a maximum of 1.2% binding and usually less than 1% binding (12). In experiments with June grass extracts, the serum pool yielded about 17% of total counts bound, and normal human serum yielded less than 1% binding (Gleich et al., in press). For testing of Alternaria extracts, the serum pool yielded binding of 10 to 13% of counts, and nonallergic serum yielded 0.4% binding (Yunginger et al., in press). In no case was serum from individuals who had recently received hyposensitization used in these serum pools.

Second, preliminary experiments are conducted in which 0.1-ml samples of each extract are tested over a range of dilutions to determine that dilution which produces approximately 50% inhibition of binding.

Third, in the actual performance of the test, 0.05 ml of the allergic serum pool, or a suitable dilution of the serum pool in RAST diluent, is added to the various inhibitors; the volume is made up to 0.5 ml with RAST diluent, and 0.5 ml of cellulose-allergen mixture (1 mg/ml) is added. The tubes are rotated for 24 h at room temperature and centrifuged at 1,500 × g at room temperature for 5 min; the solid-phase allergen is then washed twice with 1.0 ml of RAST wash solution. The cellulose particles are resuspended by mixing on a vortex mixer after addition of the wash solution. After the last wash is removed, 20 ng of affinity chromatography-purified antibody to IgE in a volume of 0.1 ml is added, and the volume is adjusted to 0.75 ml with FCS diluent. The tubes are rotated overnight at room temperature, centrifuged, and washed twice; then the quantity of radioactivity is measured in a gamma scintillation counter. If paper disks are used, one simply aspirates the wash solution from the tube; there is no need for centrifugation. Usually, the percentage of counts bound by the normal serum control is subtracted from all of the tests before analysis of the data.

The volume or quantity of allergen needed for 50% inhibition is determined from graphs in which the percent inhibition is plotted on a linear scale on the ordinate and the quantity or volume of inhibition is plotted on a log scale on the abscissa as shown in Fig. 3 and 4. Least squares regression lines are determined for the range of values from 25 to 75% inhibition. In this region the semilog plots are linear, with correlation coefficients usually greater than +0.98. Arbitrarily, we have defined the potency of an extract as 1,000 divided by the number of microliters needed to produce 50% inhibition of binding.

REAGENTS

Measurement of protein nitrogen units

The reagents for measurement of PNU are readily obtained from any of several chemical supply houses. The various procedures for measurement of nitrogen are described elsewhere. These include the Markham modifica-

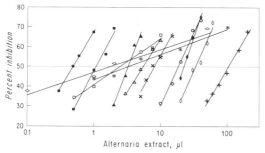

FIG. 3. *Measurement of the potency of Alternaria extracts by RAST inhibition. Correlation coefficients for the least squares regressions were +0.98 or greater. The number of microliters required for 50% inhibition in the RAST is used as a measure of potency.*

tion of the micro-Kjeldahl procedure (15), the Nessler precedure (5), and the use of an ammonia electrode (4).

Skin test end-point titration

The principal reagent needed for performance of the skin tests is an iso-osmolar buffer of physiological pH containing a protective protein. We have used a Sorenson phosphate buffer prepared by mixing 400 ml of 0.0667 M $NaH_2PO_4 \cdot H_2O$ (9.2 g per 1,000 ml of sterile water for injection, USP) and 1,600 ml of 0.0667 M $Na_2HPO_4 \cdot 7H_2O$ (35.74 g per 1,000 ml of sterile USP water). After autoclaving, 100 ml of this solution is added to 900 ml of sodium chloride for injection, USP. The resulting solution has a pH of 7.4 and is iso-osmolar, 285 mosmol per liter. Finally, 100 ml of 5% human serum albumin, available from several commercial sources, is added to yield a final solution containing approximately 0.5% albumin. The albumin is added as a stabilizing agent and to prevent glass adsorption of the proteins in dilute solutions of allergens.

Leukocyte histamine release

The reagents for leukocyte histamine release are listed elsewhere in this *Manual*.

Measurement of allergens by radial immunodiffusion

AgE from short ragweed is commercially available from Worthington Biochemical Corp., Freehold, N.J. Rye group I antigen is presently not commercially available nor are antisera to either of these purified allergens.

Reagents for performance of the radioallergosorbent test

Solid-phase supports. Paper disks (grade 595, 6.35 mm in diameter) are obtained from

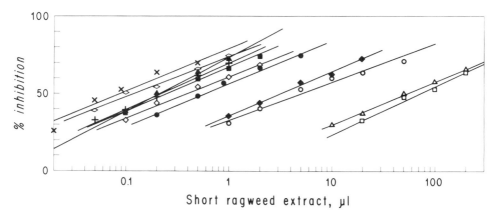

FIG. 4. *Measurement of the potency of extracts of short ragweed by RAST inhibition (12).*

Schleicher & Schuell Co., Keene, N.H. Microcrystalline cellulose is purchased from Brinkman Instruments, Inc., Westbury, N.Y. Cyanogen bromide and N,N-dimethylformamide can be purchased from any of several supply houses. RAST diluent is 0.1 M, pH 7.4, KH_2PO_4–K_2HPO_4 containing 0.2% bovine serum albumin (fraction V), 1% Tween 20, and 0.1% sodium azide. RAST wash is 0.1 M, pH 7.4, KH_2PO_4–K_2HPO_4 containing 1% Tween 20. FCS diluent consists of: 0.1 M, pH 7.5, K_2HPO_4–KH_2PO_4, 470 ml; fetal calf serum (Grand Island Biological Co., Grand Island, N.Y.), 20 ml; 10% NaN_3, 5 ml; and Tween 20, 5 ml. In comparative experiments, we found that the use of FCS diluent in the second step of the RAST resulted in lower counts associated with the normal human serum controls than use of the RAST diluent (11). RAST diluent is stable for months when kept at 4 C, whereas the FCS diluent develops slight turbidity, so that the latter reagent is usually prepared at least every month. The preparation of the solid-phase allergens has already been described. The selection of sera from sensitive subjects always presents a problem because one wishes to ensure that the IgE antibodies recognize the critical antigenic determinants associated with the allergens. In practice, one obtains as many highly potent sera as one can, at least 5 to 10, to constitute the serum pool. We select these sera because they possess considerable reactivity in the RAST and thus provide a high ratio of results with positive and negative controls in direct RAST or RAST inhibition procedures. The serum pool is stable for years at −20 C.

Perhaps the most difficult reagent to obtain for the performance of the RAST is the affinity chromatography-purified antibody to IgE. In our laboratory, we have prepared this reagent in two ways. In the first procedure we purchased specific sheep anti-IgE from Pharmacia Laboratories, Piscataway, N.J., and allowed this to react with purified IgE (PS) coupled to Sepharose 2B on a small column. The column was washed with 0.01 M K_2HPO_4–KH_2PO_4, 0.13 M NaCl, pH 7.4, and the adsorbed anti-IgE was eluted with 0.05 M, pH 3.0, glycine-HCl. An amount of borate-saline sufficient to raise the pH to near neutrality was added to every tube used to collect the glycine-HCl buffer containing the eluted anti-IgE. In this procedure, the antiserum was produced against the myeloma protein IgE (ND), and the solid-phase IgE was from myeloma patient PS. This "crossing" of IgE myeloma proteins virtually eliminates the possibility that antibodies to the individual antigenic specificities (idiotypic determinants) associated with myeloma proteins might be included in the affinity chromatography-purified antibodies.

In the second procedure we utilized only a single myeloma protein. IgE (PS) was digested with papain and fractionated on a column of Sephadex G-200 as described by Ishizaka and his associates (14). The Fc piece was recovered and used to immunize rabbits, after which the antisera were rendered specific for IgE by solid-phase immunoabsorption with a human serum deficient in IgE. The specific rabbit anti-IgE was next purified by affinity chromatography as described above with the use of a Sepharose-IgE (PS) column. Because the Fc piece does not possess the individual antigenic specificities, the resulting antiserum should not distinguish among the various IgE myeloma proteins, and indeed we have found that this reagent produces reactions of identity with different IgE myeloma proteins. At the present time, it is impossible to produce the affinity chromatography-purified anti-IgE unless the investigator has sufficient purified IgE myeloma protein to prepare a solid-phase immunoabsorbent. The only commercial source of affinity chromatography-purified antibody to IgE is Pharmacia Laboratories. They sell a ^{125}I-radiolabeled anti-IgE of high quality suitable for RAST experiments.

INTERPRETATION

At the present time, allergy extracts are only standardized by determination of PNU. However, the ability to measure the potency of short ragweed and certain grass extracts with antiserum to AgE and group I, respectively, should gradually bring about standardization of these extracts. Utilizing the RAST procedures, one can quantitate the allergens in extracts either by the direct RAST procedure or by the RAST inhibition procedure. In the case of the direct RAST procedure, various quantities of the allergenic extract are bound to paper disks or microcrystalline cellulose, and the maximal reactivity obtainable with the highest concentration of allergenic extract tested is determined. In practice, curves such as that shown in Fig. 2, are produced in which the reactivity in the RAST increased with increasing doses of allergenic extract before reaching a plateau region with the highest concentration of extract used in the test. For purposes of standardization, one can take the plateau value as 100% and then compare the extracts in terms of the number of microliters of extract needed to obtain 50% binding with the serum pool. These 50% binding values are then measures of the potency of the allergenic extract. In contrast, when one performs RAST inhibition, one obtains an additional piece of information. As shown in Fig. 3, the inhibition curves are linear between approximately 25 and 75% inhibition, and one can derive the relative potency of allergy extracts by determining that quantity of extract needed to produce 50% inhibition in the RAST. In addition, the inhibition lines have a measurable slope, and the comparison of slopes yielded by different extracts is a measure of allergenic relatedness. For example, inspection of the results shown in Fig. 3 indicates that nine of the Alternaria extracts had slopes which were quite similar and three of the extracts had slopes that were distinctly different. We would interpret these results as indicating that these nine extracts were allergenically similar, even though differing markedly in terms of their inhibitory potencies. The other three extracts had distinctly different slopes, suggesting that they possess different allergenic determinants than the first nine extracts. In the case of extracts of short ragweed, the slopes of the inhibition lines were similar, indicating that they did not differ in their content of the various allergens even though the concentration of the allergens differed by 1,000-fold (12). Thus, the RAST inhibition procedure yields two kinds of information, one relating to potency and the other relating to whether or not differences in allergenic determinants are present among the allergenic extracts. Finally, with either of the RAST procedures, one needs to analyze a standard in the same assay so that the test preparations can be compared with a reference extract. Certain reference allergens are available through the Bureau of Biologics of the Food and Drug Administration, and a series of reference extracts to many common allergens are being prepared under the auspices of the World Health Organization.

At the present time, all of this information relating to standardization of allergy extract is academic in that there is no United States standard of potency for any of the extracts. Nonetheless, the future would appear to be bright in that the means are at hand to standardize allergy extracts in terms of their potency either by measurement of their content of purified allergens, such as AgE or group I, or by measurement of their reactivity with IgE antibodies in the RAST. Thus, in the future, the labels on allergenic extracts should provide an accurate measure of the biological potency of the material in sensitive subjects. At the present time, from the results of studies by a number of investigators, it is quite clear that this situation does not obtain; therefore, the individual patient is at risk when his physician changes from one lot of extract to another,

much less from one company's to another company's product.

ACKNOWLEDGMENTS

We thank Joan May of the Food and Drug Administration for allowing us to list the procedure for PNU determination.

This work was supported by grant 223-73-1164 from the Food and Drug Administration Bureau of Biologics and Public Health Service grant 42546 from the National Institute of Allergy and Infectious Diseases. J.W.Y. is recipient of Allergic Diseases Academic Award AI 00107 from the National Institute of Allergy and Infectious Diseases.

LITERATURE CITED

1. Baer, H., H. Godfrey, C. J. Maloney, P. S. Norman, and L. M. Lichtenstein. 1970. The potency and antigen E content of commercially prepared ragweed extracts. J. Allergy 45:347–354.
2. Baer, H., C. J. Maloney, P. S. Norman, and D. G. Marsh. 1974. The potency and Group I antigen content of six commercially prepared grass pollen extracts. J. Allergy Clin. Immunol. 54:157–164.
3. Bennich, H., and S. G. O. Johansson. 1971. Structure and function of human immunoglobulin E. Adv. Immunol. 13:1–55.
4. Bremner, J. M., and M. A. Tabatabai. 1972. Use of an ammonia electrode for determination in Kjeldahl analysis of soils. Commun. Soil Sci. Plant Anal. 3:159–165.
5. Campbell, D. H., J. S. Garvey, N. E. Cremer, with D. H. Sussdorf. 1970. Methods in immunology, 2nd ed., p. 69–73. W. A. Benjamin, Inc., New York.
6. Ceska, M., R. Eriksson, and J. M. Varga. 1972. Radioimmunosorbent assay of allergens. J. Allergy Clin. Immunol. 49:1–9.
7. Clock, R. O. 1917. Comparative value of methods of preparing pollen antigen. J. Infect. Dis. 21:523–525.
8. Coombs, R. R. A., and P. G. H. Gell. 1968. Classification of allergic reactions responsible for clinical hypersensitivity and disease, p. 575–596. In P. G. H. Gell and R. R. A. Coombs (ed.), Clinical aspects of immunology. F. A. Davis Co., Philadelphia.
9. Foucard, T., H. Bennich, and S. G. O. Johansson. 1973. Studies on the stability of diluted allergen extracts using the radioallergosorbent test (RAST). Clin. Allergy 3:91–102.
10. Foucard, T., S. G. O. Johnasson, H. Bennich, and T. Berg. 1972. In vitro estimation of allergens by a radioimmune antiglobulin technique using human IgE antibodies. Int. Arch. Allergy Appl. Immunol. 43:360–370.
11. Gleich, G. J., and R. T. Jones. 1975. Measurement of IgE antibodies by the radioallergosorbent test. I. Technical considerations in the performance of the test. J. Allergy Clin. Immunol. 55:334–345.
12. Gleich, G. J., J. B. Larson, R. T. Jones, and H. Baer. 1974. Measurement of the potency of

allergy extracts by their inhibitory capacities in the radioallergosorbent test. J. Allergy Clin. Immunol. 53:158–169.

13. Ishizaka, K., and T. Ishizaka. 1968. Human reaginic antibodies and immunoglobulin E. J. Allergy 42:330–363.

14. Ishizaka, K., T. Ishizaka, and E. H. Lee. 1970. Biologic function of the Fc fragments of E myeloma protein. Immunochemistry 7:687–702.

15. Kabat, E. A., and M. M. Mayer. 1961. Experimental immunochemistry, p. 476–483. Charles C Thomas, Publisher, Springfield, Ill.

16. King, T. P., P. S. Norman, and J. T. Connell. 1964. Isolation and characterization of allergens from ragweed pollen. II. Biochemistry 3:458–468.

17. King, T. P., P. S. Norman, and N. Tao. 1974. Chemical modifications of the major allergen of ragweed pollen, antigen E. Immunochemistry 11:83–92.

18. Lichtenstein, L. M., K. Ishizaka, P. S. Norman, A. K. Sobotka, and B. M. Hill. 1973. IgE antibody measurements in ragweed hay fever. Relationship to clinical severity and the results of immunotherapy. J. Clin. Invest. 52:472–482.

19. Lichtenstein, L. M., T. P. King, and A. G. Osler. 1966. In vitro assay of allergenic properties of ragweed pollen antigens. J. Allergy 38:174–182.

20. Marsh, D. G. 1973. Purification of pollen allergens: use in genetic studies of immune responsiveness in man, p. 381–393. In Y. Yamamura, O. L. Frick, Y. Horiuchi, S. Kishimoto,

T. Miyamoto, P. Naranjo, and A. de Weck (ed.), Allergology, Proceedings of the VIII International Congress of Allergology, Tokyo, Japan, 14–20 October. American Elsevier Publishing Co., Inc., New York.

21. Osler, A. G., L. M. Lichtenstein, and D. A. Levy. 1968. In vitro studies of human reaginic allergy. Adv. Immunol. 8:183–236.

22. Parish, W. E. 1974. Skin sensitizing non-IgE antibodies. Association between human IgG S-TS and IgG$_4$, p. 19–28. In L. Brent and J. Holborow (ed.), Progress in immunology II, vol. 4. American Elsevier Publishing Co., Inc., New York.

23. Sobotka, A. K., M. D. Valentine, A. W. Benton, and L. M. Lichtenstein. 1974. Allergy to insect stings. I. Diagnosis of IgE-mediated Hymenoptera sensitivity by venom-induced histamine release. J. Allergy Clin. Immunol. 53:170–184.

24. Stull, A., R. A. Cooke, and J. A. Tennant. 1933. The allergen content of pollen extracts. Its determination and its deterioration. J. Allergy 4:455–467.

25. Wide, L., H. Bennich, and S. G. O. Johansson. 1967. Diagnosis of allergy by an in-vitro test for allergen antibodies. Lancet 2:1105–1107.

26. Yunginger, J. W., and G. J. Gleich. 1972. Measurement of ragweed antigen-E by double antibody radioimmunoassay. J. Allergy 50:326–337.

27. Yunginger, J. W., and G. J. Gleich. 1973. Seasonal changes in IgE antibodies and their relationship to the IgG antibodies during immunotherapy for ragweed hay fever. J. Clin. Invest. 52:1268–1275.

Chapter 78

Skin Testing

PHILIP S. NORMAN

INTRODUCTION

Direct reproduction of an immediate allergic reaction by introducing a small amount of extract of suspected allergen into the skin is ingrained in the practice of medicine as a diagnostic aid. A large number of tests can be done in a short time, the results appear in a matter of minutes, and the result, when positive, is striking both to the patient and to the physician. The early work of Prausnitz and Küstner showed that wheal and erythema reactions in the skin were the result of serum antibodies specific for the allergen being tested (13). Without detailing the extensive investigation of the allergic phenomenon which ensued, it resulted in the knowledge that such reactions are the result of immunoglobulin E (IgE) antibodies formed by lymphoid tissue in the organ(s) exposed to the allergen, most often the respiratory tract, but also the gastrointestinal tract, skin, and probably other tissues. IgE antibodies find specific and avid receptors on mast cells and basophils and tend to be drawn out of blood and tissue fluids to reside on the surface of these cells. The presence of IgE antibodies on mast cells and basophils sensitizes them so that a repeat contact with the allergen results in rapid (15 to 20 min) secretion of histamine, SRS-A, and other mediators, which show their characteristic activity in the skin by the development of a wheal, a sharply circumscribed localized area of edema, surrounded by a flare, a less exactly defined area of erythema surrounding the wheal (11). It was early recognized that a positive skin test simply reproduced to a minor degree, in the skin, the disease which was causing the patient's problem in other tissues. As the procedure was usually safe, it caught on rapidly in diagnosis and has been much more frequently used than direct challenges to tissues such as the respiratory tract or gastrointestinal tract, because such challenges are accompanied by a greater risk of reproducing the disease to an unpleasant or even dangerous degree.

Skin tests, however, do not always elicit a reaction when a challenge by another route will. This is seen most frequently in drug al-

lergy. For instance, in the case of penicillin, it has been shown that serum sickness, urticaria, or anaphylaxis after injection or ingestion of penicillin is often not due to penicillin itself but to metabolic products of the penicillin formed after its introduction. These metabolic products are capable of reacting with body tissues to form complete antigens which then elicit the reaction. Two skin test reagents, one an analogue of penicillin coupled to an inert polypeptide carrier, and the other a mixture of penicillin and its metabolic products, will give diagnostically helpful reactions in practically every penicillin-allergic individual, but penicillin itself will react in only a minority of sensitive individuals (1, 10). Such reagents have not been developed with other drugs, and thus skin tests are generally useless as a means of diagnosis in drug allergy. Only reproduction of disease by challenge with a full therapeutic dose will settle the issue objectively, and the hazards involved are obvious.

Furthermore, in respiratory allergy, skin tests are often said to be positive when attempts at challenge fail to reproduce the disease, and in some individuals the challenge is positive when the skin test is negative (5, 7, 15). A most careful attempt to demonstrate this phenomenon with one particularly well-characterized allergen, ragweed, showed no lack of agreement between skin tests and respiratory challenge, so that some of the differences between the two methods noted above can be ascribed to shortcomings in technique (6). The matter, however, deserves further investigation.

At a simpler level, where one does not concern oneself with reproducing the disease under observation but only with identifying the presence or absence of IgE-mediated reactions, comparisons of techniques are much easier to make. Currently, two alternatives to skin testing are available, direct estimation of serum IgE antibodies by the radioallergosorbent test (RAST), described in chapter 79 (passive transfer to skin or to cells in vitro serve the same purpose), or histamine release from peripheral blood leukocytes, described in chapter 80. Histamine release depends not only on the amount of IgE fixed to the basophils but also is subject to influences on, and variations in, the chain of intracellular events that leads to histamine secretion. Skin tests are subject not only to these influences but also to variablility from the patient's responsiveness to mediators, anatomic skin sites, drug use, hormonal state, etc.

As a practical matter, when skin tests, histamine release, and RAST are compared, the differences actually uncovered are too small to influence the final diagnostic decision, and essentially the same information is obtained by all three methods, when properly executed (12). Although RAST and histamine release are more accurate than skin tests, the physician usually has no use for the additional precision. Differences of 3- to 10-fold have no practical significance when the total range of possible results has extremes over 1 million-fold apart.

Indeed, whatever the technique, the potency and stability of the antigens or allergens employed as reagents is much more important to control than the nuances of technique in performing the test. Extracts prepared in a similar fashion from the same allergen in two laboratories may be 1 thousand-fold different in potency when subjected to biological test by skin test or histamine release or to antigenic analysis by double diffusion in gel (2, 3).

From the above analysis, one may conclude that, once a potent allergenic extract is in hand, the choice of technique for assaying a patient's sensitivity depends on such practical matters as cost and convenience rather than any innate superiority of one method over another. Although extensive efforts are being made either to automate or to simplify RAST and histamine release, the ease and simplicity of skin tests, at least for the time being, give them first place in regular diagnostic usage, despite the modest extra discomfort to the patient compared with a single venipuncture.

CLINICAL INDICATIONS

The indications for skin testing are quickly stated: any reasonable suspicion that an individual's symptoms are allergic in origin. This is a physician's decision and is based on a review of the character of the symptoms along with time and place of occurrence. This is too complicated a subject to be discussed definitively here; physicians interested in allergy must become acquainted with the multitudinous allergens in the environment, along with the timing and placement of their appearance. This lore fills whole textbooks and is constantly being supplemented. Suffice it to say that the suspicion of allergy is not an excuse to perform skin tests to all possible allergens. Skin tests should be performed only with those allergens which, from the physician's knowledge, have some likelihood of causing the individual's problem.

TEST PROCEDURES

Two procedures have stood the test of prolonged experience as providing the most consistent and interpretable results in skin testing, the intradermal test and the prick test. Each will be described and then the two will be compared.

Intradermal skin tests

While testing may be carried out by a nurse or technician, a physician should always be within easy calling distance, as generalized allergic reactions are a rare but distinctly possible occurrence. A rubber tourniquet to place above the skin test site on an extremity and 1:1,000 aqueous adrenalin should always be at hand as the first measure employed to treat a developing generalized reaction.

Sterile disposable plastic 1-ml tuberculin syringes with 26-gauge × $^{3}/_{8}$-inch needles are filled with approximately 0.1 ml of the solution to be tested. All bubbles must be carefully expelled, as these, if injected into the skin, produce "splash" reactions which reduce precision.

Tests may be performed on the volar surface of the lower or upper arm or on the back, although the arm is more convenient. If large numbers of tests are performed, the back is preferable so that the tests will not be placed too close together. The skin is cleaned with isopropyl alcohol or 70% ethyl alcohol and allowed to dry. Sites for testing are marked with an appropriate code or symbol adjacent to actual site to be employed for inserting the needle. Sites should be at least 7.6 cm apart to prevent overlap of the reactions.

If the arm is used, the skin should be stretched taut by grasping the arm from behind. The syringe is then placed at an angle of 45° to the arm, with the level of the needle *down*, facing the skin. The point of the needle is then gently inserted in a forward lifting motion as if to pick up the skin with the very tip of the needle. As the tip enters the skin, the pickup motion is gradually converted to a forward and downward pressure, while the barrel is lowered to eliminate the angle it previously formed with the skin surface. The bevel should penetrate the skin entirely and end between the layers of the skin, with the remainder of the needle outside the skin in contact with the skin surface. With the index finger, fluid is forced into the skin while the small wheal formed is observed (14). If no wheal is formed or a previously unobserved bubble of air enters the skin, the needle should be removed and a new site should be employed. About 0.02 ml of fluid will give a wheal about 3 mm in diameter. Some workers prefer to introduce 0.05 ml as an amount easier to measure on the syringe barrel. Actually, the amount introduced does not influence the size of the eventual reaction nearly so much as the concentration of allergen in the fluid.

After a series of tests are placed, about 15 min is allowed to elapse and the sites are then inspected. If fully developed wheal and erythema reactions are formed, they are ready to be measured. The occasional individual will take longer to develop a reaction; if there is no reaction or a very small reaction at 15 min, the sites should be reinspected at 30 min. When the reactions have matured, their size is measured with a millimeter rule. The greatest and the smallest diameter of the wheal and the erythema are measured. As the reactions are often oval or irregular in shape, the diameters measured are not necessarily at right angles to each other. Both diameters are recorded, summed, and divided by two. Although grading systems vary greatly from one worker to another, the grading system shown in Table 1 has been employed by us (9).

When reactions are read at 15 min, they should be reinspected at 30 min; if they are significantly larger, they should be read again and the original readings should be discarded.

Although a single concentration of a specific extract may be selected for testing and the reaction may be graded for positivity, much more information is obtained if a threshold dilution titration of skin tests is performed employing a 10-fold dilution series. In this method, a rather low concentration considered to be thoroughly safe, i.e., unlikely to produce a large reaction, is tested first. If no reaction is produced, 10-fold and 100-fold higher concentrations are then placed simultaneously. If positive, the reactions are graded; if negative, still higher concentrations are placed until either a positive reaction is elicted or the highest concentration to be tried shows a negative reaction. On the other hand, if the original test is positive, lesser concentrations are tried until a concentration is reached which gives either a trace or negative reaction. The lowest dilution required for a 1+ or 2+ reaction is considered the end point. When this end point seems to fall between two dilutions, i.e., the stronger gives a 3+ or 4+ reaction and the weaker gives a trace or negative reaction, the end point is considered to be intermediate between the two dilutions, and an interpolated value halfway (on a logarithmic scale) between the two dilutions is entered as an end point.

Prick tests

Skin tests sites are cleansed and marked as described above. Single drops of solution to be tested are applied to the sites from plastic containers containing common rubber bulb droppers. A disposable sterile 26-gauge × 0.5-inch needle is passed through the drop and inserted into the skin with the bevel *up*, facing *away* from the surface. With a slight lifting of the skin, the needle is then withdrawn. The solution is gently wiped away with a paper tissue approximately 1 min later. The prick lesion should be superficial enough not to cause bleeding. A new needle is used for each test. As described above, when fully developed, lesions are read with a millimeter rule. As the wheal and erythema is smaller by this method than by the intradermal method, the same grading system does not apply. Indeed, grading is not always done, and the mean wheal and erythema diameter are merely recorded. End-point titrations are also possible with prick tests. A prick test requires approximately 1,000-fold higher concentration of antigen than an intradermal test for a positive reaction of the same size (12).

Histamine controls may be placed to judge the quality of the technique. For the intradermal test, 0.01% histamine base solution is employed, 0.275 mg of histamine phosphate (Eli Lilly & Co., Indianapolis, Ind.) per ml of diluent. In a large group of patients, a mean wheal diameter of 11.5 mm with a standard deviation of 2.1 mm was found. For the prick test a 1% histamine solution is employed. This concentration gave a 6.4-mm mean diameter with a standard deviation of 2.1 mm in a series of controls. Failure to react to histamine raises questions as to technique or the prior use of medications (12).

A diluent control should also be employed. The rare dermographic individual will give wheal and erythema reactions to the skin trauma involved in placing the test, so that all tests will appear positive. It is sometimes possi-

TABLE 1. *Grading system for skin tests*

Grade	Erythema (mm)	Wheal (mm)
0	<5	<5
±	5–10	5–10
1+	11–20	5–10
2+	21–30	5–10
3+	31–40	10–15[a]
4+	>40	>15[b]

[a] Or with pseudopods.
[b] Or with many pseudopods.

ble to recognize reactions very much larger than the control as being true positive reactions in these people, but it may be necessary to use other methods to evaluate the patient's sensitivities.

REAGENTS

Although, many years ago, skin test materials were made directly in hospital laboratories or physician's offices by extracting pollens, dust, molds, etc., this practice has been generally abandoned and can no longer be recommended. A number of commerical suppliers collect the allergens and prepare the extracts in a fashion that is generally more satisfactory. Nevertheless, the potency of the products may vary considerably from company to company and from one lot to another in the same company, as already noted. This indicates that present methods of standardization are unsatisfactory and must be improved. This is discussed completely in a separate chapter on standardization. Until improved methods are in more general use, the physician or laboratory must approach each new batch of allergenic extract with the suspicion that it may be either considerably more or less potent than the previous lot in use. Ideally, each new lot should be compared with the old one by simultaneous testing in a few patients to determine whether the potency of the new lot is similar.

In most instances, a concentrated extract is purchased, and serial dilutions are made locally for testing. The diluting fluid may be purchased from suppliers in ready-made vials containing either 9.0 or 4.5 ml of solution. A 10-fold dilution series is then easily made by adding either 1.0 or 0.5 ml, respectively, to a vial, mixing thoroughly, withdrawing the same amount, and adding to the next vial and so on. A fresh syringe should be employed each time the mixed fluid is withdrawn, as enough material may be carried over from a syringe used for a more concentrated material to throw the concentration off considerably after several serial dilutions.

The diluting fluid is usually a phosphate-buffered physiological saline at pH 7.4 with 0.4% phenol added to inhibit bacterial growth. Recent studies indicate that this fluid is unsatisfactory in that it allows significant absorption of protein to glass, resulting in a loss of up to 90% of biological activity in the extreme dilutions required for intradermal testing. Addition of human serum albumin (0.03%) or Tween 80 (0.005%) will prevent absorption to glass (P. S. Norman, D. G. Marsh, and J. Tignall, unpublished data), but diluting fluids containing these stabilizers are not available commercially at the time of this writing. Until such diluting fluids are available, current materials will have to be used with their limitations recognized.

INTERPRETATION

As with the indications for skin tests, interpretation of results is complex. A few warnings, however, may be given.

1. Not every positive skin test means that the individual showing the reaction has actual disease to that allergen. When threshold dilution testing is employed, the higher the dilution (i.e., the less concentrated the extract) required for a positive test the greater the likelihood of clinical significance.

2. Tests may be negative when the patient is indeed sensitive. This is probably most often due to the variability of potency and stability of extracts already discussed, but it is at least possible that a few individuals may be locally sensitive and require a direct provocative test.

3. The level of sensitivity in a dilution series required to indicate clinical significance may vary considerably from allergen to allergen. In general, pollen and animal dander extracts are highly potent, whereas mold and dust extracts give positive tests only when much more protein is introduced. Presumably, this is due to a smaller proportion of the total protein in the extract being actually allergenic or, to state it conversely, extraction has removed more inert protein. Identifications of allergens and development of better methods of standardization offer a hope of making reactions to extracts a more regular and reproducible phenomenon.

ACKNOWLEDGMENTS

This work was supported by a contract with the Bureau of Biologics, Food and Drug Administration, and by Public Health Service grants AI 10304 and AI 04866 from the National Institute of Allergy and Infectious Diseases.

Publication no. 210 from the O'Neill Research Laboratories, The Good Samaritan Hospital.

LITERATURE CITED

1. Adkinson, N. F., Jr., W. L. Thompson, W. C. Maddrey, and L. M. Lichtenstein. 1971. Routine use of penicillin skin testing on an inpatient service. N. Engl. J. Med. 285:22–24.

2. Baer, H., H. Godfrey, C. J. Maloney, P. S. Norman, and L. M. Lichtenstein. 1970. The potency and antigen E content of commercially prepared ragweed extracts. J. Allergy 45:347–354.

3. Baer, H., C. J. Maloney, P. S. Norman, and D. G. Marsh. 1974. The potency and Group I content of six commercially prepared grass

pollen extracts. J. Allergy Clin. Immunol. 54:157–164.

4. Belin, L. G. A., and P. S. Norman. 1975. Diagnostic tests in the skin of and serum of workers sensitized to *B. subtilis* enzymes. J. Allergy Clin. Immunol., in press.

5. Bruce, R. A. 1963. Bronchial and skin sensitivity in asthma. Int. Arch Allergy Appl. Immunol. **22**:294.

6. Bruce, C. A., R. R. Rosenthal, L. M. Lichtenstein, and P. S. Norman. 1974. Diagnostic tests in ragweed-allergic asthma: a comparison of direct skin tests, leukocyte histamine release, and quantitative bronchial challenge 53:230–239.

7. Colldahl, H. 1952. A study of provocation tests on patients with bronchial asthma. Acta Allergol. 5:133.

8. Hjorth, N. 1958. Instability of grass pollen extracts. Acta Allergol. 12:316–335.

9. King, T. P., and P. S. Norman. 1962. Isolation studies of allergens from ragweed pollen. Biochemistry 1:709.

10. Levine, B. B., and D. M. Zolov. 1909. Prediction of penicillin allergy by immunological tests. J. Allergy 43:231–244.

11. Norman, P. S. 1975. The clinical significance of IgE. Hosp. Pract. **10**:41–49.

12. Norman, P. S., L. M. Lichtenstein, and K. Ishizaka. 1973. Diagnostic tests in ragweed hay fever. J. Allergy Clin. Immunol. 52:210–224.

13. Prausnitz, C., and H. Küstner. 1921. Studien über Überempfindlichkeit. Centralbl. Bakteriol. Abt. I Orig. **86**:160–169.

14. Scherr, M. S., W. C. Grater, H. Baer, B. A. Berman, G. Center, and R. Hale. 1971. Report of the Committee on Standardization. I. A method of evaluating skin test response. Ann. Allergy 29:30–34.

15. Stevens, F. A. 1934. A comparison of pulmonary dermal sensitivity to inhaled substances. J. Allergy 5:285.

Chapter 79

Measurement of Total Serum Immunoglobulin E and Allergen-Specific Immunoglobulin E Antibody

N. FRANKLIN ADKINSON, JR.

A. Total Serum Immunoglobulin E

INTRODUCTION: CHOICE OF METHODS

Serum immunoglobulin E (IgE) is normally present in nanogram per milliliter quantities. Methods which can be used to detect reproducibly less than 100 ng of IgE protein per ml can be divided into two groups: (i) solid-phase radioimmunoassays and (ii) radioimmunoprecipitation (double-antibody) assays (Fig. 1).

The *solid-phase methods* have in common the insolubilization of anti-IgE antibody. This insoluble antibody has been employed in a competitive binding assay using radiolabeled IgE and standards of known IgE content, or it can be used to bind serum IgE in a noncompetitive fashion with the amount bound determined by subsequent incubation with a radiolabeled anti-IgE. The competitive binding assay, commonly called the radioimmunosorbent test (RIST), is now commercially available in kit form, as are the individual reagents (Pharmacia Laboratories, Piscataway, N.J.). Like all competitive binding assays, it is subject to nonspecific inhibition by unknown serum factors when high concentrations of serum must be assayed, as for low-level IgE detection. Sensitivity (5 ng/ml) and precision (coefficient of variation [CV] $\simeq$ 18%) are moderate. This method requires the purchase (at considerable expense) or the preparation and radioiodination of the Fc portion of IgE myeloma protein. The advantages of the method include completion in a single day, lack of need of precipitating antisera, and the commercial availability of all required reagents. In clinical settings where the desire is to distinguish normal from clearly elevated levels of serum IgE in adult patients, this method is quite satisfactory. When low levels of serum IgE must be measured accurately and with precision, or when serial studies are to be performed, one of the other methods discussed below is usually preferable.

The direct (noncompetitive) radioimmunosorbent test (direct RIST) is a sandwich technique first described by Wide (11). As for the competitive binding RIST, standard and unknown sera are incubated with insolubilized anti-IgE. Unlike the RIST, however, no radiolabeled IgE is required. After the first incubation, the particles are washed, and a second incubation with radiolabeled anti-IgE is undertaken. Binding of the radiolabeled anti-IgE is directly related to the IgE content of the original sera. The advantages of this assay include increased sensitivity (as low as 10 pg of IgE) and excellent precision (CV < 5%). Such attributes are rarely needed for clinical purposes. Of greater clinical importance is that this technique is minimally affected by nonspecific serum factors which can obscure accurate assessment of low IgE levels. Thus, if maximal sensitivity and accuracy are required as for the study of young pediatric patients or immunodeficiency states, or for analysis of nonserum physiological fluids (e.g., nasal washings, gastrointestinal aspirates) in which IgE levels may be quite low, this technique may be the procedure of choice. The principal disadvantage of the assay is the necessity for a second incubation which doubles the time required to complete the test and the number of necessary technical manipulations.

Two other considerations with respect to the use of the direct RIST assay deserve mention. First, there is an additional advantage to the routine use of this method by a laboratory which also undertakes determination of specific IgE levels by the radioallergosorbent test (RAST; see below, part B). The radiolabeled anti-IgE required for the RAST may also be used in the direct RIST assay, thereby reducing the total number of radiolabeled reagents required. Furthermore, the assay avoids entirely the need for IgE myeloma protein except for purposes of immunization and affinity chromatography purification. Even these needs are eliminated if commercially available anti-IgE is employed.

Second, Johannson and Lundkuist (personal communication) have recently provided preliminary evidence that the direct RIST assay may better discriminate between atopic and nonatopic populations than do competitive binding radioimmunoassays. They attribute this im-

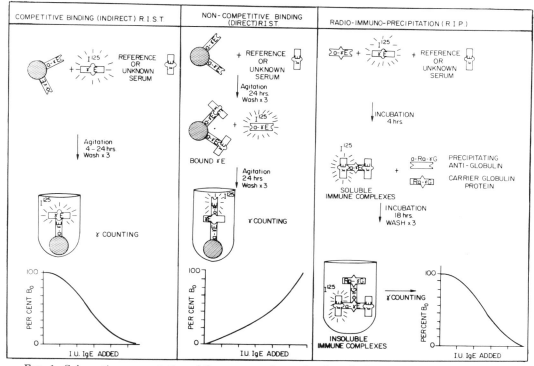

FIG. 1. *Schematic representation of three commonly employed methods for total serum IgE assay.*

proved discrimination to the minimal effects of serum inhibitory factors, which tend to increase estimates of total serum IgE protein in competitive binding assays. This observation will require independent verification, but clinical immunologists who seek to establish assays for total IgE protein in their laboratories should bear this possibility in mind when choosing an assay method. Because of these actual and potential advantages of the direct RIST assay, details of the technical performance of this test are included below as an acceptable alternative method to the radioimmunoprecipitation assay which is currently the standard method of choice.

The *radioimmunoprecipitation* (double antibody) *assay* for serum IgE protein as developed by Gleich et al. (3) is unsurpassed in precision and reproducibility. Because of widespread experience with this assay and its use in establishing the normal range for serum IgE levels, it is to be considered the usual method of choice for clinical purposes in most laboratories. Unlike solid-phase radioimmunoassays, it requires the addition of a second antibody after the completion of the competitive binding incubation in order to separate bound from free antigen (i.e., IgE). This precipitating antiserum must be available in large quantities, often at considerable cost. The assay generally requires 2 days to complete, though it can be completed in a single day if required. Its chief disadvantage is that inherent in all competitive binding assays — nonspecific interference by serum factors at high serum concentrations. For most clinical purposes, this is of little concern.

CLINICAL INDICATIONS

Some clinical situations in which a total serum IgE level may be useful diagnostically are enumerated in Table 1. Serial tests on some patients with allergic disorders may be useful to confirm the expected seasonal boost in serum IgE level regularly seen after environmental exposure to an allergen to which the patient is sensitive. In pathological conditions which are associated with high serum IgE levels (e.g., parasitism), serial assays may be useful in confirming therapeutic effectiveness, though data supporting this use of serum IgE levels are meager. Finally, the screening of young children of allergic parents may be useful in assessing the risk of future allergic problems, but by and large prospective studies of the predicative value of serum IgE levels in children have yet to be performed.

To the knowledgable physician serum IgE levels may be useful in confirming independent clinical diagnoses, and in providing supportive evidence in difficult cases of the differential diagnosis of allergic disease. However, the clinician must be wary of discounting allergy when the serum IgE level is low or normal, as well as automatically inferring allergy when the level is high. Although allergy and elevated serum IgE are positively correlated, there are patients with elevated serum IgE levels and no allergic symptoms, as well as patients with clinically unequivocal allergic problems who have normal or low serum IgE levels.

TEST PROCEDURE

Radioimmunoprecipitation assay for total serum immunoglobulin E

1. Add the following reagents in sequence to disposable 12 × 75 mm assay tubes: 0.5 ml of the standard serum or unknown serum diluted in assay buffer, 0.1 ml of the appropriate dilution of rabbit antihuman IgE, and 0.1 ml of radiolabeled IgE myeloma protein (1 to 5 ng of ^{125}I-labeled IgE per tube).

2. After gentle mixing, incubate the tubes at 37 C for 3 h.

3. To precipitate the bound IgE, add the following agents sequentially to each tube: 0.2 ml of normal rabbit serum (diluted about 1:40) or rabbit gamma globulin (50 μg/0.2 ml) and 0.2 ml of goat antirabbit gamma globulin at a dilution predetermined to produce optimal precipitation.

4. Incubation is continued at 37 C for 1 h, after which the tubes are centrifuged at 2,000 × g for 30 min at 4 C, decanted, and washed twice with 3 ml of assay buffer. Alternatively, the second incubation may be allowed to continue overnight at 4 C and then centrifuged and washed with equivalent results.

5. The tubes are then counted in a gamma counter, and the standard curve is plotted with the logarithm of added IgE as a function of maximal binding (B_0, binding observed when no unlabeled IgE is added). The unknown values are then interpolated from the standard curve, either manually or by calculation after linearization of the standard curve by suitable transformation such as the logit (Fig. 2).

Preliminary preparations

(a) Preparation of radiolabeled IgE myeloma protein or its Fc fragment. The chloramine T method is generally employed to radioiodinate the IgE, though other methods (e.g., lactoperoxidase) are also satisfactory. A brief description of a suitable chloramine T procedure fol-

TABLE 1. *Clinical conditions in which total serum IgE determinations may be useful in differential diagnoses*

Clinical condition	Usefulness
Atopic disorders: allergic rhinitis, allergic asthma, atopic dermatitis	Moderately elevated serum IgE levels positively reinforce the clinical diagnosis; however, a low or normal IgE level is not incompatible with the diagnosis.
Intrinsic (nonallergic) asthma	Normal or low serum IgE suggests that IgE-mediated mechanisms play only a minor role in the pathogenesis of the patient's asthma.
Bronchopulmonary aspergillosis	Normal serum IgE levels virtually exclude the diagnosis.
Wiskott-Aldrich syndrome	Elevated levels are commonly found in those patients who exhibit eczema.
Hypergammaglobulinemia E syndrome (elevated IgE, increased susceptibility to infection, and dermatitis)	Very high serum IgE levels are necessary for the diagnosis.
Parasitism	Many parasitic infections commonly produce extreme elevations of serum IgE levels; a very high IgE level in the absence of other explanations strongly suggests the possibility of parasitism.
Eosinophilia	A normal IgE level makes less likely the diagnosis of parasitism as a cause of eosinophilia; eosinophilia with normal serum IgE is commonly a feature of nonallergic asthma.

lows. Obtain 2 mCi of ^{125}I-labeled Na from a radiochemical supplier in aqueous solution in a volume of 0.010 to 0.015 ml in a conical reaction vial (total capacity $\simeq$ 2 ml). Working on a shielded radioactive bench, add 50 μliters of 0.5 M NaH_2PO_4, pH 7.5, to the reaction vial and gently agitate it manually. Add 25 μliters of purified IgE myeloma protein or its Fc fragment at $\simeq$2 mg/ml in phosphate-buffered saline (PBS), pH 7.5, with gentle mixing. At this point, add the 0.5 M sodium phosphate buffer to preweighed chloramine T in a light-shielded test tube to provide a fresh solution of 2 mg/ml. Add 25 μliters of this solution and begin exactly 60 s of gentle manual agitation. After 1 min, add 100 μliters of a fresh sodium metabisulfite solution (500 μg/ml) to stop the

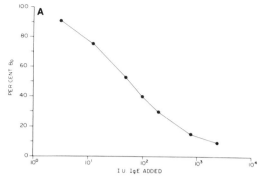

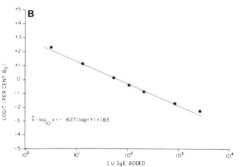

FIG. 2. *Double antibody radioimmunoassay for total serum IgE. (A) The standard curve is derived from the competition of radiolabeled IgE myeloma protein and increasing amounts of unlabeled IgE reference standard for a constant amount of rabbit anti-IgE antibody. (B) The dose-response curve may be linearized by logit transformation in order to allow direct calculation of IgE content.*

oxidation reaction. After about 20 s of further agitation, add 200 μliters of PBS solution containing KI, 8 mg/ml, and human serum albumin (HSA) or bovine serum albumin (BSA), 50 mg/ml, with additional mixing. Aspirate the entire volume of the reaction vial (about 500 μliters) into a syringe with a needle. Add two 500-μliter amounts of the KI/HSA solution to the reaction vial and then aspirate them into the syringe to wash the vial completely. The 1.5 ml-sample in the syringe is then applied directly to a 0.9 by 60 cm column of coarse Sephadex G-25, previously equilibrated with PBS, pH 7.4, containing 0.2% sodium azide and 0.2% albumin. The first radioactive peak (contained in the void volume) is collected in 1-ml samples, diluted, and counted, and the entire radioactive peak is pooled. Alternatively, the optical density at 280 nm may be used to monitor the peak of the buffering protein (HSA or BSA) which is eluted coincident with the radiolabeled IgE. Precipitation of the radiolabel by cold 10% trichloroacetic acid is determined and

should be greater than 90%. Total recovery of protein is assumed, and the specific activity is calculated. Using the method described, specific activities in the range of 50,000 to 100,000 counts per min per ng are usually achieved. With the use of about 1 ng/tube, this 25 μg of radiolabeled protein is generally sufficient for a large volume of work. Divided into portions and stored frozen at −20 C, this reagent is generally useful for several months. A new radiolabeled protein should be prepared at any time experimental results become erratic or the configuration of the standard curve changes markedly.

(b) *Choice of the appropriate dilution of rabbit anti-human IgE*. The dilution of the primary antibody (rabbit anti-human IgE) employed will determine the working range of the assay. For most clinical purposes, a useful anti-IgE dilution is that which results in 50% inhibition of maximal binding by 50 to 100 IU of IgE per ml added. This may be determined by preliminary experimentation using progressive 10-fold dilutions of the available antiserum.

(c) *Determination of appropriate dilution of goat anti-rabbit gamma globulin*. A large pool of goat anti-rabbit gamma globulin is evaluated by precipitin analysis, or more easily by a radioimmunoprecipitation technique employing a trace-labeled rabbit gamma globulin, to determine the dilution required for optimal precipitation of approximately 50 μg of rabbit gamma globulin (about 0.2 ml of a 1:40 dilution of normal rabbit serum).

(d) *Specimen requirements*. The assay is designed to measure levels of IgE protein in human serum. Heparinized or cation-chelated plasma may also be used with good results, though fibrin formation can sometimes be a problem. Respiratory secretions including saliva, nasal washings, and bronchial secretions may also be evaluated after thorough demucination, provided the sensitivity of the assay is maximized. However, at present there is no clinical utility to measurements of IgE protein in physiological fluids other than serum or plasma.

Unlike the biological activity of IgE antibody, the antigenic properties of IgE protein are maintained indefinitely when serum is stored frozen at −20 C. Allowing blood samples to clot and retract overnight at 4 C has no detectable effect on serum IgE levels. Transportation of serum specimens at ambient temperatures is not recommended, especially if the serum is also to be evaluated for specific IgE antibody (see below, part B).

(e) *Validating and standardizing the assay system*. In validating the accuracy of the assay system, it is necessary to establish the specificity of the primary antiserum for Fc_ϵ by demonstrating that cord sera and purified human immunoglobulins at a concentration of 1 mg/ml will not significantly inhibit maximal binding. The most common reason for failure to achieve good agreement between determinations derived from different dilutions of a single serum is residual cross-reactivity of the antiserum with human IgG. This effect will be maximal in sera with low serum IgE levels.

Standardization should initially be achieved by use of the World Health Organization (WHO) international reference standard for IgE (#68/341). As the supply of this reference standard is dwindling, other secondary standards are now being provided by the WHO Immunoglobulin Reference Centers. Most of these reference preparations are pools of sera which are hepatitis antigen-positive. For this reason, the international reference preparations should be employed to substandardize carefully a high-level serum pool which is available in large quantity to the laboratory performing the assay. This substandardized serum is then employed for day-to-day laboratory use, with periodic reevaluations of the international reference preparations to assure quality control.

(f) Working range, sensitivity, and reproducibility. A useful working range for clinical purposes is from 1 to 1,000 IU of IgE/ml. The range is determined in part by the dilution of the rabbit anti-IgE employed in the assay as discussed above (b). The ultimate sensitivity of the assay depends upon the affinity of the anti-IgE antibody. A sensitivity of 1 IU/ml is achievable with most antisera. The precision of the technique is excellent, with CV usually $\simeq$ 5%. Under optimal technical conditions, an interexperimental reproducibility of 10% (CV) can be achieved.

(g) Quality control. Quality control is best achieved by inclusion within each assay of three well-studied sera as external controls. One of these sera should have low serum IgE protein (<10 IU/ml) and be run at serum dilutions of 1:2 and 1:5; the second serum should have moderate IgE levels (300 to 500 IU/ml) and be evaluated at 1:5 and 1:10 serum dilutions; and the third serum should have high IgE levels (>1,000 IU/ml) and be evaluated at 1:10 and 1:20 serum dilutions. In a given assay, reproduction of acceptable estimates of the known IgE content of these sera together with good agreement between the two dilutions evaluated insure reliable results from the assay system. Statistical considerations for the use of such

quality control data are discussed elsewhere (9).

(h) Standard protocol. Triplicate determinations of B_0 (no added unlabeled antigen), N (nonspecific binding = no added serum), and each standard curve point (seven or more twofold dilutions, ranging from approximately 1,000 to 1 IU/ml) are run in each experiment. Duplicate determination of unknown sera is usually sufficient. Evaluation of each unknown serum at two dilutions increases accuracy, facilitates recognition of any inhibitory effects often seen at high serum concentrations, and increases the likelihood that one of the dilutions chosen will fall in the linear portion of the standard curve. External standard sera should also be included in each experiment (see g above).

Reagents and materials

(a) Required supplies and equipment. Disposable 12 × 75 mm test tubes (glass or plastic), micropipettes, a refrigerated centrifuge, and a gamma scintillation counter.

(b) Buffer for washing and diluting. Any isotonic buffer at pH 7 to 8 is satisfactory. Inclusion of wetting agents such as Tween 20 and/or irrelevant protein in the assay buffer often reduces nonspecific binding to the test tube. A commonly used assay buffer is PBS, pH 7.5, including 0.5% (wt/vol) sodium azide, 0.5% (vol/vol) Tween 20, and 0.2% (wt/vol) BSA. Alternatively, the assay test tubes may be preincubated for 5 min with a 0.5% solution of BSA to minimize nonspecific adherence. The coating BSA solution may be reused. If this technique is employed, Tween 20 and BSA may be omitted from the assay buffer, thereby reducing cost of reagents.

(c) A reference serum of known IgE content, preferably the WHO reference standard #68/341. Reference sera may be obtained from the WHO Immunoglobulin Reference Centers. In the United States, the address is NCI Immunodiagnostic Reference Center, 6715 Electronic Drive, Springfield, Va. 22151.

(d) Purified IgE myeloma protein. This is required both for production of anti-human IgE antibody (see below) and for radiolabeling for use in the assay itself. If accessible, serum from patients with an IgE-producing plasma cell tumor may be fractionated by diethylaminoethyl cellulose and Sephadex G-200 chromatography according to the method of Ishizaka (5). For iodination, use of the Fc fragment is preferred as it increases the specificity of the assay. This is accomplished by papain digestion (5). Alternatively, milligram quantities of IgE can be purified from myeloma serum by affinity chromatography with the use of insolubilized commercially available anti-IgE. The final alternative is the commercial purchase of IgE myeloma protein, either unlabeled or previously radiolabeled with ^{125}I (Pharmacia Laboratories, Piscataway, N.J.).

(e) Rabbit anti-human IgE (Fc$_\epsilon$ specific). This antiserum may be prepared by immunizing rabbits directly with Fc$_\epsilon$, or by immunizing with whole IgE myeloma protein followed by absorption of the antisera with Fab$_\epsilon$ fragments, light chains, and IgG, employing affinity chromatography. Satisfactory antisera will be produced by a primary immunization of 1 mg of IgE protein in complete Freund's adjuvant, followed by 100-μg booster injections 1 month and 10 days prior to subsequent bleedings. Antisera raised in sheep or goats may be unsatisfactory because of the presence of heterophile antibodies in some normal human sera which cross-react with sheep and goat gamma globulin. In such patients, the use of sheep antisera will give a falsely elevated IgE value.

(f) Goat anti-rabbit gamma globulin. Goats immunized with commercially purchased rabbit gamma globulin (Miles Laboratories, Kankakee, Ill.) by use of the schedule outlined for rabbit immunization above will produce an immune serum useful in the radioimmunoprecipitation technique without further absorption or purification. Such antisera may also be purchased commercially (Antibodies Inc., Davis, Calif.) at considerable expense. For each lot of serum, a precipitin curve or radioimmunoprecipitation technique must be employed to determine the required dilution of the antiserum for optimal precipitation (see above, Preliminary preparations, *c*). For most immune sera, the requirement is between 15 and 20 μliters of undiluted antiserum per assay tube.

ALTERNATE TEST PROCEDURE

Direct (noncompetitive) radioimmunosorbent test for total serum IgE

1. Into 12×75 mm disposable test tubes, add the following reagents sequentially: 0.5 ml of an appropriate dilution in RAST buffer of anti-IgE-sorbent (usually 0.3%, vol/vol) and 0.1 ml of serum dilution of standard or unknown sera. The standard curve is composed of 10 to 12 twofold dilutions in triplicate of a reference serum, beginning at a concentration of about 400 IU/ml. Include a reagent blank as a control for nonspecific binding and appropriate external control sera in each experiment as described above for the radioimmunoprecipitation assay. Replicates containing a 1% (vol/vol) γE-sorbent are preferably included as a control for

the immunoreactivity of the radiolabeled anti-IgE antibody (see below, description of B$_{max}$ in part B, section on Preliminary preparations, *a*).

2. Place all test tubes in a rotating rack (BBL #60448 rotator modified to hold tube racks) and rotate slowly (24 rpm) at an angle of 60° at ambient temperature for at least 4 h.

3. At the end of the first incubation, 2.5 ml of RAST buffer is added to each tube, the sorbent is pelleted by brief centrifugation ($900 \times g$ for 2 min), and all but the bottom 0.2 ml of supernatant fluid is aspirated by vacuum suction with a collared Pasteur pipette. Each test tube is subsequently washed twice more with 3.0 ml of RAST buffer in a similar fashion. After the final wash, 0.5 ml of an appropriate dilution of radiolabeled rabbit anti-IgE is added to each tube, and the tubes are again rotated at room temperature for 18 to 24 h.

4. At the end of the second incubation, all tubes except totals (tubes containing 0.5 ml of radiolabeled antibody only) are again washed in the manner described above, except that an additional wash is included (four centrifugations total).

5. All test tubes are capped and counted to statistical precision in a gamma scintillation counter. The data are processed statistically as described below for the RAST assay.

6. In the standard protocol, totals, B$_{max}$, nonspecific binding, and all standard curve points are run in triplicate. Generally, unknown samples are evaluated at two dilutions: for expected low levels (e.g., pediatric patients, immunoefficiency patients), the serum dilutions of 1:2 and 1:5 are employed; for expected high levels, 1:10 and 1:20 are suitable; for all others, 1:5 and 1:10 are useful.

Reagent preparation. The radioiodinated rabbit anti-IgE, IgE-sorbent, and RAST buffer used as diluent are prepared and evaluated as described in the RAST assay (see below, part B). The preparation of the anti-IgE-sorbent first requires the availability of about 10 mg of purified anti-IgE. The antiserum may be produced in rabbits, goats, or horses and need not be Fc$_\epsilon$ or epsilon chain specific. Purified antibody is obtained from the crude antisera by affinity chromatography with the use of an IgE-agarose column and elution with a glycine buffer, pH 2.8. Alternatively, commercially available anti-IgE antibody may also be used with satisfactory results. A 10-mg amount of purified anti-IgE antibody is coupled to 20 ml of packed Sepharose 4B by the cyanogen bromide method; 4 g of cyanogen bromide is used for agarose activation. Activation, coupling, washing, and storage are exactly as employed for preparation of the allergen-coated sorbent employed in the RAST assay. Preliminary experiments are required to determine the optimal concentration of the anti-IgE-sorbent employed in the assay. The goal is to achieve the appropriate working range for clinical use (400 IU/ml to 1 IU/ml added) while employing the lowest feasible sorbent concentration in order to minimize nonspecific binding effects and reagent use.

INTERPRETATION

Serum IgE values are preferentially expressed in international units per milliliter Laboratories working independently have now confirmed that 1 IU is equivalent to approximately 2.4 ng of IgE protein. This conversion factor may be usefully applied where weight/volume or molar concentrations are desired.

As for other Ig classes, serum IgE levels are age dependent. The IgE level of cord sera is quite low, probably less than 2 IU/ml. IgE is not known to cross the placental barrier in significant amounts. Mean serum IgE levels progressively increase with age until about 12 years of age, after which there is a modest decline to adult levels (Fig. 3).

Normative data derived from the radioimmunoprecipitation technique for healthy adults are shown in Table 2. As discussed in the Introduction, the noncompetitive solid-phase radioimmunoassay tends to give lower values than the radioimmunoprecipitation technique for serum levels below 80 IU/ml. Whether this technique will produce normal values which will better discriminate atopic from nonatopic populations remains to be established.

After the age of 12 years, serum IgE greater than 333 IU/ml (800 ng/ml) is generally considered abnormally elevated. The great majority of patients with elevated serum IgE levels have atopic disorders such as allergic rhinitis, extrinsic asthma, and atopic dermatitis. However, the overlap between atopic and nonatopic populations is considerable. For example, although the mean serum IgE level in one study of adults with allergic asthma was 1,589 ng/ml (range, 55 to 12,750 ng/ml), only about one-half of these asthmatic patients had serum IgE levels above the 800 ng/ml upper limit of normal for the nonatopic population. Atopic dermatitis is associated with very high levels of serum IgE, and only about 20% of these patients have serum IgE levels which fall within the normal range. Allergic urticaria and anaphylactic reactions are not commonly associated with elevated serum IgE levels.

Serum IgE levels are known to fluctuate as a function of exposure to relevant allergens. Patients with pollen allergies increase their basal serum IgE levels several-fold during the relevant pollen seasons. Immunotherapy with allergenic extracts also stimulates IgE production during the early phase of treatment, sometimes elevating the total serum IgE.

Basal levels of serum IgE appear to be under genetic control, with high IgE levels being inherited as a simple Mendelian recessive trait. In addition, there are numerous pathological conditions, notably parasitism, which boost, apparently in a nonspecific fashion, basal IgE production. There is increasing evidence that T lymphocytes play a role in the regulation of IgE synthesis. Elevated serum IgE levels in patients with T cell malignancies such as Hodgkin's disease have been reported. On the other hand, B cell malignancies such as chronic lymphocytic leukemia and multiple myeloma are commonly associated with very low levels of serum IgE.

As with many other laboratory tests, the total serum IgE can often be interpreted properly only with reference to pertinent clinical information. Especially important in this regard is the personal and family history of atopic disorders known to be associated with elevated IgE levels. Serum IgE determinations can often supplement and reinforce clinical diagnoses. It must be kept in mind that IgE production is but one variable in most allergic disorders. Thus, a low serum IgE level does not rule out serious allergic potential; similarly, asymptomatic individuals with high serum IgE levels are also encountered.

B. Radioallergosorbent Test for Antigen-Specific Serum Immunoglobulin E

INTRODUCTION

Thr radioallergosorbent test (RAST) was first introduced in 1968 and is now clearly established as the method of choice for serological determination of specific IgE antibody. The assay is a solid-phase radioimmunoassay variant of the earlier red cell linked-antigen-antiglobulin reaction (RCLAAR) originated by Coombs in the 1950s. In principle, the two methods are identical, the only difference bing that in the RAST the antigen of interest is coupled to an insoluble synthetic matrix rather than a red cell. Problems with allergen coupling, nonspecific agglutination, and reagent stability common to the RCLAAR have resulted in its abandonment in recent years in favor of the RAST. The only other in vitro test for specific serum IgE is radioimmunodiffusion. This test is cumbersome, time-consuming, and at best semiquantitative. This test has also been largely abandoned in favor of the RAST.

The basic principle of the RAST is quite simple. Allergen-coated particles are incubated in the serum under study, during which time specific antibody of all Ig classes is bound. The particles are then washed, and a second incubation is undertaken with a radiolabeled, highly specific anti-IgE antibody. The radioactivity bound is directly related to the specific IgE antibody content of the original serum. Since the results are compared with a standard reference serum, the exact concentrations of insolubilized allergen and the radiolabeled anti-IgE antibody are not critical. The assay generally requires 24 to 48 h (Fig. 4).

The RAST test has been subjected to numerous technical variations by a large number of

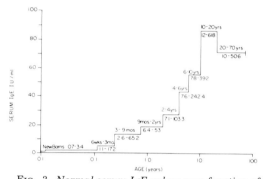

FIG. 3. *Normal serum IgE values as a function of age. Horizontal plateaus represent geometric mean values; the 95% confidence interval is shown below each plateau. Data extracted from Farmakoterapi 4: 85, 1973 (K. Aas).*

investigators. These variations have chiefly involved the use of different polymers for allergen insolubilization. Carbohydrate matrices (Sephadex, agarose, and cellulose), paper disks, and the walls of polystyrene test tubes have all been successfully employed in the RAST assay. These polymers differ with respect to their allergen-binding capacity, nonspecific adsorption properties, long-term stability, and ease of washing. The commercial supplier of RAST kits (Pharmacia, Piscataway, N.J.) has settled upon the use of allergen-coated paper disks because of the ease of washing and manipulation. For most clinical diagnostic purposes the use of paper-disk sorbents is satisfactory. However, if maximal sensitivity is required or if hyperimmunized patients with high levels of specific IgG ("blocking") antibodies are to be studied, the use of a sorbent with greater allergen-binding capacity is needed. For this reason most investigators have settled upon the use of one of the carbohydrate matrix sorbents. For a suitably equipped clinical laboratory with adequate facilities for centrifugation, aspiration, and pipetting, one of the carbohydrate matrices is to be preferred. The paper-disk sorbent will be attractive to those laboratories which would prefer not to prepare their own reagents. Polystyrene tubes are more suitable with some allergens than with others, and because of problems with quality control and reproducibility their routine use is not recommended.

The literature on RAST technique and the applications of RAST to the study of allergic disease is abundant. The reader is referred to reference 1 for detailed discussion of numerous

TABLE 2. *Normative total serum IgE levels in adults as determined by competitive radioimmunoassay (double antibody)[a]*

Reference	Population	N	Arithmetic mean	Geometric mean	Range	90% interval	95% interval
Gleich et al. (3)	Nonatopic adults[b]	95	179 (74.6)		1–2,700 (0.4–1,125)	9–539 (3.8–225)	
Nye et al. (7)	Nonatopic adults[c]	102	309 (129)	64 (26.7)	2.5–9,178 (1–3,824)	2.5–1,872 (1–780)	2.5–1,241 (1–517)
Gleich et al. (3)	Atopic adults[d]	133			55–12,750 (22.9–5,313)		
Polmar et al. (8)	Unselected adults[e]	73		105 (43.8)	6–18,951 (2.5–7,896)		5–2,045 (2.1–852)

[a] Results are given as nanograms per milliliter with international units per milliliter given in parentheses; 1 IU of IgE = 2.4 ng.

[b] Unrelated blood donors or individuals undergoing pre-employment physical examination; all denied symptoms of allergic respiratory disease and family history of asthma, allergic rhinitis, atopic dermatitis, or urticaria.

[c] Adults aged 18 to 83 years without personal or family history of asthma, eczema, allergic rhinitis. or urticaria.

[d] Patients with allergic rhinitis and/or asthma; some were receiving immunotherapy.

[e] Adult blood donors and laboratory personnel, age range, 21 to 60 years; no exclusion of allergic individuals.

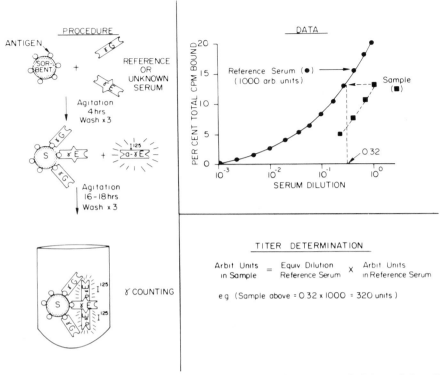

FIG. 4. *Radioallergosorbent test. The procedure is schematically represented (left) and described in the text. Data from the binding of multiple dilutions of a reference serum, as well as a sample of unknown potency, are illustrated (upper right). Note that serum dilution curves of the reference and sample sera are approximately parallel. Assuming 1,000 arbitrary units in the reference serum, the calculation of relative sample potency can be performed at any sample dilution in the parallel portion of the curve (lower right).*

technical aspects regarding RAST. Reference 6 reviews the correlation of RAST data with clinical atopic disease.

CLINICAL INDICATIONS

There is considerable controversy as to the appropriate use of the RAST for clinical diagnosis. It is generally agreed that RAST provides no further information than can be obtained by direct intradermal skin testing, using assessment of wheal and flare response at 15 to 20 min as the criterion. False-positive RAST tests are rarely a problem except for complex allergen mixtures like dust extracts which may bind IgE nonspecifically. On the other hand, when low-sensitivity RAST systems are employed, the skin test may be positive when the RAST test is negative. Whether these false-negative RAST tests are clinically significant is subject to debate. Economically, skin testing is less expensive than RAST assays. Skin testing also has the added advantage of immediate results.

There are, however, some clinical situations in which RAST assays may be preferred to direct skin testing. In young children or very apprehensive adult patients, a serum sample may be better tolerated than skin testing by patient and physician alike. In patients with dermatographism or severe dermatitis which may prevent proper interpretation of the skin test, the RAST offers an obvious advantage. Patients whose skin test results may be modified by medication such as antihistamines which for one reason or another can not be withdrawn can be evaluated by RAST. Finally, RAST assays may be useful in a few selected patients with highly suggestive clinical histories but negative skin tests, principally in order to provide independent confirmation of the absence of reaginic (IgE) antibodies.

Currently the principal disadvantage of RAST for clinical use is the difficulty of the transforming RAST results into levels of clinical sensitivity which are meaningful to the practicing physician. The correlation between RAST assay and intradermal skin testing is very good when carefully performed with the use of the same allergen extract for skin testing and for RAST assay. These ideal conditions rarely apply in actual practice. None of the commercially available RAST kits has been standardized with respect to clinical symptomatology or direct skin testing. Currently, the burden of interpretation rests entirely with the physician. The clinical laboratory desiring to provide RAST assay results should make some effort to provide physicians with a basis for interpretation. This is not easily done, as interpretative data must be gathered independently for each allergen system employed. Current research indicates that most of the disadvantages of the RAST may soon be surmountable. Methods for absolute quantitation of RAST are now available (4, 10). Attempts to relate circulating reagin levels and related parameters such as percentage of total IgE which is allergen specific to clinical status are underway. Large-volume RAST testing will allow significant reduction in average cost. In the near future, these advances may result in the RAST becoming the clear method of choice for evaluation of IgE-mediated disorders.

TEST PROCEDURE

Radioallergosorbent test for antigen-specific serum immunoglobulin E

1. Incubate 0.5 ml of appropriately diluted allergen-coated particles (usually 0.5 to 3.0%, vol/vol) and 0.1 ml of a serum dilution in duplicate in 12 × 75 mm disposable plastic test tubes. The tubes are capped and rotated at room temperature for at least 4 h. A standard reference curve is provided by including 8 to 10 twofold dilutions in triplicate of a potent reaginic sera known to contain a high titer of the allergen-specific IgE antibody of interest. A reagent blank (0.1 ml of RAST buffer) and a negative serum control are included in triplicate. A recommended option is inclusion of B_{max} replicates containing 1% (vol/vol) γE-sorbent as a control for the immunoreactivity of the radiolabeled antibody. Triplicate "total added" replicates (tubes containing 0.5 ml of radiolabeled antibody only) are provided at the beginning of the second incubation.

2. Wash the particles three times with 3.0 ml of RAST buffer using brief centrifugation (900 × g, 2 min) to sediment particles, and use a collared aspirator tube to remove all but 0.2 ml of the supernatant fluid after each wash.

3. Add 0.5 ml of ^{125}I-labeled anti-IgE to each tube, and begin a second incubation with orbital agitation for 18 to 24 h at room temperature.

4. After the second incubation (usually in the morning of the second day), wash the sorbent particles four times with 3.0 ml of RAST buffer, and count the bound radioactivity to statistical precision in a gamma scintillation counter.

The standard reference curve is plotted as the log of serum dilution versus percent maximal binding (% B_{max}) or percent total binding (% T). The reference serum may be designated 1,000 arbitrary units, and the potency of unknown sera in relative units can be estimated by interpolation from the standard curve (Fig. 4).

Preliminary preparations

(a) Preparation of radiolabeled rabbit anti-human IgE (Fc$_\epsilon$ specific). The antibody required is identical to that required for the double antibody assay for total serum IgE (see above, part A, Reagents and materials, e). Radioiodination of the purified antibody is usually by the chloramine T method, although other methods are equally satisfactory. The chloramine T procedure for radioiodination of IgE myeloma protein as described above (part A, Preliminary preparations, a) is also suitable for labeling of the anti-IgE antibody. As described, the use of 25 μliters of a 2 mg/ml rabbit anti-IgE (Fc$_\epsilon$) will usually result in specific activities in the range of 25,000 to 75,000 counts per min per ng. The use of 1 to 10 ng of ^{125}I-labeled anti-IgE per tube is generally satisfactory and provides adequate radioactivity for efficient use of gamma counting equipment. For each radiolabeled antibody preparation, I determine initial immunoreactivity and validate the useful range of antibody concentrations by incubating 10, 3, and 1 ng of ^{125}I-labeled rabbit anti-human IgE with 0.5 ml of a 1% suspension (vol/vol) of γE-sorbent employing orbital rotation at room temperature for 16 to 18 h. If the antibody immunoreactivity (i.e., maximal binding [B_{max}]) in this antigen-excess γE-sorbent system is the same at the three levels of anti-IgE evaluated, the upper portion of that range is thereby validated for use in the assay. Typically, 3 to 10 ng of anti-IgE per tube can be employed in the second stage of the assay. The immunoreactivity (B_{max}) may range from 20 to 90% depending upon antibody avidity, degree of antibody purification, and the degree of oxidative damage sustained in the iodination procedure. By monitoring B_{max} in each assay, the stability of the radiolabeled preparation can be ascertained.

(b) Preparation of the allergen-coated sorbent. Choice of the sorbent matrix to be used depends upon the needs of the laboratory. In general, the carbohydrate complexes are preferred over the use of paper disks or polystyrene tubes (see above, Introduction). Of these, the three most commonly employed are Sephadex G-25 superfine particles (Pharmacia), microcrystalline cellulose particles (E. M. Laboratories, Inc., Elmsford, N.Y.; catalogue #2331-Merck), and agarose beads (Sepharose 4B, Pharmacia). Sephadex and cellulose pellet rapidly on centrifugation and pack tightly in the pellet, thus allowing decantation. Agarose, on the other hand, is unexcelled in terms of allergen binding capacity and nonspecific adsorption properties, but requires longer centrifugation and aspiration of the supernatant fluid. The method described here employs agarose (Sepharose 4B), but the procedures may be applied identically to Sephadex and cellulose particles. Those interested in the preparation of paper-disk sorbents are referred to reference 2.

It is generally useful to couple 10 ml (packed volume) of Sepharose 4B particles at one time. For maximal sensitivity, at least 1 mg of allergen per ml of Sepharose is required. From 100 to 250 mg of cyanogen bromide/ml of Sepharose is required for activation. Description of a useful coupling procedure follows:

A 20-ml amount of a 50% (packed beads/total volume) suspension of washed Sepharose 4B in distilled water is added to a 100-ml beaker with a magnetic stirring bar. While the pH and temperature are monitored, the cyanogen bromide is added, and the pH is maintained at 11 with 2 M NaOH during the reaction. Ice is added as needed to keep the temperature at 20 C. When no clumps of cyanogen bromide remain, contents of the beaker are transferred to a coarse-filter Büchner funnel. The activated Sepharose is washed with 300 ml of cold coupling buffer (0.1 M NaHCO$_3$, 1.0 M NaCl, pH 8.5).

The bottom of the Büchner funnel is made airtight with paraffin or a stopper, and the antigen to be coupled is added in a 10-ml volume of the coupling buffer. The suspension is transferred to a 50-ml beaker and stirred *slowly* for 16 to 24 h at 4 C.

After the coupling period, the sorbent is transferred to a coarse Büchner funnel and washed with large quantities of distilled water. The sorbent is then incubated with 30 to 40 ml of 1 M ethanolamine, pH 8, for at least 2 h at room temperature. Subsequently, the sorbent is washed alternatively with low pH (0.1 M sodium acetate, 1.0 M sodium chloride, pH 4.0) and high pH (0.1 M sodium borate, 1.0 M sodium chloride, pH 8.5) buffers five times with 10-min minimal exposures to each prior to washing.

The sorbent is then washed with 100 ml of RAST buffer, resuspended in RAST buffer at a concentration of 50% (vol/vol), and stored at 4 C until used.

(c) Determination of useful sorbent concentration. If a large excess of allergen has been coupled to the sorbent, the assay binding of a given serum will diminish only slightly over a wide range of sorbent concentrations. Over this range of antigen excess, assay sensitivity is not much influenced by sorbent concentrations. In sorbent systems with little coupled antigen (or in extended dilutions of allergen-rich sorbents), increasing the sorbent concentration will often dramatically increase assay sensitivity. Thus, it is useful to evaluate each sorbent at multiple concentrations, using the most potent reference serum available, to ascertain the effect of sorbent concentration on sensitivity. In allergen-rich systems, evaluation of sorbents at 10, 3, 1, and 0.3% (vol/vol) will often result in binding which diminishes only a few percent of total. In such a system, a sorbent concentration of 1% is chosen to maximize reagent life and minimize nonspecific binding without compromising sensitivity to a significant degree. If the fall-off in binding with increasing dilutions of sorbent is steep, the need for sensitivity must be weighed against economy in choosing a sorbent concentration for the assay system. Generally, sorbent concentrations greater than 10% or less than 0.1% are technically difficult to handle.

(d) Statistical handling of RAST data. Any number of measures of ^{125}I binding may be used to plot the dilution curve of the reference sera and for interpolation of test sera results. The nonspecific binding as indicated by a negative control serum should be subtracted from the replicate means of all points on the reference curve as well as the test sera binding. Net counts per minute bound is thus an appropriate parameter for interpolation. Some investigators prefer to express the binding as a percentage of the total counts added, after nonspecific binding is subtracted from both assay tubes and totals. A useful transformation, which allows direct comparison of binding data from one experiment to the next without consideration of total counts added or radio-degradation of the label, is the use of % B$_{max}$. A 1% (vol/vol) γE-sorbent may be used to provide an estimate of maximal binding in the experiment. The use of B$_{max}$ rather than T as the denominator provides a more useful method for assessing nonspecific binding in addition to providing some comparability of binding for points on the standard

curve from experiment to experiment.

(e) Precision, accuracy, and sensitivity. The RAST is a highly sensitive assay capable of measuring picogram quantities of IgE antibody. In a well-designed system the sensitivity can equal or exceed that obtained by direct skin tests. The CV for within-experiment replicates averages 5%. The CV for results between experiments when all reagents remain constant is 10 to 15%.

(f) Quantitation and comparison of results. The RAST depends for its quantitation upon parallelism between the dilution curves of the reference serum and the sera under study. The slopes of the dilution curves are a function of the average antibody affinity. Most sera from allergic patients who have not undergone immunization may have roughly parallel serum dilution curves. Active immunization may alter antibody affinity and thus the dilution curve slopes. This fact should be kept in mind in comparing results from immunized and nonimmunized individuals, or results from a single individual at various points during his course of immunotherapy. In terms of clinical interpretation, this problem may be of little practical importance. The good correlation between RAST and other tests of reaginic activity suggests that this may be true.

Each RAST assay is tied to its own reference standard. The specific IgE content of reference sera may vary considerably. Thus, a high titer of arbitrary units of antibody against one antigen may be equivalent in terms of absolute antibody content to a relatively low titer against another antigen. To circumvent this difficulty, two approaches for absolute standardization of RAST have recently been developed. One approach involves elution of a portion of the specific IgE bound to the RAST particles, followed by measurement of the quantity of IgE eluted and the proportion eluted. This approach allows standardization of reference and test sera in weight/volume terms, usually ng/ml (10). A second approach is total depletion of specific antibody by immunoabsorption, using RAST beads and measuring the reduction of total IgE protein observed (4). The two techniques give comparable results. In both cases it appears necessary to standardize only the reference sera; test sera may be evaluated by interpolation from a standardized reference serum. These techniques hold promise that RAST results may soon be expressed in terms of absolute antibody concentration. This outcome would allow comparison of RAST results in different allergen systems, as well as facilitating interlaboratory standardization.

Reagents and materials

(a) Required supplies and equipment. Disposable 12 × 75 mm test tubes (glass or plastic), micropipettes, a centrifuge, a pH meter, a gamma scintillation counter, an aspirator bottle with collared Pasteur pipette, and a slowly rotating (~24 rpm) orbital rotator modified to hold tube racks (Baltimore Biological Laboratories, Cockeysville, Md.; #60448 rotator).

(b) Materials required for the preparation of solid-phase allergens. Sephadex G-25 superfine particles, microcrystalline cellulose particles, or Sepharose 4B particles; cyanogen bromide; ethanolamine; high- and low-pH buffers (sodium acetate, sodium borate, sodium chloride).

(c) Rabbit antisera specific for the Fc fragment of IgE (Fc$_\epsilon$), preferably purified by affinity chromatography.

(d) Radioiodinated rabbit anti-Fc$_\epsilon$, usually prepared by the chloramine T method (see above, Preliminary preparations, *a*).

(e) RAST buffer for washing and diluting. Phosphate-buffered physiological saline at pH 7.4 containing 0.2% sodium azide, 0.5% (vol/vol) Tween 20, and 0.2% (wt/vol) BSA.

INTERPRETATION

The commercial RAST kits available from Pharmacia Laboratories utilize a single birch pollen reference serum and sorbent as a single standard for all of their RAST assays. Results are expressed as negative or 1+ to 4+ depending upon binding relative to arbitrary divisions of the standard curve. This grading system is easily misinterpreted to imply corresponding severity of clinical disease. Such inference is not justified since in certain allergen systems the most sensitive individuals will not exceed 2+ on the birch pollen standard curve. Ideally, each RAST sorbent system should have its own specific reference serum drawn from the most highly sensitive patient available.

Currently, each laboratory must derive the clinical correlations necessary to give a useful interpretation to the outcome of its own RAST assay results (see Introduction). This unfortunate fact will limit the broad application of RAST technology to the clinical evaluation of allergic diseases. Standardization of RAST results in terms of absolute antibody content will help to begin to solve this problem. However, the precise clinical interpretation of specific antibody content will also have to await clinical correlation data which are not yet available.

ACKNOWLEDGMENTS

I am recipient of Allergic Diseases Academic Award AI 71026 from the National Institute of Allergy and Infectious Diseases.

Publication no. 208 from the O'Neill Research Laboratories, The Good Samaritan Hospital, Baltimore, Md.

All figures were reprinted with permission from *Clinical Immunobiology,* vol. 3, Academic Press Inc., New York, 1976.

LITERATURE CITED

1. Aalberse, R. C. 1974. Immunoglobulin E, allergens and their interaction. Rudopi N.V., Amsterdam.
2. Ceska, M., R. Eriksson, and J. M. Varga. 1972. Radioimmunosorbent assay of allergens. J. Allergy Clin. Immunol. **49**:1–9.
3. Gleich, G. J., A. K. Averbeck, and H. A. Svedlund. 1971. Measurement of IgE in normal and allergic serum by radioimmunoassay. J. Lab. Clin. Med. **77**:690–698.
4. Gleich, G. J., and G. L. Jacob. 1975. Immunoglobulin E antibodies to pollen allergens account for high percentages of total immunoglobulin E proteins. Science **190**:1106–1107.
5. Ishizaka, K., T. Ishizaka, and E. H. Lee. 1970. Biologic function of the Fc fragment of E myeloma protein. Immunochemistry **7**:687–702.
6. Johansson, S. G. O., H. H. Bennich, and T. Berg. 1972. The clinical significance of IgE. Prog. Clin. Immunol. **1**:157–182.
7. Nye, L., T. G. Merrett, J. Landon, and R. J. White. 1975. A detailed investigation of circulating IgE levels in a normal population. Clin. Allergy **1**:13–24.
8. Polmar, S. H., T. A. Waldmann, S. T. Balestra, M. D. Jost, and W. D. Terry. 1972. Immunoglobulin E in immunologic deficiency diseases. J. Clin. Invest. **51**:326–330.
9. Rodbard, D. 1974. Statistical quality control and routine data processing for radioimmunoassays and immunoradiometric assays. Clin. Chem. **20**:1255–1270.
10. Schellenberg, R. R., and N. F. Adkinson, Jr. 1975. Measurements of absolute amounts of antigen-specific human IgE by a RAST elution technique. J. Immunol. **115**:1577–1583.
11. Wide, L. 1971. Solid phase antigen-antibody systems, p. 405–412. *In* K. E. Kirkham and W. M. Hunter (ed.), Radioimmunoassay methods. E. and S. Livingstone, Ltd., Edinburgh.

Chapter 80

Histamine Release and Assay Methods for the Study of Human Allergy

REUBEN P. SIRAGANIAN

INTRODUCTION

Histamine release from the leukocytes of allergic individuals is an excellent in vitro correlate of immediate hypersensitivity. The release in this reaction is initiated by the addition of antigen to which the individual is allergic, requires Ca^{2+}, and is due to the presence of immunoglobulin E (IgE) antibody fixed to the basophil membrane. Histamine is released from the basophil, the only cell that contains histamine in human blood. Identical mechanisms are involved in the activation of human basophils by either anti-human IgE or antigen. The release of histamine from the cell is a secretory process modulated by the level of intracellular cyclic adenosine monophosphate (AMP); agents which raise intracellular levels of cyclic AMP inhibit histamine release. Similarly, both microtubules and microfilaments seem to play a role; agents that stabilize microtubules and those that cause the disruption of microfilaments enhance histamine release (17, 30).

The addition of serum or plasma is not usually essential for the release of histamine from human basophils. However, normal serum will enhance the release when reaction conditions are suboptimal, e.g., with limiting antigen concentrations (26). In rare instances, the addition of serum is essential for the release, and this should be kept in mind in using the histamine release system (41). The serum of allergic individuals also contains blocking antibodies (IgG antibodies) that compete for antigen and prevent it from reaching the IgE-sensitized basophils; the concentration of these antibodies increases as a result of hyposensitization therapy.

Histamine release from washed leukocytes has been extensively utilized for in vitro studies of allergy. However, for several reasons the technique has had only limited clinical application: (i) the histamine extraction and the fluorometric assay are cumbersome and time-consuming procedures; (ii) large amounts of blood are required; and (iii) the method is technically complicated. However, several recent technical advances have made possible the routine use of

histamine release from leukocytes as an in vitro technique for the diagnosis and study of allergy.

The extraction and assay of histamine by the fluorometric technique is an accurate and sensitive method for the determination of this biologically active molecule. The fluorometric method was originally described by Shore et al. (35) and has been modified since then to increase both its specificity and sensitivity (8, 32; reviewed in 34). The method is based on the coupling of histamine with o-phthalaldehyde at a highly alkaline pH to form a fluorescent product. The fluorescence of the histamine-o-phthalaldehyde complex is more intense and more stable at an acid pH, unlike the complex formed by some other amines. To remove other interfering compounds, the histamine is extracted prior to the condensation step. Protein is removed from the sample to be analyzed by perchloric acid precipitation; the histamine is extracted into n-butanol from the alkalinized salt-saturated solution. The histamine is recovered in an aqueous solution of dilute HCl by adding heptane. This dilute HCl solution is then used for the condensation of histamine with o-phthalaldehyde. The extraction procedure is essential to remove histidine and other interfering compounds prior to the condensation step.

Recently, a completely automated, sensitive histamine analysis system has been developed (37, 39). This method is capable of analyzing 30 samples per hour (sample volume of 0.4 to 0.6 ml) with a precision of ±1 to 2%. The system can be used with a broad range of histamine concentrations, and at the highest sensitivity is capable of analyzing samples which contain 0.05 to 5 ng of histamine (in 0.5 ml). When samples have a large amount of protein, the sensitivity is somewhat less, but samples with 0.1 to 15 ng of histamine can still be analyzed accurately. Therefore, the use of the automated histamine assay has overcome the limitations for the clinical application of the histamine release system.

An enzyme-isotopic assay for histamine has

been described which has a sensitivity of about 1 ng (44). The method has been further refined to measure histamine in the 0.1- to 2.0-ng range (11, 16, 45). The assay involves the transfer of ^{14}C-labeled methyl groups from S-adenosylmethionine to unlabeled histamine by the enzyme histamine-N-methyltransferase. The [^{14}C]-methyl histamine formed is separated from histamine by extraction into chloroform. A trace amount of [^{3}H]histamine is added to each sample to monitor the internal recovery, the ratio of ^{14}C to ^{3}H being proportional to the amount of unlabeled histamine in the sample. The sensitivity of this double-isotopic technique is in the same range as the fluorometric technique. The automated system has the further advantage of reproducibility, automation, ease of operation, and rapid analysis of a large number of samples.

Allergic reactions depend not only on circulating IgE but also on a number of other factors, including the balance between blocking antibodies and the IgE on the target cells, and the ability of basophils or mast cells to release mediators. The addition of antigen to heparinized whole blood and the measurement of the histamine released into the supernatant fluid might therefore be a better reflection of the true in vivo immunological situation. Such a system of histamine release has recently been developed and appears to be a useful correlate for the clinical status of patients (38, 40). This modification further eliminates the time-consuming procedure for the isolation of washed leukocytes.

This chapter will describe the method for histamine release from washed leukocytes and whole blood. The whole blood system should be used as a general survey method to give information on the allergic status of patients. The washed leukocyte system is used for experimental studies on the release of mediators, the effect of pharmacological agents on the release mechanism, the effect of immunotherapy on cell sensitivity, and for the measurement of blocking antibody. Both the manual and the automated fluorometric histamine assay systems are described; although the initial cost of the automated system is high, it compensates for this by its ease of operation, greater sensitivity, and reproducibility. The automated system can assay 180 to 200 samples per work day, a load which would consume the time of two technicians, at a reproducibility that cannot be matched by the manual extraction process (precision of ±5% at best manually versus ±1% automated). Furthermore, the sensitivity of the automated system is at least 5 to 10 times better than the manual extraction assay.

CLINICAL INDICATIONS

Histamine release from human basophils is a valuable tool for in vitro studies of reaginic allergy. The indications for its use are the following.

Evaluation of the allergic status of patients

In ragweed allergic individuals, there is good correlation between the severity of clinical symptoms and in vitro histamine release (19, 22–24, 29, 33). In these patients there is excellent correlation of histamine release with the skin tests, the symptom score, and the level of serum IgE specific for antigen E (19). Both the antigen concentration at which histamine is released and the percentage of histamine released are good correlates of the clinical severity of the disease. Patients who have high concentrations of ragweed specific IgE release histamine with low concentrations of antigen E ($r = 0.74$; 19). There is good correlation in ragweed and grass allergic individuals between the concentration of antigen required to release 50% histamine and the skin sensitivity as determined by intradermal tests (29). The data therefore indicate that histamine release can be used as a quantitative measure of the clinical sensitivity of a patient. Although careful skin testing with several dilutions of antigen gives quantitative data, the results are less precise.

Measurements of the blocking antibody level

The histamine release method allows the quantitation of the level of blocking antibody and measurements of the effect of hyposensitization on this antibody (12, 18, 22–24, 27).

Measurements of reaginic antibody activity

The passive sensitization of normal leukocytes allows the quantitation of the relative amounts of specific IgE antibody (13–15). The radioallergosorbent test (RAST) gives similar information and has the further advantage that it can be more easily standardized (3). However, the RAST assay requires more antigen than histamine release studies.

Studies of the purification of allergens

The purification of an antigen can be followed by determination of its ability to release histamine (10, 20, 42). Similarly, the system is very useful for studying the effect of allergen modification on its ability to release histamine.

As an alternative for skin testing

There are a number of advantages of the use of the histamine release reaction as an alternative to skin testing. The in vitro test completely avoids the possibility of an anaphylactic reaction, an important consideration for some allergens. There is also no danger of sensitizing a patient or boosting a previous immune response, as might occur during repeated skin tests. This is a remote possibility which depends on the concentration of the allergen and the frequency of skin tests. An in vitro test would also be useful in the rare patient who cannot be skin tested because of dermatological conditions and in children. In vitro tests also permit the use of antigens which have not been purified or which cannot be used clinically.

The RAST has been introduced as a useful adjunct in studies of allergic reactions (3). It can be used for the same clinical indications as leukocyte histamine release. The histamine release results compare favorably with published reports of the use of the RAST technique in allergy diagnosis (38, 40). Several reports have shown that the RAST has an overall accuracy of about 70% when correlated with a patient's clinical history (3). Preliminary data indicate that histamine release from whole blood is positive in over 90% of the patients who are allergic by clinical evaluation (38, 40). The RAST assay has the advantage of utilizing serum. This is convenient for the patient, as serum can be stored indefinitely and also can be shipped to a central location for processing. However, histamine release from whole blood is probably a more biologically meaningful index of a patient's sensitivity and might indicate the relationships existing in the patient between the different antibodies and cell control mechanisms of histamine release.

TEST PROCEDURES

Histamine release from washed human leukocytes (25, 36)

General method. (When the histamine will be analyzed by the automated technique, 1 ml of blood is sufficient for three to four reaction tubes; when histamine is analyzed manually, 1 ml of blood is required for each reaction tube.) The desired volume of blood is drawn with a plastic syringe. The blood is transferred immediately into a plastic disposable tube (e.g., 50-ml polypropylene, Falcon Plastics no. 2074) which contains 1 ml of 0.1 M ethylenediaminetetraacetate (EDTA) and 2.5 ml of dextran-dextrose solution per 10 ml of blood. The tube is mixed by inverting several times. It is allowed to sediment at room temperature for 60 to 90 min until a clear interface develops between the red cell and plasma layers. The plasma-leukocyte-platelet (top) layer is drawn off with

a 10-ml disposable plastic pipette (Falcon no. 7030) and a pipette filler (e.g., Thomas no. 7775-F10) and is transferred into another plastic tube. It is centrifuged at 1,200 rpm (PRJ or PR 600 centrifuge, I.E.C., head no. 259; $300 \times g$) for 8 min at 4 C. The supernatant fluid is carefully poured off, and 2 to 3 ml of cold Tris A-EDTA buffer (see below, Reagents) is added. The cells are resuspended by gently swirling the tube; clumps can usually be broken up in this manner, but in very difficult cases the clumps are broken up by gently drawing them up and down with a 1-ml plastic pipette. After the cells are resuspended, 40 ml of cold Tris A-EDTA buffer is added and mixed (the volume of buffer at each wash step is twice the original blood volume). The tubes are centrifuged at 1,100 rpm ($250 \times g$) at 4 C for 8 min, and the cells are resuspended in Tris A buffer (using the same technique as described above). The tubes are centrifuged at 1,100 rpm at 4 C for 8 min and finally resuspended and brought up to the desired volume of Tris ACM.

The histamine release reaction is carried out in 12×74 mm plastic tubes (Falcon no. 2052). The total volume of supernatant fluid required for histamine analysis is about 0.5 ml for the automated system and about 1.0 ml for the manual extraction. Therefore, the reaction volumes should be adjusted according to the analysis system utilized. Routinely, when the histamine is analyzed by the automated technique, the reaction tube contains 0.25 ml of antigen, buffer, or perchloric acid. In practice, 0.25 ml of Tris ACM or the allergen is added to the tubes in an ice bath. The rack of tubes is then transferred to a 37 C bath. The cells are prewarmed to the same temperature for 6 min, and then 0.25 ml is added to the tubes. The concentration of leukocytes in the reaction mixture for the histamine release reaction should be 10^6 to 4×10^6/ml. All additions are made with automatic pipettes (e.g., Oxford Sampler). In each experiment there should be several blanks, i.e., tubes which receive only cells and buffer. Perchloric acid at a final concentration of 3% is added to four or five tubes to obtain the total histamine content of the cells (completes). The tubes are mixed by shaking the racks every 10 min. At the end of 60 min, the tubes are centrifuged at 1,600 rpm ($700 \times g$) for 15 min at 4 C. The supernatant fluid is poured into 2-ml autoanalyzer cups (Technicon no. 127-0090-P01). They are conveniently stored in a plastic rack which holds 40 tubes (e.g., Elkay, Worcester, Mass.). The rack is covered with Parafilm and stored at 4 C until ready for analysis (usually within 20 h). The samples are analyzed with the automated system without dialysis and with the

0.23-ml sample uptake tube on the manifold.

If a break is desired during the leukocyte preparation procedure, the plasma-leukocyte-platelets can be drawn off and stored for several hours at 4 C without any deleterious effect on the subsequent histamine release step.

When the amount of histamine release is very low, it can be enhanced by manipulations of the reaction system. The addition of serum from normal donors will enhance histamine release, especially if the reaction conditions are suboptimal (26). In some unusual cases, the addition of serum appears to be essential for the histamine release (41). It is suggested that in such cases 10% normal serum (preferably AB Rh+) be added to the reaction mixture containing leukocytes and allergen. Similarly, some pharmacological agents enhance histamine release (6, 7). The replacement of water with heavy water (deuterium oxide – D_2O, Bio-Rad Laboratories) will in most cases increase histamine release; usually, the Tris ACM buffer should contain 30 to 50% D_2O. Occasionally, the D_2O raises the blanks to unacceptable high values (greater than 10 to 15%). Similarly, the addition of cytochalasin B to some IgE-induced reactions will enhance the histamine release; effective concentrations are usually ~10^{-5} M. Whereas cytochalasin B enhances human basophil histamine release due to C5a, D_2O has no effect (9; unpublished data). Therefore, the effects of these compounds are not uniformly observed in all situations.

In situations where the leukocyte concentrations are very low, the release reaction is performed by adding 0.1 ml of cells to 0.1 ml of buffer (or antigen). At the end of 60 min, 0.3 ml of Tris ACM is added to all the tubes, the racks are shaken, and the tubes are then centrifuged.

Blocking antibody measurements (18, 27). The above procedure can be modified to measure blocking antibody titer (antigen-neutralizing capacity) in the serum of allergic individuals (27). Donors are used for these studies whose cells release >70% histamine when challenged with the antigen under study. A full antigen-dose response curve is first determined. The following method is then used for determining the allergen-neutralizing capacity of an allergic serum. Dilutions of allergens that release 5 to 75% histamine (in the ascending portion of the curve) are mixed with a sample of normal human serum or allergic serum at a concentration of 10% (0.25 ml of allergen + 0.25 ml of 20% serum). The mixtures are then incubated for 60 min at 37 C, and the tubes are transferred to a 4 C bath; 0.25 ml of washed leukocytes is then added to the tubes. The reaction tubes are incubated at 37 C for 60 min, and

the supernatant fluids are analyzed for histamine. The addition of nonallergic serum to the controls is essential because serum may enhance the release of histamine (26, 41).

An alternative method can be utilized to determine the blocking antibody titer (18). After determining the dose response curve of an individual, a concentration of allergen is chosen which would cause 60 to 80% histamine release. To a series of tubes containing this antigen concentration, twofold dilutions of allergic (or normal) sera are added. The total serum concentration is kept constant by the addition of normal AB serum. After incubating the tubes for 60 min at 37 C, washed leukocytes are added for the usual histamine release reaction.

For these studies, normal human serum is obtained from donors who are blood type AB, who have no history of allergy, and whose leukocytes when challenged with allergen do not release histamine. The serum is stored frozen at −20 C. (The sera of allergic individuals, even those who have never received hyposensitization therapy, contain some blocking activity.)

Passive sensitization of basophils (13–15). The leukocytes (basophils) from some donors who are nonallergic can be sensitized passively in vitro for antigen-induced histamine release. Suspensions of washed leukocytes are incubated with serum from an allergic donor (as a source of IgE), washed, and then reacted with the antigen under study. Only about 20% of nonallergic subjects furnish leukocytes which can be sensitized under the conditions described. Reaginic serum from allergic individuals can be stored at −20 C and is stable on prolonged storing.

Blood is obtained and sedimented as described in the previous section. The cells are washed in Tris A-EDTA, recentrifuged, and suspended in Tris A buffer. The cells are sensitized by incubation at 37 C at a concentration of about 10^7/ml with dilutions of reaginic serum, 4 mM EDTA, and 10 μg of heparin/ml (Sigma Chemical Co.). The cells are maintained in suspension by swirling the tubes every 10 to 15 min. At the end of 2 h, the tubes are centrifuged at 1,200 rpm at 4 C for 8 min, and the cells are washed twice with cold Tris A. The cells are finally resuspended in Tris ACM for the histamine release reaction.

Histamine release from whole blood (38, 40)

(Approximately 2 to 2.5 reaction tubes can be set up per 1 ml of blood drawn). Blood is drawn with a plastic syringe and transferred into a plastic tube (e.g., Falcon, 50 ml) containing 0.5 ml of heparin (Liquemin sodium 10, 1 ml = 1,000 units, Organon Inc.) per 20 ml of blood.

The blood is kept at 4 C until used (although blood stored for 24 h is as active as when first drawn, it is usually used within 2 to 4 h). The blood is diluted about 25% with Tris ACM (5 ml to 20 ml of blood) and used directly for the histamine release reaction.

The histamine release reaction is carried out in 12 × 75 mm plastic tubes (Falcon no. 2052). A 0.5-ml amount of Tris ACM or allergen is added to the tubes in an ice bath; 0.5 ml of the diluted blood is then added to all the tubes, and the racks are transferred to a 37 C bath. The tubes are mixed by shaking the racks every 10 min. Amounts of 0.5 ml of diluted blood and 0.5 ml of 12% $HClO_4$ are added to six or seven tubes to obtain the total histamine content of the blood ("completes"). These tubes are then pooled to yield four "completes." This procedure is necessary as there is a large amount of precipitate formed, and the amount of sample (supernatant) that can be poured off for histamine analysis is less than adequate for the assay. At the end of 60 min, the reaction is stopped by transferring the tubes to an ice bath, followed by centrifugation at 2,500 rpm (1,200 × g) for 30 min at 4 C. The supernatant fluids are poured off into 2-ml autoanalyzer cups and assayed for histamine by use of the automated system with 0.32-ml sample uptake and the dialysis system.

Automated histamine assay (37, 39)

With the automated system samples are analyzed at the rate of 30 per h.

Apparatus. The following Technicon modules (Technicon Corp., Tarrytown, N.Y.) are used: sampler type II (or IV), proportioning pump II, basic system dialyzer (38 C), a fluoronephelometer, and a single pen recorder. The fluorometer is equipped with the 013-B008-01 flow cell. The primary filter is the narrow pass 7–60 (peak at 350 nm). A sharp cut filter 2A (Turner) plus a 4–72 (Corning) are used together as the secondary filter.

Procedure. The flow diagram for the system, including the size of the different manifold tubes, the connectors, and the coils used on the manifold, is shown in Fig. 1. The histamine sample is diluted with saline containing Brij and EDTA and then is dialyzed against the same solution. To the dialyzed stream, 30% NaCl is added. After mixing, butanol is added, and the stream is alkalinized to extract the histamine into butanol. In the double mixing coil, there is rapid separation into discrete segments of aqueous and organic phases. The organic phase with the air bubbles is removed by the first extractor from the upper arm. After repumping, 0.1 N HCl and n-heptane are added, and the stream is mixed. The organic-

aqueous phases are separated in the second extractor; the aqueous lower phase is removed and resegmented with air. It is then alkalinized, o-phthalaldehyde is added, and, after the optimal reaction time, the histamine-o-phthalaldehyde reaction is stopped with phosphoric acid. The stream then passes through the fluorometer. As indicated in Fig. 1, Solvaflex tubing is used for those portions of the manifold which come in contact with organic solvents.

Both extractors are placed close to the inlet side of the manifold tubes on the right side of the pump. It is crucial that the second extractor be very close to the inlet of the manifold tubes as this part of the stream is not segmented by air bubbles. It is also important that the end of the waste tubes from both extractors are kept at the level of the middle of the extractors; otherwise, a negative pressure will be applied to this part of the manifold with uneven flow characteristics. This is accomplished by connecting the "waste" ends from the extractors with a 0.100-inch inner diameter plastic tube to a length of glass tube passed through the top of a 2-liter aspirator bottle. The tip of the glass tube is at the same level as the middle of the extractors. The cork at the top of the bottle has multiple openings. The outflow from the bottle runs to the bottom of a sink which has constantly running water.

The use of nitrogen instead of air to segment the stream increases the sensitivity of the system by 30 to 50%. Nitrogen is pumped into the end of the "air" tubes from a tank with the use of several pressure reduction valves to allow gas to escape at about 10 ml/min (first valve, Matheson no. 26267-40; second valve, Matheson, model no. 620PSV with 600 tube). An overflow from the nitrogen tube allows the excess gas to escape. Although the effect of nitrogen is only on the o-phthalaldehyde-histamine reaction, the manifold in routine use has nitrogen replacing air at all the pump points.

Extractors. A special extractor was designed to separate the aqueous from the organic phase at two steps in the automated procedure (37). The extractors are constructed by using the following Technicon manifold parts: a wide-bore connector (D-3) and three nipples (N-6; Fig. 2). The diameter of the wide side arms should be close to 4 mm. The aqueous organic mixture to be separated flows in the narrow side arm with the extractor set at an angle of 110° from the horizontal. Depending on the stage of the extraction, either the aqueous or oganic phase is removed for further processing. The introduction of a 5-cm coiled thin stainless-steel wire loop in the second extractor will break up small bubbles and improve the sepa-

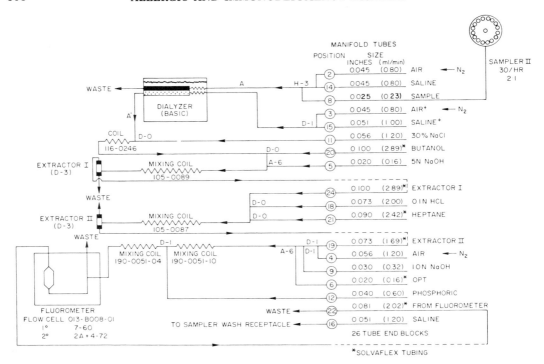

FIG. 1. *Flow diagram for histamine analysis. Manifold is shown for analysis with dialysis; for operation without dialysis, points A and A' are connected, and pump tubes marked (+) are removed. Extra sample tubes can be left on the pump at the unoccupied positions 7 (0.16 ml/min) and 10 (0.32 ml/min) for rapid changeover to analyze samples at other sensitivities. The first three coils have a 1.5-cm diameter, but, whereas coil no. 116-0246 is 10 turns with a 2.0-mm internal diameter, both coils 105-0089 and 105-0087 are 28 turns each and have an internal diameter of 2.4 mm. The last two coils (190-0051-10 is 40 turns and 190-0051-04 is 16 turns) are 3.0 cm in diameter with 2-mm internal diameter. Part numbers are listed in the Technicon Catalogue. All standard pump tubing used is of the "flow-rated" type. The end blocks are catalogue no. 113-0366-P10; they are placed on the pump using their middle holes. The o-phthalaldehyde (OPT) solution should be in a dark flask (e.g., 125-ml Erlenmeyer flask) and kept in an ice bucket. All other solutions are kept at room temperature. The aqueous solutions have a line filter between the reagent bottle and the pump (Gradko, Yonkers, N.Y.).*

ration of the two phases. The wire loop is used only in the second extractor.

Manifold changes. The flow system as described above can be modified to increase the sensitivity when analyzing histamine in samples which contain little protein. These samples are analyzed without dialysis. This modification is described in Fig. 1. The total time required for a sample to run through the manifold is 16 min with dialysis and 11 min without dialysis.

The basic manifold can easily be modified to analyze different sample volumes. In general, increasing the sample uptake volume will increase the sensitivity of the assay. The commonly used sample tubes are shown in Table 1. For routine use in assays of histamine release from washed human leukocytes, the manifold with the 0.23 ml/min sample tube is used without the dialysis step. The total volume of sample required for analysis in this system is 0.4 ml, and histamine concentrations of 5 to 10 ng/ml result in full-scale deflection. The amount of histamine that can be quantitated is usually 0.5 to 1% of the concentration that results in full-scale deflection and therefore about 100 pg/ml.

When samples are analyzed with the dialyzer, the sensitivity is decreased by about 70% (Table 1). When the histamine content of the samples is low, a larger sample is analyzed to compensate for the decreased sensitivity. With dialysis, histamine concentrations of 20 to 30 ng/ml result in full-scale deflection. The manifold with the 0.32 ml/min sample uptake tube is used with samples containing large amounts of plasma and little histamine, e.g., histamine release in whole blood. Extra sample tubes are left on the pump for rapid changeover to ana-

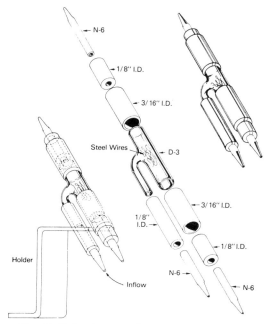

FIG. 2. *Extractor used to separate organic-aqueous phases. The ends of the N-6 should be directly in contact with the glass of the D-3 connector. The steel wire is placed only in the second extractor.*

TABLE 1. *Manifold changes for analyzing samples with and without dialysis*

Manifold	Sample uptake tube		Sample vol required[a] (ml)	Histamine concn for full-scale deflection[b] (ng/ml)
	Inner diam (inches)	Flow rate (ml/min)		
Without dialysis (protein less than 3 mg/ml)	0.025	0.23	0.4	5–10
With dialysis	0.030	0.32	0.6	20

[a] Total volume in the sample cup; actual volume analyzed is about 25% less.

[b] The readability of the graph is 0.5 to 1% of this value; therefore, the amount of histamine that can be quantitated is 25 to 100 pg.

lyze samples with different volumes (see Fig. 1).

The manifold pump tube from extractor I is changed every 20 h of machine operation time. The o-phthalaldehyde and sample uptake pump tubes are changed every 40 h, and all the manifold pump tubes are changed after 160 h of operation. These changes are important when analyzing samples at high sensitivity settings.

Operational suggestions. The fluorometer requires about 45 min for warm-up; it is suggested that the system be tested with 10 ng/ml histamine standards before analyzing any experimental samples. The aperture setting on the fluorometer is usually at 4 with damping set at 1 or 2. If the sensitivity of the system is not adequate, the 4-72 secondary filter can be removed. Similarly, if the fluorometer cannot be "blanked" at aperture setting 4, an extra secondary filter should be used to decrease the light (e.g., extra range filters; Turner). Samples on the machine are analyzed at the rate of 30/h; after every 50 to 60 samples a standard should be run to check for machine drift and also to serve as a marker on the recorder chart. It is advisable to run a sample containing only saline after analyzing samples with high histamine concentrations (e.g., completes or standards) to allow the machine to return to base line.

With use over several months, there is a decrease in the sensitivity of the system which is usually due to a decrease in the output of the ultraviolet excitation lamp in the fluorometer.

Manual histamine assay (28, 34)

Usually 48 samples are extracted at one time; this requires about 3 to 4 h. The supernatant fluids after centrifugation of the histamine release reaction are poured into 15-ml glass tubes; a 1.0-ml sample of the supernatant fluid is transferred into a 15-ml screw-cap glass culture tube (13 × 100 mm with Teflon-lined caps) containing 300 mg of NaCl (a heaping of no. 1 Coor Spatula, Thomas) and 1.25 ml of n-butanol (added with an automatic pipette, e.g., Lab Industries). After all the 1.0-ml samples are added to the butanol-NaCl tubes, 0.10 ml of 3 N NaOH is added quickly and accurately with a syringe microburette calibrated to 5 μliters/division (Micromatics Syringe). After adding the NaOH to three to five tubes, the tubes are capped and shaken for a few seconds. After all the samples are transferred, the rack is shaken for 1 min. The tubes are centrifuged at 1,500 rpm at 4 C for 5 min (600 × g). A 1.0-ml sample of the butanol (top) layer is removed by use of a pipette-filler and tranferred to a screw-cap glass tube (12 × 100 mm, 15 ml) containing 0.6 ml of 0.12 N HCl and 1.9 ml of n-heptane (add both with automatic pipettes). The tubes are capped and shaken for 1 min by rapid inversion by hand. They are allowed to stand upright for 5 min for the clear separation of the two phases. Then 0.5 ml of the 0.12 N HCl (bottom layer) is transferred into a 10 × 75 mm glass cuvette (Corning no. 99445) making sure that none of the top organic solvent layer is present. This is accomplished by placing a finger over the end of the pipette while going through the butanol-heptane, then gently blowing out before drawing up the acid layer, and wiping the outside of the pipette. The rack of tubes is transferred to an ice bath; extra tubes are added which receive either 0.12 N HCl or histamine standards of 25 to 100 ng/ml. To each tube, 100 μliters of 1 N NaOH is added with a syringe microburette (calibrated to 5 μliters/division), the tube is vortexed, immediately 25 μliters of 0.2% o-phthalaldehyde solution is added (with syringe microburette calibrated to 1 μliter/division), and the tube is vortexed again. The reaction is allowed to proceed for 40 min in an ice bath; to each tube, 50 μliters of 2 M H_3PO_4 is added (with syringe microburette); the tubes are vortexed and allowed to equilibrate to room temperature (about 15 min). The samples are then read either in a spectrofluorometer or simple fluorometer with an activation wavelength of 350 nm and a fluorescent wavelength of ~ 450 nm.

A 4-min histamine standard is run prior to analyzing the experimental samples to check the activity of the fluorophore reagents: 0.5 ml of 100 ng/ml histamine in 0.12 N HCl is allowed to react with NaOH and o-phthalaldehyde at room temperature for 4 min. After the addition of the 2 M H_3PO_4, the sample is read immediately. The fluorometer readings should be 60 to 80% of the levels of the 40-min 4 C reaction system.

Histamine is stable at an acid pH; therefore, during the extraction, tubes can be left for several hours after the transfer of the butanol samples into heptane-HCl tubes.

The extraction procedure requires modification if the samples contain appreciable amounts of protein (e.g., 10% serum); the protein should be removed by perchloric acid precipitation before proceeding with the extraction steps; e.g., to 1.0 ml of the supernatant fluid, 0.2 ml of 8% $HClO_4$ is added. The tubes are vortexed, incubated at 37 C for 30 min, and then centrifuged (1,700 rpm, 4 C, 15 min, ~ 500 × g). The supernatant fluids are poured off into glass tubes, and portions are transferred into the next step. In changing the system, care should be taken that excess NaOH is added at the first extraction step to alkalinize the aqueous phase so that histamine will be extracted into the butanol.

Calculations

The experimental results are expressed as the percentage of histamine release relative to the total cellular histamine content.

$$\text{Histamine release (\%)} = \frac{E - B}{C - B} \times 100$$

where E is the fluorometric reading of experimental sample, B is the fluorometric reading of samples with cells and buffer (and serum), and C is the fluorometric reading of complete (cells with $HClO_4$).

Cell sensitivity (HR_{50}) is the antigen concentration, expressed in micrograms, required to release 50% of the cellular histamine (25). This concentration can be determined by plotting the histamine release (as a percent) versus the antigen concentration on semilogarithmic paper. The antigen concentration on the ascending part of the curve is read from this graph. Similarly, if the histamine release is less than 50%, an HR_{30} can be determined.

Cell reactivity is the maximal amount of histamine release obtained with any amount of inducing agent (e.g., allergen or anti-IgE).

The *reaginic antibody titer* (PLS_{50}) is defined as the reciprocal of the dilution of allergic serum required for passive sensitization of normal leukocytes to release 50% of their histamine in response to the addition of antigen (15). A known standard reaginic serum is used to normalize the values.

There are several different ways of calculating the blocking antibody concentration. When antigen-dose response curves are determined in 10% normal or allergic human serum, the results are usually expressed as the *allergen neutralizing capacity (ANC)*:

$$ANC = G_{50}AHS/G_{50}NHS$$

where $G_{50}AHS$ is the antigen concentration for 50% histamine release in allergic serum and $G_{50}NHS$ is the antigen concentration for 50% histamine release in normal human serum (27). In contrast, where different dilutions of the allergic serum are tested, the *blocking antibody titer* is the reciprocal of the dilution at which the tested serum inhibits antigen-induced leukocyte histamine release by 50% (18).

REAGENTS

All solutions are made with distilled water and all chemicals are of reagent-grade purity unless otherwise specified.

Solutions for histamine release studies (25)

A 10× concentrated stock Tris buffer is prepared by dissolving 37.25 g of Preset Tris (Trizma 7.7; Sigma Chemical Co., St. Louis, Mo.), 70.15 g of NaCl, and 3.72 g of KCl in 1 liter. The pH of a 1:10 dilution of this buffer should be 7.35 at 37 C (or pH of 7.6 at 25 C). It is stored at 4 C. The human serum albumin is prepared by dissolving 3 g of human serum albumin (Behring Diagnostics, Hoechst Pharmaceuticals, Somerville, N.J.) in 0.85% saline and then brought up to 100 ml with saline. It is stored frozen (-20 C) as 5-ml portions (3% solution or 30 mg/ml solution). A 0.1 M EDTA solution is prepared by dissolving 37.23 g of disodium EDTA (Fisher) in about 600 ml of water and slowly adding 50% NaOH ($\sim$5 ml) to bring the pH to between 7.18 to 7.20. The EDTA goes into solution at that pH; the volume is then adjusted to 1 liter. This solution is stored at 4 C. Perchloric acid solutions, 12% and 6%, are prepared by diluting 200 or 100 ml of a 60% solution of $HClO_4$ (Fisher) up to 1,000 ml.

The Ca^{2+} and Mg^{2+} solutions are prepared by first drying the respective salts ($CaCl_2 \cdot 2H_2O$ and $MgCl_2 \cdot 6H_2O$) in a 50 C oven for 2 days. The stock solutions are 0.1 M each and are kept at 4 C.

The following solutions are prepared fresh daily: the dextrose-dextran solution, the Tris A, Tris A-EDTA and Tris ACM buffers. The dextrose-dextran is prepared by adding 600 mg of dextrose (Fisher) to 20 ml of sterile 6% clinical dextran (Dextran-75 with NaCl, 0.9%; Abbott Laboratories, Chicago, Ill.); 2.5 ml of this solution is added per 10 ml of blood. The Tris A buffer is prepared by diluting 10 ml of 10× stock Tris up to 100 ml and adding 1 ml of the 3% human serum albumin solution. The Tris A-EDTA is prepared by diluting 10 ml of 10× stock Tris and 4 ml of 0.1 M EDTA up to 100 ml and adding 1 ml of the 3% human serum albumin solution (4 mM EDTA). Tris ACM (1 mM Ca^{2+}, 0.5 mM Mg^{2+}) is prepared by diluting 1 ml of 0.1 M Ca^{2+} and 0.5 ml of 0.1 M Mg^{2+} up to 100 ml with the Tris A solution.

A variety of different proteins can be used as the allergens for inducing histamine release from the basophils of allergic individuals (10, 20, 42). Both purified proteins and crude extracts are effective in the histamine release reaction. The appropriate allergen dilutions are prepared in Tris ACM. There are several important considerations in the use of different types of allergens in histamine release experiments. Commercially available allergen extracts (e.g., Center Laboratories, Port Washington, N.Y.; Hollister-Stier, Yeadon, Pa.; and Greer, Lenoir, N.C.) each contain a large number of proteins, only a small fraction of which are allergenically important (e.g., crude ragweed extracts contain less than 5% antigen E, which is the important ragweed allergen). Some of these other proteins might be toxic for cells. Routinely, these allergen extracts should be tested on leukocytes from individuals known to be nonallergic to rule out nonspecific toxicity. Second, commercial allergen extracts show great variation in their content of active antigens, and there is even variation in different

lots from the same manufacturer (1, 2). Third, commercial allergen extracts are routinely not dialyzed and some contain appreciable amounts of histamine or histamine-like fluorescent material (e.g., insect whole body extracts). Fourth, commercially obtained allergen extracts contain preservatives (e.g., phenol) which at high concentrations (i.e., at higher than 0.004%) will inhibit the histamine release reaction. Fifth, dilute allergen (protein) solutions are not stable and lose their activity during storage (5). A partial solution to these problems is to dialyze the allergen extracts before use; this will effectively remove small-molecular-weight, fluorescent, inhibitory, or toxic material and preservatives. The allergen solution is then stored frozen (-20 C) in small portions. As most allergens studied so far appear to have molecular weights larger than 10,000, dialysis appears to be a practical solution. Ideally, purified, standardized allergens should be used in the histamine release reaction. At present, the only readily available allergen which fulfills that criteria is purified ragweed antigen E, the major ragweed allergen (available from Worthington Biochemical Corp., Freehold, N.J., and Research Resources Branch, National Institute of Allergy and Infectious Diseases, Bethesda, Md.).

Solutions for the automated histamine assay (37, 39)

Saline is prepared by dissolving 9.0 g of sodium chloride per liter. On the day of use, 0.5 ml of Brij-35 (30% solution, Technicon Corp.) and 15 ml of 0.1 M EDTA (prepared as in the preceding section) are added per liter. A 30% sodium chloride solution is prepared by dissolving 300 g/liter; it is filtered prior to use. The 5 N NaOH is made from a 50% solution (Fisher) by diluting 130 ml up to 500 ml; it should cool to room temperature before being used. The 1 N NaOH is prepared by diluting 100 ml of 10 N NaOH (Fisher) and 10 ml of 0.1 M EDTA up to 1 liter. The 0.1 N HCl is prepared from a 1 N stock (Fisher) by diluting 100 ml up to 1 liter. Phosphoric acid (0.73 M) is made from an 85% solution (Fisher) by diluting 50 ml up to 1 liter. The 0.5 M, pH 12.3 borate buffer is prepared by dissolving 30.95 g of boric acid (Fisher) in 900 ml of water, adjusting the pH with 50% NaOH, and bringing the solution up to 1 liter. The o-phthalaldehyde solution is prepared fresh daily by dissolving 50 mg of recrystallized o-phthalaldehyde in 2 ml of methanol (spectrophotometric grade, Fisher) and bringing it up to 100 ml with 0.5 M borate buffer, pH 12.3, in a dark Erlenmeyer flask. The solution is kept in ice in an ice bucket while being used on the analyzer. The 1-

butanol (butyl alcohol, Eastman Kodak) and *n*-heptane are reagent grade (Eastman Kodak). There is some variation in the base line with different lots of heptane.

The *o*-phthalaldehyde is recrystallized before use. A 5-g amount of crude *o*-phthalaldehyde (e.g., Sigma Chemical Co.) is added to a 125-ml Erlenmeyer flask containing 20 ml of ligroin (Eastman Kodak Co., no. 950, purified by permanganate, boiling point range 63 to 75 C). The flask is swirled under hot water (e.g., hot water tap) until the ligroin starts boiling. The supernatant fluid is poured quickly into 250-ml beakers which have been prechilled in an ice bath. To the crude residue in the Erlenmeyer flask, 20 ml of ligroin is added, and the above steps are repeated to increase the yield of recrystallized *o*-phthalaldehyde. The *o*-phthalaldehyde requires about 10 min to crystallize; the ligroin is then poured off. The beakers are allowed to evaporate at room temperature for several hours and then in a −20 C freezer overnight. The *o*-phthalaldehyde crystals are scraped off the side of the beaker into a dark bottle with a tight lid and stored at 4 C.

A histamine standard is prepared in 0.1 N HCl as 1 mg/ml solution of the base by dissolving 1.656 mg/ml of the dried histamine dihydrochloride (Fisher). The stock is kept frozen at −20 C. Standards containing 1,000, 200, 100, 50, 25, and 5 ng of histamine/ml are prepared in 2% perchloric acid and are stable at room temperature if kept tightly stoppered. All histamine standards should be kept in plastic tubes. For the human leukocyte experiments the 5 to 25 ng/ml standards are the most useful.

Solutions for the manual histamine assay (28)

The 0.12 N HCl is prepared by diluting 120 ml of 1 N HCl (Fisher) up to 1 liter; 3 N NaOH is prepared by diluting 7.8 ml of 50% NaOH (Fisher) up to 50 ml. The 2 M H_3PO_4 is prepared by diluting 12.35 ml of 85% phosphoric acid (Fisher) up to 100 ml. The 1 N NaOH is made by diluting 5 ml of 10 N NaOH (Fisher) and 2 ml of 0.1 N EDTA up to 50 ml. The 0.2% *o*-phthalaldehyde is prepared by dissolving 10 mg of recrystallized *o*-phthalaldehyde (see preceding section for method of recrystallization) in 5 ml of methanol (spectroanalyzed grade, Fisher) in a dark bottle. The *o*-phthalaldehyde and 1 N NaOH are prepared fresh daily. From a stock histamine standard of 1 mg/ml in 0.1 N HCl, standards of 10 μg/ml are prepared and kept frozen as 0.5-ml samples. For the assay the following standards are prepared fresh daily: 1,000, 100, 50, and 25 ng of histamine base per ml in 0.12 N HCl. The butanol is reagent grade

whereas the heptane is fluorometric grade (e.g., Eastman Kodak or Fisher).

INTERPRETATION

The fluorescence measured in the blank tube supernatant fluids is the sum of the histamine released from the cells and fluorescent material from the reagents. In the washed leukocyte experiments, the blank tube supernatant fluids should read less than 10% of the completes (in 41 experiments the blanks had a $\bar{X}$ 3.02%, S_x 1.36%, and a range of 0.1 to 7.1% [40]). However, in whole blood experiments the blanks are higher as a result of the fluorescent material contributed by the plasma, but the blanks still should be less than 15% of the completes (in 126 experiments $\bar{X} = 10.07\%$, $S_x = 3.52\%$, range 3.6 to 18.7% [40]). If the blanks are higher than these values, the experiment should be repeated. The experimental tubes should be in duplicate; results with the automated system indicate that release which is >10% is reproducible and significant. In contrast, with the manual extraction the errors are greater (±5%), and more duplicates are required to determine significance when the release is low. The total histamine content of blood in a group of 83 donors was $\bar{X}$ 83 ng/ml, S_x 29.5, range 39 to 209 (40).

The patient should have received no medication for 24 to 48 h prior to donating blood for histamine release studies. This is especially important if the patient is on aminophylline- or ephedrine-containing medications: basophils from such individuals are usually unreactive. As a control, it is advisable to add a few tubes of anti-IgE in all experiments; if the release is <5% at all concentrations of anti-IgE, the suspicion should be raised that the patient had taken a medication which interferes with the release or there was a technical error in the experiment.

Some compounds might contribute to the fluorescence observed in the final *o*-phthalaldehyde reaction; other compounds might quench the histamine-*o*-phthalaldehyde fluorescent complex (34, 37). Therefore, in testing the effect of compounds on the histamine release, it is prudent to test the compounds for native fluorescence in this assay. Similarly, the extraction process should be modified to determine histamine concentrations in urine because of interfering compounds (34). Allergens can contain fluorescent material and might also be toxic for cells (for a full discussion, see section on Solutions for histamine release studies).

Studies have shown that histamine release from whole blood correlates very well with release from washed leukocytes: the correlation between the maximal histamine released obtained from washed leukocytes and that from whole blood is r = 0.93 (40). The maximal release that can be obtained from whole blood, however, is usually less than the release from washed leukocytes (slope of the least square line from the correlation coefficient is 0.59 to 0.82). In patients receiving immunotherapy the antigen concentration required to give maximal histamine release is higher in whole blood than with washed leukocytes.

In most clinical studies a very close correlation has been found between the results of skin tests with ragweed pollen, antigen E, or grass pollen and histamine release (e.g., the correlation coefficient between cell sensitivity and skin test sensitivity is ~0.8 [1, 4, 29]). If skin test titrations are performed by the end-point method, they are about 10 times more sensitive than the cell sensitivity, if to a 2+ end point the methods have equal sensitivity. There is also highly significant correlation between the cell sensitivity and how symptomatic the patient is during the pollen season (12, 22–24, 29, 33). However, there are some patients with very little histamine release at any concentrations (release less than 15%) who are very sensitive by skin tests. The interpretation of this is not clear. There is also good correlation between the level of specific ragweed IgE antibody in the serum and the cell sensitivity (19, 29); however, patients with the same level of anti-ragweed serum IgE might vary in cell sensitivity by 100- to 1,000-fold. Obviously, the cell sensitivity is also measuring the effectiveness of the histamine release mechanism. These correlations appear to hold only for patients who are not on immunotherapy.

Allergic reactions depend on a number of factors, including the presence of specific IgE, the concentration of blocking antibodies, and the ability of basophils or mast cells to release mediators. The amount of histamine released when an allergen is added to whole blood in vitro is due to the interaction of all these factors. Therefore, this test more closely simulates the allergic reaction occurring in vivo than measurements of the concentration of allergen-specific IgE. Histamine release from whole blood correlates closely with a patient's skin sensitivity (38, 40). Over 90% of patients who have skin tests greater than or equal to 3+ at 100 PNU or less release significant histamine when antigen is added to whole blood. In contrast, the test is positive in less than 2% of skin test-negative patients, and most of these appear to be experimental errors.

Anti-IgE-induced release of histamine from washed leukocytes correlates to a certain extent (r = 0.42 to 0.70) with the serum IgE levels and therefore with a person's allergic history (12, 21). The cellular sensitivity determined by antigenically induced histamine release correlates significantly with that initiated by anti-IgE (12, 21). The release induced by concanavalin A has great similarities to anti-IgE-induced release, and a very close correlation exists between the histamine release induced by concanavalin A and anti-IgE (36, 43). In this reaction concanavalin A appears to react with cell-bound IgE to activate the basophil (43).

Immunotherapy of patients results in several changes in the histamine release results: there is an increase in the level of blocking antibody, a decrease in cell sensitivity and reactivity, and a progressive but slow decrease in the serum antigen specific IgE levels (12, 15, 17, 19, 22–24, 30, 31, 33). The changes in cell sensitivity and reactivity with some cells releasing no histamine are most often seen in pediatric cases (12, 31, 33). The increase in the level of blocking antibody correlates with the effectiveness of the immunotherapy. Cellular sensitivity might fall prior to seasonal exposure, and there is a postseasonal rise which appears to be less in patients on immunotherapy.

It should be emphasized that the skin test for immediate hypersensitivity using a number of common allergens and a dilution of 2+ end point is the simplest method of assessing the presence or absence of allergy. The in vitro histamine methods are useful complements to the clinical evaluation of patients and supply quantitative data on the degree of sensitivity of a patient. The automated histamine analysis system makes the assay more sensitive and far simpler to apply to routine use.

ACKNOWLEDGMENTS

I thank William A. Hook and Anne K. Sobotka for helpful discussions and Doris Light for the secretarial work.

LITERATURE CITED

1. Baer, H., H. Godfrey, C. J. Maloney, P. S. Norman, and L. M. Lichtenstein. 1970. The potency and antigen E content of commercially prepared ragweed extracts. J. Allergy 45:347–354.
2. Baer, H., C. J. Maloney, P. S. Norman, and D. G. Marsh. 1974. The potency and group 1 antigen content of six commercially prepared grass pollen extracts. J. Allergy Clin. Immunol. 54:157–164.
3. Berg, T. L. O., and S. G. O. Johansson. 1974. Allergy diagnosis with the radioallergosorbent test. A comparison with the results of skin and provocation tests in an unselected group of children with asthma and hay fever.

J. Allergy Clin. Immunol. 54:207–221.

4. Bruce, C. A., R. R. Rosenthal, L. M. Lichtenstein, and P. S. Norman. 1974. Diagnostic tests in ragweed-allergic asthma. J. Allergy Clin. Immunol. 53:230–239.

5. Center, J. G., N. Shuller, and L. D. Zeleznick. 1974. Stability of antigen E in commercially prepared ragweed pollen extracts. J. Allergy Clin. Immunol. 54:305–310.

6. Colten, H. R., and K. H. Gabbay. 1972. Histamine release from human leukocytes: modulation by a cytochalasin B-sensitive barrier. J. Clin. Invest. 51:1927–1931.

7. Gillespie, E., and L. M. Lichtenstein. 1972. Histamine release from human leukocytes: studies with deuterium oxide, colchicine, and cytochalasin B. J. Clin. Invest. 51:2941–2947.

8. Häkanson, R. A., A. L. Rönnberg, and K. Sjölund. 1972. Fluorometric determination of histamine with OPT: optimum reaction conditions and tests of identity. Anal. Biochem. 47:356–370.

9. Hook, W. A., R. P. Siraganian, and S. M. Wahl. 1975. Complement-induced histamine release from human basophils. I. Generation of activity in human serum. J. Immunol. 114:1185–1190.

10. King, T. P., P. S. Norman, and L. M. Lichtenstein. 1967. Isolation and characterization of allergens from ragweed pollen. IV. Biochemistry 6:1992–2000.

11. Kobayashi, Y., and D. V. Maudsley. 1972. A single-isotope enzyme assay for histamine. Anal. Biochem. 46:85–90.

12. Levy, D. A., L. M. Lichtenstein, E. O. Goldstein, and K. Ishizaka. 1971. Immunologic and cellular changes accompanying the therapy of pollen allergy. J. Clin. Invest. 50:360–369.

13. Levy, D. A., and A. G. Osler. 1966. Studies on the mechanisms of hypersensitivity phenomena. XIV. Passive sensitization in vitro of human leukocytes to ragweed pollen antigen. J. Immunol. 97:203–212.

14. Levy, D. A., and A. G. Osler. 1967. Studies on the mechanisms of hypersensitivity phenomena. XV. Enhancement of passive sensitization of human leukocytes by heparin. J. Immunol. 99:1062–1067.

15. Levy, D. A., and A. G. Osler. 1967. Studies on the mechanisms of hypersensitivity phenomena. XVI. In vitro assays of reaginic activity in human sera: effect of therapeutic immunization on seasonal titer changes. J. Immunol. 99:1068–1077.

16. Levy, D. A., and M. Widra. 1973. A microassay for studying allergic histamine release from human leukocytes using an enzymic-isotopic assay for histamine. J. Lab. Clin. Med. 81:291–297.

17. Lichtenstein, L. M. 1972. Allergy. Clin. Immunobiol. 1:243–269.

18. Lichtenstein, L. M., N. A. Holtzman, and L. S. Burnett. 1968. A quantitative in vitro study of the chromatographic distribution and immunoglobulin characteristics of human blocking antibody. J. Immunol. 101:317–324.

19. Lichtenstein, L. M., K. Ishizaka, P. S. Norman, A. K. Sobotka, and B. M. Hill. IgE antibody measurements in ragweed hay fever. Relationship to clinical severity and the results of immunotherapy. J. Clin. Invest. 52:472–482.

20. Lichtenstein, L. M., T. P. King, and A. G. Osler. 1966. In vitro assay of allergenic properties of ragweed pollen antigens. J. Allergy 38:174–182.

21. Lichtenstein, L. M., D. A. Levy, and K. Ishizaka. 1970. In vitro reversed anaphylaxis: characteristics of anti-IgE mediated histamine release. Immunology 19:831–842.

22. Lichtenstein, L. M., P. S. Norman, and W. L. Winkenwerder. 1968. Clinical and in vitro studies on the role of immunotherapy in ragweed hay fever. Am. J. Med. 44:514–524.

23. Lichtenstein, L. M., P. S. Norman, and W. L. Winkenwerder. 1971. A single year of immunotherapy for ragweed hay fever. Immunologic and clinical studies. Ann. Intern. Med. 75:663–671.

24. Lichtenstein, L. M., P. S. Norman, W. L. Winkenwerder, and A. G. Osler. 1966. In vitro studies of human ragweed allergy: changes in cellular and humoral activity associated with specific desensitization. J. Clin. Invest. 45:1126–1136.

25. Lichtenstein, L. M., and A. G. Osler. 1964. Studies on the mechanisms of hypersensitivity phenomena. IX. Histamine release from human leukocytes by ragweed pollen antigen. J. Exp. Med. 120:507–530.

26. Lichtenstein, L. M., and A. G. Osler. 1966. Studies on the mechanisms of hypersensitivity phenomena. XI. The effect of normal human serum on the release of histamine from human leukocytes by ragweed pollen antigen. J. Immunol. 96:159–168.

27. Lichtenstein, L. M., and A. G. Osler. 1966. Studies on the mechanisms of hypersensitivity phenomena. XII. An in vitro study of the reaction between ragweed pollen antigen, allergic human serum and ragweed-sensitive human leukocytes. J. Immunol. 96:169–179.

28. May, C. D., M. Lyman, R. Alberto, and J. Cheng. 1970. Procedures for immunochemical study of histamine release from leukocytes with small volume of blood. J. Allergy 46:12–20.

29. Norman, P. S., L. M. Lichtenstein, and K. Ishizaka. 1973. Diagnostic tests in ragweed hay fever. J. Allergy Clin. Immunol. 52:210–224.

30. Osler, A. G., L. M. Lichtenstein, and D. A. Levy. 1968. In vitro studies of human reaginic allergy. Adv. Immunol. 8:183–231.

31. Pruzansky, J. J., and R. Patterson. 1967. Histamine release from leukocytes of hypersensitive individuals. II. Reduced sensitivity of leukocytes after injection therapy. J. Allergy 39:44–50.

32. Redlich, D. V., and D. Glick. 1969. Improvements in fluorometric microdeterminations of histamine and serotonin. Anal. Biochem. 29:167–171.

33. Sadan, N., M. B. Rhyne, E. D. Mellits, E. O. Goldstein, D. A. Levy, and L. M. Lichtenstein. 1969. Immunotherapy of pollinosis in children. Investigation of the immunologic basis of clinical improvement. N. Engl. J. Med. 280:623–627.

34. Shore, P. A. 1971. The chemical determination of histamine, p. 89–97. *In* D. Glick (ed.), Analysis of biogenic amines and their related enzymes. Interscience Publishers, New York.

35. Shore, P. A., A. Burkhalter, and V. H. Cohn, Jr. 1959. A method for the fluorometric assay of histamine in tissues. J. Pharmacol. Exp. Ther. 127:182–186.

36. Siraganian, P. A., and R. P. Siraganian. 1974. Basophil activation by concanavalin A: characteristics of the reaction. J. Immunol. 112:2117–2125.

37. Siraganian, R. P. 1974. An automated continuous-flow system for the extraction and fluorometric analysis of histamine. Anal. Biochem. 57:383–394.

38. Siraganian, R. P. 1975. Automated histamine release. A method for *in vitro* allergy diagnosis. Int. Arch. Allergy Appl. Immunol. 49:108–110.

39. Siraganian, R. P. 1975. Refinements in the automated fluorometric histamine analysis system. J. Immunol. Methods 7:283–290.

40. Siraganian, R. P., and M. J. Brodsky. 1976. Automated histamine analysis for *in vitro* allergy testing. I. A method utilizing allergen induced histamine release from whole blood. J. Allergy Clin. Immunol., in press.

41. Siraganian, R. P., and B. B. Levine. 1975. Unique serum requirement for histamine release from human basophils. Int. Arch. Allergy Appl. Immunol. 48:530–536.

42. Siraganian, R. P., I. Schenkein, and B. B. Levine. 1975. Immunologic studies of a patient with seminal plasma allergy. Clin. Immunol. Immunopathol. 4:59–66.

43. Siraganian, R. P., and P. A. Siraganian. 1975. Mechanism of action of concanavalin A on human basophils. J. Immunol. 114:886–893.

44. Snyder, S. H., R. J. Baldessarini, and J. Axelrod. 1966. A sensitive and specific enzymatic isotopic assay for tissue histamine. J. Pharmacol. Exp. Ther. 153:544–549.

45. Taylor, K. M., and S. H. Snyder. 1972. Isotopic microassay of histamine, histidine, histidine decarboxylase and histamine methyltransferase in brain tissue. J. Neurochem. 19:1343–1358.

Chapter 81

Diseases of the Lung

JORDAN N. FINK

INTRODUCTION

Over the past several years, it has become apparent that any of the four types of allergic reactions (types I to IV of Gell and Coombs [5]) may be involved in the pathogenesis of immunological diseases of the lung. The most common human immunological lung disease is the atopic disease asthma, usually associated with a type I or immunoglobulin E (IgE) anaphylactic mechanism. The methods for study of this disease, including skin tests, the radioallergosorbent test (RAST), and IgE measurement, as well as assays of pharmacological mediators released by specific antigens, are covered in the chapter dealing with histamine release. The features of type II or cytotoxic reactions associated with human lung disease, especially Goodpasture's syndrome, are covered in the chapter on autoimmune diseases. The type IV or cell-mediated hypersensitivity lung diseases may be evaluated according to techniques described under the tests for cellular components, which include skin testing for cellular hypersensitivity and evaluation of lymphocyte functions by measurement of lymphokines.

Among the immunological lung diseases which may result from a type III or immune complex response are those due to the inhalation of biological dusts. Such diseases are known as hypersensitivity pneumonitis or extrinsic allergic alveolitis (7). Clinically they present as intermittent episodes of chills, fever, cough, and shortness of breath occurring 4 to 6 h after the inhalation of the specific sensitizing organic dust. Some sensitized individuals may present with only the respiratory symptoms of progressive dyspnea (3, 7). An interstitial nodular pattern can be found on chest X ray, and the pulmonary pathology is primarily a lymphocytic interstitial pneumonitis with scattered granulomas (3). Pulmonary function abnormalities include those of restriction, obstruction, and decreased gas transfer (7).

Serological studies of patients with these diseases usually demonstrate the presence of precipitating antibodies to the suspected offending dust, thus providing important information regarding (i) the diagnosis of the patient's lung disease and (ii) the possible offending antigen.

This chapter will be concerned with the techniques employed in demonstrating precipitating antibodies to a variety of organic dusts in the serum of patients suspected or known to have hypersensitivity pneumonitis. The variety of antigens involved and the disease states are shown in Table 1.

Evaluation for possible precipitating antibodies should be carried out whenever there is clinical evidence (from history or X ray) that the patient's respiratory disease may be temporally related to his environment (work, home, hobby).

METHODS OF STUDY

There are several techniques available for the detection of precipitins in the serum of patients clinically suspected to have lung disease due to one of the biological dusts. The choice of the technique described below is based on previous experience and results. The steps necessary in carrying out the test include (i) the preparation of the antigen and (ii) the use of a gel diffusion technique to detect precipitins to the antigen(s).

Preparation of antigens

Any antigen present in the patient's environment may be suspect in the pathogenesis of hypersensitivity pneumonitis. Therefore, it may be necessary to prepare crude extracts of vegetable or animal products found in the patient's environment for study. It may also be necessary to use fungal or bacterial cultures obtained from the crude materials, or from the environment.

Crude extracts. Materials such as avian droppings, vegetable compost products, wood dusts, or forced air system (humidifier) fluids should be collected from the patient's environment. A portion of the material should be saved for culture. The nonfluid material to be tested is prepared in 0.15 M NaCl on a 10% (wt/vol) basis (100 mg of material to 10 ml of 0.15 M sodium chloride), allowed to extract over 72 h with occasional gentle shaking, and filtered (1). The fluid material is used neat.

Animal sera (avian, canine, equine) may be

TABLE 1. *Some organic dust-induced lung diseases associated with serum precipitins*

Disease	Crude organic dust	Offending antigen
Farmer's lung	Moldy hay	*Micropolyspora faeni, Thermoac-*
Bagassosis	Moldy sugar cane	*tinomyces vulgaris, T. sa-*
Mushroom workers lung	Moldy mushroom compost	*charii, T. viridis,* or *T. candi-*
Forced air system disease	Contaminated forced air system	*dus*
Suberosis	Moldy cork	*Penicillium frequentans*
Maple bark lung	Moldy maple bark	*Cryptostroma corticale*
Cheese worker's lung	Cheese mold	*Penicillium caseii*
Avian handler's lung	Avian excreta	Excreted serum proteins
Pituitary snuff user's lung	Pituitary powder	Bovine and porcine serum proteins

obtained from animals or from standard suppliers (Miles Laboratories, Kankakee, Ill.) and are used on a 1:10 to 1:20 basis, diluted with buffered saline.

Extracts of cultured materials. When deemed necessary, according to the clinical history, it may be advantageous to search for precipitating antibodies in the sera of patients exposed to microorganisms present in the environment. It may be useful to determine the microflora of a sample of moldy hay (for thermophilic actinomycetes), moldy corn (for *Aspergillus* sp.), or patient's home forced air appliance water or dusts (humidifier water).

The material must initially be cultured by standard microbiological techniques, on Sabouraud medium at 20 and 37 C for saprophytic fungi and on peptone soy agar (in the case of liquids, peptone soy broth; Trypticase soy agar or broth, BioQuest, Inc., Cockeysville, Md.) at 56 C for 3 to 5 days. The cultured organisms are identified, isolated, and subcultured. They are harvested by scraping from the agar, or filtering out of the broth, are weighed where possible, and then are extracted in 0.15 M NaCl on a 10% (wt/vol) basis (1). These materials can be stored at 4 C for several weeks for use in the appropriate immunological gel diffusion test.

Gel diffusion studies

Several test procedures are available to study human sera for the presence of precipitating antibodies to a wide variety of organic dusts.

The most common method is the microscope slide modification of the Ouchterlony double-diffusion in agar (2). This test is easy to perform and requires less reagents than the other methods, but it requires 24 to 48 h of incubation. A modification of this technique by Wadsworth, using a template, requires less time to perform, but it also requires 24 to 48 h of incubation (8).

The most rapid method, that of counterimmunoelectrophoresis, requires only 90 min for results and is more sensitive than the other gel diffusion techniques (6). The major disadvantage of this method is that it lacks the reproducibility of the gel diffusion tests and may have excessive "false-positive" reactions (4). For these reasons, my laboratory has used the Wadsworth template technique for the detection of antibodies in the sera of patients suspected to have hypersensitivity pneumonitis.

PROCEDURE FOR TEMPLATE IMMUNODIFFUSION (8)

Materials

Coated glass slides. Cleaned microscope slides are dipped into 0.1% agarose solution, drained, and air-dried.

Agarose solution. Heated for 10 minutes in a boiling water bath are 80 mg of Seakem agarose (MCI BioMedical, Rockland, Mass.), 33 mg of sodium azide, and 10 ml of barbital buffer, single strength.

Barbital buffer. Store in a refrigerator as *double* strength, and dilute with an equal volume of distilled water before use: sodium barbital, 20.0 g; sodium acetate, 13.0 g; HCl (1 N), 12.88 ml; and distilled water to a final volume of 1 liter (adjusted to pH 8.6).

Slide wash solution. NaCl, 0.15 M.

Methanol-acetic acid solution for stain solvent and destaining. Absolute methyl alcohol, 450 ml; glacial acetic acid, 100 ml; and distilled water, 450 ml.

Stain. Coomassie blue R250 (Serva, Heidelberg, West Germany, or Eastman Kodak, Rochester, N.Y.), 0.2% in methanol-acetic acid solution.

Plastic templates. A sheet of Plexiglas 4.0-mm thick is cut to the size of microscope slides. Two lines of six holes each are cut along the length of the plastic tempate with a 1.5-mm drill. The distance between the holes is 8 mm. Another line of five holes is drilled between the two previous lines as shown in Fig. 1. The template is completed by enlarging the holes to

3.0 mm for three-fourths of the Plexiglas thickness.

Procedure

Cleaned, dilute agarose-dipped, and air-dried microscope slides are prepared. Hot agarose, 1.1 ml, is applied to each slide with a pipette, starting at the edges and ending in the middle. The agar is allowed to cool and harden slightly, and the template is carefully applied with the smaller hole diameter in good contact with the agarose. The slide is then placed in a moist chamber to cool and harden.

Both outer rows of wells are filled with antigen(s) or sera to be tested by means of a 1.0-ml syringe and 25-gauge needle (Fig. 2). The wells in the center row are then filled with the corresponding reagent. The slides are placed in a moist chamber, which is tightly covered and allowed to remain at room temperature for 48 h.

After 48 h, the slides are removed from the chamber, the plastic templates are carefully removed, and the slides are placed vertically in a glass stain rack and dish filled with 0.15 M

NaCl. The slides are left to wash overnight (Fig. 3).

After two changes of distilled water, 15 min each, the slides are stained in Coomassie blue R250 for 6 min. They are destained in methanol-acetic acid solution (several changes) for 10 to 15 min. They are then dried in an incubator, placed briefly into fresh methanol-acetic acid solution, and redried in the incubator. They are then labeled. (Fig. 4).

Control reagents

Control antisera are procured by testing sufficient human sera with antigens to obtain samples with adequate precipitating antibody. Alternatively, the antigens may be injected to animals to induce high-titer animal antisera for use as controls. Crude antigens cannot be adequately quality controlled.

Interpretation of the tests

Positive test (detectable precipitin bands). The demonstration of precipitin bands to the tested antigen in a given patient's serum requires interpretation. Although the intensity and number of gel diffusion bands correlates in general positively with the presence of disease, this is not always true. On occasion, asymptomatic individuals may have more intense reactions than ill patients or a patient with hypersensitivity pneumonitis to a proven organic dust may have no precipitin reaction to the dust, but these situations are unusual.

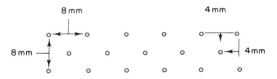

FIG. 1. *Diagram showing preparation of plastic template.*

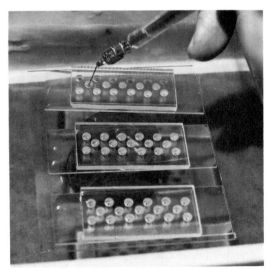

FIG. 2. *Template holes filled with reagents.*

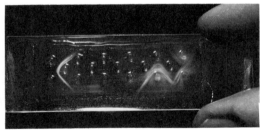

FIG. 3. *Washed slide prior to staining.*

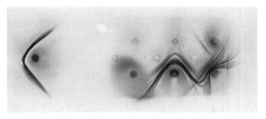

FIG. 4. *Photograph of stained slide demonstrating precipitin patterns.*

False-positive tests. False-positive reactions may occur in gel diffusion studies when C substance interacts with C-reactive protein. At times this reaction may be suppressed by adding sodium citrate to the agar gel. An additional source of false-positive reactions is the nonspecific interaction of the patient's serum with bacterial cell wall constituents, especially teichoic acid.

In serological studies of large numbers of individuals exposed to organic dust antigens, but clinically free from symptoms, up to 50% had demonstrable precipitins to the dust. Thus, the serum precipitin reaction indicates that the tested individual has made an immune response following contact with antigen. Therefore, interpretation of the results of the gel diffusion study must take into account the clinical features of the patient.

Negative tests. The lack of detectable precipitating antibody in gel diffusion tests also needs interpretation in light of the clinical picture. A wide variety of organic dust antigens have been shown to cause hypersensitivity pneumonitis, and new dust antigens are described yearly. Therefore, the tested panel of antigens may not include the pertinent one, and a sampling of the patient's environment with subsequent gel diffusion testing may be necessary.

In cases of hypersensitivity pneumonitis in which the patient has not contacted the offending antigen for some time, the previously detectable precipitating antibody may no longer be present. Thus, the lack of a reaction also needs to be interpreted in view of the clinical picture.

ACKNOWLEDGMENTS

This work was supported by National Heart and Lung Institute grant HL15389 (SCOR) and by funds from the Research Service, Veterans Administration.

LITERATURE CITED

1. Barboriak, J. J., A. J. Sosman, and C. E. Reed. 1965. Serologic studies in pigeon breeders disease. J. Lab. Clin. Med. 65:600–604.
2. Crowle, A. J. 1973. Immunodiffusion. Academic Press Inc., New York.
3. Fink, J. N. 1972. Hypersensitivity due to organic dust inhalation. N.Y. State J. Med. 72:1834–1837.
4. Flaherty, D., J. Barboriak, D. Emanuel, et al. 1974. Multilaboratory comparison of three immunodiffusion methods used for the detection of precipitating antibodies in hypersensitivity pneumonitis. J. Lab. Clin. Med. 84:298–306.
5. Gell, P. G. H., and R. R. A. Coombs. 1968. Clinical aspects of immunology. F. A. Davis Co., Philadelphia.
6. Gordon, M. A., J. Dixon, and H. A. Oberman. 1971. Diagnostic mycoserology by immunoelectroosmophoresis. Am. J. Clin. Pathol. 56:471–474.
7. Pepys, J. 1969. Hypersensitivity diseases of the lung due to fungi and other organic dusts. S. Karger, Basel.
8. Wadsworth, C. 1962. A microplate technique employing a gel chamber composed with other micro and macroplate techniques for immune diffusion. Int. Arch. Allergy 21:131–137.

Chapter 82

Immunodeficiency

RICHARD HONG

INTRODUCTION

Immunodeficiency syndromes result in increased susceptibility to infection and can be due to defects in the major systems which cooperate in the development of the normal immune responses. These systems are: (i) the T cell system and its augmentation mechanism of released mediators, (ii) the B cell system and its augmentation mechanism, the complement cascade, and (iii) the macrophage system. In addition, increased susceptibility to infection can result from deficiencies of another major defense system, the granulocyte.

With a few exceptions, there are no simple screening tests which categorically rule out major defects of a given system, so a rather extensive work-up is required in all cases of suspected deficiency. The answer to this problem is not to investigate more patients exhaustively but to be aware of the clinical symptomatology which is more likely to be associated with detectable abnormalities. Although the clinical history of the patient does not provide an absolute indicator of which system is at fault, I believe the guidelines shown in the following key are useful in directing the physician's emphasis to a given system.

Clinical Symptoms of Immunodeficiency

I. Suggest T cell defect
   A. Systemic illness following vaccination with any live virus or BCG; unusual life threatening complication following infection with ordinarily benign virus (e.g., giant cell pneumonia with rubeola; varicella pneumonia)
   B. Chronic oral candidiasis persisting after 6 months of age and resisting adequate chemotherapy
   C. Chronic mucocutaneous candidiasis
   D. Features of cartilage hair hypoplasia (fine thin hair, short-limbed dwarfism with characteristic X-ray features)
   E. Intrauterine graft-versus-host disease — most characteristic feature is scaling erythrodermia and total alopecia (absence of eyebrows quite striking)
   F. Graft-versus-host disease after blood transfusion
   G. Hypocalcemia in newborn (DiGeorge syndrome, especially with characteristic facies, ears, and cardiac lesion)
   H. Small (less than 10 μm in diameter) lymphocyte count persistently less than 1,500/mm^3; must rule out gastrointestinal loss, however

II. Suggest B cell defect
   A. Recurrent proven bacterial pneumonia, sepsis, or meningitis
   B. Nodular lymphoid hyperplasia

III. Suggest B and T cell (combined immunodeficiency disease, SCID)
   A. Features of I and II above, except I.C and II.B
   B. Features of Wiskott-Aldrich syndrome (draining ears, thrombocytopenia, and eczema)
   C. Features of ataxia telangiectasia

IV. Suggest immunodeficiency without clearly implicating T or B cell defect
   A. *Pneumocystis carinii* pneumonia
   B. Intractable eczema
   C. Ulcerative colitis in infants (less than 1 year of age)
   D. Intractable diarrhea
   E. Unexplained hematological deficiency (erythrocyte, leukocyte, platelet)
   F. Severe generalized seborrheic dermatitis (Leiner's disease) suggests C5 deficiency; seborrhea common in combined immunodeficiency disease
   G. Recurrent pyogenic infections seen in C3 deficiency

V. Suggest biochemical defect
   A. Features of combined immunodeficiency with characteristic bony lesions (adenosine deaminase deficiency)
   B. Features of Diamond-Blackfan aplastic anemia (nucleoside phosphorylase deficiency)

VI. Suggest leucocyte abnormality
   A. Primarily skin infections (if associated with asthma, eczema, coarse facies think of Buckley syndrome [3])
   B. Chronic osteomyelitis with *Klebsiella* or *Serratia* species, draining lymph nodes (chronic granulomatous disease)

VII. Suggest that the deficiency is secondary
   A. Concomitant or preceding viral infection
   B. Lymphoid malignancy (chronic lymphatic leukemia, Hodgkin's disease, myeloma)

For more detailed discussion of immunodeficiency syndromes, the reader can consult a number of recent reviews (7, 10, 25).

ASSESSMENT OF T CELLS

T cell assessment is indicated in suspected immunodeficiency states, especially when the presenting symptoms include those features listed above. At the present time, the characterization of thymic function requires many tests to define the defect fully and, until our knowledge increases greatly, multiple testing will be necessary. There is no simple single screening test which if positive categorically rules out a significant defect and if negative is diagnostic for T cell dysfunction, although skin grafts come close to fulfilling these criteria. A skin graft properly applied and vascularized cannot be retained except in some sort of T lymphocyte deficiency. However, it is not feasible to think of skin grafts as a routine T cell assessment test. Furthermore, should the patient be immunologically normal, one might be criticized for sensitizing a patient to a set of histocompatibility antigens in these times of widespread transplantation. When performed, the skin should come from an Australia antigen-negative donor and one without a history of prior hepatitis.

In vivo tests

Skin tests (see chapter 6). Skin tests are of limited value in infants because of inadequate natural sensitization and also because they are uniformly negative during the first few weeks of life regardless of antigen exposure. There is frequent transient skin anergy during viral infections and following rubeola vaccination. Of the skin tests, response to sensitization and testing with 2,4-dinitrochlorobenzene (DNCB) is the most informative.

Procedure

Apply 0.05 ml of a 30% solution of DNCB in acetone (10% for infants) to the volar surface of the forearm on a filter paper 1 cm in diameter. Apply 0.05 ml of 0.1% DNCB in acetone at another site as a presensitization control. Remove filter papers after 12 to 24 h and read the control at 48 h. It should be negative; if positive, the patient has been previously sensitized and probably has normal cellular immunity.

Test the patient 14 to 21 days later with 0.05 ml of 0.10 or 0.05% DNCB on filter paper. After 12 to 24 h, remove the paper, and assess the reaction at 48 h. In a positive reaction both erythema and induration are present under the area of the filter-paper application.

An inflammatory reaction after removal of the filter paper invalidates the test. In this event the challenge can be repeated at another site with a more dilute concentration of the testing reagent.

X ray of thymic shadow. X ray of thymic shadow is of limited value because of rapid involution during a stressful illness. A normal thymic shadow in early life with later development of the typical history of severe combined immunodeficiency disease has been observed in adenosine deaminase deficiency (suggesting an acquired defect).

Lymphoid morphology. Diphtheria and tetanus toxoids as used for childhood immunization can be injected in the medial aspect of the thigh in 0.1-ml amounts in four intradermal sites. Five to seven days later, the ipsilateral inguinal node is removed for regular histological and immunofluorescence studies. A contralateral node may be removed as a nonstimulated control, but this is not necessary.

The techniques for assessing both T and B cell systems will be described here. It is important to obtain a saggital section of the lymph node. This is done by laying the node on its side and slicing it in half along the long axis. The knife or razor blade should pass through the cortex, medulla, and hilum at the same time. The cut surface of one half is gently touched several times to each of a number of clean slides to produce imprints. Imprint slides are excellent for studies of cell morphology and for immunofluorescence studies of the cytoplasm; however, the gross structural features of the node cannot be assessed. After imprints are made, the node fragments are prepared for either frozen or paraffin sections.

For localization of reactive immunofluorescent areas, tissues prepared by the method of Sainte-Marie (26) are superior to cryostat sections. The tissue blocks can be stored for long periods of time for future studies without loss of antigenicity.

Procedure (22)

1. Cut tissues approximately 5 mm thick.

2. Immerse in 95% ethanol (precooled to 4 C) for 1 h in a jar with a screw-top lid.

3. Slice to approximately 2.5 mm thick. Put into a perforated capsule or cloth bag.

4. Fix further for 15 to 24 h in 95% ethanol.

5. Put into cold absolute ethanol. Keep off bottom of jar.

6. Put through four separate changes of absolute alcohol, 1 h each.

7. Three separate consecutive baths of cold xylene, 1 to 2 h each.

8. In the last xylene bath let the temperature come to 23 to 25 C (room temperature).

NB: At any step above specimens can be stored for 1 to 2 days in absolute alcohol or xylene at 4 C.

9. Four consecutive paraffin baths at 56 C, 1 to 2 h.

10. Embed.

11. Store blocks at 4 C. They should be cut promptly but probably can be stored for 2 to 3 months.

12. Section as usual but keep flotation time short.

13. Dry at 37 C for 0.5 h.

14. Deparaffinize in cold xylene for 10 to 15 s using gentle up and down motion; two consecutive baths.

15. Remove xylene with three consecutive cold 95% ethanol baths (10 to 15 s each).

16. Remove alcohol in three baths of cold phosphate-buffered saline (PBS), 1 min each.

17. Stain as usual.

Routine hematoxylin and eosin sections are also made; if desired, plasma cells are rendered quite prominent by using a methyl green-pyronin stain.

Procedure

Fixation: in absolute alcohol or Carnoy's.

Embedding: in paraffin.

Materials:

Pyronin Y, 05564 GT Gurr. (available from Roboz Surgical Instruments Co., Washington, D.C.).

Methyl green (available from Sargent-Welch, Skokie, Ill.).

Method:

1. Make a 2% aqueous solution of pyronin Y. Extract with chloroform until the chloroform layer becomes colorless. Make a 2% aqueous solution methyl green and extract until the chloroform layer no longer is violet.

2. Mix 12.5 ml of pyronin Y and 7.5 ml of methyl green with 30 ml of distilled water.

3. Staining:
   a. Paraffin sections must be brought to water.
   b. Stain for 6 min.
   c. Immerse in two changes of *n*-butyl alcohol, 5 min each.
   d. Xylene, 5 min.
   e. Cedar oil, 5 min.
   f. Mount in Permount.

The normal node has well-populated and clearly defined areas as shown in Fig. 1. Isolated T cell deficiency results in two major abnormalities. The T-dependent area is sparsely populated and, even though antibody formation is quite adequate, germinal centers may not be seen. The thymus-dependent paracortical zone may be replaced by histiocytes, and eosinophilia is common (Fig. 1). Isolated B cell deficiency is manifested by lack of primary follicles, germinal centers, and absence of plasma cells (Fig. 2). In combined B and T cell deficiency, nodes may not be found at all, or, if present, complete replacement by histiocytes may be seen (Fig. 3).

Thymic morphology. The thymus gland can be easily biopsied by utilizing a surgical approach through the anterior mediastinum. A small incision is made in the suprasternal notch, an endoscope is introduced, and a biopsy is taken. Nearly all knowledge of thymic histology in immunodeficiency is based upon postmortem examination, however, and subtle changes which may be present in milder T cell defects (e.g., cartilage hair hypoplasia) have not been described. The changes described here more likely represent extreme variations.

The normal thymus is a lobulated lymphoid organ with well-defined cortical and medullary areas. Scattered throughout the central medulla are Hassall's corpuscles, vestigial remnants of involuting normal thymic medullary elements.

Abnormal thymuses show three major patterns (Fig. 4–6):

1. Normal architectural features, including Hassall's corpuscles, but total mass is small (DiGeorge syndrome). These patients frequently show spontaneous improvement.

2. Embryonal (dysplastic) pattern. There is no corticomedullary differentiation; Hassall's bodies are completely lacking. The total mass of the gland is very small and seldom exceeds 1 g. Blood vessels are small and there may be much fatty infiltration. The stromal elements can be arranged in "rosettes." This is the typical pattern seen in combined B and T cell deficiency states.

3. Involuted pattern. To a lesser degree this picture can be observed following stress or extensive steroid therapy. In its most advanced form, it is very suggestive of adenosine deaminase deficiency. Blood vessels are prominent. Hassall's corpuscles are diminished in number but clearly present. Islands of differentiated epithelium are present in which the cells are larger than those seen in the embryonal forms. The nuclei are oval and the cytoplasm is eosinophilic (13).

In vitro tests (see chapter 7)

Assessment of peripheral blood. The normal small (less than 10 μm in diameter) lymphocyte count is greater than 1,500/mm^3 at any age. Frequently, T cell deficiency is associated with eosinophilia (often during a graft-versus-host reaction or *Pneumocystis carinii* pneumonia) or monocytosis. I have observed marked thrombocytosis on one occasion. Neutropenia is a common but unstressed finding in T cell deficiency.

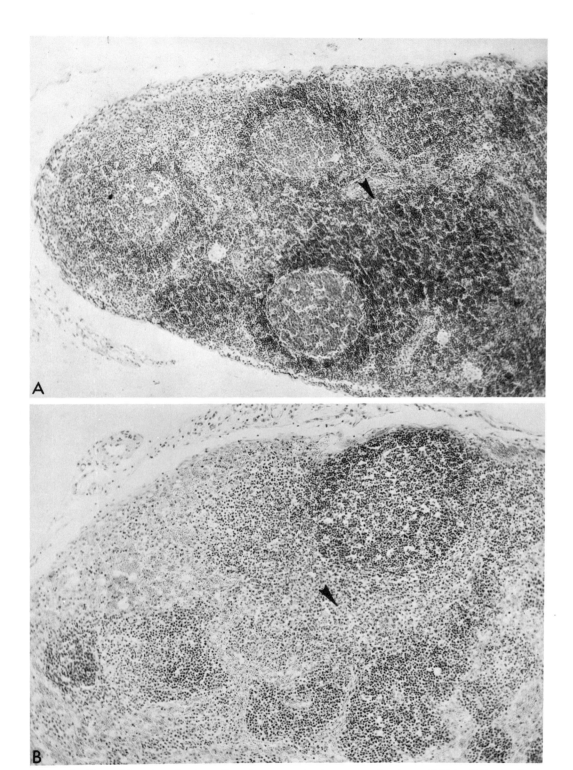

Fig. 1A. *Normal lymph node of rat. Prominent germinal centers and primary follicles following bovine albumin immunization. The T-dependent paracortical zone (arrow) is adequately populated. From Stiehm and Fulginiti (30).*

Fig. 1B. *Thymectomized rat. The paracortical zone (arrow) is depleted, but follicular development is normal. From Stiehm and Fulginiti (30). (Courtesy of B. Waksman; original magnification ×120.)*

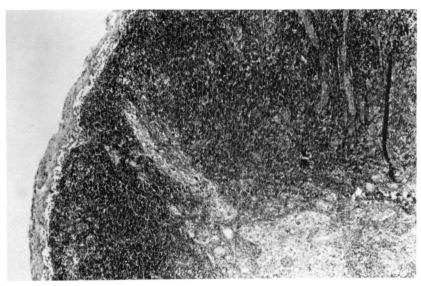

FIG. 2. *Lymph node from T cell-component B cell-deficient patient. Rich T-dependent zone but no follicular development. From Stiehm and Fulginiti (30). (Original magnification ×100.)*

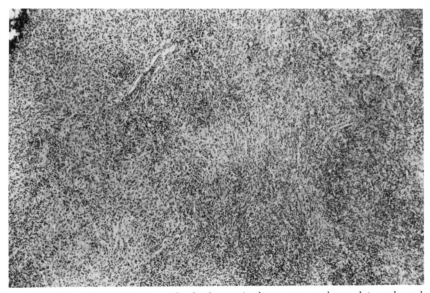

FIG. 3. *Combined T and B cell deficiency. Lack of organized structure and complete node replacement by reticulum cells and histiocytes. From Stiehm and Fulginiti (30).*

Stimulation of T lymphocytes and E rosette formation. Three major groups of stimuli are used: (i) mitogens, (ii) allogeneic cells, and (iii) antigens. E rosettes of two types can be tested—total and active. See chapter 9 of this *Manual* for details.

Lymphokine production (see chapters 10 and 11). It is usually not possible to test mediator production as the lymphocytes cannot be stimulated.

Interpretation. Patients with significant T cell deficiency can demonstrate normal responses to mitogenic and allogeneic cell stimulation and have normal numbers of total E rosettes. "Active" rosettes are more often truly representative of the functional T cell status (12). Usually, responses to all of the above stimulatory agents are decreased and the diagnosis is clear; however, certain notable exceptions exist. In Wiskott-Aldrich syndrome

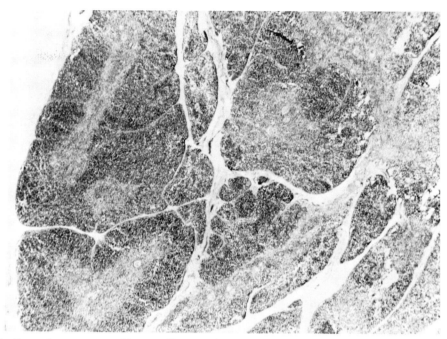

FIG. 4. *Normal thymus at ×10 magnification. Sharp corticomedullary differentiation and prominent Hassall's corpuscles can be seen.*

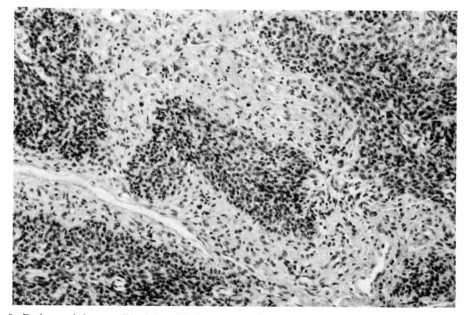

FIG. 5. *Embryonal thymus. Thick interlobular septa and small lobule consisting only of undifferentiated epithelial cells without thymocytes. (Original magnification ×100.)*

and ataxia telangiectasia there may be variable loss of T lymphocyte function depending upon the duration of the disease. To demonstrate abnormalities of some in vitro lymphocyte responses, multiple doses of stimulating agents may have to be employed. In some cases

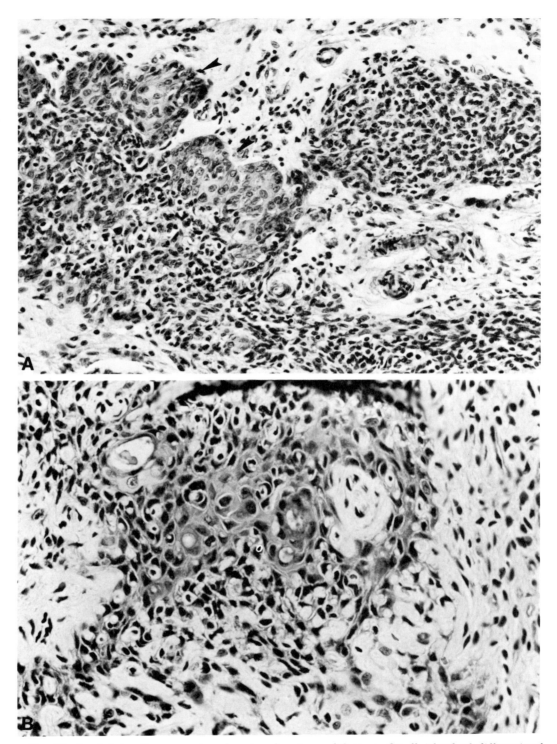

Fig. 6A. *Involuted pattern seen in adenosine deaminase deficiency. Small island of differentiated epithelium (arrow) seen in stretch of undifferentiated epithelium. (Original magnification ×100.) From Meuwissen et al. (15).*

Fig. 6B. *Higher magnification of small area of differentiated epithelium showing Hassall's body (arrow). From Meuwissen et al. (15).*

of combined immunodeficiency and in Ommen's disease (21), normal responses to phytohemagglutinin and allogeneic cells have been observed. In my experience, however, the constant in vitro abnormality in all T cell-deficient states is an inability to respond to antigens. However, thymic deficiency is not the only cause of nonreactivity to antigens, for failure to respond may be due to inadequate sensitization or to a macrophage defect. Also, any in vitro tests of T lymphocyte function may be temporarily depressed if the patient is suffering from a virus infection or has had a recent rubeola vaccination. Repeated testing must be done for confirmation.

It can be seen that assessment of the thymic system can be a complicated procedure requiring great experience and sound clinical judgment.

ASSESSMENT OF B CELLS

The key presented in the Introduction shows the clinical manifestations of B cell deficiency diseases. Assessment is in general more straightforward than for T cells. Determination of quantitative immunoglobulin (Ig) levels by the single radial diffusion method is a reliable screening technique (see section A). Immunoelectrophoretic analysis and simple protein electrophoresis are unreliable for screening and should not be employed for that purpose. There is virtually no overlap of the maximal values of truly deficient patients having primary immunodeficiency with the minimal values of normal subjects. Patients with true B cell immunodeficiency usually show deficits of all major classes of Ig's. Thus, a pattern of an abnormally low IgG (less than 2 standard deviations below mean for age) but normal IgA and IgM levels in a 4-month-old infant is still probably within normal limits. When some but not all values are low, immunodeficiency should be suspected with the finding of Ig patterns or characteristics shown in Table 1.

Uncertainty is most clearly resolved by functional assessment. Antibodies to previously administered antigens (diphtheria, tetanus, polio) can be measured, often by state or local health agencies. Isoagglutinins can be determined.

Procedure for diphtheria and tetanus antibody titration by hemagglutination (see also chapter 44)

Obtain fresh human O-positive red blood cells in ethylenediaminetetraacetate (EDTA). Cells should be washed three times in 0.9% NaCl. Resuspend the cells at a 2.5% cell sus-

TABLE 1. *Immunoglobulin (Ig) patterns in deficiency states*

Deficiency of all Ig's
  Usual type of hypogammaglobulinemia; occasionally normal IgE levels
Selective deficiencies:
  1.[a] IgA: most common primary deficiency, occurs in 70% of ataxia telangiectasia, may be associated with mild or severe T cell deficiency
  2. IgM: most common secondary deficiency
  3. IgE: deficiency of unknown significance, may occur in association with IgA deficiency, especially in ataxia telangiectasia
  4. IgG: never well documented as an isolated deficiency, IgG subgroup deficiencies are known
  5.[b] IgG and IgA: associated with elevated IgM (dysgammaglobulinemia I), elevation in part artefactual and due to 7S IgM
  6.[b] IgA and IgM: IgG normal or elevated in amounts and usually monoclonal (K or λ), single or multiple electrophoretic peaks common; associated T cell defect usually present
Unique patterns:
  1. Markedly elevated IgA and diminished IgM common in Wiskott-Aldrich syndrome (nonresponsivity to carbohydrate antigens most characteristic functional abnormality)
  2.[b] In multiple myeloma or Waldenstrom's macroglobulinemia noninvolved Ig's are usually nondetectable

[a] Serum IgA determinations usually screen for secretory IgA deficiency. Normal levels of secretory IgA with absent serum IgA have been observed but usually not the reverse.
[b] There is usually no formation of antibody in response to administered antigens despite normal or elevated levels of one or more classes of Ig in these diseases. In type 5, however, some agglutinin response has been observed.

pension in PBS, pH 7.2, and store at 0 to 4 C. Cells are good for 5 to 7 days.

Tanning procedure.

1. Prior to tanning, the cells prepared above should be washed in PBS, pH 7.2, twice.

2. Preparation of tannic acid solution: Combine 0.1 g of tannic acid and 10.0 ml of 0.9% sodium chloride. Add 0.3 ml of this solution to 49.7 ml of 0.95% saline (0.006% tannic acid).

3. To 1 volume of a 2.5% cell suspension (from above) add 1 volume of a 0.006% tannic acid solution.

4. Incubate for 15 min with shaking in a 37 C water bath.

5. Centrifuge the cells and decant the supernatant fluid. (If cells are properly tanned, they will stick to the bottom of the tube.) Cells are then washed twice in PBS, pH 7.2.

Coating procedure.

1. Prepare antigens in PBS, pH 6.4.
    a. Diphtheria toxoid: Use at 88 Lf/ml con-

centration; dilute in PBS, pH 6.4, as necessary.

b. Tetanus toxoid: Use at 150 Lf/ml concentration; dilute in PBS, pH 6.4, as necessary.

2. The tanned, washed cells from above are washed further two times in PBS, pH 6.4, and resuspended to a 2.5% concentration in this buffer.

3. Calculation of amount of cells: Each patient titration requires 0.3 ml. Since the concentration of cells used for hemagglutination is 1%, the amount of 2.5% cells coated will yield 2.5 times the starting volume for use in the final titration. For example, 17 patients × 0.3 ml = 5 ml of 1% erythrocyte solution required; therefore, start with 2 ml of 2.5% tanned cells.

4. To 1 volume of 2.5% tanned cells, add 4 volumes of the antigens as prepared above. Incubate for 10 min in a 37 C water bath. Shake well and resuspend cells every 30 s.

5. Centrifuge and remove the antigen solution. Wash once in heat-inactivated (56 C, 0.5 h) normal rabbit serum diluted 1:100 in PBS, pH 7.2. Resuspend cells to a 1% concentration in diluted normal rabbit serum.

Plating procedure. U-type plates (Cooke Laboratory Products Division, Dynatech Laboratories Inc., Alexandria, Va.) are used; wash plates with distilled water before use and dry. Plating procedure is that of Sever (27).

Scoring of plates. The method of Stavitsky (29) is used for scoring on a plus 4 to plus 1 scale. Titer recorded represents the last cup to give a plus 1 reaction.

Antibody response to ϕX174 offers a very helpful assessment of antibody response and can define many patterns of response. The virus can be obtained from Ralph Wedgwood, Department of Pediatrics, University of Washington Medical School, Seattle (telephone: 206/543-3207).

Lymphoid morphology (see above)

Surface immunoglobulins (see chapter 7)

In vitro production of immunoglobulins (see chapter 2)

In common variable immunodeficiency (B and T cell systems involved to variable degrees and deficiency state tending to be less severe than in SCID), overactivity of T suppressor cells is found in 50 to 70% of the cases.

Procedure (4, 32)

Materials (all available from Grand Island

Biological Co., Grand Island, N.Y.).

Pokeweed mitogen.

RPMI 1640, with L-glutamine and bicarbonate.

Fetal calf serum.

Penicillin-streptomycin solution, 10,000 units of each/ml.

Method:

Lymphocytes, 2×10^6 (1 ml), from a normal subject are co-cultured with 2×10^6 T cells (1 ml) obtained from a patient with common variable hypogammaglobulinemia. T cells are prepared from a Sephadex G-200 immunoabsorbent column (4; see also sections A and B). The culture is carried out in RPMI 1640 medium supplemented with glutamine, penicillin and streptomycin (10 units of each/ml), and 10% fetal calf serum. Cultures are stimulated with 10 μliters of pokeweed mitogen per tube. Non-stimulated cultures produce a mean of 212 ng of IgG, 303 ng of IgA, and 537 ng of IgM per 2×10^6 lymphocytes after 7 days of culture. Stimulated cultures produce, per 2×10^6 lymphocytes, means of 1,641, 1,698, and 3,715 ng of IgG, IgA, and IgM, respectively. When co-cultured with T lymphocyte populations having excess suppressor activity, the amount of synthesis is depressed (for all Ig's) from 40 to 100%.

Antibodies to IgA (see chapter 75)

Antibodies to IgA should be sought for in patients with selective IgA deficiency.

Procedure (23, 31)

Reagents:

1. Draw human O red cells into heparin (10 units/ml) and wash three times in 0.9% sodium chloride.

2. Chromic chloride ($CrCl_3 \cdot CH_2O$; obtained from Fisher Scientific Co., Chicago, Ill.), 10 mg in 10 ml of distilled water. Prepare fresh.

3. IgA, 2 to 2.5 mg/ml, in 0.9% sodium chloride.

4. Sodium dihydrogen phosphate, 0.15 M; titrate to pH 7.2 with 0.15 M disodium phosphate.

5. Normal rabbit serum.

6. Piperazine hydrate, 0.27 M, titrated to pH 6.5 with HCl (obtained from Sigma Chemical Co., St. Louis, Mo.).

Method:

1. Dilute stock $CrCl_3$ 1:6 in normal saline just before use.

2. Mix in a test tube in the following order:

Piperazine buffer	0.25 ml
IgA solution	0.1 ml
Red cells	0.05 ml
$CrCl_3$ solution	0.1 ml

Agitate constantly at room temperature for 5 min. Stop coating procedure immediately if macroscopic agglutination is observed.

3. Add saline to stop reaction and immediately wash three times in saline.

4. Perform hemagglutination in V-bottom microagglutination trays; use phosphate buffer containing rabbit serum diluted 1:200 for all dilutions of antisera and cells.

Normal subjects do not have antibodies against IgA.

Interpretation. The absence of marked diminution (less than 10th percentile) of all major classes virtually establishes the diagnosis of hypogammaglobulinemia. In protein-losing states IgM levels are normal to only slightly decreased; the marked diminution of albumin and transferrin confirms the true cause of the deficiency state.

A special problem arises in selective IgA deficiency. Fifty percent of these patients have antibodies to ruminant proteins. If the antiserum used for quantitation is of goat origin, there will be a detectable ring in the radial diffusion analysis. This will produce an erroneous reading of IgA presence when, in fact, deficiency exists. If such a patient's serum is used as an antibody in immunoelectrophoretic analysis and normal goat serum is used as antigen, the IgG arc of the goat will be revealed.

In interpreting Ig levels any uncertainty can be resolved by functional assessment. Measurement of the diphtheria and tetanus antibodies is a simple technique. No matter what the immunization history, one must restimulate the patient if low antibody values are initially detected before a deficiency state can be defined with certainty.

The ϕX174 responses are shown in Table 2. One advantage of testing the ϕX174 response is that a rapid presumptive diagnosis of B cell deficiency can be made at birth, since normal subjects can clear the virus immediately after birth whereas abnormal subjects show persistence of phage for more than 1 week. The antibody response will not be affected by placentally transmitted IgG since the mother would not ordinarily have antibodies to ϕX174. It has been suggested that those with type O, I, II, or III response will require IgG therapy. Patients showing type IV responses may or may not benefit from IgG, whereas those who manifest a type V response, even though they are immunodeficient, do not require IgG therapy (33).

BIOCHEMICAL TESTS

Deficiency of adenosine deaminase has been observed in nearly 20 children with combined immunodeficiency disease. The symptoms tend to occur later in infancy than other forms of SCID, and there is a suggestion that the deficiency is "acquired." Bony abnormalities are characteristic and common (16).

Gel method for screening for adenosine deaminase deficiency (20)

Materials (Important — rinse all glassware thoroughly to remove any traces of alkali):
Bromothymol blue (Sigma Chemical Co.), saturated solution made in 0.9% NaCl.
Adenosine, Baker grade (J. T. Baker Co.), 0.02 M in 0.9% NaCl.

1. Add 5 ml of bromthymol blue and 91.3 ml of adenosine to 100 ml of melted 2% agarose in saline, pH 6.0.

2. Keep mixture liquid at 45 C and fill a Linbro model 96 SC Dispotray.

3. Allow to harden.

Method:

1. Venous or capillary blood is spotted on filter paper. A 3/16-inch disk is cut through the blood drop.

2. Press disks firmly onto gel, one in the center of each well.

3. Cover tightly with clear plastic wrap (Stretch 'n Seal, Colgate Palmolive Co.) and form a seal around each well. This is used to limit diffusion of generated ammonia.

4. Incubate at room temperature under a fluorescent light (used to diminish brownish coloration due to hemoglobin).

5. Read results at 48 h. Ammonia generated

TABLE 2. *Classification of immune response to bacteriophage ϕX174*[a]

Classification	Antigen clearance	Primary response		Secondary response		Memory amplification
		Antibody amt	Ig class	Antibody amt	Ig class	
Normal	Yes	Normal	IgM	Normal	IgG	Yes
Type 0	None	None		None		None
Type I	Yes	None		None		None
Type II	Yes	Decreased	IgM	Decreased	IgM	None
Type III	Yes	Decreased	IgM	Decreased	IgM	Yes
Type IV	Yes	Decreased	IgM	Decreased	IgM IgG	Yes
Type V	Yes	Decreased	IgM	Decreased	IgG IgM	Yes

[a] From Wedgwood, Ochs, and Davis (33).

by adenosine deaminase changes the indicator from yellow to red.

Procedure for electrophoretic screening of adenosine deaminase (28)

Materials (all from Sigma Chemical Co.):
Adenosine.
MTT tetrazolium.
Phenazine methosulfate.
Nucleoside phosphorylase.
Method:
1. Draw blood into ADC containing 20 units of heparin/ml. Volume of ADC = 15% of blood drawn.
2. Centrifuge at 1,500 rpm for 15 min.
3. Remove plasma and wash red cells three times in 0.9% sodium chloride. Remove as much buffy coat as possible each time. Erythrocyte sedimentation tubes half filled with cells are convenient for this purpose.
4. Sonically treat cells for 3 minutes, or freeze and thaw cells three times to produce a lysate. The lysate is introduced into the gel on a strip of Whatman no. 3 filter paper.
5. Samples are run in 12% starch gel using this buffer system: 0.01 M PO$_4$, pH 6.5, for gel; 0.1 M PO$_4$, pH 6.5, for bridge solution.
Electrophoresis conditions: 16 h at 4 C; 3 to 3.5 V/cm.
Slice gel parallel to the surface into two equal halves.
6. Staining: Make staining gel by dissolving 40 mg of adenosine, 10 mg of MTT tetrazolium, 10 mg of phenazine methosulfate, 1.6 units of nucleoside phosphorylase, and 0.16 units of xanthine oxidase in 50 ml of 0.025 M PO$_4$, pH 7.5. Warm to 55 C and add to 50 ml of 2% special Noble agar in 0.025 M PO$_4$, pH 7.5, at 55 C. Overlay cut surface of starch with staining gel and let stand at 37 C for 1 h. Positive bands are an intense blue color.

Procedure for quantitative determination of adenosine deaminase in red blood cells (11, 28)

Materials:
Phosphate buffer, 0.05 M, pH 7.5.
Sodium chloride, 0.9%.
Adenosine, 1 mg/ml in water (Sigma Chemical Co.).
Xanthine oxidase (Sigma Chemical Co.).
Nucleoside phosphorylase (Sigma Chemical Co.).
Method:
1. Dilute lysate from preparation for electrophoresis 1:5 with water and add 50 μliters to tubes each containing 3.0 ml of 0.05 M PO$_4$, pH 7.5 (a blank tube and a reaction tube).

2. Read and record absorbance at 541 nm against a buffer blank.
3. Add 0.04 unit of xanthine oxidase and 0.4 unit of nucleoside phosphorylase to each of the tubes.
4. Allow to equilibrate at 37 C for 15 min.
5. Add 75 μliters of adenosine stock to the reaction tube only and mix well.
6. Immediately read and record the absorbance at 293 nm and start the timer (zero time).
7. Incubate the tubes at 37 C in a water bath for 10 min.
8. Read the absorbance at 293 nm again and stop the timer. Record the absorbance and time elapsed.

Notes
1. When assaying more than one sample in a group, allow the same amount of time to elapse between each sample reading in the group at the beginning of the assay and at the end as well.
2. If you are using a calibrated recording spectrophotometer, the assay may be done in cuvettes with continuous recording. Instrument must have a jacketed cuvette chamber held at 37 C. You may also calculate the change in absorbance and time from the graph as well as from the recorded absorbance and time done manually.

Calculations
The needed data for calculations are the initial and final absorbance at 293 nm, the elapsed time, and the absorbance at 541 nm.

μmol of adenosine deaminated/min

$$= \left(\frac{\Delta A_{293}}{\text{min}}\right)\left(\frac{\text{total vol}}{11.6}\right)$$

Activity is expressed as
μmol of adenosine deaminated/min
$$- \text{OD}_{541} \text{ unit}$$

Addendum: stability of adenosine deaminase activity

Erythrocytes may be kept frozen at −70 C with preservation of adenosine deaminase activity. Lysates are stable up to 1 month at −70 C. Serum appears to be stable indefinitely at −70 C. Lymphocyte lysates are unstable: activity of adenosine deaminase falls off rapidly after the cells are separated.

Procedure for electrophoretic screening of nucleoside phosphorylase (6, 28)

Materials (all from Sigma Chemical Co.):
Inosine.
Phenazine methosulfate.
Xanthine oxidase.
Method:

1. Prepare erythrocyte lysate as in steps 1–4 for electrophoretic screening of adenosine deaminase.

2. Use 11% starch gel in following buffer system.

Gel (pH 7.2): 12.4 mM tris(hydroxymethyl)-aminomethane (Tris), 3.3 mM citric acid, 3.6 mM boric acid, and 0.33 mM lithium hydroxide.

Bridge (pH 7.2): 0.44 mM boric acid and 0.04 M Tris.

Electrophoretic conditions: 4 h at room temperature; 10 V/cm for 45 min, 6 V/cm for the remainder of the time.

3. Staining: Dissolve 5 mg of inosine, 5 mg of MTT tetrazolium, 5 mg of phenazine methosulfate, and 0.04 unit of xanthine oxidase in 25 ml of 0.05 M phosphate buffer, pH 7.5. Warm to 55 C and mix with 25 ml of 2% aqueous special Noble agar at 55 C. Stain at 37 C for a few minutes. Positive bands are intense blue in color.

Procedure for quantitative determination of erythrocyte nucleoside phosphorylase (11, 28)

Materials:

Inosine (Sigma Chemical Co.), 1 mg/ml in distilled water.

NaCl, 0.9%.

PO_4, 0.05 M, pH 7.5.

Method:

1. Dilute red cell lysate prepared for electrophoresis 1:50 with water and add 50 μliters of this to two tubes, each containing 3.0 ml of 0.05 M PO_4, pH 7.5 (blank tube and reaction tube).

Steps 2, 3, and 4 are same as for quantitative adenosine deaminase determination.

5. Add 0.16 ml of inosine stock to the reaction tube, mix well, and immediately proceed to steps 6, 7, and 8, which are same as for quantitative adenosine deaminase determination.

Interpretation. Each laboratory should determine its own set of normal values from a large group of normal subjects. Deficiency of adenosine deaminase has been observed only in immunodeficiency disease (with one exception) and is probably causally related. The gel method for screening is adequate for detecting adenosine deaminase deficiency but provides less information than the electrophoretic method. Quantitative tests should be done to confirm the deficiency and to detect the heterozygous carrier state. Patients studied to date have had undetectable levels of enzyme. Most heterozygous carriers for adenosine deaminase deficiency show values less than 2 standard deviations of the normal mean. In the single case of nucleoside phosphorylase deficiency described, both parents had values less than 50% of the mean control value (8). At the present time, the complete spectrum of symptomatology associated with biochemical defects is unknown. Determinations of adenosine deaminase and nucleoside phosphorylase are indicated in all cases of severe combined immunodeficiency disease and, if facilities permit, would be of interest in all forms of immunodeficiency.

POLYMORPHONUCLEAR LEUKOCYTE ABNORMALITIES

Polymorphonuclear leukocyte (PMN) abnormalities can result in significant increased susceptibility to infection. For the PMNs to exert their full biological capability, they must perform three major functions: (i) mobilize to the area of need, (ii) phagocytize, and (iii) kill the infectious agent. The tests of neutrophil function fall into categories which measure these three basic functions.

Assessment of mobility

Epinephrine stimulation (5). Inject 0.4 ml/m² of 1:1,000 epinephrine intravenously. Capillary blood samples are taken prior to and at 5, 15, 30, 45, and 60 min after the injection of epinephrine. Normal subjects increase the total PMN count greater than 45% over the base-line values.

Cortisone stimulation (5). Hydrocortisone hemisuccinate, 100 mg, is given intravenously. Samples are drawn before and at hourly intervals after the administration of hydrocortisone. The normal response is to increase the total PMN count by 2,000 over the base-line value.

Rebuck skin window (24). A superficial abrasion is made on the volar surface of the forearm. Fine punctate capillary oozing should be seen, but frank bleeding should not be present. A sterile cover slip is covered by a small piece of cardboard cut slightly larger and held in place by adhesive tape. Cover slips are removed and new ones are placed at 2, 4, 6, 8, 12, 16, and 20 h. PMN assessment is based upon the cover slips removed at 2, 4, and 6 h, and mononuclear cell assessment is based upon the studies at 12, 16, and 20 h. Scoring is performed by counting the total number of cells on the cover slip and assigning scores as follows: 0 cells = 0; 1–10 = 1; 11–100 = 2; 101–1,000 = 3; greater than 1,000 = 4. If the total score of three slides is 6 or less, deficient migration is present.

Random mobility (2).

Materials:

Earl's balanced salt solution (from Grand Island Biological Co., Grand Island, N.Y.)

plus 0.01 mg of rabbit serum albumin/100 ml (ERA solution).

Heparin (The Upjohn Co., Kalamazoo, Mich.).

Dextran, 6% in saline (Abbott Laboratories, North Chicago, Ill.).

Preparation of leukocytes:

1. Blood is drawn into heparin-containing syringes (100 units/ml of blood).

2. Add 4 ml of dextran to each 20 ml of blood. Allow to settle for 30 to 60 min at 37 C.

3. Transfer plasma to 17 × 100 mm Falcon plastic disposable tubes and centrifuge for 5 min at 450 × g (room temperature).

4. Wash cells in ERA solution. Resuspend cells in ERA at a concentration of 5×10^6 neutrophils/ml.

Method:

1. Fill heparinized glass capillary tubes (Scientific Products, Evanston, Ill.) to approximately 70% of the total volume with the neutrophil solution.

2. Centrifuge for 20 min at 200 × g or in a microhematocrit centrifuge.

3. Incubate vertically for 4 h at 37 C.

4. Measure migration from the leading edge of packed neutrophil suspension. This can be conveniently done with a hand-held magnifier (Bausch & Lomb, catalog # 81-34-35).

Chemotaxis (see also chapter 13).

Materials:

Neuroprobe blind well chambers (# FH013BW31201).

Nuclepore chemotactic membranes, 13 mm (catalog # N 300 CPC 013 00).

Manual for use of chemotactic chambers (above available from Nuclepore Corp., Pleasanton, Calif.).

Yeast zymosan (Schwarz-Mann, Orangeburg, N.Y.).

Gey's balanced salt solution (Grand Island Biological Co.).

Method:

The studies of chemotaxis are detailed in the manual described above. A convenient attractant can be made from activated serum. For each 1 ml of fresh serum, 0.025 g of zymosan is needed. Weigh out appropriate amount of zymosan and wash with PBS. Remove PBS and add serum to zymosan precipitate. Mix well and incubate at 37 C for 30 min. Spin at 500 × g for 10 min; remove supernatant fluid and save. A mixture of 200 μliters of activated serum/ml of Gey's balanced salt solution is a good attractant solution. Various amounts of patient serum can be added to the activated serum mixture to detect inhibitors of chemotaxis. It is probably important to have the total concentration of

serum in the attractant at least 10% but no more than 20%. The effect of normal serum or plasma at various concentrations must be studied by the individual investigator.

Interpretation. For a complete assessment, all of the tests of mobility must be performed. Epinephrine stimulation measures the ability to derive leukocytes from the marginal pool. Cortisone stimulation measures the marrow reserves. The Rebuck skin window stimulates the actual neutrophil response at a local inflammatory site. Chemotactic experiments measure the ability of the PMNs to respond to a chemotactic stimulus and, furthermore, can be used to test for the presence of inhibitors of chemotaxis in the serum. Inhibitors to chemotaxis have been observed in the following conditions: Hodgkin's disease, Chediak-Higashi syndrome, diabetes mellitus, rheumatoid arthritis, elevated IgE syndromes, chronic granulomatous disease, mucocutaneous candidiasis, and as an isolated defect (1, 17). Defective chemotaxis due to intrinsic cellular abnormality of the leukocyte has been observed in Chediak-Higashi syndrome, diabetes mellitus, "lazy leukocyte syndrome," postrenal dialysis, active infection, and other diseases (1, 17).

Assessment of phagocytic capability (see also chapter 17).

Materials:

Commercial bakers' yeast

Earle's balanced salt solution (available from Grand Island Biological Co.).

Rabbit albumin (available from Sigma Chemical Co.).

Method:

1. Leukocytes prepared as above are resuspended in Earle's balanced salt solution containing 0.01 mg of rabbit albumin/100 ml (ERA) to a final concentration of 5×10^6 PMN/ml.

2. Dissolve 0.5 g of commercial bakers' yeast in 0.9% sodium chloride. Place in boiling water for 30 min.

3. Filter yeast suspension through cotton gauze.

4. Adjust yeast particles to 10^9/ml in ERA.

5. Into 13 × 150 mm screw-top tubes, place 0.1 ml of the yeast suspension and 0.1 ml of patient or control plasma.

6. Incubate mixture at 37 C for 30 min under constant rotation. Then add 0.2 ml (10^6) of PMNs. Incubate for 30 more min, removing samples at 5, 10, 15, and 30 min. Count 100 consecutive PMNs and express results as average number of yeast particles ingested per cell.

Interpretation. Phagocytosis of yeast requires C5 and is the primary defect which was observed in the Leiner's-like syndrome described by Miller (17). In another C5 deficiency with lupus symptoms and no stigmata of Leiner's disease, opsonization of yeast particles was normal, however. Phagocytosis dependent upon C1 through C5 can be assessed in the bactericidal assays (see below).

Screening tests for granulomatous disease, formazan test (9) (see also chapter 17)

Materials:

NBT dye (from Sigma Chemical Co.), 0.28 g in 100 ml of 0.9% sodium chloride; filter through ultrafine sintered-glass filter and freeze in small portions.

Safranine O (from Fisher Scientific Co., Chicago, Ill.), 1 g of Safranine O plus 100 ml of distilled water and 40 ml of glycerol.

Incubation medium: 0.5 ml of normal serum plus 0.3 ml of sterile saline plus 0.6 ml of NBT dye.

Method:

1. Collect one drop of patient's blood on a cover slip.

2. Incubate the cover slip in a humid chamber for 20 min at 37 C.

3. Carefully wash the clot off with sterile saline.

4. Invert the cover slip on a slide which contains one drop of medium.

5. Incubate for 30 min in a humid chamber at 37 C.

6. Remove cover slip from slide and air-dry rapidly.

7. Fix with absolute methanol for 60 s and wash with distilled water.

8. Stain with 0.77% safranine for 5 min; wash off with water and mount on a slide.

Interpretation. The formazan-positive cells are large and blast-like and bear no resemblance to the normal PMNs. They are filled with blue precipitate. Thirty percent or more of the granulocytes are converted to the formazan type normally. Patients with chronic granulomatous disease form no formazan cells, and this test is useful as a screen. Heterozygous carriers of the disease show less then normal conversion; however, this is not a reliable test for the carrier state.

Bactericidal killing assay

Materials (both from Grand Island Biological Co.):

Penicillin-streptomycin (5,000 units of each/ml).

Hanks balanced salt solution (HBSS).

Method (from the laboratory of Beulah Holmes, Minneapolis, Minn.):

Preparation of cells

1. Prepare leukocytes as described above.

2. Resuspend cells in HBSS at 10^7 cells/ml.

Bacterial suspension

1. Inoculate overnight culture of *Staphylococcus aureus* 502A and incubate overnight in a 37 C water-bath shaker.

2. Spin culture at $1,800 \times g$ for 10 min.

3. Wash pellet in 10 ml of normal saline.

4. Resuspend in about 7 ml of normal saline.

5. Take a Klett reading (should be about 80) or an optical density reading (should be about 0.16) at 540 nm.

6. Make a 1:50 dilution in HBSS; 0.1 ml contains approximately 10^6 bacteria.

Reaction mixture

1. Combine in a sterile disposable 12×75 mm Falcon plastic tube (prepare in duplicate if doing with and without antibiotics added): 0.3 ml of HBSS, 0.1 ml of pooled normal human serum (from five donors; stored in small portions at -70 C; DO NOT REFREEZE), 0.5 ml of white cell suspension, and 0.1 ml of bacterial suspension. Run bacterial control without white cells; substitute 0.5 ml of HBSS.

2. Incubate all tubes in a Lab-Tek Aliquot Mixer which is in a 37 C incubator.

3. Make a bacterial sample from the bacterial control tube at zero time. Sample control and all other tubes at 20 min, 1.5 h, and 3 h.

4. To one tube of each set, add 0.02 ml of penicillin-streptomycin at 20 min (5,000 units of each/ml).

Sampling of tubes without antibiotics added

1. To 9.9 ml of warm (37 C) distilled water in a 17×100 mm plastic tube, add 0.1 ml of culture mixture; cap and shake vigorously.

2. Transfer 0.1 and 1.0 ml to separate petri plates, marked for dilution of 1:1,000 and 1:100, respectively.

3. Pour into each plate the contents of a nutrient agar deep, previously melted by boiling and held at 57 C in a water bath. Mix gently by moving plate in a figure eight.

4. Incubate plates for 48 h in a 37 C incubator. Count colonies and plot results on 5-cycle semilog paper.

Sampling tubes with antibiotics added

1. Remove a 0.2-ml sample from culture mixture and pipette into 5 ml of HBSS in a sterile plastic tube.

2. Centrifuge at $450 \times g$ for 5 min. Remove supernatant fluid.

3. Wash again in HBSS and resuspend pellet in 1.9 ml of distilled water; pipette up and down vigorously.

4. Transfer 0.1 and 1.0 ml to two petri plates and pour agar as above. Plates are marked for 1:200 and 1:20 dilutions.

5. Count colonies after incubation of plates as above.

Notes

Disposable plastic pipettes are recommended to reduce sticking of bacteria and white cells (Falcon #7506). Serum from blood group AB individuals is advised for serum pool.

Interpretation. See Fig. 7.

Defective killing capacity of the leukocyte has been observed in chronic granulomatous disease, myeloperoxidase deficiency, Chediak-Higashi syndrome, glucose-6-phosphate dehydrogenase deficiency, Job's syndrome, severe burns, malignancies, Down's syndrome, iron deficiency, and to a variable degree in newborns (1, 17).

BIOCHEMICAL ASSESSMENT

Extensive biochemical analysis of the antimicrobial mechanism in PMNs is beyond the scope of this discussion. Myeloperoxidase deficiency can be detected with a simple screening test, however.

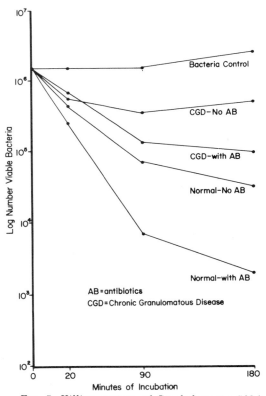

FIG. 7. *Killing pattern of Staphylococcus 502A shown by normal subject and patient with chronic granulomatous disease in presence and absence of antibiotics.*

Procedure for peroxidase stain

Fixative:

Formalin solution, 37% ...	10 ml
Absolute alcohol	90 ml

Peroxidase stain:

EDTA, 30%	100.0 ml
Benzidine dihydrochloride	0.3 g
$ZnSO_4 \cdot 7H_2O$	0.038 g
Water	1.0 ml
$NaOAc \cdot 3H_2O$	1.0 g
Hydrogen peroxide, 3% ..	0.7 ml
Add 1.0 N NaOH to adjust pH to 6.0.	

Method:

1. Fix routine blood smears, 30 s, with alcohol-formalin fixative.
2. Wash with water.
3. Stain with peroxidase stain, 30 s.

Interpretation. Peroxidase-containing cells show dense blue cytoplasmic deposits. Although myeloperoxidase deficiency has been described in five patients, only one had increased susceptibility to infection. This patient had systemic candidiasis and diabetes. He did not have a history of serious recurrent bacterial infections, even though his leukocytes killed *Staphylococcus aureus* 502A and *Serratia marcescens* at a subnormal rate.

NEUTROPENIA

There is a slight variation of PMN count with age with a prominent leukocytosis during the first 24 h of life. Generally speaking, however, persistent counts between 2,000 and 3,000 per mm^3 constitute mild neutropenia, and counts persistently below 2,000/mm^3 constitute severe neutropenia. The importance of neutropenia depends upon whether there is associated clinical symptomatology. Many children with neutropenia have no increased susceptibility to infection whatever. Neutropenia is associated with significant symptomatology and defects of mobility in the lazy leukocyte syndrome (19) and, as mentioned above, is frequently observed in T cell deficiency. All neutrophil counts show a cyclic variability. Cyclic neutropenia patients fare no worse nor better than those with persistent neutropenia.

GENERAL COMMENTS

At the present time the correlation of defects of neutrophil function with disease states is imperfect. In all assessments of host defense, it is necessary to fit the laboratory test with the clinical symptomatology, but nowhere is this more true than in assessment of neutrophil function. At the present time, a number of defects can be uncovered. Whether they appropriately explain the symptomatology or measure the in vivo processes is open to question. For extensive discussion of these problems, the reader is referred to recent reviews (14, 18).

LITERATURE CITED

1. Baehner, R. L. 1974. Molecular basis for functional disorders of phagocytes. J. Pediatr. 84:317–327.
2. Bryant, R. E., R. M. DesPrez, M. H. VanWay, and D. E. Rogers. 1966. Studies on human leukocyte motility. I. Effects of alterations in pH, electrolyte concentration, and phagocytosis on leukocyte migration, adhesiveness, and aggregation. J. Exp. Med. 124:483–499.
3. Buckley, R. H., B. B. Wray, and E. Z. Belmaker. 1972. Extreme hyperimmunoglobulinemia E and undue susceptibility to infection. Pediatrics 49:59–70.
4. Chess, L., R. P. MacDermott, and S. F. Schlossman. 1974. Immunologic functions of isolated human lymphocyte subpopulations. I. Quantitative isolation of human T and B cells and response to mitogens. J. Immunol. 113:1113–1121.
5. Deinard, A. S., I. E. Fortuny, A. Theologides, G. L. Anderson, J. Boen, and B. J. Kennedy. 1974. Studies on the neutropenia of cancer chemotherapy. Cancer 33:1210–1218.
6. Edwards, Y. H., D. A. Hopkinson, and H. Harris. 1971. Inherited variants of human nucleoside phosphorylase. Ann. Hum. Genet. 34:395–408.
7. Fudenberg, H., R. A. Good, H. C. Goodman, W. Hitzig, H. G. Kunkel, I. M. Roitt, F. S. Rosen, D. S. Rowe, M. Seligmann, and J. R. Soothill. 1971. Primary immunodeficiencies. Report of a World Health Organization committee. Pediatrics 47:927–946.
8. Giblett, E. R., A. J. Ammann, D. W. Wara, R. Sandman, and L. R. Diamond. 1975. Nucleoside-phosphorylase deficiency in a child with severely defective T-cell immunity and normal B-cell immunity. Lancet 1:1010–1013.
9. Gifford, R. H., and S. E. Malawista. 1970. A simple rapid micromethod for detecting chronic granulomatous disease of childhood. J. Lab. Clin. Med. 75:511–519.
10. Hong, R. 1974. Agammaglobulinemia and other immunologic defects, p. 1–27. In Brennemann's practice of pediatrics. Harper & Row, Publishers, Inc., Hagerstown, Md.
11. Hopkins, D. A., P. J. L. Cook, and H. Harris. 1969. Further data on the adenosine deaminase (ADA) polymorphism and a report of a new phenotype. Ann. Hum. Genet. 32:361–367.
12. Horowitz, S., T. Groshong, R. Albrecht, and R. Hong. 1975. The "active" rosette test in immunodeficiency diseases. Clin. Immunol. Immunopathol. 4:405–414.
13. Huber, J., and J. Kersey. 1975. Pathological features, p. 279–289. In H. J. Meuwissen, B. Pollara, R. J. Pickering, and I. H. Porter (ed.), Combined immunodeficiency disease and adenosine deaminase deficiency. A molecular defect. Academic Press Inc., New York.
14. Humbert, J. R. (ed.) 1975. Neutrophil physiology and pathology. Semin. Hematol. 12:1–116.
15. Meuwissen, H. J., R. J. Pickering, B. Pollara, and I. H. Porter (ed.). 1975. Combined immunodeficiency disease and adenosine deaminase deficiency. A molecular defect. Academic Press Inc., New York.
16. Meuwissen, H. J., B. Pollara, and R. J. Pickering. 1975. Combined immunodeficiency disease associated with adenosine deaminase deficiency. J. Pediatr. 86:169–181.
17. Miller, M. E. 1975. Pathology of chemotaxis and random mobility. Semin. Hematol. 12:59–82.
18. Miller, M. E. 1976. Neutrophil function. In F. H. Bach and R. A. Good (ed.), Clinical immunobiology, vol. 3. Academic Press Inc., New York, in press.
19. Miller, M. E., F. A. Oski, and M. B. Harris. 1971. Lazy-leucocyte syndrome. A new disorder of neutrophil function. Lancet 1:665–669.
20. Moore, E. C., and H. J. Meuwissen. 1975. Screening for ADA deficiency, p. 219–225. In H. J. Meuwissen, B. Pollara, R. J. Pickering, and I. H. Porter (ed.), Combined immunodeficiency disease and adenosine deaminase deficiency. A molecular defect. Academic Press Inc., New York.
21. Omenn, G. S. 1965. Familial reticuloendotheliosis with eosinophilia. N. Engl. J. Med. 273:427–432.
22. Pearse, A. G. E. 1968. Methyl-green-pyronin Y method for DNA and RNA, p. 652. In Histochemistry. Theoretical and applied, vol. 1. The Williams & Wilkins Co., Baltimore.
23. Poston, R. N. 1974. A buffered chromic chloride method of attaching antigens to red cells: use in haemagglutination. J. Immunol. Methods 5:91–96.
24. Rebuck, J. W., and J. H. Crowley. 1955. A method of studying leukocyte functions in vivo. Ann. N.Y. Acad. Sci. 59:757–805.
25. Rosen, F. S. 1972. Immunological deficiency disease, p. 271–289. In F. H. Bach and R. A. Good (ed.), Clinical immunobiology, vol. 1. Academic Press Inc., New York.
26. Sainte-Marie, G. 1962. A paraffin embedding technique for studies employing immunofluorescence. J. Histochem. Cytochem. 10:250–256.
27. Sever, J. L. 1962. Application of a microtechnique to viral serological investigations. J. Immunol. 88:320.
28. Spencer, N., D. A. Hopkinson, and H. Harris. 1968. Adenosine deaminase polymorphism in man. Ann. Hum. Genet. 32:9–14.
29. Stavitsky, A. B. 1954. Micromethods for the studies of proteins and antibodies. I. Procedure and general applications of hemagglutination-inhibition reactions with tannic acid and

protein-treated red blood cells. J. Immunol. 72:360.

30. Stiehm, E. R., and F. A. Fulginiti (ed.). 1973. Immunologic disorders in infants and children. W. B. Saunders Co., Philadelphia.

31. Vyas, G. N., L. Holmdahl, H. A. Perkins, and H. H. Fudenberg. 1969. Serologic specificity of human anti-IgA and its significance in transfusion. Blood 34:573–581.

32. Waldmann, T. A., S. Broder, R. M. Blaese, M. Durm, M. Blackman, and W. Strober. 1974. Role of suppressor T cells in pathogenesis of common variable hypogammaglobulinemia. Lancet 2:609–613.

33. Wedgwood, R. J., H. D. Ochs, and S. D. Davis. 1975. The recognition and classification of immunodeficiency diseases with bacteriophage ϕX 174, p. 331–338. In D. Bergsma, R. A. Good, and J. Finstad (ed.), Immunodeficiency in man and animals. Sinauer Associates, Sunderland, Mass.

Chapter 83

Immunological Tests for Hypersensitivity Reactions to Drugs

BERNARD B. LEVINE

Immunological tests are of great value in predicting anaphylactic allergic reactions to penicillin and are of somewhat lesser value in diagnosing other allergic reactions to penicillin. As to allergic reactions to other low-molecular-weight drugs, at the present time immunological tests generally are of only little clinical value in diagnosis or prediction of allergic reactions. The reason for this is that although we know much of the haptenic antigenic specificity of penicillin hypersensitivity, and of the various immune responses made by man to therapeutic penicillin, this kind of information is generally not available for other drugs. However, in a few cases, in vitro tests may be helpful in diagnosing cutaneous, hematological, and visceral allergic reactions to certain other drugs. This will be discussed below.

We will discuss first penicillin allergy and then allergy to other low-molecular-weight drugs. Rather than repeating the detailed methods for the tests, we will refer the reader to the original articles where the methodological details can be found.

PENICILLIN ALLERGY – TESTS FOR IGE ANTIBODIES TO PREDICT ANAPHYLACTIC REACTIONS

Humans given therapeutic penicillin produce immunoglobulin E (IgE) antibodies specific for the benzylpenicilloyl (BPO) haptenic group (8) as well as IgE antibodies specific for at least two other haptenic groups, termed "minor" haptenic groups (9, 13, 21). The chemical identity of the minor haptenic groups is not yet known. However, IgE antibodies of these specificities can be detected by dint of their reaction in immediate skin tests (wheal-and-flare reaction) with crystalline penicillin and its hydrolysis product, benzylpenicilloic acid. We used the term "minor determinant" to indicate that when penicillin reacts with tissue proteins in vivo to form hapten protein conjugates, most (perhaps 90 to 95%) of the covalently bound hapten is BPO group, whereas relatively little is covalently bound as "minor haptenic determinants."

Several tests for IgE antibodies to penicillin haptens exist: the direct immediate skin test;

Prausnitz-Kustner (P-K) reactions in man and passive transfer into the skin of nonhuman primates (as well as into tissues from nonhuman primates); radioallergoabsorbant tests (24); and direct histamine release from peripheral leukocytes and passive histamine release from peripheral leukocytes. Some comparisons of test sensitivity have been made. In most cases the direct skin test is more sensitive than P-K in man (18). For example, in penicillin hypersensitivity, in only 50 to 75% of patients with positive immediate skin tests will their sera be positive by the P-K test. Conversely, only in one unique situation has a positive P-K test been found in the absence of a positive skin test, i.e., where penicillin had been recently administered and the immune response was still evolving. In this situation, sufficient time for skin fixation might not yet have occurred, or alternatively, a temporary state of skin desensitization might have existed (12). Where P-K tests in man and in various primates have been compared, the P-K test in man is almost always more sensitive (D. M. Zolov and B. B. Levine, unpublished data). We are not aware of any rigorous comparisons between the direct skin test and radioallergoabsorbant test or histamine release in vitro. Although clear data do not exist, we provisionally believe that the direct skin test is generally more sensitive than are the other tests as presently done.

BPO-specific skin tests are done by using as the eliciting reagent, BPO-polylysine (3, 4, 8, 12, 15, 17). The best materials available are of relatively low molecular weight and are maximally conjugated.

Minor-determinant specific immediate reactions are elicited by a mixture of penicillin and other chemicals derived from penicillin. The latter are benzylpenicilloate, benzylpenilloate, and benzylpenicilloylamines (of various aliphatic amines) (13). A mixture of benzylpenicillin and benzylpenicilloate can be used as a minor-determinant mixture (MDM). In doing this, one gains in simplicity of this mixture, but gives up a certain amount of reaction intensity in some patients (13).

The two-component MDM, i.e., penicillin and benzylpenicilloate, is used at a 10^{-2} M concentration for each component in a weak phosphate-buffered saline at pH 7.2. The benzylpenicilloate is relatively unstable and the solution should be used immediately. It is convenient to lyophilize and reconstitute just before use. No commercial preparation of MDM is currently available.

We recommend that skin tests be done as follows (see reference 15 for details). First a prick test is done; i.e., droplets of BPL, MDM, and a diluent control are placed on the volar aspect of the forearm, and a prick is made through each droplet by pressing a no. 26 needle at an acute angle into the skin through the droplet. The sites are inspected at 8 min for a wheal-and-flare response. A negative reaction shows nothing or only a puncture mark. A positive is a wheal with a surrounding erythematous flare. In most cases the prick test will be negative, since it is positive only when the patient is very highly sensitive. The role of the prick test is to screen out the very highly hypersensitive individual so that the definitive intradermal test will not be done on these patients. If the prick test is positive, the intradermal test (with that reagent) should not be done. The prick test appears to give a reaction equivalent to an intradermal test done with about 1/1000th that concentration. If the prick test is negative, the intradermal tests are done with the three reagents. The lateral aspect of the midportion of the arm is used. The three solutions were originally drawn up into three tuberculin syringes with a no. 26 intradermal needle. Quantities of approximately 0.01 ml of the reagents are injected about 1.5 inches (3.8 cm) apart into the skin. Blebs of about 1 mm in diameter result. Please note that 0.01 ml is injected, not 0.1 ml as is used for a tuberculin test. The test sites are read in 15 min. In reading the test sites, the BPL and MDM sites are compared with the control site. If the test is negative, the three sites should be identical, i.e., poorly defined blebs, 1 to 3 mm in diameter, without surrounding erythema. A positive reaction is a well-defined wheal, distinctly larger than the control, with sharply defined margins, and almost always surrounded by a zone of homogenous erythema. The size of the wheal, in a very rough way, is a measure of the intensity of the reaction. Most positive reactions (moderate positive) give wheals between 6 and 10 mm (with erythema of about 20 to 35 mm in diameter, edge to edge). Intense reactions are wheals that are more than 10 mm in diameter, frequently with pseudopodia. Weak reactions are distinct wheals 3 to 6 mm in diameter with some surrounding erythema.

When a patient gives a history of having had an anaphylactic reaction in the past, we recommend starting the tests with more dilute solutions. In this case we dilute the BPL and MDM 1:100 (i.e., 0.1 ml of reagent plus approximately 10 ml of saline), perform the prick test with the dilute materials, and, if the test is negative, then proceed with the test as outlined above. The extra step, a prick test with the 1:100 dilution of the standard reagents, will detect most of those extremely rare individuals who might react with a constitutional reaction to the prick test with the undiluted reagents.

A false negative reaction may be obtained in people whose skin cannot express a wheal-and-flare reaction. Most often this will occur in patients taking antihistaminic drugs (particularly hydroxyzine) and β-adrenergic agonists such as ephedrine in high dosage, or in elderly debilitated patients with atrophic skin. In general, a positive control (e.g., histamine at a concentration of 10 μg of histamine base per ml in saline) should be done in immediate skin testing. In the hospital setting, when we are dealing with acutely ill or chronically ill people, or people taking drugs that may inhibit histamine effect, we have used the histamine control. We found that only in patients on hydroxyzine and in elderly and debilitated patients is the histamine control significantly reduced in intensity. Accordingly, for most patients we have dispensed with the histamine control. Also, in patients without prior history of penicillin allergy, it may not be necessary to do a prick test before the intradermal test, which would speed up the procedure. The probability of a generalized reaction to the test, when done as outlined above, is very small. We have not had such a reaction in our 12 years of testing. Nevertheless, epinephrine should be kept at hand when skin tests are done, and the tester should be prepared to treat an anaphylactic reaction should one develop.

The clinical significance of the skin test for IgE antibodies is as follows:

(i) Clinically, the most important use of these tests is to screen out the potential allergic reaction (particularly the anaphylactic reactor) to penicillin in patients who are about to receive penicillin therapy. These tests may be used in both history (of penicillin allergy)-positive and history-negative patients. Patients with prior histories of penicillin allergy should receive penicillin only when it is believed that the β-lactam antibiotics would be significantly better than others. In these situations, several studies demonstrated (1, 15, 22) that approximately 85% of history-positive patients were currently negative to skin tests with BPL and MDM, and that the skin test-negative patients tolerated penicillin therapy without immediate allergic reaction. In our study on 218 consecutive patients with past histories of penicillin allergy who needed penicillin therapy for serious infectious diseases, 185 were skin test negative (to BPL *and* MDM). All 185 patients were given penicillin therapy without premedication and without attempts at desensitization. None had immediate reaction, one had an accelerated reaction (due to an anamnestic IgG response at 72 h), and 6 of the 185 (3.2%) had late reactions (exanthematic reactions). By contrast, 11 patients who were skin test positive and who had major indications for penicillin therapy were premedicated with benadryl, and penicillin therapy was started by a desensitization program. Eight of 11 had urticaria or diffuse flush (IgE-mediated reactions) during or shortly after desensitization, and 3 of the 11 patients (27%) had, in addition, late allergic reactions (urticaria, exanthematic reactions, and Coombs-positive hemolytic anemia).

At the present time, based on published data (1, 15, 22), it appears that a negative skin test to BPL and to MDM indicates little or no risk of immediate allergic reaction (including anaphylaxis). A positive test indicates the presence of IgE antibodies, and accordingly a risk of IgE-mediated allergic reaction. In practice, this risk of a clinical allergic reaction varies with the intensity of the positive test, the haptenic determinant to which the patient reacts, and the dose of penicillin given. Where very large doses of penicillin are given (10 to 30 million units/day), the incidence of allergic reactions in skin test positive patients is high, perhaps 80 to 90%. Also, positive tests to the minor determinants appear to be associated with high risk of immediate allergic reaction even to relatively small doses of penicillin (1, 14, 15, 22).

PENICILLIN ALLERGY TESTS FOR IgG AND IgM ANTIBODIES

The direct diagnostic value of these tests appears to be in the diagnosis of some exanthematic skin rashes, possibly of the rare case of penicillin-induced agranulocytosis and of penicillin-induced Coombs-positive hemolytic anemia (see chapter 72). In about one-fourth to one-third of the cases of penicillin-associated exanthematic rashes, high titers of IgM antibodies specific for BPO were found. For example, 103 patients who had recent penicillin therapy without allergic reaction had IgM antibody titers averaging 64, and none of these 103 controls had a titer over 1,000. By contrast, about 30% of patients who developed maculopapular reactions while on penicillin therapy had IgM BPO-specific antibody titers of 2,000 to 12,000

(14). The one patient with penicillin-induced agranulocytosis had an IgM antibody titer of 1:12,000, the highest we have ever seen (unpublished data). Penicillin-induced hemolytic anemia is associated with IgG antibodies specific for the BPO hapten and also for an unknown haptenic group (10, 11).

We recommend a hemagglutination (HA) assay for BPO-specific IgG and IgM antibodies. Details of the method are given in the literature (5, 6). Basically, human O+ erythrocytes are reacted with penicillin under defined conditions to yield erythrocytes with haptenic groups coupled covalently onto their surface. The use of a diluent containing dextran (average molecular weight = 75,000) and fetal calf serum resulted in a marked increase in the sensitivity of the test and also permitted a proportionality between HA titers and antibody concentration as measured by quantitative precipitation reaction. Using known rabbit anti-BPO sera, it was found that the sensitivity of the HA system was 0.0003 to 0.0006 μg of antibody protein per ml. The sensitivity of this assay for human BPO-specific IgG antibody appears to be about the same. The sensitivity is modified by antibody binding affinity; low-affinity antibodies show lower sensitivity than do antibodies of high-binding affinity (7) in this system.

Hapten specificity is proved by showing specific inhibition of agglutination with a univalent BPO hapten, BPO-*n*-propylamine (diasterioisomeric mixture) (5, 6), in low concentrations.

PENICILLIN ALLERGY – OTHER TESTS

Delayed hypersensitivity tests of tuberculin type (19) as well as lymphocyte blastogenesis in vitro (2, 20, 23) can be elicited by penicillin. The methods and findings in various populations of patients are detailed in the literature (2, 19, 20, 23). Suffice it to say here that when patients having recent penicillin therapy were tested, a significantly higher percentage of those having had clinical allergic reactions than those that did not have allergic reactions had manifestations of cellular hypersensitivity. Also, delayed hypersensitivity to penicillin correlated with other manifestations of the immune response to penicillin (19). It is possible that cellular hypersensitivity may mediate some exanthematic skin reactions.

TESTS FOR ALLERGY TO OTHER DRUGS – IMMEDIATE SKIN TESTS

The literature on drug allergy contains several isolated reports on positive immediate skin tests to other simple chemical drugs found in suspected cases of immediate allergic reaction to these drugs. These include local anesthetics, tetracycline, bromsulfophthalein, salicylates, and others. The significance of the tests is unclear because of technical factors and inadequate controls. For higher-molecular-weight drugs such as peptide and protein hormones (insulin, pitressin) and tetanus toxoid, positive immediate skin reactions are obtained in patients having immediate allergic reactions, and are clinically significant when the concentration of the drug used for testing is appropriately small, e.g., for insulin, 10^{-6} M or lower.

LYMPHOCYTE BLASTOGENESIS

Lymphocyte blastogenesis has been suggested as an effective or at least promising diagnostic test for allergic drug reactions (2, 16, 20, 23). It has had little or no trial as a predictive test. The method involves incubation of peripheral blood lymphocytes from a patient with suspected drug allergy with the offending drug at several concentrations and monitoring the effect upon blastogenesis as compared with suitable controls. Blastogenesis was measured in early reports by morphological means, blast transformation, and subsequently by incorporation of radio-tagged DNA precursors into DNA. The detailed methodology is given in the literature (2, 16, 20, 23) and also in chapter 9.

The reader should be aware of several caveats. First, the clinical significance of both negative or positive tests is not clear. It appears that many patients truly allergic to a drug may not give a positive blastogenesis test to that drug. The actual antigenic mechanisms whereby a simple chemical drug can elicit the lymphocyte blastogenesis reaction in vitro is not understood. We do not know whether metabolic conversion of the drug to a chemically reactive pro-antigen is required as an initial step, or whether, in some cases, a drug might bind to a cell membrane by hydrophobic forces, thus forming an antigenic particle. In the former case, one might construct an argument that for certain drugs (e.g., isonicotinic acid hydrazide or p-aminosalicylic acid) to induce and elicit an allergic reaction, they must first be metabolized by oxidative enzymes of liver microsomes to form a chemically reactive intermediate (such as epoxide, a quinone, or a free radical) which then covalently binds to protein to form the complete antigen. Or a different enzymatic reaction capable of finally coupling the drug to proteins may be involved. Continuing this argument, when the drug is added to the lymphocyte culture in vitro, the culture may or may not contain the requisite enzymatic machinery for this reaction. If not, the test

would be negative despite the presence of specifically sensitized T-lymphocytes.

Second, it is not necessarily true that a positive response to a drug would mean that the clinical allergic reaction was due to that drug. For example, we (19) found that 3 of 45 patients (7%) recently (7 to 21 days before) completing a course of penicillin therapy without clinical allergic reaction had positive tuberculin-type skin tests for cellular hypersensitivity to penicillin. Thus the mere detection of cellular hypersensitivity some time after a course of drug therapy is not necessarily synonymous with a past allergic reaction to that drug. The time factor may be important here. Thus, it is conceivable that while the drug is still being given, or for one or 2 days after the drug is discontinued, a very low percentage of patients not manifesting an allergic reaction to that drug will manifest cellular hypersensitivity. Subsequently, as the drug and its metabolic products are eliminated, a higher percentage of patients will manifest cellular hypersensitivity. For example, in the penicillin system, as stated above, only 7% of nonallergic patients with very recent penicillin therapy manifested cellular hypersensitivity to penicillin; by contrast, among such patients who had not received therapeutic penicillin for more than 1 year, 24 or 114 (21%) manifested cellular hypersensitivity to penicillin (19). Thus, although a positive or negative lymphocyte blastogenesis test to the drug would be some help, one's clinical judgment would be needed to place these data into perspective. Further work on this test will be needed to improve it and to define its clinical usefulness as a diagnostic test.

LITERATURE CITED

1. Adkinson, N. F., Jr., W. L. Thompson, W. C. Maddrey, and L. M. Lichtenstein. 1971. Routine use of penicillin skin testing on an inpatient service. N. Engl. J. Med. 285:22–24.
2. Halpern, B. N. 1972. Antibodies produced by drugs and methods for their detection, p. 113–147. In M. Samter (ed.), International encyclopedia of pharmacology and therapeutics, vol. 1. Pergamon Press, New York.
3. Levine, B. B. 1964. The preparation of penicilloyl-polylysine; skin test reagents for the clinical evaluation of penicillin hypersensitivity. J. Med. Chem. 7:675–676.
4. Levine, B. B. 1964. Studies on antigenicity. The effect of succinylation of amino groups on the antigenicity of benzylpenicilloyl-poly-L-lysine conjugates in random bred and in strain 2 guinea pigs. Proc. Soc. Exp. Biol. Med. 116:1127–1131.
5. Levine, B. B., M. J. Fellner, and V. Levytska. 1965. Benzylpenicilloyl-specific serum antibodies to penicillin in man. I. Development of

a sensitive hemagglutination assay method and hapten specificities of antibodies. J. Immunol. **96**:707–718.

6. Levine, B. B., E. C. Franklin, M. J. Fellner, V. Levytska, and N. Alisberg. 1965. Benzylpenicilloyl specific serum antibodies to penicillin in man. II. Sensitivity of the assay method, molecular classes of antibodies, and antibody titres of random patients. J. Immunol. **96**:719–726.

7. Levine, B. B., and V. Levytska. 1967. A sensitive hemagglutination assay method for DNP-specific antibodies. Effect of antibody binding efficiency on titers. J. Immunol. **98**:648–652.

8. Levine, B. B., and Z. Ovary. 1961. Studies on the mechanism of the formation of the penicillin antigen. III. The N-(D-α-benzylpenicilloyl) group as an antigenic determinant responsible for hypersensitivity to penicillin G. J. Exp. Med. **114**:875–904.

9. Levine, B. B., and V. H. Price. 1964. Studies on the immunological mechanisms of penicillin allergy. II. Antigenic specificities of allergic wheal-and-flare responses in patients with histories of penicillin allergy. Immunology **7**:542–556.

10. Levine, B. B., and A. P. Redmond. 1967. Immune mechanism of penicillin induced Coombs positivity in man. J. Clin. Invest. **46**:1085.

11. Levine, B. B., and A. P. Redmond. 1967. Immune mechanism of penicillin induced immunohemolytic anemia. Int. Arch. Allergy Appl. Immunol. **21**:594–606.

12. Levine, B. B., and A. P. Redmond. 1968. The nature of the antigen-antibody complexes initiating the specific wheal-and-flare reaction in sensitized man. J. Clin. Invest. **47**:556–566.

13. Levine, B. B., and A. P. Redmond. 1969. Minor haptenic determinant-specific reagins of penicillin hypersensitivity in man. Int. Arch. Allergy Appl. Immunol. **35**:445–455.

14. Levine, B. B., A. P. Redmond, M. J. Fellner, H.

E. Voss, and V. Levytska. 1966. Penicillin allergy and the immune response of man to penicillin. J. Clin. Invest. **45**:1895–1906.

15. Levine, B. B., and D. M. Zolov. 1969. Prediction of penicillin allergy with immunological tests. J. Allergy **43**:231–244.

16. Mathews, K. P., P. M. Pan, and J. H. Wells. 1972. Experience with lymphocyte transformation tests in evaluating allergy to aminosalicylic acid, isoniazid and streptomycin. Int. Arch. Allergy Appl. Immunol.

17. Parker, C. W., and J. A. Thiel. 1963. Studies in human penicillin allergy: a comparison of various penicilloyl-polylysines. J. Lab. Clin. Med. **62**:482–491.

18. Redmond, A. P., and B. B. Levine. 1967. The relationship between immediate skin tests and passive transfer tests in man. J. Allergy **39**:51–56.

19. Redmond, A. P., and B. B. Levine. 1968. Delayed skin reaction to benzylpenicillin in man. Int. Arch. Allergy Appl. Immunol. **33**: 193–206.

20. Sakarny, I. 1967. Lymphocyte transformation in drug hypersensitivity. Lancet **1**:743–745.

21. Siegel, B. B., and B. B. Levine. 1964. Antigenic specificities of skin sensitizing antibodies in the sera from patients with immediate septemic allergic reactions of penicillin. J. Allergy **35**:488–498.

22. Van Dellen, R. G., and G. J. Gleich. 1970. Penicillin skin tests as predictive and diagnostic aids in penicillin allergy. Med. Clin. North Am. **54**:997–1007.

23. Vickers, M. R., and E. S. K. Assem. 1974. Tests for penicillin allergy in man. I. Carrier effect on response to penicilloyl conjugates. Immunology **26**:425–440.

24. Wide, L., and L. Juhlin. 1971. Detection of penicillin allergy of the immediate type by radioimmunoassay of reagins (IgE) to penicilloyl conjugates. Clin. Allergy **1**:171–177.

Section H

AUTOIMMUNE DISEASES

Chapter 84

Introduction

The beginning chapter of this section is a description of a test for the detection of antibodies to nuclear antigens (ANA) with the use of the immunofluorescence technique. This is quite appropriate because, together with the much longer established tests for rheumatoid factor, assays for ANA are the most commonly used tests for detection of autoantibodies in human disease. Indeed, hundreds of clinical laboratories throughout the country have the capacity to perform these tests and already are using them. At present, there is no agreement on a standard method which could be used by all laboratories, and, in fact, there is probably no method that is superior in all respects to any other method. The method described in this section is that used in a laboratory engaged in both research and clinical service in immunological diseases.

With the rapidly advancing knowledge concerning immunological specificities of ANA, clinicians have been asking for more characterization of ANA according to their immunological specificities. This is particularly so because it has been clearly shown that antibodies of certain specificities appear to be more or less restricted to certain diseases, and, moreover, antibodies of certain specificities, particularly antibody to deoxyribonucleic acid (DNA), can be related to pathogenetic events associated with immune complex vasculitis. For these reasons, the next three chapters are devoted to tests which describe methods that characterize ANA according to their immunological specificities. They include a radioimmunoassay method for detection of antibodies to DNA and hemagglutination methods for detection of antibodies to DNA and deoxyribonucleoprotein. Both of these methods have been presented because the expertise available in clinical laboratories may be limited to one or the other method. In the fourth chapter in this group of papers, a hemagglutination method for detection of antibodies to two nuclear acidic proteins, the Sm antigen and nuclear ribonucleoprotein, is described. Antibodies to Sm antigen appear to be highly specific for systemic lupus erythematosus, and antibodies to ribonucleoprotein, although not specific, when present in high

titer are diagnostic of the new clinical syndrome, mixed connective tissue disease.

In the next chapter, tests for the detection of rheumatoid factor are described in meticulous detail. In addition to the commonly used latex agglutination method, a method is described in which aggregated immunoglobulin G (IgG) is used in a precipitin test. The interpretation of positive tests and the so called "false-positive" tests is explained.

It has only been in the past decade that immune complexes in the autoimmune diseases have been detected, and they are now receiving increasing attention. One of the earliest assays for detection of immune complexes in human sera was that using the C1q component of serum complement. Very rapidly thereafter, it was found that anti-IgG (rheumatoid factor) either of the monoclonal or of the polyclonal variety was a useful reagent for detection of circulating immune complexes. Many modifications using these two reagents have been reported. All these different methods for detection of immune complexes with the use of C1q or rheumatoid factors are described in detail in this chapter, and the sensitivities of the different methods are compared. The next chapter describes another important method for the detection of immune complexes in which complement receptors on a human lymphoblastoid cell line (Raji cells) are used. As described by the authors, this method has been quantitated in terms of immune complexes expressed as equivalent of aggregated IgG. This method is extremely sensitive and may be the method of choice in laboratories where tissue culture cell lines are readily available.

In the next chapter, tests are described for detection of tissue-specific antigens. These include antibodies to thyroid, adrenal, parathyroid, mitochondria, smooth muscle, and gastric parietal cells. Obviously, these antibodies appear to be restricted to certain disease states. Some of the tissue-specific antibodies have been useful in the diagnosis of certain diseases, especially those associated with thyroid diseases, primary biliary cirrhosis (anti-mitochondrial antibodies) and chronic active hepatitis (anti-smooth muscle antibodies). The type of staining of these tissues is described and illustrated, and the interpretation of these tests is discussed.

The next two chapters of this section deal with the immunohistopathology of the kidney and the skin. It has become quite clear to many workers in the field that there is a continuous thread which ties together the observations of circulating autoantibodies, the detection of circulating immune complexes, and finally the finding of reactants (immunoglobulins or complement) in the tissues. As explained in these two chapters, this can result either from direct reaction of antibodies with tissue components or the entrapment of immune complexes. Indeed, it might be stated that a complete histopathological examination of kidney or skin tissue in these times might be considered inadequate without immunofluorescence study. In these two chapters, techniques for preparing tissues and reagents for immunofluorescence microscopy are described in detail, and, more importantly, the findings and the interpretations of what can be observed are discussed in great detail and clarity. The last chapter describes a number of tests for detection of antibodies to human sperm. This field of work is becoming increasingly important not only in searching for causes of spontaneously occurring infertility, but also in evaluating possible immunological sequelae of vasectomy.

Although the tests described in this section are by no means a complete repertoire of all the available tests which can be offered by a laboratory for help to the clinician interested in autoimmune diseases, they provide a good cross-section of these tests. In the area of autoimmunity, it might be expected that, in the next few years, the assays will be aimed more and more at recognizing the immunological specificities of the many types of autoantibodies present in these diseases. Such assays might be expected to develop in diseases such as Sjögren's syndrome, scleroderma, and myasthenia gravis. In the detection of immune complexes, it might be anticipated that future tests may be able to zero in on defining the specificity of immune complexes. However, what is currently available to the clinical immunologist already represents a powerful array of diagnostic tests to help him in the recognition and in certain instances guide him in the therapy of patients with autoimmune diseases.

Chapter 85

Detection of Antibodies to Nuclear Antigens by Immunofluorescence

NAOMI F. ROTHFIELD

INTRODUCTION

The detection of antinuclear antibodies by immunofluorescence has become an extremely valuable clinical tool. This technique allows all antinuclear antibodies to be demonstrated since all antibodies that react with nuclei or components of nuclei are detected. In addition, the technique is extremely sensitive. Thus, the immunofluorescence technique is frequently positive, whereas tests for precipitating or complement-fixing antinuclear antibodies are negative. On the other hand, the high sensitivity of the test leads to the detection of antinuclear antibodies in a wide variety of diseases, in elderly individuals without disease, and in about 10% of normal nonelderly individuals.

There is very little variation in the immunofluorescence techniques used for detecting antinuclear antibodies. The method here described in which mouse liver is used as a substrate has been found to yield consistent results during the past 12 years (9). Others have used peripheral blood leukocytes (4). The latter technique has one advantage in that sera from certain individuals contain leukocyte-specific antinuclear antigens which are missed using tissue sections (5).

CLINICAL INDICATIONS

The major indication for ordering the fluorescence test for antibodies to nuclear antigens (ANA) is to rule out a diagnosis of active systemic lupus erythematosus (SLE). A negative ANA in a patient whose clinical features suggest SLE essentially rules out the diagnosis of active SLE. Thus, an ANA should be ordered on all patients suspected of having SLE. Patients receiving drugs which are known to induce SLE, such as procainamide and hydralazine, should be tested for a positive ANA if symptoms suggestive of SLE occur (1). Such patients may merely complain of joint pains, but the ANA as well as the lupus erythematosus (LE) preparation may be positive. As discussed below, it is important in such patients to determine the pattern and titer of ANA since low titers may occur in 36% of normal elderly individuals (3). Patients with chronic active hepatitis should be tested since the ANA is most frequently positive in those patients without detectable hepatitis associated antigen (2). All children with juvenile rheumatoid arthritis should have ANA testing since it has been shown that there is a significant correlation between a high titer of ANA and the presence of iridocyclitis (12, 13). Although positive ANA is found in many diseases (see below, Interpretation), the clinical significance in patients with these diseases has not been clarified. For example, the presence of high-titer speckled or nucleolar ANA in patients with progressive systemic sclerosis has been found to have no practical clinical significance, since there is no correlation with any clinical parameter of the disease (10).

Thus, the test should be used clinically to rule out the diagnosis of SLE. In patients with SLE, the test is of great clinical value in that the pattern and titer may reflect clinical disease activity (6).

One advantage of the ANA over other tests for antinuclear antibodies is its ease of performance and interpretation; in addition, it is less time-consuming to perform than an LE cell test. The same data cannot be obtained by use of other techniques for detection of antinuclear antibodies because the other techniques are incapable of detecting all antinuclear antibodies present in the patient's serum to the same degree of sensitivity as the ANA technique. For example, anti-deoxyribonucleic acid (DNA) antibodies, while more specific for active SLE patients, are usually not present in SLE patients in remission. Therefore, although more specific for active SLE, anti-DNA antibodies are less sensitive as a diagnostic technique since many SLE patients in remission have no anti-DNA antibodies whereas their ANA is positive.

TEST PROCEDURES

Sera should be tested undiluted. If positive, serial dilutions should be carried out. The pattern should be noted on neat sera and for each titer.

647

Make a stock solution of phosphate-buffered saline (PBS) containing 85 g of NaCl, 10.7 g of Na_2HPO_4, and 3.9 g of NaH_2PO_4. Add up to 1 liter of distilled water, and adjust the pH to 7.0. The stock buffer is diluted 1:10 for use in the test. Diluted buffer is kept at 4 C.

Preparation of tissue

Kill a young mouse (Ajax mice, Jackson Laboratories, Bar Harbor, Me.) by breaking its neck. The mouse should be between 4 and 8 weeks old. Immediately open the abdominal cavity and remove the liver. Cut the liver into 0.5-cm squares, place on a cryostat specimen holder, and quick freeze for 2 min in a cryostat. Cut sections of the liver 4 μm thick and store in a freezer for no longer than 3 weeks. (One hundred sections may be cut in 20 min and then stored.)

Test for antibodies to nuclear antigens

1. Remove the slides from the freezer, number them with a diamond pencil, and immediately place them in a staining rack in a staining dish in acetone for 10 min (Fisher Scientific Co., Fair Lawn, N.J.; A-18 70087).

Note: A histological staining dish with a holder of a capacity of about 30 slides should be filled with no more than 10 slides.

2. Remove the slide holder from the acetone and immediately place it in a staining dish filled with buffer. Wash slides for 2 min with agitation (Rotating Apparatus; A. H. Thomas Co., Philadelphia, Pa.). Slides should be able to rock back and forth slightly during the wash.

3. Remove the dish from the shaker.

4. Remove one slide at a time from the buffer and quickly blot dry the slide surrounding the tissue with bibulous paper. Do not allow the tissue to dry out. Place one drop of serum over the tissue and place the slide flat in a moist chamber for 30 min at room temperature. A moist chamber can be made of a closed chamber which is level and which has moist blotting paper on the bottom. Pipettes are used to place the slides on. Slides must be placed flat so that the serum remains on the tissue during the entire incubation period. Timing starts at the time the last slide has been placed in the chamber.

5. Remove one slide at a time, tip the slide to allow serum to run off into a piece of bibulous paper, and immediately place the slide in a slide holder placed in a staining dish filled with buffer. Repeat for each slide.

6. Place the staining dish on a rotating apparatus and wash for 5 min. Remove the slide holder with slides and immediately place in another staining dish filled with buffer. Place the staining dish on a rotating apparatus and wash for 5 min.

7. Remove the staining dish from the rotating apparatus.

8. Remove one slide at a time; blot around the tissue as before.

9. Place one drop of fluorescein isothiocyanate (FITC) antiserum over the tissue.

10. Place the slide in a moist chamber.

11. Repeat the process for each slide and set a timer for 30 min.

12. After the 30-min incubation, remove slides one by one, drain off excess FITC antiserum as before, and immediately place the slide in a slide holder in a staining dish filled with buffer.

13. When all slides are in the buffer, place the staining dish on a rotating apparatus and wash with agitation for 5 min.

14. Remove the slide holder from the staining dish and immediately place it in another staining dish containing buffer.

15. Place the staining dish on a rotating apparatus and wash for 5 min with agitation.

16. Remove the staining dish from the rotating apparatus.

17. Remove one slide; blot dry around the tissue. Place one drop of glycerol-buffer solution (nine parts glycerol to one part PBS) over the tissue and place a cover slip over the tissue (Gold Seal Cover Glass, size 22 × 22 thin 1).

18. The slide should be wiped dry on the bottom.

19. The slide is ready for viewing within 1 h. Slides can be kept at 4 C for up to 4 h.

Note: Slides to be kept longer must be sealed with clear nail polish and kept at 4 C until used. Slides used are precleaned Gold Seal Micro slides (size 3 × 1; thickness, 0.97 to 1.07 mm).

General considerations

It is very important that the tissue be covered at all times by fluid; i.e., the tissue must not dry out. Therefore, slides must be left in buffer until ready to be blotted, and the blotting must be performed rapidly, leaving a moist area over the tissue. Similarly, slides must be incubated in a chamber with wet blotting paper, and the drop of serum or conjugate on top of the tissue must not roll off during incubation.

Conjugate

A goat or rabbit FITC-conjugated anti-human immunoglobulin should be used. This may be obtained commercially from Antibodies, Inc., Davis, Calif., or from other commercial sources. The method for preparation of such antisera is described in detail by Johnson and Holborow (7).

All conjugates, whether prepared in the laboratory of the user or obtained commercially, should be evaluated prior to use for suitability in the ANA test. Physicochemical characterization should include determination of fluorescein to protein ratio, antibody content, and analysis of other proteins present (7). Performance testing should be conducted in each laboratory prior to using each lot of conjugate. This provides information on the dilution of conjugate to be employed in the ANA test. Performance testing should include checkerboard titration in which a positive ANA serum is serially diluted and each dilution is tested for ANA against a series of dilutions of the conjugate (7).

Controls

The following controls should be set up each time the test is performed: (i) a negative control serum plus conjugate; (ii) a positive control serum with conjugate; and (iii) buffer plus conjugate. Only the positive control serum plus conjugate should be positive. An additional positive control which produces a peripheral pattern should be set up for each run.

INTERPRETATION

About 10% of the normal healthy population below the age of 60 years have low titers of antinuclear antibodies. Thus, titers of 1:16 or less are not infrequently found in healthy individuals. It is important to test sera undiluted in order to note the pattern. The peripheral pattern is not infrequently noted in dilutions up to

TABLE 1. *Pattern and titer of antibodies to nuclear antigens (ANA) in various diseases*

Disease	Most frequent pattern	Incidence of positive ANA (%)	
		Neat sera	1:16 or >
Systemic lupus erythematosus			
Active	Peripheral	100	99
Remission	Diffuse	95	90
Rheumatoid arthritis	Diffuse	66	40
Juvenile rheumatoid arthritis	Diffuse	61	24
Progressive systemic sclerosis	Speckled or nucleolar	83	60
Chronic discoid lupus	Diffuse	76	19
Normal healthy individuals (< age 60)	Fine speckles	10	2

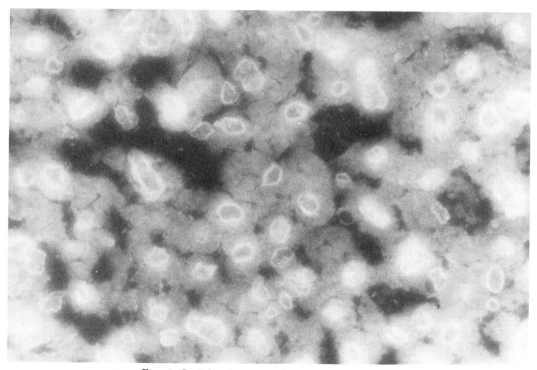

FIG. 1. *Peripheral pattern of nuclear fluorescence.*

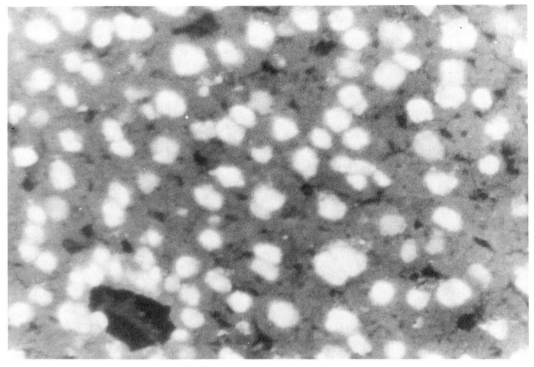

FIG. 2. *Diffuse pattern of nuclear fluorescence.*

1:16 or 1:32, at which dilution the pattern changes to a mixed diffuse and peripheral pattern and then with further dilution to a diffuse pattern. Sera producing each of the major patterns, i.e., fine speckles, diffuse, peripheral, or nucleolar, should be available for each laboratory. The interpretation of the patterns should be on the basis of clinical knowledge of the patients tested. Thus, sera from acutely ill SLE patients should be obtained to establish titers and patterns in this group of patients. Each laboratory should have sera from patients with established rheumatoid arthritis, patients with systemic sclerosis, elderly individuals, juvenile rheumatoid arthritis patients, and other clinical groups, to establish for the laboratory the incidence of positive tests, the titers, and the patterns for each disease (see Table 1).

The peripheral pattern of nuclear fluorescence (Fig. 1) is produced by sera which contain antibodies to double-stranded DNA (4, 11, 14), although SLE sera which produce a diffuse pattern (Fig. 2) may also have such antibodies (8). Sera producing a speckled or nucleolar pattern do not have antibodies to double-stranded DNA (8). The diffuse pattern may also be produced by sera containing antibodies to deoxyribonucleoprotein. Multiple antibodies may produce speckled patterns, including antibodies to a phosphate buffer extract of nuclei which may be directed to ribonucleoprotein and to an antigen, Sm (15).

LITERATURE CITED

1. Alarcon-Segovia, D. 1969. Drug induced lupus syndromes. Mayo Clin. Proc. 44:664-681.
2. Bulkley, B. H., S. E. Goldfinger, W. D. Heizer, K. J. Isselbacher, and N. R. Shulman. 1970. Distinctions in chronic active hepatitis based on circulating hepatitis-associated antigen. Lancet 1:1324-1326.
3. Cammarata, R. J., G. P. Rodnan, and R. H. Fennell. 1967. Serum anti-gamma globulin and antinuclear factors in the aged. J. Am. Med. Assoc. 199:455-458.
4. Casals, S. P., G. J. Friou, and P. O. Teague. 1963. Specific nuclear reaction pattern of antibody to DNA in lupus erythematosus sera. J. Lab. Clin. Med. 62:625-631.
5. Faber, V., and P. Elling. 1966. Leukocyte-specific antinuclear factors in patients with Felty's syndrome, rheumatoid arthritis, systemic lupus erythematosus and other diseases. Acta Med. Scand. 179:257-267.
6. Gonzalez, E. N., and N. F. Rothfield. 1966. Immunoglobulin class and pattern of nuclear fluorescence in systemic lupus erythematosus. N. Engl. J. Med. 274:1333-1338.
7. Johnson, G. D., and E. J. Holborow. 1973. Immunofluorescence, p. 18.1-18.20. *In* D. Weir (ed.), Immunochemistry, vol. 1. Handbook of

experimental immunology. Blackwell Scientific Publications, Oxford.

8. Luciano, A., and N. F. Rothfield. 1973. Patterns of nuclear fluorescence and DNA-binding activity. Ann. Rheum. Dis. 32:337–341.

9. Rothfield, N. F., B. Frangione, and E. C. Franklin. 1965. Slowly sedimenting mercaptoethanol-resistant antinuclear factors related antigenically to M immunoglobulins in patients with systemic lupus erythematosus. J. Clin. Invest. 44:62–72.

10. Rothfield, N. F., and G. P. Rodnan. 1968. Serum antinuclear antibodies in progressive systemic sclerosis (scleroderma). Arthritis Rheum. 11:607–617.

11. Rothfield, N. F., and B. D. Stollar. 1967. The relation of immunoglobulin class, pattern of anti-nuclear antibody and complement-fixing antibodies to DNA in sera from patients with systemic lupus erythematosus. J. Clin. Invest. 46:1785–1794.

12. Rudnicki, R. D., M. Ruderman, E. Scull, A. Goldenberg, and N. Rothfield. 1974. Clinical features and serologic abnormalities in juvenile rheumatoid arthritis. Arthritis Rheum. 17:1007–1015.

13. Schaller, J., C. Kupfer, and R. Wedgwood. 1969. Iridocyclitis in juvenile rheumatoid arthritis. Pediatrics 44:92–100.

14. Tan, E. M. 1967. Relationship of nuclear staining patterns with precipitating antibodies in SLE. J. Lab. Clin. Med. 70:800–812.

15. Tan, E. M., and H. G. Kunkel. 1966. Characteristics of a soluble nuclear antigen precipitating with sera of patients with systemic lupus erythematosus. J. Immunol. 96:464–471.

Chapter 86

Radioimmunoassay for Antibodies to Deoxyribonucleic Acid

NORMAN TALAL AND RAO PILLARISETTY

INTRODUCTION

Under normal circumstances, deoxyribonucleic acid (DNA) is a very poor immunogen. Indeed, normal animals have a remarkable tolerance to DNA and are only capable of making antibodies to single-stranded DNA when the latter is complexed to methylated albumin and presented in Freund's adjuvant. Double-stranded DNA does not produce antibodies in experimental animals under any circumstances. The greater immunogenicity of single-stranded compared with double-stranded DNA is true clinically as well. A number of disease states are associated with the formation of antibodies to single-stranded DNA. The formation of antibodies to double-stranded DNA, however, is generally confined to systemic lupus erythematosus alone. The only other situation in which antibodies to double-stranded DNA appear with any frequency is in the disease of hybrid New Zealand black mice (NZB/NZW F_1) (5).

These mice are an inbred strain genetically predisposed to develop lupus erythematosus cells (LE cells), antinuclear factor, and immune complex glomerulonephritis. They are considered a laboratory model for human systemic lupus erythematosus. Immunological and virological factors, as well as genetic influences, are involved in their disease. The homozygous New Zealand black mouse has a Coomb's positive autoimmune hemolytic anemia as the predominant clinical manifestation. In the hybrid NZB/NZW F_1 mouse, a spontaneous immune complex glomerulonephritis with LE cell formation is the major clinical picture. As in human systemic lupus erythematosus, this disease is worse in female NZB/NZW F_1 mice, who develop severe disease earlier in life compared with males (2).

The kidneys of patients dying from systemic lupus erythematosus and those from NZB/NZW F_1 mice have been studied by immunofluorescence and by elution methods to determine the antibody nature of the immunoglobulins present in the glomerular deposits. In both the human and the mouse disease, a large percentage of these deposits are made up of antibodies to nuclear material and especially to DNA. Thus, the significance of antibodies to double-stranded DNA is twofold: (i) such antibodies are frequently associated with systemic lupus erythematosus and are therefore useful diagnostically, and (ii) their presence is also associated with severe active lupus and the presence of immune complex glomerulonephritis. Therefore, the development of tests to specifically identify antibodies to DNA was a major step forward in the field of antinuclear antibodies.

A wide variety of techniques is available for measuring the presence and concentration of antibodies to DNA. These techniques include hemagglutination, immunoprecipitation in agar, complement fixation, counterimmunoelectrophoresis, bentonite flocculation, and radioimmunoassay. The last is preferred because it measures the direct interaction of DNA with antibody, is extremely sensitive and reliable, and yet is relatively easy to perform.

CLINICAL INDICATIONS

The most important fact to remember about a positive LE cell test or assay for antinuclear factor is that these findings are not diagnostic of systemic lupus erythematosus. Although a positive LE cell test is considered one of the 14 major diagnostic features of systemic lupus (4 of these features are required for a definite diagnosis), LE cells and antinuclear factor are also found in a number of other diseases which include rheumatoid arthritis, discoid lupus erythematosus, scleroderma, dermatomyositis, Sjogren's syndrome, and drug-induced lupus. They are occasionally seen in chronic or lupoid hepatitis.

LE cells and antinuclear factor occur in about 25% of patients with rheumatoid arthritis, particularly those with the most severe disease. LE cells and antinuclear factor are often associated with complications of rheumatoid arthritis such as vasculitis, peripheral neuropathy, leukopenia and splenomegaly (Felty's syndrome), and the sicca complex (Sjogren's syndrome). The appearance of LE cells or antinuclear factor in a patient who otherwise has rheumatoid arthritis should not alter the diagnosis. Glomerulonephritis is not seen in such patients.

Discoid lupus erythematosus is part of the general spectrum of lupus in which skin manifestations predominate. About 35% of patients with the discoid variety have antinuclear factor and about 8% have LE cells.

Drugs that are frequently associated with LE cells, antinuclear factor, and a lupus-like syndrome include procainamide, hydrolazine, isoniazid, various anticonvulsants, phenothiazines, and oral contraceptives. The serological abnormalities and symptoms are generally dose and time related and reversible in days to weeks following discontinuation of the drug. Antibodies to double-stranded DNA and immune complex nephritis are generally not seen in drug-induced lupus. The mechanism of this phenomenon is not understood.

Antibodies to single-stranded DNA are only slightly more specific for systemic lupus erythematosus than is antinuclear factor. They are seen in a variety of related rheumatic diseases including Sjogren's syndrome and rheumatoid arthritis. By contrast, antibodies to double-stranded DNA are highly correlated with systemic lupus erythematosus. As shown in Table 1, even when anti-double-stranded DNA occurs in other conditions, it is present in extremely low concentrations. A rising titer of antibodies to DNA, particularly when associated with a fall in serum complement, may be a sign of an incipient lupus crisis or episode of glomerulonephritis.

We employ a radioimmunoassay to measure the direct binding of radioactive DNA to antibody. The radioactive antigen-antibody immune complexes are collected on cellulose ester filters. The amount of radioactivity retained on the filter is a direct measure of serum antibody concentration (1).

One of the problems with this assay method is the source, strandedness, and specificity of the radioactive DNA. Since from an immunochemical standpoint all DNA is structurally similar, the source of the DNA should not be of great consequence. In fact, antibodies from systemic lupus are equally reactive with DNA from human normal or leukemic leukocytes, salmon sperm, calf thymus, and pneumococcus. More important, however, is the degree to which the DNA is truly double or single stranded. Single-stranded DNA is highly negatively charged and can bind nonspecifically to basic groups on serum proteins. Such binding, even if it occurs to gamma globulins, would not be immunologically specific (i.e., through specific antigen binding sites on the Fab fragment of the immunoglobulin). The filter cannot distinguish specific from nonspecific binding, and so there is always some retention of radioactivity even with normal serum. This problem is minimized by working at a pH of 8.0. This "background" radioactivity can be quite high with some preparations of DNA, possibly because a large amount of single-stranded material is present.

Nevertheless, after determination of DNA binding by a panel of normal sera, an arbitrary upper limit of normal can be established (generally 2 standard deviations above the mean for the normal group). Sera from patients with systemic lupus erythematosus and from NZB/NZW F_1 mice frequently bind more DNA than this, indicating anti-DNA antibodies. In the mice, the concentration of such antibody increases progressively with age. In patients, high binding correlates with low serum complement, active disease, and a markedly abnormal urinary sediment. These are signs of active lupus with nephritis. Low binding is associated with normal serum complement, clinical remission, improved urinary sediment, and improved renal function.

Antibodies to ribonucleic acid (RNA) can also be detected by the filter radioimmunoassay method with the use of either radioactive viral or synthetic RNAs. The former is preferred but is not yet commercially available. The two most studied synthetic polyribonucleotides are poly-inosinic·polycytidylic acid [poly(I)·poly(C)] and polyadenylic·polyuridylic acid [poly(A)·poly(U)], both of which are available commercially (Miles Chemical Co.). We have recently studied the binding of [^{14}C]poly(I)·poly(C) and [^{3}H]poly(A)·poly(U) by lupus sera which were first fractionated by sucrose density

TABLE 1. Antibodies to [^{14}C]KB DNA detected by the cellulose ester filter radioimmunoassay[a]

Serum tested	No. tested	No. positive	Per cent positive	Counts/min	
				Mean	Range
Systemic lupus erythematosus	50	38	76	119	7–269
NZB/NZW F_1 mice	29	15	52	64	10–143
Sjogren's syndrome	45	0	0	18	7–35
Rheumatoid arthritis and Sjogren's syndrome	24	2	8	23	10–65
Rheumatoid arthritis	21	1	5	20	8–56
Normal	44	1	2	29	16–83

[a] Radioactivity added = 280 counts/min (positive > 55 counts/min).

gradient ultracentrifugation. We found that poly(A)·poly(U) was always bound in the regions of the gradient corresponding to the distribution of immunoglobulins (either 7S or 19S, or both). However, poly(I)·poly(C) was sometimes bound to very light fractions smaller than 7S and presumably not immunoglobulin. For this reason, we believe that nonspecific binding may occur more readily with poly(I)·poly(C). We prefer poly(A)·poly(U) to detect anti-RNA antibodies when viral RNA is not available (3, 4).

TEST PROCEDURE

Antibodies to DNA can be detected by all of the standard immunological techniques that measure an antigen-antibody interaction. Methods employing immunoprecipitation, complement fixation, hemagglutination, bentonite flocculation, and counter-immunoelectrophoresis are all in use.

The ideal test should be sensitive, specific, reproducible, and quantitative. The precipitin test is generally performed as an Ouchterlony double diffusion assay in dilute agarose gel. It is relatively insensitive and only detects antibodies to DNA in a limited number of lupus patients. The complement-fixation test is more sensitive and detects between 50 and 70% of lupus patients as positive. However, it is somewhat difficult to perform as a routine assay procedure and cannot be used with anticomplementary sera. Since many lupus sera are anticomplementary, this is a serious limitation. The passive hemagglutination test, in which DNA is absorbed onto the surface of tanned formalinized erythrocytes, is a useful and sensitive assay procedure employed in many research laboratories. However, we favor the radioimmunoassay method because it detects the primary interaction between radioactive DNA and antibody rather than depending on a secondary phenomenon such as hemagglutination.

The DNA can be made radioactive in one of two ways. It can be complexed with radioactive actinomycin, which binds strongly to DNA, or it can be internally labeled by growing tissue culture cells or bacteria in the presence of radioactive thymidine (labeled with either ^{14}C or ^{3}H), which gets incorporated into DNA. The cells or bacteria are then lysed, and the radioactively labeled DNA is chemically purified and isolated. A human tumor cell line called KB is frequently used for this purpose. Radioactive DNA can now also be purchased from several commercial sources.

The serum to be studied for antibodies is heated to 56 C for 30 min to destroy complement components, which can bind some nucleic acids nonspecifically. Next, the serum is incubated with the radioactive DNA at 37 C for 30 min and then at 4 C for at least 60 min. Essentially all of the antigen binding and formation of radioactive immune complexes take place during this time period, but longer incubations in the cold may be used if one wishes. An overnight incubation at this point is sometimes convenient.

The ractioactive immune complex can be detected in several ways. In a Farr-type assay, the complex is precipitated by 50% saturated ammonium sulfate, which brings down the gamma globulin. Any radioactive DNA bound to gamma globulin is precipitated, whereas free unbound DNA is soluble in the ammonium sulfate. The separation of precipitate and supernatant fluid is accomplished by centrifugation. Since the volumes are generally small and the precipitate is easily disturbed, great care must be exercised in removing a sample of supernatant fluid for determination of radioactivity. The amount of radioactive antigen bound can be calculated from this determination.

The Farr assay is time-consuming and cannot be used with some radioactive nucleic acids. For these reasons, it has been replaced in our laboratory by the cellulose ester filter method for detecting radioactive immune complexes. In this assay procedure, the antigen-antibody immune complexes are collected on cellulose ester (Millipore) filters, whereas free DNA passes through the filter. The filters are then processed for determination of radioactivity by scintillation counting. The amount of radioactivity retained on the filter is a direct measure of serum antibody concentration. Results are generally expressed as counts per minute rather than percentage of antigen bound. The mean and two standard deviations for a panel of normal sera are determined for each new preparation of radioactive DNA. High binding is found with most lupus sera.

Antibodies to RNA or to DNA:RNA hybrid nucleic acids can be determined in much the same way with the filter radioimmunoassay method. Radioactive antigens currently used in our laboratory include [^{3}H]reovirus RNA, [^{14}C]-poly(I)·poly(C), [^{3}H]poly(A)·poly(U), [^{3}H]poly-(A), and [^{14}C]polydeoxythymidylic·polyriboadenylic acid. Many of these are commercially available, and it is hoped that more will become available as these assays become more routine.

An additional advantage of the radioimmunoassay method is the ability to study the specificity of the antinucleic acid antibody by inhibition of binding with the use of nonradioactive antigens in a competive manner. The relative specificity of anti-RNA antibodies for viral RNA was established in part by such a procedure (4). The exact procedure used in our laboratory is as follows.

Radioimmunoassay for anti-RNA and anti-DNA antibodies

1. Collect sera from 5 ml or more of peripheral blood.

2. Set up protocols for anti-DNA and anti-RNA antibody, giving the patient's name, the date, and the amount of serum, borate buffer, and radioactive DNA or RNA.

3. Number 10 × 75 Kimble disposable culture tubes to correspond with the number of sera being assayed.

4. Place in wire racks in numerical order.

5. Carefully pipette 10 μliters of serum and 80 μliters of borate buffer (pH 8.0) into the tubes.

6. Place racks in a 56 C water bath for 30-min incubation.

7. Add isotope (10 μliters of radioactive DNA or RNA), mix well by gentle shaking, and incubate in a 37 C water bath.

8. Place at 4 C for 30 min or more.

9. If many samples are being assayed, set up a filter manifold (e.g., #3025 Millipore Sampling Manifold); use a cellulose ester filter (02500, 0.45 μm, 25 mm) to cover each hole as needed; wet the filter with borate buffer to avoid breakage of the filter; place top on the manifold and lock.

10. Wash each tube twice with borate buffer (pH 8.0).

11. Remove the manifold top and dry the filter under a sun lamp for 8 to 10 min; label scintillation vials and remove cap vials.

12. Place the dry filter in a bottle, and add 10 ml of scintillation fluid (42 ml of Liquifluor and 1 liter of toluene).

13. Place scintillation vials in a beta scintillation counter; determine radioactivity for 10 min/sample; subtract background and record counts per minute.

14. *Preparation of borate buffer*: Add 168.3 g of NaCl and 2 to 2.6 g of H_3BO_3 to an 18-liter vessel, and titrate to pH 8.0 with concentrated NaOH (requires about 35 ml); store at 4 C until used.

The above quantities can be scaled down to needed volume.

ACKNOWLEDGMENTS

This work was supported by Public Health Service grant AM16140 from the National Institute of Arthritis, Metabolism, and Digestive Diseases and by research support from the Veterans Administration.

LITERATURE CITED

1. Attias, M. R., R. A. Sylvester, and N. Talal. 1973. Filter radioimmunoassay for antibodies to reovirus RNA in systemic lupus erythematosus. Arthritis Rheum. 16:719–725.
2. Talal, N. 1974. Autoimmunity and lymphoid malignancy in New Zealand black mice. Clin. Immunol. 2:101–120.
3. Talal, N., and R. J. Pillarisetty. 1976. IgM and IgG antibodies to DNA, RNA and DNA:RNA in systemic lupus erythematosus. Clin. Immunol. Immunopathol. 4:24–31.
4. Talal, N., A. D. Steinberg, and G. G. Daley. 1971. Inhibition of antibodies binding polyinosinic·polycytidylic acid in human and mouse lupus sera by viral and synthetic ribonucleic acids. J. Clin. Invest. 50:1248–1252.
5. Talal, N., and A. D. Steinberg. 1974. The pathogenesis of autoimmunity in New Zealand black mice. Curr. Top. Microbiol. Immunol. 64:79–103.

Chapter 87

Hemagglutination Tests for Detection of Antibodies to Deoxyribonucleic Acid and Nucleoprotein

Y. H. INAMI AND R. M. NAKAMURA

INTRODUCTION

The indirect immunofluorescence test is a practical screening test for the presence of antinuclear antibodies. However, the indirect immunofluorescence test will detect the presence of many antinuclear antibodies and is of limited value in identifying the important and pathogenic antibodies in systemic lupus erythematosus (SLE). The presence of significant amounts of anti-deoxyribonucleic acid (DNA) antibodies and anti-soluble nucleoprotein (sNP) antibodies is characteristic of SLE. The hemagglutination tests for the detection of DNA and soluble nucleoprotein (sNP) antibodies are helpful in the diagnosis of SLE and in monitoring the therapy of SLE. Positive hemagglutinating DNA antibodies have been demonstrated in patients who show no detectable precipitating antibodies by the agar double diffusion test.

MATERIALS AND EQUIPMENT

Preparative and test equipment

Refrigerated centrifuge (Sorvall, model RC-2B with SS-34 rotor).
Tissue homogenizer (Waring blender, model 5010S).
Sonifier (Branson Sonic Power Sonifier, model 9110).
Rotator (Scientific Industries Inc.; multipurpose).
Microdiluters (Cooke Engineering Co.; 25-μliter delivery).
Micropipette droppers (Cooke Engineering Co.; 25-μliter delivery).
Test Reading Mirror (Cooke Engineering Co.).
Disposable V-shaped plates (Linbro of the Pacific, Los Angeles, Calif.).
Micropipette (Eppendorf, 25 μliters).

Materials

Fresh type O Rh-negative blood (blood bank or live donor).
DNA, calf thymus (Worthington Biochemical Corp.).
Bovine albumin, 30% (Hyland Laboratories or Spectra Biologics), inactivated at 56 C for 30 min.
sNP (extracted from fresh calf thymus, see below).
Acetaldehyde, Baker grade (J. T. Baker Chemical Co.).
Biuret reagent (Technicon SMA 12/60 biuret reagent).
Human serum, Versatol, assayed (General Diagnostics).
Dialysis tubing (Union Carbide Corp.; 20/32 inch).
Test sera from patients (inactivated at 56 C for 30 min).
Control sera from normal people (inactivated at 56 C for 30 min).
All other chemicals are Baker Analyzed Reagents (J. T. Baker Chemical Co.).

Reagents

Phosphate-buffered saline (PBS)
PBS(I): 0.075 M potassium phosphate, 0.075 M sodium chloride, pH 7.3.
PBS(II): 0.01 M potassium phosphate, 0.15 M sodium chloride, pH 7.3.
PBS(III): 0.01 M potassium phosphate, 0.1 M sodium chloride, pH 7.3.
McIlvaine buffer: 0.05 M citric acid, 0.1 M disodium hydrogen phosphate, pH 4.9.
Tannic acid (0.05% or 1:20,000), freshly diluted with PBS(II).

Antigens

Native DNA (1 mg/ml N-DNA). Calf thymus DNA is dissolved in McIlvaine buffer or PBS(II) by gentle mixing on a vertical rotating wheel.
Single-stranded DNA (1 mg/ml SS-DNA). SS-DNA is prepared fresh daily by heating N-DNA in a boiling-water bath for 10 min and cooling immediately in an ice-water bath.
Sonically treated DNA (1 mg/ml So-DNA). N-DNA is placed in an ice bath and sonically disrupted for 2 min, at 1-min intervals, with a power Sonifier.
sNP.
Preparation. sNP is prepared from fresh calf

thymus nuclei according to the method of Robitaille and Tan (6) in which the thymocyte nuclei are obtained by the method described by Allfrey, Littau, and Mirsky (1). All preparative steps are performed at 4 C. Six to eight thymuses obtained from freshly killed calves are transported to the laboratory packed in ice, washed in cold 0.25 M sucrose solution containing 0.003 M calcium chloride, trimmed free from blood clots and connective tissues, cut into bite-size pieces, and washed to remove remaining blood. Amounts of 50 g of thymus and 450 ml of sucrose solution are homogenized in a Waring blender at low speed for 4 min. The homogenate is filtered through cheese cloth, and the filtrate is centrifuged at $200 \times g$ for 10 min to sediment the nuclei. Two volumes of cold PBS(II) are added to the precipitate. The nuclei are disrupted in a Waring blender operated at high speed for 4 min and extracted by slow stirring for 30 min. The homogenate is centrifuged at $12,000 \times g$ for 30 min. The sedimented nuclear material is extracted overnight by stirring in three to four times its volume of 1 M NaCl, and the resulting viscous solution is separated from the undissolved material by centrifugation at $27,000 \times g$ for 60 min. The supernatant fluid is decanted and made 0.12 M in NaCl by addition of water, and the precipitate is sedimented at $2,000 \times g$. This precipitate is redissolved in 1 M NaCl. This cycle is repeated two more times, and the final 1 M NaCl solution is stored at -20 C. Further purification steps involve dialysis against decreasing ionic strength buffers to isotonicity with 0.015 M NaCl-0.0015 M sodium citrate, pH 7.0, according to the procedure described by Huang, Bonner, and Murray (3). This consists of dialysis against 0.4 M NaCl for 4 h, 0.3 M NaCl for 1 h, 0.15 M NaCl for 1 h, and 0.015 M NaCl-0.0015 M sodium citrate overnight. The solution is cleared by centrifugation at $27,000 \times g$ for 1 h, and the supernatant fluid is stored at 4 C with 0.1% NaN_3 or lyophilized.

Determination of protein in sNP. The protein content of sNP is measured by the biuret method (8), with assayed human serum as a standard. Protein standards ranging from 50 to 2,000 μg/ml are prepared in saline. sNP is diluted 1:5 and 1:10 in 0.015 M NaCl. Amounts of 1 ml of each standard and each sNP solution are mixed with 2 ml of biuret reagent and incubated for 30 min at 37 C. The absorbances of these solutions are determined at 555 nm with the use of a reagent blank consisting of 2 ml of biuret reagent and 1 ml of saline in the reference cuvette. A calibration curve is plotted. The absorbance value for each sNP sample is used to read the protein concentration from the calibration curve.

Determination of DNA in sNP. The DNA content of sNP is estimated by the diphenylamine method (2). With N-DNA solution as a standard, DNA standards of 5, 10, 20, and 40 μg/ml and sNP dilutions of 1:100 and 1:200 are prepared in 10% perchloric acid solution. A 2-ml amount of 4% diphenylamine freshly prepared in glacial acetic acid is mixed with 2 ml of each standard, test solution, and 10% perchloric acid solution, followed by addition of 100 μliters of aqueous 1.6 mg/ml acetaldehyde solution. After incubation overnight at 30 C, the absorbances at 595 and 700 nm are determined against the reagent blank and the difference $A_{595} - A_{700}$ is calculated. By use of the absorbance difference for the test solution, the DNA content of sNP is read from the curve plotted for the standards ($A_{595} - A_{700}$ versus DNA concentration). The protein to DNA ratio ranges from 0.9 to 1.1.

Formalinization of human erythrocytes

Human erythrocytes are formalinized at 37 C and used to provide DNA-coated cells (4). Attempts to coat these cells with sNP are not successful. However, with the use of cells formalinized at 30 C, sNP-coated cells having high sensitivity and good specificity to sNP and DNA antibodies are consistently obtained (5). Some hemolysis of the cells occurs on standing.

Fresh human type O Rh-negative blood is centrifuged at $800 \times g$ for 4 min, and the cells are washed four times, each time with 7 to 10 volumes of PBS(I), taking care to remove any buffy coat observed on the surface of the cells. After the fourth washing, the cells are suspended to a concentration of 10% in PBS(I), and an equal volume of 3.7% formaldehyde in PBS(I) is added. The suspension is allowed to stand, with occasional stirring, at room temperature for 4 to 6 h. After this preincubation period, the suspension is continuously stirred and incubated at either 30 or 37 C for 14 to 18 h. The formalinized cells are washed four times, each time with 10 volumes of PBS(I), and stored as a 10% suspension in PBS(I) at 4 C. Smaller quantities of cells are formalinized at 30 C because these cells tend to hemolyze on storage, whereas cells treated at 37 C show no hemolysis even after standing for 6 months.

Preparation of sonically treated DNA- and soluble nucleoprotein-coated cells

Formalinized cells are centrifuged and washed once with PBS(II). Usually, 0.5 ml of packed cells is suspended in 25 ml of 1:20,000 tannic acid dissolved in PBS(II) and incubated for 45 min at 37 C, with intermittent mixing. The cells are washed three times, each time with 20 volumes of PBS(II). Final wash is carried out with McIlvaine buffer. The tanned cells are suspended in 12 ml of McIlvaine buffer to which is added either 0.5 ml of sNP (5.3 mg/ml) in 0.015 M NaCl-0.0015 M sodium citrate or 0.62 ml of So-DNA (1.0 mg/ml) in McIlvaine buffer. The suspension is incubated for 1 h at 37 C with intermittent mixing. Cells are packed, washed three times with PBS(II) containing 0.07% bovine serum albumin, and suspended in the BSA-buffer solution to a cell concentration of approximately 1%.

TEST PROCEDURE

Diluents

PBS(III) with 0.07% BSA is used with the sNP-coated cell system, and PBS(III) with 0.2% BSA is used with the So-DNA coupled cells.

Determination of antibodies

With a micropipette (Eppendorf), 25 μliters of sNP (500 μg/ml) is transferred to the first well of the second row. Similarly, 25 μliters of So-DNA (200 μg/ml) is placed in the first well of the third row. In each of the remaining empty wells of rows 1 to 3, a drop of diluent is delivered from a micropipette dropper. With a microdiluter, 25 μliters of serum is added to the first well of each row and serially diluted. After a 15-min incubation at room temperature, one drop of sNP-coated cells is added to each well; the plates are tapped, covered, and allowed to stand at room temperature for 1 h before reading the hemagglutination. With each run known positive and negative controls are included. Hemagglutination titers are given by the last well showing a positive agglutination pattern as indicated by a smooth mat of cells at the bottom of the wells. Negative results are designated by a clearly defined button of cells centered at the bottom of the wells. Intermediate reactions show some properties characteristic of both a positive and negative reaction.

Since sNP is a complex of DNA and histones, agglutination of the sNP-coated cells by the test serum could be caused by antibodies reacting to the DNA moiety of sNP or to the DNA-histone complex. Thus, hemagglutination tests with and without inhibitors give rise to one of three possible patterns exemplified in Table 1. Serum A contains only antibody to DNA. Serum B contains antibodies to sNP, but antibody to DNA cannot be excluded because it may be

TABLE 1. *Possible hemagglutination patterns with sNP-coated cells*

Inhibitor	Hemagglutination titer		
	Serum A	Serum B	Serum C
None	1:128	1:512	1:256
sNP	0	0	0
So-DNA	0	1:512	1:32

present in lower titer. Serum C contains antibodies to DNA and sNP; the titer of sNP antibody is 1:32. Since non-SLE serum may exhibit titers of 1:2, antibody titers of 1:4 and greater are significant. The DNA antibody titer for serum B and C is readily determined from hemagglutination tests with DNA-coated cells. The titration procedure outlined for sNP-coated cells is applicable. DNA antibody specificity obtained by performing hemagglutination-inhibition experiments with So-DNA, SS-DNA, and N-DNA. Nonspecific agglutination may be encountered occasionally, and these agglutinins are removed by prior absorption of the serum with uncoated formalinized cells.

INTERPRETATION

The detection of DNA and sNP antibodies is helpful in the diagnosis of SLE. The pathogenic antibody is the DNA antibody. When DNA is released into the circulation and combines with DNA antibodies, immune complexes are formed with the development of clinical symptoms (7).

sNP is a complex of DNA and histones, and the hemagglutination test utilizing sNP coated cells will detect two antibodies, one showing reactivity to the DNA moiety of sNP and the other to the DNA-histone complex of sNP. Significant antibody titers are 1:4 or greater. Antibody specificity can be determined by inhibition experiments on sera with added DNA or sNP. The anti-sNP antibodies are related to the serum lupus erythematosus factor associated with the lupus erythematosus cell phenomenon (5). The DNA-coated red cell hemagglutination test is more sensitive for detection of native DNA antibodies than the sNP-coated cells.

LITERATURE CITED

1. Allfrey, V. G., V. C. Littau, and A. E. Mirsky. 1964. Methods for the purification of thymus nuclei and their application to studies of nuclear protein synthesis. J. Cell Biol. 21:213–231.
2. Giles, K. W., and A. Myers. 1965. An improved diphenylamine method for estimation of deoxyribonuclei acid. Nature (London) 206:93.
3. Huang, R. C., J. Bonner, and K. Murray. 1964.

Physical and biological properties of soluble nucleohistones. J. Mol. Biol. 8:54–64.

4. Inami, Y. H., R. M. Nakamura, and E. M. Tan. 1973. Microhemagglutination tests for detection of native and single-strand DNA antibodies and circulating DNA antigen. J. Immunol. Methods 3:287–300.

5. Inami, Y. H., R. M. Nakamura, and E. M. Tan. 1975. Microhemagglutination test for the detection of nucleoprotein antibody in systemic lupus erythematosus. Am. J. Clin. Pathol. 64:65–74.

6. Robitaille, P., and E. M. Tan. 1973. Relationship between deoxyribonucleoprotein and deoxyribonucleic acid antibodies in systemic lupus erythematosus. J. Clin. Invest. 52:316–323.

7. Tan, E. M., and H. G. Kunkel, 1966. Characteristics of a soluble nuclear antigen precipitating with sera of patients with systemic lupus erythematosus. J. Immunol. 96:464–471.

8. Weischselbaum, T. E. 1964. An accurate and rapid method for the determination of proteins in small amounts of blood serum and plasma. Am. J. Clin. Pathol. 16:40–49.

Chapter 88

Quantitation of Antibodies to Sm Antigen and Nuclear Ribonucleoprotein by Hemagglutination

E. M. TAN and C. PEEBLES

INTRODUCTION

Antibodies to deoxyribonucleic acid and to deoxyribonucleoprotein were the antinuclear antibodies which were the earliest to be identified by their immunochemical specificities. Subsequently, studies by many investigators demonstrated that antibodies were present in sera of patients with autoimmune diseases which reacted with nuclear antigens of other chemical specificities. In this chapter, a hemagglutination technique is described which will detect antibodies to two saline-soluble nuclear antigens, one called Sm and the other, nuclear ribonucleoprotein (RNP).

Antibody to Sm antigen was first described and the nuclear antigen was partially characterized in 1966 (8). Antibody to nuclear RNP has been described by a number of investigators (1, 2, 4, 5). Antibody to Sm antigen is present almost exclusively in systemic lupus erythematosus, and the suggestion has been raised that antibody to Sm might be a marker antibody for this disease (3). Antibody to nuclear RNP occurs in a number of systemic rheumatic diseases, including systemic lupus erythematosus, discoid lupus, and progressive systemic sclerosis (3, 6). However, antibody to nuclear RNP was first identified in patients who appeared to have an "overlap" syndrome, with symptoms of systemic lupus erythematosus, systemic sclerosis, and dermatomyositis (6). This clinical entity was called the "mixed connective tissue disease" (MCTD) syndrome. Characteristic features have now become apparent in the MCTD syndrome — presence of extremely high concentrations of antibodies to nuclear RNP, relatively low prevalence of renal disease, and good response to treatment with corticosteroids (6).

The nuclear antigens Sm and RNP are only two of many nuclear antigens which are saline soluble and easily extracted from the nucleus. The Sm antigen is a nonhistone nuclear protein which is devoid of nucleic acids. Its antigenicity is not destroyed by treatment with ribonuclease (RNase). On the other hand, nuclear RNP is thought to consist of a complex of ribonucleic acid and protein, and the antigenicity of RNP is destroyed by digestion with RNase. Sensitivity (RNP) or resistance (Sm) to RNase is the basis for distinguishing between antibodies to RNP and Sm in the hemagglutination test.

The earlier literature has referred to ENA (extractable nuclear antigen) and to RNase-sensitive and RNase-resistant ENA. This has been a source of some confusion, and it would be preferable to refer directly to Sm or RNP systems. In the hemagglutination assay described below, with few exceptions, the antibodies detected are against Sm and RNP. The assay system utilizes lyophilized rabbit thymus as the source of antigens. This is convenient because the antigens can be obtained commercially, which makes it unnecessary to isolate calf thymus nuclei to obtain the antigens in the manner originally described (2, 6).

HEMAGGLUTINATION ASSAY

Principle

Tanned sheep erythrocytes are coated with an extract of rabbit thymus containing Sm and RNP antigens. A portion of the treated cells is incubated with RNase to selectively remove the RNP antigen. A passive hemagglutination test is performed in a microtiter system with the use of parallel dilutions of the patient's serum against both the untreated and treated cells. A positive hemagglutination with both the untreated and treated cells indicates antibody to Sm antigen. A positive hemagglutination with the untreated and a negative hemagglutination with the treated cells indicates antibody to RNP.

Reagents

Phosphate-buffered saline (PBS): 0.01 M PO$_4$, 0.15 M NaCl, pH 7.2.

McIlvaine's buffered saline, pH 7.8: 0.02 M Na$_2$HPO$_4$, 0.15 M NaCl; adjusted to pH 7.8 with 0.1 M citric acid.

Tannic acid, 0.005% (wt/vol): prepared *fresh* just prior to use.

Normal calf serum (NCS), 1% (vol/vol), in PBS. See below, Serum preparations.

RNase solution (Worthington Biochemical Co.): 1 mg of RNase in 1 ml of 1% NCS will treat cells for one set of plates.

Rabbit thymus acetone powder (Pel-Freez Biologicals, Rogers, Ark.).

Sheep erythrocytes in Alsever's solution (Colorado Serum Co.).

Serum preparations

Control sera:

Serum positive for antibody to Sm antigen.

Serum positive for antibody to RNP antigen.

Normal human serum.

1. Prepare a 1:10 (vol/vol) dilution of the patients' sera and control sera in PBS (0.05 ml of serum + 0.45 ml of PBS).

2. Inactivate samples at 56 C for 30 min.

3. Inactivate calf serum (neat) at 56 C for 30 min.

4. Absorb samples for 30 min at room temperature with equal volumes of packed sheep erythrocytes that have been washed four times with PBS. See below, Cell preparation (0.5 ml of sample + 0.5 ml of packed sheep erythrocytes). The calf serum is absorbed a second time with packed sheep erythrocytes.

5. Centrifuge samples in a serofuge and remove supernatant serum for use in testing.

Note: The sample preparation may be done 1 or 2 days before testing. Extra absorbed calf serum may be stored frozen at −20 C for future use.

Rabbit thymus extract preparation

1. To each 60 mg of rabbit thymus powder add 1 ml of PBS.

2. Extract for 4 h at 4 C on a magnetic stirrer using a low speed to avoid denaturation.

3. Centrifuge at 10,000 × g (Brinkman microcentrifuge) for 2 min.

4. Determine the protein concentration of the supernatant fluid. This varies from 8 to 10 mg of protein per ml.

5. This saline extract of rabbit thymus which contains Sm and RNP antigens can be stored in small portions at −20 C and is stable for at least 10 weeks. The extract containing antigens is always cleared by centrifugation prior to use for coupling to erythrocytes.

Note: Care must be taken to keep reagents cold to avoid enzymatic digestion of the antigens.

Cell preparation

1. Prepare enough cells in suspension to make 0.1 ml of packed cells for each set of four microtiter plates. Add another 0.05 ml of packed cells for control cells.

2. Centrifuge at 2,300 rpm for 6 min (IEC PR2 centrifuge), standard speed and time.

3. Wash cells four times with PBS with gentle resuspension.

4. Resuspend the cells after the final wash to give a 2.5% (vol/vol) suspension in PBS. An easy method is to use 0.3 ml of packed sheep erythrocytes + 11.7 ml of PBS.

Tanning of cells

1. Mix gently equal volumes of a 2.5% suspension of sheep erythrocytes and 0.005% tannic acid in PBS which has been warmed to 37 C.

2. Incubate for 15 min in a 37 C water bath with gentle swirling at 5 and 10 min.

3. Centrifuge.

4. Wash two times with PBS. (This should be at least 20 times the volume of packed sheep erythrocytes.)

5. Resuspend to 2.5% suspension and remove a 2-ml sample for cell control. The rest of the cells are to be coated with antigen and will be designated test cells.

Coupling of antigens to sheep erythrocytes

Erythrocytes are coated at an antigen concentration of 1 mg of rabbit thymus extract for each 0.05 ml of packed sheep erythrocytes.

1. Prepare sufficient antigen in McIlvaine's saline buffer to have 1 mg of rabbit thymus extract in 2 ml. Each 2-ml amount will coat 0.05 ml of packed sheep erythrocytes.

2. Centrifuge washed cell samples.

3. Resuspend the tanned cells with 10 ml McIlvaine's saline buffer for each 0.05 ml of packed cells in both test cells and control. (If a large number of cells are to be sensitized, this step should be done in an Erlenmeyer flask.)

4. Add 2 ml of McIlvaine's saline buffer to the tube containing the control cells.

5. Add 2 ml of antigen solution to the test cells for each 0.05 ml of packed sheep erythrocytes.

6. Cap and mix gently.

7. Incubate at 37 C for 1 h. Swirl or shake gently at 10-min intervals for even coating of cells.

8. Centrifuge.

9. Wash cells three times with 1% NCS. Wash sides of the tubes carefully to remove any free antigen.

10. Add 5 ml of 1% NCS for each 0.05 ml of packed sheep erythrocytes to the control cells and *one half* of the *test cells*. These cells are ready to use.

11. Add 4 ml of 1% NCS and 1 ml of ribonuclease solution containing 1 mg of ribonuclease/ml for each 0.05 ml of packed sheep erythrocytes to the *other half* of the *test cells*.

12. Incubate at 37 C in the water bath for 30 min with gentle mixing at 10-min intervals. These RNase-treated cells are now ready for use.

Performance of hemagglutination test
  Materials.

Pipette droppers: 0.025-ml calibration (Cooke Engineering).

Microdiluters: 0.025-ml calibration (Cooke Engineering).

Disposable V-shaped microtiter plates (Cooke Engineering).

Diluent: 1% (vol/vol) NCS in PBS.

Sera for titration: see section on Serum preparations.

Cells:

  Control cells.

  Test cells coated with rabbit thymus extract.

  Test cells coated with thymus extract and treated with RNase.

Controls:

  Serum positive for Sm antibody.

  Serum positive for RNP antibody.

  Normal human serum

  Antibody controls—patient's serum + tanned sheep erythrocytes.

  Cell controls—diluent + cells.

  Procedure.

1. Label four plates for each set of eight sera to be tested. Two plates are for test cells and two plates are for RNase-treated test cells. Sera are titered to 22 wells. The next to the last vertical row of the second plate is labeled antibody control. The three wells of the last vertical row on the test plate containing the serum controls are labeled for cell control—tanned cells, test cells, RNase-treated test cells.

2. Add with the pipette dropper 0.025 ml of diluent to each well.

3. Add with a diluter 0.025 ml of patient and/or control serum to the proper antibody control well.

4. Mix well by twirling about 10 times.

5. Remove and blot.

6. Add 0.025 ml of the patient and/or control serum to the first well of the plate using the same diluter.

7. Repeat this procedure until all sample diluters are in the first wells.

8. Make serial dilutions of the eight samples stimultaneously.

9. Mix well by twirling about 10 times in each well.

10. Blot the loops when the dilutions are finished, rinse several times in distilled water, flame to incandescence, and plunge into distilled water. Dry and use again.

11. Add 0.025 ml of the control cells with a pipette dropper to the row of antibody control wells and to the cell control for tanned sheep cells.

12. Add 0.025 ml of the test cells with a pipette dropper to each of the appropriate serum dilutions and to the cell control labeled for test cells.

13. Add 0.025 ml of RNase-treated cells with a pipette dropper to each of the appropriate serum dilutions and to the cell control labeled for RNase test cells.

14. Tap plates gently to mix. Examine and remove bubbles on the bottom of the wells. (Toothpicks work well for this.)

15. Cover with plate sealers.

16. Allow cells to settle for at least 2 h at room temperature and observe hemagglutination reaction. The plates may be left overnight before reading with no appreciable change in results.

Results

Positive: A smooth mat of cells covering the bottom of the well (+).

Negative: A clearly defined button in the bottom of the well (−).

Intermediate: Incomplete settling of cells with no clearly defined button. The reactions are noted (±) but not reported.

End point: Highest dilution giving a positive reaction.

INTERPRETATION

An illustration of the results which can be obtained with the hemagglutination test is presented in Fig. 1.

Serum EB is positive to well 8 with test cells and with RNase-treated test cells to well 9. This difference of one well is not significant, and the results essentially demonstrated that EB has antibody to Sm antigen to a titer of 1:1,280. Note that antibody to RNP, if present in lower titer than 1:1,280, would not have been detected.

Serum BN is positive with test cells to well 12, but with RNase-treated test cells the titer dropped to less than 1:10. Serum BN contains only antibody to RNP to a titer of 1:20,480.

Serum PH is positive with test cells to well 12, but with RNase-treated test cells the titer dropped partially to well 6. This serum contains antibody to RNP to a titer of 1:20,480 and antibody to Sm to a titer of 1:640.

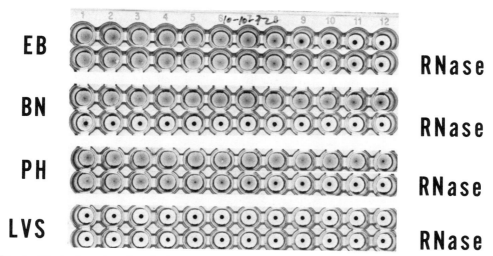

FIG. 1. *Illustration of results which might be obtained in hemagglutination tests for antibodies to Sm and nuclear RNP. Serum EB contained only antibody Sm, the titer remaining about the same before and after RNase treatment. BN had antibody only to nuclear RNP. PH had antibodies to both Sm and RNP, with antibody to RNP present in higher concentration than antibody to Sm. LVS was a negative control.*

Serum LVS is negative for antibodies to Sm or RNP.

All cell controls and antibody control wells should be negative. If a positive result occurs in the antibody controls, the serum was not sufficiently absorbed with sheep erythrocytes. If any of the cell controls are positive, then nonspecific agglutinations cannot be ruled out.

There are several steps in the procedure that affect the sensitivity and specificity of the test. Stavitsky (7) reported that the cell concentration and the antigen concentration to be coupled were of definite significance. With increased cell concentration, there is a decrease in sensitivity. Too great an excess of antigen to be coupled to the cells results in nonspecific agglutination, reducing the specificity. Serum which has been inactivated and absorbed with sheep erythrocytes is used to prevent nonspecific agglutination due to complement or heterophile antibodies. Serum is always used, as various anticoagulants may give different results which are not comparable (7). Other factors which influence the results are the pH of the coupling buffer and the RNase used for digestion. The pH of 7.8 gives optimal coating of both Sm and RNP, and the concentration of the RNase allows for proper digestion of the RNP for differentiation.

Since there are so many variables involved in hemagglutination, there are important limitations to these methods. Stavitsky mentioned occasional lack of reproducibility, qualitative rather than quantitative in nature, and occasional nonspecificity. These variables are largely due to variations in the erythrocytes with prolonged in vitro storage. This can be overcome by using fresh blood or blood in Alsevers' solution. To account for these variables, it is necessary to test simultaneously standard samples with known agglutination titers.

In spite of the variables, with proper adherence to the technique, this test can identify specific antinuclear antibodies which are valuable to proper diagnosis, prognosis, and treatment.

ACKNOWLEDGMENTS

This work was supported by Public Health Service grants AM 12198 and AI 10386.

LITERATURE CITED

1. Koffler, D., R. Carr, V. Agnello, R. Thoburn, and H. Kunkel. 1971. Antibodies to polynucleotides in human sera: antigenic specificity and relation to disease. J. Exp. Med. 134:294–312.
2. Northway, J. D., and E. M. Tan. 1972. Differentiation of antinuclear antibodies giving speckled staining patterns in immunofluorescence. Clin. Immunol. Immunopathol. 1:140–154.
3. Notman, D., N. Kurata, and E. M. Tan. 1975. Profiles of antinuclear antibodies in systemic rheumatic diseases. Ann. Intern. Med. 83:464–469.
4. Reichlin, M., and M. Mattioli. 1972. Correlation of a precipitin reaction to an RNA protein antigen and a low prevalence of nephritis in patients with systemic lupus erythematosus. N. Engl. J. Med. 286:908–911.

5. Sharp, G. C., W. S. Irvin, R. L. Laroque, C. Velez, V. Daly, A. D. Kaiser, and H. R. Holman. 1971. Association of autoantibodies to different nuclear antigens with clinical patterns of rheumatic disease and responsiveness to therapy. J. Clin. Invest. 50:350–359.

6. Sharp, G. C., W. S. Irvin, E. M. Tan, R. G. Gould, and H. R. Holman. 1972. Mixed connective tissue disease—an apparently distinct rheumatic disease syndrome associated with a specific antibody to an extractable nuclear antigen (ENA). Am. J. Med. 52:148–159.

7. Stavitsky, A. B. 1954. Micromethods for the study of proteins and antibodies. I. Procedure and general applications of hemagglutination and hemagglutination-inhibition reactions with tannic acid and protein-treated red blood cells. J. Immunol. 72:360–367.

8. Tan, E. M., and H. G. Kunkel. 1966. Characteristics of a soluble nuclear antigen precipitating with sera of patients with systemic lupus erythematosus. J. Immunol. 96:464–471.

Chapter 89

Tests for Detection of the Rheumatoid Factors

ROBERT WINCHESTER

INTRODUCTION

The term "rheumatoid factors" refers to a diverse group of immunoglobulins found most notably in patients with rheumatoid arthritis. These antibodies react specifically with the Fc regions of immunoglobulin G (IgG) molecules; thus, they are more properly, but less commonly, referred to as anti-IgG or antigamma globulins. There are a number of tests available, each with advantages and limitations. The primary test selected for presentation is the latex test originally described by Singer and Plotz, in which human fraction II is used as the antigen (7). This test is widely used because of its reliability and simplicity and the ready availability of reagents. In addition, a second simple technique of aggregated IgG precipitation of particular use in special situations will be discussed.

The principle of all the commonly used methods for the demonstration of rheumatoid factors involves the use of an indicator system containing a large number of IgG molecules. The IgG is either bound to carrier particles, such as latex, bentonite, or erythrocytes, or IgG molecules are simply aggregated by heat denaturation or other means. The presence of rheumatoid factor is recognized by agglutination, flocculation, or precipitation of the respective indicator system (9). Serial dilutions of the serum provide an estimate of the quantity of the rheumatoid factor in terms of titer.

The basis of agglutination of precipitation of rheumatoid factors with aggregated IgG on indicator particles was debated for many years. Available evidence now indicates that the aggregated IgG does not contain new antigenic determinants for rheumatoid factors, but that the positive reactions depend on the antigenic multivalency of IgG achieved by aggregation of these molecules.

Although rheumatoid factors occur in each major immunoglobulin class, most systems primarily reflect the amount of IgM rheumatoid factor because of the efficacy of IgM molecules in agglutination reactions, attributed to the pentavalence of these molecules. Furthermore, all tests for rheumatoid factors are inhibited by serum IgG to some degree. Indeed certain IgM

rheumatoid factors are so strongly inhibited by serum IgG that they can be detected only if IgG is completely removed, for example, by gel filtration in acid buffers. Rheumatoid factors detectable in this manner have been termed "hidden rheumatoid factors" (1).

IgG rheumatoid factors are usually difficult to demonstrate by conventional and easily performed assays, although they are sometimes the dominant class of rheumatoid factor in a patient. The poor detectability of the IgG rheumatoid factors primarily arises because they are bivalent and usually have on their Fc regions the antigenic determinant to which their antibody specificity is directed. Thus, they preferentially self-associate to form complexes of several IgG rheumatoid factors that are demonstrable by analytic ultracentrifugation as the "intermediate complexes."

CLINICAL INDICATIONS

The most common use of an assay for rheumatoid factors is to seek support for a diagnosis of rheumatoid arthritis in a patient with inflammatory arthritis. Less commonly, in situations where chronic inflammatory disease is suspected, such as bacterial endocarditis, tuberculosis, leprosy, etc., a positive test may be a useful adjunct to diagnosis. Knowledge of the amount of the rheumatoid factors is also useful, along with other tests in this section, in establishing a profile of the abnormal immune response in the various diseases with autoimmune features.

Sjögren's syndrome, often with an associated cryoprecipitate, and benign hyperglobulinemic purpura of Waldenström require strongly positive tests to support their diagnosis. Patients with diffuse interstitial pulmonary fibrosis and those with subacute pericarditis should also be tested for the possibility of unsuspected rheumatoid disease or related pathological processes. Along with a search for a cryoprecipitate, rheumatoid factors should be assayed in adult patients with vasculitis, purpura, and petechial rashes (particularly when limited to the legs), nephritis, and malignancies of the lymphoid system. Here, one is concerned with uncovering what may prove to be a monoclonal rheumatoid factor that is responsible for the findings.

TEST PROCEDURES

Latex-human IgG (fraction II) slide agglutination

Materials.

Serological slide with divided wells.
Glycine-buffered saline (GBS).
Latex-human IgG reagent.
Standard positive serum and normal serum.

Method.

1. Heat-inactivate serum for 30 min at 56 C, and dilute 1:20 using 0.1 ml of serum and 1.9 ml of GBS.
2. In a slide with divided wells, add one big drop of diluted serum (0.04 ml) and one drop of undiluted latex-human IgG. Mix completely with a separate piece of applicator stick.
3. Read after 5 min of incubation at room temperature by inspection against a black background. Score as trace or 1+ to 4+ positive, with 4+ designating the agglutination of all the latex reagent into a few large clumps.
4. With each group of samples, include a normal serum control.

Latex-human IgG (fraction II) tube dilution of Singer and Plotz

Materials.

Test tubes, 10 × 75 mm; pipettes, 2 ml.
GBS.
Latex-F_{II} reagent.
Centrifuge: A Serofuge (Clay Adams Co., Inc.) is suitable.
A simple photometer capable of measuring the density of suspension of latex by nephelometry.

Method.

1. Heat-inactivate serum for 30 min at 56 C, and dilute 1:20 using 0.1 ml of serum and 1.9 ml of GBS in a 10 × 75 mm test tube.
2. Place 1.0 ml of GBS into eight additional tubes, and serially dilute with 1.0 ml from the first tube, discarding 1.0 ml from the last tube.
3. Add 1.0 ml of latex-human IgG reagent as prepared below to each tube and to an additional control tube containing 1 ml of GBS. Incubate for 30 min at 4 C, for 90 min at 56 C, and for 5 min in the Serofuge.
4. Centrifuge.
5. Read by tapping the bottom to dislodge the flocculate and view against a black background; score each tube as positive (+) or negative (−). The highest tube dilution showing

agglutination defines the titer of rheumatoid factor.

Aggregated IgG precipitin test (4)

Materials.

Microhematocrit capillary tubes and clayboard.
Heat-aggregated IgG solution at a concentration of 15 mg/ml.
Control positive and normal serum.

Method.

1. Heat-inactivate serum for 30 min at 56 C, and, if turbid, clarify by centrifugation.
2. Draw some aggregated IgG solution into a 1-ml pipette and lay it horizontally at the bench edge.
3. Avoiding fingerprints on the tube by gripping only a tip, dip the microhematocrit tube into the serum to load it with a column about 1 cm in length. Wipe off excess serum on the outside of the capillary.
4. Without allowing the serum to run up the tube and thus leave an interposed air bubble, fill 1 to 2 cm of the capillary with the aggregated IgG solution.
5. Insert the capillary, serum end down, in the clayboard, and observe for precipitation against a black background with oblique illumination.
6. The intensity of the reaction is readily assessed by a simple scale. A 4+ positive reaction is evident as immediate gross flocculation; weaker reactions appear as a band at the interface over several minutes. A 3+ reaction begins to appear in 0.5 min, and a 1+ reaction appears by 5 to 10 min. Observation is not usually continued past 30 min.

REAGENTS

Latex-human IgG (fraction II)

Slide test. For the slide test, a commercial preparation such as Hyland Laboratories latex globulin reagent is preferable because the longer shelf life justifies the added cost. This is particularly important if the assay is performed on one or two sera per day.

Tube dilution method. The reagent for the tube dilution method is prepared as follows:

1. Make a stock solution of Cohn fraction II human IgG such as that sold by Difco (250 mg per ampoule). Layer the lyophilized fraction II on 40 ml of GBS and centrifuge for 10 min at 500 to 1,000 × g; dilute to 250 ml with GBS. This is stable at 4 C for several months if a preservative is added.
2. Add 1.0 ml of 0.81-μm latex spherules (Difco latex) to 100 ml of GBS, adjust the con-

centration of the spherules using a photometer (Klett, red filter, reading 250 ± 5, or a lumetron red, 20%) to guide in addition of slightly more buffer or latex. Add 5.0 ml of fraction II solution and incubate at 37 C for 90 min. The final reagent should be prepared fresh on the day used.

Glycine saline buffer

In a 2-liter volumetric flask, add 15 g of glycine HCl and 20 g of sodium chloride. Add nearly 2 liters of distilled water and adjust the pH to 8.20 using 3.6 to 4.0 ml of 1.0 N NaOH. Bring final volume to 2,000 ml, and store at 4 C.

Soluble aggregated fraction II IgG

Dissolve 150 mg of fraction II IgG in 10 ml of unbuffered 0.85% sodium chloride as described above. Some preparations of IgG containing glycine, etc., should be dialyzed overnight to remove the stabilizer since it interferes with aggregation. Heat the fraction II IgG in a water bath, monitoring the temperature of the solution so it remains between 62.5 and 63.5 C for 10 to 12 min; render 0.02% sodium azide, and store at 4 C. The useful life of the preparation is several months. Some preparations of fraction II are unsuitable for heat aggregation because their particular treatment alters the manner in which they aggregate, causing either complete precipitation or no significant aggregation.

INTERPRETATION

A properly performed latex fixation test has very few factors that might cause a false-positive reaction. Incompletely heat-inactivated C1q, especially if present at elevated levels, unusual hyperlipidemic states, and bulky cryoglobulins are potential reasons for false-positive results. Occasionally, in earlier reports, the term "false positive" was applied to instances of rheumatoid factors being found in the absence of rheumatoid arthritis, but this usage is obsolete.

Since increased levels of rheumatoid factors may accompany certain acute immune responses such as infectious mononucleosis and may also be found in a considerable percentage of elderly individuals, the interpretation of the clinical significance of a positive test result must be made with caution. Extremely high titers usually present no problem in interpretation, but titers of 1:20 to 1:80 raise considerable questions, since such titers may be found in early rheumatoid arthritis as well as in situations mentioned above.

It should be remembered that in diseases such as sarcoidosis, systemic lupus erythematosus, and Sjögren's syndrome the arthritis is not considered to be rheumatoid arthritis despite the positive test for rheumatoid factor. The marked elevation of IgG characteristic of these diseases suggests that a disease other than rheumatoid arthritis is responsible for the rheumatoid factors, since marked hyperglobulinemia is not common in patients with rheumatoid arthritis.

The common rheumatoid factors found in rheumatoid arthritis are polyclonal and rarely, if ever, precipitate with native IgG at 4 C. However, another variety termed "cold-reactive rheumatoid factor" is more frequently monoclonal and forms mixed cryoprecipitates with native IgG (2). This latter variety occurs in some patients with systemic lupus, Sjögren's syndrome, and infectious mononucleosis, but most notably in vasculitis associated with a lymphoid malignancy. In some instances, the cold-reactive rheumatoid factor has had a pH optimum around 6.8 and is poorly reactive at the higher pH and ionic strength of the latex system (5, 6). The recognition of this type of rheumatoid factor is perhaps most easily made through the use of aggregate precipitation methods. The cryoprecipitate or serum containing a cryoprecipitate should be solubilized by incubating at 37 C, and debris and fibrin should be removed by centrifugation. Laboratories that expect to detect frequently rheumatoid factors of this variety should use an agglutination system that favors their ready detection. The human anti-Rh antibody "Ripley" coated erythrocytes provide the best indicator system for cold-reactive rheumatoid factors, but other methods of coating IgG on erythrocytes should prove equally acceptable (2, 5, 8), since the "Ripley" serum is available in limited quantities.

IgG rheumatoid factors are found in abundance in many patients with rheumatoid arthritis as well as Sjögren's syndrome. In younger women with extreme hypergammaglobulinemia and positive rheumatoid factor tests, the syndrome. of the hypergammaglobulinemic purpura of Waldenström should be considered (3). This interesting condition presents clinically with nonpruritic petechial lesions on the legs, characteristically appearing after prolonged sitting or standing. These patients uniformly have abundant IgG rheumatoid factor with varying amounts of IgM rheumatoid factor. One test that readily distinguishes this condition from other states of hypergammaglobulinemia is the formation of a turbid precipitate on diluting the serum with 15 volumes of distilled water. This is due to precipitation of the self-associated IgG rheumatoid factor complexes. Any sera with high levels of IgM will also form similar precipitates (Sia test).

Seronegative rheumatoid arthritis is a term that designates patients who meet the ARA diagnostic criteria for rheumatoid arthritis but in whom the rheumatoid factor test is negative. In some instances, the tests for rheumatoid factors are negative because circulating immune complexes are present in such quantity that they compete with the particulate system for the rheumatoid factors. In most instances, however, no rheumatoid factor, even of the "hidden" variety, can be found. These patients also fail to exhibit a number of other laboratory findings such as lowered joint fluid complement and immune complexes usually found in rheumatoid arthritis patients.

LITERATURE CITED

1. Allen, J. C., and H. G. Kunkel. 1966. Hidden rheumatoid factors with specificity for native γ globulin. Arthritis Rheum. 9:758-768.
2. Capra, J. D., R. J. Winchester, and H. G. Kunkel. 1969. Cold-reactive rheumatoid factors in infectious mononucleosis and other diseases. Arthritis Rheum. 12:67-73.
3. Capra, J. D., R. J. Winchester, and H. G. Kunkel. 1971. Hypergammaglobulinemic purpura. Studies on the unusual anti-γ-globulins characteristic of the sera of these patients. Medicine 50:125-138.
4. Edelman, G. M., H. G. Kunkel, and E. C. Franklin. 1958. Interaction of rheumatoid factor with antigen-antibody complexes and aggregated gamma globulin. J. Exp. Med. 108:105-120.
5. Kritzman, J., H. G. Kunkel, J. McCarthy, and R. C. Mellors. 1961. Studies of a Waldenstrom-type macroglobulin with rheumatoid factor properties. J. Lab. Clin. Med. 57:905-917.
6. Logothetis, J., W. R. Kennedy, A. Ellington, and R. C. Williams. 1968. Cryoglobulinemic neuropathy: incidence and clinical characteristics. Arch. Neurol. 19:389-397.
7. Singer, J. M., and C. M. Plotz. 1956. The latex fixation test. I. Application to the serologic diagnosis of rheumatoid arthritis. Am. J. Med. 21:888-892.
8. Waller, M. V., and J. H. Vaughan. 1956. Use of anti-Rh sera for demonstrating agglutination activating factor in rheumatoid arthritis. Proc. Soc. Exp. Biol. Med. 92:198-200.
9. Ziff, M. 1957. The agglutination reaction in rheumatoid arthritis. J. Chronic Dis. 5:644-667.

Chapter 90

Detection of Immune Complexes

VINCENT AGNELLO

INTRODUCTION

In recent years, the development of a variety of new procedures for detecting immune complexes has facilitated the accumulation of evidence which now indicates that antigen-antibody complexes have a pathological role in a wide variety of diseases. The techniques currently available for detecting circulating immune complexes have recently been reviewed (11). There are a number of physiochemical and biological techniques which have been employed for the detection of circulating immune complexes in human diseases. However, these for the most part are research laboratory procedures. At present, a clinically well-proven, simple, sensitive assay for all types of immune complexes is not available.

The physiochemical methods currently used are unsuitable for adaptation to routine clinical tests because of the elaborate equipment and time required for their performance. Among the biological techniques, a major approach to the detection of immune complexes in pathological fluids has been the use of reagents which will react with complexes of immunoglobulins (Ig's) but not monomeric Ig molecules. Two such reagents are the C1q component of complement and monoclonal anti-IgG. This chapter will be concerned with methods for detecting immune complexes which utilize these two reagents, since at present this appears to be the most promising approach for development of standard clinical methods for detection of circulating complexes. Those techniques which are well tested and with which I have experience will be described in detail in a laboratory manual format. Radioimmunoassays which have only recently been described and have not been widely tested will be described here only in general terms for the purpose of discussion which may aid in further development. In addition, another biological approach which has been used in recent years, the detecting of complexes by aggregation of platelets, will be briefly considered.

The C1q molecule, a subunit of the first component of complement, binds with monomeric IgG1, IgG2, IgG3, and IgM (12). However, the binding is greatly enhanced by aggregation of these Ig's (6), and, under proper conditions, soluble Ig aggregates can be precipitated by C1q (13). This direct reaction of C1q with aggregated Ig can be demonstrated in a gel diffusion system (Fig. 1) and forms the basis for a qualitative assay for aggregated Ig or antigen-antibody complexes that react with complement (4). More recently, methods employing radioisotope-labeled C1q have been developed for quantitative determination of immune complexes (14, 18), making the potential clinical usefulness of this approach to detection of immune complexes considerably greater.

The 19S anti-IgG, or rheumatoid factor (RF) as it is more commonly called, can be used in a similar way to the C1q molecule for detection of complexes (20). In gel diffusion it precipitates with aggregated IgG (Fig. 1) but not monomeric IgG or other Ig's. Monoclonal 19S anti-IgG (mRF) shows a greater ability for precipitating complexes than does polyclonal anti-IgG (pRF) found in rheumatoid arthritis (20). Also, it precipitates with small heat aggregates of IgG that escape precipitation by most pRFs or C1q (Fig. 2).

Precipitin reactions with mRF in free solution are more sensitive in detecting complexes than in gel diffusion, but it now appears that both these methods will be supplanted by techniques using radioisotope-labeled anti-IgG similar to the one recently reported (10).

The platelet aggregate reaction for detection of immune complexes is based on the phenomenon of interaction of complexes with the surface of platelets which causes alteration of the platelets, resulting in platelet aggregation. The aggregation is not based on cross-linking of platelets by complexes but is due to changes in the adhesive properties of the platelets. Viable platelets must be used in the reaction since the surface alteration in the presence of immune complexes is dependent on metabolic state. The technique has been used mainly in detecting immune complexes involving known viral antigens (15, 21) but can be used as well to detect immune complexes when the antigen is unknown (19).

669

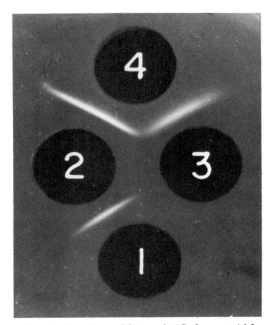

FIG. 1. *Reactions of C1q and 19S rheumatoid factors with aggregated Ig. The effect of reduction and alkylation on the reaction of aggregated Ig and C1q is shown. (1) Purified C1q; (2) aggregated Ig; (3) aggregated Ig reduced and alkylated; (4) purified rheumatoid factor. Reprinted from Agnello et al. (4), with permission.*

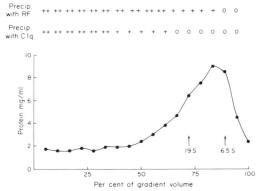

FIG. 2. *Sucrose density gradient fractionation of aggregated Ig. Precipitation of various size aggregates with C1q or RF in gel diffusion is indicated at the top. The positions of the 19S and 6.5S markers are indicated.*

CLINICAL INDICATIONS

Immune complexes have been implicated in the pathological process in systemic lupus erythematosus (SLE), rheumatoid arthritis, hypocomplementemia glomerulus nephritis, derma-

titis herpetiformis, pemphigus, and a variety of syndromes associated with infectious states such as hepatitis, subacute bacterial endocarditis, and leprosy. However, the clinical usefulness of detection of circulating complexes or levels of complexes in other body fluids has not as yet been well assessed. Part of the reason for this has been the lack of a simple methodology which could be widely applied. In SLE and rheumatoid synovitis, immune complexes have been shown to correlate with disease activity and depression of complement. But even in these diseases, which are probably the most extensively studied immune complexes in humans, it is not established whether detection of immune complexes affords any advantage over hemolytic complement determination alone. These questions remain to be answered by clinical immunology laboratories with large populations of patients that can be screened, perhaps by use of some of the newer methods described in this chapter.

At present, there are not sufficient comparative data on the methods described here to indicate selective advantages of a given method for specific disease, with the following exceptions. Methods utilizing the C1q reagent can be applied only to complexes that activate the complement system. Monoclonal 19S anti-IgG is the reagent of choice in studying small complexes such as the intermediate-sized ones found in the serum of some patients with rheumatoid arthritis.

TEST PROCEDURES

Methods utilizing C1q

A. Gel diffusion
Preparation of 0.6% agarose gel in pH 7.2 0.05 M phosphate-0.01 M ethylenediaminetetraacetate (EDTA):

1. Dilute 12.3 ml of 0.5 M KH_2PO_4 and 11.3 ml of 1.0 M Na_2HPO_4 to 800 ml with distilled water.

2. Add 8.0 ml of 1.0 M (Na_4)EDTA and adjust the solution to pH 7.2 with 1.0 N HCl (approximately 4.8 ml).

3. Add 4.8 g of agarose (Sea Kem Agarose; Marine Colloids, Inc.) and 0.08 g of NaN_3.

4. Heat in a boiling-water bath; then filter through a 10-cm Büchner funnel with Whatman no. 2 filter paper. Preheat the filter and suction flask first by pouring boiling distilled water through.

5. Divide into 100-ml batches and store at 4 C.

6. Pour gels just before use. Pipette 22 ml into a 9-cm petri dish to give a 5 mm thick gel.

Wells are cut 9 mm in diameter with a center to center distance of 12 mm.

Wells have a capacity of approximately 0.15 ml. Specimens to be tested are diffused against a solution of C1q at 200 μg/ml. Plates are incubated at 22 C for 48 h. Precipitin lines obtained can then be further intensified by incubation at 0 C for up to 72 h. Pathological sera are initially screened undiluted. Positive specimens are then tested in twofold dilution to 1:16. A normal serum and positive control are routinely run with each batch of unknowns.

B. Radioimmunoassay methods

Radiolabeled C1q binding test utilizing polyethylene glycol (14):

This method is based on two phenomena, the binding of C1q by antigen-antibody complexes and precipitation of antigen-antibody complexes by polyethylene glycol (9). The test specimens are heated at 56 C for 30 min, and 200 μliters is incubated with C1q labeled with ^{125}I. Polyethylene glycol is then added to a final concentration of 2.5% to precipitate gamma globulin complexes. Trace amounts of C1q bound by complexes can then be quantitated by measuring the radioactivity in the precipitate.

C1q deviation test (18):

This method is based on the inhibition by immune complexes of radiolabeled C1q uptake by sheep erythrocytes coated with antierythrocyte IgG. A 50-μliter amount of serum is diluted fivefold so that the conductance of the final solution is 7 mmho/cm. The solution is then heated at 56 C for 30 min, [^{125}I]C1q is added, and the mixture is incubated for 15 min at 20 C. Sensitized erythrocytes are then added, and another 15-min incubation at 20 C is performed. Cells are then separated from the fluid phase in 40% sucrose. The uptake of [^{125}I]C1q by cells with and without the test specimen is determined, and the percent inhibition is calculated.

Methods utilizing monoclonal anti-immunoglobulin G

A. Gel diffusion

Preparation of 0.6% agar gel in pH 7.2 0.05 M phosphate-buffered saline:

1. Dilute 12.3 ml of 0.5 M KH_2PO_4 and 11.3 ml of 1.0 M Na_2HPO_4 to 800 ml with distilled water, and add 7.0 g of NaCl.

2. Add 4.8 g of purified agar (Baltimore Biological Laboratory, Baltimore, Md.) and 0.08 g of NaN_3.

3. Heat in a boiling-water bath; then filter through a 10-cm Büchner funnel with Whatman no. 2 filter paper. Preheat the filter and

suction flask first by pouring boiling distilled water through.

4. Divide into 100-ml batches and store at 4 C.

5. Pour gel just before use. Pipette 22 ml into a 9-cm petri dish to give a 5 mm thick gel. Wells are cut 9 mm in diameter with a center to center distance of 12 mm.

Wells have a capacity of approximately 0.15 ml. Specimens tested are diffused against a solution of isolated monoclonal 19S anti-IgG at 1 mg/ml. Plates are incubated at 25 C for 48 h. Positive specimens are then tested in twofold dilutions to 1:16. A normal serum and positive control are run routinely with each batch of unknowns.

B. Quantitative precipitins

Monoclonal 19S anti-IgG is used to measure complexes of IgG in pathological specimens by classical precipitin methods (20). A precipitin curve is constructed by adding 50 μliters of serum containing mRF to tubes containing increasing amounts of the test specimen up to 500 μliters. The volume is equalized to 500 μliters with phosphate-buffered saline and incubated at 22 C for 2 h. The precipitates are collected, washed, and quantitated. Controls for each point without the addition of RF are used to correct the precipitin curve. Greater sensitivity of the method can be obtained by using larger volumes of the specimen and mRF.

C. Solid-phase radioimmunoassay utilizing mRF conjugated to microcrystalline cellulose (10)

This method is based on the inhibition by immune complexes of the reaction of mRF with ^{125}I-labeled heat-aggregated Ig. Since monomeric IgG causes some inhibition as well, specimens are diluted to a final concentration of 60 μg/ml. A one-step inhibition assay is performed by incubating 0.5 ml of the unheated diluted specimen at 37 C for 1 h and then for 12 h at 4 C. The solid-phase mRF is then collected by centrifugation and washed, and the radiolabeled bound Ig aggregates are measured. The amount of immune complexes in the specimen is determined by comparison with a standard curve prepared with each assay by adding known amounts of aggregated IgG to the inhibition system.

Method utilizing polyclonal rheumatoid factor (8)

This method is based on the inhibition by immune complexes of the reaction of pRF with ^{125}I-labeled aggregated Ig. The bound ^{125}I-labeled aggregates are determined by precipitating the RF with an anti-IgM reagent and measuring the radioactivity in the precipitate. The tests are performed in a two-step inhibition procedure. A 200-μliter specimen is diluted, and the appropriate amount of pRF is added as a rheumatoid serum diluted in carrier IgM. The solution is refrigerated at 4 C for 24 h. ^{125}I-labeled aggregated Ig is added, and the tubes are refrigerated for another 24 h. The third day, antihuman IgM is added, and the tubes are refrigerated for an additional 24 h. On the fourth day, the precipitated radiolabeled aggregates are counted. The amount of immune complexes in the specimen is determined by comparison with a standard curve. The assay can detect 125 μg of soluble immune complexes.

Method utilizing platelet aggregation (21)

Human platelets are isolated, washed, and adjusted to a count of about 200,000/mm^3. A pool of platelets from three donors is collected and must be used the same day as drawn. Reactivity of each batch must be tested with known antigen-antibody solutions. Test sera are inactivated at 56 C for 30 min. Several twofold dilutions beginning with a 1:10 dilution are made with a microtiter pipette in U plates. To each well, 50 μliters of the platelet suspension is added, and the plates are incubated overnight at 5 to 8 C. The titers are determined by the highest dilution showing a positive pattern of sedimentation. Amounts of complexes are estimated by comparison with titers of solutions of known concentrations of immune complexes.

REAGENTS

Preparation of C1q

Several methods are now available for isolating C1q (4, 5, 7, 8, 16, 22). The method used in my laboratory, which has been successfully used over the past 5 years in a number of other laboratories as well, utilizes the precipitation of C1q with deoxyribonucleic acid (DNA). This reaction is based on the unique cationic properties of the C1q molecule.

Pooled normal serum or recalcified plasma is dialyzed overnight at 4 C against 0.025 M Veronal-0.01 M EDTA buffer, pH 8.6. The pH and conductance are checked to determine completion of dialysis. The dialyzed serum is then spun at 1,000 $\times$ g for 30 min at 4 C to remove nonspecific precipitate. A precipitin curve is made of the reaction of the serum and DNA (Worthington Biochemical Corp.) to determine maximal precipitation. The optimal amount of DNA, usually 25 μg per ml, is then added to the pooled serum, stirred at room temperature for 1

h, and kept at 4 C for 24 h. The solution is spun at 1,000 $\times$ g for 30 min, and the precipitate obtained is washed four times with 0.05 M phosphate buffer, pH 6.9. The precipitate, which has a weak gel-like consistency, is then adjusted to 0.003 M MgCl$_2$. A 0.1-ml amount of deoxyribonuclease I (Worthington Biochemical Corp.) at 1 mg/ml in 0.05 M phosphate buffer-0.003 M MgCl$_2$, pH 6.9, is added per ml of suspension. The suspension is then stirred at 37 C for 1 h and dialyzed against the suspending buffer until most of the precipitate is dissolved. The solution is spun at 100,000 $\times$ g for 30 min. The supernatant fluid contains approximately 70% C1q and is further purified by column chromatography (7) with the use of G-200 Sephadex in pH 5.3, 0.3 M phosphate buffer (75.35 g of NaH$_2$PO$_4$ and 35.0 ml of 0.5 M Na$_2$HPO$_4$ are dissolved in 2 liters of distilled water; 1.6 ml of a 2% solution of chloramphenicol in ethanol is added as a preservative). The deoxyribonuclease and deoxyribonuclease digestion products are eliminated in this step. C1q is present in the exclusion volume. Fractions containing C1q are pooled and precipitated by adding 28% (NH$_4$)$_2$SO$_4$. The precipitate after 5 h at 4 C is collected, dissolved in pH 7.0, 0.1 M phosphate buffer, and dialyzed overnight. Undissolved precipitate is removed by spinning at 100,000 $\times$ g for 30 min. The clear solution is divided into portions and stored at -70 C. The column-purified material contains greater than 90% C1q and is sufficiently pure for use in the gel diffusion method.

To obtain the highly purified C1q needed for radiolabeling, preparative electrophoresis is used (7). A 50-cm block of Pevikon C-870 (Mercer Consolidated Corp., Yonkers, N.Y.) in pH 6.0 phosphate buffer, 0.1 ionic strength, is used. Buffer is prepared as follows: 1,050 ml of 1 M NaH$_2$PO$_4$ and 336 ml of 0.5 M Na$_2$HPO$_4$ are diluted to 15 liters. The ammonium sulfate-precipitated C1q from the column chrotomatography step is dissolved in enough buffer to give a total volume of 5 to 6 ml, transferred to $^8/_{32}$-inch Visking tubing, and dialyzed against the same buffer. The sample is applied to the Pevikon block 20 cm from the anodal end. Electrophoresis is carried out at 4 C for 40 h at a potential gradient of 4 V/cm. The C1q band can then be detected by placing two 0.5-cm filter-paper strips (2043B, 1 $\times$ 23 inch strips, Schleicher & Schuell Co., Keene, N.H.) on the block immediately after electrophoresis and staining strips with bromophenol blue (1% bromophenol blue in ethyl alcohol; saturate with mercuric chloride). After staining for 10 min, the strips are decolored with 5% acetic acid. The C1q band once located is cut out, packed into a Büchner funnel with coarse fritted disk, and eluted twice with 10 ml of phosphate buffer, pH 6.0, ionic strength 0.2 (35.0 ml of 1 M NaH$_2$PO$_4$ and 9.0 ml of 0.5 M NaH$_2$PO$_4$ diluted to 500 ml with distilled water). The C1q band is usually found about 12 cm to the cathode side of the origin. If the concentration of the band is not high enough for detection by the staining method, the block must be cut into 1.25-cm segments, and each segment is eluted until the peak is found (7). The eluted C1q is concentrated and prepared for storage as described above for the column chromatography product.

Preparation of 19S monoclonal rheumatoid factor

mRFs are most usually obtained from certain patients with lymphoproliferative diseases or idiopathic mixed cryoglobulinemia and can generally be isolated in sufficiently pure state for precipitin studies by column chromatography in dissociating buffers. Generally, pH 4.0, 0.1 M acetate buffer is sufficient for good dissociation; however, with certain RFs stronger dissociating conditions are needed, in which case pH 3.0, 0.1 M glycine HCl buffer is used. When the RF is not a cryoglobulin, the serum is dialyzed against pH 4.0, 0.1 M acetate buffer overnight and applied to a Sephadex C-200 column in the same buffer. The exclusion volume, which contains the isolated RF, is pooled and dialyzed against phosphate-buffered saline. When the RF is a cryoglobulin, the serum is clotted at 37 C, and the cryoprecipitate is prepared by refrigerating at 4 C for 24 h. The precipitate is collected by centrifugation, washed quickly with phosphate-buffered saline at 4 C, and then dissolved in the column buffer. The remainder of the preparation is the same as that for RF from whole serum.

INTERPRETATION

The methods utilizing C1q are useful in detecting and quantitating immune complexes of the IgG or IgM type in sera and other body fluids. However, the investigator must be well aware of the fact that a positive C1q test does not always indicate the presence of immune complexes. Two major factors must be considered in interpreting the results of these tests.

1. Neither the precipitin reaction in gels nor the radioimmunoassays differentiate reactions due to immune complexes from those due to nonspecificially aggregated Ig, such as those that might occur in vivo with physical alteration of Ig (as has been postulated in rheumatoid arthritis) or in vitro artifact. The latter can occur by freezing and thawing sera or on storage; hence, fresh sera should be used in these tests. Surprisingly, heating normal sera at 56 C for 30 min does not appear to produce false-positive C1q reactions. Since heating normal sera will produce artifactual precipitin lines with mRF, it may be that this treatment produces only small complexes of Ig that are detected by mRF but not C1q, which reacts best with complexes larger than 19S (Fig. 2). The enhanced reactivity of pathological sera with heating which has been observed (18) may be due either to the phenomenon of release of C1q as has been postulated or to the enlargement of smaller complexes present. The data at present do not favor one or the other possibility.

2. Substances other than complexes of Ig will react with C1q. These are mainly polyanionic molecules, including some that may occur in pathological fluids such as double-stranded and single-stranded DNA, double-stranded and single-stranded polyribonucleotides, endotoxin lipopolysaccharide, and meningococcal group A polysaccharides (1). Heparin when added to serum will also give a reaction with C1q (2, 17). In addition, low-molecular-weight substances that precipitate with C1q have been detected in sera of patients with SLE (1) and SLE-like syndromes (3). In general, these substances can readily be differentiated from Ig complexes by their persistence after reduction and alkylation, a treatment which eliminates reactivity of Ig complexes (Fig. 1). In additon, immune complexes can be differentiated from small reactive substances such as those found in certain SLE sera by determining size of the reactant on sucrose density gradient analysis (1).

Defining the C1q reactants in pathological sera is of basic importance and interest, but from a clinical standpoint quantitation of C1q reactants alone may be worthwhile since in some instances they appear to correlate with disease activity. This seems to be the case for the low-molecular-weight C1q reactants found in SLE and those recently reported in dengue (18). Hence, even without knowing the nature of substances reacting with C1q, these tests may prove of practical use.

The use of monoclonal RF, although limited to the detection of immune complexes of the IgG type, affords some distinct advantages over other methods described here. In the other methods, the maximal sensitivity is for large complexes, generally larger than 19S, and this sensitivity decreases with greater degrees of antigen excess and the consequent diminished complex size. Since in immune complex disease the complexes which persist in the circulation are the smaller, soluble ones, a reagent which will detect complexes in this range is most desirable. Another advantage of these reagents is that they provide greater specificity for complexes of Ig since they do not react with nonimmune substances, as do C1q and platelets. In additon, they are not inhibited by pRF.

To a great extent, however, the successful use of these reagents in detecting immune complexes depends on the mRF selected. There is marked variation in the amount of monomeric IgG which will inhibit the reaction of different mRF with complexed IgG. The greater the affinity of RF for complexed IgG, the more sensitive the method will be when done in the presence of large amounts of IgG. In general, the noncryoglobulin type of mRF is best in this respect.

A possible limitation of the mRF methods is that there may be a selectivity for complexes present in rheumatoid arthritis. The results obtained with both gel diffusion (20) and the radioimmunoassay (10) show a much greater incidence of complexes in the rheumatoid sera than in the SLE sera screened. This may just be a quantitative difference resulting from the persistence of the intermediate-size complexes in the serum in rheumatoid arthritis, whereas there may actually be considerably less circulating complexes in SLE. A more sensitive assay may resolve this question.

COMMENT

The sensitivities of the various methods described are shown in Table 1. Reactivity with heat-aggregated IgG was chosen to compare sensitivities because these data provided the best comparative information on these tests currently available. The gel methods, although simple, lack the sensitivity and the quantitative capacity needed for wide application. The

TABLE 1. *Minimal concentration of soluble heat-aggregated Ig detectable by various immune complex tests*

Test	Aggregated Ig(μg/ml)
C1q gel diffusion	100
C1q-polyethylene glycol raidoimmunoassay	50
C1q deviation	5
mRF gel diffusion	100
mRF quantitative precipitins	1
mRF radioimmunoassay	25
pRF radioimmunoassay	0.35[a]
Platelet aggregation	1

[a] Soluble tetanus toxoid-antitoxoid complexes; no data available for heat-aggregated Ig.

quantitative precipitin method using mRF can detect minute amounts of immune complexes but only when relatively large amounts of reagents are used. In addition, the procedure is so time-consuming that it is not suited for routine testing of large numbers of specimens. The platelet aggregation test is also sensitive and has been very useful in studying immune complexes in the research laboratory, but the need for obtaining and standardizing the key reagent daily makes this impractical at present as a routine clinical test. In addition, it has been shown that RF will inhibit the aggregation reaction, so that pathological sera containing RF most likely cannot be assayed by this method.

The pRF method provides the greatest sensitivity of the tests currently available; however, sera containing RF have been shown to interfere, making the method ineffective in testing specimens of patients with rheumatoid arthritis and other diseases where RFs occur.

The C1q radioimmunoassay methods have considerably greater quantitative capacity than the C1q gel method and have greater sensitivity, although the potential enhanced sensitivity afforded by radioimmunoassay has not been realized thus far. One factor which may decrease the sensitivity of these tests at present is that C1q tends to aggregate easily when iodinated, thus limiting the effective specific activity. This is not a major problem in the C1q deviation test since the binding properties of the protein are not significantly altered, but in the C1q-polyethylane glycol method aggregates of C1q which are not removed at $7,000 \times g$ tend to precipitate more readily in polyethylene glycol, raising the background and diminishing sensitivity.

Additional technical refinement is needed before these assays will be of practical clinical use, but the work done so far appears to provide a solid base for further development. The C1q reagent provides the basis for detecting complement-fixing immune complexes as well as certain other biological substances occurring during pathological states and related to hypocomplementemia. The use of selected monoclonal rheumatoid factors is the best method currently available for detection of small complexes of IgG. Radioimmunoassay appears to be the best approach to a sensitive quantitative method, and at present the competitive-inhibition technique with precipitating antibody (8) appears to offer the greatest sensitivity.

LITERATURE CITED

1. Agnello, V., D. Koffler, J. W. Eisenberg, R. J. Winchester, and H. G. Kunkel. 1971. C1q pre-

cipitins in the sera of patients with systemic lupus erythematosus and other hypocomplementemic states: characteristic of high and low molecular weight types. J. Exp. Med. 134:228S–241S.

2. Agnello, V., D. Koffler, and H. G. Kunkel. 1973. Immune complex systems in the nephritis of systemic lupus erythematosus. Kidney Int. 3:90–99.

3. Agnello, V., S. Ruddy, R. J. Winchester, C. C. Christian, and H. G. Kunkel. 1975. Hereditary C_2 deficiency in systemic lupus erythematosus and acquired complement abnormalities in an unusual SLE-related syndrome. Birth Defects Orig. Artic. Ser. 9:312–317.

4. Agnello, V., R. J. Winchester, and H. G. Kunkel. 1970. Precipitin reactions of the C1q component of complement with aggregated γ globulin and immune complexes in gel diffusion. Immunology 19:909–919.

5. Assimeh, S. N., D. Bing, and R. H. Painter. 1974. A simple method for the isolation of the subcomponents of the first component of complement by affinity chromatography. J. Immunol. 13:225–234.

6. Augener, W., H. M. Grey, N. R. Cooper, and H. J. Müller-Eberhard. 1971. The reaction of monomeric and aggregated immunoglobulins with C1. Immunochemistry 8:1011–1020.

7. Calcott, M. A., and H. J. Müller-Eberhard. 1972. The C1q protein of human complement. Biochemistry 11:3443–3450.

8. Cowdery, J. S., P. E. Treadwell, and R. B. Fritz. 1975. A radioimmunoassay for human antigen-antibody complexes in clinical material. J. Immunol. 114:5–9.

9. Creighton, W. D., P. H. Lambert, and P. A. Miescher. 1973. Detection of antibodies and soluble antigen-antibody complexes by precipitation with polyethylene glycol. J. Immunol. 111:1219–1227.

10. Luthra, H. S., F. C. McDuffie, G. G. Hunder, and E. A. Samayoa. 1975. Immune complexes in sera and synovial fluids of patients with rheumatoid arthritis: radioimmunoassay with monoclonal rheumatoid factor. J. Clin. Invest. 56:458–466.

11. Mannik, M., A. O. Haakenstad, and W. P. Arend. 1974. The fate and detection of circulatory immune complexes, p. 91–101. In L. Brent and J. Holboron (ed.), Progress in immunology II, vol. 5. North Holland Publishing Co.

12. Müller-Eberhard, H. J., and M. A. Calcott. 1966. Interaction between C1q and γ globulin. Immunochemistry 3:500.

13. Müller-Eberhard, H. J., and H. G. Kunkel. 1961. Isolation of a thermolabile serum protein which precipitates γ globulin aggregates and participates in immune hemolysis. Proc. Soc. Exp. Biol. Med. 106:291–295.

14. Nydegger, U. E., P. H. Lambert, H. Gerber, and P. A. Miescher. 1974. Circulating immune complexes in the serum in systemic lupus erythematosus and in carriers of hepatitis B antigen. Quantitation by binding to radiolabeled C1q. J. Clin. Invest. 54:297–309.

15. Penttinen, K., G. Myllylä, O. Mäkelä, and A. Vaheri. 1969. Soluble antigen-antibody complexes and platelet aggregation. Acta Pathol. Microbiol. Scand. 77:309–317.

16. Reid, K. B. M., D. M. Lowe, and R. R. Porter. 1972. Isolation and characterization of C1q, a subcomponent of the first component of complement, from human and rabbit sera. Biochem. J. 130:749–763.

17. Rent, R., N. Ertel, R. Eisenstein, and H. Gewurz. 1975. Complement activation by interaction of polyanions and polycations. I. Heparin-protamine induced consumption of complement. J. Immunol. 114:120–124.

18. Sobel, A. T., V. A. Bokisch, and H. J. Müller-Eberhard. 1975. C1q deviation test for the detection of immune complexes, aggregates of IgG, and bacterial products in human serum. J. Exp. Med. 142:139–150.

19. Wager, O., K. Penttinen, J. A. Räsänen, and G. Myllylä. 1973. Inhibition of IgG complex-induced platelet aggregation by antiglobulin-active cryoglobulin IgM components. Clin. Exp. Immunol. 15:393–408.

20. Winchester, R. J., H. G. Kunkel, and V. Agnello. 1971. Occurrence of γ-globulin complexes in serum and joint fluid of rheumatoid arthritis patients; use of monoclonal rheumatoid factors as reagents for their demonstration. J. Exp. Med. 134:286S–295S.

21. World Health Organization. 1970. Viral hepatitis and tests for the Australia (hepatitis-associated) antigen and antibody. Bull: W.H.O. 42:980–982.

22. Yonemasu, K., and R. M. Stroud. 1971. C1q: rapid purification method for preparation of monospecific antisera and for biochemical studies. J. Immunol. 106:304–313.

Chapter 91

Complement Receptors on Raji Cells as In Vitro Detectors of Immune Complexes in Human Sera

A. N. THEOFILOPOULOS AND F. J. DIXON

INTRODUCTION

Human and animal diseases, in most instances, appear to be associated with immunologically induced tissue injury. Evidence drawn from a variety of investigations indicates that antigen-antibody immune complexes (IC) are frequently pathogens involved in damaging tissues (7). By using immunofluorescence and electron microscopy, deposits of such IC can be found in a characteristic pattern on limiting basement membranes of renal glomeruli, arteries, and choroid plexi (22, 29). Moreover, IC can be eluted from the diseased tissue, and the antigen and antibody can be recovered, identified, and quantitated (22).

There is increasing interest in detecting IC directly in biological fluids, and numerous attempts have been and are being made to develop immunological techniques, reliable and sensitive enough, for their demonstration and quantitation (1, 3, 5, 10, 11, 13–15, 19–21, 23, 30). Human bone marrow-derived (B) lymphocytes as well as human lymphoblastoid cells in continuous culture (HCL) with B cell characteristics can bind IC via receptors for Fc and receptors for C3b (8, 16, 26). Therefore, these cells can be used as in vitro detectors of IC in biological fluids. HCL have an advantage over peripheral B lymphocytes in that they represent a relatively homogeneous and easily accessible cell population. Studies with several HCL with B cell characteristics have shown that they carry some or all of the following: membrane-bound immunoglobulin (MBIg), receptors for IgGFc, receptors for C3 and C3b, receptors for C1q, and receptors for C4b (2, 26; A. T. Sobel and V. A. Bokisch, Fed. Proc. 34:965, 1975). The Raji cell line, among the several studied, was found to be the most suitable for use as an in vitro detector of IC since it is devoid of MBIg, has IgGFc receptors of low avidity, and has a large number of receptors for C3-C3b, C3d (26), and C1q (Sobel and Bokisch, Fed. Proc. 34:965, 1975). Consequently, complement receptors on Raji cells were used in an immunofluorescence assay for the detection of complement-fixing IC in experimental animal and human sera (27).

However, this assay had the disadvantage of not being quantitative. We have modified this method and now present the technical details used to demonstrate IC in human sera and quantitate them by measuring uptake of radioactive antibody by IgG in the IC bound to cells (28).

TEST PROCEDURES

Preparation of materials

Lymphoblastoid cell line. Raji cells, which are derived from Burkitt's lymphoma (24), are cultured in Eagle's minimal essential medium (MEM) as has been described (17, 26). The cell number is determined with a standard-type hemacytometer, and cell viability, by trypan blue exclusion.

Aggregated human gamma globulin (AHG) and 7S IgG. Human IgG is obtained from Cohn fraction II after fractionation on a diethylaminoethyl (DEAE)-52 cellulose column with a 0.01 M phosphate buffer, pH 7.3. This IgG in phosphated-buffered saline (PBS) is freed from AHG by centrifugation at 35,000 rpm for 90 min; the upper third of the supernatant fluid (deaggregated or 7S IgG) is removed, and the protein concentration is determined by an automated micro-Kjeldahl method (9). The 7S IgG is divided into amounts of 0.1 ml (6.5 mg/ml) and stored at -70 C. AHG is freshly made each day after heating a portion of 7S IgG in a water bath at 63 C for 30 min. Preliminary studies with sucrose density gradients have shown that AHG prepared from day to day under the same conditions varies little in the pattern of protein distribution along the gradient. However, to ensure uniformity in the size of AHG in later experiments, we prepare a large batch of AHG and store 0.1-ml portions of this preparation at -70 C. AHG is used in the assay described below as an in vitro model of human IC, since it has been shown to possess many of their properties (4, 12) and binds to the same Fc and complement receptors on cell surfaces (6, 26).

Antisera. Antiserum to human IgG is prepared in rabbits, and the IgG fraction of this antiserum is isolated on a DEAE-52 column as above and brought to a concentration of 5 mg/ml of PBS.

Radioiodination of protein. The IgG fraction of the rabbit antihuman IgG serum is iodinated with ^{125}I according to the procedure of McConahey and Dixon (18) and brought to a concentration of 1 mg/ml of PBS. The specific activity is 0.3 μCi per μg of protein.

Raji cell radioimmune assay for detecting and quantitating immune complexes in human sera

1. A 1-ml amount of a Raji cell suspension is removed from a 72-h-old culture (cell density $\sim$ 10^6 cells/ml). Two drops of trypan blue are added and mixed with a Pasteur pipette, after which the cell number and viability are assessed with a hemacytometer.

2. The total number of Raji cells needed for a group of tests is calculated by knowing that 2×10^6 cells are required for each test. Each test serum is run in duplicate or triplicate, and each point of the standard curve (see below) is run in duplicate. Cells are removed from the culture flask and poured into 50-ml conical tubes.

3. The cells are centrifuged at 1,800 rpm for 10 min. Supernatant fluids are removed, and pellets are combined and resuspended in Spinner's medium to a volume of 2×10^6 cells per 200 μliter.

4. Amounts of 2×10^6 cells (200 μliters) are placed into 1.5-ml plastic Eppendorf conical tubes (Brinkman Instruments, Los Angeles, Calif.); 1 ml of Spinner's medium is added to each tube, and the cells are centrifuged at 1,800 rpm for 10 min.

5. Supernatant fluids are removed by using an aspirator, and the pellets are resuspended in 50 μliters of Spinner's medium.

6. Serum to be tested for IC is diluted 1:4 with 0.15 M NaCl (physiological saline), and 25 μliters added to the Raji cells

7. After an incubation period of 45 min at 37 C with gentle shaking (every 5 to 10 min by hand), cells are washed three times with Spinner's medium. For the first wash, 1 ml of Spinner's medium is added, and the cells are centrifuged at 1,800 rpm for 10 min. Supernatant fluids are aspirated and discarded. The second and third washings are identical; 200 μliters of Spinner's medium added to the cell pellet is mixed carefully with an Eppendorf pipette, and then 1 ml of Spinner's medium is added. Cells are centrifuged as above and supernatant fluids are removed.

8. The washed cells are allowed to react (30 min, 4 C), under gentle shaking (every 5 to 10 min by hand), with an optimal amount (see below, Results) of the ^{125}I-rabbit antihuman IgG diluted 1:2 with Spinner's medium containing 1% human serum albumin (HSA).

9. After incubation, the cells are washed three times as in step 7, with the exception that the Spinner's medium contains 1% HSA.

10. The supernatant fluid is removed as close to the cell pellet as possible, and radioactivity associated with the pellet is determined in a gamma counter.

11. The amount of uptake (mean of duplicates or triplicates) expressed as absolute counts or as a percentage of the input is then referred to a standard curve of radioactive antibody uptake by cells incubated with normal human serum (NHS) containing various amounts of AHG (standard curve).

The standard curve is obtained as follows: 50 μliters of AHG (40 μg of protein) is serially diluted in 11 twofold dilutions in saline. Subsequently, to each dilution of AHG, 50 μliters of a 1:2 dilution of fresh NHS, NHS stored at -70 C, or NHS from a pool of 20 sera (sources of complement) is added, mixed, and incubated at 37 C for 30 min. Thereafter, 25 μliters of each mixture is added to 2×10^6 cells in duplicates (1:4 final dilution of serum containing from 10 μg to 10 ng of AHG), and incubation, washes, and counting are performed as with the test sera (steps 6 to 10).

A base line of radioactive antibody uptake (background) by cells incubated with 25 μliters of a 1:4 dilution of an individual NHS or of pooled NHS, which were used as complement sources in the above reference curve, is also established.

Experimental sera. Sera from patients with various disorders and from normal subjects are obtained after their blood has clotted at room temperature for 30 min and at 4 C for 30 min, and are subsequently centrifuged. Sera to be tested are used immediately or after being frozen at -70 C and thawed once.

RESULTS

Detection of aggregated human gamma globulin in normal human serum by measuring Raji cells' uptake of radioactive antibody to human immunoglobulin G

The efficiency of Raji cells in detecting IC in sera is first tested by incubating them with NHS containing various concentrations of AHG and then measuring their uptake of radioactive antihuman IgG. As shown in Fig. 1, cells incubated with only 40 ng of AHG in 25 μliters of 1:4 serum (6 μg/ml) take up considerably more radioactive antibody than cells incubated with NHS without AHG. The amount of radioactive antibody taken up by the cells is directly related to the amount of AHG present in the serum. The addition of similar amounts of AHG in heated (56 C, 30 min) or 7S IgG in NHS does not increase uptake of radioactive antihuman IgG by the cells over that observed with serum alone (Fig. 1).

Titration of radiolabeled antihuman immunoglobulin G for the demonstration of aggregated human gamma globulin in serum

Raji cells that have been allowed to react with NHS bind IgG only via Fc receptors. In contrast, Raji cells incubated with sera containing IgG complexes with fixed complement bind native 7S IgG via Fc receptors and complexed IgG via complement receptors (26). To detect the difference in radioactive antibody uptake between cells incubated in sera with or without IC, an excess of that amount of antibody needed to react with the molecules of native 7S IgG bound via Fc receptors must be offered to the cells. As in Fig. 2, when 15 μg of radioactive antibody is added to cells incubated with 25 μliters of 1:4 NHS in saline alone or containing 10 μg of AHG, uptake by the latter is ninefold greater. However, with 10 times less antibody,

the uptake by the cells incubated with NHS or NHS containing AHG is equivalent. The use of more than 15 μg of antibody does not increase the difference in uptake between NHS alone and NHS containing AHG, indicating that 15 μg of the radioactive antibody saturates both 7S IgG bound via Fc receptors and AHG bound via complement receptors.

Detection and quantitation of immune complexes in human sera

Since Raji cells efficiently bind AHG that has been allowed to react with serum, these cells are used in a radioimmune assay system for the detection and quantitation of circulating IC in humans. Accordingly, cells are incubated with the serum to be tested (25 μliters of 1:4 dilution in saline) and then allowed to react with an optimal amount of radioactive antibody to human IgG (15 μg). Subsequently, the uptake is determined and referred to a standard curve of radioactive antibody uptake by cells previously incubated with various amounts of AHG in serum. The amount of IC present in serum is readily equated to an amount of AHG after correcting for the dilution factor. Thus, the estimated amount of IC in each serum tested is

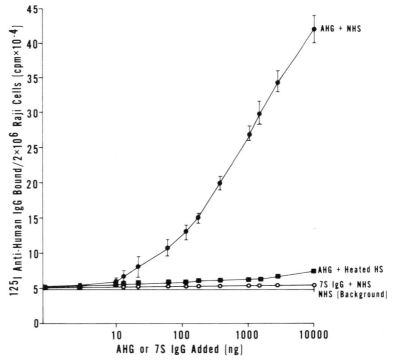

FIG. 1. *Raji cell uptake of* ¹²⁵I-*labeled antihuman IgG after incubation with increasing amounts of AHG in fresh or heated (56 C, 30 min) human serum, and 7S IgG in NHS. Each point of the AHG + NHS curve represents the mean ± standard deviations of duplicate samples run in 3 consecutive days.*

expressed as micrograms of AHG equivalent per milliliter of serum. Using this method, we were able to detect more than 12 μg of AHG equivalent, a level exceeding the upper limits of normal, in sera of patients with acute hepatitis with or without hepatitis surface antigen (HB$_s$-Ag), systemic lupus erythematosus, vasculitis, subacute sclerosing panencephalitis, dengue hemorrhagic fever, and malignancies (Table 1). In detailed studies on these sera, the

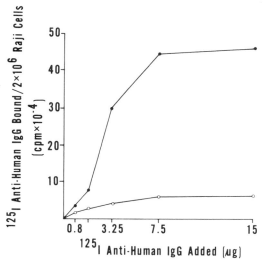

FIG. 2. *Titration of* [125]*I-labeled antihuman IgG for the demonstration of AHG in serum. Amounts of 2 × 10⁶ Raji cells were incubated (37 C, 45 min) with 25 μliters of 1:4 final dilution of NHS which had been first incubated (37 C, 30 min) with or without 10 μg of AHG. The washed cells were reacted (4 C, 30 min) with increasing amounts of* [125]*I-labeled antihuman IgG, and the radioactivity in the washed cell pellets was counted.*

results obtained by the Raji cell assay correlated well with disease activity (28).

DISCUSSION

In a radioimmune assay, uptake of radioactive antihuman IgG by Raji cells previously incubated with sera of patients with various disorders is used to identify and quantitate their circulating IC. The assay is based on the ability of Raji cells to bind much more IgG from a serum containing IgG-type IC with fixed complement than from NHS. This higher binding can be explained by postulating that there is a larger number or greater affinity of Raji cells' complement receptors than that of Raji cells' Fc receptors for their ligand molecules. Since much more IgG binds to Raji cells when it has been altered so that it can fix complement, the presence of IgG-type IC in human sera can be quantitated by measuring uptake of radioactive antihuman IgG. Our experiments have shown that uptake of radioactive antibody is proportional to the quantity of AHG bound to cells, which in turn is proportional to the quantity of AHG present in the serum.

In the Raji cell assay, to differentiate between NHS and serum containing IgG complexes, one must add radioactive antibody in excess of the amount needed to saturate the monomeric 7S IgG bound to cells via Fc receptors. In experiments presented elsewhere (28), the Raji cell assay efficiently detected IC even of 18 to 11S. Furthermore, the same experiments demonstrated that excess complement had little inhibitory effect on the binding of IC containing complement to C3-C3b, C3d, and possibly C1q receptors on Raji cells (28).

Results from the Raji cell radioimmune assay have been reproduced repeatedly. Thus, when

TABLE 1. *Raji cell radioimmune assay for immune complexes in human sera*

Diagnosis	No. of cases	No. positive	Percent positive	Amt (μg) of AHG equivalent/ml	
				Mean	Range
Serum hepatitis (with or without HB$_s$-Ag)	34	18	52.9	65	24–212
Systemic lupus erythematosus	13	13	100	327	24–1,100
Vasculitis[a]	25	14	56	155	25–1,000
Subacute sclerosing panencephalitis	6	3	50	58	24–100
Dengue hemorrhagic fever	24	15	62	62	25–225
Malignancies[b]	104	43	41	68	20–383
Hospitalized patients[c]	60	5	8.3	39	20–100
Normal subjects	120	4	3.3	21	12–30

[a] Eight sera from patients with idiopathic vasculitis, seven from rheumatoid vasculitis, and ten from Sjögren's syndrome-cryoglobulinemia-vasculitis.

[b] Fifty-five sera from patients with solid tumors and forty-nine sera from patients with lymphoid tumors.

[c] Patients with no suspected immune complex disease (hypertension, heart failure, diabetes, obstructive pulmonary disease).

30 different human sera containing IC were subjected to replicate examination, the coefficient of variation was 3.9%. In order to obtain reproducible results in the Raji cell radioimmune assay, the following should be observed:

1. Use the same number of cells (same number of available receptor sites) per test at each examination. It is known that the amount of IC bound to complement receptors is linearly related to the cell number (8).

2. For obtaining the standard reference curve, use only one preparation of AHG or preparations containing the same or similar distributions of aggregate sizes. Larger aggregates or IC fix more complement than smaller ones, and AHG or IC having more complement bind best to complement cellular receptors (8, 26).

3. Use the same radioactive antibody throughout.

The sensitivity of the Raji cell radioimmune assay is significantly greater than that of other tests utilizing C1q for the detection of soluble IC. Whereas C1q precipitation in gel (1) and radiolabeled C1q-polyethylene glycol precipitation (21) detect AHG at minimal concentrations of approximately 100 μg/ml, the Raji cell assay allows the detection of 6 μg/ml. However, a C1q deviation test was developed recently and reportedly was about as sensitive as the Raji cell assay (25). Nevertheless, the Raji cell test may be more specific for IC than the tests utilizing C1q, since C1q is known to react not only with IC and AHG but also with non-Ig substances such as endotoxin and deoxyribonucleic acid (1, 25). It is also noteworthy that a very small amount of serum (25 μliters of 1:4 dilution) is sufficient for one determination by the Raji cell assay. Furthermore, Raji cells fixed with limited concentrations of glutaraldehyde, which preserves the complement receptors (unpublished data), are presently being investigated. The use of fixed cells may allow the routine performance of this test in clinical laboratories. The relationship of the results obtained by the Raji cell radioimmune assay in detecting IC in sera of patients with various disorders and the results obtained by other methods, as well as other clinical and experimental data supporting the specificity of the test, have been discussed elsewhere (28).

The possible disadvantages of the Raji cell radioimmune assay are, first, that cultures of Raji cells must be maintained. This potential difficulty is offset by the laboriousness of many methods used to isolate substances for other IC tests, whereas Raji cells are easy to grow. Second, antilymphocyte antibodies in certain sera (31, 32) may interfere with the test. However,

under the conditions used for our assay (interaction of test serum with cells at 37 C), antilymphocyte antibodies, which are mainly if not exclusively of the cold-reactive IgM type (32), are not absorbed by Raji cells.

Apart from the ability of Raji cells to detect IC in vitro, it should be pointed out that these cells, which can concentrate antigen-antibody complexes on their surfaces, may provide the tool by which antigens involved in IC diseases will be identified and antisera against them will be raised.

ACKNOWLEDGMENTS

This is Publication No. 1011 from Scripps Clinic and Research Foundation, La Jolla, Calif. This work was supported by contract DADA 17-73-C-3137 from the U.S. Department of the Army, by Public Health Service grant AI-07007 from the National Institute of Allergy and Infectious Diseases, and by contract NO1-CB-53592 from the National Cancer Institute.

LITERATURE CITED

1. Agnello, V., R. J. Winchester, and H. G. Kunkel. 1970. Precipitin reactions of the C1q component of complement with aggregated-γglobulin and immune complexes in gel diffusion. Immunology 19:909–919.

2. Bokisch, V. A., and A. T. Sobel. 1974. Receptor for the fourth component of complement on human B lymphocytes and cultured human lymphoblastoid cells. J. Exp. Med. 140:1336–1347.

3. Brouet, J. C., J. P. Caluvel, F. Danon, M. Klein, and M. Seligmann. 1974. Biologic and clinical significance of cryoglobulinemias. Am. J. Med. 57:775–788.

4. Christian, C. L. 1960. Studies of aggregated γ-globulin. I. Sedimentation, electrophoretic and anticomplementary properties. J. Immunol. 84:112–116.

5. Creighton, W. D., P. H. Lambert, and P. A. Miescher. 1973. Detection of antibodies and soluble antigen-antibody complexes by precipitation with polyethylene glycol. J. Immunol. 111:1219–1227.

6. Dickler, H. B. 1974. Studies of the human lymphocyte receptor for heat-aggregated or antigen-complexed immunoglobulin. J. Exp. Med. 140:508–522.

7. Dixon, F. J. 1973. Immune complex diseases. J. Invest. Dermatol. 59:413–415.

8. Eden, A., C. Bianco, and V. Nussenzweig. 1973. Mechanism of binding of soluble immune complexes to lymphocytes. Cell. Immunol. 7:459–473.

9. Ferrari, A. 1960. Nitrogen determination by a continuous digestion and analysis system. Ann. N.Y. Acad. Sci. 87:792–800.

10. Franklin, E. C., H. R. Holman, H. J. Müller-Eberhard, and H. G. Kunkel. 1957. An unusual protein component of high molecular weight in the serum of certain patients with

rheumatoid arthritis. J. Exp. Med. 105:425–438.

11. Heimer, R., and J. L. Abruzzo. 1972. A latex test for the detection of human IgG aggregates and IgG anti-IgG antibody. Immunochemistry 9:921–931.

12. Ishizaka, K. 1963. Gamma globulin and molecular mechanisms of hypersensitivity reactions. Prog. Allergy 7:32.

13. Jewell, D. P., and I. C. M. MacLennan. 1973. Circulating immune complexes in inflammatory bowel disease. Clin. Exp. Immunol. 14:219–226.

14. Koffler, D., V. Agnello, R. Thoburn, and H. G. Kunkel. 1971. Systemic lupus erythematosus: prototype of immune complex nephritis in man. J. Exp. Med. 134:169s–179s.

15. Koffler, D., R. Carr, V. Agnello, R. Thoburn, and H. G. Kunkel. 1971. Antibodies to polynucleotides in human sera: antigenic specificity and relation to disease. J. Exp. Med. 134:294–312.

16. Lay, W. H., and V. Nussenzweig. 1968. Receptors for complement on leukocytes. J. Exp. Med. 128:991.

17. Lerner, R. A., and L. D. Hodge. 1971. Gene expression in synchronized lymphocytes: studies on the control of synthesis of immunoglobulin polypeptides. J. Cell. Physiol. 77:265.

18. McConahey, P. J., and F. J. Dixon. 1966. A method of trace iodination of proteins for immunologic studies. Int. Arch. Allergy Appl. Immunol. 29:185–189.

19. Mowbray, J. F., A. V. Hoffbrand, E. J. Holborow, P. P. Seah, and L. Fry. 1973. Circulating immune complexes in dermatitis herpetiformis. Lancet 1:400–402.

20. Myllylä, G. 1973. Aggregation of human blood platelets by immune complexes in the sedimentation pattern test. Scand. J. Haematol. Suppl. 19:1–55.

21. Nydegger, U. E., P. H. Lambert, H. Gerber, and P. H. Miescher. 1974. Circulating immune complexes in the serum in systemic lupus erythematosus and in carriers of hepatitis B antigen. Quantitation by binding to radiolabeled C1q. J. Clin. Invest. 54:297–309.

22. Oldstone, M. B. A. 1975. Virus neutralization and virus-induced immune complex disease. Virus-antibody union resulting in immunoprotection or immunologic injury — two sides of the same coin. Prog. Med. Virol. 19:84–119.

23. Onyewotu, I. I., E. J. Holborow, and G. D. Johnson. 1974. Detection and radioassay of soluble circulating immune complexes using guinea pig peritoneal exudate cells. Nature (London) New Biol. 248:156–159.

24. Pulvertaft, R. J. V. 1965. A study of malignant tumors in Nigeria by short-term tissue culture. J. Clin. Pathol. 18:261–273.

25. Sobel, A. T., V. A. Bokisch, and H. J. Müller-Eberhard. 1975. C1q deviation test for the detection of immune complexes, aggregates of IgG and bacterial products in human sera. J. Exp. Med. 142:139–150.

26. Theofilopoulos, A. N., F. J. Dixon, and V. A. Bokisch. 1974. Binding of soluble immune complexes to human lymphoblastoid cells. I. Characterization of receptors for IgG Fc and complement and description of the binding mechanism. J. Exp. Med. 140:877–894.

27. Theofilopoulos, A. N., C. B. Wilson, V. A. Bokisch, and F. J. Dixon. 1974. Binding of soluble immune complexes to human lymphoblastoid cells. II. Use of Raji cells to detect circulating immune complexes in animal and human sera. J. Exp. Med. 140:1230–1244.

28. Theofilopoulos, A. N., C. B. Wilson, and F. J. Dixon. 1976. The Raji cell radioimmune assay for detecting immune complexes in human sera. J. Clin. Invest. 57:169–182.

29. Wilson, C. B., and F. J. Dixon. 1974. Diagnosis of immunopathologic renal disease. Kidney Int. 5:389–401.

30. Winchester, R. J., H. G. Kunkel, and V. Agnello. 1971. Occurrence of γ-globulin complexes in serum and joint fluid of rheumatoid arthritis patients: use of monoclonal rheumatoid factors as reagents for their demonstration. J. Exp. Med. 134:286s–295s.

31. Winchester, R. J., J. B. Winfield, F. Siegal, P. Wernet, Z. Bentwich, and H. G. Kunkel. 1974. Analyses of lymphocytes from patients with rheumatoid arthritis and systemic lupus erythematosus; occurrence of interfering cold reactive anti-lymphocyte antibodies. J. Clin. Invest. 54:1082–1092.

32. Winfield, J. B., R. J. Winchester, P. Wernet, S. M. Fu, and H. G. Kunkel. 1975. Nature of cold reactive antibodies to lymphocyte surface determinants in systemic lupus erythematosus. Arthritis Rheum. 18:1–8.

Chapter 92

Tests for Antibodies to Tissue-Specific Antigens

P. E. BIGAZZI AND N. R. ROSE

INTRODUCTION

Sera from patients with chronic thyroiditis (Hashimoto's disease) may contain several types of antibody to thyroid antigens. Antibodies to thyroglobulin or to microsomal antigen of the thyroid are most commonly detected by routine diagnostic procedures; antibodies to the colloid antigen (called "second antigen of the colloid" or "CA2") and cytotoxic antibodies to an antigen of the thyroid cell surface are less frequently observed.

In addition to chronic thyroiditis, these antibodies may be found in other thyroid disorders, such as primary myxedema, hyperthyroidism, colloid goiter, nodular goiter, and thyroid tumors (22). Thyroid antibodies have also been observed in sera of patients with pernicious anemia, adrenal insufficiency, diabetes mellitus, and other conditions. Finally, antithyroid antibodies have been observed in normal subjects (22).

ANTIBODIES TO THYROGLOBULIN

Thyroglobulin antibodies can be demonstrated by several procedures, such as precipitation in agar, indirect immunofluorescence (IF), passive agglutination of cells coated with thyroglobulin, and radioimmunoassay. Precipitation in agar is simple to perform, but of low sensitivity, so that it detects only antibodies present in relatively large amounts. On the other hand, recently developed radioimmunoassay procedures for thyroglobulin antibodies are highly sensitive, but not yet widely used (21, 23). At present, passive hemagglutination and indirect IF are the most commonly employed tests. Both have advantages and disadvantages. Passive hemagglutination tests with the use of tanned red cells (tanned cell hemagglutination, TCH) or chromic chloride-treated red cells (chromic chloride hemagglutination, CCH) are very sensitive and thus detect antibodies to thyroglobulin in a variety of conditions other than thyroiditis, a possible disadvantage from the diagnositc point of view. Indirect IF is less sensitive, but reportedly can detect nonagglutinating antibodies that are missed by other procedures (25). It can also detect antibodies to CA2, which are undetectable by hemagglutination. Therefore, until radioimmunoassays are fully elaborated, it seems advisable to employ both hemagglutination and IF.

Tanned cell hemagglutination test for antibodies to thyroglobulin

Erythrocytes treated with tannic acid are capable of adsorbing protein antigens on their surface. When added to serial dilutions of a patient's serum, they will react with the appropriate antibody, if present, with a visible agglutination reaction. Tanned red cells coated with thyroid extract or purified thyroglobulin are employed to detect antibodies to thyroglobulin. The test may be performed in tubes, but more commonly a microtitration method is used, in which the process of titration is accomplished with minute amounts of reagents. Special plastic plates, containing small cups with a conical bottom, are used instead of racks of test tubes. Specially calibrated "loops," capable of picking up constant volumes of fluid and transferring them for serial dilutions, are used instead of standard pipettes, and special pipette droppers, calibrated to deliver accurate volumes of fluid, are used to fill the cups.

Materials.

Phosphate-buffered saline solution (PBS), pH 7.2 ± 0.05:

Sodium chloride .... 13.20 g
Disodium phosphate (Na_2HPO_4) 2.96 g
Monopotassium phosphate
(KH_2PO_4) .... 0.86 g
Dissolve salts in 2 liters of distilled water.

Tannic acid solution in PBS: Dissolve 0.1 g of tannic acid in 20 ml of distilled water. This stock solution is considered a 1:200 dilution and may be kept at room temperature for 1 week. Dilute 1:125 or more in PBS before use in the test.

Normal rabbit serum (NRS) diluent: Heat-inactivated pooled normal rabbit serum, diluted 1:100 in PBS.

Human group O red blood cells, tanned, coated with human thyroid extract:
1. Wash human erythrocytes three times in

PBS; then prepare a 4% suspension in PBS.

2. Mix 5 ml of 4% erythrocyte suspension with 5 ml of tannic acid solution (1:25,000 in PBS) and allow to stand at room temperature for 30 min.

3. Wash three times in PBS.

4. In a 50-ml tube, mix 0.1 ml of human thyroid extract (prepared by mincing thyroid tissue in PBS, incubating overnight in the cold, and then centrifuging at 64,000 × g for 45 min) with 5.0 ml of PBS. (Alternatively, purified thyroglobulin can be prepared by precipitation with 1.60 to 1.70 M ammonium sulfate followed by filtration through Sephadex G-200. The first peak should be separated and concentrated. It can be lyophilized or stored frozen. It is used in a 10 μg/ml solution.) Place in boiling water for exactly 2 min. Cool the tube under running water, and add 15 ml of cold PBS.

5. Prepare 10 ml of a 2% suspension of tanned erythrocytes. Add 5 ml of tanned cells and 5 ml of the 1:200 dilution of thyroid extract, mix, and let stand at room temperature for 30 min. Wash three times in NRS diluent, and after washing prepare 10 ml of 1% cell suspension in NRS diluent.

6. Prepare uncoated tanned cells by mixing 5 ml of tanned erythrocytes with 5 ml of NRS diluent. Incubate, wash, and prepare as for coated tanned cells.

Test sera, positive and negative control sera.
Plates, pipettes, loops, tubes, etc.

Procedure.

1. Prepare 1:5 dilutions of sera to be tested, including control sera, using NRS diluent.

2. Using a pipette dropper, place 0.025 ml of NRS diluent in wells 1 to 12.

3. Using a 0.025-ml microtitration diluter, take a loopful of 1:5 serum dilution and place it in the first well. Mix and transfer to the next well, and so on until well 9.

4. Using a 0.025-ml microtitration diluter, take a loopful of 1:5 serum dilution and place it in well 11. Mix and transfer to well 12.

5. Repeat these steps for all sera to be tested, including positive and negative control sera.

6. Add 0.025 ml of tanned, coated red cells to wells 1 and 10. Add 0.025 ml of tanned, uncoated cells to wells 11 and 12.

7. Gently shake the plate to mix.

8. Incubate plates at room temperature until cells settle (usually 1 h) and then overnight at 4 C. To avoid evaporation, plates are stacked up on top of one another, and the topmost plate

is covered with plastic or another empty plate.

9. Read the patterns of sedimentation on the button of the wells.

As shown in Fig. 1, strong agglutination usually gives an even mat over the bottom of the well. Weaker reactions give doughnut-shaped patterns, whereas no agglutination gives a compact button of cells in the center of the well.

Chromic chloride hemagglutination test for antibodies to thyroglobulin

Chromic chloride can be used to couple thyroglobulin to red blood cells, providing an alternative to the tannic acid method. It appears to be comparable in sensitivity and specificity. The method of microtitration is given.

Materials.

Normal saline (1.5 g of NaCl in 1 liter of double distilled water).
NRS diluent: Heat-inactivated NRS is diluted 1:100 in saline.
Chromic chloride solution:
1. Stock
   0.125 g of CrCl₃·6H₂O
   10 ml of saline
2. Wash solution
   0.1 ml of stock
   100 ml of saline
3. Coating solution (0.1% solution made up fresh)
   0.8 ml of stock solution
   9.2 ml of saline
Human thyroglobulin, prepared as for TCH.
Human group O red blood cells:
1. Collect 10 ml in 3.8% sodium citrate.
2. Use up to 10 days.
Inactivated test sera, positive and negative control sera.
Plates, pipettes, loops, tubes, etc.

Procedure.

1. Wash human group O erythrocytes three times with the chromic chloride wash solution. Pack.

2. Pipette 0.2 ml of packed erythrocytes into a 12-ml graduated centrifuge tube.

3. In the centrifuge, combine: 0.2 ml of packed erythrocytes, 0.2 ml of 0.19 M CrCl₃ solution, and 0.2 ml of diluted thyroglobulin (or 1:200 NRS for control cells). Mix with an applicator stick and incubate for 4 min at room temperature.

4. Add 10 ml of saline to stop reaction. Centrifuge.

5. Wash twice in NRS diluent.

6. After the last wash, resuspend in 9.8 ml of NRS diluent to make a 2% suspension.

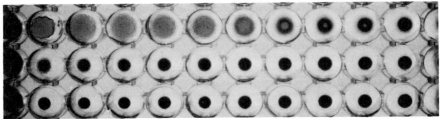

FIG. 1. *Tanned cell hemagglutination test for antibodies to thyroglobulin. The upper row contains serial dilutions (1:5 through 1:1,280) of patient's serum mixed with tanned erythrocytes coated with purified human thyroglobulin. Tubes 1–5 are strongly positive (note the folding of the mat evident in the first tube) and tubes 6–9 are weakly positive. Tube 10 is negative. The middle row shows serial dilutions of normal human serum mixed with tanned and coated erythrocytes. In row three are dilutions of the patient's serum mixed with tanned erythrocytes that were not coated with thyroglobulin.*

7. Set up test, proceeding as with the TCH test.

8. The test is read like the TCH test.

Interpretation of hemagglutination test results

At present, the TCH test is the most commonly employed technique for the detection of antibodies against thyroglobulin. The incidence of these antibodies detectable by the TCH test is 75% in patients with chronic thyroiditis, 75% in myxedema, and 40% in Graves' disease and in thyroid tumors.

Approximately 30% of patients with chronic thyroiditis have TCH titers ranging from 1,000 to 2,500,000. Such high titers are found in only about 10% of patients with Graves' disease. Low titers of thyroglobulin antibodies may be found in normal individuals. The incidence of such antibodies in subjects without overt thyroid disease is higher in women. The incidence also increases with age, so that 18% of women over 40 years have antibodies to thyroglobulin.

Indirect immunofluorescence for antibodies to thyroglobulin

Indirect IF performed on sections of human or monkey thyroid can demonstrate antibodies to thyroglobulin, CA2, microsomes of thyroid epithelial cells, and antinuclear antibodies. Tests for these antibodies may be performed on unfixed sections, but in most laboratories IF for antibodies to thyroglobulin and CA2 is performed on methanol- or acetone-treated sections. The pattern of staining that is obtained when methanol-fixed sections are used with thyroglobulin antibodies is characteristic and has a floccular, "puffy" appearance (Fig. 2). The less commonly observed CA2 pattern has been described as diffuse, with a "ground-glass" appearance.

Materials.

PBS, pH 7.2.

Rabbit or goat antiserum to human immunoglobulins, conjugated with fluorescein isothiocyanate (FITC-conjugate). This may be a commercial preparation, as long as the company provides adequate information on its characteristics, i.e., immunoelectrophoretic analysis of conjugate to show its specificity, antibody concentration, protein and fluorescein concentration, and fluorescein to protein ratio. When a commercial conjugate is obtained, the lot number should be recorded, and the optimal dilution should be first checked by testing several dilutions in a chess-board titration. The same lot should then be used as long as available.

Buffered glycerol: Mix 9 volumes of glycerol with 1 volume of phosphate buffer, pH 7.2.

Procedure.

1. Prepare 1:10 dilutions in PBS of all sera to be tested (unknown, positive and negative controls). Sera may be screened at 1:10 dilutions or titrated in serial twofold dilutions until the end point is reached.

2. Incubate diluted sera with cryostat sections of monkey or human thyroid (previously fixed in absolute methanol at 56 C for exactly 3 min) in a humid chamber at room temperature for 30 min.

3. Wash slides in PBS for 30 min at room temperature. More efficient washing can be obtained by gently stirring with a magnetic stirrer and changing washes three times.

4. Incubate sections with diluted FITC-conjugate to human immunoglobulin in a humid chamber at room temperature for 30 min.

5. Wash again for 30 min as previously described.

6. Mount cover slips with buffered glycerol and read under an ultraviolet (UV) microscope.

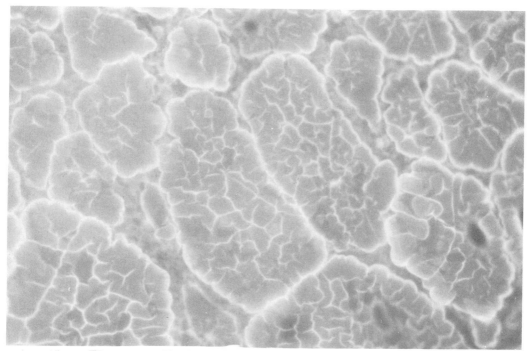

FIG. 2. *Immunofluorescence test for antibodies to thyroglobulin. Monkey thyroid sections, 4 μm thick, were fixed in methanol at 56 C for 10 min, covered with patient's serum, washed, and covered with goat antihuman gamma globulin labeled with fluorescein ("FITC-conjugate"). A floccular or crazed pattern of colloid staining can be seen. ×770.*

Interpretation of immunofluorescence test results

The same considerations apply for results of the IF test as for the hemagglutination tests, with the difference that the sensitivity of IF seems to be less. One of the advantages of the IF test is that it allows the detection of antibodies to CA2 (3, 13, 25). Such antibodies have been reported present in 40 to 70% of patients with thyroiditis and in smaller percentages of patients with thyrotoxicosis, nontoxic goiters, and other thyroid diseases (3, 13, 25). The sera of 5 to 8% of thyroiditis patients, negative by other procedures, contain antibodies to CA2. The nature of CA2 is still obscure, and recently it has been hypothesized that the "diffuse" pattern of staining characteristic of CA2 antibodies may be due to complexes of thyroglobulin and antibodies to thyroglobulin (5).

ANTIBODIES TO MICROSOMAL ANTIGENS OF THYROID EPITHELIAL CELLS

Antibodies to microsomal antigens of thyroid epithelial cells may be detected either by complement fixation or indirect IF. The latter, performed on unfixed thyroid sections, is the more sensitive test; serum titers obtained by this procedure are 4 to 10 times higher than those obtained by complement fixation and may reach 1,200 or higher.

The antibodies to the microsomal antigens belong predominantly to the immunoglobulin G (IgG) class and, when detected by indirect IF, stain the cytoplasm of thyroid cells (Fig. 3). The nucleus is unstained.

Indirect immunofluorescence test

Materials.

The same reagents described above for the IF test for antibodies to thyroglobulin are used.

Procedure.

1. Prepare 1:10 dilutions in PBS of all sera to be tested (unknown, positive and negative controls). Sera may be screened at 1:10 and 1:30 dilutions or titrated in serial twofold dilutions until the end point is reached.

2. Incubate diluted sera with cryostat sections of monkey or human thyroid (unfixed, air-dried) in a humid chamber at room temperature for 30 min.

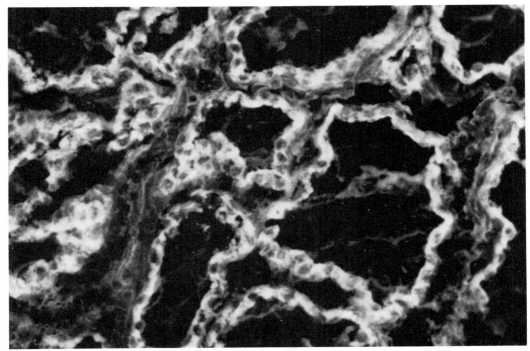

FIG. 3. *Immunofluorescence test for antibodies to thyroid microsomes. Monkey thyroid sections, 4 μm, unfixed, were air-dried, covered with patient's serum, washed, and covered with FITC-conjugate. Only the cytoplasm of the thyroid epithelial cells has stained.* ×770.

3. Wash slides in PBS for 30 min at room temperature. More efficient washing can be obtained by gently stirring with a magnetic stirrer and changing washes three times.

4. Incubate sections with diluted FITC-conjugate to human immunoglobulins in a humid chamber at room temperature for 30 min.

5. Wash again as in step 3.

6. Mount in buffered glycerol and read under a UV microscope.

Interpretation of test results

The indirect IF test for antibodies to microsomal antigens of thyroid epithelial cells is positive in approximately 70 to 90% of patients with chronic thyroiditis. It is also positive in 64% of patients with primary hypothyroidism, 50% with thyrotoxicosis, 10% with simple goiters, and 17% with thyroid tumors (9).

ANTIBODIES TO ADRENAL ANTIGENS

Patients with idiopathic Addison's disease have circulating antibodies to adrenal antigens. Such antibodies have been detected by a variety of procedures (2, 8, 17), but the most commonly used method is indirect IF. Antibodies detected by IF stain the cytoplasm of cells of the adrenal cortex and are directed to an anti-

gen associated with the microsomes of these cells. They belong predominantly to the IgG class and, in general, have rather low titers (not higher than 100).

Indirect immunofluorescence test

Materials.

The same reagents previously described for the IF test for antibodies to thyroglobulin are used.

Procedure.

1. Prepare 1:10 dilutions in PBS of all sera to be tested (unknown, positive and negative controls). Sera may be screened at a 1:10 dilution or titrated in serial twofold dilutions. Usually, it is not necessary to dilute higher than 1:80.

2. Incubate diluted sera with cryostat sections of monkey adrenal (either unfixed or after a 30-s fixation in cold acetone) in a humid chamber at room temperature for 30 min.

3. Wash slides in PBS for 30 min at room temperature. More efficient washing can be obtained by gently stirring with a magnetic stirrer and changing washes three times.

4. Incubate sections with diluted FITC-conjugate to human immunoglobulins in a humid chamber at room temperature for 30 min.

5. Wash again for 30 min as previously described.

6. Mount in buffered glycerol and read under a UV microscope.

Interpretation of test results

Antibodies to adrenocortical cells are detected in the serum of 38 to 60% of patients with idiopathic Addison's disease (22). They are present in 7 to 18% of patients with tuberculous Addison's disease and in 1% of normal subjects. The presence of antibodies to adrenocortical cells is a good indication that the disease is idiopathic and not of tubercular or other nature.

Different patterns of staining have been observed: most sera stain the whole cortex, with a brighter fluorescence in the glomerulosa zone, but a few sera stain only the fasciculata and reticularis zones, and not the zone glomerulosa (Fig. 4). The latter pattern has been reported with sera that also stain the interstitial cells of the testis and the theca interna cells of the ovary (see next section).

ANTIBODIES TO ANTIGENS OF OVARY, TESTIS, AND PLACENTA

Antibodies staining the cytoplasm of cells of the theca interna, interstitial cells and corpus luteum cells of the ovary, interstitial cells of the testis, and the trophoblast of placenta have been detected in the sera of patients with Addison's disease and patients with premature ovarian failure (1, 6, 16).

The antigens involved have not been very well characterized, and the test itself at present is more of research than diagnostic interest. It is performed on unfixed cryostat sections of ovary, testis, and placenta.

ANTIBODIES TO PARATHYROID ANTIGENS

Sera from patients with idiopathic hypoparathyroidism (IHP) contain antibodies to antigens of parathyroid cells. Such antibodies have been detected by indirect IF on sections of normal human parathyroid tissue obtained at autopsy (7). They are not directed against parathyroid hormone, but to cytoplasmic antigens of parathyroid cells.

Indirect immunofluorescence test
Materials.

The same reagents are used as for the other IF tests.

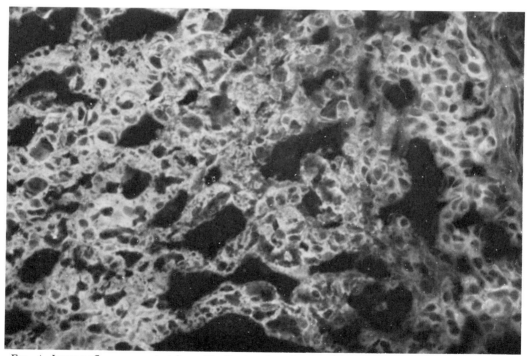

Fig. 4. *Immunofluorescence test for antibodies to adrenal cortex. Monkey adrenal sections, unfixed, were air-dried, covered with patient's serum, washed, and covered with FITC-conjugate. All layers of the cortex are stained. ×770.*

Procedure.

The test is performed like the other indirect IF tests previously described, with the difference that unfixed cryostat sections of parathyroid are used as substrate.

Interpretation of test

Antibodies to parathyroid cells are found in the serum of approximately 38% of patients with IHP, 26% of patients with idiopathic Addison's disease, 12% of patients with chronic thyroiditis, and 6% of controls.

Since approximately 60% of patients with IHP do not have demonstrable parathyroid antibodies, a negative test does not obviously exclude this condition. On the other hand, a positive test, while indicative of IHP, is not necessarily diagnostic, in that the patient might have adrenal insufficiency or thyroiditis, or a combination of these disorders.

ANTIBODIES TO MITOCHONDRIAL ANTIGENS

Sera from patients with primary biliary cirrhosis contain antibodies to mitochondrial antigens that are detectable by indirect IF (10, 11,

20). They belong to the IgG, IgA, and IgM classes. The mitochondrial antibodies stain the cytoplasm of epithelial cells from different organs, such as thyroid or kidney, giving a granular pattern of staining (Fig. 5).

Indirect immunofluorescence test

Materials.

See above.

Procedure.

The test is performed as previously described, with the difference that unfixed cryostat sections of rat kidney (the most commonly used substrate) are employed.

Interpretation of test

Mitochondrial antibodies are detected in 90 to 94% of patients with primary biliary cirrhosis. They are also observed in 25 to 28% of patients with active chronic hepatitis and 25 to 30% of patients with cryptogenic cirrhosis. They are only seldom observed in patients with extrahepatic biliary tract obstruction and occur very rarely (less than 1%) in normal subjects. Titers of mitochondrial antibodies observed in

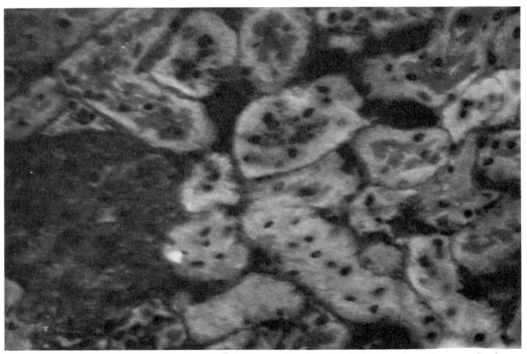

FIG. 5. *Immunofluorescence test for antibodies to mitochondria. Rat kidney sections, 4 μm, unfixed, were air-dried, covered with patient's serum, washed, and covered with FITC-conjugate. The cytoplasm of the tubular epithelium has stained.* ×770.

primary biliary cirrhosis are in the range of 10 to 6,000, with approximately 50% of the positive cases having titers of 200 to 6,000. However, there does not seem to be a correlation between titers of mitochondrial antibodies and severity or duration of liver disease.

ANTIBODIES TO SMOOTH MUSCLE ANTIGENS

Sera from patients with chronic active hepatitis contain antibodies to smooth muscle antigens that are detectable by indirect IF and stain the smooth muscle of several organs, such as the stomach (Fig. 6; 14, 19, 26, 27). They belong mainly to the IgG class, but can also be found in the IgM class.

Indirect immunofluorescence test

Materials.

See above.

Procedure.

The test is performed as previously described, with the difference that unfixed cryostat sections of rat stomach are used as substrate.

Interpretation of test

Smooth muscle antibodies are detected in 40 to 70% of patients with active chronic hepatitis, 50% with primary biliary cirrhosis, and 28% with cryptogenic cirrhosis. They are also found in patients with acute viral hepatitis, infectious mononucleosis, asthma, yellow fever, and malignant tumors (carcinomas of the ovary, malignant melanoma). They have been found in less than 2% of the normal population. Antibody titers are in the range of 80 to 320 in active chronic hepatitis and are much lower, rarely over 80, in the other conditions listed above.

ANTIBODIES TO GASTRIC PARIETAL CELLS

Circulating autoantibodies to intracytoplasmic antigens of gastric parietal cells (parietal cell antibodies), to the B12 binding site of intrinsic factor, and to the intrinsic factor-B12 complex occur with high frequency in patients with pernicious anemia (4, 12, 15, 18, 24). Antibodies to intrinsic factor may be detected by several radioassay procedures. However, these methods are not yet regularly performed in most hospitals. Parietal cell antibodies may be detected by indirect IF or by complement fixation. Since complement fixation is less sensi-

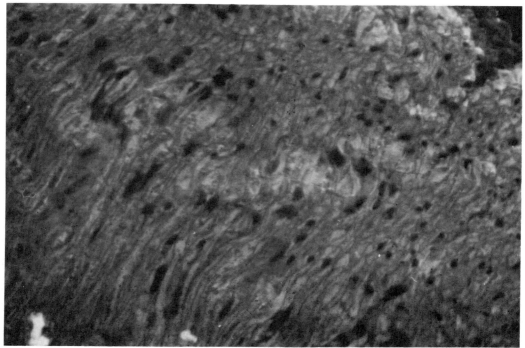

FIG. 6. *Immunofluorescence test for antibodies to smooth muscle. Rat stomach sections, 4 μm, unfixed, were covered with patient's serum, washed, and covered with FITC-conjugate. Only the submucosal muscle layer stained.* ×770.

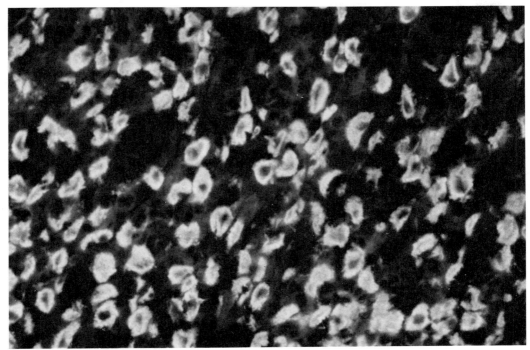

FIG. 7. *Immunofluorescence test for antibodies to gastric mucosa. Rat stomach transverse sections, 4 μm, unfixed, air-dried, were covered with serum of patient with pernicious anemia, washed, and covered with FITC-conjugate. Some of the mucosal cells show fluorescence in the cytoplasm. ×770.*

tive, IF is the method chosen in most clinical laboratories. Parietal cell antibodies, when detected by indirect IF, stain the cytoplasm of parietal cells of the gastric fundal mucosa of humans and various animals, like monkeys, rats, and guinea pigs (Fig. 7).

Indirect immunofluorescence test

Materials.

The same materials are used as described above.

Procedure.

The test is performed as previously described, with the difference that unfixed sections of rat stomach (gastric mucosa) are used as substrate.

Interpretation of test

Parietal cell antibodies are found in 90% or more of patients with pernicious anemia. They are also present in a number of other conditions, such as chronic thyroiditis (33%), Sjögren's sicca syndrome (15%), atrophic gastritis (60%), gastric ulcer (22%), etc. They are also found in the normal population, with an incidence that varies according to age, i.e. from 2%

in subjects below 20 years to 16% in subjects older than 60 years. They are more common in women than men.

LITERATURE CITED

1. Anderson, J. R., R. B. Goudie, K. Gray, and D. A. Stuart-Smith. 1968. Immunological features of idiopathic Addison's disease: an antibody to cells producing steroid hormones. Clin. Exp. Immunol. 3:107–117.
2. Andrada, J. A., P. E. Bigazzi, E. Andrada, F. Milgrom, and E. Witebsky. 1968. Serological investigations on Addison's disease. J. Am. Med. Assoc. 206:1535–1541.
3. Balfour, B. M., D. Doniach, I. M. Roitt, and K. G. Couchman. 1961. Fluorescent antibody studies in human thyroiditis: autoantibodies to an antigen of the thyroid colloid distinct from thyroglobulin. Br. J. Exp. Pathol. 43:307–316.
4. Bernhardt, H., L. L. Burkitt, M. L. Fields, and J. Killan. 1965. The diagnostic significance of the parietal cell immunofluorescent test. Ann. Intern. Med. 63:635–641.
5. Beutner, E. H., W. L. Hale, R. J. Nisengard, T. P. Chorzelski, and K. Holubar. 1973. Defined immunofluorescence in clinical immunopathology, p. 197–247. *In* E. H. Beutner, T. P. Chorzelski, S. F. Bean, and R. E. Jordan (ed)., Immunopathology of the skin: labeled antibody studies. Dowden, Hutchison & Ross,

Inc., Stroudsburg, Pa.

6. Bigazzi, P. E., J. A. Andrada, E. Andrada, E. H. Beutner, and E. Witebsky. 1968. Immunofluorescence studies on Addison's disease. Int. Arch. Allergy 34:455–469.

7. Blizzard, R. M., D. Chee, and W. Davis. 1966. The incidence of parathyroid and other antibodies in the sera of patients with idiopathic hypoparathyroidism. Clin. Exp. Immunol. 1:119–128.

8. Blizzard, R. M., D. Chee, and W. Davis. 1967. The incidence of adrenal and other antibodies in the sera of patients with idiopathic adrenal insufficiency (Addison's disease). Clin. Exp. Immunol. 2:19–30.

9. Delespesse, G., P. A. Bastenie, L. Vanhaelst, and P. Neve. 1972. Thyroid autoimmunity, p. 39–67. In P. A. Bastenie and A. M. Evans (ed.), Thyroiditis and thyroid function. Pergamon Press, Oxford.

10. Doniach, D., I. M. Roitt, J. G. Walker, and S. Sherlock. 1966. Tissue antibodies in primary biliary cirrhosis, active chronic (lupoid) hepatitis, cryptogenic cirrhosis and other liver diseases and their clinical implications. Clin. Exp. Immunol. 1:237–262.

11. Doniach, D., J. G. Walker, I. M. Riott, and P. A. Berg. "Autoallergic" hepatitis. N. Engl. J. Med. 282:86–88.

12. Goldberg, L. S., and H. H. Fudenberg. 1969. The autoimmune aspects of pernicious anemia. Am. J. Med. 46:489–494.

13. Hjort, T. 1963. The occurrence of antibody against "second colloid antigen" (CA-2 antibody) in patients with and without thyroid disease. Acta Med. Scand. 174:147–154.

14. Holborow, E. J. 1972. Smooth-muscle antibodies, viral infections and malignant disease. Proc. R. Soc. Med. 65:481–484.

15. Irvine, W. J. 1963. Gastric antibodies studied by fluorescent microscopy. Q. J. Exp. Physiol. 48:427–438.

16. Irvine, W. J. 1971. Adrenalitis, hypoparathyroidism and associated diseases, p. 1214–1227. In M. Samter (ed.), Immunologic diseases,

vol. 2. Little Brown & Co., Boston.

17. Irvine, W. J., A. G. Stewart, and L. Scarth. 1967. A clinical and immunological study of adrenocortical insufficiency (Addison's disease). Clin. Exp. Immunol. 2:31–69.

18. Jeffries, G. H. 1971. Pernicious anemia and atrophic gastritis, p. 1228–1239. In M. Samter (ed.), Immunologic diseases, vol. 2. Little Brown & Co., Boston.

19. Johnson, G. D., E. J. Holborow, and L. E. Glynn. 1965. Antibody to smooth muscle in patients with liver disease. Lancet 2:878–879.

20. Lam, K. C., S. P. Mistilis, and M. Perrott. 1972. Positive tissue antibody tests in patients with prolonged extrahepatic biliary obstruction. N. Engl. J. Med. 286:1400–1401.

21. Peake, R. L., D. B. Willis, G. K. Asimakis, and W. P. Deiss. 1974. Radioimmunologic assay for antithyroglobulin antibodies. J. Lab. Clin. Med. 86:907–919.

22. Rose, N. R., and P. E. Bigazzi. 1974. The autoimmune diseases, p. 765–794. In A. I. Laskin and H. A. Lechevalier (ed.), Handbook of microbiology, vol. 4. CRC Press, Cleveland.

23. Salabe, G. B., S. Fontana, and M. Andreoli. 1972. Radioimmunoassay for human antithyroglobulin antibodies. I. The relationship between tanned cell hemagglutination and a double antibody technique. Hormones (Basel) 3:1–13.

24. Strickland, R. G., S. Baur, L. A. E. Ashworth, and K. B. Taylor. 1971. A correlative study of immunological phenomena in pernicious anemia. Clin. Exp. Immunol. 8:25–36.

25. Tung, K. S. K., C. V. Ramos, and S. D. Deodhar. 1974. Antithyroid antibodies in juvenile lymphocytic thyroiditis. Am. J. Clin. Pathol. 61:549–555.

26. Whitehouse, J. M. A., and E. J. Holborow. 1971. Smooth muscle antibody in malignant disease. Br. Med. J. 4:511–513.

27. Whittingham, S., J. Irwin, I. R. Mackay, and M. Smalley. 1966. Smooth muscle autoantibody in "autoimmune" hepatitis. Gastroenterology 51:499–505.

Chapter 93

Immunohistopathology of the Kidney

CURTIS B. WILSON

INTRODUCTION

Immunofluorescence is the mainstay among immunohistochemical techniques used in identifying the immunopathogenesis of renal disease (20, 23). Enzyme-conjugated antibodies helpful in electron microscopy have not yet found wide use in light microscopy (6). Immunological renal injury may follow, first, if antibodies react with the renal basement membranes, either glomerular or tubular (GBM, TBM), and, second, if antibodies combine with nonglomerular antigens in the circulation to form nephritogenic immune complexes that lodge in the glomerular filter or renal interstitium (20, 25). With immunofluorescence, one can then identify these antibody deposits which initiate renal injury. Since anti-GBM or anti-TBM antibodies react all along the GBM or TBM, they appear as smooth linear deposits of immunoglobulin (Ig). Immune complexes depositing at random in the renal vasculature, predominantly the glomeruli, produce a granular, irregular accumulation of Ig. Either type of antibody reaction in the kidney can lead to activation of mediators of immunological injury, such as complement, which can also be characterized by immunofluorescence. The recent recognition of two pathways of complement activation (classical and alternative) has led to wider use of immunofluorescence in detecting components of each pathway bound in glomeruli. Indeed, complement activation in the absence of antigen-antibody reaction may represent a third mechanism of glomerular injury. Other possible mediators of immunological injury, such as coagulation proteins, i.e., fibrinogen and related antigens (FRA), can also be detected with the immunofluorescence technique. Immunofluorescence has also been used to identify and enumerate the cells in inflammatory infiltrates when specific antisera were available.

Satisfactory immunofluorescence study requires adequate tissue sections, optimal fluorescent-antibody reagents, adequate fluorescence microscopic equipment, and a good deal of experience in interpreting the findings. Portions of this chapter are directed toward each of these points, and a detailed description of tissue processing, fixation, and staining is included.

TISSUE PROCESSING AND SECTIONING

Renal tissue is usually obtained at biopsy by either an open or closed technique. Renal specimens taken at autopsy usually have an inordinate amount of background accumulation of serum proteins which make subsequent interpretation of immunologically specific deposits difficult. The tissue should be frozen as rapidly as possible. The method of choice is immersion in liquid nitrogen. Dry ice-organic solvent (acetone, alcohol) baths for snap-freezing have a distinct disadvantage since the organic solvents may inadvertently penetrate the tissue, rendering it soft and unsectionable at cryostat temperatures. The useful life of the frozen specimen is limited by the rate at which it desiccates. Desiccation can be retarded by freezing the specimen in isopenthane or in one of the commercial cryostat compounds, such as O.C.T. (Ames Co., Division of Miles Laboratories, Inc., Elkhart, Ind.). For the latter method, immerse the tissue fragment in a drop of O.C.T. placed on a thin slice (3 to 5 mm) of an appropriately sized cork. The cork, O.C.T., and tissue are then immersed in liquid nitrogen with a long forceps (Fig. 1). I prefer this method since the cork-mounted frozen specimen can be affixed directly on the cryostat chuck without any handling or danger of thawing. Thawing and refreezing of tissue for immunofluorescence study are often accompanied by loss of structural detail and increased nonspecific background staining. Refrozen tissue often does not adhere properly to microscopic slides, greatly increasing technical difficulties. The tissue should be stored in a small, sealed container with a chip of ice to increase humidity and placed in a nonfrost-free compartmentalized freezer. The freezer should be reserved for the frozen specimens and opened as infrequently as possible. A temperature of -70 C is optimal, although -30 C is usually satisfactory. No matter how much care is taken, the specimens will deteriorate with time, so sections should be obtained as soon as possible after tissue procurement.

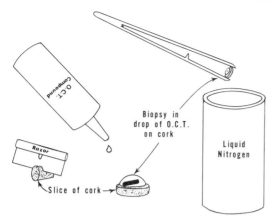

FIG. 1. *Preparation of renal biopsy tissue for immunofluorescence study. Biopsy specimens are placed in a drop of O.C.T. compound on a thin slice of cork. The cork, O.C.T. and biopsy are snap-frozen by immersion in liquid nitrogen with a long forceps.*

Several types of cryostats are available to house microtomes for sectioning frozen tissue. The open top models are most common and offer relative ease in operation. They have the disadvantage of rather poor temperature stability at the level of the knife blade, which may result in thawing of the very small needle biopsy fragments usually sectioned. I prefer the closed cabinet type of cryostat in which the operator works with fleece-lined gauntlets. The small needle biopsy specimens then may be handled at leisure without danger of thawing. I have been pleased with the Harris cryostat (Harris Manufacturing Co., Cambridge, Mass.) which, when used in combination with the British Slee microtome (Slee International, Inc., Pennsauken, N.J.), has enabled us routinely to obtain sections less than 3 μm thick. Techniques have also been described for preparing paraffin-embedded tissue for immunofluorescence study (17, 18).

FIXATION AND STAINING

Cryostat sections are routinely washed, fixed, and stained as outlined below. It should be noted, however, that there are several alternative ways of processing the sections, particularly in regard to fixation, so that it is wise to study the effects of each step on the end result. Certain antigens may be soluble in phosphate-buffered saline (PBS) or in solvents used in fixation, so that these steps may need to be modified accordingly. For example, we have observed that the patterns of fluorescent reactants may differ when acetone or methanol, rather than ether-ethanol, fixation is used. Direct immunofluorescence techniques have suffi-

cient sensitivity for renal studies and require fewer controls than the indirect method. The procedure used in my laboratory for routine renal immunofluorescence processing is listed below.

1. Cryostat sections are air-dried on slides with easily labeled frosted ends.

2. The dried tissue sections are surrounded by a ring of Tri-Chem liquid embroidery (Tri-Chem and Co., Belleville, N.J.) that forms a well to hold the fluorochrome-conjugated reagent and that simplifies locating the tissue fragment during examination with the fluorescence microscope.

3. The tissue sections are washed by immersion in a histological staining dish for 2 to 3 min in PBS (0.01 M sodium phosphate-buffered 0.15 M NaCl, pH 7.0) to remove unbound serum proteins.

4. The PBS-washed sections are immersed in ether-95% ethyl alcohol (50:50) for 10 min and ethyl alcohol (95%) for 20 min for fixation.

5. After fixation, the sections are washed in three changes of PBS to remove the fixative. The excess PBS is then wiped from the slide, and the still moist tissue section is transferred to a level moist chamber for staining.

6. For fluorescence staining, 20 μliters of the appropriate fluorochrome-conjugated reagent is delivered to the section with a mechanical pipette. The staining reaction is carried out in a moist chamber for a minimum of 30 min.

7. After staining, the sections are again washed in three changes of PBS to remove any unbound reagent.

8. Cover slips are next mounted over the sections with 0.01 M Tris-buffered glycerol [1 part tris(hydroxymethyl)aminomethane, 9 parts glycerol], pH 9.6. The high pH increases and stabilizes the luminescence of fluorescein.

9. Sections fixed and stained in this manner can be stored flat in folders in the cold for months and even years.

FLUORESCENT REAGENTS

The quality of the final fluorescence slides depends for the most part on the quality of the fluorochrome-labeled reagent. Optimal fluorescence reactions should be bright with virtually no background staining. Background staining usually results when antibody molecules are heavily labeled with fluorochrome, which causes them to adhere nonspecifically to tissue. Fluorescein-conjugated antibodies prepared commercially often have this fault. To obtain optimal reagents, I have found it most efficient to perform the fluorescein conjugation in my own laboratory. The specific antibodies of interest may be obtained commercially or pre-

pared by immunizing animals. Fluorescein isothiocyanate (FITC) and tetramethyl rhodamine
(10) are the most commonly used fluorochromes, with the former generally employed
for immunofluorescence studies of kidneys. I
have found that FITC-labeled IgG fractions of
antisera (specific for the antigen of interest
when tested by immunodiffusion and immunoelectrophoresis) provide satisfactory agents if,
after labeling, they are chromatographed to
select populations of molecules containing optimal FITC to protein ratios (26). Specific fluorochrome-labeled antibody fractions can also be
prepared by affinity chromatography (7). A
procedure for preparing FITC-conjugated
reagents for use in renal immunofluorescence
is listed below.

1. A crude gamma globulin fraction of the
antiserum of interest is first prepared from the
raw antiserum by ammonium sulfate precipitation at 50% saturation.

   a. The raw antiserum is diluted 1:2 with 0.1
      M borate buffer, pH 8.6.

   b. An equal volume of filtered and pH-ad-
      justed (NH_4OH, pH 8.6) saturated ammo-
      nium sulfate (0 C) is added slowly and
      stirred into the diluted antiserum.

   c. Precipitation is allowed to proceed for 30
      min at 4 C.

   d. The gamma globulin-rich precipitate is
      separated by centrifugation (3,000 rpm for
      30 min).

   e. The precipitate is then dissolved in borate
      buffer and reprecipitated a second time,
      following a similar procedure.

   f. The resultant second precipitate is dis-
      solved in a minimal amount of PBS and
      dialyzed extensively in PBS to remove the
      ammonium sulfate.

2. The gamma globulin fraction is dialyzed
against 0.01 M potassium phosphate buffer (pH
7.6) in preparation for diethylaminoethyl
(DEAE) cellulose chromatography equilibrated
with a similar buffer. The IgG fraction which
voids from this column is concentrated to 10
mg/ml by using negative pressure dialysis.

3. The IgG (10 mg/ml) fraction thus obtained
is fluorescein-conjugated by dialysis (3), with
the use of 0.025 M carbonate buffer (pH 9.6)
with FITC dissolved at a concentration of 0.1
mg/ml. A sufficient volume of FITC-containing
carbonate buffer is used to provide 1 mg of FITC
per 10 mg of IgG. The fluorescein conjugation
process takes 18 to 24 h of dialysis at 4 C. The
conjugated protein is then freed from unbound
FITC by further dialysis in PBS (24 to 48 h).

4. Finally, the dialyzed FITC-conjugated IgG
is reequilibrated in 0.01 M potassium phosphate buffer, pH 7.6, by dialysis so that it can
be rechromatographed on DEAE cellulose.

   a. The non-fluorescein-conjugated IgG in the
      sample which voids from the DEAE col-
      umn equilibrated at 0.01 M potassium
      phosphate (pH 7.6) is discarded since it
      would serve as a blocking antibody.

   b. By step elution, populations of Ig mole-
      cules with increasing amounts of FITC per
      molecule can be eluted. A 0.05 M potas-
      sium phosphate (pH 7.6) step fraction is
      ideal for tissue staining. A 0.1 M potas-
      sium phosphate (pH 7.6) step fraction may
      also be recovered which, although having
      somewhat higher background staining, is
      usually useful for tissue fluorescence.
      When fluorescence reagents of higher
      FITC to protein ratios are required, for
      example, to detect cell surface Ig, 0.2 or 0.3
      M fractions may be obtained from a simi-
      lar column.

   c. The fluorescein-conjugated IgG fractions
      thus obtained from DEAE cellulose chro-
      matography are concentrated or diluted
      until appropriate staining of a known posi-
      tive target tissue is observed. The specific-
      ity controls outlined below are then car-
      ried out.

5. The reagents are frozen at -30 C in small
portions until used. The useful life of the reagent may be prolonged by adding a small
amount of carrier such as bovine serum albumin to increase the protein concentration. The
stored reagent should always be tested on a
known positive target tissue before use.

IMMUNOFLUORESCENCE CONTROLS

Two types of specificity controls are needed in
interpreting immunofluorescence results.
First, the specificity of the fluorochrome-labeled antibody must be assessed at the level of
sensitivity of fluorescence. The best way to do
this is to absorb the reagent with its specific
antigen. This is done most easily by using the
antigen in an insoluble form so that fluorescein-conjugated, soluble, and potentially reactive immune complexes do not form in the reagent. One of the easiest ways to make the
antigen insoluble is to affix it to a particle such
as Sepharose activated with cyanogen bromide
(5). An alternative control, that of blocking
positive staining by prior reaction with a non-
fluorescein-conjugated antibody, has been suggested, but does not clearly establish the specificity of either the conjugated or nonconjugated
blocking antibody. Once the immunological
specificity of the fluorochrome-labeled reagent
has been established, a second set of specificity
controls must be employed to determine the

immunological specificity of any observed positive reaction. This addresses the question of whether the deposits of protein detected by the fluorescein-conjugated reagent are present because of an immunological reaction or are merely trapped within the tissue for nonimmunological reasons. A fibrin coagulum, for example, can nonspecifically entrap serum proteins which are not easily removed by washing. These controls include the use of reagents specific for nonimmunological serum proteins, such as transferrin and albumin to detect serum trapping. The true immunological nature of an Ig deposit can be shown by removing the Ig by elution in a buffer known to dissociate antigen-antibody bonds (23). The eluted Ig can be studied in vitro to determine its specificity.

FLUORESCENCE MICROSCOPES, LIGHT SOURCES, AND VIEWING PROCEDURES

The fluorescence-stained sections are next viewed with a fluorescence microscope (10). Two methods of providing illumination are available. For maximal intensity at the magnifications utilized in studying renal biopsies (100 to 600 ×), the light is transmitted to the section via an immersed cardioid dark-field condenser. Recently, vertical illumination employing dichroic mirrors with selective, reflective properties (16) has been introduced as an alternative system which provides good illumination at very high magnification since the objective serves as its own condenser. However, the light provided by this system at lower magnifications is much less than that obtained by the more conventional systems. High-pressure mercury or xenon light sources provide the best illumination. Halogen-quartz light sources have been introduced as a cheaper source of illumination which can be used with the new interference filter systems. This latter light source, however, does not provide sufficient light to utilize other filter systems which are helpful in determining specificity.

Three filter systems are commonly used in immunofluorescence study of renal biopsies (10). Each system utilizes an exciter filter to provide light of a certain wavelength to excite the fluorochrome and a second barrier filter to exclude the exciting light, allowing transmission of only the secondary and longer wavelength fluorescent illumination. For example, fluorescein is maximally excited around 490 nm and emits a fluorescent light of 517 nm (10). The different filter systems available have different intensities as well as providing different hues of background fluorescence which are helpful in determining the specificity of the reaction. For example, the UG 1 exciter system transmits light maximally at 365 nm and, when viewed with a 410-nm barrier filter, imparts an intense blue-white autofluorescence to the elastica of arterial walls. In contrast, the FITC interference filter transmits maximally between 400 and 500 nm and, when viewed with a 500-nm barrier filter, gives a yellow autofluorescence to the elastica. This yellow color must be differentiated from the yellow-green fluorescence of FITC. However, the FITC interference filter transmits a great deal more light and may increase the detection of small quantities of fluorescent material which might be missed by the less intense UG 1 or BG 12 filter systems (13). We usually view sections with both the UG 1 and FITC interference systems to obtain the advantages of both, namely, sensitivity and specificity.

The stained sections should be viewed in a standard way so the glomeruli, tubules, vessels, and interstitium are evaluated on each slide. The pattern and amount rather than the intensity of fluorescence (a property of the reagent) should be noted. Serum proteins in tubular casts and reabsorption droplets within tubular epithelium must be distinguished from immune deposits. Autofluorescent cellular granules as well as connective tissue and vascular elastic lamina must not be confused with specific fluorescent deposits. However, attention should be paid to any unusual autofluorescent material; calcium deposits, for example, may emit a striking autofluorescence. An adequate number of glomeruli must be examined because presumed immune complex (granular) deposits may be quite "focal" and involve only a few glomeruli in the biopsy. On the other hand, granular deposits of immune complexes associated with membranous glomerulonephritis (GN), or linear deposits in anti-GBM antibody-induced GN, are usually uniform from glomerulus to glomerulus, so that a single glomerulus may be adequate for diagnosis.

ROUTINE IMMUNOFLUORESCENCE STUDY OF RENAL BIOPSIES

Each biopsy is routinely stained for IgG, IgA, IgM, IgE, Clq, C3, C4 and C5, C6, C8, properdin, and C3 activator, as well as FRA. Reagents specific for albumin and/or transferrin are included to evaluate nonspecific entrapment of serum proteins within the tissue. Additional reagents for other Ig classes or subclasses, complement-related proteins, and coagulation factors are utilized when indicated. Light chain antisera are useful in detecting amyloid deposits which may not be visualized with Ig heavy chain class-specific antisera. Antisera specific for suspected immune complex antigens are also being used with increasing regularity.

INTERPRETATION OF IMMUNOFLUORESCENCE STUDIES ON RENAL BIOPSIES

A detailed discussion of the interpretation of immune reactants in the kidney is beyond the scope of this technical chapter; however, a few points merit mention. Linear deposits of Ig suggesting anti-GBM antibodies are found along the GBM in about 5% of kidney studied in my laboratory (22). Early in the course of anti-GBM GN, the linear deposits are very smooth, continuous, and uniform (Fig. 2A); however, as damage progresses, the GBM becomes disrupted, compressed, and corrugated, with corresponding changes in the pattern of Ig deposits (Fig. 2B). As the kidney with anti-GBM GN reaches end stage, little recognizable deposition may remain to be seen by immunofluorescence; however, anti-GBM antibodies can often still be eluted from the specimen (23). IgG is the predominant Ig in anti-GBM GN (22). Rarely, linear deposits of IgA are encountered. IgM is more frequently found, but it is usually present in an irregular granular distribution instead of as a linear deposit. C3 is present in about two-thirds of specimens (22), but it is often less intense than Ig and may only be irregular or segmental. When present, the C3 is usually accompanied by initial components of the complement cascade, suggesting classical complement pathway activation (19). FRA deposits are often found in areas of crescent formation.

Detection of linear deposits of Ig should be only the first step in making the diagnosis of anti-GBM GN. Normal kidneys perfused for transplantation, one-fourth to one-half of kidneys at autopsy, and kidneys from patients with diabetes mellitus and possibly lupus erythematosus may have nonimmunological linear deposits of IgG (23). In addition, roughly 10% of often minimally damaged kidneys have linear accentuation of the GBM when stained for IgG; this deposition probably represents the roughly 2% of IgG normally present in the GBM (23). Therefore, elution studies or detection of circulating anti-GBM antibodies (indirect immunofluorescence or radioimmunoassay) is essential for confirming the immunological specificity of any observed linear deposits.

About 70% of kidneys from patients with anti-GBM GN also have linear deposits of IgG along the TBM (Fig. 2E). In far advanced cases, this may be the only remaining immune deposit. The alveolar basement membrane often has evidence of linear deposition in the Goodpasture's syndrome form of anti-GBM GN (pulmonary hemorrhage and GN), and linear deposits as well can be observed along the basement membrane of the choroid plexus in this form of disease. Linear TBM deposits may also be found occasionally in renal transplants, in patients with tubulo-interstitial nephritis, in methicillin-associated nephrotoxicity, and in association with immune complex-induced GN (11).

Upwards of 80% of GN seems to be induced by immune complex deposition in glomeruli typified by granular deposits of IgG and complement early in the course of disease. At end stage, minimal amounts of Ig and often only C3 deposits may remain. In evaluating immunofluorescence-stained sections, one should characterize deposits according to the size (fine, coarse) and distribution (mesangial, GBM, diffuse, confluent, segmental, etc.). The deposition is graded 0 to 4+, depending on the extent of deposition, not its intensity (21).

Immune complexes can lead to a wide spectrum of histological forms of GN, with the immune deposits corresponding in general to the severity of the disease as determined from the light microscopic appearance (Table 1). Diffuse proliferative GN usually has diffuse deposits, whereas focal GN generally has segmental GBM or mesangial deposits. Membranous GN is typified by uniform granularity all along the GBM (Fig. 2C). Immune complexes of apparently similar composition cause the multiple histological forms of GN seen in systemic lupus erythematosus. Again, the amount of granular deposits corresponds in general to the degree of histological change, and, if appropriate specimens are available, one should be able to see that deposits precede evidence of histological damage.

In immune complex GN, IgG is the most common Ig identified. It is often accompanied by IgM and less frequently by IgA. In systemic lupus erythematosus GN, IgA and IgM are commonly observed with IgG. IgA is also frequent in Henoch-Schönlein purpura, in which it may predominate over IgG in a mesangial distribution. Mesangial deposits of IgA and IgG or IgM and IgG are also observed in patients with recurrent benign hematuria and focal GN (Fig. 2D). A summary of the Ig, complement, and FRA deposits in several forms of immune complex-induced GN is presented in Table 1. Some overlap is observed in the various histological forms of immune complex GN, both in Ig pattern and in Ig class, so that, although these generalizations are helpful, they cannot be

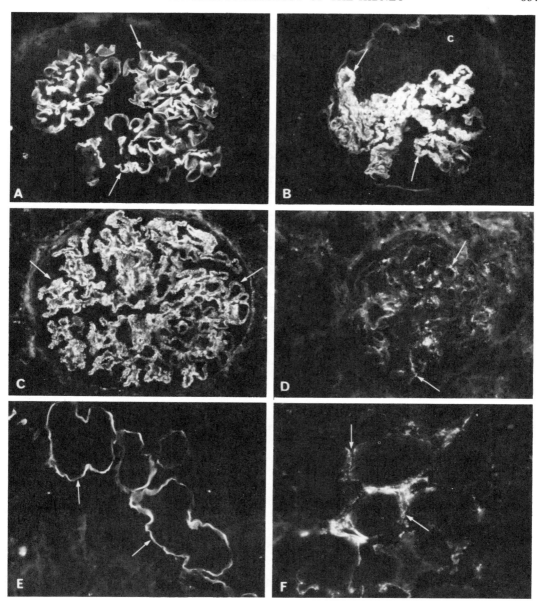

FIG. 2. (A) Smooth, continuous linear deposits of IgG (arrows) are present along the GBM from a patient with anti-GBM GN with minimal glomerular architectural derangement. (B) Heavy IgG deposits (arrows) are present along the corrugated and crumpled GBM from a patient with far advanced anti-GBM GN. A large portion of Bowman's space is occupied by crescent (c) formation. (C) Heavy granular deposits of IgG (arrows) are present all along the GBM from a patient with immune complex-induced membranous GN. (D) Focal, segmental granular deposits of IgG (arrows) are present along the GBM from a patient with focal GN. (E) Smooth, linear deposits of IgG (arrows) are present along the TBM of a renal biopsy from a patient with anti-GBM GN. (F) Irregular, granular deposits of IgG (arrows) are present along the TBM of a renal biopsy from a patient with systemic lupus erythematosus. Direct immunofluorescence staining fluorescein isothiocyanate-conjugated rabbit antihuman IgG antiserum. Original magnification: A, B, C, and D × 250; E and F × 400.

TABLE 1. *Renal immunofluorescence in human glomerulonephritis (GN)*[a]

Pathogenesis	Glomerular immunofluorescence findings
I. Anti-GBM GN	
Goodpasture's syndrome and rapidly progressive GN	Linear IgG, infrequent linear IgA, irregular IgM. C3 present in 70%, usually irregular. FRA prominent in crescents.
II. Presumed immune complex GN	
Diffuse proliferative GN, including poststreptococcal	Diffuse granular IgG. Variable presence of granular IgA and IgM. C3 usually present and may be seen in absence of Ig. FRA usually absent.
Rapidly progressive GN	Granular IgG, C3, variable IgA, IgM. FRA prominent in crescents.
Focal proliferative GN	Segmental granular and mesangial IgG, C3 often with prominent mesangial IgA or IgM. FRA variable.
Membranous GN	Diffuse granular IgG, C3, with variable IgA and IgM all along the GBM. FRA variable.
Membranoproliferative GN	Coarse granular C3. IgG with variable IgA, IgM frequent in subendothelial deposit form. FRA variable.
Focal glomerulosclerosis	Segmental granular IgG, IgM, C3. IgA, FRA usually absent.
GN of systemic disease	
Systemic lupus erythematosus	Granular IgG, IgA, IgM, and C3 in diffuse, segmental or mesangial pattern. FRA variable.
Henoch-Schönlein purpura	Segmental and mesangial IgG, IgA, C3, FRA. IgM variable.
III. Unclear immune pathogenesis	
Minimal change lesion (lipoid nephrosis)	No IgG, IgA, IgM, C3, FRA deposits.
Hereditary nephritis (Alport's syndrome)	Usually no IgG, IgA, IgM, C3, FRA deposits.
Coagulopathies (hemolytic uremic syndrome, eclampsia, etc.)	Prominent FRA. Little or no IgG, IgA, IgM, or C3.

[a] Useful references: 1, 2, 4, 9, 11, 12, 14, 15, 19, 20, 22, 23.

used unqualifiedly to predict histological or clinical classification.

Of course, granular deposits of Ig and complement must only be presumed to represent immune complexes. To confirm the immune complex nature of the deposit, its antigenic content must be identified. This can sometimes be done with immunofluorescence by using fluorescein-conjugated antisera specific for the suspected antigen. In some instances, partial elution of the Ig portion of the immune complex (8) enhances detection of residual antigen(s). Elution of antibody for subsequent specificity studies also aids in identification of antigen-antibody systems in kidneys suspected of harboring immune complexes. The following are examples of antigen-antibody systems which can lead to formation of nephritogenic immune complexes in humans.

Foreign (exogenous) antigens
    Foreign serum proteins, drugs, toxoids
    Bacterial antigens: nephritogenic streptococci, *Streptococcus albus*, *Diplococcus pneumoniae*, enterococcus, *Salmonella typhosa*, *Treponema pallidum*
    Parasitic antigens: *Plasmodium malariae*, *P. falciparum*, *Schistosoma mansoni*, *Toxoplasma gondii*
    Viral antigens: hepatitis B, measles, Epstein-Barr, oncornavirus
Self (endogenous) antigens
    Nuclear materials, thyroglobulin, renal tubular brush border, carcinoembryonic antigen, other tumor antigens, Ig (cryoglobulins)

Granular Ig (presumed immune complex) deposits (19) are usually accompanied by C3 with complement components suggestive of classical complement pathway activation. As immune complex GN progresses, only C3 and terminal complement components (C5 to C9) may remain, suggesting continued complement activation via the alternative complement pathway. In about 10% of kidneys with GN, complement but not Ig is observed. Whether this represents end-stage immune complex GN or primary nephritogenic nonimmune complement activation via the alternative (properdin) complement pathway is unknown. Immunofluorescence is being employed to differentiate the pathways of complement activation. The reagents used are specific for complement components, properdin, and other proteins of the alternative complement pathway, including the C3 activating substance (C3 NeF), isolated from patients with membranoproliferative GN. The latter patients have drawn considerable interest recently because of associated complement abnormalities. Two histological variants now identified have some differences in immunofluorescence findings. The subendothelial dense deposit variety of membranoproliferative GN has Ig and complement deposits suggestive of immune complexes, whereas the intramembranous dense deposit form generally has only complement deposits, suggestive of nonimmunological complement activation.

Granular deposits of Ig and complement indicative of immune complexes may occur in extraglomerular renal tissue. About 70% of biopsies from patients with systemic lupus erythematosus-associated GN have granular deposits in vessels, the renal interstitium, and TBM (Fig. 2F). In systemic lupus erythematosus, staining of cellular nuclei can also occasionally be visualized, indicating the presence of antinuclear antibodies. Whether the antinuclear reaction occurs in vivo or is an artifact induced in vitro during tissue processing is unclear. Vascular deposits of Ig, complement, and FRA may be identified in vessels of patients with vasculitis and also in patients with malignant hypertension. Complement deposits without Ig are quite common in vessels, renal interstitium, and TBM in kidneys from patients with advanced GN; however, the immunopathological significance of these deposits is not yet clear.

Limited information regarding immunofluorescence studies is available on other forms of renal disease. Glomeruli from patients with minimal change or "lipoid nephrosis" are generally free from deposits, as are glomeruli from patients with hereditary nephritis (Alport's syndrome). The GBM and TBM from diabetics often contain Ig; however, the Ig in the thickened diabetic basement membrane does not appear to denote an immune reaction. Renal biopsies from patients with dysproteinemia may show accumulations of the abnormal protein within glomerular capillaries. Amyloid deposits generally do not stain with heavy chain specific anti-Ig antisera but may be detected in some patients with light chain antisera. In renal lesions associated with coagulopathies (hemolytic uremic syndrome, thrombotic thrombocytopenic purpura, eclampsia, etc.), FRA may accumulate in glomeruli without Ig and complement.

In renal allografts, both anti-GBM and immune complex GN may recur, resulting in immunofluorescence pictures similar to those seen in the patients' native kidneys. Both antibasement membrane (GBM and TBM) and immune complex forms of renal injury may also develop de novo in renal allografts, with immunofluorescence findings similar to those described for their counterparts in native kidneys. Vascular deposits of Ig, particularly IgM, and complement are also frequently encountered in renal allografts.

Immunofluorescence studies are then of primary importance in differentiating the immunopathogenesis of renal injury, which cannot be readily discerned by using routine light microscopy. Indeed, the former techniques provide the simplest and most direct approach for identifying the presence of antibasement membrane or immune complex antibodies which can induce the wide variety of clinical and histological forms of GN seen in the practice of nephrology. Therefore, immunofluorescence evaluation should be included in the meaningful interpretation of any renal biopsy.

ACKNOWLEDGMENTS

This work was supported by Public Health Service contract AI-42505 and Public Health Service grant AI-07007 from the National Institute of Allergy and Infectious Diseases.

Publication No. 1027 from the Department of Immunopathology, Scripps Clinic and Research Foundation, La Jolla, Calif.

LITERATURE CITED

1. Andres, G. A., and R. T. McCluskey. 1975. Tubular and interstitial renal disease due to immunologic mechanisms. Kidney Int. 7:271–289.

2. Berger, J., H. Yaneva, and N. Hinglais. 1971. Immunohistochemistry of glomerulonephritis. Adv. Nephrol. 1:11–30.

3. Clark, H. F., and C. C. Shepard. 1963. A dialysis technique for preparing fluorescent antibody. Virology 20:642–644.

4. Cochrane, C. G., and D. Koffler. 1973. Immune complex disease in experimental animals and man. Adv. Immunol. 16:186–264.

5. Cuatrecasas, P. 1970. Protein purification by affinity chromatography. Derivatizations of agarose and polyacrylamide beads. J. Biol. Chem. 245:3059–3065.

6. Dujovne, I., V. E. Pollak, C. L. Pirani, and M. G. Dillard. 1972. The distribution and character of glomerular deposits in systemic lupus erythematosus. Kidney Int. 2:33–50.

7. Edgington, T. S. 1971. Dissociation of antibody from erythrocyte surfaces by chaotropic ions. J. Immunol. 106:673–680.

8. Edgington, T. S., R. J. Glassock, and F. J. Dixon, 1967. Autologous immune complex pathogenesis of experimental allergic glomerulonephritis. Science 155:1432–1434.

9. Germuth, F. G., and E. Rodriguez. 1973. Immunopathology of the renal glomerulus: immune complex deposit and antibasement membrane disease. Little, Brown and Co., Boston.

10. Goldman, M. 1968. Fluorescent antibody methods. Academic Press Inc., New York.

11. Lehman, D. H., C. B. Wilson, and F. J. Dixon. 1975. Extraglomerular immunoglobulin deposits in human nephritis. Am. J. Med. 58:765–786.

12. McCluskey, R. T. 1971. The value of immunofluorescence in the study of human renal disease. J. Exp. Med. 134:242s–255s.

13. Markham, R. V., J. C. Sutherland, and M. R. Mardiney, Jr. 1973. The ubiquitous occurrence of immune complex localization in the renal glomeruli of normal mice. Lab. Invest. 29:111–120.

14. Michael, A. F., N. G. Westberg, A. J. Fish, and R. L. Vernier. 1971. Studies on chronic membrano-proliferative glomerulonephritis with hypocomplementemia. J. Exp. Med. 134:208s–227s.

15. Morel-Maroger, L., A. Leathem, and G. Richet. 1972. Glomerular abnormalities in nonsystemic diseases: relationship between findings by light microscopy and immunofluorescence in 433 renal biopsy specimens. Am. J. Med. 53:170–184.

16. Ploem, J. S. 1967. The use of a vertical illuminator with interchangeable dichroic mirrors for fluorescence microscopy with incident light. Mikrosk. Technik 68:129–142.

17. Post, R. S. 1965. A technique for cutting thin sections from solvent-substituted paraffin embedded tissues. Cryobiology 1:261–269.

18. Saint-Marie, G. 1962. A paraffin embedding technique for studies employing immunofluorescence. J. Histochem. Cytochem. 10:250–256.

19. Verroust, P. J., C. B. Wilson, N. R. Cooper, T. S. Edgington, and F. J. Dixon. 1974. Glomerular complement components in human glomerulonephritis. J. Clin. Invest. 53:77–84.

20. Wilson, C. B. 1975. Immunofluorescence in differentiating the immunopathogenesis of renal disease. Ariz. Med. 32:283–289.

21. Wilson, C. B., and F. J. Dixon. 1970. Antigen quantitation in experimental immune complex glomerulonephritis. I. Acute serum sickness. J. Immunol. 105:279–290.

22. Wilson, C. B., and F. J. Dixon. 1973. Anti-glomerular basement membrane antibody induced glomerulonephritis. Kidney Int. 3:74–89.

23. Wilson, C. B., and F. J. Dixon. 1974. Diagnosis of immunopathologic renal disease. Editorial. Kidney Int. 5:389–401.

24. Wilson, C. B., and F. J. Dixon. 1974. Immunopathology and glomerulonephritis. Annu. Rev. Med. 25:83–98.

25. Wilson, C. B., and F. J. Dixon. 1976. The renal response to immunologic injury, p. 838–940. In B. M. Brenner and F. C. Rector, Jr. (ed.), The kidney. W. B. Saunders Co., Philadelphia.

26. Wood, B. T., S. H. Thompson, and G. Goldstein. 1965. Fluorescent antibody staining. III. Preparation of fluorescein-isothiocyanate-labeled antibodies. J. Immunol. 95:225–229.

Chapter 94

Immunohistopathology of the Skin

ROBERT E. JORDON

INTRODUCTION

Immunohistochemical methods have provided the dermatologist, as well as the clinical immunologist, with valuable histological and serological techniques for both research and diagnosis. These methods are of particular value in the diagnosis, classification, and management of patients with vesiculobullous skin diseases and cutaneous forms of lupus erythematosus and vasculitis.

By far the most popular of the immunohistochemical methods are the immunofluorescence (IF) procedures, which include indirect, direct, modified indirect, and mixed IF staining, and in vitro complement staining. Ferritin-, tritium-, and peroxidase-labeling methods are basically research tools and are difficult to perform. These techniques, therefore, are not practical routine procedures. Only the IF methods have gained widespread popularity in dermatology as diagnostic tests. In this chapter, I shall present a brief review of the IF methods as we are presently using them in our laboratories for both investigative and diagnostic purposes. More specific information, including a review of all phases of research and methodology, is recorded in two recent monographs (4, 5).

LABELED ANTISERA

Labeled antisera used in IF testing vary, depending upon the diagnostic or investigational problem. In current use are antisera to various immunoglobulins (IgG, IgA, IgM, IgD, and IgE), complement components (Clq, C4, C3, factor B, and properdin), and fibrin. Details of the preparation of these antisera will not be presented here since such a review would exceed the limitations of this chapter. With the exception of anti-properdin, however, all of the above antisera are available commercially (Hyland Division, Travenol Laboratories, Costa Mesa, Calif. 92626; and Behring Diagnostics, American Hoechst Pharmaceuticals, Sommerville, N.J. 08876).

TISSUE HANDLING

The handling of tissues used in the various IF staining procedures is as critical as is the qual-ity of the conjugated antisera. In addition, different tissues are currently being used in the different IF tests.

For indirect IF testing of pemphigus and bullous pemphigoid sera, monkey esophageal tissue provides the best antigen source. The esophagus should be removed immediately after the rhesus monkey is killed, cut into small segments suitable for mounting, and quick-frozen in liquid nitrogen. Tissues are stored at −70 C until sectioned. Rhesus monkey esophagus may also be purchased (Gibco Inc., Div. of Mogul Corp., Grand Island, N.Y. 14072).

Skin biopsies for immunopathological investigation are handled in a similar manner. Skin specimens are obtained by punch biopsy or surgical excision and are quick-frozen in liquid nitrogen and stored at −70 C. This is by far the best method for handling skin biopsy specimens.

An alternative to the above-mentioned procedure, however, has recently been developed. A fixative, called Michel's solution (4) may be used to ship biopsy material when liquid nitrogen or dry ice is not available. The composition of this fixative is as follows: $(NH_4)_2SO_4$, 3.12 M; N-ethylmaleimide, 0.0005 M; $MgSO_4$, 0.0005 M; and citrate, 0.025 M. Upon receipt of the biopsy in the fixative, the specimen should be washed three times for 10 min in a buffer with the following composition: 2.5 ml of 1 M K citrate buffer (pH 7.0), 5.0 ml of 0.1 M $MgSO_4$, 5.0 ml of 0.1 M N-ethylmaleimide, and 87.5 ml of water; adjust to pH 7.0 with 7 M KOH. After this rinse, the biopsy specimens should be frozen at −20 C and may then be processed for IF staining.

IMMUNOFLUORESCENCE PROCEDURES

Indirect immunofluorescence staining

Indirect IF staining is by far the most popular of the IF test procedures used in immunodermatology. This technique is used to detect intercellular substance antibodies in patients with pemphigus and basement membrane zone reactive antibodies in patients with bullous pemphigoid (4–8, 14, 26, 34, 51). First described by Weller and Coons (52), the indirect IF is a two-step serological procedure for the detection of circulating antibodies and is a valuable screening procedure.

Unfixed frozen sections of stratified squamous epithelium, usually monkey esophageal tissue, are cut in a cryostat at −30 C. These sections on microscopic slides are then flooded with one or two drops of dilutions of test serum. The specimens are allowed to incubate for 30 to 45 min at room temperature. After a saline rinse, the sections are treated with an antihuman, IgG antiserum labeled with fluorescein isothiocyanate. After a second buffered saline rinse, the slides are mounted and examined. Figure 1 depicts the steps of the indirect IF staining method.

Direct immunofluorescence staining

A modification of the direct IF method originally outlined by Coons and Kaplan (16) is used to detect bound immunoreactants in skin lesions from patients with bullous skin diseases, lupus erythematosus, or cutaneous vasculitis. The test is not a true serological procedure but is a histological technique for the localization of Igs, complement components, and fibrin in tissues. Direct IF should be interpreted with this reservation in mind.

Unfixed sections of skin, also cut in a cryostat at −30 C, are treated with fluorescein-conjugated antisera to human Igs (IgG, IgA, IgM, IgD, and IgE), C3, and fibrin. The slides are incubated in moist chambers at room temperature for 30 to 45 min and are mounted and examined as described above.

Modified indirect immunofluorescence staining

Trace proteins, such as early complement components (Clq and C4) and properdin pathway components (properdin and factor B), have recently been identified in skin lesions of patients with bullous diseases by a modified indirect IF method (30, 31, 36, 38). In this modified procedure, tissues are first treated with rabbit antisera to Clq, C4, properdin, and factor B. After an appropriate incubation period (30 to 45 min), the tissues are rinsed and treated with a labeled goat antirabbit IgG antiserum. The modified indirect IF test is illustrated in Fig. 2.

In vitro complement staining

These methods are true serological procedures for the detection of antibodies capable of complement fixation (4, 5, 27, 28). As such, these tests are valuable tools for immunopathological investigation, although they are of less importance in diagnosis and treatment at the present time.

Serum samples to be tested are first heat-inactivated at 56 C for 30 min to destroy remaining complement activity. Samples are then reconstituted with a fresh human complement source (usually fresh normal human serum), and serial dilutions of the reconstituted samples are prepared in the routine manner. Unfixed sections of normal stratified squamous epithelium are used as the antigen source, as in the indirect IF staining procedure. Sections are incubated with a few drops of reconstituted serum for 30 to 45 min at 37 C. The slides are then rinsed with saline and treated with labeled antisera to various complement components (Clq, C4, and C3). Positive reactions will be similar to those of indirect IF but will be apparent only when a complement-fixing antibody system is under investigation. The in vitro complement staining method is illustrated in Fig. 3.

OBSERVATIONS IN DISEASE STATES

Pemphigus

Numerous indirect IF studies have confirmed the presence of autoantibodies specific for an intercellular substance of skin and mucosa (Fig. 4A) in serum from patients with pemphigus (6–8, 34, 51). These antibodies occur in all forms of true pemphigus, including pemphigus vulgaris, pemphigus foliaceus, pemphigus erythematosus (Senear-Usher syndrome), and Brazilian pemphigus foliaceus or "fogo selvagem" (9), and react precisely at the site of the primary histopathological lesion. The presence of these antibodies in serum is, therefore, helpful diagnostically, especially in an early stage of the disease. Titers of pemphigus antibodies often reflect the disease activity and may be used in the assessment of therapy (15, 39).

Intercellular reactive antibodies are considered disease specific, although some exceptions to this rule must be considered. Szulman (45), Grob and Inderbitzen (23), and Ablin et al. (1) have reported that the intercellular staining patterns of esophageal mucosa with strong anti-A and anti-B blood group sera are similar to those with pemphigus serum. Absorption of the anti-A and anti-B sera with AB substance will prevent the positive intercellular staining, but similar absorption of pemphigus serum will not (1, 23).

"Pemphigus-like antibodies" have been reported in approximately 20% of burn patients (1, 24). Such activity is usually detectable between 12 and 30 days after an extensive burn. Absorption of these sera with AB substance does not inhibit intercellular staining, similar

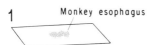

1 Monkey esophagus

Cryostat cut sections
on slide air dryed
for 15 minutes

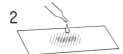

2

Section treated with
serum dilution

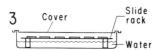

3 Cover   Slide rack

Water

Slide placed on rack
in moist incubation
chamber for 30 minutes

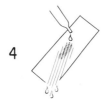

4

Serum dilution rinsed
from slide with PBS

5

Slide placed in Coplin jar
for 15 minute wash in PBS

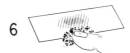

6

Excess PBS wiped from slide

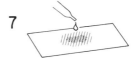

7

Section treated with
conjugated antiserum (IgG)

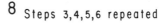

8 Steps 3,4,5,6 repeated

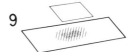

9

Slide mounted with
buffered glycerol

FIG. 1. *Steps of the indirect immunofluorescence staining procedure. Modified from Beutner, Chorzelski, and Jordon (5).*

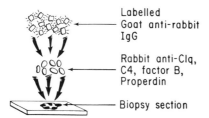

Labelled
Goat anti-rabbit
IgG

Rabbit anti-Clq,
C4, factor B,
Properdin

Biopsy section

FIG. 2. *Modified indirect immunofluorescence staining.*

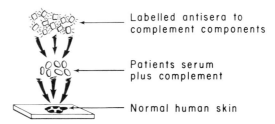

Labelled antisera to
complement components

Patients serum
plus complement

Normal human skin

FIG. 3. *In vitro complement staining.*

to the situation in true pemphigus. Fellner et al. have detected pemphigus-like antibodies in the serum of patients with morbilliform eruptions caused by penicillin (M. J. Fellner et al., Clin. Res. **19**:359, 1971); thus far, these findings have not been comfirmed. More recently, Cram and associates (19) reported pemphigus-like an-

tibodies in two cases of cicatricial pemphigoid despite other immunological findings suggestive of that diagnosis.

Despite these relatively rare exceptions, however, the presence of antibodies reactive to intercellular substance strongly suggests a diagnosis of pemphigus.

By direct IF testing, IgG deposition localized

to the intercellular areas occurs in most pemphigus skin lesions, including oral lesions (31, 33). This test, therefore, may also contribute diagnostically, again especially early in pemphigus. C3 deposition (Fig. 4B) is present mainly in skin lesions prior to initiation of corticosteroid therapy (18, 31, 50). Deposition of early complement components (Clq and C4), in addition to C3, is also present in early acantholytic lesions of pemphigus, suggesting that the complement system may contribute to the pathogenesis of pemphigus (31, 50). In addition, we have recently demonstrated factor B and properdin deposition in some early pemphigus lesions (31). By in vitro C3 IF staining, however, we have not been able to demonstrate that pemphigus antibodies will fix complement (29).

Bullous pemphigoid

Differentiation of bullous pemphigoid from other subepidermal bullous dermatoses, especially dermatitis herpetiformis, is often difficult. By indirect IF staining, autoantibodies reactive with the basement membrane zone of skin and mucosa (Fig. 5A) are found in the serum of most patients (approximately 70%) with bullous pemphigoid (4, 5, 7, 14, 26, 34). As in pemphigus, bullous pemphigoid antibodies also react precisely with their primary histopathological site, the basement membrane zone area, which may explain the subepidermal location of the bullae. Because of the disease-specific nature of these autoantibodies, their presence is of considerable diagnostic importance. However, pemphigoid antibody titers do not appear to fluctuate with disease activity and therefore are not good indexes of therapeutic efficacy (39).

By direct IF staining, basement membrane zone deposition of IgG and C3 (Fig. 5B) has been demonstrated consistently in almost all skin lesions examined to date (4, 5, 13, 33), including those in patients with active disease but without circulating antibodies. The direct IF pattern is identical with the indirect pattern and, in the absence of circulating pemphigoid antibodies, is also of considerable diagnostic importance (4, 5).

Using both direct and modified indirect IF methods, Provost and Tomasi (36, 38) found that factors associated with the properdin pathway are present in bullous pemphigoid skin lesions. Deposition of properdin and factor B was noted in addition to deposition of Clq, C4, and C3. We have recently been able to confirm these interesting observations (30) which are compatible with local complement activation by both the classical and properdin pathways in bullous pemphigoid skin lesions.

By in vitro complement staining methods, we had previously shown that most serologically positive bullous pemphigoid sera fix complement (C3) to the basement membrane zone (28). We have recently extended those studies and have demonstrated that bullous pemphigoid antibodies will fix Clq and C4 in addition to C3 (27).

Cicatricial pemphigoid

Cicatricial pemphigoid or benign mucous membrane pemphigoid is a well-defined clinical entity characterized by blistering, erosive, and often scarring lesions of the mucosal surfaces and ocular membranes. The histopathological hallmark of this disease, subepidermal bulla formation, is identical to that of bullous pemphigoid.

Recent IF investigations suggest that an etiological relationship may exist between true bullous pemphigoid and cicatricial pemphigoid. That is, basement membrane zone localization of IgG in oral, epidermal, and conjunctival lesions of cicatricial pemphigoid has been reported (2, 3, 20, 22, 25). The direct IF pattern is linear and therefore identical to that observed in true bullous pemphigoid. In a few recently reported cases (2, 21, 46), circulating basement membrane zone antibodies were found in the serum, suggesting further that some overlapping of cicatricial pemphigoid and true bullous pemphigoid must exist.

Basement membrane zone deposition of C3 has been demonstrated in addition to Ig deposition (2, 25). We have also recently demonstrated deposition of Clq, C4, factor B, and properdin in cicatricial pemphigoid lesions, suggesting, as in true bullous pemphigoid, local activation of both the classical and alternate complement pathways (R. S. Rogers III and R. E. Jordon, Clin. Res. 23:231A, 1975).

Dermatitis herpetiformis

Like bullous pemphigoid and cicatricial pemphigoid, dermatitis herpetiformis is also a subepidermal bullous dermatosis that may be an immunologically mediated disease. First described by van der Meer in 1969 (49), the deposition of IgA at the dermal-epidermal junction both in uninvolved skin and in skin adjacent to lesions is now well established (12, 24, 43). The positive direct IF pattern usually has a granular or fibrillar appearance in the upper dermis and dermal papillae (Fig. 6A). Occasionally, the positive IgA staining will be a continuous linear band along the basement membrane zone (12), identical to the IgG deposition observed in bullous pemphigoid.

Complement deposition also occurs in lesions

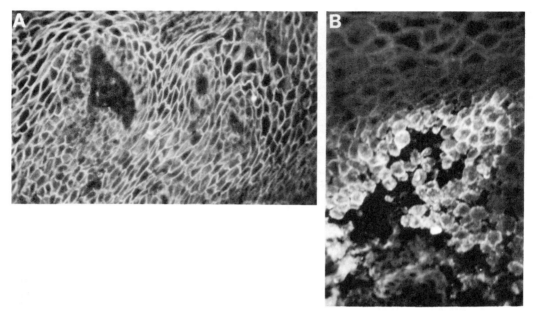

FIG. 4. *Immunofluorescence (IF) studies in pemphigus. (A) Indirect IF staining of monkey esophagus with pemphigus serum. Staining of the intercellular substance (ICS) is evident. × 200. (B) Direct IF staining of a pemphigus skin lesion demonstrating ICS deposition of C3. × 200.*

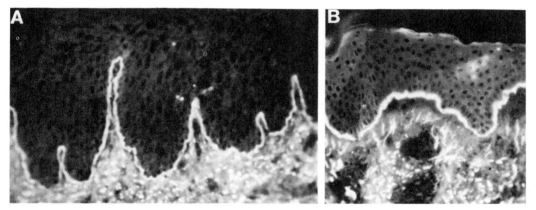

FIG. 5. *Immunofluorescence (IF) studies in bullous pemphigoid. (A) Indirect IF staining of monkey esophagus with bullous pemphigoid serum. Basement membrane zone (BMZ) staining is evident. × 200. (B) Direct IF staining of a bullous pemphigoid skin lesion showing linear BMZ deposition of C3. × 200.*

of dermatitis herpetiformis. Holubar et al. (24) first reported that C3 deposition is found in the skin immediately adjacent to vesicular lesions. Seah et al. (42) reported that C1q deposition was not present in most early dermatitis herpetiformis skin lesions despite IgA and C3 deposition, findings which suggested alternate pathway activation. Provost and Tomasi, in a recent study (37), found factor B deposition in four of seven patients, although properdin deposition was seen in only one. All seven patients had typical

IgA deposition. Although all of these studies suggest alternate pathway activation, further studies are needed to substantiate these conclusions.

Herpes gestationis

An uncommon vesiculobullous dermatosis of pregnancy and the postpartum period, herpes gestationis has recently been added to the list of bullous skin diseases with specific immunopathological findings. IF studies of two such

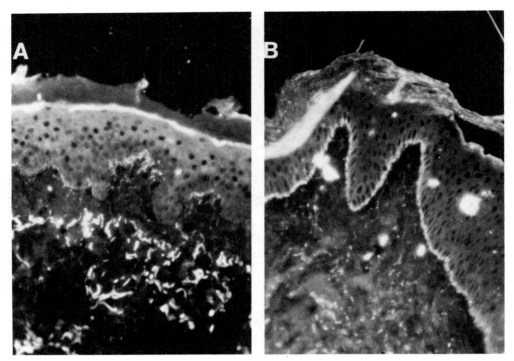

FIG. 6. *Immunofluorescence (IF) studies of dermatitis herpetiformis and herpes gestationis. (A) Direct IF staining of a dermatitis herpetiformis skin lesion demonstrating deposition of IgA in the dermal papillae.* ×
200. (B) In vitro complement (C3) staining of normal human skin using herpes gestationis serum. Basement membrane zone staining is evident. × *200.*

patients were recently reported by Provost and Tomasi (36). One patient's skin lesion showed basement membrane deposition of C3, C5, and properdin but without similar deposition of Clq and Igs. The second patient demonstrated only C3 deposition. Basement membrane antibodies were not present in the serum of either patient, but a heat-labile humoral factor, capable of precipitating C3 on normal skin basement membrane, was present.

A patient with herpes gestationis but who had IF findings similar to those of bullous pemphigoid was recently described by Bushkell, Jordon, and Goltz (11). This patient had circulating IgG antibodies to the basement membrane zone and deposition of IgG and Clq in skin lesions in addition to properdin and C3. This case suggests that herpes gestationis and bullous pemphigoid may be pathogenetically related, but the immunological findings appear to be the exception, although a patient with similar findings has recently been reported (H. Yaoita, K. Hertz, and S. Katz, J. Invest Dermatol. 64:203, 1975).

We have recently had the opportunity to study seven additional cases of herpes gesta-tionis by IF methods (unpublished data). Deposition of C3 and properdin was apparent in skin lesions of all seven patients. Minimal Clq deposition occurred in two, but Igs (IgG, IgA, IgM, and IgE) were absent. In addition, the serum of these seven patients did not contain circulating basement membrane zone antibodies. The heat-labile factor capable of precipitating C3 (Fig. 6B) on normal skin basement membrane zone was detected in serum samples from all seven patients and in cord serum samples from three patients so studied. The presence of this factor, therefore, may be of some value in the diagnosis of herpes gestationis.

Lupus erythematosus

In addition to serum antinuclear factors (described in chapter 85) deposition of IgG and IgM at the dermal-epidermal junction in both diseased and clinically normal skin has become a diagnostic hallmark of systemic lupus erythematosus (10, 17, 35, 47). Similar deposition of the Igs in diseased skin occurs in discoid lupus erythematosus, but not in the uninvolved areas (17). Direct IF, therefore, is a useful test in differentiating between systemic and discoid

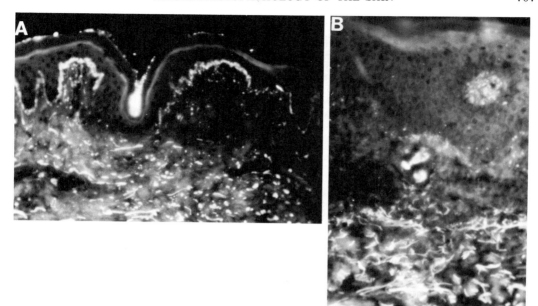

FIG. 7. *Immunofluorescence (IF) studies of lupus erythematosus (LE) and vasculitis. (A) Direct IF staining of a systemic LE skin lesion demonstrating granular IgM deposition at the dermal-epidermal junction. × 200. (B) Direct IF staining of a vasculitis skin lesion showing deposition of C3 in the superficial cutaneous vessels. × 200.*

lupus erythematosus. The pattern of staining observed is usually coarse and more granular than the thin linear pattern observed in bullous pemphigoid.

In our experience IgM is the more frequently encountered Ig in lupus erythematosus skin, particularly in uninvolved areas in systemic lupus erythematosus (32). Occasionally, IgM may be the only Ig found at the dermal-epidermal junction. Complement components (Clq, C4, C3, factor B, and properdin) are often encountered in a similar pattern but more frequently in lesional skin (32, 36). Typical granular deposition of IgM at the dermal-epidermal junction in a skin lesion of a patient with systemic lupus erythematosus is illustrated in Fig. 7A.

Cutaneous vasculitis

Various forms of vasculitis have long been considered to be cutaneous expressions of immune complex disease. This assumption is based primarily upon recent IF findings although more conclusive investigations are currently underway in several laboratories.

We have studied by various IF techniques patients with acute necrotizing (40), lividoid (41), and rheumatoid vasculitis (A. L. Schroeter, D. L. Conn, and R. E. Jordon, J. Invest. Dermatol. 62:346, 1974) for Ig and complement

deposition. IgG, IgM, and C3 are often apparent in involved dermal vessels and perivascular spaces in most cases of necrotizing vasculitis (40, 44). Fresh, early lesions, however, must be studied, as the positive fluorescence is apparent for only a short time. In lividoid vasculitis (the vasculitis of atrophie blanche), IgG and IgM deposition is apparent within walls of diseased vessels in the upper and middle dermis. Similar deposition of Clq, C3, and properdin, in addition to Igs has also been noted in diseased vessels of lividoid vasculitis (41). Similar deposits of IgM, IgG, Clq, and C3 have been noted within vessel walls of patients with rheumatoid arthritis and vasculitis (Schroeter et al., J. Invest. Dermatol. 62:346, 1974). Whether or not such deposits represent immune complexes must be investigated further. In any event, the demonstration of dermal vessel fluorescence is a useful diagnostic aid in the diagnosis of various types of cutaneous vasculitis. Typical vessel deposition of C3 in a skin lesion of a patient with lividoid vasculitis is illustrated in Fig. 7B.

LITERATURE CITED

1. Ablin, R. J., F. Milgrom, K. Kano, E. H. Beutner, and F. Rapaport. 1969. Pemphigus-Like antibodies in patients with skin burns. Vox Sang. 16:73-75.
2. Bean, S. F. 1974. Cicatricial pemphigoid: immu-

nofluorescent studies. Arch. Dermatol. 110:552–555.

3. Bean, S. F., M. Waisman, B. Michel, C. I. Thomas, J. M. Knox, and M. Levine. 1972. Cicatricial pemphigoid: immunofluorescent studies. Arch. Dermatol. 106:195–199.

4. Beutner, E. H., T. P. Chorzelski, S. F. Bean, and R. E. Jordon (ed.). 1973. Immunopathology of the skin: labeled antibody studies. Dowden, Hutchinson and Ross, Inc., Stroudsburg, Pa.

5. Beutner, E. H., T. P. Chorzelski, and R. E. Jordon. 1970. Autosensitization in pemphigus and bullous pemphigoid. Charles C Thomas, Publisher, Springfield, Ill.

6. Beutner, E. H., and R. E. Jordon. 1964. Demonstration of skin antibodies in sera of pemphigus vulgaris patients by indirect immunofluorescent staining. Proc. Soc. Exp. Biol. Med. 117:505–510.

7. Beutner, E. H., R. E. Jordon, and T. P. Chorzelski. 1968. The immunopathology of pemphigus and bullous pemphigoid. J. Invest. Dermatol. 51:63–80.

8. Beutner, E. H., S. F. Lever, E. Witebsky, R. E. Jordon, and B. Chertock. 1965. Autoantibodies in pemphigus vulgaris: response to an intercellular substance of epidermis. J. Am. Med. Assoc. 192:682–688.

9. Beutner, E. H., L. S. Prigenzi, W. L. Hale, C. A. Lerve, and O. G. Bier. 1968. Immunofluorescent studies of autoantibodies to intercellular areas of epithelia in Brazilian pemphigus foliaceus. Proc. Soc. Exp. Biol. Med. 127:81–86.

10. Burnham, T. K., T. R. Neblett, and G. Fine. 1963. The application of the fluorescent antibody technic to the investigation of lupus erythematosus and various dermatoses. J. Invest. Dermatol. 41:451–456.

11. Bushkell, L. L., R. E. Jordon, and R. W. Goltz. 1974. Herpes gestationis: new immunologic findings. Arch. Dermatol. 110:65–69.

12. Chorzelski, T. P., E. H. Beutner, S. Jablonska, M. Blaszczyk, and C. Triftshauser. 1971. Immunofluorescent studies in the diagnosis of dermatitis herpetiformis and its differentiation from bullous pemphigoid. J. Invest. Dermatol. 56:373–380.

13. Chorzelski, T. P., and R. H. Cormane. 1968. The presence of complement bound in vivo in the skin of patients with pemphigoid. Dermatologica 137:134–138.

14. Chorzelski, T., S. Jablonska, M. Blaszczyk, and M. Jarzabek. 1968. Autoantibodies in pemphigoid. Dermatologica 136:325–334.

15. Chorzelski, T. P., J. V. von Weiss, and S. F. Lever. 1966. Clinical significance of autoantibodies in pemphigus. Arch. Dermatol. 93:570–576.

16. Coons, A. H., and M. H. Kaplan. 1950. Localization of antigen in tissue cells. II. Improvements in method of detection of antigen by means of fluorescent antibody. J. Exp. Med. 91:1–13.

17. Cormane, R. H. 1964. Bound globulin in the skin of patients with chronic discoid lupus erythematosus and systemic lupus erythematosus. Lancet 1:534–535.

18. Cram, D. L., and K. Fukuyama. 1972. Immunochemistry of ultraviolet-induced pemphigoid lesions. Arch. Dermatol. 106:819–824.

19. Cram, D. L., M. R. Griffith, and K. Fukuyama. 1974. Pemphigus-Like antibodies in cicatricial pemphigoid. Arch. Dermatol. 109:235–238.

20. Dabelstein, E., S. Ullman, K. Thomsen, and J. Rygaard. 1974. Demonstration of basement membrane autoantibodies in patients with benign mucous membrane pemphigoid. Acta Derm.-Venereol. 54:189–192.

21. Dantzig, P. 1973. Circulating antibodies in cicatricial pemphigoid. Arch. Dermatol. 108:264–266.

22. Griffith, M. R., K. Fukuyama, D. Tuffanelli, and S. Silverman, Jr. 1974. Immunofluorescent studies in mucous membrane pemphigoid. Arch. Dermatol. 109:195–199.

23. Grob, P. J., and T. M. Inderbitzen. 1967. Pemphigus antigen and blood group substances A and B. J. Invest. Dermatol. 49:285.

24. Holubar, K., M. Doralt, and G. Eggerth. 1971. Immunofluorescence patterns in dermatitis herpetiformis. Br. J. Dermatol. 85:505–510.

25. Holubar, K., H. Hönigsman, and K. Wolff. 1973. Cicatricial pemphigoid: immunofluorescence investigations. Arch. Dermatol. 108:50–52.

26. Jordon, R. E., E. H. Beutner, E. Witebsky, G. Blumental, W. L. Hale, and W. F. Lever. 1967. Basement zone antibodies in bullous pemphigoid. J. Am. Med. Assoc. 200:751–756.

27. Jordon, R. E., J. M. Nordby, and H. Milstein. 1975. The complement system in bullous pemphigoid. III. Fixation of Clq and C4 by pemphigoid antibody. J. Lab. Clin. Med. 86:733–740.

28. Jordon, R. E., W. M. Sams, Jr., and E. H. Beutner. 1969. Complement immunofluorescent staining in bullous pemphigoid. J. Lab. Clin. Med. 74:548–556.

29. Jordon, R. E., W. M. Sams, Jr., G. Diaz, and E. H. Beutner. 1971. Negative complement immunofluorescence in pemphigus. J. Invest. Dermatol. 57:407–410.

30. Jordon, R. E., A. L. Schroeter, R. A. Good, and N. K. Day, 1975. The complement system in bullous pemphigoid. II. Immunofluorescent evidence for both classical and alternate pathway activation. Clin. Immunol. Immunopathol 3:307–314.

31. Jordon, R. E., A. L. Schroeter, R. S. Rogers III, and H. O. Perry. 1974. Classical and alternate pathway activation of complement in pemphigus vulgaris lesions. J. Invest. Dermatol. 63:256–259.

32. Jordon, R. E., A. L. Schroeter, and R. K. Winkelmann. 1975. Dermal-epidermal deposition of complement components and properdin in systemic lupus erythematosus. Br. J. Dermatol. 92:263–271.

33. Jordon, R. E., C. T. Triftshauser, and A. L.

Schroeter. 1971. Direct immunofluorescent studies of pemphigus and bullous pemphigoid. Arch. Dermatol. 103:486–491.

34. Peck, S. M., K. E. Osserman, L. B. Weiner, A. Lefkovits, and R. S. Osserman. 1968. Studies in bullous diseases: immunofluorescent serologic tests. N. Engl. J. Med. 279:951–958.

35. Pohle, E. L., and D. L. Tuffanelli. 1968. Study of cutaneous lupus erythematosus by immunohistochemical methods. Arch. Dermatol. 97:520–526.

36. Provost, T. T., and T. B. Tomasi, Jr. 1973. Evidence for complement activation via the alternate pathway in skin diseases. I. Herpes gestationis, systemic lupus erythematosus and bullous pemphigoid. J. Clin. Invest. 52:1779–1787.

37. Provost, T. T., and T. B. Tomasi, Jr. 1974. Evidence for the activation of complement via the alternate pathway in skin diseases. II. Dermatitis herpetiformis. Clin. Immunol. Immunopathol. 3:178–186.

38. Provost, T. T., and T. B. Tomasi, Jr. 1974. Immunopathology of bullous pemphigoid: Basement membrane deposition of IgE, alternate pathway components and fibrin. Clin. Exp. Immunol. 18:193–200.

39. Sams, W. M., Jr., and R. E. Jordon. 1971. Correlation of pemphigoid and pemphigus antibody titres with activity of disease. Br. J. Dermatol. 84:7–13.

40. Schroeter, A. L., P. W. M. Copeman, R. E. Jordon, W. M. Sams, Jr., and R. K. Winkelmann. 1971. Immunofluorescence of cutaneous vasculitis associated with systemic disease. Arch. Dermatol. 104:254–259.

41. Schroeter, A. L., J. L. Diaz-Perez, R. K. Winkelmann, and R. E. Jordon. 1975. Livido vasculitis (the vasculitis of atrophy blanche): immunohistopathologic study. Arch. Dermatol. 111:188–193.

42. Seah, P. P., L. Fry, M. R. Mazaberi, J. F. Mowbray, A. V. Hoffbrand, and E. J. Holborow. 1973. Alternate-pathway complement fixation by IgA in the skin in dermatitis herpetiformis. Lancet 2:175–177.

43. Seah, P. P., L. Fry, J. S. Stewart, B. L. Chapman, A. V. Hoffbrand, and E. J. Holborow. 1972. Immunoglobulins in the skin in dermatitis herpetiformis and coeliac disease. Lancet 1:611–614.

44. Stringa, S. G., C. Bianchi, A. M. Casala, and O. Bianchi. 1967. Allergic vasculitis Gougerot-Ruiter syndrome: immunofluorescent study. Arch Dermatol. 95:23–27.

45. Szulman, A. E. 1960. The histological distribution of blood group substances A and B in man. J. Exp. Med. 111:785.

46. Tagami, H., and S. Imamura. 1974. Benign mucous membrane pemphigoid: demonstration of circulating and tissue-bound basement membrane antibodies. Arch. Dermatol. 109:711–713.

47. Tan, E. M., and H. G. Kunkel. 1966. An immunofluorescent study of the skin lesions in systemic lupus erythematosus. Arthritis Rheum. 9:37–46.

48. Thivolet, J., and A. J. Beyvin. 1967. Anticorps antiepiderme dans le dermatoses bulleuses. Document cliniques et experimentaux. Bull. Soc. Fr. Dermatol. Syphiligr. 74:300–304.

49. van der Meer, J. B. 1969. Granular deposits of immunoglobulin in the skin of patients with dermatitis herpetiformis: an immunofluorescent study. Br. J. Dermatol. 81:493–503.

50. van Joost, T., R. H. Cormane, and K. W. Pondman. 1972. Direct immunofluorescent study of the skin on occurrence of complement in pemphigus. Br. J. Dermatol. 87:466–474.

51. Waldorf, D. S., C. W. Smith, and A. J. L. Strauss. 1966. Immunofluorescent studies in pemphigus vulgaris: confirmatory observations and evaluation of technical considerations. Arch. Dermatol. 93:28–33.

52. Weller, T. H., and A. H. Coons. 1954. Fluorescent antibody studies with agents of varicella and herpes zoster propagated in vitro. Proc. Soc. Exp. Biol. Med. 86:789–794.

Chapter 95

Human Sperm Antibodies and Their Detection

SIDNEY SHULMAN

INTRODUCTION

It has become well established in recent years that certain people—both women and men—are producers of antibodies to human sperm cells. Since there is also considerable evidence that these antibodies may play a role in causing or exacerbating spontaneous infertility, and since infertility is a problem that afflicts about 15% of couples, it will be of increasing importance that the detection of these antibodies can be dependably and reliably made. In addition to spontaneous infertility, a second area of concern is that of vasectomy, a surgical procedure that is frequently followed by production of sperm autoantibodies.

SURVEY OF USEFUL METHODS

The most useful methods are those based on the agglutination or immobilization of spermatozoa. Other methods of interest are cytotoxicity and immunofluorescence, but these are much less frequently reported. Precipitation methods are not available, but hopefully they will evolve in the future as suitable soluble antigens are developed. Therefore, I will discuss only the agglutination and immobilization methods in detail. The methods have been described and discussed in a number of review articles (1, 3, 5, 7, 10, 11, 14, 19, 20). An international workshop meeting was held in Aarhus, Denmark, in June 1974, for discussions of these methods in great detail (8).

PROCEDURES OF SPERM AGGLUTINATION

There are several quite distinct techniques for performing each of the methods. In the category of agglutination, there are at least five techniques. A widely used macro-scale technique is the Kibrick method (the gelatin agglutination test), published by Kibrick et al. in 1952 (6). In this method (using tiny test tubes), we not only see whether the serum is positive or negative, but we can also study a dilution series and thus obtain a titer for the sperm antibody activity.

Reagents and containers

The reagents needed are Baker's buffer (17), saline, and gelatin.

Baker's buffer has the following composition: glucose, 30.0 g; $Na_2HPO_4 \cdot 7H_2O$, 4.6 g (or, alternatively, $Na_2HPO_4 \cdot 12H_2O$, 6.0 g); NaCl, 2.0 g; KH_2PO_4, 0.1 g; with water to 1,000 ml; pH 7.7.

The gelatin (Difco) is a 10% solution in Baker's buffer, conveniently made up in 250-ml quantities, with storage in 5-ml portions; each portion will generally be suitable for one day's work.

The gelatin and the buffer are to be kept in the refrigerator until needed. Neither reagent should become more than 2 months old.

The Kibrick tubes are most readily prepared from glass tubing of 3-mm inner diameter, which is cut into 3-cm lengths. One end is sealed in a flame. To provide a test-tube rack, it is convenient to obtain a block of styrofoam or similar plastic of comfortable dimensions for holding in the hand, such as $9 \times 9 \times 5$ cm in height. In the top surface of such a block, a pattern of short holes can be drilled to accommodate these tubes.

Detailed test procedure of the gelatin agglutination test (Kibrick method)

1. The serum samples should be inactivated by heating at 56 C for 30 min. Dilutions are prepared, using serological pipettes and tubes, and using Baker's buffer as diluent.

2. A fresh semen sample is diluted with Baker's buffer to 40×10^6 cells/ml. The original semen sample should preferably have a sperm count of at least 80×10^6 cells/ml and a motility of at least 50%.

3. A suitable volume of the sperm suspension is warmed to 37 C and mixed with an equal volume of a 10% gelatin solution in Baker's buffer, also at 37 C.

4. A volume of 0.2 ml of each serum sample or of each dilution (beginning with the 1:4 dilution) is placed in a clear serological tube.

5. A volume of 0.2 ml of the semen-gelatin mixture is added to each tube, and the contents are gently mixed.

6. Each mixture is then transferred to a Kibrick tube.

7. The tubes are incubated at 37 C, and the results are observed and recorded at 1 and 2 h.

8. Agglutination is seen as the appearance of

white floccules (or sparkling threads), along with a clearing of the intervening medium.

Comments on the procedure

1. A fresh semen sample must be used in order to have maximum motility. Also, the donor should be selected (if a donor is being used) so that there is very little of other cells and debris, and there is a count of at least 100×10^6 cells/ml. Motility and count must therefore be measured. Washing is not to be done; the semen is merely diluted. It is not known how much difference the percent motility or the unwashed status really makes. If a husband's semen is being studied, rather than using a selected donor, we should know how urgent these criteria really are. In our laboratory, we accept a motility as low as 50% and a sperm count as low as 40×10^6 cells per ml in some cases, but we generally repeat the test with better semen.

2. The gelatin and the buffer should be fresh, and care should be taken to avoid microbial growth. Older samples of gelatin may become less viscous and may show a decreased pH. The pH must be kept above 7 to avoid spontaneous agglutination of the sperm cells.

3. The serum is inactivated, at 56 C for 30 min. It is diluted 1:4, or to higher dilutions, with Baker's buffer. Equal volumes of diluted serum and of semen-gelatin are mixed; this must be done with calibrated pipettes and not by counting drops, because the two mixtures have quite different surface tensions. We usually use 0.2 ml of each. Each mixture is then transferred to a Kibrick tube. It is not known whether larger (or smaller) tubes would be suitable.

4. The Kibrick tubes are incubated at 37 C for 2 h; they are carefully read after 1 h and again after 2 h. There seems to be no advantage in incubating them longer, although there are only sparse data on this question.

5. Control sera must be included in every test. One should always use a positive control and a negative control for each semen sample. If they do not both give the expected result, the test results must be discarded. A saline solution should not be used as a negative control (although it may be an extra control); a negative serum is needed. A positive serum control for Kibrick tests may well be a different serum from that used as a positive control in other techniques.

6. The semen source may be completely unimportant. In a detailed study, it was found that in the vast majority of cases the same results were obtained for each serum, whether the semen was autologous (from the man of the couple) or homologous (from a donor) (15).

7. The ABO blood group status of the semen source has no influence on the results.

8. The mode of agglutination may be of interest. From other kinds of observation, we know that clumping may occur in head-to-head, tail-to-tail in the main part of the tail, tail-tip-to-tail-tip, and head-to-tail, (or tangled) modes. However, it is not clear which modes occur under Kibrick conditions. Nor is it yet clear which mode correlates better with other phenomena. There is still a large question as to the nature and number of reactive antigenic determinants on the sperm cells, with regard to agglutination. There may even be several determinants for the same region, as in the head-to-head attachment.

9. Several studies have shown that the Kibrick type of agglutination is caused by immunoglobulin. This can be either IgG or IgM, although the IgG class is more common.

10. Application can be made to other fluids. The Kibrick test can, and should, be applied to seminal plasma and to cervical mucus. Regarding seminal plasma one may find lower or higher titers than in serum, or no activity at all (12). We must emphasize that a lack of activity does not necessarily mean that antibody is absent, since it may well be that the semen antibody has adhered to the sperm cells without showing any agglutination or immobilization. We need to develop a technique to test such suspected sperm by means of an indirect agglutination procedure. Sperm antibody in cervical mucus has been discussed elsewhere in some detail (16, 18, 21).

11. The tissue specificity has been explored. Positive sera have been tested against erythrocytes, leukocytes, and platelets; these were always negative. Various other clinical sera, containing antibodies to these three types of white blood cells, were tested against spermatozoa; these were always negative, also. Hence, it has been concluded that the Kibrick-positive sera are specific for spermatozoa (9, 13).

PROCEDURES OF SPERM IMMOBILIZATION

The fact that some antibodies to spermatozoa can cause the immobilization of sperm cells, as long as the system contains complement, gave rise to the very first method that was developed for the detection of sperm antibody. An approach to an immobilization method for clinical purposes is that reported by Isojima and his colleagues (4).

PERFORMANCE OF THE SPERM IMMOBILIZATION TEST

1. Human sperm cells of at least 70% motility and good forward progression are diluted to

60×10^6 cells per ml, in Baker's buffer.

2. As a source of complement, pooled fresh rabbit normal serum is used. Human and guinea pig serum may also be used.

3. As a positive control serum, an appropriate dilution is used of rabbit antihuman sperm serum, such that it will immobilize about 90 to 95% of the sperm cells in 1 h in the presence of complement.

4. As a negative control serum, a negative human serum (having no immobilizing activity) is used.

5. The control and test sera are inactivated at 56 C for 30 min.

6. To a small tube, add:

0.25 ml of inactivated test serum or a control serum,

plus 0.05 ml of complement solution,

plus 0.025 ml of fresh human semen dilution.

7. There should also be a mixture for detecting any non-specific sperm-immobilizing activity of the test serum; this consists of 0.25 ml of test serum plus the semen sample. There should be no immobilization in this mixture.

8. Incubate the mixtures at 37 C for 1 h.

9. Examine a drop of each mixture on a microscope slide, at $100\times$ to $250\times$, studying several fields for a reliable estimate. Measure the percentage of motility. Positive results are those mixtures that have motilities of one-half or less that of the negative control mixture.

10. The initial study of each test serum is made at full concentration; those which are positive are then titrated, for example, from 1:2 to 1:128, or more.

DIAGNOSTIC APPLICATION

Several principles have evolved for the guidance of the testing in clinical applications to infertile couples (22). Both members of the couple should have their blood serum analyzed. This should be explored in any long-standing case of infertility, even in the absence of indicating factors in either person. The use of a single type of test is not adequate, since many studies have shown that each test has a different incidence of positive results in an infertile population; studies have in fact shown that various parts of test procedures will at times give different results for a particular serum sample. In our Laboratory we always apply both the Kibrick and the Franklin-Dukes (F-D) agglutination methods; on some occasions, the immobilization method is also used. Undiluted serum seems almost certain to give many false-positive results, that is, non-specific positive results. Each serum sample should be tested more than once by each method; this allows an

evaluation of the semen sample and of other technical factors. Sperm motility above 50 or 60% is desirable. The only method that does not require a good motility count is the capillary method. Positive and negative control sera must be included in each test. In general, the semen used as the reagent can come from almost any man, provided that it has adequate count and motility. Hence, a donor semen (termed, homologous semen) can be used, and it is not essential to use the semen from the test couple. On the other hand, it may be well also to use the semen from the patient or the patient's husband (termed, autologous semen) if it has adequate quality. The results will generally be the same (15).

An apparent difference between a husband-semen and a donor-semen may be genuine, but on the other hand, one must not be misled as to the interpretation; such a difference, if found, may simply reflect individual differences as might be found between any two donors. The husband's status per se might have no relationship to the semen property as a test reagent.

INCIDENCE OF SPERM ANTIBODIES

A very large number of infertile couples have been analyzed in our laboratory by use of these methods. In the great majority of cases, the couples had unexplained infertility. A small number had organic causes for infertility. Table 1 shows totals of antibody incidence for an accumulated total of about 400 infertile couples. We had positive findings for the Kibrick method in 18% of the women and 9% of the men and, for the F-D method, in 15% of women and 5% of men.

We can also consider the control study that was done in our laboratory. Serum samples were obtained from about 100 fertile women at our hospital, including pregnant, that is, ante-partum, patients and immediate-post-partum patients. The Kibrick and F-D methods were applied to these sera, and in most cases we were including infertility samples at the same time. We found only 3% to be positive in Kibrick and 3% in F-D (22).

TABLE 1. *Incidence of positive results in serum samples from infertile couples: results from 409 couples*

Method	No. of patients	No. positive	% Positive
Kibrick			
Females	409	72	17.6
Males	381	33	8.7
F-D			
Females	389	58	14.9
Males	347	17	4.9

It should be emphasized that weak reactions in the Kibrick techniques have been taken as positive by us. This may explain why some other laboratories have reported a lower incidence of Kibrick-positive results in infertile women than we have, although the incidence of positive results in men has been very similar in several other laboratories, notably that of Fjällbrant (2). We may speculate that men generally develop a strongly agglutinating sperm antibody, if they develop any activity, whereas women develop a spectrum of intensities in this activity. An actual Kibrick test is shown in Fig. 1. It should be kept in mind that the observer must acquire experience with many tests and must decide how to compare the appearances of the negative control mixtures with the various test mixtures. In this way, it will be possible to establish a minimal dilution that can be taken as a significant positive result.

The immobilization method should also be evaluated in terms of the incidence of positive results. According to Isojima et al. (4), positive findings were made in 18% of a group of 74 women from couples with unexplained infertility, whereas the incidence was zero in a group of 83 pregnant women. On the other hand, Vaidya and Glass (23) also applied this method, and they found positive results in 2.5% of a group of 40 women from infertile couples. Admittedly, this is too small a group, but it may be important to have further studies of the results of this method on a number of large groups of various types of population.

ACKNOWLEDGMENTS

This work was aided by a Public Health Service contract (N01-HD-4-2428) from the National Institute of Child Health and Human Development, a Public Health Service General Research Support grant (RR-05398), and by the Sperm Antibody Laboratory Fund.

LITERATURE CITED

1. Behrman, S. J. 1961. Immunologic aspects of infertility. Int. J. Fertil. 6:349.
2. Fjällbrant, B. 1974. Incidence of sperm antibodies in males with regard to age, p. 36. *In* A. Centaro and N. Carretti (ed.), Immunology in obstetrics and gynecology, Proceedings of the 1st International Congress, Padua, Italy, 1973. Excerpta Medica, Amsterdam.
3. Hekman, A., and P. Rümke. 1976. Auto- and iso-immunity against spermatozoa. *In* P. A. Miescher and H. J. Müller-Eberhard (ed.), Textbook in immunopathology, 2nd ed. Grune and Stratton, New York, in press.
4. Isojima, S., K. Tsuchiya, K. Koyama, C. Tanaka, O. Naka, and H. Adachi. 1972. Further studies on sperm-immobilizing antibody found in sera of unexplained cases of sterility in women. Am. J. Obstet. Gynecol. 112:199.
5. Jones, W. R. 1974. The use of antibodies developed by infertile women to identify relevant antigens, p. 376. *In* Karolinska Symposia on Research Methods in Reproductive Endocrinology, 7th Symposium, Immunological Approaches to Fertility Control, July 1974. Karolinska Institutet, Stockholm.
6. Kibrick, S., D. L. Belding, and B. Merrill. 1952. Methods for the detection of antibodies against mammalian spermatozoa. II. A gelatin agglutination test. Fertil. Steril. 3:430.
7. Li, T. S. 1974. Sperm immunology, infertility and fertility control. Obstet. Gynecol. 44:607.
8. Rose, N. R., T. Hjort, P. Rümke, M. J. Harper, and O. Vyazov. 1976. Workshop on techniques for detection of iso- and auto-antibodies to human spermatozoa. Clin. Exp. Immunol. 23:175–199.
9. Rümke, P. 1959. Auto-antibodies against spermatozoa in sterile men, p. 145. *In* Immunopathology, 1st International Symposium. Basel/Seelisberg, 1958, Benno Schwabe and Co., Basel.

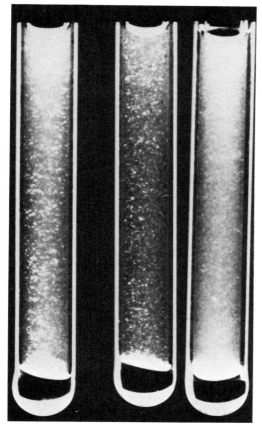

FIG. 1. *The gelatin agglutination test (the Kibrick method), illustrating two positive tubes on the left and a negative tube on the right.*

10. Rümke, P. 1969. Antigenicity of spermatozoa, p. 665. *In* P. A. Miescher and H. J. Müller-Eberhard (ed.), Textbook of immunopathology. Grune and Stratton, New York.

11. Rümke, P. 1969. Immunity to sperm, p. 669. *In* P. A. Miescher and H. J. Müller-Eberhard (ed.), Textbook of immunopathology. Grune and Stratton, New York.

12. Rümke, P. 1974. The origin of immunoglobulins in semen. Clin. Exp. Immunol. 17:287.

13. Rümke, P., and G. Hellinga. 1959. Auto-antibodies against spermatozoa in sterile men. Am. J. Clin. Pathol. 32:357.

14. Shulman, S. 1971. Antigenicity and autoimmunity in sexual reproduction: a review. Clin. Exp. Immunol. 9:267.

15. Shulman, S. 1973. Antibodies to spermatozoa. IV. Human spermagglutinating activity in different tests with variation in semen source. Am. J. Obstet. Gynecol. 117:233.

16. Shulman, S. 1974. Sperm antibodies in the serum and cervical mucus of women, p. 87. *In* A. Centaro and N. Carretti (ed.), Immunology in obstetrics and gynecology, Proceedings of the 1st International Congress, Padua, Italy, 1973. Excerpta Medica, Amsterdam.

17. Shulman, S. 1975. Reproduction and antibody response. CRC Press, Cleveland.

18. Shulman, S. 1976. Sperm antibodies in serum of men and women in cervical mucus. *In* Proceedings of the 8th World Congress on Fertility and Sterility, Buenos Aires, Argentina, 1974. Excerpta Medica, Amsterdam, in press.

19. Shulman, S. 1976. Agglutination of spermatozoa. *In* C. A. Williams and M. W. Chase (ed.), Methods in immunology and immunochemistry, vol. 4. Academic Press Inc., New York, in press.

20. Shulman, S. 1976. Sperm immunity and human infertility – problems and progress. *In* K. Bratanov (ed.), Immunology and reproduction, Proceedings of the 3rd International Symposium, Varna, Bulgaria, 1975. Bulgarian Academy of Sciences Press, Sofia, in press.

21. Shulman, S., and M. R. Friedman. 1975. Antibodies to spermatozoa. V. Antibody activity in human cervical mucus. Am. J. Obstet. Gynecol. 122:101.

22. Shulman, S., H. Jackson, and M. L. Stone. 1975. Antibodies to spermatozoa. VI. Comparative studies of spermagglutination activity in groups of infertile and fertile women. Am. J. Obstet. Gynecol. 2:139.

23. Vaidya, R. A., and R. H. Glass. 1971. Sperm-immobilizing and agglutinating antibodies in the serum of infertile women. Obstet. Gynecol. 37:546.

Section I

TUMOR IMMUNOLOGY

Chapter 96

Introduction

ROBERT S. SCHWARTZ

In its present state of development, tumor immunology must be considered largely experimental. As such, it is not yet ready for routine clinical application. This view is not meant to dismiss the importance of tumor immunology. On the contrary, movement is so rapid that it is the relatively leisurely field of clinical immunology that needs to catch up.

Consider, for example, the following: cytotoxic tests for cellular immunity against tumor cells; assays for blocking factors; preparation of soluble tumor antigens; and in vitro sensitization of lymphocytes against tumor cells. All of these procedures are in current use, but their role in diagnostic or prognostic testing remains unsettled. Therefore, the description of these and similar procedures in a manual of clinical immunology may be premature. Some may even consider that the inclusion of a section on carcinoembryonic antigen (CEA) in this manual is controversial. However, the care taken by the authors of this section to sift through the numerous variables and caveats required for performance and interpretation of the tests amply justifies its publication here. If properly done in selected patients, this test has clinical value. And, like all other tests, when it is improperly done or when interpreted out of context, the results are meaningless. There is, unfortunately, no "cancer test."

Another area of considerable progress is the classification and diagnosis of malignant lymphoproliferative disorders. Much of this is due to the application of cell marker techniques and the correlation of the results with pathological findings. Although the classification of these disorders is still evolving, the battery of diagnostic techniques that can be used in the diagnosis of lymphoproliferative disorders has come

into widespread use. These techniques have already found application not only in the differential diagnosis of various lymphomas, but also in distinguishing between reactive (polyclonal) and neoplastic (monoclonal) lymphoproliferation. The association between certain cell markers and prognosis, as appears to be emerging in acute lymphoblastic leukemia, may add a new dimension to the value of these methods. And the suggestion from recent studies that the blast crises of chronic myelogenous leukemia may in some cases be characterized by the proliferation of *lymphoblasts* indicates how these techniques may bring about radical shifts in our concepts of certain malignancies.

The work-up of an "M" spike—the monoclonal gammopathy—demonstrates how beautifully research techniques were adapted and standardized for clinical investigation. Kyle and his associates have meticulously adapted the methodology of analytical immunochemistry to this problem. Their experience in the differential diagnosis of monoclonal gammopathies is among the most extensive in the world. The diagnostic criteria they employ are based on the analysis of thousands of sera, combined with thorough clinical evaluation and long-term follow-up. As in the case with all laboratory tests, the interpretation of results in the *clinical context* is all important. The users of this manual should contemplate the potential usefulness of combining the techniques used in the diagnosis of monoclonal immunoglobulins in serum with those used in the identification of monoclonal immunoglobulins on cell surfaces. Combination of these methods may increase considerably the resolving power of the diagnostic laboratory.

Chapter 97

Diagnosis of Hematopoietic, Mononuclear, and Lymphoid Cell Neoplasms

R. D. COLLINS, J. H. LEECH, J. A. WALDRON, J. M. FLEXNER, AND A. D. GLICK

INTRODUCTION

The hematopoietic system, mononuclear phagocyte system (MPS), and lymphoid system are responsible for the production of formed elements of the blood and the development of immunity. Many functions and sites of action are shared by these systems, and in the adult the bone marrow is the site of production of the basic elements of all three systems. Since their origin, sites of action, and functions are shared and since their diseases may be similar both clinically and pathologically, there is considerable practical and conceptual advantage in discussing these systems and their diseases in a unified fashion.

Techniques for diagnosing neoplasms of the hematopoietic system, MPS, and lymphoid system have changed dramatically in the past few years, as the complexities of these systems have become more apparent. It is now clear that precise categorization of their neoplasms requires an integrated approach in which histopathological, immunological, and histochemical techniques are used. The specific items of information which have probably had the greatest influence in changing our diagnostic methodology are as follows:

1. Distinct subpopulations of lymphocytes and macrophages have been demonstrated and have been shown to interact in many immune functions and diseases.

2. Techniques for recognition of some normal lymphocyte and macrophage subpopulations are becoming widely available and may also be used to recognize neoplastic derivatives of these populations (8, 13, 14, 16, 19, 23, 27). For lymphocytes, functional assessments of membrane characteristics of living cells are often necessary for subpopulation identification. For derivatives of the MPS, histochemical or ultrastructural techniques seem essential for recognition.

3. Lymphocytes may undergo striking morphological changes in vitro after mitogenic stimulation and in vivo during immune responses, changing from small "mature" or "well-differentiated" lymphocytes to large blasts.

This information has forced conceptual as well as technological changes in our approach to neoplasms of the hematopoietic system, MPS, and lymphoid system. Previous classifications of lymphomas have been based primarily on cell size and growth pattern. Recently, Lukes and Collins (21, 22) proposed the use of a combined functional and structural analysis to classify these neoplasms by presumed cell of origin. The latter approach facilitates interchange of information gained by studying normal, deficient, or neoplastic cells and follows the general principles used to classify most other malignant neoplasms. Such an approach requires that we have as basic information details about normal cell lines, including their sites of action, structure, and functions, and secondly that we have techniques for recognition of normal cell lines and capacities to measure their functions. This information and methodology may then be used to group neoplasms (and deficiencies) of the hematopoietic system, MPS, and lymphoid system on the basis of comparison of abnormal and normal cells.

LYMPHOCYTE SUBPOPULATIONS

It is presently postulated that there are two major functional subpopulations of lymphocytes. The thymus-dependent or T cell system is responsible for cell-mediated immunity. The bursal equivalent or B cell system is responsible for the production of immunoglobulins. Both of these subpopulations are derived from lymphoid precursors (lymphoid stem cells) originating in the marrow.

Techniques for recognition (see chapter 7)

T cells may be identified most easily by their capacity to form nonimmune rosettes (E rosettes) with sheep erythrocytes (17). B cells may be identified by demonstrating immunoglobulin (Ig) on the cell surface or in the cell, by use of fluoroscein-labeled antisera (1, 24). This fluorescence technique has the advantage of identifying clonality in subpopulations of B cells, but concurrent cytological examination is very difficult. B cells may also be identified by their receptors for complement and aggregated IgG.

Lymphoid precursor cells (stem cells) may be identified by the absence of T and B cell markers, coupled with a characteristic histochemical appearance. Lymphoid cells without markers are frequently called null cells, or undefined (U) cells.

MONONUCLEAR PHAGOCYTE SYSTEM AND HEMATOPOIETIC SUBPOPULATIONS

Members of the MPS are derived from bone marrow cells and apparently share a common stem cell with the hematopoietic cell lines. Both circulating and tissue members of the MPS are derived from this marrow-based stem cell (29). There are probably several different subpopulations of macrophages; one subpopulation (often found in the skin) has a strikingly folded nucleus and contains specific cytoplasmic organelles called Langerhan's granules. It is not known whether subpopulations of macrophages have different functions.

Granulocytes, erythrocytes, and megakaryocytes have a common stem cell—a stem cell probably shared with the MPS.

Techniques for recognition

Identification of the members of these cell lines is accomplished by histochemical stains of air-dried imprints or smears and ultrastructural evaluation. Ultrastructural features of particular value include demonstration of cytoplasmic organelles such as granules. MPS cells may also be identified by binding of suitably marked immune complexes to surface receptors for the Fc fragment of IgG (26).

DIAGNOSIS OF NEOPLASMS BY USE OF COMBINED METHODOLOGY

Our approach is to establish the diagnosis of neoplasia on the basis of histopathological and cytological criteria and then to determine the cell line involved by correlating functional and morphological studies. The diagnosis of neoplasia must be based primarily on traditional morphological methodology. Functional studies are used principally for more precise categorization of cell lines involved, and their interpretation should not supersede the evaluation based on morphology.

Since most neoplasms are composed of mixtures of neoplastic cells and reacting, non-neoplastic components, interpretation of functional studies depends on identification of the

neoplastic cell in relationship to the marker used. When most of the cells tested may be presumed to be neoplastic on the basis of their cytological features or by comparison with sections of tissue from which they were obtained, and when most of the cells either mark or fail to mark, the functional typing is self-evident. If, instead, few cells mark, the marking cells must be examined cytologically to determine whether they appear neoplastic. When a small percentage of cells may be presumed to be neoplastic, the marking cells must again be examined cytologically to determine whether they appear neoplastic.

Accurate morphological evaluation of neoplasms of the hematopoietic system, MPS, and lymphoid system requires adequate and representative biopsies, properly fixed, sectioned, and stained. Similar techniques must be applied to all tissues. A protocol for handling tissue specimens is given below under Test Procedures. Sophisticated functional methodology is no substitute for properly prepared, representative histopathological material.

Generally, the most reliable criterion for establishing that a process is a malignant neoplasm is the demonstration in histopathological sections of a mass lesion containing a homogeneous population of immature-appearing cells. Normally, hematopoietic, MPS, and lymphoid cells are intermingled, and homogeneous populations tend to be neoplastic. The establishment of homogeneity of a cell product (e.g., Ig) or the demonstration of a clonal population of lymphocytes by functional studies supports the possibility of a neoplastic disorder.

Mass lesions containing homogeneous populations of immature-appearing cells are usually seen in the acute leukemias, multiple myeloma, malignant histiocytoses, and malignant lymphomas composed of transformed lymphocytes. Proliferations of small lymphocytes may be more difficult to recognize as neoplastic. Hodgkin's disease may be difficult to diagnose because it contains mixtures of neoplastic and reacting cells, often with neoplastic cells in the minority.

Cytological features which help establish a diagnosis of malignant neoplasm include dysplasia and cytoplasmic structures such as Auer rods. Karyotypic demonstration of abnormal chromosomal features (e.g., aneuploidy) may be helpful.

SIGNIFICANCE OF TERMS LEUKEMIA AND LYMPHOMA

The term leukemia refers to neoplasms of bone marrow origin, often with involvement of the peripheral blood. Leukemias include bone marrow neoplasms originating from the hematopoietic system and MPS, as well as from some lymphoid cell lines.

Most lymphoid neoplasms of nodal or extramarrow lymphoid sites are called lymphomas. Lymphomas are customarily divided into Hodgkin's disease and non-Hodgkin's lymphomas because their tissue reactions are so different.

Lymphoid neoplasms often have leukemic phases. It is difficult, with traditional methodology, to determine in these cases whether the leukemic cells have arisen from a marrow-based neoplasm or a node-based neoplasm, and functional studies of blood and node may be required to determine the source of the circulating neoplastic lymphocytes.

DEFINITION AND CRITERIA FOR DIAGNOSIS OF NEOPLASMS

Neoplasms of the hematopoietic system, MPS, and lymphoid system are listed below in relationship to their presumed cell of origin. Definitions, specific histopathological criteria, and immunological features are given for the more important neoplasms.

Malignant Neoplasms of the Hematopoietic, Mononuclear Phagocyte, and Lymphoid Systems, in Relationship to the Presumed cell of Origin
(modified from Lukes and Collins [21,22])

Stem cell neoplasms
  Acute lymphoblastic leukemias
Hematopoietic precursor neoplasms
  Acute granulocytic leukemia
  Chronic granulocytic leukemia
  Erythroleukemia
MPS neoplasms
  Acute myelomonocytic leukemia
  Malignant histiocytoses
T cell neoplasms
  T cell acute lymphoblastic leukemia
  T cell chronic lymphocytic leukemia
  Thymic lymphoma (convoluted lymphocytic lymphoma)
  Node-based T cell lymphoma (immunoblastic sarcomas of T cells)
  Mycosis fungoides and Sézary syndrome
B cell neoplasms
  B cell acute lymphoblastic leukemia
  B cell chronic lymphocytic leukemia
  Follicular center cell lymphomas including Burkitt's lymphoma
  B cell neoplasms with plasmacytic differentiation (Waldenstrom's macroglobulinemia, multiple myeloma)
  Immunoblastic sarcomas of B cells

Neoplasms with cell of origin uncertain
  Leukemic reticulendotheliosis
  Hodgkin's disease

Acute lymphoblastic leukemias

Definition. Acute lymphoblastic leukemias (ALL) are bone marrow-derived neoplasms, possibly arising from stem cells able to produce any hematopoietic, MPS, or lymphoid cell line. ALL is almost certainly heterogeneous, as cases differ clinically, morphologically, histochemically, and by immunological function studies.

Criteria for diagnosis. The marrow shows sheets of blasts with high nuclear-cytoplasmic ratios and no Auer rods. ALL blasts are negative for Sudan black and significant esterase activity. Periodic acid-Schiff (PAS) reaction is present (in a few or often many cells) as coarse granules or blocks against a negative background. Electron microscopy shows primitive cells with nuclear folding, cytoplasmic microfilaments, and few granules.

Immunological characteristics. In most cases of ALL, B or T characteristics are not detected on the surface of leukemic cells (7). In some series cytotoxicity assays with anti-T cell antisera show killing of leukemic cells in 30 to 60% of cases (7, 18). Some cases of T cell ALL are probably thymus-based neoplasms, as thymic lymphomas often involve the marrow early and produce a hematological picture similar to the more common marrow-based ALL. Rarely, ALL blasts may be shown to bear monoclonal surface immunoglobulins.

Acute granulocytic leukemia

Definition. Acute granulocytic leukemia (AGL) is a bone marrow-derived neoplasm, composed of blasts and cells differentiating into granulocytes. Cell of origin is a granulocytic precursor cell.

Criteria for diagnosis. The marrow is infiltrated by blasts and promyelocytes. Young cells are Sudan black positive. Auer rods may be present. PAS reaction shows diffuse tinge with superimposed granules, and chloroacetate esterase reaction is positive in young cells. Very few (1 to 2%) monocytic cells are present. Electron microscopy shows primitive blasts and cells with specific types of lysosomal granules. The promyelocytic variant of AGL is composed primarily of promyelocytes with numerous azurophilic granules and stacked Auer rods.

Chronic granulocytic leukemia

Definition. Chronic granulocytic leukemia (CGL) is a bone marrow-derived neoplasm composed principally of granulocytic cells in various stages of maturation. The cell of origin is probably a stem cell which can differentiate into hematopoietic or MPS cells.

Criteria for diagnosis. White blood cell counts are usually greater than 50,000/mm³ with a marked left shift, and leukocyte alkaline phosphatase is absent or low. The marrow is solidly cellular. A Philadelphia chromosome is present in bone marrow cells in 90% of the cases. Granulocytes stain with Sudan black, PAS, and chloroacetate esterase stains. In blastic crisis of CGL, the predominant cell may resemble, by histochemistry and morphology, primitive myeloid, monocytic, or lymphoid cells.

Erythroleukemia

Definition. Erythroleukemia is a bone marrow-derived neoplasm of hematopoietic stem cells in which abnormal erythroid precursor cells predominate.

Criteria for diagnosis. The marrow and blood show excessive numbers of erythroid precursors which stain with granular or diffuse PAS activity and often show diffuse α-naphthyl acetate esterase activity. Megaloblastic changes, nuclear atypia, and ring sideroblasts may be seen. There is usually an associated proliferation of young granulocytic or monocytic cells. Auer rods may be present. Electron microscopy shows glycogen clumps in erythroblasts, and ferruginous micelles may be seen in erythroid mitochondria. Erythroleukemia may change to a picture indistinguishable from AGL or AMML.

Acute myelomonocytic leukemia

Definition. Acute myelomonocytic leukemia (AMML) is a bone marrow-derived neoplasm composed primarily of blasts, promonocytes, monocytes, and some granulocytic precursors. The cell of origin is a precursor cell of the MPS and may be a stem cell shared with the hematopoietic system.

Criteria for diagnosis. The marrow is infiltrated by variable numbers of monocytic cells and some granulocytic cells. Cells of the MPS usually make up greater than 50% of the total. The young cells may have Auer rods and stain with Sudan black and α-naphthyl acetate esterase (Fig. 1). PAS reaction is diffuse with superimposed small granules. Electron microscopy shows characteristic lysosomal granules, nuclear convolutions, and microfilaments. Muramidase activity is often increased in urine and serum.

Malignant histiocytoses

Synonyms: histiocytosis X, histiocytic medullary reticulosis, familial hemophagocytic reticulosis

Definition. This group includes several neoplasms derived from the tissue phase of the MPS; therefore, the neoplastic cells resemble macrophages or histiocytes. These neoplasms may begin unifocally in skin and soft tissue or multifocally, with involvement of lymph nodes, spleen, lungs, and often bone.

Criteria for diagnosis. Infiltrating cells have

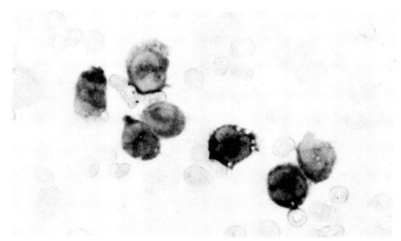

FIG. 1. *Esterase stain of bone marrow smear in acute myelomonocytic leukemia, demonstrating diffuse cytoplasmic staining for α-naphythyl acetate esterase in all but one cell.* ×781.

folded nuclei and abundant cytoplasm, and they uniformly stain positively for diffuse PAS and α-naphthyl acetate esterase activity. Neoplastic cells often demonstrate phagocytic activity. Electron microscopy shows typical lysosomal granules and sometimes Langerhan's structures. Eosinophil accumulations are often present.

Thymic lymphoma

Synonym: convoluted lymphocytic lymphoma

Definition. Thymic lymphoma is believed to arise from immature thymic lymphocytes and is characteristically a neoplasm of children and young adults. Although the blood and bone marrow are initially uninvolved, dissemination occurs quickly, with progressive nodal, visceral, and marrow involvement and development of a leukemic phase. The disseminated disorder may be confused with ALL.

Criteria for diagnosis. Histologically, thymic lymphoma presents infiltrative masses of poorly cohesive cells with scant (non-pyroninophilic) cytoplasm (3). Tumor cells vary greatly in size and show finely distributed chromatin and small nucleoli. Nuclei of the larger cells have complex convolutions. Mitoses are generally numerous, and scattered clear macrophages frequently impart a "starry sky" appearance.

Immunological features. The T cell nature of the neoplasm is readily established by immunological function studies, in which most tumor cells form very tight rosettes with sheep erythrocytes (Fig. 2).

Node-based T lymphomas

Synonym: immunoblastic sarcomas of T cells

Definition. These lymphomas are incompletely described, but they appear to arise from T cells in lymph nodes and are seen principally in adults. Superficial, retroperitoneal, and mediastinal lymphadenopathy are generally present. The bone marrow and peripheral blood are initially uninvolved, but early dissemination to pleura, lung, and bone marrow usually occurs.

Criteria for diagnosis. Histologically, nodes show diffuse involvement by a pleomorphic infiltrate of cells varying in size and degree of transformation. Slight nuclear folding may be detected; multinucleated cells are frequent, and mitotic figures are numerous. Scattered macrophages are generally present, and they may have an epithelioid appearance. These lymphomas are rather heterogeneous histologically because of variation from case to case in the size of the predominant cell.

Immunological features. Node-based T lymphomas are identified primarily by immunological function studies, in association with sections showing a pleomorphic, diffuse lymphoma. The larger cells in these lymphomas tend to form fragile, easily disrupted E rosettes. When large cells predominate, only a few large cells may be found in rosettes in cytocentrifuge preparations. In all cases, however, rosette formation by lymphocytes in various stages of transformation can be demonstrated. Lymphocytes with surface Ig (SIg) are present in low numbers, and no evidence of monoclonality of SIg should be present.

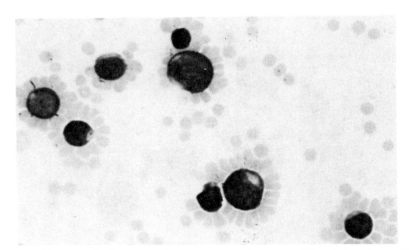

FIG. 2. *E rosette Giemsa-stained cytocentrifuge preparation from case of thymic lymphoma. Both large and small lymphoid cells are seen in rosettes. Note red cell elongation, useful for recognition of rosettes in cytocentrifuge preparations.* ×730.

Mycosis fungoides, Sézary syndrome

Definition. Mycosis fungoides (MF) is a cutaneous T cell proliferative disorder with an indolent but progressive course frequently spanning many years and typically evolving into an overt lymphoma, with dissemination to lymph nodes, viscera, and bone marrow. Patients with the related Sézary syndrome have generalized pruritic erythroderma and characteristic lymphocytes in the peripheral blood. The origin of these lymphomas and their prolonged localization in skin suggests that they arise from immunocompetent T cells specialized to provide cutaneous immunity. This hypothesis is supported by the particular morphological resemblances of MF lymphocytes to lymphocytic elements in a variety of benign dermatoses.

Criteria for diagnosis. Skin biopsies during the later stages of MF show extensive involvement of the dermis and to a lesser degree the epidermis by a pleomorphic lymphocytic infiltrate. Lymph nodes biopsied after dissemination of MF may show residual areas of dermatopathic lymphadenopathy. The neoplastic infiltrate is diffuse in pattern and is composed of lymphocytic elements of intermediate to large size which characteristically show complex nuclear folding. Mitoses are generally numerous, and scattered large macrophages are also present.

Immunological features. Neoplastic cells in blood or node may be identified as T lymphocytes by the formation of E rosettes (6).

Chronic lymphocytic leukemias

Definition. Chronic lymphocytic leukemias (CLL) are a heterogeneous group of diseases in which there is proliferation of small lymphocytes usually of the B type. Cells of origin may be marrow based and include B cells with potential to become follicular center cells (FCCs), as well as non-FCC lymphocyte-plasma cell systems.

Criteria for diagnosis. CLL is usually recognized when white counts are greater than 30,000/mm^3 with a predominance of small lymphocytes. Marrow may show diffuse or focal infiltrates, and nodes contain diffuse growths often with pale areas interspersed ("mounding").

Immunological features. Many patients with CLL have been studied. Virtually all cases show evidence of a clonal B cell proliferation, although occasional cases have been biclonal, and rare cases (3%) are T derived rather than B (7). The SIg is usually IgM, or IgM+D, with a single light chain. The amount of surface fluorescence in CLL is very slight and may be difficult to detect. Cases are accepted as B cell CLL in our laboratory only when the amount of SIg is slight. Cases having brighter surface fluorescence are called small cell B cell neoplasms, until more specific differential criteria are established.

In some cases of CLL, there is no detectable SIg and the cells do not form E rosettes. Surface receptors for aggregated IgG have been demonstrated in many of these cases (10) and may represent a more sensitive marker of B lymphocytes than SIg.

Follicular center cell lymphomas

Synonyms: general—follicular lymphoma, lymphosarcoma, histiocyte lymphoma; cleaved FCC—poorly differentiated lymphocytic lymphoma; transformed FCC—histiocytic lymphoma, reticulum cell sarcoma

Definition. FCC lymphomas comprise a complex group of malignant lymphomas arising from follicular (germinal) centers and are, therefore, of B cell origin. FCC lymphomas usually develop in superficial or retroperitoneal nodes. FCCs have been divided into four cell types, presumably representing the morphological variations of a single cell line during in vivo transformation (20). The four cell types are small and large cleaved FCC and small and large noncleaved or transformed FCC; neoplastic counterparts have been recognized for each of these types.

Criteria for diagnosis. Malignant lymphomas may be assumed to be FCC in origin, if any of the following histopathological features (19) are demonstrated:

1. Production of follicular nodules by the neoplasm (Fig. 3).
2. Diffuse growth of cleaved FCCs or mixtures of cleaved FCCs and noncleaved, transformed cells.
3. Diffuse growth of noncleaved or transformed cells, if a previous biopsy showed neoplastic follicular nodules.

These criteria are restrictive, by excluding presumed FCC neoplasms such as Burkitt's lymphoma or other transformed lymphocytic B cell neoplasms which do not have neoplastic follicular nodules or a significant admixture of cleaved FCCs.

Immunological features. We have studied 47 patients with lymphomas assumed to be FCC in origin by light microscopy. In a few of these cases, SIg was not demonstrated or the SIg pattern was not monoclonal. However, the great majority showed a monoclonal pattern of

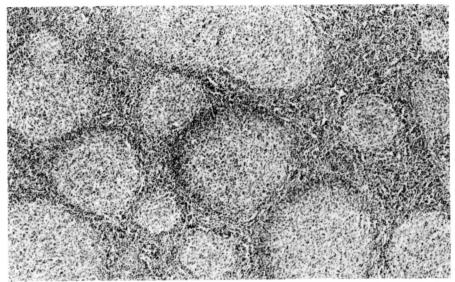

FIG. 3. *Neoplastic follicular nodules in follicular center cell lymphoma. Hematoxylin and eosin.* ×157.

SIg, with IgD+M, IgM, and IgG the usual predominant heavy chains. IgD+M and IgM were usually associated with cleaved FCC neoplasms; IgG was usually associated with transformed or noncleaved FCC neoplasms. In most FCC lymphomas, Ig-bearing cells made up more than 40% of the cells at test, and E rosette-forming cells were less than 27% of the total. The rare lymphomas with IgA as the predominant SIg were usually associated with involvement of the bowel.

The pattern of surface fluorescence in FCC lymphomas was uniform from cell to cell, with distinct positivity. Rare cases had intracellular Ig in lymphoid-appearing cells.

Jaffe et al. used a frozen section technique to demonstrate complement receptors on the neoplastic cells in follicular lymphomas (16).

Burkitt's lymphoma (see chapter 56)

Definition. Burkitt's lymphoma is a B cell neoplasm, probably arising from small noncleaved FCCs; it is a distinct clinical pathological entity and is most frequent in Africa.

Criteria for diagnosis. For accurate diagnosis, tissue sections must be well fixed (B5 or equivalent), and impression smears are useful. The neoplastic cells are small transformed lymphocytes, very uniform in size and shape (4). Nuclei are round and regular, and two to five nucleoli are usually present. Methyl green pyronin stain shows a small amount of positively staining cytoplasm. Mitoses and macrophages are abundant, with the macrophages producing the nonspecific "starry sky" appearance.

Immunological features. Relatively few cases have been studied by immunological function techniques. The neoplastic cell is a B cell, and IgM seems to be the usual SIg.

Waldenstrom's macroglobulinemia (see chapter 3)

Definition. Waldenstrom's macroglobulinemia (WM) is a widespread neoplasm characterized by bone marrow proliferation of lymphocytes and plasma cells, frequent involvement of nodes and other lymphoid tissues, and a striking increase in serum IgM. Cell of origin may be in non-FCC lymphocyte-plasma cell system.

Criteria for diagnosis. Marrow examination shows: nodules or sheets of small cells with intermixed "plasmacytoid lymphocytes" and typical, benign-appearing plasma cells; strongly PAS-positive cytoplasmic material in plasma cells; and PAS-positive intranuclear inclusions (Dutcher bodies) in lymphoid cells.

Lymph node examination shows: extensive infiltration by a lymphocytic-plasmacytic infiltrate similar to that in marrow and partial to almost complete loss of nodal architecture with some sparing of follicular centers.

Immunological features. Lymphocytic and plasmacytic components of WM usually have SIg with the same heavy and light chain found in the serum M component (25). Similar membrane patterns of SIg are found on most of the blood lymphocytes, although the peripheral counts are usually not elevated. Amounts and distribution of fluorescence seem to show considerable variation from cell to cell in individual cases, in contrast to the more homogeneous patterns of fluorescence in other lymphoid neoplasms (25).

Rare patients with the typical morphological features of WM have IgG or IgA serum components and similar cellular Ig patterns. Nonsecreting forms of WM have also been demonstrated (25).

Mixed patterns of serum and cellular Ig have occasionally been found, indicating biclonal populations of lymphocytic and plasmacytic elements. Occasional patients with mixed Ig patterns apparently produce monoclonal IgM with anti-IgG activity.

Multiple myeloma (see chapter 3)

Definition. Multiple myeloma (MM) is a plasmacytic neoplasm primarily involving the bone marrow with minimal significant extension to extra-osseous sites. Cell of origin may be in a marrow-based B cell system.

Criteria for diagnosis. Changes diagnostic of MM include massive replacement of marrow by homogeneous sheets of plasma cells or the presence of homogenous nodules of plasma cells one-half high-power field or greater in diameter in marrow particle sections (9; Fig. 4).

Changes strongly suggestive of MM include: presence of broad or band infiltrates of plasma cells in marrow particles, preponderance of immature forms in plasma cell infiltrates, progressive rise in paraprotein levels, multiple lytic lesions of bone associated with a paraprotein spike.

Immunological features. Plasma cells from patients with MM generally bear the same heavy and light chains as present in the M component. However, monoclonal populations of plasma cells may also occur in benign monoclonal gammopathy. Peripheral blood lymphocytes from patients with MM may have a SIg identical to the serum M component or the Ig in neoplastic plasma cells, whereas lymphocytes with other Ig specificities are regularly decreased in number (25).

Leukemic reticuloendotheliosis

Synonym: hairy cell leukemia

Definition. Leukemic reticuloendotheliosis (LRE) particularly affects marrow and spleen and often has a leukemic phase. The cell of origin is not known. Proliferating cells have features of both B lymphocytes and monocytes.

Criteria for diagnosis. Wright's stained smears of peripheral blood or marrow show characteristic lymphoid-monocytoid cells, which on phase microscopy have typical hair-like projections. If possible, the diagnosis of LRE should be confirmed by histochemistry (31) or electron microscopy.

Immunological features. Hairy cells have features of both B lymphocytes and monocytes.

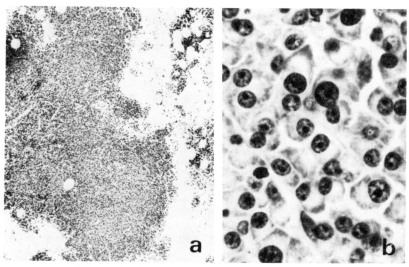

FIG. 4. *Bone marrow particles section in multiple myeloma. (a) Note replacement of normal marrow by nodules of cells. Two uninvolved particles are present on the right. PAS. ×125. (b) Higher power of cells in noddules, showing characteristic appearance of plasma cells with large nucleoli. PAS. ×742.*

Most studies have demonstrated SIg; IgD has been predominant in a high percentage of cases. Capping of the SIg-anti-Ig complex produces a distinctive globular cap that is unique to LRE in our experience (Fig. 5).

Some cases of LRE have had SIg in a mixed, rather than a monoclonal, distribution when fresh cells were studied with conventional antisera. Fu et al. showed that preincubation of cells in artificial media and staining with antiserum composed of Fab fragments revealed a monoclonal distribution of SIg (12). We have found that hairy cells from several patients resynthesize SIg after trypsinization.

Jaffe et al. have demonstrated an Fc, but not a complement receptor, on hairy cells (16), and others have shown that hairy cells from many patients are capable of phagocytizing latex beads. Esterase and Sudan black stains are generally negative.

Hodgkin's disease

Definition. Hodgkin's disease (HD) is a neoplastic disease or diseases primarily affecting lymph nodes, with later involvement of liver, spleen, bone marrow, and lung. Proliferating cells seem to be mononuclear Reed-Sternberg cells (MRS cells) and possibly binucleate or multinucleated types of Reed-Sternberg cells (RS cells). Cell of origin is probably lymphoid (28) because:

1. RS and MRS cells resemble (by routine and electron microscopy) transformed and dysplastic lymphocytes.
2. RS and MRS cells show only slight esterase positivity (11).
3. Aneuploidy found in RS and MRS cells has also been demonstrated in cells resembling transformed lymphocytes.

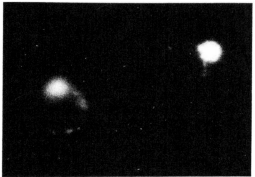

FIG. 5. *Hairy cell in leukemic reticuloendotheliosis stained with fluorescein-conjugated antiserum to human Ig. Note the characteristic nodular cap formation.* ×1,760.

In nodular sclerosing HD, T lymphocytes have been proposed as the cell of origin, as the thymus is often involved, disease often affects thymus-dependent areas of node initially, and defects in cell-mediated immunity develop.

Immunological features. MRS and RS cells are difficult to study in vitro, in part because nodes from patients with HD are difficult to disrupt into single-cell suspensions. Although the morphological and histochemical studies cited above indicate that MRS and RS cells are lymphoid, more precise characterization of the neoplastic cell has not been reported. Intracellular Ig has been demonstrated in a few patients with mixed-cellularity HD.

TEST PROCEDURES

All tissue specimens from patients with hematopoietic, MPS, and lymphoid neoplasms should be examined by protocol. The following procedures are essential components of our protocol:

1. Fresh material is brought to the laboratory and processed immediately.
2. Microscopic sections are made of all tissues, including marrow. B5 (5) is the standard fixative. Periodic acid-Schiff-hematoxylin (PAS) and methyl green pyronin (MGP) stains are routinely prepared.
3. Impression smears of tissues, or smears of marrow and peripheral blood, are prepared routinely and are available for histochemical stains including PAS, Sudan black, and combined esterase stains.
4. Single-cell suspensions are prepared from node, marrow aspirate, peripheral blood, or body fluids for immunological function studies. For accurate interpretation, such preparations should be high in viability and should be shown to be representative by comparison with tissue sections and smears.
5. Portions of all tissues are fixed in glutaraldehyde and sectioned for electron microscopy if necessary.

The techniques described below are those with which we have had extensive experience. References to other techniques are given below in the section Comments on Methods. We have listed the materials and sources which we have used; in nearly every case, other satisfactory sources are available.

Initial processing of tissue

Materials.

Media for cell culture: Roswell Park Memorial Institute 1640 (RPMI-1640) and phosphate-buffered saline (PBS; Grand Island Biological Co., Grand Island, N.Y.).

Fetal calf serum (FCS; Grand Island Biological Co.).

Petri dishes (Falcon Plastics, Los Angeles, Calif.).

Sterile gauze, 15-gauge needles with syringes.

Conical centrifuge tubes, 50 and 15 ml (Falcon Plastics).

Ficoll-Hypaque: combine 24 parts of 9% Ficoll (Pharmacia Laboratories) with 10 parts of 34% Hypaque-M (Winthrop Laboratories). Then Millipore-filter the mixture into autoclaved bottles. Store at 4 C.

Sterile pipettes.

Trypan blue, 0.5%.

Refrigerated centrifuge.

5% CO_2 incubator.

Vortex mixer.

Filtrator coffee paper (Filtrator Coffee Apparatus Co., New York, N.Y.).

Solid tissue (lymph node, spleen, thymus, mass lesions). Nodes are cut across the long axis with razor blades, and the central portions are used for histopathology. Focal lesions and areas of necrosis are often present in nodes, and tissue sections should be selected accordingly. The node poles are used for cultures, immunological function studies, impression smears, and electron microscopy. Other solid tissues are sliced at 1-cm intervals, examined for lesions, and then processed.

Proper fixation requires that slice thickness be no greater than 3 mm, that large volumes of fixative be used in proportion to volume of tissue, and that tissue slices not be stacked in the fixative.

Impression smears are prepared from thin slices of tissue immobilized on absorbent cytocentrifuge pads. Glass slides should be touched to the surface with a slightly rolling motion.

1. Preparation of cell suspensions for immunological studies: Immediately place fresh tissue in cold RPMI-1640 in a petri dish and disrupt into small fragments with sterile tweezers. Gently pipette the fragments through a 15-gauge needle to aid in dispersion, and filter the suspension through 4-ply sterile gauze into a sterile 50-ml conical centrifuge tube. Admixed granulocytes and erythrocytes (often present in splenic tissue) can be removed by centrifugation on a Ficoll-Hypaque gradient (see below).

2. Wash cells three times by Vortexing in 50 ml of RPMI-1640 followed by centrifugation at $400 \times g$ for 6 to 10 min. After the final wash, resuspend cells in RPMI-1640 by Vortexing and pipetting.

3. Cell count and viability assay: Add 0.1 ml of 0.5% trypan blue to 0.5 ml of cell suspension. After 5 min, count in a hemacytometer. Dead cells will not exclude trypan blue.

4. This is the basic cell preparation used for immunological function studies. For the next procedure, see sections on immunofluorescence and E rosette techniques below.

Bone marrow. Several techniques are available for preparing sections of aspirated marrow fragments. We use filtration to collect the marrow particles (9), and the filtrate is thereby available for immunological function studies or cytocentrifuge preparations. Particles not used for smears may be collected for electron microscopy in a small clot or by slicing 1 mm off the marrow biopsy core. If necessary, impression smears for special stains may be made off the biopsy core.

1. Centrifuge marrow filtrate on a Ficoll-Hypaque gradient (see below) to remove erythrocytes and granulocytes.

2. Wash cells three times, count, and assay viability.

Blood.

1. Dilute 1 volume of blood with 3 volumes of PBS, at 20 C.

2. Pipette 10 ml of Ficoll-Hypaque into a sterile 50-ml centrifuge tube. Carefully layer 40 ml of diluted blood onto the Ficoll-Hypaque.

3. Centrifuge at $400 \times g$ for 30 min at 20 C.

4. Aspirate mononuclear cells from the Ficoll-Hypaque–PBS interface. A bright light behind the tube makes the interface more visible.

5. Wash three times, count, and assay viability.

Body fluids (cerebrospinal fluid, pleural fluid, peritoneal fluid).

1. Centrifuge fluid at $400 \times g$ for 30 min, and resuspend cells in RPMI-1640.

2. Layer the cell suspension onto Ficoll-Hypaque in a 50-ml tube, centrifuge, and collect cells at the interface as described above. This step is unnecessary for cerebrospinal fluid.

3. Wash three times, count, and assay viability.

Histochemical techniques

Materials.

Pararosanilin hydrochloride: Sigma Chemical Co. #P3750.

Sodium nitrite (F.W. 69.0): Fisher Scientific Co. #S-347.

Fast blue BB base: Sigma #F 0125.

2 N HCl: Fisher #SO-A-431.

α-Naphthyl acetate: Sigma #N-6750.

Naphthol AS-D chloroacetate: Sigma #N 3000.

N,N-dimethylformamide, 99 mol% pure: Fisher #D-133.

2-Methoxyethanol (F.W. 76.10): Fisher #E-182.

Giesma staining solution: Giemsa-Losung Chroma Roboz #2 E 040.

Methyl green GA: C.I. 42590 Roboz #1A442.

Sudan black B: C.I. 26150 Roboz #11595.

Nuclear fast red: C.I. 60760 Roboz #1A402.

Aluminum sulfate (crystals): Mallinckrodt Chemical Works #3268.

Phenol crystals: Mallinckrodt #0028.

Solutions for esterase stains.

Fixative (store in refrigerator)

Weigh: 20 mg of Na_2HPO_4, 100 mg of KH_2PO_4.

Add: 30 ml of water, 45 ml of acetone, 25 ml of formalin (39%).

The pH should be 6.6.

Buffer (store in refrigerator)

Weigh: 27.6 g of NaH_2PO_4; dilute to 1 liter of water

28.3 g of Na_2HPO_4; dilute to 1 liter of water.

For pH 7.6: 13 ml of NaH_2PO_4 (0.2 M), 87 ml of Na_2HPO_4 (0.2 M), 100 ml of water.

Pararosanilin

Weigh: 5.0 g of pararosanilin hydrochloride powdered dye.

Add: 100 ml of water, 25 ml of concentrated HCl.

Mix and filter. Can be stored indefinitely at room temperature.

Sodium nitrite (store in refrigerator; discard after 1 week)

Weigh: 4 g of $NaNO_2$.

Mix with: 100 ml of distilled water.

Fast blue BB (make immediately before using)

Weigh: 80 mg of fast blue BB.

Mix with: 2.0 ml of 4% sodium nitrite, 2.0 ml of 2 N HCl.

Allow to bubble for 1 min.

Substrate 1 (store in refrigerator; discard after 1 week)

Weigh: 200 mg of α-naphthyl acetate (store in freezer).

Mix with: 10 ml of 2-methoxyethanol.

Substrate 2 (store in refrigerator; discard after 1 week)

Weigh: 20 mg of naphthol chloroacetate (store in freezer).

Mix with: 10 ml of N,N-dimethylformamide (do not use plastic).

Esterase staining method.

1. Fix slides with cold fixative.
2. Wash with distilled water, and allow to dry.

3. Mix well 2.0 ml of pararosanilin and 2.0 ml of 4% sodium nitrite. Let bubble for 1 min. This is dye mixture 1.

4. Mix appropriate volume of buffer, dye mixture 1, and substrate 1:

10 ml = 8.9 ml of buffer, 0.6 ml of dye mixture 1, 0.5 ml of substrate 1

30 ml = 26.7 ml of buffer, 1.8 ml of dye mixture 1, 1.5 ml of substrate 1

60 ml = 53.4 ml of buffer, 3.6 ml of dye mixture 1, 3.0 ml of substrate 1

5. Stain for 45 min, and wash well with distilled water.

6. Mix 2.0 ml of sodium nitrite and 2.0 ml of 2 N HCl, followed by 80 mg of fast blue BB. Let bubble for 1 min. This is dye mixture 2.

7. Mix appropriate volume of buffer, dye mixture 2, and substrate 2:

10 ml = 9.1 ml of buffer, 0.4 ml of dye mixture 2, 0.5 ml of substrate 2

30 ml = 27.3 ml of buffer, 1.2 ml of dye mixture 2, 1.5 ml of substrate 2

60 ml = 54.6 ml of buffer, 2.4 ml of dye mixture 2, 3.0 ml of substrate 2

8. Stain for 10 min, and wash well with distilled water.

9. Counterstain with 1% methyl green for 2 to 10 min.

Solutions for Sudan black B.

1. Dissolve 0.3 g of Sudan black B in 100 ml of absolute ethanol.

2. Prepare buffer by dissolving 16 g of crystalline phenol in 30 ml of absolute ethanol. Add to 100 ml of distilled water containing 0.3 g of $Na_2HPO_4 \cdot 12H_2O$.

3. Prepare working stain by mixing 40 ml of buffer and 60 ml of Sudan black B solution; filter by suction. Stain may be stored for 2 to 3 months.

4. Dissolve by heating 0.1 g of nuclear fast red in 100 ml of a 5% solution of aluminum sulfate. Cool; filter. Add grain of thymol as preservative.

Sudan black B staining method.

1. Fix air-dried smears in formalin vapor for 5 to 10 min.

2. Wash in running tap water for 10 min.

3. Immerse in working stain in a Coplin jar for 1 h.

4. Wash with 70% ethanol for 2 to 3 min to remove excess dye. Watch timing.

5. Wash with tap water for 2 min. Watch timing.

6. Blot dry and counterstain with nuclear fast red for 10 min.

Immunological techniques: detection of SIg by direct immunofluorescence (see chapter 7)

Materials.

Fluorescein-conjugated antisera to human Ig. Antisera include:

Specific antisera to heavy chains G, M, A, and D

Antisera to light chains K and λ

Polyvalent antiserum, with activity against several heavy chains and both light chains (PV antiserum)

We have purchased antisera from Meloy, Inc., and have routinely used a dilution of 1:8 to 1:10 to enhance specificity. Specificity of antisera must be established in individual laboratories, since many antisera contain contaminant activities and may contain aggregates or immune complexes capable of binding to Fc receptors on monocytes and lymphocytes. Only conjugates with protein to fluorochrome ratios between 2 and 3 should be used. Immunoelectrophoresis of specific antisera should show activity against only a single heavy chain class or light chain type. Staining of washed, fixed bone marrow cells from patients with MM and WM should only demonstrate positivity with antisera of the same specificity as the serum monoclonal Ig. Living cells from patients with known monoclonal lymphocytic proliferations such as CLL and WM should also stain in a monoclonal distribution. Normal thymus cells are useful negative controls. Methods for raising, absorbing, and conjugating specific antisera for use with living cells are given in several sources (2, 23).

Microscope equipped for incident light fluorescence. We use a Leitz orthoplan microscope and an HbO 100 light source (Osram) with 2KP490 exciter filters, a BG38 red suppression filter, and K510-K530 barrier filters.

Mixture of PBS and glycerol in 1:1 ratio.

Alcohol-cleaned glass slides and cover slips.

Method.

1. Pellet 4×10^6 washed cells in a 15-ml plastic centrifuge tube at $400 \times g$. Resuspend by Vortexing with diluted antiserum. Final volume, 0.1 ml.

2. Incubate for 45 min at 4 C.

3. Wash twice with PBS at 4 C. (Note: centrifuge at 4 C.)

4. Resuspend washed cells in 2 drops of PBS-glycerol (4 C) and prepare slides. Keep slides at 4 C until examined.

5. Examine slides at $1,000\times$ and determine the percentage of positive cells by counting oil-immersion fields alternately by light and fluorescence microscopy.

Detection of intracellular immunoglobulin by immunofluorescence

Materials.

Cytocentrifuge (Shandon Southern Instruments, Inc., Sewickley, Pa.).

Acetone.

Method.

1. Dilute washed cells to 0.5×10^6 to 1.0×10^6/ml with RPMI-1640 with 10% FCS.

2. Prepare slides using 0.5 ml of cell suspension per cytocentrifuge block.

3. Fix for 10 min in acetone. Store slides at -70 C.

4. Stain by covering cell button with diluted antiserum and incubating slide in a humidified incubator for 30 to 45 min.

5. Wash slides in a PBS bath with three changes of PBS.

6. Place a drop of PBS-glycerol on cell button, cover with a cover slip, and examine by fluorescence microscopy.

E rosette technique (see chapter 7)

Materials.

Sheep erythrocytes. Sheep erythrocytes in Alsever's solution may be obtained from Baltimore Biological Laboratory, Cockeysville, Md. We discard batches after 2 weeks. Just before use, sheep erythrocytes should be washed and diluted in RPMI-1640 to make a 1% suspension.

Sheep erythrocyte-absorbed FCS. Serum should be absorbed at 37 C for 30 to 45 min with an equal volume of washed sheep erythrocytes. Freeze serum in small portions and store at -20 C.

Cytocentrifuge (Shandon Southern Instruments, Inc.).

Method.

1. Concentrate washed cells to 10×10^6/ml in RPMI-1640.

2. Combine 0.1 ml of cell suspension, 0.1 ml of 1% sheep erythrocyte suspension, and 0.1 ml of the absorbed FCS in a 15-ml plastic centrifuge tube. Prepare in duplicate.

3. Incubate on a slow rotator for 30 min at 37 C in a 5% CO_2 incubator.

4. Centrifuge at $200 \times g$ and 4 C for 10 min, and keep overnight at 4 C.

5. Add 0.1 ml of 0.5% trypan blue and very gently resuspend cells by flicking tube with finger.

6. Place a drop of suspension in a hemacytometer and determine by phase microscopy the percentage of living cells forming rosettes. Cells binding three or more sheep erythrocytes are scored as positive.

7. Cytocentrifuge slides. Dilute the duplicate E rosette preparation kept overnight at 4 C to a total volume of 5 to 10 ml with RPMI-1640. Use about 0.5 ml per cytocentrifuge block. Slides may be stained with Giemsa or Wright's stain.

COMMENTS ON METHODS

Representative single-cell suspensions with viability averaging more than 90% may usually be prepared from blood, marrow filtrate, and body fluids. However, solid tumors, especially if they contain fibrous tissue, may be difficult to disperse into single-cell suspensions. Enzymatic digestion may be useful in such cases, but we have not had extensive experience with this method. A disproportionate number of small cells may be obtained from neoplasms containing both large and small cells, as the larger cells seem more fragile and are less easily freed as single cells. Also, solid tumors occasionally yield suspensions low in viability, as a result of difficulties with disruption or necrosis in the original tumor mass. Viability of suspensions from solid tumors has ranged from 0 to 100% (average 80%). Suspensions with viability below 60% should be interpreted with caution.

Specimens received late in the day may usually be dispersed, washed, and maintained overnight at 4 C at a concentration of 2×10^6/ml of RPMI with 10% FCS. Immunological studies can then be performed the next day.

Monocytes and macrophages are often present in cell suspensions prepared from pleural fluid and some solid tumors, and they collect at the Ficoll-Hypaque interface along with lymphocytes. Because MPS cells often carry cytophilic antibody, they may contribute significantly to the percentage of Ig-positive cells. Contamination by MPS cells can be evaluated by α-naphthyl acetate esterase-stained cytocentrifuge slides. Alternatively, the suspension can be incubated with latex particles so that phagocytic cells can be identified during the counting procedure. Most techniques for removal of phagocytic cells also simultaneously remove lymphocytes, with possible distortion of the lymphocyte population.

Histochemical studies

Sudan black and esterase stains are most useful for differentiating granulocytic or monocytic cells from lymphoid cells (15). Granulocytic cells, even when very immature, usually stain with Sudan black. Monoblasts and promonocytes are often Sudan black positive and show α-naphthyl acetate esterase positivity, but a few cases of monocytic leukemia, ultimately identified by electron microscopy, have not had positive staining. In both granulocytic and monocytic leukemia, there may be great variation in the frequency of staining cells, and occasionally only 5 to 10% of leukemic cells will be positive. Auer rods are more easily seen with Sudan black-stained than Wright's-stained preparations.

Immunofluorescence techniques

Immunofluorescence studies are designed to detect Ig on the surface of living cells or in the cytoplasm of fixed cells. The reliability of these studies is dependent on use of specific antisera and excellent fluorescence microscopy equipment. SIg usually represents an intrinsic membrane protein synthesized by the cell but may be derived from several other sources. Circulating antibodies against lymphocytes may bind in vivo to the cell surface. Immune complexes and IgG aggregates in plasma or in reagents can bind to Fc receptors. SIg with rheumatoid factor activity may bind to plasma IgG. Staining due to any of these situations may produce an immunofluorescence result in which individual lymphocytes appear to carry multiple heavy and light chains. In neoplasms the presence of a single type of light chain on the majority of cells suggests that the SIg is an intrinsic membrane protein synthesized by the cells at test, as exogenous antibody is associated with a light chain mixture. Production of Ig by neoplastic cells is the most reliable indicator that the malignant cells are B cells. However, removal of SIg by trypsin with resynthesis is a difficult method to incorporate into laboratories, because trypsin stripping of Ig is erratic. Prolonged incubation of lymphocytes with membrane turnover is technically much simpler than trypsinization and often distinguishes between antibody produced by test cells and cytophilic antibody (12, 19, 30).

Most tissues involved by neoplasms contain a mixture of neoplastic cells and reactive cells. In lymphoid neoplasms, it may be difficult to differentiate by phase microscopy between neoplastic and reactive lymphocytes. Cell size may differentiate reactive from neoplastic cells, assuming that the larger cells are more likely to be neoplastic. With immunofluorescence, B cell neoplasms should show an increase above normal tissues in the percentage of positive cells, with a monoclonal distribution of heavy and light chains.

The percentages and distribution of Ig-bearing cells are known for normal peripheral blood but have not been well established for other tissues. Normal values for SIg-bearing cells in peripheral blood are as follows: IgM, 5 to 25% (mean 13%); IgG, 1 to 7% (mean 4%); IgA, 0.5 to 4% (mean 2%); IgD (see below); K, 10 to 16% (mean 13.5%); λ, 2 to 7% (mean 5%); PV, 10 to 30% (mean 20%). There is evidence that IgD is a common SIg on blood lymphocytes and is usually present on the same cells as IgM. The D and M heavy chains appear to be attached to identical light chains. The number of Ig-bearing cells in non-neoplastic lymph node and spleen varies with the immunological reactivity of the tissue. Normal and reactive lymph nodes usually contain low numbers (<35%) of Ig-bearing cells, compared with B cell lymphomas, but they may contain 80% or more Ig-bearing cells, especially in cases with intense follicular hyperplasia. Normal spleen usually contains 40 to 50% Ig-bearing cells. In our experience, the B cell population in reactive tissue is usually polyclonal.

Examination of immunofluorescence preparations should determine the percentage of positive cells, the intensity and distribution of fluorescence, and whether the intensity is constant or variable from cell to cell. Most of this information is useful in interpretation of immunological function studies, as indicated above in the section on specific neoplasms.

E rosette technique

Two pieces of information may be derived from E rosette studies: the percentage of cells forming rosettes and the kind of cell in the rosette. In contrast to immunofluorescence, the E rosette technique does not determine the clonality of T cell populations. An advantage of the E rosette technique is that slides of the E rosette preparations may be used to evaluate the cytological appearance and staining characteristics of cells in rosettes. However, the cytocentrifuge procedure may disrupt rosettes, and cells at the edges of cytocentrifuge preparations often appear artifactually surrounded by several layers of red cells. A rosette-forming cell is most easily recognized on cytocentrifuge preparations when the adjacent red cells are elongated and surround the cell.

We have used many batches of sheep erythrocytes, presumably from different animals, without significant change in results. Others have reported that different lots of FCS may cause variation in E rosette results.

Normal values for E rosette-forming cells in blood are 50 to 80% (mean 65%). Normal and reactive lymph nodes usually contain a high percentage of E rosette-forming cells. Normal values for most tissues and fluids are not well established.

Other techniques

B cells can also be detected by their surface receptors for complement, for aggregated IgG, and for Epstein-Barr virus. The complement receptor technique permits cytological examination of positive cells. Functional studies on frozen tissue sections allow evaluation of the marking system in relationship to architectural features of the neoplasm but are difficult to interpret in diffuse growths. None of these techniques, however, gives an estimate of the clonality of B cell populations.

Antisera to thymocytes and to T lymphocytes have been prepared in several laboratories. Most rely on a cytotoxicity assay in which the percentage of cells killed by the antiserum plus complement reflects the percentage of T lymphocytes present. This method appears to be flawed by varying specificity, and it is very difficult to assess cytologically the cells being killed.

It now appears that some neoplasms are composed of cells which have membrane characteristics of several different normal cell lines. The significance of such cases is not completely known but demonstrates the need for great caution in interpreting immunological function studies, especially when few techniques are used.

CONCLUSIONS

The studies outlined above clearly show that techniques for identification of normal hematopoietic, MPS, and lymphoid populations may be routinely applied to the neoplasms of these systems. Although these investigations are somewhat preliminary in scope and limited in case number, some conclusions seem justified:

1. Hematopoietic, MPS, and lymphoid neoplasms may be categorized more precisely by using a combination of functional and structural investigations.

2. Most lymphoid neoplasms are derived from B cells. However, several different neoplasms of

T cells have recently been recognized by a combination of morphological and functional studies.

3. Neoplasms of large cells ("histiocytic lymphoma" or "reticulum cell sarcoma") are usually composed of transformed lymphocytes and include both B and T cell neoplasms.

4. MPS malignant neoplasms are rare, with the exception that many monocytic elements are found in most cases of acute leukemia in adults.

5. Diseases such as ALL, CLL, and blastic phases of CGL have been shown to be distinctly heterogeneous by combined methodology.

6. The term lymphosarcoma has become so nonspecific as to be virtually meaningless.

Relatively specific functional and structural criteria may now be enumerated for most hematopoietic, MPS, and lymphoid neoplasms. Uniform application of these criteria by investigative centers will greatly facilitate communication and seems essential for refinement of clinical protocols. The methodology described in this chapter was chosen in part because it seems adaptable to most laboratories. More sophisticated methods are now being developed and should lead to even greater specificity in categorization of neoplasms of the hematopoietic system, MPS, and lymphoid system.

LITERATURE CITED

1. Aisenberg, A. C., and K. J. Bloch. 1972. Immunoglobulins on the surface of neoplastic lymphocytes. N. Engl. J. Med. **287**:272–276.

2. Aiuti, F., J. C. Cerottini, R. R. A. Coombs, M. Cooper, H. B. Dickler, S. Fröland, H. H. Fudenberg, M. F. Greaves, H. M. Grey, H. G. Kunkel, J. Natvig, J. L. Preud'homme, E. Rabellino, D. S. Rowe, M. Seligman, F. P. Siegal, J. Stjërnsward, W. D. Terry, and J. Wybran. 1974. Identification, enumeration and isolation of B and T lymphocytes from human peripheral blood. Report of a WHO sponsored workshop on human B and T cells. Scand. J. Immunol. **3**:521.

3. Barcos, M. P., and R. J. Lukes. 1975. Malignant lymphoma of convoluted lymphocytes: a new entity of possible T cell type, p. 147–177. Conflicts in Childhood Cancer. Progress in clinical and biological research, vol. 4. Alan R. Liss, Inc., New York.

4. Berard, C., G. T. O'Connor, L. B. Thomas, and H. Torloni. 1969. Histopathological definition of Burkitt's tumour. Bull. WHO **40**:601–607.

5. Bowling, M. C. 1967. Histopathology laboratory procedures of the Pathologic Anatomy Branch of the National Cancer Institute. U.S. Government Printing Office, Washington, D.C.

6. Brouet, J. C., G. Flandrin, and M. Seligmann. 1973. Indications of the thymus-derived nature of the proliferating cells in six patients with Sézary's syndrome. N. Engl. J. Med. **289**: 341–344.

7. Brouet, J. C., J. L. Preud'homme, and M. Seligmann. 1975. The use of B and T membrane markers in the classification of human leukemias, with special reference to acute lymphoblastic leukemia. Blood Cells **1**:81–90.

8. Brown, G., M. F. Greaves, T. A. Lister, N. Rapson, and M. Papamichael. 1974. Expression of human T and B lymphocyte cell-surface markers on leukaemic cells. Lancet **2**:753–755.

9. Canale, D. D., and R. D. Collins. 1974. Use of bone marrow particle sections in the diagnosis of multiple myeloma. Am. J. Clin. Pathol. **61**: 382–392.

10. Dickler, H. B., F. P. Siegal, Z. H. Bentwich, and H. G. Kunkel. 1973. Lymphocyte binding of aggregated IgG and surface Ig staining in chronic lymphocytic leukaemia. Clin. Exp. Immunol. **14**:97–106.

11. Dorfman, R. F. 1964. Enzyme histochemistry of normal, hyperplastic and neoplastic lymphoreticular tissues. Symp. Lymph Tumours in Africa, Paris, 1963, p. 304–326.

12. Fu, S. M., R. J. Winchester, K. R. Rai, and H. G. Kunkel. 1974. Hairy cell leukemia: proliferation of a cell with phagocytic and B-lymphocyte properties. Scand. J. Immunol. **3**:847–851.

13. Glick, A. D., and R. G. Horn. 1974. Identification of promonocytes and monocytoid precursors in acute leukaemia of adults: ultrastructural and cytochemical observations. Br. J. Haematol. **26**:395–403.

14. Glick, A. D., J. H. Leech, J. A. Waldron, J. M. Flexner, R. G. Horn, and R. D. Collins. 1975. Malignant lymphomas of follicular center cell origin in man. II. Ultrastructural and cytochemical studies. J. Natl. Cancer Inst. **54**: 23–36.

15. Hayhoe, F. G. J., and J. C. Cawley. 1972. Acute leukaemia: cellular morphology, cytochemistry and fine structure. Clinics in Hematology **1**:49–94.

16. Jaffe, E. S., E. M. Shevach, E. H. Sussman, M. Frank, I. Green, and C. W. Berard. 1975. Membrane receptor sites for the identification of lymphoreticular cells in benign and malignant conditions. Br. J. Cancer **31**:107–120, Suppl. II.

17. Jondal, M., G. Holm, and H. Wigzell. 1972. Surface markers on human T and B lymphocytes. I. A large population of lymphocytes forming nonimmune rosettes with sheep red blood cells. J. Exp. Med. **136**:207–215.

18. Kersey, J., M. Nesbit, H. Hallgren, A. Sabad, E. Yunis, and K. Gajl-Peczalska. 1975. Evidence for origin of certain childhood acute lymphoblastic leukemias and lymphomas in thymus-derived lymphocytes. Cancer **36**:1348–1352.

19. Leech, J. H., A. D. Glick, J. A. Waldron, J. M. Flexner, R. G. Horn, and R. D. Collins. 1975. Malignant lymphomas of follicular center cell origin in man. I. Immunologic studies. J. Natl. Cancer Inst. **54**:11–21.

20. Lukes, R. J., and R. D. Collins. 1973. New

observations on follicular lymphoma. Gann Monogr. 15:209–215.

21. Lukes, R. J., and R. D. Collins. 1974. Immunologic characterization of human malignant lymphomas. Cancer 34:1488–1503.

22. Lukes, R. J., and R. D. Collins. 1975. New approaches to the classification of the lymphomata. Br. J. Cancer 31:1–28, Suppl. II.

23. Preud'homme, J. L., and M. Seligmann. 1972. Surface bound immunoglobulins as a cell marker in human lymphoproliferative diseases. Blood 40:777–794.

24. Raff, M. C. 1970. Two distinct populations of peripheral lymphocytes in mice distinguishable by immunofluorescence. Immunology 19:637–650.

25. Seligmann, M., J. L. Preud'homme, and J. C. Brouet. 1973. B and T cell markers in human proliferative blood diseases and primary immunodeficiencies, with special reference to membrane bound immunoglobulins. Transplant. Rev. 16:85–113.

26. Shevach, E. M., E. S. Jaffe, and I. Green. 1973. Receptors for complement and immunoglobulin on human and animal lymphoid cells.

27. Smith, J. L., G. P. Clein, C. R. Barker, and R. D. Collins. 1973. Characterisation of malignant mediastinal lymphoid neoplasm (Sternberg sarcoma) as thymic in origin. Lancet 1:74–77.

28. Tindle, B. H., J. W. Parker, and R. J. Lukes. 1972. "Reed-Sternberg cells" in infectious mononucleosis? Am. J. Clin. Pathol. 58:607–617.

29. VanFurth, R., Z. A. Cohn, J. G. Hirsch, J. H. Humphrey, W. G. Spector, and H. L. Langevoort. 1972. The mononuclear phagocyte system: a new classification of macrophages, monocytes, and their precursor cells. Bull. WHO 46:845.

30. Winchester, R. J., J. B. Winfield, F. Siegal, P. Wernet, Z. Bentwich, and H. G. Kunkel. 1974. Analyses of lymphocytes from patients with rheumatoid arthritis and systemic lupus erythematosus. J. Clin. Invest. 54:1082–1092.

31. Yam, L. T., C. Y. Li, and H. E. Finkel. 1972. Leukemic reticuloendotheliosis: the role of tartrate-resistant acid phosphatase in diagnosis and splenectomy in treatment. Arch. Intern. Med. 130:248–256.

Transplant. Rev. 16:3–28.

Chapter 98

Diagnosis of Monoclonal Gammopathies

ROBERT A. KYLE

INTRODUCTION

The monoclonal gammopathies are a group of disorders characterized by proliferation of a single clone of plasma cells that produce a homogenous, monoclonal (M) protein. A monoclonal immunoglobulin (Ig) consists of two heavy polypeptide chains of a single class and subclass and two light polypeptide chains of a single type (Table 1). Thus, it contrasts with a polyclonal Ig increase, which consists of one or more heavy-chain classes and both light-chain types.

Monoclonal gammopathies are synonymous with plasma cell dyscrasias (25), immunoglobulinopathies (6), gammopathies (44), and dysproteinemias.

The different kinds of monoclonal Ig are designated by capital letters that correspond to the class of their heavy chains, which are designated by Greek letters: γ in IgG, α in IgA, μ in IgM, δ in IgD, and ϵ in IgE. Their subclasses are IgG1, IgG2, IgG3, IgG4, or IgA1 and IgA2; and their light-chain types are kappa or κ and lambda or λ (not K or L, because L and H are used for light and heavy chains).

Classification of Monoclonal Gammopathies

I. Malignant monoclonal gammopathies
  A. Multiple myeloma (IgG, IgA, IgD, IgE, and free light chains)
    1. Solitary plasmacytoma of bone
    2. Extramedullary plasmacytoma, solitary and multiple
    3. Plasma cell leukemia
    4. Nonsecretory myeloma
  B. Waldenström's macroglobulinemia, primary macroglobulinemia (IgM)
  C. Heavy-chain diseases (HCD)
    1. γ (gamma) HCD
    2. α (alpha) HCD
    3. μ (mu) HCD
  D. Amyloidosis
    1. Primary
    2. With myeloma
    3. Secondary
    4. Localized
    5. Familial
II. Monoclonal gammopathies of unknown significance
  A. Benign (IgG, IgA, IgD, IgM, and, rarely, free light chains)
  B. Associated with malignant lymphoma
  C. Associated with neoplasms of cell types not known to produce monoclonal proteins

In this chapter on the monoclonal gammopathies, I shall review briefly the structure of immunoglobulins, relate normal immunoglobulins to myeloma and macroglobulinemia, discuss the nature of monoclonal proteins, and then describe laboratory methods for the recognition and study of monoclonal proteins.

TABLE 1. *Classification of immunoglobulins of normal human serum*

Immuno-globulin	Synonyms	Heavy-chain		Light-chain types	Molecular formula	Designation
		Classes	Subclasses			
IgG	γ, $7S\gamma$, γ_2, γG	γ	IgG1, IgG2, IgG3, IgG4	κ	$\gamma_2\kappa_2$	IgG κ
				λ	$\gamma_2\lambda_2$	IgG λ
IgA	βx, β_2A, γ_1A, γA	α	IgA1, IgA2	κ	$\alpha_2\kappa_2{}^a$	IgA κ
				λ	$\alpha_2\kappa_2{}^a$	IgA λ
IgM	γ_1, $19S\gamma$, β_2M, γ_1M, γM	μ	—	κ	$(\mu_2\kappa_2)5$	IgM κ
				λ	$(\mu_2\lambda_2)5$	IgM λ
IgD	γD	δ	Ja, La	κ	$\delta_2\kappa_2$	IgD κ
				λ	$\delta_2\lambda_2$	IgDλ
IgE	γE	ϵ	—	κ	$\epsilon_2\kappa_2$	IgE κ
				λ	$\epsilon_2\lambda_2$	IgE λ

^{a} May form polymers.

IMMUNOGLOBULIN STRUCTURE

Prior to 1960, the term "gamma globulin" was used for any protein that migrated in the gamma mobility region (toward the cathode) of the electrophoretic pattern. Now these proteins are referred to as "immunoglobulins," and the five groups presently recognized and their properties are listed in Table 2. Several reviews of immunoglobulins have been published (3, 11, 18, 19, 24, 27, 29, 38, 45).

Immunoglobulin G (see chapter 2)

Three-fourths of the Ig in normal serum is of the IgG class, and this is the type most thoroughly investigated. It has a molecular weight of 150,000 and a sedimentation coefficient of 6.7S. Its electrophoretic mobility ranges from slow gamma (cathodal area) to alpha-2. Many antibodies to both bacteria and viruses are of the IgG class.

A reducing agent such as mercaptoethanol disrupts the disulfide bonds linking the polypeptide chains of the IgG molecule. If the reduced protein is alkylated with iodoacetamide and fractionated in the presence of a solvent (such as guanidine or urea) capable of dissociating noncovalent bonds, two kinds of polypeptide chains can be recovered (Fig. 1): heavy (H) and light (L).

Heavy chains. Both heavy chains of the IgG molecule are of the γ class, and the two light chains are alike—both kappa or both lambda. The γ chains have a molecular weight of approximately 55,000, and their structure comprises 440 to 450 amino acids. They have variable (V) regions in which there are many amino acid substitutions from one IgG molecule to the next and constant (C) regions in which there are very few amino acid differences from one γ chain to the next. The variable region of the γ chain consists of approximately 110 amino acid residues beginning at the amino terminal of the chain. The constant regions of the γ chains consist of 310 to 330 amino acids arranged linearly, adjacent regions having homologies with the constant portion of the light chain and also with each other. These portions of the γ heavy chain are called "homology regions" or "domains" and are designated $C_{\gamma 1}$, $C_{\gamma 2}$, and $C_{\gamma 3}$. The first homology region of the constant portion ($C_{\gamma 1}$) corresponds to the constant part of the Fd fragment (Fig. 1) and runs from about amino acid 110 to 210–220. The sec-

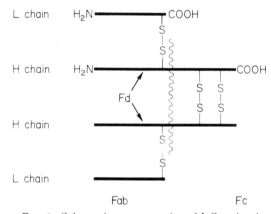

FIG. 1. *Schematic representation of IgG molecule, with cleavage by papain into Fab and Fc fragments. Modified from Kyle et al. (18).*

TABLE 2. *Properties of immunoglobulins of normal human serum[a]*

Property	IgG	IgA	IgM	IgD	IgE
Electrophoretic mobility	Gamma to alpha-2	Gamma to beta	Gamma to gamma-2	Gamma to beta	Gamma to beta
Sedimentation coefficient	6.7S	7–15S^b	19S	7S	8S
Molecular weight	150,000	170,000–500,000^b	900,000	180,000	200,000
Carbohydrate, %	2.6	5–10	9.8	10–12	11
T ½, days	23	5.8	5.1	2.8	2.3
Serum concentration, mean mg/ml	11.4	1.8	1.0	0.03	0.0003
Total serum immunoglobulin, %	74	21	5	0.2	0.002
Total body pool in intravascular space, %	45	42	76	75	51
Intravascular pool catabolized per day, % (normal)	6.7	25	18	37	89
Normal synthetic rate, mg per kg per day	33	24	6.7	0.4	0.02
Fixes complement	Yes	Alternate pathway	Yes	No	No
Crosses placenta	Yes	No	No	No	No

[a] Modified from Kyle et al. (18).

[b] Tends to form polymer of the monomer form.

ond homology region ($C_{\gamma 2}$) is in the amino (NH_2)-terminal half of the Fc fragment and extends from 210 to 220 up to position 330 to 340, and the third homology region ($C_{\gamma 3}$) extends to the carboxy terminus.

Immunological analysis of myeloma proteins has disclosed four distinct subclasses of IgG heavy chains designated IgG1, IgG2, IgG3, and IgG4. The IgG1 subclass constitutes 64 to 70% of normal IgG molecules; IgG2, 23 to 28%; IgG3, 4 to 7%; and IgG4, 3 to 4% (35). Normal serum pools contain the following concentrations of IgG subclasses (mg/100 ml): IgG1, 5.1 to 8.1; IgG2, 2.5 to 3.6; IgG3, 0.55 to 0.70; and IgG4, 0.35 to 0.40.

The molecular weight of IgG1, IgG2, and IgG4 heavy chains is 54,200; that of IgG3 is 60,950. The average biological half-life of IgG1, IgG2, and IgG4 myeloma proteins injected into patients with malignancies is 21 days, whereas IgG3 has a half-life of 7 to 8 days. Although many antigens evoke an antibody response within the IgG subclasses proportional to their distribution in normal serum, others produce antibodies mainly within one subclass. For example, almost all antibodies to factor VIII (found in hemophiliacs, postpartum women, and elderly patients) are of the IgG4 subclass (37). Without predilection, only 3 to 4% of the antibodies would be of this subclass. A high proportion of antibodies to dextran, levan, and teichoic acid is limited to the IgG2 subclass. IgG1 and IgG3 fix complement readily; IgG2 does so less well. It has been shown that aggregates of IgG4b, but not IgG4a, fix complement via the alternate pathway (9).

Light chains. In 1962, Edelman and Gally (4) demonstrated that light chains prepared from a serum IgG myeloma protein and the Bence Jones protein in the same patient's urine behaved identically: that is, they precipitated when heated to between 40 and 60 C, dissolved on boiling, and reprecipitated when cooled to between 40 and 60 C. The light chains have a molecular weight of 22,500 and contain approximately 214 amino acids. Analysis of Bence Jones proteins (urinary light chains) and light chains prepared from myeloma proteins revealed two antigenic types, kappa and lambda. Approximately 70% of serum IgG myeloma immunoglobulins are of the kappa type and about 30% are lambda; the proportion among light chains of normal IgG is similar.

Amino acid sequence analyses of individual light chains of each type have disclosed a remarkable fact: although the region of the chain from approximately position 107 to the carboxy terminus at position 214 is virtually identical in light chains of the same type (κ or λ), the region from the amino (NH_2) terminus (position 1) to position 107 has been different in every light chain thus far analyzed. Consequently, these two are termed the constant (C_L) and variable (V_L) portions of the light (L) chains. Both constant and variable portions contain a loop consisting of approximately 60 amino acid residues. In the variable portion there are many amino acid differences, whereas in the constant portion differences exist at one or two sites only.

Bence Jones proteins are synthesized de novo and are not degradation products. They are catabolized by the renal tubular cells (48) or, when present in excess, excreted promptly in the urine. Approximately 75% of human IgG myeloma tumors produce an excess of light chains, but not all of the patients have light chains in their urine.

Fab and Fc fragments. The relation of the heavy and light chains in the structure of the Ig molecule is inferred from the effect of certain proteolytic enzymes (Fig. 1). Papain, by breaking the heavy chains, cleaves the molecule into three pieces: an Fc fragment (so named because in certain species it can be crystallized) and two Fab fragments (so named because of their ability to combine with antigen, i.e., an antibody).

The Fc fragment consists of the C-terminal portion of both heavy chains, still linked to each other by disulfide bonds. Other designations of this fragment are fast, B, and III; its molecular weight is 48,000. Biological activities of the Fc fragment include fixation of complement, passive cutaneous anaphylaxis (PCA), binding with rheumatoid factors, binding with receptors on macrophages and lymphocytes, reaction with staphylococcal A protein, and transfer across the placenta. Isotypic specificity—specificity for γ, α, μ, δ or ϵ—resides in the Fc fragment. The Fc piece is devoid of antibody activity.

Each Fab fragment is the N-terminal portion of a heavy chain and the complete light chain. Other designations are slow, A, C, I, or II. The molecular weight is 52,000. The Fab fragment contains the antigen-combining site which is composed of perhaps 15 to 20 amino acid residues, some being in the heavy-chain portion and others in the light-chain portion.

Immunoglobulin A

IgA, which was first described by Heremans et al. in 1959 (42), is composed of two heavy α chains and two light chains, both κ or λ (Fig. 2, left). IgA has a molecular weight of 170,000 and a sedimentation coefficient of 7S but has a propensity to form polymers. Its catabolic rate of 5.8 days (T ½) is greater than that of IgG. Containing antibodies to bacteria as well as to viruses, IgA promotes phagocytosis, particularly by monocytes. Aggregated IgA can fix the late components of complement, beginning with C3 (alternate pathway; 9). There are two subgroups of the α chain, α_1 and α_2, resulting in IgA1 and IgA2 proteins (43). Almost 95% of monoclonal IgA proteins are of the IgA1 class. IgA2 molecules are unique among the immunoglobulins in that the light chains are bound to the α_2 chains by noncovalent forces instead of disulfide bonds (10).

The IgA monomer, whose sedimentation coefficient is 7S, has a propensity to form polymers with sedimentation coefficients of 9 to 15S. In one study of 13 monoclonal IgA1 myeloma proteins, the major component in six patients was 9S (polymer) rather than 7S (8). Occasionally, two discrete electrophoretic spikes, one of 7S monomer and the other of polymers, may be seen in a monoclonal IgA protein.

The IgA polymers are linked covalently by disulfide bonds and joining (J) chains. The J chain is a non-Ig with a molecular weight of approximately 15,000. It is found in polymers of IgA and the pentamer structure of IgM (15).

Secretory IgA. Secretory IgA (SIgA) is found in high concentration in the secretions of many glands lining the respiratory and gastrointestinal tracts as well as in tears, colostrum, and urine. SIgA has a sedimentation coefficient of 11S and a molecular weight of 390,000. As shown in Fig. 2 (right), it is composed of two IgA molecules attached by disulfide bonds to a glycoprotein (molecular weight, 60,000) called the "secretory piece" (or "S piece"). The secretory piece is synthesized in mucosal epithelial cells. The secretory piece increases the resistance of the molecules against digestion by trypsin and pepsin (20).

Immunoglobulin M

A third Ig, IgM (Fig. 3), consists of 7S subunits linked by disulfide bonds and J chains (23). It constitutes 5 to 10% of the total serum Ig in the normal human. Approximately three-fourths of this Ig is intravascular because of its high molecular weight. Its catabolic rate is greater than that of IgG and IgA, and its synthetic rate is less.

The heavy chain (μ) of IgM has a molecular weight of approximately 70,000; the subunits, composed of two heavy chains and two light chains, each have a molecular weight of approximately 180,000 to 190,000. Since the molecular weight of IgM is approximately 900,000, it

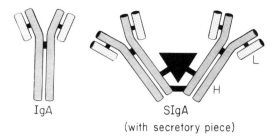

FIG. 2. *Scheme of IgA and SIgA molecules (L = light chain; H = heavy chain). Modified from Kyle et al. (18).*

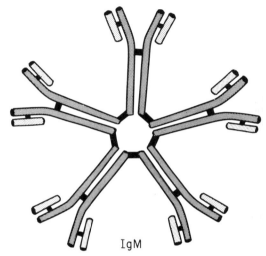

FIG. 3. *IgM molecule. From Kyle et al. (18).*

evidently comprises five subunits. The μ chain, recently sequenced, consists of one variable (V_H) and four constant ($C_{\mu 1}$, $C_{\mu 2}$, $C_{\mu 3}$, $C_{\mu 4}$) domains. V_H and $C_{\mu 1}$ are in the Fd piece, $C_{\mu 2}$ is in the hinge region, and $C_{\mu 3}$ and $C_{\mu 4}$ are in the Fc fragment (32).

IgM has a sedimentation coefficient of 19S, but more rapidly sedimenting molecules of 22S (composed of dimers of the 19S molecule) and 35S also occur. In addition, low-molecular-weight IgM (sedimentation coefficient 7S) has been found in patients with various pathological conditions, including lupus erythematosus, macroglobulinemia, other lymphoproliferative processes, and cirrhosis (1). The low-molecular-weight IgM is most likely synthesized as such, rather than being a breakdown product of 19S IgM.

IgM antibodies are the first produced in a primary immune response. Cold agglutinins, isoagglutinins, rheumatoid factor, and heterophile and Wasserman antibodies, as well as antibodies to various bacteria, are of the IgM class. Approximately 80% of IgM monoclonal proteins are of kappa type, in contrast to two-thirds of IgG and IgA monoclonal proteins.

Immunoglobulin D

In 1965, Rowe and Fahey (34) found a myeloma protein containing a heavy chain unlike those of the other immunoglobulins. This class, named IgD, is present in low concentrations in normal serum, is rapidly catabolized, and has a serum half-life of 2.8 days. Approximately 75% of IgD is intravascular, a distribution that may be due to the shape of the molecule. Of patients with IgD myeloma, 80% have λ light chains, in contrast to the 30% of patients with IgG myeloma. In addition, the monoclonal IgD protein peak is small and not readily seen on the serum protein electrophoretic pattern. Although antigen-combining activity associated with IgD has been reported, the functions of the molecule that are attributable to the heavy chain have remained obscure. It has been reported that IgD is frequently found on the surface of lymphocytes. Antigenic heterogeneity has been reported in IgD heavy chains and may be indicative of subclasses of IgD (Ja and La).

Immunoglobulin E (see chapter 79)

A fifth class of Ig, IgE, has been purified from the serum of allergic patients (12); four cases of IgE myeloma have been reported. IgE has a molecular weight of 200,000 and a sedimentation coefficient of 8S. The combination of a short biological half-life of 2.3 days and a very low synthesis rate results in an extremely low serum concentration in normal persons.

IgE mediates the wheal-and-flare reaction associated with reaginic allergies and binds to basophils. IgE is fixed on normal human target cells, and histamine is released when the cell-fixed IgE reacts with the allergen. IgE is often increased in patients with extrinsic asthma, hay fever, and parasitic infections (13, 49). As expected, the serum IgE level is reduced in patients with B-cell diseases, such as chronic lymphocytic leukemia and multiple myeloma. But the IgE level increases in patients with Hodgkin's disease, with which abnormalities of cellular immunity and disorders of T cell function are associated (46).

RELATION OF MYELOMA PROTEINS AND MACROGLOBULINS TO NORMAL IMMUNOGLOBULINS

Although myeloma proteins and macroglobulins have long been considered abnormal, studies during the past several years strongly suggest that they are only normal immunoglobulins in excessive quantities. The striking feature of myeloma proteins and macroglobulins that led investigators to consider them as abnormal is their homogeneity. Whereas normal IgG in human serum is electrophoretically heterogeneous, with mobility ranging from the alpha-2 to the slow gamma regions, IgG myeloma proteins are localized sharply in their electrophoretic migration.

Kunkel (17) showed that each light-chain type and heavy-chain subclass in myeloma proteins has its counterpart among normal immunoglobulins and also among antibodies. After the discovery of the two types of light chains (κ and λ) in myeloma proteins in a ratio of approximately 2:1, these same light chains were detected in essentially the same ratio among normal immunoglobulins. Similarly, the IgG and IgA subclasses and IgD class were discovered among myeloma proteins and then found as normal serum components. These identifications have gradually weakened the belief that the myeloma proteins and macroglobulins are abnormal and have suggested that they represent the overproduction of a normal product by an abnormally functioning cell. However, many of the heavy chains found in the heavy-chain diseases (HCD) show significant deletions of amino acids; thus, they are abnormal immunoglobulins.

Even the antigenic determinants (also termed "individual antigenic specificities" or "idiotypic specificities" [24] thought to be associated uniquely with myeloma proteins) have been shown to occur among antibodies. Conversely, studies of highly purified antibodies have revealed a homogeneity approaching that seen in myeloma proteins. In some instances, after primary immunization with a carbohydrate antigen, monoclonal immunoglobulins consisting of a single light-chain type and single IgG heavy-chain subclass have been seen (16).

The possibility expressed by Kunkel (17) that myeloma proteins are individual antibodies and are products of the individual plasma cells arising from a single clone of malignant cells has been supported by their antigen-combining activity (5, 30). Monoclonal antibody activity in humans has been associated with cold agglutinin disease as well as with a wide variety of bacterial antigens, including streptolysin O, staphylococcal protein, klebsiella polysaccharides, and brucella (36).

Transient monoclonal proteins have been seen in young children with immunodeficiency and infections. These proteins are modest in amount and disappear within 2 months. Since infections may produce transient monoclonal proteins, it seems likely that the homogeneity of myeloma proteins and macroglobulins reflects the homogeneity associated with highly purified antibodies—namely, that resulting from their production by a single clone of Ig-synthesizing cells. It is almost certain that more monoclonal human proteins will be found to have antibody activity. Indeed, it has been postulated that all myeloma proteins may have antibody activity (26).

In this view, as illustrated in Fig. 4, the heterogenous normal collection of IgG molecules comprises minute amounts of highly homogenous proteins from many diverse single clones of plasma cells and so is polyclonal. If a single clone escapes the normal controls over its multiplication, it reproduces excessively and

(A) Polyclonal

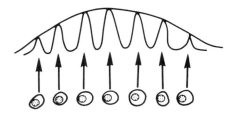

(B) Monoclonal

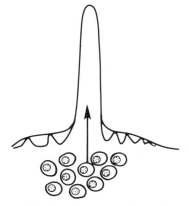

FIG. 4. *Polyclonal and monoclonal electrophoretic patterns. (A) Broad outline comprising small peaks of many different homogenous proteins (each represented here in normal amount, related by arrow to its peak) that have been produced by many different plasma cell clones (polyclonal). (B) Tall, narrow peak of homogenous protein (single heavy-chain and single light-chain type), which is excessive output of single clone (monoclonal). Modified from Kyle and Gleich (19).*

synthesizes an excess of antibody-like protein of a single heavy-chain class and subclass and single light-chain type. This monoclonal protein often is associated with a neoplastic process. Support for the once-cell, one-Ig concept comes from studies of the cellular localization of these proteins. Experiments performed with antisera to light chains have shown that nearly all individual plasma cells contain either κ or λ light chains but not both.

Patterns of overproduction

Normally, plasma cells produce heavy chains and a slight excess of light chains that spill over into the urine. In IgG myeloma, about three-fourths of patients have an excess of light chains that may be excreted into the urine (Bence Jones proteinuria) or catabolized (2). This small excess of light-chain production could be due to imbalance in translation or transcription within occasional clones or a possible suppression of heavy-chain synthesis in such clones. In other instances, no heavy chain is produced by the plasma cell and only excessive quantities of light chains are detected ("light-chain disease"; 39). Finally, a small proportion of myeloma cells do not secrete either heavy or light chains to excess, whether because of a simple failure of production or blocking of secretion; these are called "nonsecretory."

PROCEDURES FOR STUDYING MONOCLONAL PROTEINS

Analysis of the serum or urine for monoclonal proteins requires a sensitive, rapid, dependable screening method to detect the possibility of a monoclonal protein and a specific assay to identify it according to heavy-chain class and light-chain type.

The basic principle of electrophoresis is that charged particles in solution migrate according to their charge—albumin toward the anode (positive pole). The pH of the buffer is selected to give the best separation of the individual components. In 1937, Tiselius used electrophoretic techniques to separate serum globulins into three components, which he designated α, β, and γ (40). Two years later, Tiselius and Kabat localized antibody activity in the gamma globulin fraction of the plasma proteins (41). They noted that antibodies to egg albumin or to pneumococcus type I were found in the area of gamma mobility in rabbit serum, but antibodies to pneumococcal organisms migrated between beta and gamma in horse serum. Electrophoretic techniques, applied in the study of multiple myeloma proteins by Longsworth et al. (21), demonstrated the tall, narrow-based spike. The method was cumbersome and difficult, so electrophoresis was not readily available until the early 1950s when filter paper was introduced as a supporting medium (for zone electrophoresis). More recently, cellulose acetate has largely supplanted filter paper in electrophoresis for detection of monoclonal immunoglobulins (14).

After such screening, immunoelectrophoresis should be employed to confirm the presence of a monoclonal protein and to distinguish the Ig class and light-chain type of which it is made.

Serum electrophoresis (see chapter 3)

Serum protein electrophoresis should be done in all cases in which multiple myeloma, macroglobulinemia, or amyloidosis is suspected. In addition, this test is indicated by any unexplained weakness or fatigue, anemia, elevation of the erythrocyte sedimentation rate (ESR), back pain, osteoporosis or osteolytic lesions or fractures, Ig deficiency, hypercalcemia, Bence Jones proteinuria, renal insufficiency, or recurrent infections. It is an excellent screening test because it is easy and rapid to perform.

The advantages of *cellulose acetate membrane* over filter paper for electrophoresis include lessened absorption of serum on the supporting medium. This makes it possible to use a very small quantity of serum (0.7 μliter), and it also results in less tailing and a sharper separation of protein bands. On acetate, alpha-1 globulin is well separated from albumin, whereas in filter paper patterns alpha-1 globulin frequently is found in the trailing edge of the albumin peak. Such sharper separation provides superior sensitivity, which is a very important advantage. Although myeloma, macroglobulinemia, and benign monoclonal gammopathy are associated with discrete bands or peaks, these may be small, particularly in benign monoclonal gammopathy, amyloidosis, and heavy-chain diseases, and thus not readily detected on filter paper. When I compared the results from electrophoretic analysis of 134 sera on filter paper and on cellulose, significant, detectable differences in more than a third of the cases proved the superiority of cellulose acetate membrane. In addition, separation occurs in less than 20 min, in contrast to 15 h on filter paper.

However, use of this membrane has its shortcomings and disadvantages also. Despite the sensitivity of electrophoresis on cellulose acetate, a small quantity of monoclonal protein may be obscured in the beta or gamma band and escape notice. Also, a band on the cellulose pattern, though somewhat discrete, may yet have some fuzziness, so that one cannot tell whether it is monoclonal or polyclonal. Monoclonal light chains (Bence Jones proteinemia) usually are not detected with electrophoresis. Obviously one cannot determine the type of light chain or heavy chain in a cellulose acetate tracing. Another problem is that a monoclonal band may run and contaminate the adjacent sample from another patient.

Determination of total protein.

Biuret stock solution
    180 g of sodium potassium tartrate $\cdot$ 4H$_2$O
    60 g of CuSO$_4$ $\cdot$ 5H$_2$O
    20 g of KI
    Make up to 4 liters with 0.2 N NaOH.
Diluting solution
    20 g of KI
    32 g of NaOH
    Make up to 4 liters with water.
Biuret working solution
    400 ml of biuret stock solution
    Make up to 2 liters with diluting solution.

A Beckman DSA (discrete sample analyzer) is used for determination of total protein. In each of two vials, 20 μliters of serum is placed; 500 μliters of diluting solution is added to the first vial and 500 μliters of biuret working solution is added to the second. Incubation is at room temperature, and protein concentration is provided by teletypewriter printout. The unit is calibrated with 2, 4, 6, 8, and 10 g/100 ml standards (New England Reagent Laboratory, Bovine Albumin, Fraction V). An alternative is the AutoAnalyzer method using Weichselbaum's biuret reagent without any blank corrections except for turbid sera (47).

Many instruments are available for serum protein electrophoresis (Beckman Instruments, Fullerton, Calif.; Helena Laboratories, Beaumont, Tex.). My colleagues and I use a Sepratek electrophoresis chamber, Sepratek multiapplicator, Drummond microdispenser, Sepraphore III cellulose polyacetate electrophoresis strips, Ponceau S protein stain, tris(hydroxymethyl)aminomethane-barbital-sodium barbital buffer (pH 8.8), and a Digiscreen "C II" scanner and computer from Gelman Instrument Co., Ann Arbor, Mich.

Procedure.

1. Soak the Sepraphore strips in the buffer tray for at least 6 days prior to use.

2. Fill the Sepratek electrophoresis chamber with 230 ml of buffer solution, and equalize the buffer levels in the two compartments.

3. Use a Drummond microdispenser to place 2

μliters of the specimen on the matted surface of each sample well.

4. Place the applicator onto the applicator block to pick up the sample and then apply it to the cellulose polyacetate membrane.

5. Set the power supply at 200 V and run for 16.5 min.

6. Place the cellulose polyacetate membrane in Ponceau S stain for 10 min. Decolorize the membrane by rinsing in five successive baths of aqueous 5% acetic acid until the background is again white. Place the strip in dehydrating solution (100% methanol) for 1 min and then in the clearing solution (15 ml of CH_3COOH in 85 ml of CH_3OH) for 1 min. Dry the membrane in an oven (92 to 95 C) until clear.

7. Place the cellulose polyacetate membrane in the Digiscreen scanner for densitometric quantitation.

Ordinarily, *controls* are not needed for performance of electrophoresis; if the laboratory does need them, it is advisable to run a serum specimen known to contain a large amount of monoclonal protein and one known to have a normal electrophoretic pattern. Quality control should be maintained by utilizing sera in which the size of the components is agreed upon by several laboratories. Instrument *standardization* is also important, and linearity of response may be checked by use of densitometric standards such as a stepwedge. *Normal values* for serum electrophoresis are given in Table 3.

Interpretation. The first peak at the anodal (positive) end of the serum electrophoretic pattern is albumin, and the next peak is alpha-1 globulin, which contains alpha-1 antitrypsin, alpha-1 lipoprotein, and alpha-1 acid glycoprotein (orosomucoid). The next peak, alpha-2 globulin, is composed mainly of alpha-2 macroglobulin, alpha-2 lipoprotein, haptoglobin, ceruloplasmin, and erythropoietin. Beta lipoprotein, transferrin, plasminogen, complement, and hemopexin are the major components of the beta globulin peak. Fibrinogen (in plasma) appears as a discrete band between the beta and gamma peaks. Immunoglobulins (IgG, IgA, IgM, IgD, and IgE) make up the gamma component, but it must be emphasized that immunoglobulins are found in the beta region also and that IgG extends to the alpha-2 region.

A decrease in albumin and increases in alpha-1 and alpha-2 globulins and occasionally in gamma globulin are nonspecific findings, seen in inflammatory processes (tissue inflammation and destruction) such as infections or metastatic malignancy. Gamma globulin increases are seen in chronic infections, connective-tissue diseases, or liver disease. Rarely, two albumin bands (bisalbuminemia) may be found. This is a familial abnormality and produces no symptoms.

Hypogammaglobulinemia is characterized by a definite decrease of the gamma component, and the diagnosis should be confirmed by quantitative determination of the Ig levels. Hypogammaglobulinemia may be congenital (such as Bruton's sex-linked or "Swiss-type" combined deficiency) or acquired (idiopathic or related to nephrotic syndrome, multiple myeloma, chronic lymphocytic leukemia, lymphosarcoma, or treatment with corticosteroids). The presence of a modest increase in the beta band associated with a decrease in gamma raises the possibility of multiple myeloma or amyloidosis. In this situation, proteinuria of the Bence Jones type is often present, and immunoelectrophoresis of the serum and urine is necessary.

A marked decrease of the alpha-1 globulin component is usually due to a congenital deficiency of alpha-1 anti-trypsin and is often associated with recurrent pulmonary infections and chronic obstructive lung disease.

After electrophoresis, a monoclonal protein usually appears in the gamma, beta, or alpha-2 regions as a narrow peak, like a church spire in the densitometry tracing (Fig. 5), or as a dense, discrete band on the cellulose membrane (Fig. 6). In contrast, a polyclonal excess of Ig makes a broad-based peak (Fig. 7) or broad band (Fig. 8) and usually is limited to the gamma region. Whereas a polyclonal peak consists of increased Ig of one or more heavy-chain types with both κ and λ light chains, a monoclonal protein contains a single light-chain type and a single heavy-chain class. An occasional serum contains two monoclonal proteins of different Ig classes, and this situation is designated "biclonal gammopathy."

A tall, narrow homogenous peak or a discrete band is most suggestive of myeloma, Waldenström's macroglobulinemia, or benign monoclonal gammapathy, but monoclonal peaks may

TABLE 3. *Serum protein electrophoresis: normal values (180 cases)*

Fraction	Normal values (g/100 ml)[a]
Total protein	6.6–7.9
Albumin	3.5–4.7
Alpha-1 globulin	0.2–0.5
Alpha-2 globulin	0.5–0.8
Beta globulin	0.7–1.3
Gamma globulin	0.8–1.6

[a] The 2.5 to 97.5 percentile.

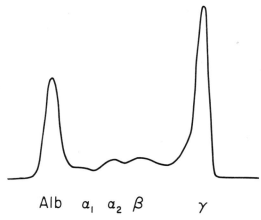

Alb α₁ α₂ β   γ

FIG. 5. *Tall, narrow-based monoclonal peak of gamma mobility on serum electrophoresis of patient with multiple myeloma. From Kyle et al. (18).*

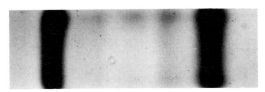

FIG. 6. *Cellulose acetate electrophoretic pattern. The anode is on the left. The dense band on the right represents a monoclonal protein. From Kyle and Bayrd (17a).*

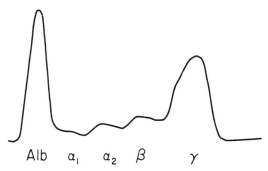

Alb α₁ α₂ β   γ

FIG. 7. *Broad-based polyclonal peak of gamma mobility. From Kyle et al. (18).*

occur also in amyloidosis and in lymphoma. It is appropriate at this point to consider the electrophoretic patterns of certain other conditions. The nephrotic syndrome is distinguished by a distinctive serum pattern featuring low albumin and gamma globulin and an increased amount of alpha-2 and beta globulins (Fig. 9, left). The increased alpha-2 or beta globulin may look like a monoclonal peak of rapid mobility and might be mistaken for a myeloma protein. The urinary

pattern consists mainly of albumin (Fig. 9, right). Similarly, an increased concentration of transferrin or haptoglobin may be mistaken for a monoclonal peak. Chronic infections, connective-tissue diseases, and chronic liver diseases may be characterized by large, broad-based polyclonal patterns. This is particularly true in chronic active hepatitis (Fig. 10), where the gamma component may be 4 or 5 g/100 ml. Occasionally, a monoclonal protein appears as a broad band on cellulose acetate and is mistaken for a polyclonal increase in Ig. Presumably it is due to the presence of aggregates or polymers, and immunoelectrophoresis is required for identification.

It must be emphasized that a patient can have a monoclonal protein when the total protein concentration and the beta and gamma globulin concentrations are within normal limits. In certain cases of IgD myeloma, the monoclonal protein may appear slight or not be evident at all on the cellulose acetate membrane. Often the presence of a monoclonal protein in the heavy-chain diseases is not apparent. In fact, the serum protein electrophoretic pattern is normal in half the cases of alpha heavy-chain disease (α HCD), and an unimpressive broad band in the alpha-2 or beta region is the only electrophoretic abnormality among the rest. The characteristic sharp band or peak suggestive of a monoclonal protein is never seen. In μ HCD, the electrophoretic pattern usually is normal except for hypogammaglobulinemia, and the presence of a dense band is exceptional. In γ HCD, there usually is a band in the beta-gamma area, but often it is broad, appears heterogenous, and is more suggestive of a polyclonal than a monoclonal protein. Furthermore, a small monoclonal peak may be concealed among the beta or gamma components and therefore be missed. As mentioned above, a serum monoclonal light chain is rarely seen in the cellulose acetate tracing. Thus, a normal value for the components of the electrophoretic

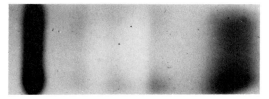

FIG. 8. *Cellulose acetate electrophoretic tracing. There is an increase in the gamma globulin fraction on the right side (cathode) of the slide. The band is broad, and both the advancing and trailing edges are diffuse. This represents a polyclonal increase in immunoglobulins. From Kyle and Bayrd (17a).*

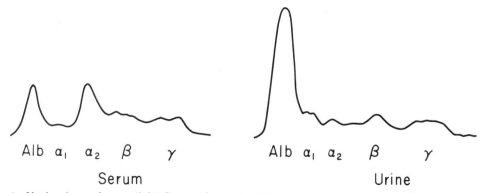

FIG. 9. *Nephrotic syndrome. (left) Serum electrophoretic pattern: note decreased albumin and gamma globulin and increased α₂-globulin components. (right) Urinary electrophoretic pattern: most of the protein is albumin. From Kyle et al. (18).*

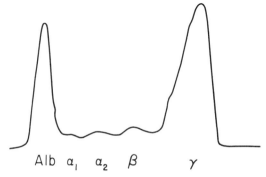

FIG. 10. *Serum electrophoretic pattern of chronic active hepatitis. From Kyle et al. (18).*

pattern or a normal-appearing pattern may hide a monoclonal protein. In this situation, immunoelectrophoresis is crucial.

If there is a small but discrete band between beta and gamma in the cellulose pattern, we add 30 μliters of bovine thrombin (1,000 U/100 ml) to 100 μliters of the sample. Prompt development of a clot indicates the presence of fibrinogen. It may be detected also by immunodiffusion (Ouchterlony) utilizing fibrinogen antisera. Fibrinogen may be present because the sample has not clotted sufficiently; if the patient has received heparin or coumadin, the sample is actually plasma rather than serum. If no evidence of fibrinogen is found, immunoelectrophoresis should be done because the beta-gamma band might represent a small monoclonal protein. If fibrinogen is present, addition of thrombin produces a clot and will leave no evidence of the beta-gamma band when electrophoresis on cellulose acetate is repeated. Another clue to the possibility of fibrinogen is the spontaneous formation of a clot in the specimen.

Serum immunoelectrophoresis for identification (see chapter 3)

Immunoelectrophoresis is used to identify the heavy-chain class and light-chain type of the monoclonal protein. The serum specimen is placed in a well on a microscope slide covered with 1% agar or agarose and subjected to electrophoresis to separate the various serum proteins. A trough is cut into the agar, parallel to the line of migration of the components, and the trough is filled with specific antisera. Proteins from the sample that has undergone electrophoresis (antigen) and from the antisera (antibody) are allowed to diffuse toward each other and to form precipitin lines or arcs along the line of contact between the antigen and the antibody.

Immunoelectrophoresis should be performed in all cases where a sharp peak or band is found in the cellulose acetate tracing or where myeloma, macroglobulinemia, amyloidosis, or a related disorder is suspected. It is particularly helpful in determining whether a solitary plasmacytoma is localized or not. After tumoricidal radiation therapy, a monoclonal protein should disappear. Its persistence suggests disseminated myeloma. Immunoelectrophoresis is essential in the differentiation of a monoclonal from a polyclonal increase of Ig. It is essential to use monospecific antisera to determine whether the increase of a heavy-chain class is associated with an increase of either κ or λ light chain if the excess protein is monoclonal protein or an increase of both light-chain types if the excess is polyclonal. Polyclonal increases of Ig are usually associated with an inflammatory process, and a monoclonal protein is usually associated with a neoplastic or potentially neoplastic proliferation.

There are *difficulties* in application of this method. The agar must be free from bubbles and other impurities because they will produce distortions in the precipitin arcs. The agar must be of uniform depth throughout the plate because unequal depth of agar can cause aberrations of the arcs. Drying or freezing of the agar plates will prevent satisfactory electrophoresis and diffusion of the samples in the agar. In cutting and removing the agar from the wells and troughs, great care must be taken to avoid any irregularities or splitting of the agar, because this will allow the antiserum to produce bowing or asymmetry of the arcs and suggest a monoclonal protein. One must avoid pulling the agar away from the microscope slide, because antiserum can run under the agar. During electrophoresis, the wicks must maintain a good contact between the slide holder and the microscope slides and the buffer, or electrophoresis of the serum will be irregular. Inadvertent dropping of antiserum on the agar slide will produce artifactitious distortion of the arcs and make interpretation very difficult.

Reagents.

Barbital buffer
205.3 g of barbital sodium
    36.8 g of barbital (must be dissolved in hot distilled water)
These reagents are placed in a 5-liter volumetric container and diluted to 20 liters with distilled water. The buffer (pH 8.2, 0.03 M) is stored at 4 C until use.

Noble agar (1%)
Mix 4 g of Noble agar with 400 ml of barbital buffer. Heat to dissolve. Add 9 drops of 1% thimerosal (Merthiolate).

Procedure. A plastic slide holder is used to place six glass microscope slides. The electrophoresis chamber will hold three slide holders, so that six sera can be run at one time.

1. Place six new clean microscope slides in a slide holder and put the slide holder on a table previously leveled.

2. Apply several drops of warm agar (1% Noble agar in barbital buffer) to the microscope slides to make a seal between the slides and at both ends of the row of slides to prevent excess loss of agar.

3. After allowing the agar seal to cool, apply a total of 10 ml of warm agar to one row of three slides.

4. Add 10 ml of warm agar to the second row of three slides.

5. Allow the slides to cool at 4 C in a

humidity chamber until needed. They should be poured at least 0.5 h before use.

6. Record the name and number of the patient whose serum will be placed in the wells. This is best done by stamping an outline of the six troughs on a sheet 21.5 by 28 cm, where the arcs can be drawn and results of interpretation can be recorded.

7. Punch the well-trough pattern, using an LKB die with a 1-mm trough and a diffusion distance of 5.1 mm from the trough (Fig. 11).

8. Remove the agar from the wells only with gentle suction.

9. Using Fisher capillary tubes, fill the wells with serum. The top wells of five slides in the holder are filled with the same patient's serum and the bottom well of each slide is filled with the serum of a different patient.

10. Add a small quantity of indicator dye (1% Evans blue in 0.15 NaCl) to the patient's serum in the first slide.

11. Fill the wells of two more slide holders with the sera of four additional patients, and place the three slide holders in the electrophoresis chamber. Be certain that the wicks are in good contact with the agar on all three slide holders. Set the voltage at 150, which produces approximately 30 mA.

12. The current is applied continuously until the indicator dye has migrated 15 to 20 mm. This takes approximately 1.5 h.

13. Shut the current off and take the slide holders from the electrophoresis chamber.

14. Remove the agar gently from the troughs with suction.

15. Fill the troughs with monospecific antisera to IgG, IgA, IgM, κ, and λ (Fig. 11).

16. Store the slide holders in a humidity chamber at room temperature for 24 h.

17. Read the immunoelectrophoretic patterns in a view box. Photograph the abnormal patterns with a Polaroid camera.

Interpretation. Potent antiserum to whole human serum produces nearly 30 precipitin arcs and causes difficulty in interpretation. Therefore, I use and recommend monospecific antisera to IgG, IgA, IgM, IgD, and IgE, and κ and λ

o Anti IgA	o Anti IgG	o Anti IgM
o	o	o
o Anti Kappa	o Anti Lambda	Extra slide
o	o	

o Patient serum

FIG. 11. *Immunoelectrophoresis: arrangement of six slides in holder, with different antisera in troughs of five.*

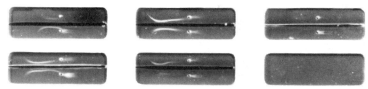

Fig. 12. *Immunoelectrophoretic patterns in myeloma. Trough of each slide contains monospecific antiserum. Upper row: Antiserum to IgA in first, to IgG in second, and to IgM in third. Lower row: Antiserum to kappa in first and to lambda in second (no slide in third position). Serum from first patient, placed in upper well of each slide, has produced thickening and bowing of IgG and lambda arcs, indicating presence of IgG λ monoclonal component. Serum from second patient, placed in lower well of each slide, has produced thickening of IgA arc and bowing of kappa arc, indicating IgA κ monoclonal component. From Kyle and Bayrd (17a).*

light chains. In addition to its monospecificity, the antisera must be potent. It is most important for each laboratory to test its antisera. For example, to ascertain the specificity and strength of IgG antiserum, it should be run against known IgA κ, IgA λ, IgM κ, and IgM λ monoclonal sera, against several known IgG κ and IgG λ monoclonal sera, and against urine containing only κ or λ light chains. It is always useful to have antisera of various sources available when typing monoclonal proteins, because the antigenic determinants of some monoclonal proteins are so restricted that they will not be recognized by all antisera.

The monoclonal protein appears as a localized thickening or bowing of a heavy-chain arc and a similar thickening or bowing of the light-chain arc. The alterations in the heavy-chain and light-chain arcs should be approximately the same distance from the well. Occasionally, a thickened arc will appear to be cut off abruptly near the trough. This may be due to overwhelming of the antisera by the antigen or by formation of a soluble antigen-antibody complex. Immunoelectrophoresis should be repeated with the serum diluted 1:5 or 1:10 by normal saline. This usually results in the formation of an arc that can be interpreted readily. Lesser concentrations of antigen will produce an arc nearer the well. Most precipitin arcs form within 24 h (Fig. 12). If one allows the diffusion to continue more than 24 h, the arcs become diffuse and exaggerated, making interpretation very difficult.

In multiple myeloma, antisera to IgG, IgA, IgD, or IgE produce a thickening, bowing, or asymmetry of the precipitin arc over a narrow range of mobility (Fig. 13–16). In Waldenström's macroglobulinemia, IgM antisera produce a similarly localized arc (Fig. 17). Additionally, in multiple myeloma and in macroglobulinemia, one must see a similar deflection from thickening and bowing of the arc by antisera to either κ or λ light chains, but not both. The corresponding thickening and bowing of the heavy-

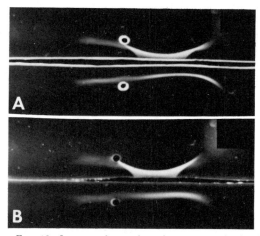

Fig. 13. *Immunoelectrophoretic patterns obtained in myeloma. (A) With antiserum to IgG, showing markedly thickened arc from patient's serum in upper well; for comparison, normal arc from normal serum in lower well. (B) With antiserum to kappa chains, showing thickened arc (top); for comparison, normal arch from normal serum (bottom), indicating monoclonal protein from patient's serum is IgG, κ type. From Kyle et al. (18).*

chain and light-chain arcs indicate the presence of a monoclonal protein. As IgG has a wide range of electrophoretic mobility, extending from the slow gamma through the alpha-2 globulin region, the bowing of the IgG precipitin arc may occur anywhere within that range.

The serum protein electrophoretic pattern may be relatively broad based, suggesting a polyclonal increase of Ig, as in Fig. 18 (upper). Immunoelectrophoresis with monospecific antisera in the illustrated case revealed impressive thickening and bowing of the arc with IgA antisera and a similar thickening and bowing with kappa antisera, indicating the presence of a monoclonal IgA κ protein (Fig. 18, middle and lower). The tendency of IgA monoclonal protein to produce polymers may be the reason for the broadness of the peak.

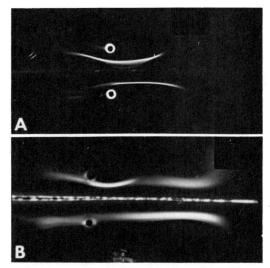

FIG. 14. *Myeloma: results of immunoelectrophoresis.* (A) *With antiserum to IgA, showing thickened arc from patient's serum in upper well, compared with normal arc from normal serum in lower well.* (B) *Results from testing same sera with antiserum to kappa chains. These studies indicate monoclonal protein of IgA, κ type. From Kyle et al. (18).*

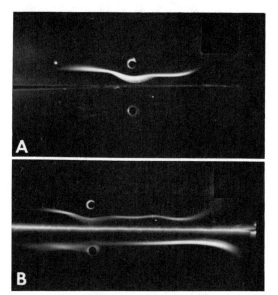

FIG. 15. *Myeloma and plasma-cell leukemia.* (A) *Immunoelectrophoresis with antiserum to IgE: markedly thickened arc from patient's serum in upper well and absence of arc from normal serum in lower well.* (*IgE serum was a gift of O. R. McIntyre, Hanover, N.H.*). (B) *Immunoelectrophoresis with antiserum to lambda chains: same patient's serum in upper well and normal serum in lower well. Results indicate IgE, λ type, monoclonal protein. From Kyle et al. (18).*

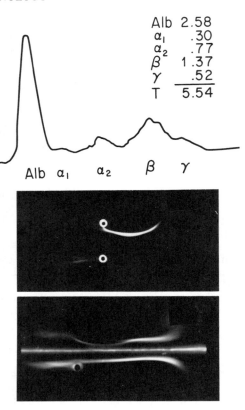

Alb	2.58
α_1	.30
α_2	.77
β	1.37
γ	.52
T	5.54

FIG. 16. *Myeloma and amyloidosis. Upper: Electrophoretic pattern on paper of patient's serum, showing only modestly increased beta globulins. Middle: Immunoelectrophoretic response to IgD antiserum is sharp arc from patient's serum (upper well) and absence of arc from normal serum (lower well). Lower: Immunoelectrophoretic responses to lambda chain antiserum by same patient's serum (upper well) and by normal serum (lower well), confirming presence of an IgD monoclonal protein in patient. From Kyle et al. (18).*

Thickening of the IgG arc occurs in many cases of polyclonal increase of Ig (Fig. 19). In this situation, the thickening occurs over a wide range and is not restricted. Further, there is an increase in both the κ and λ light-chain arcs. One must find a localized increase of one—and only one—light-chain arc before accepting the presence of a monoclonal protein.

Occasionally, one sees a dense, localized band on the cellulose acetate electrophoresis membrane, but only a dense IgM arc without an accompanying light-chain arc on immunoelectrophoresis. The inability to identify a light-chain component suggests the possibility of μ HCD. Treatment of the serum with a reducing agent, such as dithiothreitol or 2-mercaptoetha-

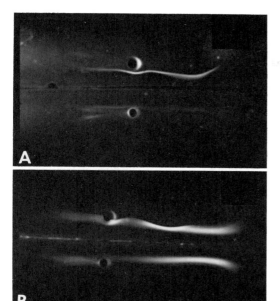

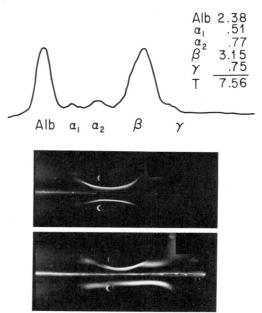

economical to screen the sera of all our patients by Ouchterlony immunodiffusion, using antisera to IgD and IgE against each patient's serum. The central well is filled with a mono-

FIG. 17. *Macroglobulinemia. (A) Immunoelectrophoresis with antiserum to IgM: thickened arc from patient's serum in upper well and very faint arc from normal serum in lower well. (B) Immunoelectrophoresis with antiserum to kappa chains: response of patient's serum in upper well confirms presence of IgM, κ type. From Kyle et al. (18).*

FIG. 18. *Results of electrophoresis and immunoelectrophoresis of serum of patient with multiple myeloma. Upper: Serum electrophoretic pattern on paper with rather broad β peak appearing polyclonal but consisting of monoclonal IgA κ protein. Middle: Result of immunoelectrophoresis of patient's serum (top well) and normal serum (bottom well) with IgA antiserum in center trough; note patient's thickened IgA arc. Lower: Result of immunoelectrophoresis, showing reaction to kappa chain antiserum: prominent arc from patient's serum (upper well) and elongated arc without localized thickening from normal serum (lower well). These results confirm presence of monoclonal IgA κ protein. From Kyle et al. (18).*

nol, produces a preparation that may be readily identified as IgM κ or IgM λ monoclonal proteins when immunoelectrophoresis is repeated.

It must be emphasized again that the densitometer tracing of a monoclonal protein may be very small, or the monoclonal protein may be concealed in the normal beta or gamma band and not be discovered until immunoelectrophoresis is done. IgD myeloma frequently produces only a small peak or band. The α and μ HCD sera never show a dense band or sharp peak on electrophoresis and can be detected only with immunoelectrophoresis; γ HCD often produces a broad band on electrophoresis, and the diagnosis is not made until immunoelectrophoresis is done. Thus, immunoelectrophoresis is necessary for the diagnosis of these diseases. A densitometer tracing of a serum electrophoretic pattern, the bands on the cellulose acetate strip, and the localized arc resulting from immunoelectrophoresis of a monoclonal protein are shown in Fig. 20.

Detection of immunoglobulin D and E monoclonal proteins

All sera should be screened for the possibility of IgD or IgE myeloma proteins. We find it

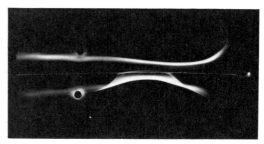

FIG. 19. *Immunoelectrophoresis with antiserum to IgG: polyclonal arc (dense but without localized thickening) from serum in top well, thickened precipitin arc from monoclonal protein in lower well. From Kyle et al. (18).*

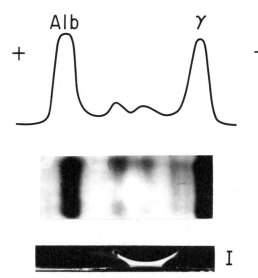

FIG. 20. *Corresponding determinations of monoclonal serum protein. Upper: Densitometer tracing of electrophoretic separation on cellulose acetate membrane. Middle: Band separated electrophoretically on cellulose acetate. Lower: Localized arc from immunoelectrophoresis. From Kyle and Bayrd (17a).*

Quantitation of immunoglobulins in serum

Quantitation of immunoglobulins also aids in the assessment of gammopathies. Usually this is performed by radial immunodiffusion (7). With this method, antiserum to the specific Ig (IgG, IgA, IgM, or IgD) is mixed with agar and layered on a plate. Known concentrations of a specific Ig and the unknown serum are placed in wells. The size of the precipitin zones that develop about the wells is proportional to the antigen in the test serum, so the precipitin zone surrounding each well is measured and compared with known standards.

Excess lipids in the serum sample may obscure the precipitin ring, so the serum should be obtained when the patient is fasting. Overfilling or underfilling of the wells must be avoided. Fluctuation of the temperature during immunodiffusion can produce double rings. High concentrations of Ig may produce soluble, invisible complexes, leaving the appearance of no Ig. The serum then must be diluted to make the precipitin zone visible. Low-molecular-weight ($7S$) IgM produces a spuriously elevated IgM value because its rate of diffusion is greater than that of the $19S$ IgM used as a standard.

Satisfactory quantitative immunodiffusion plates and reference standards may be obtained commercially (Meloy Laboratories, Inc., Springfield, Va.; Kallestad Laboratories, Inc., Chaska, Minn.; Hyland Laboratories, Costa Mesa, Calif.; Behring Diagnostics, Somerville, N.J.), or the technician may make his own immunodiffusion plates.

Both the immunodiffusion plates and the

specific IgD or IgE antiserum, and each surrounding well is filled with undiluted serum from each patient. Dense precipitin bands form if the patient has an increased concentration of IgD or IgE protein (Fig. 21). All sera forming a precipitin band are then studied further by immunoelectrophoresis with monospecific antisera to IgD, IgE, kappa, and lambda (Fig. 15 and 16). As the majority of sera produce no reaction on immunodiffusion, immunoelectrophoresis is not necessary. Since four to six sera can be screened with 7 or 8 μliters of IgD or IgE antisera by immunodiffusion, but 60 μliters of antisera is needed to perform immunoelectrophoresis on two sera, prior screening by immunodiffusion saves a significant amount of antisera.

Immunodiffusion (Ouchterlony).

1. Microscope slides are coated with 1% agar as described for immunoelectrophoresis, except that agar is dissolved in 0.01 M potassium phosphate-0.15 M sodium chloride.
2. Wells are punched as in Fig. 21. One may use a die that makes six or eight wells around the central well rather than four.
3. The center well is filled with IgD or IgE monospecific antisera. One of the peripheral wells is filled with the serum of a patient with known IgD or IgE myeloma as a control. The sera to be tested are placed in the other wells.

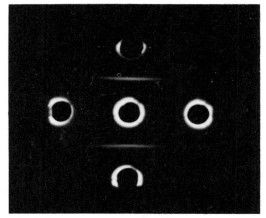

FIG. 21. *Immunodiffusion with antiserum to IgD in central well and serum of two patients with IgD myeloma in upper and lower wells. Dense precipitin bands confirm presence of IgD protein. From Kyle et al. (18).*

reference standards should be stored at 2 to 5 C and then be allowed to reach room temperature before use. Sera from each patient and three dilutions of the pooled standardized human sera are placed in the wells. The plate is incubated for 16 to 24 h, and the diameter of the precipitin ring is measured. The plates should be viewed against a dark background. The standard concentrations are plottted on the Y axis of semilog paper and the ring diameters are plotted on the X axis. When a line is drawn through the points, the concentration of the patient's serum can be determined. Specimens whose ring diameters are greater than the standards should be diluted with isotonic saline and reassayed. If the concentration of the specimen falls below the lowest reference standard, a "low-level" plate may be used to determine its level. Normal values for quantitative Ig are in Table 4, and low ranges of immunodiffusion plates are as follows (mg/100 ml): 71 for IgG, 12 for IgA, and 9 for IgM (Meloy low-level plates).

Immunodiffusion is done on IgG, IgA, and IgM plates. Polymeric IgA will produce low values because the standards consist of $7S$ IgA. Therefore, if secretory IgA is to be assayed, one must use polymeric IgA standards. It should be pointed out again that $7S$ IgM will produce spuriously high levels because the standard consists of $19S$ IgM. Quality control with laboratory standards (human serum pools) run daily for measurement of variance is important, and participation in interlaboratory proficiency studies is very important.

If the laboratory performs a large number of quantitative tests for Ig, an automated immunoprecipitin system (Technicon Instrument Corp., Tarrytown, N.Y.) is practical (22). In this system the basis for measurement is the degree of turbidity produced by antigen-antibody interaction with the use of nephelometry in the near ultraviolet region. Monospecific antisera are appropriately diluted (usually about 1:40) with a 40 g/liter polyethylene glycol 6000 solution in 0.9% NaCl containing 0.3 ml of Tween 20. Serum samples are diluted 1:200 in

TABLE 4. *Serum concentrations of immunoglobulins in adults: normal (95%) ranges (mg/100 ml)[a]*

Group	IgG	IgA	IgM
Caucasian			
Males	635–1,400	60–297	41–248
Females	645–1,300	48–295	59–280
Black			
Males	816–1,654	53–378	47–275
Females	950–1,580	96–295	54–265

[a] Meloy Laboratories.

normal saline. The automated system introduces diluted samples into a continuously flowing stream of diluted antibody. Interaction produces turbidity, which is measured and recorded, and a standard calibration curve is used to convert turbidity to milligrams per milliliter. The average time per sample is about 4 min. Since the method is not affected by molecular size of the antigen (as is radial immunodiffusion), the nephelometric technique is capable of accurately measuring $7S$ IgM.

Other tests for serum protein abnormalities

Serum viscometry. I recommend serum viscometry in every case with more than 2.0 g of IgM monoclonal protein or more than 4.0 g of monoclonal IgA or IgG protein per 100 ml and in any patient with oronasal bleeding, blurred vision, or neurological symptoms suggestive of the hyperviscosity syndrome.

An Ostwald-100 viscometer is a satisfactory instrument for this purpose. Distilled water and serum, separately, are made to flow through a capillary tube, and the quotient of the flow duration (serum/water) is the viscosity value. For normal serum the value is 1.6 or less, but symptoms of hyperviscosity are rare unless the value is greater than 4. In fact, some patients with a value of 10 or more do not have symptoms of hyperviscosity.

A Wells-Brookfield viscometer (Brookfield Engineering Laboratories, Inc., Stoughton, Mass.) is preferred because it is more accurate and requires less serum (about 1.0 ml). In addition, determinations can be made much more rapidly than with the Ostwald viscometer, especially if the viscosity of the serum sample is high. This instrument allows one to determine the viscosity at different shear rates and at different temperatures. In a series of 100 samples from normal blood bank donors, we found that 95% had a value of 1.8 centipoises or less, determined at a shear rate of $23 \ s^{-1}$ (6 rpm).

Cryoglobulins. Each serum sample should be tested for the presence of cryoglobulins. Blood is allowed to clot at room temperature, without any refrigeration. The serum is poured to fill a disposable Wintrobe hematocrit tube to the 10 mark, care being taken to allow no air bubbles in the tube. The hematocrit tube is incubated at 0 C (in an ice bath in a cold room) for 24 h. Then, if a precipitate or gel is seen, the tube is warmed at 37 C for 30 min. Dissolution of the precipitate indicates a cryoglobulin. In that event, the tube is placed in the ice bath for another 24 h, then centrifuged at 2,000 rpm for 30 min at 1 C, and the cryocrit is read. Because the precipitate in some instances is very dense after centrifugation and will not dissolve readily when warmed, one should warm the sample to 37 C before determining the cryocrit.

When filling the hematocrit tube, all portions of clot should be excluded because fibrin will produce a precipitate that will not dissolve with heating. If an excess of lipid is present, a small cryoglobulin may be missed. Cryoglobulins of the mixed type may require up to a week to precipitate.

Pyroglobulins. Pyroglobulins are proteins that precipitate irreversibly when heated to 56 C and do not dissolve when cooled. They usually are discovered when serum is inactivated for the Venereal Disease Research Laboratory test. Pyroglobulins resemble Bence Jones protein in that both precipitate when heated to 60 C, but the two can be distinguished easily by immunoelectrophoresis with appropriate antisera.

Sia test. The Sia test for euglobulins is performed by adding a drop of serum to a tube of distilled water. A positive result is the formation of a precipitate or flocculant as the serum is diluted by the water. This test has been recommended for the diagnosis of macroglobulinemia, but many false-positive and false-negative reactions are seen. In a study, the Sia test did not distinguish IgM monoclonal proteins from IgG or IgA monoclonal proteins, nor did it separate monoclonal sera as a group from polyclonal sera at the 5% level (33). The Sia test is largely of historic interest; I do not recommend it.

Analysis of urine for protein

In studying patients who have gammopathies, analysis of urine is essential. Sulfosalicylic acid (Exton's test) is best for the detection of protein. Albustix often does not detect Bence Jones protein and should not be used as a routine screening test for Bence Jones proteinuria.

A simple heat test for detection of Bence Jones protein consists of mixing 4 ml of centrifuged urine with 1 ml of 2 M acetate buffer (pH 4.9) and heating at 56 C in an incubation bath for 15 min. Formation of a precipitate that disappears after 3 min in a 100 C bath but reappears with cooling indicates the presence of Bence Jones protein (31). Occasionally, the result of a heat test is positive even though the patient has no evidence of myeloma or macroglobulinemia and his urine provides no sharp peak in the electrophoretic pattern or evidence of a monoclonal light chain on immunoelectrophoresis. Such false-positive results occur in cases of connective tissue disease, renal insufficiency, or malignancy (28). Conversely, in some cases of myeloma, urine containing large amounts of monoclonal proteins has given negative results on the heat test. Thus, there are serious shortcomings of the heat test for Bence Jones proteinuria.

Electrophoresis and immunoelectrophoresis of urine. In all cases of monoclonal proteinemia, electrophoresis and immunoelectrophoresis of urine should be performed. Additionally, both tests should be applied to urine in all instances of multiple myeloma, macroglobulinemia of Waldenström, amyloidosis, benign monoclonal gammopathy, heavy-chain diseases, or suspicion of these entities.

To determine total protein, prepare biuret solution (900 ml of 23% NaOH added to 300 ml of 1% $CuSO_4 \cdot 5H_2O$) and tungstic acid (100 ml of 10% $Na_2WO_4 \cdot 2H_2O$ added to 800 ml of 0.083 N H_2SO_4; add 0.1 ml of H_3PO_4). Add 1 ml of urine to 5 ml of tungstic acid, and allow to sit for 5 min; then centrifuge. Dissolve the precipitate in 5 ml of saline and 5 ml of biuret solution. After 10 min, read at 545 nm in a Coleman Junior spectrophotometer. Optical density $\times$ 22.7 $\div$ 10 = g/100 ml.

For electrophoresis of urine, a sample of the 24-h urine specimen must first be concentrated. We prefer ultrafiltration with a Minicon-B15 concentrator (Amicon Corp., Lexington, Mass.). A 5-ml amount of urine is added to the concentrator; when the volume has decreased, 3 ml more of urine is added. The volume of urine is reduced to 0.1 ml ($\times$80). The urine concentrate is placed on the cellulose polyacetate membrane with the Drummond microdispenser and applicator (just as with serum). The number of applications depends on the protein concentration of the urine: one of 6.5 g or more/100 ml, two of 4.0 to 6.5 g/100 ml, three of 2.0 to 4.0 g/100 ml, four of 1.0 to 2.0 g/100 ml, and five of concentrations less than 1 g/100 ml.

Immunodiffusion is performed with κ and λ antisera on unconcentrated urine. Immunoelectrophoresis is performed with κ and λ antisera on concentrated urine. This can be done on the sixth microscope slide in each slide holder. If the monoclonal protein concentration in the urine is high, the precipitin arc may overwhelm the antisera or form a soluble, invisible arc. Consequently, immunoelectrophoresis should then be repeated with unconcentrated urine. Occasionally the monoclonal light-chain content of the urine is so high that the unconcentrated urine must be diluted to make an arc visible. If electrophoresis of the urine reveals a globulin spike and one is unable to demonstrate a monoclonal light chain on immunoelectrophoresis, one must suspect the possibility of heavy-chain disease. Immunoelectrophoresis of concentrated urine should then be done with antisera to IgG, IgA, and IgM (γ, α, and μ heavy chains). A 24-h collection of the urine must be made for determination of the total amount of protein excreted per day.

Although the heat test for Bence Jones protein is useful clinically, one must remember its shortcomings mentioned above. Electrophoresis and immunoelectrophoresis of an adequately concentrated specimen are the methods of choice for demonstrating a monoclonal light chain in the urine.

LITERATURE CITED

1. Bush, S. T., H. A. Swedlund, and G. J. Gleich. 1969. Low molecular weight IgM in human sera. J. Lab. Clin. Med. **73**:194–201.
2. Buxbaum, J. N. 1973. The biosynthesis, assembly, and secretion of immunoglobulins. Semin. Hematol. **10**:33–52.
3. Capra, J. D., and J. M. Kehoe. 1975. Hypervariable regions, idiotypy, and the antibody-combining site. Adv. Immunol. **20**:1–40.
4. Edelman, G. M., and J. A. Gally. 1962. The nature of Bence-Jones proteins: chemical similarities to polypeptide chains of myeloma globulins and normal γ-globulins. J. Exp. Med. **116**:207–227.
5. Eisen, H. N., J. R. Little, C. K. Osterland, and E. S. Simms. 1967. A myeloma protein with antibody activity. Cold Spring Harbor Symp. Quant. Biol. **32**:75–81.
6. Engle, R. L., Jr., and L. A. Wallis. 1969. Immunoglobulinopathies: immunoglobulins, immune deficiency syndromes, multiple myeloma and related disorders. Charles C Thomas, Springfield, Ill.
7. Fahey, J. L., and E. M. McKelvey. 1965. Quantitative determination of serum immunoglobulins in antibody-agar plates. J. Immunol. **94**:84–90.
8. Fine, J. M., P. Lambin, and D. Frommel. 1973. Size heterogeneity of human IgA myeloma proteins: relationships between polymers and "J" chain. Biomedicine **18**:145–151.
9. Götze, O., and H. J. Müller-Eberhard. 1971. The C3-activator system: an alternate pathway of complement activation. J. Exp. Med. **134**:90S–108S.
10. Grey, H. M., C. A. Abel, W. J. Yount, and H. G. Kunkel. 1968. A subclass of human γA-globulins (γA2) which lacks disulfide bonds linking heavy and light chains. J. Exp. Med. **128**:1223–1236.
11. Hopper, J. E., and A. Nisonoff. 1971. Individual antigenic specificity of immunoglobulins. Adv. Immunol. **13**:58–99.
12. Ishizaka, K., T. Ishizaka, and M. M. Hornbrook. 1966. Physicochemical properties of reaginic antibody. V. Correlation of reaginic activity with γE-globulin antibody. J. Immunol. **97**:840–853.
13. Johansson, S. G. O. 1967. Raised levels of a new immunoglobulin class (IgND) in asthma. Lancet **2**:951–953.
14. Kohn, J. 1957. A cellulose acetate supporting medium for zone electrophoresis. Clin. Chim. Acta **2**:297–303.
15. Koshland, M. E. 1975. Structure and function of the J chain. Adv. Immunol. **20**:41–69.
16. Krause, R. M. 1970. The search for antibodies with molecular uniformity. Adv. Immunol. **12**:1–56.
17. Kunkel, H. G. 1968. The "abnormality" of myeloma proteins. Cancer Res. **28**:1351–1353.
17a. Kyle, R. A., and E. A. Bayrd. 1976. The monoclonal gammopathies. Charles C Thomas, Springfield, Ill.
18. Kyle, R. A., R. C. Bieger, and G. J. Gleich. 1970. Diagnosis of syndromes associated with hyperglobulinemia. Med. Clin. North Am. **54**:917–938.
19. Kyle, R. A., and G. J. Gleich. 1972. Syndromes associated with hyperglobulinemia, p. 1–37. In R. G. Slavin (ed.), Tice's practice of medicine, vol. 1. Harper & Row, Hagerstown, Md.
20. Lindh, E. 1975. Increased resistance of immunoglobulin A dimers to proteolytic degradation after binding of secretory component. J. Immunol. **114**:284–286.
21. Longsworth, L. G., T. Shedlovsky, and D. A. MacInnes. 1939. Electrophoretic patterns of normal and pathological human blood serum and plasma. J. Exp. Med. **70**:399–413.
22. Markowitz, H., and A. R. Tschida. 1972. Automated quantitative immunochemical analysis of human immunoglobulins. Clin. Chem. **18**:1364–1367.
23. Metzger, H. 1970. Structure and function of γM macroglobulins. Adv. Immunol. **12**:57–116.
24. Natvig, J. B., and H. G. Kunkel. 1973. Human immunoglobulins: classes, subclasses, genetic variants, and idiotypes. Adv. Immunol. **16**:1–59.
25. Osserman, E. F., and T. Isobe. 1972. Lymphoreticular disorders: malignant proliferative response and/or abnormal immunoglobulin synthesis—plasma cell dyscrasias, p. 950–956, 977–984. In W. J. Williams, E. Beutler, A. J. Erslev, and R. W. Rundles (ed.), Hematology. McGraw-Hill Book Co., New York.
26. Osterland, C. K., and L. R. Espinoza. 1975. Biological properties of myeloma proteins. Arch. Intern. Med. **135**:32–36.
27. Park, B. H., and R. A. Good. 1974. Principles of modern immunobiology: basic and clinical, p. 91–107. Lea & Febiger, Philadelphia.
28. Perry, M. C., and R. A. Kyle. 1975. The clinical significance of Bence Jones proteinuria. Mayo Clin. Proc. **50**:234–238.
29. Porter, R. R. 1967. The structure of antibodies. Sci. Am. **217**:81–90.
30. Potter, M. 1971. Myeloma proteins (M-components) with antibody-like activity. N. Engl. J. Med. **284**:831–838.
31. Putnam, F. W., C. W. Easley, L. T. Lynn, A. E. Ritchie, and R. A. Phelps. 1959. The heat precipitation of Bence Jones proteins. I. Op-

timum conditions. Arch. Biochem. Biophys. **83:**115–130.

32. Putnam, F. W., G. Florent, C. Paul, T. Shinoda, and A. Shimizu. 1973. Complete amino acid sequence of the mu heavy chain of a human IgM immunoglobulin. Science **182:**287–291.

33. Ritzmann, S. E., R. E. Wolf, M. C. Lawrence, J. S. Hart, and W. C. Levin. 1969. The Sia euglobulin test: a re-evaluation. J. Lab. Clin. Med. **73:**698–705.

34. Rowe, D. S., and J. L. Fahey. 1965. A new class of human immunoglobulins. I. A unique myeloma protein. J. Exp. Med. **121:**171–184.

35. Schur, P. H. 1972. Human gamma-G subclasses. Prog. Clin. Immunol. **1:**71–104.

36. Seligmann, M., and J. C. Brouet. 1973. Antibody activity of human myeloma globulins. Semin. Hematol. **10:**163–177.

37. Shapiro, S. S. 1975. Characterization of Factor VIII antibodies. Ann. N.Y. Acad. Sci. **240:**350–360.

38. Solomon, A., and C. L. McLaughlin. 1973. Immunoglobulin structure determined from products of plasma cell neoplasms. Semin. Hematol. **10:**3–17.

39. Stone, M. J., and E. P. Frenkel. 1975. The clinical spectrum of light chain myeloma: a study of 35 patients with special reference to the occurrence of amyloidosis. Am. J. Med. **58:**601–619.

40. Tiselius, A. 1937. Electrophoresis of serum globulin. II. Electrophoretic analysis of normal and immune sera. Biochem. J. **31:**1464–1477.

41. Tiselius, A., and E. A. Kabat. 1939. An electrophoretic study of immune sera and purified antibody preparations. J. Exp. Med. **69:**119–131.

42. Tomasi, T. B., Jr. 1968. Human immunoglobulin A. N. Engl. J. Med. **279:**1327–1330.

43. Vaerman, J.-P., and J. F. Heremans. 1966. Subclasses of human immunoglobulin A based on differences in the alpha polypeptide chains. Science **153:**647–649.

44. Waldenström, J. 1961. Studies on conditions associated with disturbed gamma globulin formation (gammopathies). Harvey Lect. **56:**211–231.

45. Waldmann, T. A. 1969. Disorders of immunoglobulin metabolism. N. Engl. J. Med. **281:**1170–1177.

46. Waldmann, T. A., J. M. Bull, R. M. Bruce, S. Broder, M. C. Jost, S. T. Balestra, and M. E. Suer. 1974. Serum immunoglobulin E levels in patients with neoplastic disease. J. Immunol. **113:**379–386.

47. Weichselbaum, T. E. 1946. An accurate and rapid method for the determination of proteins in small amounts of blood serum and plasma. Am. J. Clin. Pathol. (Tech. Sect.) **16:**40–49.

48. Wochner, R. D., W. Strober, and T. A. Waldmann. 1967. The role of the kidney in the catabolism of Bence Jones proteins and immunoglobulin fragments. J. Exp. Med. **126:**207–221.

49. Yuninger, J. W., and G. J. Gleich. 1973. Seasonal changes in IgE antibodies and their relationship to IgG antibodies during immunotherapy for ragweed hay fever. J. Clin. Invest. **52:**1268–1275.

Chapter 99

Summary of Clinical Use and Limitations of the Carcinoembryonic Antigen Assay and Some Methodological Considerations

NORMAN ZAMCHECK AND HERBERT Z. KUPCHIK

INTRODUCTION

Thomson and Gold's initial studies (58) of serum carcinoembryonic antigen (CEA) in patients with colon cancer reported 97% positivity (Table 1). Such findings were confirmed by the 1970 study of patients with "overt" colon cancer from this laboratory (43), many of whom had metastases, and by studies of other workers (32, 48). In an expanded study, however, patients with earlier diseases were included, and the percent positivity fell to 72% (13, 42). The positivity rate fell further to 59% in patients seen preoperatively, but rose to 96% in those who had evidence of metastases following surgery. These findings have been widely confirmed.

TABLE 1. *Carcinoembryonic antigen in colonic cancer: variations in positivity from series to series*

Study	Year	Method[a]	Percent "positivity"
Montreal General Hospital (58)	1969	T	97
Boston City Hospital		T	
Initial series (43)	1970	T	91
Expanded series (42)	1971	T	72
Later series (13)	1972	T	
Preoperative (all stages)			59
Postoperative with known tumor recurrence			96
New York – Nutley (32)	1971	H	86
Buffalo – Roswell Park (48)	1972	H	83
London – Chester Beatty (30)	1972	E	67
Joint NCI/ACS Study, preoperative cases (25)	1972	T	62
Lausanne – Inst. Biochem. (34)	1974	M	
All stages			71
Localized tumor			63

[a] T = Thomson-Gold (58); H = Hansen (32); E = modified Egan-Todd (15); M = Mach's modified Thomson-Gold method (34).

The combined Canadian National Cancer Institute-American Cancer Society Study reported 62% positivity in patients studied preoperatively using the original Thomson-Gold assay (25).

Thus, the CEA assay is a better indicator of widespread disease, particularly of metastases to the liver, than it is of early colon cancer. A preoperatively negative assay does not exclude the diagnosis of cancer, but it makes the diagnosis of metastases less likely. In patients with known colon cancer, it suggests, but does not guarantee, a localized lesion and a favorable prognosis. Generally, the higher the level of CEA, the poorer is the prognosis. Markedly elevated preoperative CEA determinations are consistent with metastases.

NONSPECIFICITY OF THE CARCINOEMBRYONIC ANTIGEN ASSAY

None of the present assays for CEA is specific for colon cancer or for digestive tract cancer. The high rates of positivity initially reported in patients with pancreatic cancer were very likely due to the fact that pancreatic cancer is usually diagnosed late in its course. Approximately 52% positivity was reported in unselected patients with breast cancer, 40% in prostatic cancer, 33% in bladder cancer, and 72% in cancer of the bronchus (68).

CARCINOEMBRYONIC ANTIGEN IN BENIGN DISORDERS

With the exception of some heavy cigarette smokers, 97% of healthy normal individuals have normal blood CEA levels (23). Values as high as 10 ng/ml, however, have been reported by Hansen. Perhaps more than any other common benign clinical condition, liver disease may give elevated CEA levels, especially severe alcoholic cirrhosis (6, 26, 41). Some patients with benign obstructive jaundice may also have CEA elevations, which are usually reversed on release of the obstruction, provided persistent biliary inflammation or liver abscess does not supervene (33). Ulcerative colitis of long duration is known to predispose to colonic cancer. But there is no convincing evidence yet available that CEA levels will detect early colon cancer in this disease. "Active" inflammatory bowel disease may be associated with transient elevation.

SCREENING

Thus, although "malignancy" may be differentiated from "nonmalignancy," in part by the circulating CEA levels, there is no sharp threshold between the two. A high proportion of patients with "early" colonic cancer have negative CEA values. These two facts militate against successful screening for early cancer by use of the CEA assay alone.

The higher the threshold level applied, the more reliable is the detection of cancer; however, the more advanced are the cancers detected. Thus, screening for advanced cancer is presently feasible.

The majority of patients with benign disease have normal CEA levels, and elevations, when observed, are usually modest. Quantitation by dilution (without prior perchloric acid extraction) has revealed very high levels of CEA (above 1,000 ng/ml) in some patients with advanced cancer; such levels are not reported in benign diseases.

SERIAL ASSAYS IN THE ASSESSMENT OF COLON CANCER

Many laboratories (13, 30, 32, 34, 42, 48) confirmed Thomson and Gold's initial report (58) that preoperatively elevated assay levels fell to normal levels after complete resection of colonic cancers. A single negative postoperative CEA level, however, did not exclude the presence of residual tumor, as was initially hoped. Rising CEA levels following tumor resection correlated with residual, recurrent, or metastatic tumor.

The use of serial determinations has increased the clinical usefulness of the CEA assay. (It is not possible to summarize all clinical applications in this brief report. References 23, 30, and 65 are useful sources.)

The case summarized in Fig. 1 exemplifies the use of serial CEA values in a 76-year-old man who had an abdominal-perineal resection of a Dukes C adenocarcinoma. His initial CEA level was undetectable preoperatively, postoperatively, and again 18 months after resection. When he returned to the clinic, rising CEA values were noted. He was examined carefully for evidence of metastases by X ray, colonoscopy, and liver scan, but none was found. He was admitted to the hospital, and again complete examinations were done to no avail. Sev-

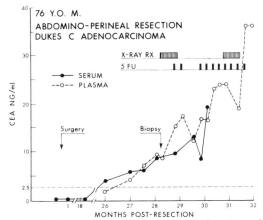

FIG. 1. *Use of serial CEA assays in detection of recurrence of colonic cancer in a 76-year-old man. From Sorokin et al. (54) (copyright 1974, American Medical Association), with permission.*

eral months later, however, a small node in the neck was found positive for cancer. CEA levels rose further, and the patient continued to do poorly despite chemotherapy and radiation therapy.

To determine whether serial CEA assays would help to detect recurrence after resection, Sorokin et al. studied prospectively 102 patients who had undergone potentially curative resection for colorectal cancer (54). When first studied, none had detectable metastases or evidence of recurrent cancer. Eighteen patients showed CEA levels greater than 2.5 ng/ml. Six of these had progressively rising CEA levels; all six subsequently developed recurrent cancer. Holyoke et al. (24), Mach et al. (34), Dykes et al. (5), and Mackay et al. (37) reported similar series of patients, whose rising CEA levels preceded clinical evidence of tumor recurrence by 2 to 18 months. Despite this general agreement that serial assays help detect recurrent colon cancer in asymptomatic patients, Ravry and co-workers at the Mayo Clinic reported that tumor recurrence was readily detected by "other clinical means" in such patients (47). Sugarbaker et al. also showed that careful symptom review and clinical examination is indispensable in assessing such patients, especially since some colonic cancers (as well as many other cancers) may produce no CEA (P. H. Sugarbaker, N. Zamcheck, and F. D. Moore, unpublished data).

Mach et al., at Lausanne, Switzerland (34), reported eight patients who had recurrent colonic cancer after apparently complete tumor resection (Fig. 2). Note that all patients had elevated values (greater than 5 ng/ml) preoperatively and that some fell to "normal"

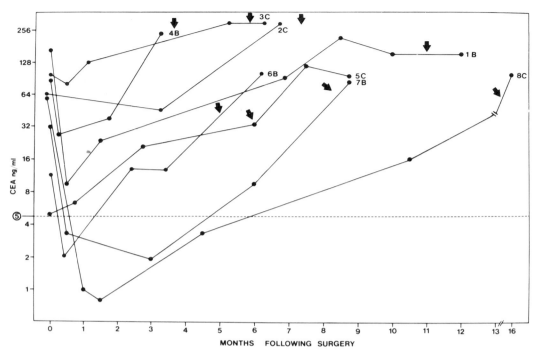

FIG. 2. *Variations of CEA level in eight patients who showed a relapse of their carcinoma after what was considered as a macroscopically complete tumor resection. The increased CEA level was apparent between 2.5 and 10 months before clinical evidence of tumor relapse (arrows). After the final CEA determination, the case number and the letter corresponding to the Dukes classification are indicated. From Mach et al. (34), with permission.*

levels postoperatively, whereas others did not fall at all or very much. All had rising levels thereafter. The arrows in Fig. 2 indicate that clinical evidence of recurrence was observed 2.5 to 10 months later.

In contrast, flat serial CEA levels were observed in eight patients after complete tumor resection who had no evidence of recurrence at the time of Mach's report (34). As can be seen in Fig. 3, the preoperative levels tended to be lower than those seen in the first group, and all fell and remained below 5 ng/ml during the follow-up studies.

The serial CEA levels in six symptom-free patients slowly rose after apparently complete tumor resection, but there was no evidence of tumor recurrence at the time of the report (Fig. 4). It is necessary to determine whether such asymptomatic patients, with no other evidence of recurrence, can be benefited by second-look surgery or prophylactic chemotherapy, radiation therapy, immunotherapy, or possibly combinations thereof. Martin and Minton have successfully used rising CEA trends as an indication for second-look surgery (personal communication).

The use of serial CEA levels as a *monitor of*

chemotherapy for *colon cancer* is also under active investigation (24, 44, 47, 52). Rising serial CEA levels in patients with metastatic gastrointestinal cancer being treated with chemotherapy generally indicated disease progression (52). Persistently low CEA levels (i.e., less than 2 to 3 ng/ml) and, particularly, undetectable CEA levels were generally favorable prognostically in patients with colon cancer—but not invariably, since some tumors apparently produce no CEA.

CHEMOTHERAPY FOR METASTATIC CANCER OF THE COLON

Almost all patients did poorly who had rising CEA levels or stable elevated values (52). The rises often preceded clinical evidence of deterioration. A few patients with consistently normal CEA levels had no evidence of progressive tumor metastases. CEA levels decreased only in the few patients with colon carcinoma who showed a remission with chemotherapy. Elevated CEA levels may remain stable despite progressive disease. The relative ineffectiveness of the available chemotherapy for gastrointestinal cancer precluded drawing any

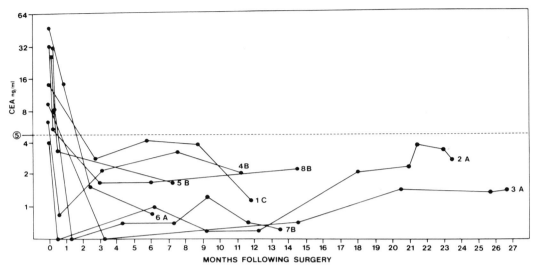

FIG. 3. *Variation of CEA level in eight patients who, after macroscopically complete tumor resection, showed a fall of CEA and whose CEA value subsequently remained below 5 ng/ml. None showed any evidence of tumor recurrence. From Mach et al. (34), with permission.*

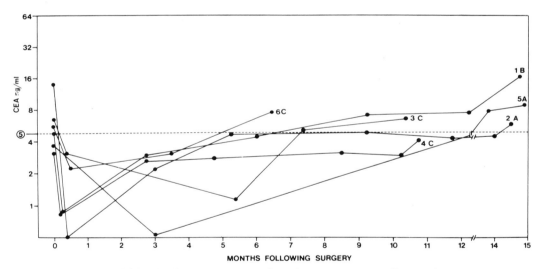

FIG. 4. *Variation of CEA level in six patients who, after a macroscopically complete tumor resection, showed an initial fall and a subsequent moderate increase in CEA levels above 5 ng/ml. None of these patients had shown any clear evidence of tumor relapse. From Mach et al. (34), with permission.*

firm conclusions regarding the use of CEA levels as a monitor.

Figure 5 illustrates the course of a 60-year-old man who underwent sigmoid resection for adenocarcinoma associated with chronic occult bleeding. A solitary hepatic metastasis was present as well as metastases to two of four regional lymph nodes. When first evaluated for chemotherapy 18 weeks postoperatively, hepatomegaly, diffuse abdominal masses, and ascites

were present. During the first 8 weeks of therapy, his clinical status was stable with little decrease in measurable tumor. He appeared to be improving, but an irregular and progressive rise in serial CEA levels heralded advancing metastatic disease. CEA increased threefold before the widespread progressive disease was apparent clinically.

A 52-year-old woman presented with weight loss, abdominal pain, and diarrhea (Fig. 6).

Barium enema revealed an annular lesion of the left transverse colon. Hemicolectomy and ileotransverse colostomy were performed. At surgery she had omental and ovarian metastases. The preoperative CEA level was 9.5 ng/ml and it fell to 2.8 ng/ml 2 days postoperatively. Chemotherapy was initiated 5 weeks postoperatively and was continued on an intermittent basis. Initially, the liver scan showed a large focal defect compatible with metastatic disease. Repeated liver scan at 45 weeks showed no evidence of metastases. The initial fall in CEA reflected the surgical removal of gross tumor, and the continuing fall to normal

may have been the result of chemotherapy, especially in view of the reversal of the abnormal liver scan. No other evidence of disease was apparent 45 weeks after surgery. The significance of the fluctuating low CEA level was uncertain. However, CEA increased to 18 ng/ml 82 weeks after surgery, and the diagnosis of metastatic disease was made.

These findings give hope that serial CEA measurement will be helpful in monitoring when more effective therapy for colon cancer becomes available.

These are all preliminary findings, however, and longer follow-up is needed before firm conclusions can be drawn. It has not yet been shown that the changes in CEA levels occur early enough to permit beneficial change of chemotherapy.

BREAST CANCER

Patients with metastatic breast cancer show a better response to chemotherapy than do those with gastrointestinal cancer. Accordingly, 13 patients with metastases undergoing chemotherapy and/or hormonal therapy were studied for 3 to 18 months (mean of 14 months) with serial CEA estimations (55). Falling serial CEA appeared to correlate with response to treatment, and rising levels correlated with nonresponse. However, Chu and Nemoto and others did not feel that serial CEA levels provide an adequate monitor for breast cancer (8).

LUNG CANCER

Vincent and Chu reported that the CEA assay is capable of indicating successful resection

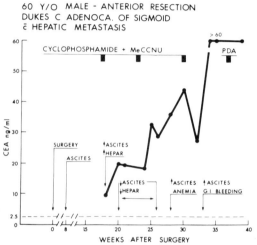

FIG. 5. *Use of serial CEA assays in monitoring unsuccessful treatment of sigmoid cancer metastatic to the liver. From Skarin et al. (52), with permission.*

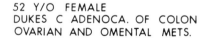
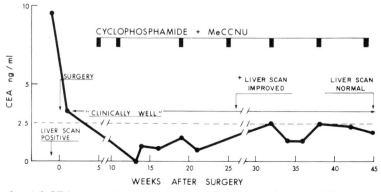

FIG. 6. *Use of serial CEA assays in monitoring initially apparently successful treatment of metastatic colonic cancer in a 52-year-old woman. From Skarin et al. (52), with permission.*

of lung cancer and of confirming clinical response to either radiotherapy or chemotherapy (61). They noted that CEA levels anticipated clinical evidence of disease progression by several months.

LIVER STATUS

Highest CEA levels are reported in metastatic disease of the liver. Terminal "failure" of the liver to metabolize and/or excrete CEA in the face of an increasing load of tumor antigen may contribute to the rapid rises in circulating levels often observed. It would seem unlikely that such elevations are caused solely by a rapid increase in production of CEA by the tumor masses. Whether liver toxicity by chemotherapeutic agents contributes to elevated CEA levels in some patients also needs study. Thus, concomitant monitoring of liver function may be useful for the correct interpretation of CEA levels. Among useful liver function tests are phosphohexose isomerase, alkaline phosphatase, gamma-glutamyl transpeptidase, lactate dehydrogenase, and serum glutamic oxalacetic transaminase (68). More study of this matter is needed.

Munjal and co-workers (45) compared plasma CEA levels with serum enzyme levels of phosphohexose isomerase, gamma-glutamyl transpeptidase, and lactate dehydrogenase in 147 patients with cancer. Elevations of CEA and of all three enzymes were most frequent in patients with hepatic metastases. Enzyme measurement did not increase the detection of metastatic gastrointestinal cancer over that achieved by CEA alone, whereas it did increase the detection of metastatic breast cancer and, to a lesser extent, metastatic lung cancer. Cooper et al. (11), on the other hand, found that the use of gamma-glutamyl transpeptidase in addition to CEA did result in earlier determination of liver metastases in some patients.

McIntire et al. (36) showed that the combined measurement of alpha-fetoprotein and CEA detected more patients with gastric cancer than either alone, although alpha-fetoprotein measurement did not help detect more colon cancers.

Several groups (67, 68) are actively studying combinations of different markers in the same patient in the effort to improve further the usefulness of the CEA assay. Such tumor markers include enzymes such as alkaline and acid phosphatase, phosphohexose isomerase, gamma-glutamyl transpeptidase, 5-nucleotidase, and aldolase, and ectopic hormones such as adrenocorticotropic hormone, human chorionic gonadotropic hormone, and gastrin and parathormone among many others.

CARCINOEMBRYONIC ANTIGEN ACTIVITY IN OTHER BODY FLUIDS

CEA and/or *CEA-like substances* have been identified in extracts of—in addition to gastrointestinal tract cancer—normal fetal and adult gastrointestinal tract, lung, and lactating breast, as well as in extracts of tumors of nongastrointestinal origin such as lung, breast, and ovary (28, 63). CEA-active substances have been measured in saliva (39), meconium (20, 49), feces (17), urine (22), seminal fluid (J. P. Vandevoorde et al., Fed. Proc. 32:1007, 1973), pancreatic and duodenal secretions (R. P. McCabe et al., Fed. Proc. 34:845, 1975; V. L. W. Go et al., Clin. Res. 22:489A, 1974), pleural effusions, and ascitic fluid (31). In general, these studies have indicated some quantitative correlation between the level of CEA activity in each of the tissues or fluids and the presence or absence of malignancy, thus supporting their potential clinical usefulness.

SOME METHODOLOGICAL CONSIDERATIONS

The available methods for measuring CEA cannot be considered as the usual "routine" clinical chemistry methods. Experience has demonstrated the need for carefully standardized reagents and meticulous technical procedure. The assay was initially applied clinically as a qualitative test differentiating "positive" from "negative" values in the vain hope that it would serve as a screening test for colon cancer. This application was soon replaced clinically by its quantitative use in determining trends of serial levels. The interesting evolution of the early development of the assays for CEA and their clinical application is reported in detail elsewhere (67). A previous report (28) and a recent detailed review by Fuks et al. (18) summarize in greater detail many of the methodological and immunochemical considerations not possible in this present summary because of limited space. A technical comparison of the initial Thomson, Hansen, and Egan assay methods was published by Fleischer et al. (16). The following sections summarize material selected largely from these and other papers.

Table 2 summarizes some of the methods which have been developed for the clinical measurement of circulating CEA (67). Radioimmunoassays for CEA differ primarily in the methods used for (i) preparing blood samples for analysis and (ii) separating antigen-antibody complexes from free labeled antigen in order to determine the amount of inhibition due to the test sample.

The *indirect* methods use preliminary per-

TABLE 2. *Comparison of some clinical immunoassays for carcinoembryonic antigen (CEA)*[a]

Reference	Extraction[b]	Coprecipitation	Sample and time needed[c]	Normal level (ng/ml)
Thomson (58)	PCA, 1.0 M	Ammonium sulfate, 50%	Serum, 5 ml; 5 days	<2.5
Smith (53)	PCA, 1.0 M	Ammonium sulfate, 50%	Serum or plasma, 1 ml; 3 days	<1.3
Mach (34)	PCA, 1.0 M	Ammonium sulfate, 50%	Plasma, 2 ml; 4 days	<5.0
Hansen[d] (23)	PCA, 0.6 M	Z-gel	Plasma, 0.5 ml; 1 day	<2.5
Lange (29)	PCA, 0.55 M	Hemagglutination inhibition[e]	Serum, 2.5 ml; 1 day	<5.0
Martin (40)	Immunoprecipitation plus PCA	Ammonium sulfate, 50%	Serum, 5 ml; 6 days	<4.0
Egan (15)	None	Anti-IgG antibody	Buffer, 0.2 ml; 1 day	2.5[f]
Laurence[g] (30)	None	Anti-IgG antibody	Plasma, 0.2 ml; 2 days	<12.5[h]
MacSween (38)	None	Anti-IgG antibody	Serum, 25 μliters; 3 days	<5.0
Searle (51)	None	Anti-IgG antibody	Plasma, 0.5 ml; 2 days	<2.5
Go (19)	None	Z-gel	Plasma, 0.1 ml; 2 days	<2.0
McPherson[i]	None	Tube solid phase	Serum or plasma, 1 ml; 5 days	<2.5
Coller (10)	None	RIEP binding[j]	Serum, 10 μliters; 2 h	—[k]
Edgington (14)	None[l]	Anti-IgG antibody	Serum, 0.33 ml; 2 days	—[m]

[a] Update of table from Zamcheck and Kupchik (65).
[b] PCA = perchloric acid.
[c] Volumes shown are for single determinations (duplicates required).
[d] Reported by LoGerfo et al. (32).
[e] Non-isotope technique.
[f] No clinical data reported; normal levels reported by Coligan et al. (9).
[g] Modification of Egan's double-antibody assay.
[h] Normal range for blacks was reported to be up to 30 ng/ml.
[i] T. A. McPherson, P. R. Bank, N. A. Hyde, and V. Paturadham, Can. Fed. Biol. Soc., p. 361, 1972.
[j] RIEP = radioimmunoelectrophoretic.
[k] Samples assessed qualitatively only.
[l] Serum clarified at 7,000 × g for 10 min.
[m] Reported as 14 units of CEA-S/ml; CEA equivalent unclear.

chloric acid extraction to separate the carbohydrate-rich proteins (including CEA) from the carbohydrate-poor proteins. The *direct* methods do not use this preliminary "purification" and in general require smaller volumes of serum or plasma.

There are several methods for precipitating the antigen-antibody complex. Coprecipitation may be achieved with ammonium sulfate, zirconyl phosphate gel, a second antibody, or with solid-phase immunoabsorbents.

The definition of "normal" serum or plasma CEA levels depends not only on the assay technique but also on the construction of standard curves, which vary in different laboratories (28). Some standard curves are prepared with whole or perchloric acid-extracted normal human serum or plasma; others use phosphate-buffered saline or ethylenediaminetetraacetate buffer as diluent. "Normal" levels may vary

markedly from 0 to 12.5 ng/ml or higher. As the clinical importance of serial determinations has become increasingly apparent, the significance of "cut-off" or threshold levels between "positive" and "negative" levels has properly diminished.

The Roche "indirect" assay, perhaps the most widely used method at present, measures plasma CEA concentrations reliably up to approximately 20 to 25 ng/ml. Specimens with CEA concentrations greater than 20 ng/ml must then be reassayed by a "direct" method (*without* perchloric acid extraction). Madsen et al. (Clin. Res. 23:115A, 1975), using split samples, noted that the direct assay gave higher levels than did the indirect at levels (indirect) less than 20 ng/ml. Kupchik et al. have found that the direct method measures a variable amount (31 ± 11 ng/ml) of additional CEA activity at indirect levels between 15 and

30 ng/ml (unpublished observations).

In serial assays, an abrupt jump to 40 to 60 ng/ml may occur when concentrations rise above 20 ng/ml as the indirect assay is switched to the direct; this abrupt rise does not necessarily imply tumor growth or dissemination. Conversely, declining levels may abruptly fall from the range of 40 to 60 ng/ml to levels less than 20 ng/ml as the indirect assay replaces the direct, without implying tumor regression. Thus, physicians using the assays should be aware that changes in reported CEA concentrations spanning the range of 20 to 60 ng/ml may not necessarily be "clinically significant." Interpretation of values in this transitional zone, especially serial levels, must be made with this in mind (M. S. Loewenstein, H. Z. Kupchik, and N. Zamchek, N. Engl. J. Med., in press).

Clinicians need to bear in mind that methodological differences in technical performance of the CEA assay in differing laboratories may also influence the values reported.

HETEROGENEITY OF CARCINOEMBRYONIC ANTIGEN

Characterization of the physicochemical properties of CEA by various investigators (1, 18, 50, 57, 60) has yielded several consistent findings in addition to evidence of heterogeneity (Table 3). CEA has been shown to be soluble in perchloric acid, water, and 50% saturated ammonium sulfate and insoluble in ethanol. Investigators agree that CEA is at least partially stable to heating at 100 C and has a sedimentation coefficient of 7 to 8S, a β mobility, and a molecular weight of approximately 200,000. However, the carbohydrate to protein ratio can range from 1:1 in preparations from colonic cancer tissue to 5:1 in those from gastric cancer tissue (4), and differences have been noted on polyacrylamide gel electrophoresis (4) and on isoelectric focusing of preparations from different sources (50).

The review by Terry et al. (57) of the charac-

TABLE 3. *Some properties of carcinoembryonic antigen*[a]

Carbohydrate to protein ratio, 3(1–5):1
Soluble in perchloric acid or water
Soluble in 50% saturated ammonium sulfate
Insoluble in ethanol
Heat stable
Sedimentation coefficient of 7 to 8S
β mobility on agar electrophoresis at pH 8.6
Single polydisperse band on polyacrylamide gel electrophoresis
Molecular weight of 200,000 ± 20,000
Isoelectric points of <3 and 3.75 ± 0.25

[a] Modified from Fuks et al. (18), with permission.

TABLE 4. *Materials cross-reacting with carcinoembryonic antigen*

Antigen	Investigator
Nonspecific cross-reacting antigen[a]	von Kleist et al. (62)
Normal glycoprotein[a]	Mach and Pusztaszeri (35)
Colonic carcinoembryonic antigen-2[a]	Turberville et al. (59)
Breast carcinoma glycoprotein[a]	Kuo et al. (27)
Colon carcinoma antigen-III[a]	Newman et al. (46)
Colon carcinoma antigen-II	Newman et al.[b]
Nonspecific cross-reacting antigen-II	Burtin et al. (7)
Fetal sulfoglycoprotein antigen	Hakkinen (21)

[a] Glycoproteins of 50,000 to 60,000 molecular weight with β electrophoretic mobility, presumably similar or identical.
[b] E. S. Newman, S. E. Petras, J. G. Hamilton, H. J. Hager, and H. J. Hansen, Fed. Proc. 31:639, 1972.

terization of CEA pointed out the need for more complete chemical characterization of CEA and related glycoproteins before a precise CEA nomenclature could be established.

Numerous *cross-reacting materials* share antigenic determinants with CEA (Table 4). Preliminary studies indicate that nonspecific cross-reacting antigen, normal glycoprotein, colonic carcinoembryonic antigen-2, breast carcinoma glycoprotein, and colon carcinoma antigen-III may be identical (12, 28, 57) and that they do not cross-react in radioimmunoassays for CEA performed on perchloric acid extracts (46). These substances should be termed "CEA-like" and their radioimmunoassay measurement should be expressed as "CEA-activity" until their chemical structures are more clearly established and the CEA nomenclature is accordingly revised.

Several investigators have begun to characterize the *chemical and physical properties* of several preparations of purified CEA and associated molecules (18, 57). The carbohydrate (Table 5) and protein (Table 6) moieties are being analyzed to determine the exact chemical composition of CEA as well as their antigenic components.

Although the monosaccharide N-acetylglucosamine did not inhibit ^{125}I-labeled CEA–anti-CEA binding, Banjo et al. (3) suggested that N-acetylglucosamine was a major component of the cancer-specific antigenic site of CEA. More recent studies by the same investigators (18) showed that aspartic acid bound to N-acetylglu-

TABLE 5. *Carbohydrate composition of carcinoembryonic antigen*[a]

Monosaccharide	Percent[b]			
	A[c]	B	C	D
Fucose	11.3	12.0	15.2	21.0
Mannose	12.8	21.7	14.3	11.3
Galactose	19.9	15.6	17.9	26.6
Sialic acid	8.1	7.9	10.7	3.9
N-acetylgalactosamine .	2.6	NS[d]	1.8	1.1
N-acetylglucosamine ...	43.3	42.3	40.2	35.7

[a] From Fuks et al. (18), with permission.
[b] Gas liquid chromatography weight of monosaccharide/weight of total carbohydrate × 100.
[c] (A) Banjo et al. (3, 4); (B) Hansen, as reported by Kupchik et al. (28); (C) J. E. Coligan, W. C. Schnute, M. L. Egan, and C. W. Todd (U.S. Atomic Energy Commission Report Conf. 73114, 1974); (D) Westwood (64).
[d] Not significant.

TABLE 6. *Amino acid composition of carcinoembryonic antigen purified from hepatic metastases of colonic carcinoma*[a]

Amino acid	Percent[b]			
	A[c]	B	C	D
Aspartic acid	14.1	16.6	15.0	14.7
Glutamic acid	11.3	12.4	11.6	10.6
Serine	8.4	10.5	8.1	10.4
Threonine	8.0	8.6	7.9	9.6
Isoleucine	6.0	5.8	5.0	4.7
Leucine	10.3	9.4	9.0	8.2
Proline	6.5	4.6	10.0	8.4
Glycine	3.3	4.2	3.1	5.5
Alanine	3.8	3.9	4.1	6.2
Valine	5.8	6.6	6.3	7.3
Tyrosine	3.6	5.8	5.6	3.6
Phenylalanine	3.3	2.7	3.8	2.2
Lysine	2.9	2.9	3.4	2.8
Histidine	2.0	1.8	2.4	1.8
Arginine	4.6	4.2	4.9	3.3
Cysteine	0.0	0.0	0.0	0.8
Methionine	0.0	0.0	ND[d]	Trace
Tryptophan	ND	ND	ND	ND

[a] From Fuks et al. (18), with permission.
[b] Weight of amino acid/weight of total protein × 100.
[c] (A) Banjo et al. (3, 4) and Terry et al. (56); (B) Hansen, as reported by Kupchik et al. (28); (C) Coligan et al. (9); (D) J. H. Westwood, P. Thomas, and A. B. Foster (Biochem. Soc. Trans. 2:1250, 1974).
[d] Not determined.

cosamine via an N-acetylglycosylamine-type linkage was capable of weak inhibition of ^{125}I-labeled CEA–anti-CEA binding (Table 7). Thus, their results suggested that the carbohydrate moiety was involved in the immunodominant tumor site and that the protein moiety also contributed to the specific im-

munochemical site. More recently, Anderson et al. (2) reported that one of the immunodeterminant structures of CEA involved two N-acetylglucosamine residues in $\beta 1 \rightarrow 4$ linkage plus a second β anomeric configuration. They suggested the di-N-acetylchitobiose-to-asparagine type of linkage described in several glycoproteins.

Banjo et al. (4) showed that despite the heterogeneity within the same CEA preparation and between different CEA preparations, purified CEA of colonic cancer origin manifested several consistent features including (i) the carbohydrate/protein ratio, (ii) the concentration of various amino acids, (iii) the high concentration of N-acetylglucosamine, (iv) the low concentration or absence of N-acetylgalactosamine, (v) the range and mean molecular weight of the material, and (vi) the charge characteristics of CEA before and after treatment with neuraminidase. The variations reported by various investigators may be due in part to differing tissue sources of CEA, damage of the molecule due to autolysis and/or purification procedures, or differences in purification techniques.

To date, most of the appropriately *absorbed anti-CEA antisera* prepared against different preparations of CEA have been immunochemically indistinguishable. One exception to this may be the reported isolation of a species of CEA called CEA-S by Edgington and Plow (14), which was *biochemically* similar to conventional CEA but demonstrated quantitative immunochemical differences when studied with

TABLE 7. *Substances inhibiting binding of carcinoembryonic antigen (CEA) by absorbed anti-CEA antiserum*[a]

Substance	Relative inhibitory wt[b]
CEA	1
Asparagine-N-acetylglucosamine ...	1.2 × 10⁶
CEA-derived glycopeptides	10–330
IgM glycopeptide	ND[c]
Blood group A	3.3 × 10³
	1.3 × 10³
Blood group B	2.6 × 10³
Blood group Le^a	73.3 × 10³
Blood group H	1 × 10³
Pneumococcus type XIV substance ..	ND
Gastric mucosa A substance	4.6 × 10⁵
Streptococcal group A antigens	ND
Alpha-acid glycoprotein	ND
Ovomucoid	ND
Ovarian cyst fluid material	1 × 10³

[a] From Fuks et al. (18), with permission.
[b] Weight of substance relative to weight of purified CEA needed to achieve 50% inhibition.
[c] Not determined.

their antisera in their radioimmunoassay (Table 2). When these workers used their assay system to test patients' sera, they found it to be as sensitive as CEA in detecting digestive tract cancer while yielding fewer elevated CEA-S values with other cancers and with nonmalignant diseases of the digestive tract. Whether this is truly a more specific test for digestive tract cancer or a manifestation of differences in *quantitation* between CEA-S and CEA remains to be determined.

Vrba et al. (63) recently suggested that CEA consists of multiple antigenic determinants or a family of different "isoantigens" and results of radioimmunoassays currently used for CEA measurements reflect the binding of a particular CEA-isoantigen(s) to a given polyvalent anti-CEA antiserum.

The need for more specific markers of colonic and other cancers has stimulated workers to seek new methods for the extraction of malignant tissues with more gentle reagents than perchloric acid. As these become refined, a continuing development of methods of CEA assay, or modifications of existing assays, can be expected. Each new assay method will have to be put through the same time-consuming process of clinical evaluation that has been required of the present CEA assay. The availability of serum and plasma banks of carefully characterized patients with staged diseases and histologically classified malignancies should expedite the process.

In summary, for the first time an opportunity has been made available to study the use and limitations of assays for one tumor-associated macromolecule, CEA. The need for close collaboration among chemists, clinicians, and pathologists has become apparent. CEA values can never be used as a substitute for complete clinical and laboratory work-up of the patient. Physicians using the assays must become familiar with the variability of the methods. We can expect rapid progress in the development of this field.

ACKNOWLEDGMENTS

This work was supported by Public Health Service grant CA-04486 from the National Cancer Institute, grant IM-18C from the American Cancer Society, and contract NIH-NCI N01 CP-33264 from the National Cancer Institute.

This paper is an up-dated and revised version of papers previously published from this laboratory, especially references 28 and 65–67.

We wish to thank A. Fuks for his critical review of the manuscript.

LITERATURE CITED

1. Abeyounis, C. J., and F. Milgrom. 1972. Studies on carcinoembryonic antigen. Int. Arch. Allergy Appl. Immunol. 43:30–38.
2. Anderson, B., A. Jameson, A. A. Hirata, J. W. Safford, and J. T. Tomita. 1975. Carcinoembryonic antigen – identification of a tri-N-acetylchitotriosyl type structure as an immunodeterminant group. Immunochemistry 12:577–580.
3. Banjo, C., P. Gold, S. O. Freedman, and J. Krupey. 1972. Immunologically active heterosaccharides of carcinoembryonic antigen of human digestive system. Nature (London) New Biol. 238:183–185.
4. Banjo, C., J. Shuster, and P. Gold. 1974. Intermolecular heterogeneity of the carcinoembryonic antigen. Cancer Res. 34:2114–2121.
5. Booth, S. N., G. C. Jamieson, J. P. G. King, J. Leonard, G. D. Oates, and P. W. Dykes. 1974. Carcinoembryonic antigen in management of colorectal carcinoma. Br. Med. J. 2:183–186.
6. Booth, S. N., J. P. G. King, J. C. Leonard, and P. W. Dykes. 1973. Serum carcinoembryonic antigen in clinical disorders. Gut 14:794–799.
7. Burtin, P., G. Chavanel, and H. Hirsch-Marie. 1973. Characterization of a second antigen that cross reacts with CEA. J. Immunol. 111:1926–1928.
8. Chu, T. M., and T. Nemoto. 1973. Evaluation of carcinoembryonic antigen in human mammary carcinoma. J. Natl. Cancer Inst. 51:1119–1122.
9. Coligan, J. E., P. A. Henkart, C. W. Todd, and W. D. Terry. 1972. Isolation and characterization of carcinoembryonic antigen. Immunochemistry 9:377–386.
10. Coller, J. A., R. W. Crichlow, and L. K. Yin. 1973. Radioimmunoelectrophoretic binding assay for the detection of carcinoembryonic antigen. Cancer Res. 33:1684–1688.
11. Cooper, E. H., R. Turner, L. Steele, A. M. Neville, and A. M. Mackay. 1975. The contribution of serum enzymes and carcinoembryonic antigen to the early diagnosis of metastatic colorectal cancer. Br. J. Cancer 31:111–117.
12. Darcy, D. A., C. Turberville, and R. James. 1973. Immunological study of carcinoembryonic antigen (CEA) and a related glycoprotein. Br. J. Cancer 28:147–154.
13. Dhar, P., T. L. Moore, N. Zamcheck, and H. Z. Kupchik. 1972. Carcinoembryonic antigen (CEA) in colonic cancer: use in pre- and postoperative diagnosis and prognosis. J. Am. Med. Assoc. 221:31.
14. Edgington, T. S., R. W. Astarita, and E. F. Plow. 1975. Association of an isomeric species of carcinoembryonic antigen with neoplasia of the gastrointestinal tract. N. Engl. J. Med. 293:103–107.
15. Egan, M. L., J. T. Lautenschleger, J. E. Coligan, and C. W. Todd. 1972. Radioimmunoassay of carcinoembryonic antigen. Immunochemistry 9:289–299.
16. Fleischer, M., H. F. Oettgen, E. Besenfelder, and M. K. Schwartz. 1973. Measurement of carcinoembryonic antigen. Clin. Chem. 19:1214–1218.
17. Freed, D. L. J., and G. Taylor. 1972. Carcinoem-

bryonic antigen in faeces. Br. Med. J. 1:85–87.

18. Fuks, A., C. Banjo, J. Shuster, S. O. Freedman, and P. Gold. 1974. Carcinoembryonic antigen (CEA): molecular biology and clinical significance. Biochim. Biophys. Acta 417:123–152.

19. Go, V. L. W., A. J. Schutt, C. G. Moertel, W. H. J. Summerskill, and H. R. Butt. 1972. Radioimmunoassay of carcinoembryonic antigen (CEA). A modified method and clinical evaluation. Gastroenterology 62:754.

20. Goldenberg, D. M., N. G. O. Tchilinguiran, H. J. Hansen, and J. P. Vandevoorde. 1972. Carcinoembryonic antigen present in meconium: the basis of a possible new diagnostic test of fetal distress. Am. J. Obstet. Gynecol. 113:66–69.

21. Hakkinen, I. 1972. Immunological relationship of the carcinoembryonic antigen and the fetal sulfoglycoprotein antigen. Immunochemistry 9:1115–1119.

22. Hall, R. R., D. J. R. Laurence, D. Darcy, U. Stevens, R. James, S. Roberts, and A. M. Neville. 1972. Carcinoembryonic antigen (CEA) in the urine of patients with urothelial carcinoma. Br. Med. J. 3:609–611.

23. Hansen, H. J., J. J. Snyder, E. Miller, J. P. Vandevoorde, O. M. Miller, L. R. Hines, and J. J. Burns. 1974. Carcinoembryonic antigen (CEA) assay. A laboratory adjunct in the diagnosis and management of cancer. J. Hum. Pathol. 5:139–147.

24. Holyoke, E. D., G. Reynoso, and T. Chu. 1972. Carcinoembryonic antigen in patients with carcinoma of the digestive tract, p. 215–219. In N. G. Anderson, J. H. Coggin, E. B. Cole, and J. W. Holleman (ed.), Embryonic and fetal antigens in cancer, vol. 2. USAEC Report CONF-720208, Department of Commerce, Springfield, Va.

25. Joint National Cancer Institute of Canada/ American Cancer Society Investigation. 1972. A collaborative study of a test for carcinoembryonic antigen (CEA) in the sera of patients with carcinoma of the colon and rectum. Can. Med. Assoc. J. 107:25–33.

26. Khoo, S. K., N. L. Warner, J. T. Lie, and I. R. Mackay. 1973. Carcinoembryonic antigenic activity of tissue extracts: a quantitative study of malignant and benign neoplasms, cirrhotic liver, normal adult and fetal organs. Int. J. Cancer 11:681–687.

27. Kuo, T., J. Rosai, and T. W. Tillack. 1973. Immunological studies of membrane glycoproteins isolated from human breast carcinomas. Int. J. Cancer 12:532–542.

28. Kupchik, H. Z., N. Zamcheck, and C. A. Saravis. 1973. Immunochemical studies of carcinoembryonic antigens: methodologic considerations and some clinical implications. J. Natl. Cancer Inst. 51:1741–1749.

29. Lange, R. D., A. I. Chernoff, T. A. Jordan, and J. R. Collmann. 1971. Experience with a hemagglutination inhibition test for carcinoembryonic antigen. Preliminary report, p. 379–386. Proc. 1st Conference and Workshop on Embryonic and Fetal Antigens in Cancer.

Oak Ridge National Laboratory, Oak Ridge, Tenn.

30. Laurence, D. J. R., U. Stevens, R. Bettelheim, D. Darcy, C. Leese, C. Turberville, P. Alexander, E. W. Johns, and A. M. Neville. 1972. Evaluation of the role of plasma carcinoembryonic antigen (CEA) in the diagnosis of gastrointestinal, mammary and bronchial carcinoma. Br. Med. J. 3:605.

31. Loewenstein, M. S., R. A. Rittgers, H. Z. Kupchik, A. E. Feinerman, and N. Zamcheck. 1975. Improved detection of malignant ascites and pleural effusions by combined assay of fluid CEA and cytology. Clin. Res. 23:596A.

32. LoGerfo, P., J. Krupey, and H. J. Hansen. 1971. Demonstration of an antigen common to several varieties of neoplasia. N. Engl. J. Med. 285:138.

33. Lurie, B. B., M. S. Loewenstein, and N. Zamcheck. 1975. Elevated carcinoembryonic levels and biliary tract obstruction. J. Am. Med. Assoc. 233:326–330.

34. Mach, J. P., P. H. Jaeger, M. M. Bertholet, C. A. Ruegsegger, R. M. Loosli, and J. Pettavel. 1974. Detection of recurrence of large bowel carcinoma by radioimmunoassay of circulating carcinoembryonic antigen (CEA). Lancet 2:535–540.

35. Mach, J. P., and G. Pusztaszeri. 1972. Carcinoembryonic antigen (CEA): demonstration of a partial identity between CEA and normal glycoprotein. Immunochemistry 9:1031–1034.

36. McIntire, K. R., T. A. Waldmann, V. L. W. Go, C. G. Moertel, and M. Ravry. 1974. Simultaneous radioimmunoassay for carcinoembryonic antigen (CEA) and alpha-fetoprotein (alpha-FP) in neoplasms of the gastrointestinal tract. Ann. Clin. Lab. Sci. 4:104–108.

37. Mackay, A. M., S. Patel, S. Canter, U. Stevens, D. J. R. Laurence, E. H. Cooper, and A. M. Neville. 1974. Role of serial plasma CEA assays in detection of recurrent and metastatic colorectal carcinoma. Br. Med. J. 4: 383–385.

38. MacSween, J. M., N. L. Warner, A. D. Bankhurst, and I. R. Mackay. 1972. Carcinoembryonic antigen in whole serum. Br. J. Cancer 26:356–360.

39. Martin, F., and J. Devant. 1973. Carcinoembryonic antigen in normal human saliva. J. Natl. Cancer Inst. 50:1375–1379.

40. Martin, F., C. Kleppine, and J. Guerrin. 1976. Dosage radioimmunologique de l'antigene carcino-embryonnaire circulant. Extraction immuno-perchlorique du serum. Arch. Mal. Appar. Dig. Mal. Nutr., in press.

41. Moore, T. L., P. Dhar, N. Zamcheck, A. Keeley, L. Gottlieb, and H. Z. Kupchik. 1972. Carcinoembryonic antigen(s) in liver disease. I. Clinical and morphological studies. Gastroenterology 63:88–94.

42. Moore, T. L., P. Dhar, N. Zamcheck, and H. Z. Kupchik. 1971. Carcinoembryonic antigen (CEA) in diagnosis of digestive tract cancer, p. 393–400. Proc. 1st Conference and Workshop on Embryonic and Fetal Antigens in

Cancer. Oak Ridge National Laboratory, Oak Ridge, Tenn.

43. Moore, T. L., H. Z. Kupchik, N. Marcon, and N. Zamcheck. 1971. Carcinoembryonic antigen assay in cancer of the colon and pancreas and other digestive tract disorders. Am. J. Dig. Dis. 16:1.

44. Mulcare, R., and P. LoGerfo. 1972. Tumor associated antigen in the chemotherapy of solid tumors. J. Surg. Oncol. 4:407–417.

45. Munjal, D., P. L. Chawla, J. J. Lokich, and N. Zamcheck. 1975. Combined measurement of carcinoembryonic antigen, phosphohexose isomerase, gammaglutamyl transpeptidase, and lactate dehydrogenase in G. I., lung and breast cancer patients. Cancer, in press.

46. Newman, E. S., S. E. Petras, A. Georgiadis, and H. J. Hansen. 1974. Interrelationship of carcinoembryonic antigen and colon carcinoma antigen-III. Cancer Res. 34:2125–2130.

47. Ravry, M., V. L. W. Go, A. J. Schutt, and C. G. Moertel. 1973. Usefulness of serial serum carcinoembryonic antigen (CEA) during anticancer therapy or long term follow-up of gastrointestinal cancer. Cancer Chemother. Rep. 57:111.

48. Reynoso, G., T. M. Chu, D. Holyoke, E. Cohen, L. A. Valensuela, T. Nemoto, J. J. Wang, J. Chuang, P. Guinan, and G. P. Murphy. 1972. Carcinoembryonic antigen in patients with different cancers. J. Am. Med. Assoc. 220:361–365.

49. Rule, A. H. 1973. Carcinoembryonic antigen (CEA): activity of meconium and normal colon extracts. Immunol. Commun. 2:15–24.

50. Rule, A. H. and C. Golesky-Reilly. 1973. Carcinoembryonic antigen (CEA): separation of CEA-reacting molecules from tumor, fetal gut, meconium and normal colon. Immunol. Commun. 2:213–226.

51. Searle, F., A. C. Lovesey, B. A. Roberts, G. T. Rogers, and K. D. Bagshawe. 1974. Radioimmunoassay methods for carcinoembryonic antigen. J. Immunol. Methods 4:113–125.

52. Skarin, A. T., R. Delwiche, N. Zamcheck, J. J. Lokich, and E. Frei III. 1974. Carcinoembryonic antigen: clinical correlation with chemotherapy for metastatic gastrointestinal cancer. Cancer 33:1239–1245.

53. Smith, H. J., P. H. Figard, P. J. O'Neill, and M. Gookcen. 1973. Carcinoembryonic antigen (CEA): radioimmunoassay using highly purified CEA and ^{125}I-CEA. Res. Commun. Chem. Pathol. Pharmacol. 5:573–583.

54. Sorokin, J. J., P. H. Sugarbaker, N. Zamcheck, M. Pisick, H. Z. Kupchik, and F. D. Moore. 1974. Serial CEA assays: use in detection of recurrence following resection of colon cancer. J. Am. Med. Assoc. 228:49–53.

55. Steward, A. M., D. W. Nixon, N. Zamcheck, and A. Aisenberg. 1974. Carcinoembryonic anti-

gen in breast cancer patients: serum levels and disease progress. Cancer 33:1246–1252.

56. Terry, W. D., P. A. Henkart, J. E. Coligan, and C. W. Todd. 1972. Structural studies of the major glycoprotein in preparations with carcinoembryonic antigen activity. J. Exp. Med. 136:200–204.

57. Terry, W. D., P. A. Henkart, J. E. Coligan, and C. W. Tood. 1974. Carcinoembryonic antigen: characterization and clinical applications. Transplant. Rev. 20:100–129.

58. Thomson, D. M. P., J. Krupey, S. O. Freedman, and P. Gold. 1969. The radioimmunoassay of circulating carcinoembryonic antigen of the human digestive system. Proc. Natl. Acad. Sci. U.S.A. 64:161.

59. Turberville, C., D. A. Darcy, D. J. Laurence, E. W. Johns, and A. M. Neville. 1973. Studies on carcinoembryonic antigen (CEA) and a related glycoprotein, CCEA-2. Preparation and clinical characterization. Immunochemistry 10:841–843.

60. Turner, M. D., T. A. Olivares, L. Harwell, and M. S. Kleinman. 1972. Further purification of perchlorate-soluble antigens from human colonic carcinomata. J. Immunol. 108:1328–1339.

61. Vincent, R. G., and T. M. Chu. 1973. Carcinoembryonic antigen in patients with carcinoma of the lung. J. Thorac. Cardiovas. Surg. 66:320–328.

62. von Kleist, S., G. Chavenel, and P. Burtin. 1972. Identification of an antigen from normal human tissue that cross-reacts with carcinoembryonic antigen. Proc. Natl. Acad. Sci. U.S.A. 69:2492–2494.

63. Vrba, R., E. Alpert, and K. Isselbacher. 1975. Carcinoembryonic antigen (CEA). N. Engl. J. Med. (correspondence) 293:877–878.

64. Westwood, J. H., E. M. Bessell, M. A. Bukhari, P. Thomas, and J. M. Walker. 1974. Studies on the structure of the carcinoembryonic antigen. I. Some deductions on the basis of chemical degradations. Immunochemistry 11:811–818.

65. Zamcheck, N. 1974. Carcinoembryonic antigen: quantitative variations in circulating levels in benign and malignant digestive tract disease. Adv. Intern. Med. 19:413–433.

66. Zamcheck, N. 1975. The present status of CEA in diagnosis, prognosis, and evaluation of therapy. Cancer 36:2460–2468.

67. Zamcheck, N., and H. Z. Kupchik. 1974. The interdependence of clinical investigation and methodological development in early evolution of assays for carcinoembryonic antigen. Cancer Res. 34:2131–2136.

68. Zamcheck, N., and G. Pusztaszeri. 1975. CEA, AFP and other potential tumor markers. Ca 25:204–214.

Chapter 100

Alpha-Fetoprotein

K. R. McINTIRE and T. A. WALDMANN

BACKGROUND

The presence of alpha-fetoprotein (AFP) in adult serum has come to have significance beyond the diagnosis of hepatocellular carcinoma, for which it once appeared to be quite specific. The detection of serum AFP by relatively insensitive techniques such as double diffusion in agar may be of help in the diagnosis of clinically suspected hepatocellular carcinoma in regions of high incidence, but does not allow the following of a dynamic disease process that is available by the quantitative measurement of AFP. There are excellent methods, both radioimmunoassay and enzymoimmunoassay, for the sensitive quantitation of AFP (7, 10) that allow the measurement of normal, physiological levels of AFP. This chapter will review primarily studies which have used these sensitive and quantitative assays.

DESCRIPTION OF ANTIGEN

Alpha-fetoprotein is synthesized by the fetal liver and yolk sac and is one of the main serum proteins during early development of the human fetus. The molecular weight of AFP is 65,000 to 70,000, and the isoelectric point is 4.75; it is a glycoprotein with 4% carbohydrate (11). Some electrophoretic heterogeneity of AFP has been ascribed to variation in sialic acid content. There is antigenic cross-reactivity between the fetal AFP of a variety of mammalian species and antigenic identity between human AFP from different sources, i.e., fetal, hepatocellular carcinoma, germ cell neoplasms, pancreatic carcinoma, etc.

The biological function of AFP during fetal development is not yet known. Several functions have been suggested and include the suppression of both cellular and humoral immune responsiveness, binding or transport of hormones, and as a precursor of serum albumin. Since a homologue of AFP has been demonstrated in birds and sharks in addition to a large number of mammals, it would appear that an ancestral homologue of this protein has existed since before the development of mammals (4).

Elevations of serum AFP occur with certain neoplasms and some diseases of hepatic origin (probably due to increased production of AFP). Three possible explanations have been offered (1): (i) increased numbers of specialized cells which synthesize AFP; (ii) increased numbers of cells in a certain stage of differentiation which synthesize AFP ("dedifferentiation"); (iii) induction of AFP synthesis secondary to other changes, similar to the induction of enzyme synthesis ("derepression").

COLLECTION AND STORAGE OF SPECIMENS

Serum should be separated and frozen at −20 C until assayed. AFP is resistant to degradation or denaturation upon standing at room temperature for up to 48 h or after freezing and thawing. However, freezing or other manipulation may cause aggregation of AFP which does not seem to interfere with immunoprecipitability.

NORMAL LEVELS

There has been universal agreement from many independent laboratories that there is a normal range of measurable AFP in the serum of healthy adults. The level of AFP in fetal serum reaches a peak at around 13 to 15 weeks after conception and diminishes to 1/100 to 1/1,000 of that level by the 40th week of gestation (4, 8). The level continues to fall during the neonatal period, and by 6 to 24 months of age it has reached the normal adult level. Ruoslahti and Seppälä have demonstrated that this normal AFP is indistinguishable from fetal and hepatoma AFP. The lower limit of the concentration of AFP in normal sera has not been well established but is probably less than 1 ng/ml; the upper limit varies between 10 to 30 ng/ml depending upon the laboratory performing the assay. Healthy individuals appear to have stable levels of AFP so that variations even within the normal range have the potential for reflecting a disease process. At the present time the understanding of serum AFP variation comes primarily from studies on synthesis by neoplasms; further studies are needed to define the transient changes seen in non-neoplastic diseases.

HEPATOCELLULAR CARCINOMA

AFP is synthesized and secreted by hepatocellular carcinoma cells and a high percentage of these tumors are associated with elevated serum levels of AFP. The incidence of elevated AFP is close to 70% in Europe and North America and is 80 to 90% or higher in hepatocellular carcinoma patients in Africa and Asia (1). The range of AFP levels varies over six logs of concentration (Fig. 1) but appears to remain fairly stable for any one patient in the absence of treatment (6). This plateau of AFP concentration in untreated patients may be indicative of the diminished growth of tumor cells (or increased catabolism) in the terminal stages of this disease. Screening for early detection of hepatocellular carcinoma has been attempted using assays for AFP considerably less sensitive than the radioimmunoassay; these have been performed in areas where the incidence of liver cancer is high. In a serial study of nearly

10,000 men in Dakar, Senegal (expected hepatoma incidence rate, 45/100,000 per year) screened by double diffusion AFP assays every 4 months, only one-third of the nine cases of primary liver cancer had elevated AFP before the diagnosis was clinically evident, and these all died in less than 4 months after discovery. A sensitive RIA for AFP in Bantu (expected hepatoma incidence rate, 36/100,000 per year) failed to find a single early case in a study of over 5,000 subjects.

Elevated serum AFP is found more frequently in hepatocellular carcinoma patients under the age of 30 and is found less frequently in patients over age 60, but there is no significant correlation of AFP elevation with length of clinical symptoms before diagnosis, degree of cellular differentiation in the tumor, size of tumor, or length of survival time from diagnosis.

The most valuable use of serum AFP measurement in hepatocellular carcinoma is for following the effectiveness of therapy. With effective therapy and reduction in tumor size (most often by surgical resection) there is a corresponding decrease in the serum AFP level (Fig. 2). A later increase in serum AFP has been shown to precede the recurrence of clinical tumor by up to several months (6).

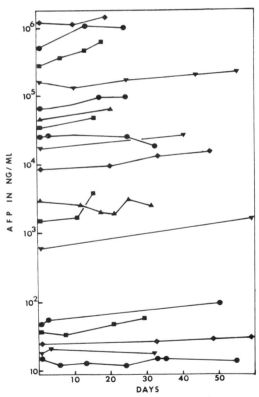

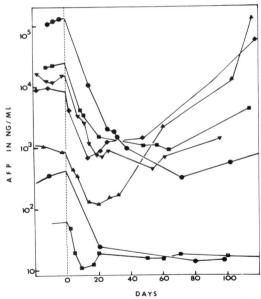

FIG. 1. *Serial values of serum AFP in 18 individual patients with proven hepatocellular carcinoma. All sera were collected before the start of therapy. Note the wide range of variation between individuals and the tendency for values to remain stable or rise only slightly in the late stage of the disease.*

FIG. 2. *Serial serum AFP values after surgical resection (day 0) of hepatocellular carcinoma. All seven resections were incomplete and clinical evidence of recurrent tumor was preceded by a rise in serum AFP in five; the other two were not followed long enough.*

GERM CELL TUMORS

Germ cell tumors of gonadal, retroperitoneal, or mediastinal origin are frequently associated with elevated levels of serum AFP. Between 50 and 70% of such tumors demonstrate elevated AFP, and are usually those containing embryonal cell or endodermal sinus tumor elements. The levels of AFP seen in germ cell tumors show considerable overlap with those seen in hepatocellular carcinoma (Fig. 3), and the protein itself appears to be antigenically identical in both conditions.

The absolute levels of AFP in sera of germ cell tumor patients do not correlate with tumor size, nor do they provide prognostic information which correlates with expected survival or responsiveness to therapy. However, serial determinations of AFP appear to provide a dynamic reflection of the progression or regression of tumor. Successful therapy which reduces tumor size will cause a fall in serum AFP level; complete clinical remission will be accompanied by serum AFP levels within the normal range.

In germ cell tumors human chorionic gonadotropin (hCG, see chapter 25) is also synthesized by a high percentage and provides a second circulating tumor marker when measured by RIA specific for the β chain of hCG. In a series of over 100 germ cell neoplasms of the testis, both markers were elevated in 58%, AFP alone was elevated in 17%, hCG alone was elevated in 14%, and both were normal in only 11% (13). Serum hCG parallels AFP in diminishing with decreasing tumor size. Recurrent tumor may synthesize both markers or may show a discordant synthesis of only one (3). There is no evidence available to indicate synthesis of a marker in metastatic disease that was not present with the primary tumor, but it is possible to have recurrent tumor with no associated rise in serum AFP or hCG despite the presence of either or both markers in the primary tumor.

OTHER MALIGNANCY

Serum AFP elevation has been reported in

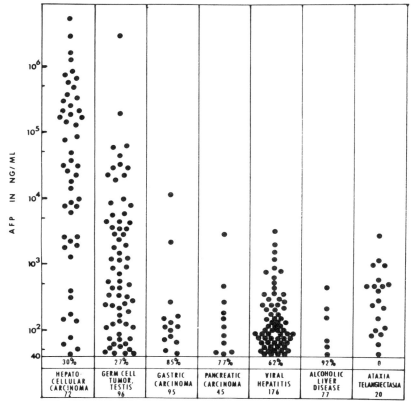

FIG. 3. *Comparison of serum AFP levels in four types of neoplasms, two varieties of nonmalignant liver disease, and ataxia telangiectasia. The percentage figure indicates the percentage of patients within the normal range for AFP, <40 ng/ml (13). The number of patients in each group is in parentheses.*

association with a number of other neoplastic diseases; patients with carcinoma of the pancreas, stomach, and biliary system are those where AFP is found with greatest frequency (Fig. 3) and where AFP might be a useful marker for following the disease process (6). Patients with carcinoma of the kidney, lung, colon, and prostate have also had rare reports of elevated AFP. Only in gastric carcinoma, in addition to hepatocellular carcinoma and germ cell neoplasms, has actual synthesis of AFP been demonstrated.

NON-NEOPLASTIC LIVER DISEASE

Until sensitive assays for AFP became available, it was generally considered that elevated serum levels in adults were indicative of neoplastic disease (or pregnancy). Early work with experimental animals demonstrated elevations of serum AFP after partial surgical removal of the liver or damage to the liver with chemical toxins. The timing of the rise in serum AFP in experimental animals led to the assumption that it indicated regeneration of the liver.

In patients with non-neoplastic liver disease, the frequency of elevated serum AFP is greater in those diseases with marked necrosis and inflammation of the hepatic parenchyma than in those where portal inflammation and cholestasis are the predominant lesions. The highest levels are seen in viral subacute hepatic necrosis where about 10% of patients had serum AFP above 500 ng/ml and 52% were above normal levels (2). Up to 30% of patients with other liver diseases may have elevated serum AFP, but none are likely to be higher than 500 ng/ml (Fig. 3). Less than 1% of patients with other acute and chronic gastrointestinal diseases have elevated serum AFP. In patients with viral hepatitis, the elevated levels of serum AFP do not correlate with the presence of hepatitis B antigen, nor do they correlate with the usual liver function tests (SGOT, serum bilirubin and alkaline phosphatase). Serial serum studies show AFP elevation begins as SGOT levels are falling, which could be related to hepatic regeneration following parenchymal damage by hepatitis virus.

It has been noted that all or very nearly all patients with the immunodeficiency disease ataxia telangiectasia have elevations of serum AFP, and there is a correlation between the AFP elevation and the severity of recurrent infections. The elevated serum AFP is probably directly related to the basic disease disorder rather than as a secondary phenomenon, since elevations in ataxia telangiectasia occur without evidence of hepatic disease and other immunodeficiency conditions have no elevation of serum AFP. Synthesis of a fetal protein of hepatic origin suggests incomplete development of the liver and supports the hypothesis that patients with ataxia telangiectasia have a defect in tissue differentiation that affects both thymus and liver.

OBSTETRIC CONDITIONS

AFP synthesized by the fetal liver and yolk sac appears to be at its highest concentration in the amniotic fluid in the early stages of pregnancy, whereas AFP in the fetal serum reaches a peak at the beginning of the second trimester; both then diminish in concentration through the remainder of gestation (Fig. 4). AFP crosses the placenta and increases in the maternal circulation until the third trimester, when it also begins to decrease (5). Seppälä and Ruoslahti showed the association of fetal intrauterine death with maternal serum AFP levels higher than normal for the specified time of pregnancy. Brock and Sutcliffe noted elevated levels of AFP in amniotic fluid of fetuses with various neural tube defects; others have reported elevated levels with other congenital defects, i.e., esophageal and duodenal atresia, hydrocephaly, and congenital nephrosis and omphalocele. The use of sensitive AFP measurement has been suggested as a means of screening for neural tube defects, but there is disagreement as to whether the levels in maternal serum are sensitive enough to the changes occurring in

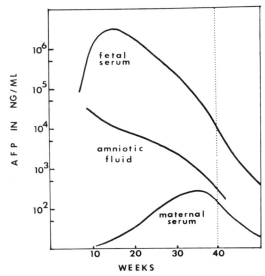

FIG. 4. Comparison of AFP levels during pregnancy in fetal serum (4), amniotic fluid, and maternal serum.

the amniotic fluid. There is need for further study with appropriate ancillary tests (sonography and amniography) before conclusions are reached regarding the usefulness of AFP measurement for the diagnosis of neural tube defects or fetal distress.

WORLD STANDARD

The International Agency for Research on Cancer has established a pool of human cord serum that has been designated by the World Health Organization as "International Reference Preparation for AFP." Aliquots of this preparation have been lyophilized and have an assigned activity of 100,000 international units of AFP per ampoule. Ampoules are supplied free of charge upon application to: International Agency for Research on Cancer, Interdisciplinary Programme and International Liaison, 150 Cours Albert Thomas, 69008 Lyon, France (12).

LITERATURE CITED

1. Abelev, G. I. 1971. Alpha-fetoprotein in ontogenesis and its association with malignant tumors. Adv. Cancer Res. 14:295–358.
2. Bloomer, J. R., T. A. Waldmann, K. R. McIntire, and G. Klastskin. 1975. α-Fetoprotein in nonneoplastic hepatic disorders. J. Am. Med. Assoc. 233:38–41.
3. Braunstein, G. D., K. R. McIntire, and T. A. Waldmann. 1973. Discordance of human chorionic gonadotropin and alpha-fetoprotein in testicular teratocarcinomas. Cancer 31:1065–1068.
4. Gitlin, D. 1975. Normal biology of α-fetoprotein. Ann. N.Y. Acad. Sci. 259:7–16.
5. Harris, R., R. F. Jennison, A. J. Barson, K. M. Laurence, E. Ruoslahti, and M. Seppälä. 1974. Comparison of amniotic-fluid and maternal serum alpha-fetoprotein levels in the early antenatal diagnosis of spina bifida and anencephaly. Lancet 1:429–433.
6. McIntire, K. R., C. L. Vogel, A. Primack, T. A. Waldmann, and S. K. Kyalwazi. 1976. Effect of surgical and chemotherapeutic treatment on alpha-fetoprotein levels in patients with hepatocellular carcinoma. Cancer 37:677–683.
7. Maiolini, R., B. Ferrua, and R. Masseyeff. 1975. Enzymoimmunoassay of human alpha-fetoprotein. J. Immunol. Methods 6:355–362.
8. Masseyeff, R., J. Gilli, B. Krebs, A. Calluaud, and C. Bonet. 1975. Evolution of α-fetoprotein serum levels throughout life in humans and rats, and during pregnancy in the rat. Ann. N.Y. Acad. Sci. 259:17–28.
9. Purves, L. R., C. Manso, and F. O. Torres. 1973. Serum α-fetoprotein levels in people susceptible to primary liver cancer in southern Africa. Gann Monogr. 14:51–66.
10. Ruoslahti, E., and M. Seppälä. 1971. Studies of carcino-fetal proteins. III. Development of a radioimmunoassay for α-fetoprotein. Demonstration of α-fetoprotein in serum of healthy human adults. Int. J. Cancer 8:374–383.
11. Ruoslahti, E., H. Pihko, and M. Seppälä. 1974. Alpha-fetoprotein: immunochemical purification and chemical properties. Expression in normal state and in malignant and nonmalignant liver disease. Transplant. Rev. 20:38–60.
12. Sizaret, P., N. Breslow, S. G. Anderson, and twelve other participants. 1975. Collaborative study of a preparation of human cord serum for its use as a reference in the assay of alpha-fetoprotein. J. Biol. Stand. 3:201–223.
13. Waldmann, T. A., and K. R. McIntire. 1974. The use of a radioimmunoassay for alpha-fetoprotein in the diagnosis of malignancy. Cancer 34:1510–1515.

Chapter 101

Cellular and Humoral Immune Responses in Neoplasia

YOSEF H. PILCH AND SIDNEY H. GOLUB

INTRODUCTION

The science of tumor immunology is barely more than a decade old, but it has expanded at a virtually logarithmic rate. Thus, any review of methods in this field must of necessity begin with a series of disclaimers. No attempt is made to provide a complete compendium of information in this field, as that is beyond the scope of this *Manual*. Instead, we attempt to evaluate different approaches for the study of immune reactions to tumors. It is our predominant purpose to describe which approaches are most likely to yield the most information and the pitfalls inherent in studies in this area.

There is a plethora of data in the literature dealing with various aspects of immunological function in cancer patients. Immunocompetence has been evaluated by determination of serum immunoglobulin levels, lymphocyte responses to mitogens, mixed lymphocyte culture reactivity, delayed cutaneous hypersensitivity to common recall antigens, cutaneous hypersensitivity reactions to contact allergens or other skin-sensitizing agents, and measurement of specific antibody production. All of these approaches can be useful in evaluating the status of the immune system, but they do not measure specific responses to tumor-associated antigens. Many of these studies have indicated that diminished immunological function is often associated with a poor clinical prognosis. It is also apparent that the frequency with which defects in immune function are found will depend on both the population of cancer patients studied and the assays employed (19). However, none of these approaches poses the fundamental question of whether an effective immune response is generated against the antigens of the tumor. For this reason, the rest of our discussion is focused on immune reactions which are specific for tumor-associated antigens. We note in passing, however, that determination of immunocompetence is a closely related area and may prove to be most useful as a guide to extent of disease and/or prognosis. Moreover, the immunocompetence of a given cancer patient may prove to be a deciding factor in the choice of an immunotherapeutic modality.

METHODS FOR ASSESSMENT OF CELL-MEDIATED IMMUNITY IN CANCER

Even casual perusal of the literature in the area of cell-mediated immunity to tumors will disclose that there are almost as many techniques for the measurement of these interactions as there are researchers in the field. This indicates either that scientists in this field are inordinately creative or that no one technique has been able to answer all the pertinent questions. Unfortunately, the latter is probably the case. A recent symposium comparing many of these techniques provides an excellent reference source for the procedures, pitfalls, and advantages of each of them (29). We shall not attempt to evaluate the different methods, many of which are presented in other sections of this *Manual*, but shall only attempt to point out the types of information that one can and cannot obtain from each.

Lymphocyte-mediated cytotoxicity (see chapter 12)

By far the most common technique used for the study of cell-mediated reactions against tumor-associated antigens is the lymphocyte-mediated cytotoxicity assay. This assay is based upon the ability of lymphocytes to lyse target tumor cells. A variation of this approach is to assess inhibition of growth of target tumor cells rather than cell death. In either case, the purpose is to determine whether the putatively immune lymphocyte will damage the tumor cells being tested. Assessment of the damage can be accomplished either by visual observation or by the use of a radioactive isotope to label the target cell. Visual observation was the original approach in this area and still is widely used (25, 51). The Hellströms first reported that lymphocytes from cancer patients could inhibit colony formation by tumor cells recently explanted into tissue culture (24). Since colony inhibition is a time-consuming assay and the criteria used for the designation of a colony may be difficult to establish, most laboratories have abandoned colony inhibition in favor of the various microcytotoxicity assays. Visual observation or counting is time-consuming and may become a limiting factor in the performance of cytotoxicity assays. One alternative approach is to read the results electronically, but this technology is not available to most laboratories (52). Therefore, isotopic labels have been developed to permit the automated enumeration of labeled target cells. Much of the work on cell-mediated immunity to histocompatibility antigens has been accomplished by use of ^{51}Cr-labeled target cells (7, 9). Unfortunately, this potentially useful cytotoxicity assay has been difficult to adapt to human tumor target cells. The test requires a target cell which will readily bind the isotope, will not release it spontaneously in appreciable amounts, and will promptly release sufficient quantities of the label upon cytolysis by immune lymphocytes. These requirements are well fulfilled by any number of mouse ascites tumor cell lines, but are only marginally, if at all, fulfilled by cells from human solid tumors. Thus, only in studies of human leukemia and lymphoid neoplasms has the chromium release assay been exploited (46).

The problems associated with the chromium release assay led to attempts to find more suitable isotopic markers for target cells. Among the most promising markers now in use are [^{125}I]-iododeoxyuridine (^{125}IDU; 11) and tritiated compounds, [^{3}H]thymidine, [^{3}H]uridine, and [^{3}H]proline (5, 31, 37). The ^{125}IDU assay has the clear-cut advantage of simplicity of counting, as ^{125}I, being a gamma emitter, can be counted more readily than can tritium, which requires liquid scintillation counting. However, IDU is toxic to the target cells, whereas the tritiated labels are more innocuous. Of course, it is possible that cell damage induced by the labels may enhance the sensitivity of the assay by making partially damaged cells more susceptible to lymphoid cell-mediated cytolysis. In any case, it appears that there is little fundamental difference among the various radioisotopic assays, and researchers continue to use the one with which they feel most comfortable.

The technical problems associated with cytotoxicity assays have consumed much of the discussion about their use. This has tended to obscure a more fundamental question. What does lymphocyte-mediated cytotoxicity measured in vitro really mean? Does it, in fact, reflect a phenomenon which is pertinent to tumor immunity in vivo? There is an obvious appeal to the conceptual correlation of tumor rejection and the ability of a lymphoid cell to kill a tumor cell in vitro. However, hard evidence that the cell that mediates cytolysis in vitro is identical to the cell that mediates tumor rejection in vivo is difficult, if not impossible, to obtain. It is hard to imagine that the presence

within an organism of lymphoid cells that have the ability to kill tumor cells can be harmful. But even this simple logic has been challenged by the work of Prehn (45), who has suggested that a weak immune response which is insufficient to destroy the tumor may enhance or promote its growth. In human solid tumors, the nearly universal finding has been that lymphocytes from cancer patients evidence cytotoxic activity against tumor cells of the same histological type as the lymphocyte donor. Since almost all patients, irrespective of the stages of their malignancies, appear to produce cytotoxic lymphocytes, much work has centered about the interactions of cytotoxic lymphocytes with serum factors that block or interfere with lymphocyte-mediated cytotoxicity. This has tended to obscure the very real possibility that quantitative differences in numbers or efficiency of cytotoxic lymphocytes may greatly influence the progression of the disease. To a large extent, this difficulty is due to inability to quantitate lymphocyte-mediated cytotoxicity accurately, and most work has tended simply to classify lymphocytes as cytotoxic or noncytotoxic. More recent data, in studies of melanoma patients, have suggested that the magnitude of the cytotoxic response does, indeed, bear some relationship to the clinical course of the disease (28, 50). If this is the case, then it provides strong indirect evidence that cytotoxic lymphocytes are not simply an in vitro phenomenon, but do play an important role in tumor-host interactions.

Blastogenesis (see chapter 9)

Cytotoxicity reflects the final event in a series of cellular reactions. The earlier phases of the initiation of immune responses to tumors, i.e., the interaction between lymphoid cells and tumor antigens, may be of equal importance. The most convenient tool for the study of recognition of tumor antigens by lymphoid cells is the blastogenesis assay. In this test, lymphocytes are cultivated in the presence of tumor antigens, in the form of either intact tumor cells or extracts of tumor cells, and deoxyribonucleic acid synthesis or some other aspect of lymphocyte proliferation is measured. The major conceptual difficulty with blastogenesis assays is the question of what the blastogenic response represents. Does it indicate prior sensitization to tumor antigens, or does it simply indicate an antigenic disparity between the responding cell and that antigen? The evidence, albeit indirect, would seem to favor the former. It is well known that lymphocytes cannot be stimulated by soluble antigens, such as purified protein derivative (PPD) or mumps antigen, without prior exposure of the host to these antigens. However, one cannot be absolutely certain whether this is the case in humans, since lymphocytes obtained prior to tumor development are not available. Thus, some investigators resist using blastogenesis as a measure of "cell-mediated immunity," although it probably represents the detection and recognition of tumor-associated antigens.

The blastogenesis test has been remarkably useful in the study of immune responses to lymphoid tumors. Leukemia cells and cultured lymphoblastoid cells, obtained from lymphomas, leukemias, or the peripheral blood of patients with mononucleosis or normal individuals, have been shown by many laboratories to have remarkable stimulating properties when tested against responder lymphocytes of the same donor. The blastogenic response by remission-phase lymphocytes to leukemic cells has been reported to have clinical significance. Moreover, the presence in the serum of a leukemic patient of antibodies that can inhibit his blastogenesis has also been reported to be a good prognostic sign (23).

One of the major drawbacks to the blastogenesis assay is that it is hard to determine the nature of the stimulating antigen and the specificities involved. Golub and associates (20) have attempted to circumvent this problem by correlating the cytotoxic activity of lymphocytes with blastogenic responses in vitro, using lymphocytes from patients who have Burkitt's lymphoma. In this system, lymphocytes could be stimulated very effectively with mitomycin-treated lymphoblastoid cells derived from autochthonous tumors. In these experiments, the lymphocytes responding (by blastogenesis) to the lymphoblastoid cell antigens were then recovered and tested for cytotoxicity in a colony inhibition assay. The results indicated that Burkitt tumor-derived target cells were effectively killed by responder lymphocytes, whereas control target cells were not. This approach permits the determination of the specific antigens involved in the blastogenesis assay.

The blastogenesis assay has also been used for the estimation of cellular immune responses to solid tumors. Immune responses to human sarcomas and malignant melanoma have been detected with the blastogenesis assay (38, 42, 56). In these studies, lymphocytes from tumor-bearing patients or from patients "cured" of tumors by surgical resection have been shown to undergo blastogenesis upon exposure to tumor cells or solubilized tumor antigens. There is suggestive evidence that the degree of lymphocyte stimulation may correlate with prognosis and/or extent of disease. In some of these studies, sera from tumor-bearing patients have been shown to block this blastogenic response. (Blastogenesis provides another method for assaying serum "blocking factors.") In contradistinction to the observations of Gutterman and colleagues in leukemia patients (23), the detection of serum blocking activity in these cases was correlated with a poor prognosis and/or with extensive disease.

The fact that soluble extracts of tumor tissue (presumably containing solubilized tumor-associated antigens) have been shown to stimulate lymphocytes from cancer patients to undergo blastogenesis is of considerable significance. The blastogenesis assay may provide a "bioassay" for detecting the presence of solubilized tumor antigens and may prove extremely useful for monitoring the isolation and purification of tumor-associated antigens.

Detection of lymphokines (see chapters 10 and 13)

Some humoral substances are elaborated by specifically sensitized lymphocytes upon contact with antigen. These substances are collectively called "lymphokines." Two of these have been utilized for the detection of cellular immune responses to tumor-associated antigens. The first of these is migration inhibition factor (MIF). The inhibition of macrophage migration by the products of sensitized lymphocytes has been one of the best of in vitro correlates of delayed hypersensitivity. In the usual MIF assay, antigen and putatively sensitized lymphocytes are allowed to interact, and the supernatant fluid containing MIF is tested on normal macrophages (usually guinea pig peritoneal exudate cells) for the inhibition of migration. There have been studies in animal model systems in which tumor-specific immunity has been detected by the generation of MIF from sensitized lymphocytes in the presence of tumor cells (33, 54).

Given the background of positive results in animals and the good correlations known to exist between MIF production and delayed cutaneous hypersensitivity reactions as measured by skin tests, it is obvious that this would be an assay with considerable potential for the study of tumor immunity in humans. This is especially true with the advent of skin testing for tumor-associated antigens in humans. However, with few exceptions (30, 58) attempts to use the usual "indirect" type of MIF assay described above for the detection of human tumor-associated antigens have been unsuccessful. Most of the success in this field has resulted from a "direct" assay in which leukocytes from cancer patients are tested for their migration in the presence or absence of tumor cell extracts. Presumably, the mechanism of inhibition of leukocyte migration is similar to that of inhibition of macrophage migration.

This leukocyte inhibition of migration assay (the so-called "LIF" assay) has been used by Andersen et al. in a study of immune responses to human breast carcinoma antigens (2). Perhaps the most effective exploitation of this technique has been in the studies of Cochran and co-workers of immune responses to malignant melanoma (10). These studies are particularly interesting because the authors were able to correlate variations in the quantitative extent of cellular immunity, as detected by this technique, with the clinical stage of disease. As has been mentioned earlier, most studies involving the determination of lymphocyte-mediated cytotoxicity have found little correlation between the absolute level of cytotoxicity and prognosis or clinical stage.

The migration inhibition assays have the distinct advantage of speed. These assays are usually complete the day after initiation of the experiment. This certainly compares favorably with the several days to a week required for cytotoxicity or blastogenesis assays. The equipment required is minimal, and the technique can be readily standardized. The amount of migration inhibition usually observed with tumor-associated antigens is small (of the order of 30 to 40%), and difficulties due to nonspecific toxicity of some of the antigen preparations may be encountered. Unfortunately, little is known of the relationship between leukocyte migration inhibition and other cell-mediated immune reactions, and comparison of results obtained with this assay and results obtained with other assays is difficult. It is clear that leukocyte migration along with the blastogenesis assay may prove useful for the analysis of antigenic extracts of a tumor, and preliminary evidence would seem to indicate that it may prove useful for the analysis of cell-mediated immunity in the cancer patient as well. Whether it will be as useful as cytotoxicity assays for the analysis of interactions between immune lymphocytes and serum blocking factors remains to be determined.

The second lymphokine of possible significance in tumor immunology is known as "lymphotoxin." This substance (or substances), like MIF, is also elaborated by sensitized lymphocytes upon exposure to antigen. Lymphotoxin is considered by many investigators to be responsible for the cytotoxic effects exerted by lymphocytes. Cytotoxic effects can be generated either by specifically sensitized lymphocytes stimulated with antigens to which the lympho-cytes are immune or by lymphocytes nonspecifically stimulated with mitogens (21, 47). In either case, the cytotoxic effect is on a third party or "bystander" cell and is nonspecific. Presumably, activation of specifically immune lymphocytes by tumor-specific antigens produces cytotoxic effects upon tumor cells by a similar mechanism. This concept is consistent with data suggesting that cytotoxicity is a two-stage phenomenon, the first stage being immunologically specific activation by antigen, and the second being a nonspecific cytotoxic event (12). However, this leaves the problem of specificity open, and it remains difficult to explain why tumor cells are killed preferentially by the lymphotoxins and normal cells are not. This may be due, at least in part, to differential sensitivities to lymphotoxins (48).

Delayed hypersensitivity reactions (see chapter 6)

Perhaps no single reaction of cellular immunity is so simple and so readily estimated as the delayed cutaneous hypersensitivity responses. Because of their simplicity, safety, and ease and rapidity of elicitation, skin test responses to a variety of antigens have been extensively studied in a variety of animal tumor-host systems and in many human cancer patients. Delayed cutaneous hypersensitivity responses in cancer patients have been more extensively studied than any other immunological aspect.

The vast majority of these studies have dealt with the evaluation of skin test reactivity to nonspecific antigens (i.e., antigens unrelated to any tumor-associated antigen) in order to evaluate the immunocompetence of cancer patients, or, rather, in order to evaluate the competence of the cellular immune responses of cancer patients. Two general groups of antigens have been employed. The first group are common "recall" antigens, antigens to which all or most adults may be expected to have been sensitized. These include tuberculin (PPD), monilia, mumps, trichophyton, and the streptococcal antigens streptokinase and streptodornase (Varidase). The second group consists of organic chemical haptens which do not exist in nature and which are potent sensitizing haptens when applied to human skin. Sensitization occurs when the hapten combines with proteins in the skin. When a challenging dose of the same hapten is applied 2 weeks later, a delayed cutaneous hypersensitivity response results in most immunocompetent subjects. On the assumption that exposure of the host to the tumor-associated antigens of a newly established tumor constitutes a primary stimulus to a new antigen, it has been widely held that testing with such haptenic antigens may be of peculiar value in immunocompetence testing of cancer patients. In addition, these haptens have the unquestioned advantage of testing antigen recognition and processing (the afferent arc of the immune response), as well as effector responses. The most widely employed haptenic agent for such testing has been dinitrochlorobenzene (DNCB), to which approximately 95% of normal, immunocompetent adults will become effectively sensitized.

The incidences of skin test reactivity to "recall" antigens and to DNCB have been correlated with prognosis and/or the extent of disease in a wide variety of human neoplasms. A number of studies have suggested that tests of delayed cutaneous sensitivity to such antigens may be a guide to prognosis and may, perhaps, eventually lead to the identification of groups of cancer patients who, because of their poor prognosis, should receive adjuvant therapies.

Another application of such tests of immunocompetence may be to influence the selection of immunotherapeutic modality most appropriate for each patient. Active immunization may not be a suitable approach for an anergic cancer patient. Anergic patients may be better served by passive or adoptive forms of immunotherapy.

Delayed cutaneous hypersensitivity reactions to extracts of human tumor cells have also bee elicited in cancer patients. It is hoped that such responses may reflect tumor-specific cellular immunity of the host, since there is suggestive evidence that positive skin test reactions to tumor antigens may correlate with a favorable prognosis. Recently, two types of tumor extracts have been particularly promising as skin test reagents for studying tumor-specific cutaneous responses. One is a tumor cell membrane extract (43) which has been utilized to elicit skin reactions in patients with mammary cancer (1), malignant melanoma (16), Burkitt's lymphoma (15), and cervical carcinoma (57). The second is a solubilized antigen preparation produced by extracting tumor cells with hypertonic 3 M potassium chloride (38). This type of extract has been used to elicit cutaneous reactions in patients with leukemia and melanoma. Of considerable interest is the fact that this type of antigen preparation will also induce lymphocytes from tumor-bearing patients to undergo blastogenic responses in vitro. If such extracts do indeed contain solubilized tumor-associated antigens (and it appears that they do), it is to be hoped that these antigens may eventually be isolated in purified form from such preparations.

METHODS FOR ASSESSMENT OF HUMORAL IMMUNITY

In discussing humoral immune responses to tumor-associated antigens, it is appropriate to consider humoral factors in their broader rather than narrower sense so as to include not only a consideration of serum antibodies directed against tumor antigens but also other serum factors related to tumor-specific immune responses which interact with the cellular reactions discussed above. Such serum factors can be divided into two groups: (i) serum "blocking" factors which impede or block lymphocyte-mediated cytotoxic immune responses and (ii) serum factors which promote lymphocyte-mediated cytotoxicity.

All of these serum factors are estimated by variations of the methods for assessing lymphocyte-mediated cytotoxic immune reactions discussed above. Serum is incubated with either target cells or lymphocytes prior to the cocultivation of lymphocytes and target cells in the cytotoxicity assays. The enhancement or diminution of cytotoxic activity produced by the serum is compared with the undisturbed cytotoxic activity of the same lymphocytes incubated in control serum.

Serum "blocking" factors

Two types of interactions which would result in inhibition of the cytotoxic effect of lymphocytes upon tumor cells can be envisioned. The first type of "blocking" activity is assumed to affect the efferent limb of the immune response by the masking of antigenic determinants on the target tumor cells by immunoglobulins, which prevent recognition of tumor cells by immune lymphocytes and therefore abort subsequent cytotoxic effects.

Many of our current concepts of serum blocking activity in human tumor systems are related directly to the findings of the Hellströms. Their pioneering work indicated that most cancer patients have lymphocytes which are cytotoxic for tumor cells of the same histopathological type as the tumor of the patient. The presence of cytotoxic lymphocytes seemed to be a relatively constant finding in all patients except those with extremely advanced disease and, with that exception, appeared to be unrelated to the clinical status of the patient. However, they found a strong correlation between the presence of blocking factors in the sera of patients and the clinical status of their disease. Patients who had progressive disease had a much higher incidence and much higher levels of serum factors which would inhibit lymphocyte cytotoxic activity than did patients who were apparently "cured" or tumor-free. Sera from such patients manifested little or no blocking activity (27). Since blocking activity could be absorbed with tumor cells and could clearly be demonstrated in the immunoglobulin fraction of the serum, it was assumed to represent tumor-specific antibody. However, the mechanism of blocking was not immediately apparent. Although it was possible that tumor-specific antibodies would mask the antigenic determinants on the tumor cells and thereby protect the tumor cell from the action of the cytotoxic lymphocyte, this did not explain the rapid disappearance of the blocking activity in patients following resection of the tumor. Why the production of tumor-specific antibodies should cease following extirpation of a tumor was not known. However, later findings by Sjögren and co-workers (49) suggested that the blocking activity was due to antigen-antibody complexes rather than antibody alone. Obviously, the antigen-antibody ratio must be less than that required to saturate all antibody-combining sites, as the complexes can be absorbed out with tumor cells (3). Antigen-antibody complexes would provide a bifunctional type of blocking agent that could block efferent cytotoxic activity at the level of the tumor cell by masking the antigenic sites on the tumor cell surface or at the level of the effector cell, by reacting with receptors for tumor antigen on the surface of the immune lymphocyte. Under both circumstances the lymphocyte is prevented from interacting properly with the target tumor cell.

A different form of blocking in which antibody apparently plays no role has been described. This type of blocking is apparently due to circulating soluble antigen, perhaps shed from the cell membrane by metabolic turnover, which interacts with receptors on the surfaces of immune lymphocytes and renders these cells noncytotoxic. Recent work has suggested that it plays an important role in tumor-specific immune reactions, as found in animal tumor-host systems by Sjögren, by Alexander, and by Baldwin. Baldwin, in a rat hepatoma system, has measured the effect of the quantity of antigen and has studied the interactions of antigen with antibody in a very elegant fashion. He has shown the importance of the ratio of antigen and antigen-antibody complex in inhibiting lymphocyte cytotoxicity. Recent work has suggested that this type of blocking plays an important role in cell-mediated immunity to human melanomas. Currie and Basham have shown that lymphocyte-bound tumor-associated antigens can inhibit the cytotoxic activity

of lymphocytes and may be quantitatively correlated with the tumor burden in the patient (13).

Serum factors which promote cytotoxicity

Two types of serum effects which promote cytotoxicity have been described. The first, termed "unblocking" by the Hellströms (26), is thought to represent the interaction of free antibody with blocking complexes. The Hellströms found that sera from patients who were disease-free or ostensibly "cured" seldom contained blocking activity. Moreover, when such serum samples were mixed with serum samples from patients with progressive disease which manifested significant blocking activity in vitro, the blocking activity was abrogated. Furthermore, Bansal and Sjögren have shown that "unblocking" activity in vitro is correlated with enhanced tumor immunity (tumor regression responses) in vivo (4).

A number of possible mechanisms for unblocking can be envisioned, although definitive evidence for the mechanism is lacking. One possibility, not favored by the proponents of unblocking, is that unblocking is merely cytotoxic antibody which in the presence of complement can yield cytolysis of target tumor cells. Although the addition of complement is not necessary to demonstrate unblocking activity in vitro, it is at least conceivable that small amounts of complement synthesized by the cells added to the culture, along with heat-stable components in the serum, could yield the effect. However, the kinetics of the reaction argue against cytotoxicity. It seems more likely that unblocking serum is antitumor antibody which saturates the available antigen sites in the soluble antigen-antibody complexes and thereby prevents their interaction with immune lymphocytes. If this is the case, then this would argue against any significant role for blocking by antibody alone due to masking of antigen sites on the target tumor cells. The final hypothesis is that unblocking activity is the equivalent of antibody-dependent cellular cytotoxicity, which is discussed below. If that is the case, then it is possible that one type of cytotoxicity can continue in the presence of an inhibition of a second type of cytotoxicity.

The second form of serum-promoted or -enhanced cytotoxicity is what has been termed "antibody-dependent cellular cytotoxicity" (ADCC). This phenomenon has also been described as lymphocyte-dependent antibody, "arming" antibody, and synergistic cytotoxicity. A proliferation of descriptive titles for a phenomenon invariably indicates a failure to understand the phenomenon, and ADCC is no exception. It has been intensively investigated recently, primarily by Perlmann and Mac-Lennan (36, 44). The phenomenon basically consists of cytotoxicity mediated by nonimmune lymphoid cells in the presence of antibody specific for the target cell. The reaction represents a nonphagocytic type of cytotoxicity, and, although sera from a number of different species have been utilized, it has been reported that only immunoglobulin G (IgG) fractions are active in promoting this form of cytotoxicity. The cytotoxicity is completely independent of complement. The antibodies must have an intact Fc fragment, which appears to indicate that the Fc fragment of the IgG molecule attaches to the lymphoid cell and the combining site then attaches to the target cell (34). The result is an event which is cytotoxic to the target cell. It is of interest that only certain types of lymphoid cells can be activated or "armed" in this fashion. Thymus-derived lymphocytes (T cells) are completely inactive in this assay, whereas bursal equivalent-derived lymphocytes (B cells) are active (55). Mononuclear and polymorphonuclear cells have been reported to be active, as well as "null cells" (lymphocytes which are neither T cells nor B cells) (22). The lymphocytes which act as killer cells in the ADCC reaction have been called K-

cells (killer cells) and contain Fc receptor on their membranes.

Thus, tumor immunology is obviously a multicomponent system (Fig. 1). Assuming at most 10 components (which is obviously insufficient since this would group all lymphokines as one component, complement as a single component, all immunoglobulin classes as one component, etc.), this could lead to 10^{10} possible interactions. Any single experiment cannot hope to examine more than one small aspect of the larger picture.

Methods for measurement of antitumor antibodies

The first method employed in the late 1950s and early 1960s to detect the presence of antitumor antibodies was tanned red cell hemagglutination with the use of either fresh or formalinized sheep erythrocytes. Although a number of significant studies resulted from the use of this technique, problems resulting from spontaneous agglutination of sheep red cells by the crude, aqueous extracts of tumor tissue employed as antigens resulted in these methods being larely forsaken for newer methods described below. Although tanned red cell hemagglutination remains a very important method for assessing antibodies to a variety of antigens, this technique is now rarely used in

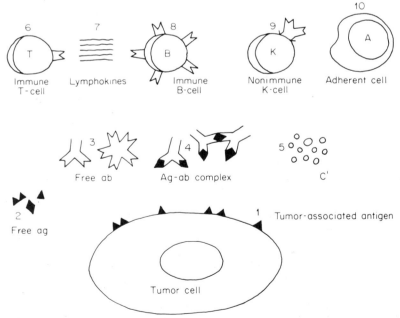

FIG. 1. *Components of tumor-specific immunity: (1) the tumor cell with tumor-associated antigens on its surface, (2) free tumor antigen, (3) free antibody to tumor antigen, (4) antigen-antibody complexes, (5) complement, (6) specifically immune T lymphocytes, (7) the lymphokines, (8) specifically immune B lymphocytes, (9) nonimmune K lymphocytes, (10) adherent cells, ? macrophages.*

measuring antibodies to tumor antigens.

Perhaps the most widely utilized test for the detection of antitumor antibodies is immunofluorescence. Two types of immunofluorescence techniques are available. In one, which employs living tumor cells, membrane immunofluorescence is detected by fluorescent "dots and spots" on the tumor cell surface. The second method employs frozen sections of tumor tissue or air-dried acetone-fixed smears or "touch" preparations of tumor cells. In this instance, cytoplasmic fluorescence is detected within the dead fixed cells. Both the membrane immunofluorescence and cytoplasmic immunofluorescence tests may be further subdivided into direct and indirect tests. In the direct tests, immunoglobulins from the serum to be tested are conjugated with fluorescein prior to application to the tumor cells (18). In the indirect test, which is much more widely used, a "sandwich" technique is employed. The serum to be tested is first allowed to react with the tumor cells, after which the cells are washed and a fluorescein-labeled antiglobulin is applied as a "developing reagent." By using antiglobulin reagents directed against specific subclasses of immunoglobulins, the particular immunoglobulin class to which the antitumor antibody belongs may be elucidated (32). These methods have been particularly useful in demonstrating antibodies reactive with human tumor antigens in the sera of cancer patients (40, 41, 53).

A variation of the indirect immunofluorescence test on living tumor cells is the so-called radiolabeled antiglobulin binding test (8). In this test, the serum to be tested is allowed to react with living tumor cells. After a number of washes, an antiglobulin is applied which has previously been labeled with ^{125}I instead of fluorescein. Then, instead of examining the tumor cells under the fluorescence microscope for evidence of immunofluorescence, the tumor cells are counted in a gamma counter. The number of counts bound to the cells is an indirect measure of the amount of antitumor antibody bound to the tumor cell surface. This test has the advantage of being more amenable to quantitation than immunofluorescence and also provides the potential for defining the specific immunoglobulin class of the antibody. However, nonspecific adherence of the radiolabeled antiglobulin to the tumor cells is often a problem and frequently results in high nonspecific reactivity.

Another method for estimating antitumor antibody is complement fixation (14, 39). It is thought that antibodies which fix complement may be directed against tumor antigens on the cell surface and may be potentially clinically relevant cytotoxic-type antibodies (since complement is required for antibody-mediated immune cytolysis). There is some evidence that levels of complement-fixing antibodies may correlate with the clinical course of neoplastic disease in humans (39). These complement-fixation tests are usually performed as a micromethod in microtiter plates. Although intact tumor cells have been employed as antigens in these tests, it is more common to employ solubilized extracts of tumor cells. A problem which has prevented wide acceptance of the complement-fixation test centers on the fact that many of the antigen extracts are anticomplementary, particularly at higher concentrations.

Finally, a variety of methods exist for measuring the cytotoxic effects of antisera on tumor cells in the presence of complement (6, 17, 35, 59). Any of the methods for assessing lymphocyte-mediated cytotoxicity described above may be, and have been, modified to measure complement-dependent cytotoxic antibody activity by simply substituting antibody and complement for lymphocytes. Rabbit complement is usually employed and must be carefully absorbed to eliminate nonspecific reactions. These tests have the advantage of being quantitative and of providing information regarding the functional activity of the antibody. Antibodies measured by these techniques are of particular interest because it is attractive to postulate that such antibodies may have antitumor cytotoxic effects in vivo and may therefore be of clinical significance. It may be hazardous, however, to assume that antibodies which mediate cytotoxic reactions against tumor target cells in vitro are cytotoxic to tumor cells in vivo.

LITERATURE CITED

1. Alford, C., A. C. Hollinshead, and R. B. Herberman. 1973. Delayed cutaneous hypersensitivity reactions to extracts of malignant and normal human breast cells. Ann. Surg. 178:20–24.

2. Andersen, V., O. Bjerrum, G. Bendexin, T. Schiødt, and I. Dissing. 1970. Effects of autologous mammary tumor extracts on human leukocyte migration in vitro. Int. J. Cancer 5:357–363.

3. Baldwin, R. W., M. R. Price, and R. A. Robins. 1972. Blocking of lymphocyte-mediated cytotoxicity by tumour-specific antigen-antibody complexes. Nature (London) New Biol. 238:185–187.

4. Bansal, S. C., and H. O. Sjögren. 1972. Counteraction of the blocking of cell-mediated tumor immunity by inoculation of unblocking sera and splenectomy: immunotherapeutic effects on primary polvoma tumors in rats. Int. J. Cancer 9:490–509.

5. Bean, M. A., H. Pees, G. Rosen, and H. F.

Oettgen. 1973. Prelabeling target cells with ^{3}H-proline as a method for studying lymphocyte cytotoxicity. Natl. Cancer Inst. Monogr. 37:41–48.

6. Bloom, E. T. 1970. Quantitative detection of cytotoxic antibodies against tumor specific antigens of murine sarcomas induced by 3-methylcholanthrene. J. Natl. Cancer Inst. 45:443–453.

7. Brunner, K. T., J. Mauel, J.-C. Cerottini, and B. Chapuis. 1968. Quantitative assay of the lytic action of lymphoid cells on ^{51}Cr labelled allogeneic target cells in vitro: inhibition by isoantibody and by drugs. Immunology 14: 181–190.

8. Burdick, J. F., A. M. Cohen, and S. A. Wells. 1973. A simplified isotopic antiglobulin assay: detection of tumor-cell antigens. J. Natl. Cancer Inst. 50:285–289.

9. Canty, T. G., and J. R. Wunderlich. 1970. Quantitative in vitro assay of cytotoxic cellular immunity. J. Natl. Cancer Inst. 45:761–772.

10. Cochran, A. J., W. G. S. Spilg, R. M. Mackie, and C. E. Thomas. 1972. Postoperative depression of tumour-directed cell-mediated immunity in patients with malignant disease. Br. Med. J. 4:67–70.

11. Cohen, A. M., J. F. Burdick, and A. S. Ketcham. 1971. Cell-mediated cytotoxicity: an assay using ^{125}I-iododeoxyuridine-labeled target cells. J. Immunol. 107:895–898.

12. Cohen, I. R., and M. Feldman. 1971. The lysis of fibroblasts by lymphocytes sensitized in vitro: specific antigen activates a nonspecific effect. Cell. Immunol. 1:521–535.

13. Currie, G. A., and C. Basham. 1972. Serum mediated inhibition of the immunological reactions of the patient to his own tumor: a possible role for circulating antigen. Br. J. Cancer 26:427–438.

14. Eilber, F. R., and D. L. Morton. 1970. Sarcoma-specific antigens: detection by complement fixation with serum from sarcoma patients. J. Natl. Cancer Inst. 44:651–656.

15. Fass, L., R. B. Herberman, and J. Ziegler. 1970. Delayed cutaneous hypersensitivity reactions to autologous Burkitt-lymphoma cells. N. Engl. J. Med. 282:776–780.

16. Fass, L., J. L. Ziegler, R. B. Herberman, and J. W. M. Kiryabwire. 1970. Cutaneous hypersensitivity reactions to autologous extracts of malignant melanoma cells. Lancet 1:116–118.

17. Fritze, D., D. H. Kern, and Y. H. Pilch. 1974. Brief communication. Quantitation of cytotoxic antitumor antibody in vitro: a microassay with ^{125}I-iododeoxyuridine as a tumor cell label. J. Natl. Cancer Inst. 53:1403–1407.

18. Goldstein, G., G. Klein, G. Pearson, and P. Clifford. 1969. Direct membrane immunofluorescence reaction of Burkitt's lymphoma cells in culture. Cancer Res. 29:749–752.

19. Golub, S. H., T. X. O'Connell, and D. L. Morton. 1974. Correlation of in vivo and in vitro assays of immunocompetence in cancer patients. Cancer Res. 34:1833–1837.

20. Golub, S. H., E. A. J. Svedmyr, J. F. Hewetson, G. Klein, and S. Singh. 1972. Cellular reactions against Burkitt lymphoma cells. III. Effector cell activity of leukocytes stimulated in vitro with autochthonous cultured lymphoma cells. Int. J. Cancer 10:157–164.

21. Granger, G. A., and W. M. Kolb. 1968. Lymphocyte in vitro cytotoxicity: mechanisms of immune and non-immune small lymphocyte mediated L-cell destruction. J. Immunol. 101:111–120.

22. Greenberg, A. H., L. Hudson, L. Shen, and I. M. Roitt. 1973. Antibody-dependent cell-mediated cytotoxicity due to a "null" lymphoid cell. Nature (London) New Biol. 242: 111–113.

23. Gutterman, J. U., R. D. Rossen, and W. T. Butler. 1973. Immunoglobulin on tumor cells and tumor-induced blastogenesis in human acute leukemia. N. Engl. J. Med. 288:169–175.

24. Hellström, I. 1967. A colony inhibition (CI) technique for demonstration of tumor cell destruction by lymphoid cells in vitro. Int. J. Cancer 2:65–68.

25. Hellström, I., K. E. Hellström, G. E. Pierce, and J. P. S. Yang. 1968. Cellular and humoral immunity to different types of human neoplasms. Nature (London) 220:1352–1354.

26. Hellström, I., K. E. Hellström, H. O. Sjögren, and G. A. Warner. 1971. Serum factors in tumor-free patients cancelling the blocking of cell-mediated tumor immunity. Int. J. Cancer 8:185–191.

27. Hellström, I., H. O. Sjögren, G. Warner, and K. E. Hellström. 1971. Blocking of cell-mediated tumor immunity by sera from patients with growing neoplasms. Int. J. Cancer 7: 226–237.

28. Hellström, I., G. A. Warner, K. E. Hellström, and H. O. Sjögren. 1973. Sequential studies on cell-mediated immunity and blocking serum activity in ten patients with malignant melanoma. Int. J. Cancer 11:280–292.

29. Herberman, R. B., and C. E. Gaylord. 1973. Conference and workshop on cellular immune reactions to human tumor-associated antigens. Natl. Cancer Inst. Monogr. no. 37.

30. Hilberg, R. W., S. P. Balcerzak, and A. F. Lo Buglio. 1973. A migration inhibition factor assay for tumor immunity in man. Cell. Immunol. 7:152–158.

31. Jagarlamoody, S. M., J. C. Aust, R. H. Tew, and C. F. McKhann. 1971. In vitro detection of cytotoxic cellular immunity against tumor-specific antigens by a radioisotopic technique. Proc. Natl. Acad. Sci. U.S.A. 68:1346–1350.

32. Klein, G., P. Clifford, E. Klein, and J. Stjernswärd. 1966. Search for tumor specific immune reactions in Burkitt lymphoma patients by the membrane immunofluorescence reaction. Proc. Natl. Acad. Sci. U.S.A. 55:1628–1635.

33. Kronman, B. S., H. T. Wepsic, W. H. Churchill, Jr., B. Zbar, T. Borsos, and H. J. Rapp. 1969. Tumor-specific antigens detected by inhibi-

tion of macrophage migration. Science 165: 296–297.

34. Larsson, A., and H. Perlmann. 1972. Study of Fab and F(ab')₂ from rabbit IgG for capacity to induce lymphocyte mediated target cell destruction *in vitro*. Int. Arch. Allergy Appl. Immunol. 43:80–88.

35. Lewis, M. G., R. L. Ikonopisov, R. C. Nairn, T. M. Phillips, G. H. Fairley, D. C. Bodenham, and P. Alexander. 1969. Tumour-specific antibodies in human malignant melanoma and their relationship to the extent of the disease. Br. Med. J. 3:547–552.

36. MacLennan, I. C. M., G. Loewi, and B. Harding. 1970. The role of immunoglobulins in lymphocyte mediated cell damage *in vitro* I. Comparison of the effects of target cell specific antibody and normal serum factors on cellular damage by immune and non-immune lymphocytes. Immunology 18:397–404.

37. MacPherson, B. R., and Y. H. Pilch. 1972. Cellular cytolysis *in vitro*: mechanisms underlying a quantitative assay for cellular immunity. J. Natl. Cancer Inst. 48:1619–1627.

38. Mavligit, G. M., U. Ambus, J. U. Gutterman, and E. M. Hersh. 1973. Antigen solubilized from human solid tumours: lymphocyte stimulation and cutaneous delayed hypersensitivity. Nature (London) New Biol. 243:188–190.

39. Morton, D. L., F. R. Eilber, R. A. Malmgren, and W. C. Wood. 1970. Immunological factors which influence response to immunotherapy in malignant melanoma. Surgery 68:158–164.

40. Morton, D. L., R. A. Malmgren, E. C. Holmes, and A. Ketcham. 1968. Demonstration of antibodies against human malignant melanoma by immunofluorescence. Surgery 64:233–240.

41. Muna, N., S. Marcus, and C. Smart. 1969. Detection by immunofluorescence of antibodies specific for human malignant melanoma cells. Cancer 23:88–93.

42. Nagel, G. A., G. St. Arneault, J. F. Holland, D. Kirkpatrick, and R. Kirkpatrick. 1970. Cell-mediated immunity against malignant melanoma in monozygous twins. Cancer Res. 30:1828–1832.

43. Oren, M. D., and R. B. Herberman. 1971. Delayed cutaneous hypersensitivity reactions to membrane extracts of human tumor cells. Clin. Exp. Immunol. 9:45–56.

44. Perlmann, P., and H. Perlmann. 1970. Contactual lysis of antibody-coated chicken erythrocytes by purified lymphocytes. Cell. Immunol. 1:300–315.

45. Prehn, R. T. 1972. The immune reaction as a stimulator of tumor growth. Science 176:170–171.

46. Rosenberg, E. B., R. B. Herberman, P. H. Levine, R. H. Halterman, J. L. McCoy, and J. R. Wunderlich. 1972. Lymphocyte cytotoxicity reactions to leukemia associated antigens in

identical twins. Int. J. Cancer 9:648–658.

47. Ruddle, N. H., and B. H. Waksman. 1968. Cytotoxic effect of lymphocyte-antigen interaction in delayed hypersensitivity. Science 157:1060–1062.

48. Singh, J. N., E. Sabbadine, and A. H. Sehon. 1973. Detection of nonspecific cytotoxicity in graft-versus-host reaction as a function of target cell type. Cell. Immunol. 8:280–289.

49. Sjögren, H. O., I. Hellström, S. C. Bansal, and K. E. Hellström. 1971. Suggestive evidence that the "blocking antibodies" of tumor-bearing individuals may be antigen-antibody complexes. Proc. Natl. Acad. Sci. U.S.A. 68: 1372–1375.

50. Sulit, H., D. Chee, and M. Mastrangelo. 1972. *In vitro* assays of cellular and humoral immunity during a clinical trial of immunotherapy in human melanoma. Proc. Am. Assoc. Cancer Res. 13:21.

51. Takasugi, M., and E. Klein. 1970. A microassay for cell-mediated immunity. Transplantation 9:219–227.

52. Takasugi, M., M. R. Mickey, and P. Terasaki. 1973. Quantitation of the microassay for cell-mediated immunity through electronic image analysis. Natl. Cancer Inst. Monogr. 37:77–84.

53. Tevethia, S. S., M. Katz, and F. Rapp. 1965. New surface antigen in cells transformed by simian papovavirus SV40. Proc. Soc. Exp. Biol. Med. 119:896–901.

54. Vaage, J., R. D. Jones, and B. W. Brown. 1972. Tumor-specific resistance in mice detected by inhibition of macrophage migration. Cancer Res. 32:680–687.

55. van Boxel, J. A., J. D. Stobo, W. E. Paul, and I. Green. 1972. Antibody-dependent lymphoid cell-mediated cytotoxicity: no requirement for thymus-derived lymphocytes. Science 175: 194–196.

56. Vanky, F., J. Stjernswärd, G. Klein, and V. Nilsonne. 1971. Serum-mediated inhibition of lymphocyte stimulation by autochthonous human tumors. J. Natl. Cancer Inst. 47:95–103.

57. Wagner, H., and M. Rollinghoff. 1973. *In vitro* induction of tumor-specific immunity. I. Parameters of activation and cytotoxic reactivity of mouse lymphoid cells immunized *in vitro* against syngeneic and allogeneic plasma cell tumors. J. Exp. Med. 138:1–15.

58. Wolberg, W. H., and M. L. Goelzer. 1971. *In vitro* assay of cell mediated immunity in human cancer: definition of leukocyte migration inhibitory factor. Nature (London) 229:632–634.

59. Wood, W. C., and D. Morton. 1970. Microcytotoxicity test: detection in sarcoma patients of antibody cytotoxic to human sarcoma cells. Science 170:1318–1320.

Section J

TRANSPLANTATION IMMUNOLOGY

Chapter 102

Introduction

EDMOND J. YUNIS AND L. J. GREENBERG

We have attempted in the various sections of this *Manual* to provide the reader with detailed accounts of methods routinely in use for clinical tissue typing as it relates to allotransplantation, blood transfusion, and, more recently, the study of disease. Some methods (capillary leuko-agglutination and the leukocyte aggregation test), although not in routine use, have been included since they offer novel approaches to the diagnosis of allograft rejection. It should also be pointed out that some tests have not been included, not because they are unimportant but because they either are not applicable for routine testing or are still being evaluated for their specificity.

The human major histocompatibility complex, designated the HLA region and located on chromosome 6, includes several genetic loci having different classes of product and probably different functions. At present, four genetic loci designated HLA-A, HLA-B, HLA-C, and HLA-D have been described. The products of the HLA-A and HLA-B loci, formerly designated the 1st and 2nd loci, have been studied extensively, and serological tests for the detection of most of the specificities are in routine use.

The HLA-C and HLA-D loci are less well defined. HLA-C reputedly produces a product of different chemical composition which may be less stable than the HLA-A and HLA-B gene products. Like the HLA-A and HLA-B products, the HLA-C antigens are believed to be present on all lymphoid cells. This is not necessarily true of the HLA-D. The HLA-D gene is responsible for the ability of lymphocytes to stimulate allogeneic lymphocytes in mixed culture. As stimulation is largely or wholly a function of B lymphocytes, the HLA-D product is probably expressed mainly on the B lymphocyte, and, since vascular endothelial cells can also stimulate, presumably is also expressed on these cells.

Typing of HLA-A, -B, and -C specificities is done either by lymphocyte microcytotoxicity or by platelet complement-fixation texts not routinely used. The composite description of the HLA antigens of one person is called the phenotype. Although the HLA linkage group is not a single genetic locus, a large group of alleles can identify the segregation of paternal and maternal antigens by the serological reactions transmitted to the children. Therefore, only six genotypes could be found in a given family. The paternal genes are usually designated as A and B and the maternal as C and D. There are four possible genotypes in the children: AC, BD, AD, and BD. Two haplotypes (composite alignment of two or more loci in one chromosome) form one genotype (Table 1). The genes controlling the production of these alloantigens are codominant, since they are expressed in each member of the family. The inheritance of HLA haplotypes defined by HLA antisera can be corroborated by the mixed lymphocyte culture (MLC) since, in most families, the children inheriting identical haplotypes fail to stimulate in MLC. Studies of families have revealed several examples of recombination between HLA-A and HLA-B of the maternal or paternal haplotypes.

The genetic control of stimulation in MLC has been studied in families in which there are children with recombination between HLA-A and HLA-B or between HLA-B and HLA-D. These studies revealed that siblings differing at HLA-B and not HLA-A produce mutual stimulation of lymphocyte blastogenesis. Furthermore, the observation that some haploidentical siblings are not stimulatory whereas HLA identical siblings are mutually stimulatory suggested the existence of a locus (HLA-D) independent of and outside of HLA-B.

Several other genetic loci are believed to be more loosely linked to HLA. These include immune response genes controlling responsiveness to allogeneic lymphocytes and genes controlling responsiveness to a variety of bacterial and other natural product antigens. Structural genes for several enzymes and for C'2 and C'3b components of complement have also been located on the same chromosome as HLA. The mapping of human genes has been greatly facilitated through the development of techniques for somatic-cell hybridization, i.e., the fusion of human somatic cells with cells of other mammals. When human cells are fused with mouse or hamster cells under appropriate culture con-

TABLE 1. *Inheritance of HLA antigens*

Antisera		♂ AB	♀ CD	Siblings					Chromosome marker
				1	2	3	4	5	
Anti	HLA-A	+	−	+	−	+	−	+	A
	HLA-B	+	−	+	−	+	−	+	
Anti	HLA-A	+	−	−	+	−	+	−	B
	HLA-B	+	−	−	+	−	+	−	
Anti	HLA-A	−	+	+	−	−	+	+	C
	HLA-B	−	+	+	−	−	+	+	
Anti	HLA-A	−	+	−	+	+	−	−	D
	HLA-B	−	+	−	+	+	−	−	

GENOTYPES

Paternal haplo-types	A Ⓐ B / A Ⓑ B	A Ⓐ B / A Ⓑ B	A Ⓐ B / A Ⓑ B	A Ⓐ B

Maternal haplotypes: A Ⓒ B / A Ⓓ B   A Ⓒ B / A Ⓓ B   A Ⓓ B   A Ⓒ B / A Ⓒ B

ditions, the rodent genetic material is retained intact while the human chromosomes are selectively lost. Cells retaining the C′6 chromosome have been found to express HLA as well as several enzyme markers (Fig. 1).

Although the full biological significance of the genes of the HLA region is not yet fully understood, the direct proof that HLA antigens (HLA-A and HLA-B) are important in transplantation comes from the observation that allografts are rejected in an accelerated manner when performed in the presence of alloantibody specific to the antigen(s) of the donor. The cross-match test is, therefore, the most important test indicated before allotransplantation. Similarly, the presence of ABO incompatible isoagglutinins in the recipient eliminates one particular donor for transplantation. The importance of the human HLA antigens themselves in transplantation in the absence of immunization is difficult to ascertain. However, HLA typing has its main clinical indication in the selection of the best possible match for organ transplantation, since HLA antigens could be the markers for closely linked genes that express determinants necessary for the initiation of a first set phenomenon (HDR hypersensitivity delayed reaction locus).

Triggering of an allogeneic response in vitro and the resulting cellular differentiation might enable us to study cellular events leading to the rejection of a graft and possibly the basis of a graft-versus-host reaction. A mixture of allogeneic leukocytes differing at HLA-D results in proliferation of lymphocytes measured in the MLC reaction and also the generation of killer lymphocytes as measured by cell-mediated lysis (CML). Both tests have immunological specificity, as demonstrated by the fact that the primed lymphocytes produced display allogeneic memory. The clinical application of primed lymphocytes is preliminary. The proliferative phase is initiated by differences at determinants genetically controlled by genes closely linked to HLA-B, now named HLA-D. The determinants initiating the production of killer cells as well as those involved in the lysis of the target are not known but are probably genetically controlled by genes linked to HLA-A and HLA-B and different from HLA-D (HDR as CML-S). Matching at HLA-D is important in the prevention of graft-versus-host reaction in bone marrow transplantation. MLC identical siblings are the best match for bone marrow transplantation, to treat immunodeficiencies, aplastic anemia, and leukemias. In the absence of HLA-D identical siblings, HLA-D typing is indicated in the donor selection. Since HLA-D typing, at present, is performed with lymphocytes that are homozygous for different HLA-D determinants, the maintenance of a library of frozen lymphocytes as typing reagents is of prime importance. Equipment for freezing and storing lymphocytes in liquid nitrogen is a necessary

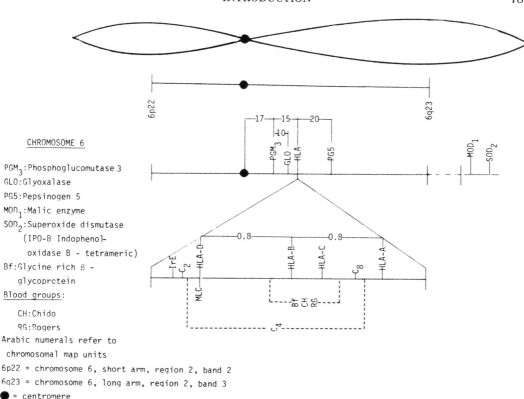

CHROMOSOME 6

PGM$_3$:Phosphoglucomutase 3

GLO:Glyoxalase

PG5:Pepsinogen 5

MOD$_1$:Malic enzyme

SOD$_2$:Superoxide dismutase
   (IPO-B Indophenol-
      oxidase B - tetrameric)

Bf:Glycine rich B -
   glycoprotein

Blood groups:

  CH:Chido

  RG:Rogers

Arabic numerals refer to
 chromosomal map units

6p22 = chromosome 6, short arm, region 2, band 2

6q23 = chromosome 6, long arm, region 2, band 3

● = centromere

FIG. 1. *Chromosomal linkage to HLA.*

part of the clinical transplantation laboratory. Since only six HLA-D specificities were identified during the VI Histocompatibility Workshop, HLA-D typing is not sufficiently developed to select unrelated donors matched at HLA-D. In some cases, it has been possible to identify HLA-D identical unrelated donors by simply performing MLC between the recipient and several potential donors who share the HLA-B determinants. This procedure can work in situations where the HLA-B antigens in question are in genetic linkage disequilibrium with the more common HLA-DW specificities: HLA-BW35, -B7, -B8, and -B12. However, approximately 65% of recipients at present do not have compatible donors. A new method (primed lymphocyte test: PLT) may prove to be useful in selection of donors. When the stimulator cell in an MLC has only one HLA-D difference from the responding cells (family members: father, mother, or haploidentical sibling), the primed lymphocytes produced sharing one HLA-D with the stimulating cells can be used against unrelated donors to identify HLA-D identical unrelated donors. Although the typing of B cell alloantigens is still in preliminary stages, this approach has the most promise for the rapid and efficient screening of compatible donors for bone marrow transplantation. Thus far, we have considered the importance of cross-matching HLA antigens and ABO in transplantation. Although the CML (cell-mediated lysis) and LDA (ABCIL) (lymphocyte-dependent antibody-mediated lysis) tests are not as yet practical in the routine laboratory, both tests will probably be important adjuncts of the cross-match. By way of example, it is conceivable that transplantation performed in a recipient not producing cytotoxic antibodies or killer cells could lead to hyperacute rejection or the absence of a bone marrow take. In fact, there have already been reports of shortened allograft survival in patients with a negative cross-match and negative cytotoxic cells against the donor but who had specific lymphocyte-dependent antibody-mediated lysis against the donor cells.

It would be inappropriate to discuss the HLA system without including one of its most important and rapidly growing applications, i.e., HLA and disease. Although there is a degree of association between certain HLA specificities and wide variety of diseases, the strongest association has been with HLA-B27 and certain arthritides such as ankylosing spondylitis, Reiter's syndrome, and anterior uveitis group.

Less powerful, but nonetheless significant, are the HLA-B8-associated endocrinopathies: myasthemia gravis, chronic active hepatitis, adult sprue, and dermatitis herpetiformis. Typing of diseases with HLA-D homozygous test cells has demonstrated an increased incidence of the following DW specificities and disease: DW2, multiple sclerosis and C2 deficiency; DW3, juvenile diabetes and Addison's disease; DW4, adult rheumatoid arthritis. The association of ragweed allergy and sensitivity to ragweed antigen E has led to the tentative mapping of immune response gene E (IrE) outside of HLA-D. Finally, an in vitro study describing the association of HLA-B5 with immune responsiveness to streptococcal antigen may have relevance to the study of streptococcal disease.

Our goal in assembling this *Manual* has been not only to provide the transplantation surgeon, the medical staff, and laboratory technicians with an introductory manual of accepted procedures critical for successful transplantation but also to acquaint the reader with some of the far-reaching ramifications of the HLA region, a genetic system containing many clues of diverse function which are involved in differentiation, regulation of immunity, disease, and possibly natural selection.

ACKNOWLEDGMENTS

E.J.Y. is supported by Public Health Service grants from the National Institutes of Health (NIAID, NCI, and HL).

The expert editorial assistance on this section of the *Manual* by Margery Knutson is gratefully acknowledged.

Chapter 103
Perspectives in Transplantation Immunology and Immunogenetics

JEAN DAUSSET

The development of the field into which the readers are about to enter is both so extraordinary and so rapid that it could serve as a model in biology.

The story began in 1936 when P. Gorer discovered what he thought to be another blood group system in the mouse. The following year, he established the identity of one gene of this system (governing the antigen II) with a gene for tumor resistance. The immunological theory of tumor transplantation was then formulated and confirmed experimentally.

Research with mice always preceded that with humans. A great advance was the initiation by G. Snell of the first congenic line in which a histocompatibility complex was introduced into the genome of another strain. Thanks to this marvelous tool, the laws of histocompatibility were formulated, and, besides the main histocompatibility complexes (H-2), many other H loci were discovered.

The serology of H-2 is astonishingly similar to that of the human HLA. There is an obvious analogy between the mouse and the human antigenic determinants as shown by multiple cross-reactions between them. They both bear "private" as well as "public" specificities. Both species contain public specificities which are shared by the two main loci (interlocus specificities). Even the biochemical composition and structure are analogous.

Moreover, in both species, the whole complex appears to have the same gene sequence as those governing the proliferation in the mixed lymphocyte reaction, the immune response, the specific structures on the B lymphocyte, and several components of complement, leading to C3 activation, and probably even more.

It is therefore recommended to newcomers in the HLA field to make a parallel study of the H-2 system and the so-called H-2 supergene. Indeed, it is remarkable that these small chromosomal segments are not composed of adjacent and completely independent genes. On the contrary, there is a close relationship between them. They seem to be associated in the same chromosomes, and fulfill a precise biological

function which is now beginning to emerge.

Scientists are very grateful to the few devoted workers who have made history of H-2. It is, however, only right to say that HLA, owing to its different biological material (larger populations of unrelated subjects), is trying, with some success, to pay its debt to H-2.

Curiously enough, the beginnings of HLA were not inspired by H-2. The approach was quite different, since the first technique used in man, leuko-agglutination, was devised to detect a state of autoimmunization.

It was very quickly realized that the antibodies thus detected were allo-antibodies since they only reacted with a certain percentage of unrelated blood leukocytes. The first antigen was called Mac from the initial letters of a nonagglutinated blood donor. This same antigen was described independently by using complement fixation on platelets. Only at this point did H-2 and HLA actually meet, and the implication of HLA in transplantation was postulated.

A very important contribution was the independent discovery of the frequent existence of anti-leukocyte antibodies in multiparous women, and the introduction of computer analysis to unravel the extreme serological complexity. The serological entities 4a and 4b behaved almost like well-described alleles. Subsequently, the two first allelic antigens LA1 and LA2 (LA2 being similar to Mac) were defined.

It is not possible to give a detailed account of the contribution of all the pioneers in the field. Let us say, however, that they showed an unusual scientific spirit. Collaborative work under the name of "workshops" began in 1965 in Durham, N.C., and these have been followed at regular intervals by other workshops. The story of these very fruitful endeavors deserves to be told.

Ten years have gone by since, at the suggestion of Bernard Amos, the small group of pioneers gathered round Rose Payne in Durham. During this first workshop, working together on the bench, we compared our techniques. The results were so contradictory that

787

we did not even dare to publish them. However, we all knew that we were on the threshold of important discoveries and we were not discouraged. Another meeting was held the following year in Leiden, organized by Jon van Rood. This time the results were satisfactory. It became very clear that different tissue types could be recognized.

Are these differences inborn, passed down from father to son? During the third workshop, held in Turin under the auspices of Ruggero Ceppellini, their heredity was studied by using Italian families. The results were clear-cut. Mendelian laws applied perfectly.

These conclusions could not have been drawn without extraordinary collaborative work, unique, probably, in the annals of biology. But we did not stop there. Two years later, Paul Terasaki welcomed us to Los Angeles, Calif., for the Fourth Workshop, during which, thanks to an extensive serological study of 300 families, the human major histocompatibility system was definitely established. All participants will remember the enthusiasm with which each brought his bricks for the building of the common house.

Soon we felt sufficiently sure of ourselves to venture outside of our own populations and to extend our studies to all mankind. A vast anthropological investigation covering 54 populations throughout the world was the object of the Fifth Workshop, which I had the pleasure of organizing in France, with the help of Walter Bodmer. Disguising ourselves as explorers, we penetrated the thickest jungles, climbed the highest mountains, and sailed to the most forsaken islands to collect samples of blood. Thus we learned that the genetic laws we had worked out were true in all populations. Fortunately, the biological map of humanity was drawn before the modern mixture of populations, which will soon obscure all the differences.

Progress, however, calls for more progress. Scientists may not rest on their laurels, for each victory is only one step forward. Soon, other human cell characteristics, governed by neighboring genes on the same chromosome, began to emerge. The serologists, as we all were, became cellular immunologists. Reactive cells, often found in children of consanguine marriages, became badly needed. Once again, it was necessary to band together and sally forth into isolated places where marriages between first cousins are not infrequent. The lucky ones obtained the list of dispensations for such marriages from their Catholic Archbishops.

The last workshop, organized by Fleming Kissmeyer-Neilsen in Aarhus, allowed us to determine the first six alleles of the HLA-D locus, which govern the mixed lymphocyte reaction, and to confirm, without any ambiguity, the existence of the third HLA-C locus.

Too often scientists make discoveries and never know how valuable they will prove. We, however, are already harvesting the first fruits of our labors and know the pride of seeing their usefulness.

Hundreds of researchers are even now making use of HLA markers whose importance to human biology is continually increasing.

On a basic scientific level, the HLA complex is without doubt the best known linkage group, enabling us to undertake systematic study of recombination over the shortest known chromosomal distance, and, above all, of the ontogenic and phylogenic development of molecules of the various main histocompatibility complexes in different species. Certain structures seem to be indispensable since they are found to be practically identical in all vertebrates studied so far. Because of the extraordinary polymorphism of the HLA system, we have been able to draw important anthropological conclusions on human origins and migrations.

But what is perhaps even more amazing is that the relationships between different genes in the main histocompatibility complexes have remained unchanged throughout evolution (for maybe 300×10^6 years, according to studies on the toad *Xenopes laevis*). The latter appear to be functional units, as all the genes known at the present time are involved, to a greater or lesser extent, in the immune response. We can, in fact, find coding genes for making a specific immunological response, for cellular cooperation between T and B lymphocytes, for different components of the complement, and, finally, for the targets composed of transplantation antigens. So, like all main histocompatibility complexes, the HLA complex is the real nerve center of the organisms immunological defense.

The allogenic response is certainly the most studied, since any further knowledge can be promptly and usefully applied to therapeutics, that is, transplantation. As is often the case in history, scientific knowledge has followed empirical usage. We can now predict the future of an organ graft with ever-increasing accuracy, thanks to HLA compatibility, and many patients benefit daily from the fact that we can choose a donor who will be the most compatible for them. But much remains to be done to improve the long-term prognosis of grafts. Although the process of donor selection could be refined still further, it is unlikely to provide the ultimate solution to the problem of transplantation. For this we must look to the specific tolerance for the donor's antigens. But here again, development at will of such a tolerance requires a greater understanding of transplantation antigens, and of the delicate balance mechanism which is formed between forces of rejection (effector cells and specific antibodies) and forces of unresponsiveness (suppressor cells, facilitating antibodies, or antigen/antibody complexes). Certainly, the HLA region plays a crucial part in maintaining this balance.

More recently, biologists have turned their interest to another fascinating aspect of the HLA complex — the associations of numerous diseases with certain antigens of the HLA system. Although it has not yet been formally proved, these associations are very probably connected with the immunological functions of the HLA region. The discovery of the precise mechanism of these associations will mark the opening of a new chapter in pathology. As a matter of fact, we do not yet know the causes of all these diseases, but they do have a certain hereditary characteristic and are usually accompanied by immunological disorders such as lymphocytic infiltration in the target organ.

This poses a major problem for clinicians, biologists, and, in particular, geneticists and virologists.

We can foresee great progress being made as much on the clinical level (especially for nosology, diagnosis, prognosis, and prevention) as on a fundamental level, such as comprehension of selection forces, allowing the spread of a gene, the constitution, and then the maintenance of the polymorphism.

The HLA system is a very small link in the chain constituted by the HLA complex. It is now beginning to be exploited on a large scale. With the help of the cohort of young researchers who will be reading this book, its contribution to science will surely be even more significant than it has been until now.

Chapter 104

Screening Sera for HLA Antibodies

W. E. BRAUN AND D. E. KAYHOE

INTRODUCTION

A critical component of accurate histocompatibility testing for HLA antigens is well-characterized antiserum. Throughout the world numerous investigators have been successful to various degrees in finding antiserum of high quality which can duplicate the identification of already-known HLA antigens as well as detect new specificities. It is clear that the simpler task is that of finding sera capable of detecting antigen specificities that are already known. In contrast, characterizing antisera for specificities still undefined requires a good deal more sophistication.

In this chapter, we have attempted to describe simple ways of identifying potentially good serum donors, of constructing lymphocyte panels for evaluating sera, of collecting blood from the HLA antibody producers, and of characterizing the antiserum specificity. Methods for shipping, processing, freeze-drying, cataloging, and dispensing of serum specimens are also described. For more complex procedures for serum analysis, both descriptive and computer-assisted, one may refer to recent publications in this area (2, 6).

SELECTION OF DONORS

Women who have had pregnancies that have gone to term or lasted into the third trimester are the most rewarding group to study for HLA antibodies with the potential to be quality typing reagents. In general, the more recent the pregnancy the more likely one is to find an antibody, if it has been present at all. However, several investigators have had the experience of finding excellent reagents in women who have not had a pregnancy for more than 15 years. Although primiparas may as a group have a lower incidence of antibody than the approximately 20% frequency in those with two or more pregnancies, they do in fact have a frequency of antibody formation sufficient to warrant investigating them. However, in the primiparous population it seems that the antibody does not persist as long and the antibody must be obtained, as all should, as soon as possible after detection. In a recent study of 300 primiparas, it was found that 8% formed antibody; that anti-HLA-A5 and HLA-B14 were formed significantly more often than other antibodies, implying that these antigens were more immunogenic than others; and that antibodies were produced against either series of antigens but not against both (9). However, in general, only about 2% of all parous females make an antibody sufficiently specific to be a typing reagent.

Usually, one obtains serum from healthy females during or shortly after their hospitalization for delivery. We request the woman's written permission for the venipuncture and the serum screening procedure (Table 1) and compile basic information including name, age, address, telephone number, race, number of pregnancies, number of children, age of youngest child, number of blood transfusions, ABO and Rh, and age and race of the immunizing father (and ideally his HLA antigens). However, to find other highly motivated women who may be willing to donate serum, one may also use free advertisements provided by resources such as local suburban newspapers, clubs, or benevolent associations.

Other sources of antiserum that have been worthwhile have been patients who have rejected kidney allografts. Although this seems to vary quite a bit from center to center, in our experience some excellent reagents have been obtained. If these patients are stable, they can undergo plasmapheresis while being dialyzed. In contrast, multiply transfused individuals in almost everyone's experience have been poor sources of antibody. It may be, however, that multiply transfused individuals who receive their blood from a single donor, such as now is being done in some of the platelet matching programs, may provide excellent reagents if the recipients are well enough to be serum donors. Serum obtained by planned immunization of human volunteer or paid donors appears to be done only rarely in the United States. Certain soluble antigens, particularly the more abundant circulating HLA-A9, derived from human plasma have been used to produce HLA xenoantibodies in rabbits.

Typing sera may be improved with respect to

TABLE 1. *Authorization for drawing 10 ml of venous blood for white cell antibody study*

Date _____

I voluntarily authorize approximately 10 ml of my blood to be taken by standard aseptic venipuncture techniques and examined for the possible occurrence of white blood cell antibodies. I understand that if such antibodies are found I may be requested to donate additional blood, either as a volunteer or a paid donor, at some future date in accordance with accepted Blood Banking Criteria.

Signed _____

(Patient or person authorized to consent for patient)

Witness _____

Doctor in Charge _____

History Number _____

specificity, i.e., "cleaned up," by (i) diluting out weaker specificities, (ii) using platelet absorption to remove a second specificity of a different segregant series (12), and (iii) using human spleens to absorb several lower-titer, secondary specificities (D. Cross, Proc. Am. Assoc. for Clinical Histocompatibility Testing, Birmingham, Ala., 29 April 1975).

After collection, sera are stored at 4 C until placed on trays. A master tray of the sera to be tested is prepared, and from it 60 or more identical 72-well trays can be made and stored at −70 C. If serum is not going onto trays within a few days, it should be stored at −70 C.

To improve efficiency in antiserum screening, one could do a cross-match of a postpartum female's serum against her husband's or child's lymphocytes so that those women without antibody can be separated and so that the specificity can be at least suggested by the husband's immunizing antigens. However, in many places, as in our own case, it is not possible to do immediate cross-matches, and we must embark on a screening program which will be outlined below. Since about 75% of peripheral lymphocytes are T cells, sera that are cytotoxicity negative with these cells may still have non-HLA cytotoxicity when tested against appropriate cells (i.e., B cells).

In some centers a program has been developed in which all blood being donated at a blood bank by postpartum females is screened for HLA antibody before being released for transfusion purposes. In this way any antibody that is found is already accompanied by a large serum donation. This avoids the problems of losing a good serum because of a waning antibody titer from delays in plasmapheresis of the donor or of encountering an uncooperative antibody former who refuses to give any further specimens. In addition, it may protect the potential transfusion recipient from a donor-HLA antibody recipient-white cell transfusion reaction.

CONSTRUCTING A LYMPHOCYTE PANEL FOR EVALUATING SERA

An ideal lymphocyte panel to be used for serum screening may be made up from random or selected fresh cells and selected frozen cells stored in bulk or on trays. It should utilize genotyped families with blanks, as well as saturated phenotypes, different races, T-rich (standard peripheral blood preparations) and B-rich (chronic lymphocytic leukemic cells or enriched preparations) testing, and carefully standardized complement and technique.

Lymphocyte cell panels may be composed of fresh or frozen lymphocytes, or both. In laboratories without facilities for freezing cells, it will be possible to test the unknown sera only against random fresh cells as they arrive for typing. This approach may miss certain antigens unless one also has a "walking" panel of rarer specificities that can be brought in any time a group of sera is to be screened in order to have all antigens in the panel. Another approach is to use as the screening cell panel frozen lymphocytes carefully selected to include all antigen specificities. In some laboratories lymphocytes comprising the panel are frozen on trays for a more rapid screen. The third possibility is to use a combination of fresh and frozen cells so that random cells are used up to the point of rare specificities, and then rare specificities are utilized from the frozen cell panel. To get at least three representations of all specificities, generally 20 to 30 cells are necessary at a minimum. The higher number appears necessary when screening for C series antigens also.

It is worthwhile to have in one's cell panel not only those with a saturated phenotype but also genotyped individuals who have less than a four-antigen HLA typing and in which homozygosity is not the explanation. These individuals, then, with a "verified blank" may help to define previously unknown specificities. On the other hand, reactions of lymphocytes homozygous for an HLA antigen may be anomalous, and the reaction of such cells should be studied separately.

When sera are acquired from either Caucasian or non-Caucasian women the father of whose child(ren) is non-Caucasian and thus the potential possessor of uncommon antigens, lymphocytes from a person of the father's race should also be used to test those women's sera.

In screening sera for HLA antibodies, lymphocytes from peripheral blood are almost always used. These lymphocytes are approximately 75% T cells. Sera negative by cytotoxicity with these T cells may still have antibody reactive with B cells. Although these "B cell" antibodies are poorly described at present, their ultimate value may well exceed that of HLA in areas of immune responsiveness and disease associations. Therefore, if a commitment is made to screening sera for HLA antibodies, it would probably be worthwhile to screen these sera, especially those negative for HLA, against B cells derived by enrichment techniques, or from cultured cell lines, chronic lymphocytic leukemias, or beta-2 microglobulin "stripped" cells.

In the cytotoxicity assay the complement should be carefully standardized to avoid missing or creating reactions that will frustrate efforts to define any serum's specificity (7).

It has been shown that certain sera are "technique dependent." Such technique dependency has been attributed in some cases to anticomplementary factors, not specifically defined, which can depress cytotoxicity but can be eliminated in the two-stage technique (1, 3). On the other hand, there is an opposite type of problem with possibly excessive reactivity when the antiglobulin technique is used (4).

BLOOD COLLECTION FROM HLA ANTIBODY PRODUCERS

As soon as one finds a parous woman who is an antibody producer, arrangements should be made to collect a large serum specimen. This is usually accomplished no later than the woman's 6-week postpartum check-up. The specimen should be rechecked for activity and titer, but one should not postpone obtaining the plasmapheresis donation.

Having used both a cell separator and a plasmapheresis program to obtain plasma from serum donors, we would note that the cell separator has been more of a discomfort to the patient and a more time-consuming method of obtaining plasma than has been the double-bag plasmaphereses. Consequently, at the present time, we have obtained our collections with double-bag (about 450 ml) plasmaphereses in ACD solution and have used a method of recalcification to produce the serum (11). A few drops of thrombin will accelerate and solidify the clot, which can be obtained most easily by using a glass rod and gently stirring the plasma. The clot will be wrapped around the glass rod and easily removed. Additional amounts of serum may be expressed from this clot. A repeat plasmapheresis may be worthwhile in 1 month if a repeat assay of the sera still shows suitable reactivity.

CHARACTERIZATION OF THE ANTISERUM SPECIFICITY

The identification of the specificity of an unknown serum may be made by testing it against lymphocytes with known antigens or by comparing the reactions of an unknown serum with those of known sera and using 2×2 chi square analyses. In reality, however, since the definition of any HLA antigen is based on antibody reactions at some point in time, the use of previously typed cells is still a form, albeit indirect, of serum-to-serum comparison for identification. If the reactions of an unknown serum deviate from those of known antigens or if the serum is not reacting, one should note the racial origin of the serum producer and of the immunizer (father) and attempt to resolve differences in the pattern of reaction by including lymphocytes from the same race as the immunizer having both blanks and saturated phenotypes. Finally, a segregation pattern of reactivity should be sought in families which would be informative for this antigen in order to confirm a "split" or a new specificity. A recent example of this is the detection of Hs as a B series antigen by a primiparous Chinese woman's serum that failed to react against a Caucasian panel of cells (10).

The analysis of antisera can be done in two ways, manually and by computer. The major advantage of computer analysis seems to be primarily with large serum screening programs (more than 1,000 sera per year) or with patterns of reactions from a constant group of antisera tested against hundreds or thousands of individuals. The complexities of this approach are summarized in recent publications (2, 6). Frequently, all of the fundamental specificities of an antiserum can be detected manually by a highly experienced person comparing the reactions of the unknown sera with those of the existing typing sera on a selected lymphocyte panel. These are laid out on a checkerboard type paper with the cells arranged along an upper horizontal axis. Along the vertical axis each HLA antigen is noted and its reaction pattern (as determined by the existing typing sera) is displayed horizontally. Each individual reaction pattern of an unknown serum is placed below. Simply by lining up, for example, the pattern given by cells that react with the known HLA-A2 antisera and looking for the same pattern among the unknown sera, the new HLA-A2 sera can be identified. In a 2×2 chi square analysis ideally all of the reactions would be concordant $++$ or $--$, and none would be $+-$ or $-+$. Obviously this clear-cut distinction is too frequently not the case, and additional reactions may be produced by the serum. To help in this problem, a different colored marking pencil may be used to paint out the reactions unique to each suspected specificity so that two or possibly three antibodies are then apparent. The occurrence of cross-reactions must be considered (8). This, it must be emphasized, is a very basic but very useful approach when modest numbers of sera are screened.

For examining a large number of sera or complex sera, a more discriminating descriptive approach (6) or an elaborate inclusion analysis (2) may be used to assign the primary specificity and to define additional specificities. The inclusion analysis computer program used for the 1972 and 1975 International Workshops uses a 2×2 table to compare a serum's reactions with a set of known antigens and to select the most significant antigen recognized by the serum. All cells with this antigen are then excluded from the analysis. The remaining cells which contain ideally all the other known antigens are used to identify any additional antigen specificities. As each additional specificity is identified, the cells with those antigens are dropped from the analysis until the residual positive reactions ("tail") are zero or fail to yield significant specificities according to a preset end point. The most significant antigen is the one giving the highest chi-squared value with the serum (i.e., the greatest concordance of reactions either $++$ or $--$ and the least discordant reactions either $+-$ or $-+$).

However, this method does not recognize subgroups of a specificity unless their existence has previously been assumed. Consequently, for very discriminating analyses a descriptive analysis may be necessary. The definition of subspecificities or new ones may require testing against lymphocytes of other races in which the suspected antigen is more clearly expressed and can obtain confirmation in families.

The question frequently occurs as to whether weak reactions should be included in a serum evaluation. With properly controlled test conditions, especially the complement, such weak reactions may indicate a true antigen specificity found perhaps only on a minority of peripheral lymphocytes (e.g., B cells), a point discussed earlier.

SERUM PREPARATION

With the current need for antisera to rare, low-frequency antibodies, a number of laboratories now collect sera from non-Caucasian donors. In many cases, this involves the operation of programs among remote, exotic population groups. Sera are then forwarded to the research laboratory for testing. Procedures for field processing of sera to be shipped should be kept simple. Limitations in the availability of equipment and the maintenance of sterility and the prevention of spoilage may present almost insurmountable problems. Sera obtained with great difficulty in the field may arrive back at the testing laboratory in poor condition.

There should be a minimum of handling of the sera in the field. Blood should be collected from fasted donors to lessen the problems with lipemic sera and should be kept cool to prevent lysis and bacterial growth.

SHIPPING CONTAINERS

Blood should be shipped in well-labeled sterile plastic containers. Commercially available 300-ml blood bags have proved most satisfactory. These withstand freezing and do not present the problems of breakage seen with glass bottles. When small volumes are to be shipped, the 125-ml bags may be used. Sufficient empty space should be left in the bags to allow for expansion with freezing. An identification tag should be securely tied to each bag, and waterproof labels and ink should be used (A. W. Faber Feltstik #750 or Sanford's Sharpie #3000). Cellophane or plastic tapes may fall off when frozen and should be avoided. A packing slip should be included in each box, listing the contents of each bag and the destination of the shipment.

For an outside container, use well-constructed insulated boxes with sturdy protective cardboard covers and sufficient insulation to maintain the serum in a frozen state for 48 to 96 h (TC-34 insulation boxes with covers, available from E. R. Hitchcock and Associates, Washington, D.C. 20006). Although these are expensive, they may be reused many times and are more efficient than the coolers used to store beverages or food. Sera should be frozen before packing and then placed in the container with cardboard bracing to prevent the shifting of serum bags during shipment. The insulated box should then be filled with large pieces of dry ice. Small chips evaporate rapidly and will not maintain prolonged freezing. The packing should be completed just prior to shipment to assure the maximal amount of cold protection en route. Details concerning the routing of shipments, choice of carriers, etc. should be worked out in advance. Large "Frozen Shipment" labels should be prominantly displayed on three sides of each box. The consignee should be notified by telephone or Telex of shipping plans, and at this time a check should be made concerning special instructions, whom to call in the event of missed shipments, etc. International shipments usually require that some sort of a statement be placed on the box to indicate the contents. A label which states that the package contains "scientific research reagents—of no commercial value" has proved useful for customs purposes. Some countries have special regulations and forms which must be filled out to obtain customs clearance. Laboratories making frozen air shipments in the United States should be aware of the provisions of the Federal Standard 42 CFR 72.25(C) and affix to each package the appropriate label indicating compliance.

In our program we have utilized the services of commercial forwarding companies who provide door-to-door service, arrange for customs processing, and add dry ice. We mark the boxes to indicate the time at which they should be re-iced. Care should be taken to avoid shipments which will arrive on weekends or holidays.

PROCESSING OF
HISTOCOMPATIBILITY ANTISERA

Upon receipt, bags of frozen serum should be repackaged into containers which will permit convenient storage in a stable form for eventual use in the laboratory. Bulk sera containers should be carefully checked for signs of damage as soon as they are received; if cracked or broken, they should be placed, while still frozen, into large plastic bags which are then sealed, labeled, and placed in frozen storage until ready for processing. All sera should be stored at −70 C in an alarm-equippped, horizontal, mechanical freezer.

In handling antisera, thawing and refreezing should be avoided whenever possible. Sera which have thawed should be retested to see if they have lost activity. In the majority of cases, high-titer sera will not be damaged by brief periods of thaw. Sodium azide (0.1%) has been suggested as a serum preservative (11). Since cell membranes may be altered by a variety of chemicals, we prefer to use no preservatives.

All blood products should be considered capable of transmitting hepatitis, and precautions should be taken to prevent accidental infection. Personnel should not eat or smoke in the laboratory.

The frozen serum containers are placed in large clean beakers and are thawed in a constant-temperature 35 to 37 C water bath. A magnetic stirrer facilitates rapid thawing. The serum should be kept at 4 C for the remainder of the processing.

A modification of the procedure described by Perkins (11) can be used to remove additional fibrin. Thrombin (Thrombin, topical, Parke-Davis #NDC 0071-1355-01) is added, 1 unit per min, to 5 ml of serum. If any clotting occurs, the serum is returned to the original pool, and 1 unit of thrombin is added to each 1 ml of serum, allowing for the thrombin already added to the sample. The serum should be placed in a refrigerator (4 C) overnight, and the fibrin is then removed by cold centrifugation at 5,000 rpm for 20 min. The serum is then recentrifuged at 15,000 rpm for 30 min, and any lipoid material is carefully skimmed off. Serum is passed through a coarse filter (Millipore #AP2004700) and then through clean 1.2-, 0.45-, and 0.22-μm membrane filters (RAWP, HAWP, and GSWP). A gentle pressure (2 to 4 lb/in²) of nitrogen is used to push the sera through the filters. Final sterilization is accomplished by 0.22-mm filtration. A 1-ml amount of serum is transferred into a sterile 3-ml type 1 borosilicate vial (T.C. Wheaton Co., #S-104E), stoppered with a flange-type butyl rubber stopper (West Co., #124-0), and sealed with a triple aluminum seal (West Co., #13-30). To avoid mislabeling, only one serum is bottled at a time and labels are affixed immediately. We use Avery #S-1623 P4 Flex Labels which adhere well to glass at −70 C.

Following completion of the bottling and labeling, the antisera are packed into well-marked boxes which fit into metal racks and are stored in a horizontal −70 C freezer. A cataloging system has been used which makes it possible to locate any of 288 boxes within several seconds.

FREEZE-DRYING OF HISTOCOMPATIBILITY ANTISERA

In the operation of a large serum distribution program, it may be desirable to freeze-dry sera. This is a complicated procedure requiring special equipment. Freeze-dried sera can be stored at −20 C in a walk-in cold room. This facilitates inventory control and permits shipment at ambient temperatures, with a very considerable saving in costs. After receipt in the laboratory, sera should be stored at −20 C until reconstituted with sterile distilled water (no preservatives). They must then be stored at −70 C. The process we use has been described (5).

1. Vials, 3 ml (see above), containing 1 ml of serum are loosely stoppered with fluted gray butyl stoppers (Wheaton #23637). These are especially designed for freeze-drying. Vials containing frozen serum are placed into a freeze-dryer which has been precooled to −60 C. (External condensers are maintained at −75 C or lower throughout the entire drying cycle).

2. After loading, the shelf is kept at −40 C or lower for 10 or more h until the chamber pressure equilibrates at 10 μm or lower (McLeod gauge).

3. The serum temperature is then manually raised at a rate of 2 C per hour until it reaches 20 C. Vials are stoppered in the chamber while still under vacuum. They are removed and triple aluminum sealed (see above). Test sample residual moisture should be 0.8 to 1.9%. Sera drier than 0.5% are difficult to dissolve, whereas those with a moisture content in excess of 2% may be unstable with prolonged storage.

Because of limited observation time, we have no information to indicate that freeze-drying results in a prolongation of serum activity over that observed at −70 C storage. In accelerated degradation studies, a single serum studied had no loss of activity after storage for 14 days at 50 C.

DISPENSING OF SERUM IN THE LABORATORY

One milliliter of serum should be adequate to perform over 800 microcytotoxicity tests. Most laboratories need only a fraction of this amount for 1 day's typings. Although we found no loss of cytotoxic titer after 25 thaw-freeze cycles with a single high-titered multispecific serum, we believe that refreezing should be avoided whenever possible. Small samples of sera should be placed in microtubes (Beckman

#314326), labeled, stored in the minus 70 C freezer, and thawed as needed. Unused residual sera can usually be safely refrozen several times until the tube is used up.

An alternate means for dispensing sera for daily laboratory use is the preloaded multiwell typing tray (Cooke 72-well tray #236-72 or Falcon 60-well tray #3034).

During the past 4 years, we have distributed over 90,000 preloaded trays to 125 U.S. typing laboratories. Care must be exercised in filling the wells to be sure that 1 μliter of serum is placed under the microdroplet of mineral oil that is used to prevent evaporation. Trays should be carefully examined before and after freezing to be sure that all wells have been filled. They should be stored and shipped at −70 C or colder. Because certain sera seem to lose potency after prolonged exposure in the trays to carbon dioxide, trays are shipped in sealed air-tight metal cans. Users should avoid exposing preloaded trays to carbon dioxide fumes.

We have been unsuccessful in our attempts to develop a preloaded tray containing freeze-dried sera. Although lyophilization is a relatively simple process, the problem of preventing subsequent absorption of atmospheric water has proven insurmountable.

CATALOGING AND UPDATING OF SERUM INFORMATION

During the past 10 years, there has been a remarkable growth in knowledge of the antigens involved in the recognition of histocompatibility. Early studies seemed to indicate that there were a relatively small number of antigens involved. We now realize that the HLA system involves a very large number of antigens in at least three segregant series. Sera which were thought to be operationally monospecific may now be found to contain a variety of antibodies. Many sera which were thought to be worthless because they did not seem to "fit" any reactivity pattern when used to type for the old two-segregant HLA system should now be tested to see if they contain antibodies to new locus histocompatibility antigens. As new populations are studied and more tests are done, there is a continued acquisition of information on sera. Reagents which work well by one technique may not work or may produce weakly positive reactions when used by another laboratory with different procedures. For this reason, continuing programs of data collection must be used to obtain current information needed in the interpretation of test results. Much to the concern of many laboratories, we have avoided stating unequivocally that a serum has a certain specificity. We prefer listing the reactions reported by individual laboratories. Information is given concerning panel size and composition and the testing techniques used. The immunologist then learns of the vagaries of the various sera and is in a better position to select reagents which are likely to work with the procedures that he uses in the populations that he is studying.

We do not believe that a single set of sera will do a complete job of identifying histocompatibility antigens in all patients. Most laboratories report using 120 or more sera for "routine typing," and when questions arise they fall back on additional special sera. Despite this, on some occasions it is impossible to identify correctly all of the histocompatibility antigens. This is a particular problem when typing non-Caucasians. The National Institute of Allergy and Infectious Diseases (NIAID) Serum Bank periodically requests that users provide information concerning their experiences with the reactions of sera in a variety of racial groups. This information is published in the periodic updating of the NIAID Serum Catalog (National Institutes of Health, Bethesda, Md.).

SOURCES OF REAGENTS AND SUPPLIES

Filters: Millipore Corp., Bedford, Mass. 01730

Labels: Avery Label Systems, Washington, D.C. 20007

Microtubes: Beckman Instruments, Chamblee, Ga.

Thrombin: Parke, Davis & Co., Detroit, Mich. 48323

Trays: Cooke Engineering, Alexandria, Va., or Falcon Plastics, Los Angeles, Calif.

Vial stoppers: Wheaton Scientific, Millville, N.J. 08332

LITERATURE CITED

1. Amos, D. B. 1974. Cytotoxicity testing, p. 23–26. *In* J. G. Ray, Jr., D. B. Hare, P. D. Pedersen, and D. E. Kayhoe (ed.), Manual of tissue typing techniques. Publication no. (NIH) 75-545, U.S. Department of Health, Education, and Welfare, Washington, D.C.

2. Bodmer, J. G., W. F. Bodmer, and A. Piazza. 1975. An inclusion analysis of Fifth Histocompatibility Testing Workshop sera in 25 populations. Tissue Antigens 5:315–366.

3. Ferrone, S., R. M. Tosi, and D. Centis. 1967. Anticomplementary factors affecting the lymphocytotoxicity test, p. 357–364. *In* E. S. Curtoni, P. L. Matting, and R. M. Tosi (ed.), Histocompatibility testing 1967. The Williams & Wilkins Co., Baltimore.

4. Johnson, A. H. 1974. Antiglobulin microcytotoxicity test, p. 110–113. *In* J. G. Ray, Jr., D. B. Hare, P. D. Pedersen, and D. E. Kayhoe (ed.), Manual of tissue typing techniques. Publication. no. (NIH) 75-545, U.S. Department of Health, Education, and Welfare, Washington, D.C.

5. Kroener, C. A., V. P. Perry, J. L. Martin, and J. C. Sasso. 1975. Freeze drying of histocompatibility serum. Cryobiology 12:397–404.

6. Lepage, V., L. Degos, and J. Dausset. 1975. Descriptive serological analysis. Tissue Antigens 5:301–314.

7. MacQueen, J. M. 1974. Some practical experiences with rabbit complement in the cytotoxicity test, p. 149–153. *In* J. G. Ray, Jr., D. B. Hare, P. D. Pedersen, and D. E. Kayhoe (ed.), Manual of tissue typing techniques. Publication no. (NIH) 75-545, U.S. Department of Health, Education, and Welfare, Washington, D.C.

8. Mittal, K. K., and P. I. Terasaki. 1974. Serological cross-reactivity in the HL-A system. Tissue Antigens 4:146–156.

9. Oh, J. H., and L. D. Maclean. 1975. Comparative immunogenicity of HL-A antigens: a study in primiparas. Tissue Antigens 5:33–37.

10. Payne, R., R. Radvany, and C. Grumet. 1975. A new second locus HL-A antigen in linkage disequilibrium with HL-A2 in Cantonese Chinese. Tissue Antigens 5:69–71.

11. Perkins, H. 1974. Conversion of plasma to serum, p. 147–148. *In* J. G. Ray, Jr., D. B. Hare, P. D. Pedersen, and D. E. Kayhoe (ed.), Manual of tissue typing techniques. Publication no. (NIH) 75-545, U.S. Department of Health, Education, and Welfare, Washington, D.C.

12. Rodey, G. E., B. Sturm, and R. H. Aster. 1973. Cross-reactive HL-A antibodies. Separation of multiple HL-A antibody specificities by platelet absorption and acid elution. Tissue Antigens 3:63–69.

Chapter 105

HLA Typing

D. BERNARD AMOS AND PAMELA POOL

INTRODUCTION

The HLA antigens are glycoproteins present on the membranes of most nucleated cells. Antigen concentrations are especially high on lymphocytes and blood platelets, but the antigens are also found on fibroblasts, epidermal cells, and kidney parenchyma cells. All of these cell types have been used in antigen assays.

The genetic control of HLA resides in the human C6 chromosome. The HLA region or haplotype occupies an area of undetermined extent on this chromosome and includes a minimum of four genetic loci. The various loci are closely linked and are thus usually inherited as a genetic unit; but the loci have been separated by recombination and so are known to be distinct entities.

The best-known antigens belong to the HLA-A and HLA-B series. These were previously known as the first- or LA and second- or FOUR locus antigens. Those specificities which are universally accepted are designated by Arabic numerals—thus, HLA-A1, HLA-B5, etc. Specificities that are less well defined are given provisional status and indicated by the prefix "W" before the numeral; examples are HLA-AW32 and HLA-BW35. A list of specificities and their former designations is given in Table 1. The antigenic products of the A and B loci have a molecular weight of about 56,000 and are made up of two chains that are noncovalently bound. The smaller chain of 11,000 daltons corresponds to β_2-microglobulin found in serum and urine. The heavy chain of 45,000 daltons has two domains, each with an internal disulfide bond. The heavy-chain molecule is inserted into the membrane through a hydrophobic fragment of about 10,000 daltons, which is cleared from the rest of the molecule by papain.

The nature of the antigenic site(s) is at present unknown. It has been suggested that each molecule includes more than one site, one site being highly specific and constituting a private specificity, with the other sites being more widely distributed and constituting a broadly reactive or public specificity. The designated HLA-A and HLA-B specificities, e.g., HLA-A2, would be private specificities, and the "anti-gens" 4a and 4b of van Rood and van Leeuwen would be broadly reactive (11).

Whatever its basis, cross-reactivity is the bane of tissue typing. Cross-reactions occur only between specificities on the same locus. For example, most antisera primarily directed against HLA-A3 also react against cells carrying HLA-A11 and sometimes even HLA-A1; antisera reacting with HLA-B7 almost invariably react against HLA-B27 and often against HLA-BW22, and so on. A list of common cross-reactions is given in Fig. 1.

The reaction of an antiserum is strongest with its homologous antigen; e.g., in a cytotoxic reaction more cells will be killed and at a greater dilution of serum than in a cross-reaction. To minimize cross-reactivity, many antisera are therefore diluted so that only the homologous reaction is detected. The distinction between cross-reactive specificities, such as HLA-A3 and A11, is quite sharp. The distinction between some other cross-reactive series is often quite difficult. Even highly experienced workers may, on occasion, have difficulty in distinguishing between highly cross-reactive specificities such as HLA-AW30 and AW31, or AW25 and AW26. P. I. Terasaki analyzed the results of identification of the antigens of a number of donor cells distributed to a large number of laboratories (personal communication). Almost all laboratories agreed on the identification of well-defined specificities such as HLA-A2, but there were many discrepancies in the characterization of certain W specificities.

There are many methods for the detection of HLA specificities, and for each category of procedure there are many variants. Many major centers have standardized on a particular procedure that is then used by other laboratories in the same region or those using the same antisera.

The first method to gain wide acceptance was leukoagglutination. The procedures of van Rood and van Leeuwen (12), Dausset (5), or Amos and Peacocke (2) are still occasionally employed. The principle of each was similar. Dausset believed that the results were influenced by the presence or absence of free diva-

TABLE 1. *Antigenic specificities of HLA*[a]

New terminology	Old terminology	New terminology	Old terminology	New terminology	Old terminology	New terminology	Old terminology
HLA-A	1st segregant series, 1st-locus or LA series antigens	HLA-B	2nd segregant series, 2nd- or FOUR series antigens	HLA-C	3rd segregant series, 3rd- locus or AJ series antigens	HLA-D	MLR-S1, LAD, or LD determinant
HLA-A1	HL-A1	HLA-B5	HL-A5	HLA-CW1	T1	HLA-DW1	LD101
HLA-A2	HL-A2	HLA-B7	HL-A7	HLA-CW2	T2	HLA-DW2	LD102
HLA-A3	HL-A3	HLA-B8	HL-A8	HLA-CW3	T3	HLA-DW3	LD103
HLA-A9	HL-A9	HLA-B12	HL-A12	HLA-CW4	T4	HLA-DW4	LD104
HLA-A10	HL-A10	HLA-B13	HL-A13	HLA-CW5	T5	HLA-DW5	LD105
HLA-A11	HL-A11	HLA-B14	W14			HLA-DW6	LD106
HLA-A28	W28	HLA-B18	W18				
HLA-A29	W29	HLA-B27	W27				
HLA-AW23	W23	HLA-BW15	W15				
HLA-AW24	W24	HLA-BW16	W16				
HLA-AW25	W25	HLA-BW17	W17				
HLA-AW26	W26	HLA-BW21	W18				
HLA-AW30	W30	HLA-BW22	W22				
HLA-AW31	W31	HLA-BW35	W5				
HLA-AW32	W32	HLA-BW37	—				
HLA-AW33	W19.6	HLA-BW38	W16.1				
HLA-AW34	—	HLA-BW39	W16.2				
HLA-AW36	—	HLA-BW40	W10				
HLA-AW43	—	HLA-BW41					
		HLA-BW42					

[a] Adapted from W. J. Williams, E. Beutler, A. J. Erslev, and R. W. Rundles (ed.), 1975, *Hematology*, 2nd ed., McGraw-Hill Book Co., New York, in press.

lent cations. In all procedures, one or more drops of buffy-coat lymphocytes, freed from red cells and platelets by Amos and Peacocke (2), were mixed with serum in small test tubes, incubated at room temperature, and read microscopically after mixing. Most other workers lysed any residual red cells with acetic acid before reading (5, 14). The procedures gave about 95% reproducibility with cells from most subjects, but were unsuitable for cells from severely ill donors. Also, the cells could not be stored; therefore, they could not be shipped. Microagglutination methods were developed by Payne (10) and others, but never came into widespread use for the same reasons that the semimicro methods were dropped; all forms of agglutination have given way to the microcytotoxicity test (8). Other procedures, such as complement consumption (3) or platelet agglutination (6), have also been largely discontinued. Platelet complement fixation is a precise procedure giving excellent results in experienced hands (4). Its use is, however, restricted to a very few laboratories, largely because of difficulties in obtaining antisera.

The advantages of the microcytotoxicity test are the minute (1.0 µliter or less) volumes of antiserum required and a concomitantly small requirement for target cells, development of procedures for sending cell suspensions live (9) or frozen (16) by mail, applicability to cadaveric lymphocytes from blood or lymph node, and reproducibility (15). Even though the reproducibility is not 100%, day-to-day agreement often exceeds 98%, and this is considered acceptable. Although the test is readily described, there are many difficulties in tissue typing. Some of the technical considerations are discussed by Ward et al. (15). Questions of antigenic specificity and definition of antigens occupy many volumes and have been the subject of several international workshops (7).

TEST PROCEDURE

Two procedures will be described. The most widely used procedure is the cytotoxicity test developed by Terasaki and standardized in agreement with the National Institute of Allergy and Infectious Disease. This procedure is generally known as the NIH technique (14). The other procedure, that of Amos and his col-

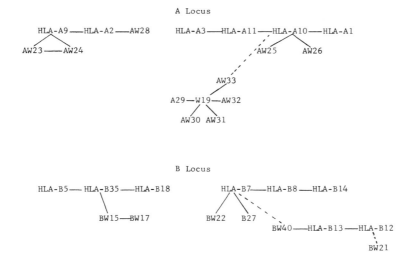

FIG. 1. *Cross-reacting groups. (Adapted from D. B. Amos and F. E. Ward, 1975, Immunogenetics of the HL-A system, Physiol. Rev. 55:206–246).*

leagues, is similar to the NIH technique but with the important difference of a wash step being introduced, which greatly increases the sensitivity of the test (1).

I. Cell Preparation: Preparation of Lymphocytes from Whole Peripheral Blood Using a Ficoll-Hypaque Gradient

1. Six to eight glass beads are added to each 10 ml of blood immediately upon drawing. The blood is then immediately defibrinated by continuously inverting the tube for approximately 5 min.

2. The blood is then diluted 1:3 with barbital buffer (BB) (1 part blood to 2 parts BB).

3. Measure 2 ml of Ficoll-Hypaque solution into a 16 × 100 mm glass tube and, with a Pasteur pipette, carefully layer up to 6 ml of diluted blood onto the solution, being careful not to cause mixing at the interface.

4. Spin tubes in a table centrifuge at 400 × g (2,000 rpm) for 30 min.

5. Remove supernatant down to a thin layer of cells. The thin cell layer is removed and placed in a 10 × 75 mm tube. This tube is nearly filled with BB, mixed, and spun at 1,000 rpm (120 × g) for 6 min.

6. The supernatant is discarded. If red blood cells are not present, proceed to step 8. If red blood cells are present, 1 ml of Tris-buffered NH_4Cl is mixed with the cells.

7. The cells are placed in a 37 C water bath for 10 min and then spun at 800 rpm for 6 min. Discard supernatant.

8. The cells are reconstituted in BB to desired concentration for testing (2.0 × 10^6 to 2.5 × 10^6 cells/ml).

II. Donor Panel

It is important to select reliable donors who will be available when required. Cells may be stored frozen in bulk or on trays, or may be prepared on the day required. It is customary to characterize the antigens of 60 or more individuals. In an outbred Caucasian population, most of the specificities will be represented at least once. It may be necessary to recruit additional subjects to cover some rare specificities. These may be from subpopulations, e.g., Nordic or Mediterranean, and some specificities are best characterized in subjects of Oriental or Negro origins.

From the full panel, a screening panel of 20 subjects representing all available specificities may be selected. This is adequate for the screening of new sera, especially if the husband of the multiparous donor can also be used as a donor of test cells. Obviously, it is desirable to have each specificity represented more than once. For more detailed testing, the full donor panel should be used.

III. Collection of Antisera

About one in three multiparous women has detectable levels of anti-HLA antibody. Some of the antibodies are lost soon after delivery, and others persist for long periods and sometimes for many years. The highest incidence of antibody producers is thus found in the first few days after delivery, and some antibodies (antisera) are collected at the time of discharge from the hospital. Most anti-HLA sera, however, are provided by blood donors. Serum from multiparous blood transfusion donors is screened for anti-HLA activity against lymphocytes from a typed panel that includes all known specificities. It is useful to screen with serum prediluted to 1:4 or 1:8 since sera that react only weakly are of little value.

Most of the sera that react will be broadly reactive; that is, they will react with panel cells carrying different specificities. If the serum reacts with one first- and one second-locus specificity, and especially where one or both of the specificities are rare, the serum may be valuable. Otherwise, only sera that give highly specific reactions are retained.

It is advisable to have the pattern of reactivity checked by a collaborating laboratory. If the serum is found to be specific, it is divided into smaller quantities and frozen. Several sizes of container are useful, especially those holding about 8 to 10 ml, 1 ml, and 400 μliters. Most donors are later re-bled and may be plasmaphoresed. The sera are stored frozen in the dark; -30 C appears to be a suitable temperature, although colder temperatures may also be used. Sera slowly deteriorate at -20 C, but may retain activity for as long as 10 years. Many laboratories prefer to lyophilize sera either in bulk and to weigh out small quantities for reconstitution, or in 1-ml quantities. Reconstitution is done with distilled water. The pH should be adusted to near neutrality. Sera should not be kept for more than 24 h in contact with CO_2 vapor. Serum (or cells) in contact with CO_2 vapor for any length of time becomes very acidic and deteriorates. This is most marked with small volumes as in the microtiter plates. Some sera are extremely sensitive, whereas others are more resistant. This adds to the danger, since a plate may seem to be intact yet some of the sera may have become inactivated. Precious sera may be stored in liquid nitrogen.

Additional sera may be obtained from commercial sources in the U.S. or abroad, by exchange with other laboratories, or from the NIH serum bank. The serum bank maintains a collection of several thousand lyophilized sera for investigative purposes, including the characterization of lymphocyte donor panels.

IV. Loading Microtiter Plates

It is frequently convenient to load microtiter plates with sera and to keep them frozen at -80 C or colder. Two methods are used to prevent evaporation. A small quantity of lightweight mineral oil (Atlas or Squibb), usually 1 or 2 μliters (although the amount is not critical), is placed in the well with a multiple dispenser. The serum is then dispensed through the oil. The second method relies on saturation of the air inside the microtiter plate. Collars of bibulous paper are prepared. Each collar is U-shaped and approximately 7 mm wide. The collar fits on three sides of the moat surrounding the wells, leaving the fourth side free for ease in identifying the rows. The paper is saturated with buffer or saline. The top of the microtiter plate is kept in place as much as possible during filling (Fig. 2A). Plates made in this manner slowly dry out in about 2 months, but appear to retain good potency.

Before loading, the plates are labeled with the batch number and date, using a Markette Thin-Rite Marker. For loading, a Hamilton dispenser, single- or six-place, is used. It is necessary when loading a six-place dispenser to have made a block with holes drilled to hold serumfilled microtubes so that the tubes have the same spacing as the wells in the row of the plate (Fig. 2B). Sixty microtubes containing sera are placed in the block. The syringes are filled with the sera in row one, and 50 plates are filled by pressing the button once for each plate. Several batches of 50 plates may be filled sequentially. The first row of serum-filled tubes is then discarded to avoid the possibility of error, and the Hamilton syringes are then washed 10 times with BB or saline to avoid the slightest possibility of serum carry-over. The danger of carry-over cannot be overemphasized, especially if one of the sera is particularly strong. It is usual to include a negative control (normal human group AB serum) and a positive control (antilymphocyte serum diluted to the point where it just gives 100% kill) in each plate.

A little dye, trypan red or neutral red, added to the serum before dispensing aids in quality control checking that all the wells are indeed filled. A blocked needle may prevent even dispensing. This can be detected by checking the residual serum before discarding the serum tube and by inspecting the wells in the filled plate. The trays are then placed in the bottom of a Revco Ultra Low freezer, the colder the better. They are removed from the freezer only 5 min before use.

V.(A) NIH Technique

1. One microliter of cells is dispensed into Falcon plastic microtiter plates (preloaded with oil or collars and serum as in section IV) with a

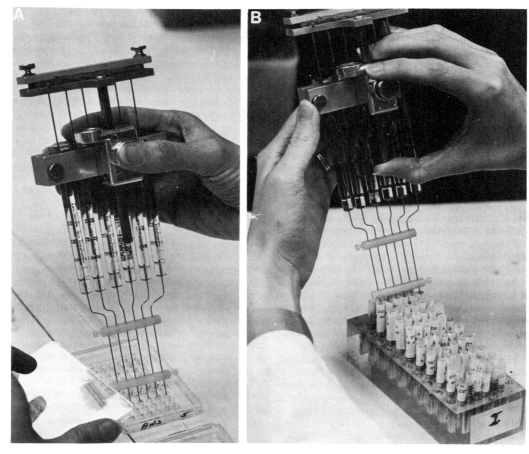

Fig. 2. *Loading of microtiter plates. (A) Position of microtiter plate during filling. (B) Block for holding serum-filled microtubes.*

Hamilton dispenser. A single-place dispenser is most frequently used.

2. The cells and sera are mixed by placing the microplate against a Yankee pipette shaker (or similar vibrator) and are left to incubate at room temperature for 30 min.

3. Five microliters of rabbit complement is then added to each well. (A few microliters of eosin, 1% trypan red, or neutral red in the complement serves as a marker.) The plates are then left to incubate at room temperature for 60 min.

4. Using a multiple dispenser, 3 μliters of 5% aqueous eosin is added to each well. Two minutes is allowed to elapse to allow the dead cells to stain.

5. The wells are then filled with formalin (pH 7.2), and a cover glass (50 × 75 mm) is placed over the wells in order to flatten the top of the droplet.

(B) Wash Step or Flick Procedure

1. One microliter of cells is dispensed into Falcon plastic microtiter plates (preloaded with oil or collars and serum as in section IV) with a Hamilton dispenser.

2. The cells and sera are mixed by placing the microplate against a Yankee pipette shaker (or similar vibrator) and are left to incubate at room temperature (approximately 20 to 22 C) for 30 min.

3. The wells are filled with BB, using a finely drawn Pasteur pipette employing a gentle swirling action to allow thorough mixing. The cells are left to settle for 8 to 10 min or gently centrifuged, using a suitable plate holder (many different forms exist).

4. Excess fluid is removed by inverting the plate over a sink or large waste container with a snapping motion of the wrist (flick). This

procedure is difficult to describe but is rapidly learned. The motion resembles that used by some red-cell serologists to remove supernatants from red-cell pellets. Early learning attempts may result in the loss of some cells from some of the wells, but proficiency soon comes with practice. Alternatives are to blot off or pipette off excess fluid, but these are time consuming and may also cause loss of the cells.

5. Five microliters of rabbit complement is then added to each well with a 0.250-μliter Hamilton syringe. Incubation is for 60 min at room temperature.

6. The plates are then flicked as in step 4.

7. Wells are filled with 0.3% trypan blue in EDTA, and plates are allowed to stand for 8 to 10 min or centrifuged as before.

8. The plates are flicked to remove excess trypan blue and permit better visualization of the cells.

9. The wells are filled with BB, and 2 drops of formalin is applied to the collar or margin of the plate for preservation of the cells. The lid is replaced. If trays are not to be read immediately, they should be refrigerated at 4 C.

VI. Reading

1. Determinations of incidence of staining are made by placing the plate under a standard (wash step technique) or inverted (NIH technique) microscope at $\times 150$ ($\times 10$ objectives, $\times 15$ oculars) (Table 2). The degree of staining is usually by estimation, but stained and unstained cells may also be counted.

2. The most frequent sources of error or difficulty in determining the degree of staining test cells are as follows: (i) Uneven distribution of cells. In some wells, cells may accumulate on the walls; these are most likely to be live cells. Centrifugation or mixing may be required. (ii) Clots in the wells. This is often due to improperly clotted serum. (iii) Debris in solutions used accumulating in the wells or dust in the wells before the serum was introduced. Solutions should be centrifuged and only the supernatants retained. Dusty plates can be cleaned before filling with an air jet. (iv) No cells in some wells. This may be from several causes: faulty dispenser (usually worn mechanical parts), uneven flicking, or over-lysis. Over-lysis may be corrected in subsequent tests by diluting the serum or by retitrating and diluting the complement. (v) Contamination of the lymphocyte suspension with granulocytes. This is a special problem with some cadaver donors, granulocytic leukemia patients, and patients with infections. The granulocytes often remain unstained, but may stain after exposure to some antisera.

3. Background level of staining is determined from the well containing AB serum. The proportion of stained cells rarely exceeds 5%. Causes of high background are: (i) cells are prepared too long before testing; (ii) cells are improperly handled (pH or isotonicity of solutions is incorrect); (iii) there are reactions of xenoantibodies in rabbit complement (this is especially a problem with cells from leukemic donors; preabsorption of complement with spleen cells or leukemic lymphocytes is advisable for use with leukemic cells); (iv) cells that have been stored frozen usually have higher than normal backgrounds; (v) occasionally, for no apparent reason, the control well contains a high proportion of stained cells whereas many wells containing antiserum give clear negative results. With due caution, the background may then be based on the negative reactions.

VII. Materials

1. Barbital buffer	Consolidated Laboratories, Inc., Chicago Heights, Ill.; Oxoid Barbitone C.F.T. diluent, 100 tablets.
2. Tris-NH$_4$Cl	Mix 1 part Tris buffer (a) in 9 parts NH$_4$Cl (b). (a) Tris buffer Trisma base, Sigma Chemical Co., or Tris buffer, General Biochemicals, Laboratory Park, Chagrin Falls, Ohio, 3$\times$ crystallized. Use 20.6 g of Tris per 1,000 ml of distilled water. Make up a flask $\frac{1}{2}$ to $\frac{3}{4}$ volume and adjust pH with concentrated HCl to pH 7.2 to 7.4 (starting pH will be about pH 11.0). Do at room temperature. Transfer to volumetric flask and added distilled water to desired volume. (b) Use 0.83 g of NH$_4$Cl per 100 ml of distilled water.
3. Mineral oil	Atlas Mineral Oil or Squibb Light Weight Mineral Oil, E.R. Squibb & Sons, Inc.

TABLE 2. *Two techniques for incidence of staining*

Wash step scoring system		NIH scoring system	
% Lysis	Scoring	% Lysis	Scoring
0–14	1	(Same as	
15–19	2	negative	
20–29	3	control)	1
30–59	4	10–19	2
60–94	5	20–39	4
95–100	6	40–79	6
		80–100	8

4.	Ficoll-Hypaque	24 ml of 9% Ficoll and 10 ml of 34% Hypaque should have a final specific gravity of 1.078 to 1.080. Store at 4 C. (a) Ficoll. Sigma Chemical Co.; 500 g/bottle. F4375 – 9% solution, 9 g of Ficoll per 100 ml of distilled water. (b) Hypaque. Hypaque sodium, 50% (wt/vol) 50-ml vials, Winthrop Labs. Use 6.8 ml of Hypaque and 3.2 ml of distilled water to make a 34% solution, or a commercially prepared gradient may be purchased. See 5, below.
5.	Lymphocyte separation medium (LSM solution)	Bionetics Lab Productions, Litton Bionetics Inc., Kensington, Md., catalogue no. 8410-01, 500 ml/carton.
6.	Trypan blue	K & K Laboratories, Inc., Plainview, N.Y., or Harleco, Hartman-Leddon Co., Philadelphia. 1 g per 100 ml of distilled water, filtered = 1% stock solution. For daily use: dilute 3 ml of 1% stock solution with 7 ml of 2% EDTA solution (see 7) = 0.3% trypan blue in EDTA. Stock solution may need occasional filtration.
7.	EDTA	Disodium ethylenediaminetetraacetate #S-311. Fisher Scientific Co., Fairlawn, N.Y. 2% EDTA is made: 20 g of EDTA in 1,000 ml of barbital buffer solution adjusted with NaOH to pH 7.0 to 7.4.
8.	Microplates	Falcon Plastics, Los Angeles. Microtest plates #3034; 1 case = 100 units.
9.	Rabbit complement	Pel Freeze Biologicals, Rogers, Ark. Nonpooled complement. Test each rabbit for cytotoxicity, and then titer in varying dilutions against antiserum with a known titer to determine which are strong enough to pool and use.
10.	Hamilton dispenser, syringe	Hamilton Co., Inc., Whittier, Calif.; 50-μliter capacity, #705-N. Repeating dispenser, PB-600-1, Terasaki dispenser with six 705 SN syringes, 0.050 ml, #83726.

LITERATURE CITED

1. Amos, D. B., R. Corley, D. Kostyu, Y. Delmas-Marsalet, and M. Woodbury. 1972. The serologic structure of HL-A as indicated by cross reactivities: the inclusion of HL-A loci into major histocompatibility complex H-1, p. 359–366. *In* J. Dausset, and J. Colombani (ed.), Histocompatibility testing 1972. Munksgaard, Copenhagen.

2. Amos, D. B., and N. Peacocke. 1963. Leucoagglutination. A modified technique and preliminary results of absorption with tissues, p. 1132–1140. *In* H. Lüdin (ed.), Proc. 9th Cong. Eur. Soc. Hematol. S. Karger, Basel/New York.

3. Chudomel, V., Z. Jezkova, and J. Libansky. 1958. Detection of leukocyte antibodies by the complement consumption test, p. 30–64. *In* Ha. Videbaek (ed.), Proc. 6th Cong. Soc. Eur. Hematol. 1957. S. Karger, Basel/New York.

4. Colombani, J., M. Colombani, A. Benajam, and J. Dausset. 1967. Leucocyte platelet antigens defined by platelet complement fixation test, p. 413–418. *In* E. S. Curtoni, P. L. Mattuiz, and R. M. Tosi (ed.), Histocompatibility testing 1967. Munksgaard, Copenhagen.

5. Dausset, J. 1956. Technique for demonstrating leukocyte agglutination, p. 147. *In* National Academy of Sciences Research Council (ed.), Histocompatibility testing. Government Printing Office publ. 1229, Washington, D.C.

6. Dausset, J., and G. Malinvaud. 1954. The effect of shaking on thrombocyte-agglutination. Its use in the study of thrombo-agglutinins and for the performance of the Coombs platelet test. Sang 25:847–850.

7. Kissmeyer-Nielsen, F. (ed.). 1976. Histocompatibility testing 1975. Munksgaard, Copenhagen, in press.

8. Mittal, K. K., M. R. Mickey, D. P. Singal, and P. I. Terasaki. 1968. Serotyping for homotransplantation. XVIII. Refinement of microdroplet cytotoxicity test. Transplantation 6:913–927.

9. Park, M. S., and P. I. Terasaki. 1974. Storage of human lymphocytes at room temperature. Transplantation 18:520–524.

10. Payne, R., as quoted by C. M. Zmijewski, R. L. St. Pierre, J. L. Fletcher, S. F. Wilson, W. Cannady, and H. Zmijewski. 1967. A comparison of two microagglutination tests, p. 389–405. *In* E. S. Curtoni, P. L. Mattuiz, and R. M. Tosi (ed.), Histocompatibility testing 1967. Munksgaard, Copenhagen.

11. Rood, J. J. van, and A. van Leeuwen. 1963. Leukocyte grouping. A method and its application. J. Clin. Invest. 42:1382–1390.

12. Rood, J. J. van, and A. van Leeuwen. 1965. An agglutination technique for the demonstration of leucocyte antigens in man using leucocytes from EDTA blood, p. 153. *In* National Academy of Sciences Research Council (ed.), Histocompatibility testing. Government Printing Office publ. 1229, Washington, D.C.

13. Terasaki, P., J. D. McClelland, M. S. Park, and B. McCurdy. 1973. Microdroplet lymphocyte cytotoxicity test, p. 54–61. *In* Manual of tissue typing techniques, DHEW publ. (NIH) 74–

545. Government Printing Office, Washington, D.C.

14. Walford, R. 1960. Leukocyte antigens and antibodies, p. 21. Grune & Stratton, New York/London.

15. Ward, F. E., D. B. Amos, W. B. Bias, J. C. Pierce, and R. D. Stulting, Jr. 1971. Report of three histocompatibility testing workshops in the Southeast regional procurement program. Transplantation 12:392–398.

16. Wood, N., H. Bashir, J. Greally, D. B. Amos, and E. J. Yunis. 1972. A simple method of freezing and storing live lymphocytes. Tissue Antigens 2:27–31.

Chapter 106

Transplantation Antigens Studied by Complement-Fixation Methods

J. COLOMBANI AND MONIQUE COLOMBANI

INTRODUCTION

In most cases, immune complexes formed by human histocompatibility antigens (HLA) and their specific antibodies activate the complement sequence. When HLA determinants are carried by the plasma membrane of a living cell, this activation leads to the killing of the cell. The most common application of this phenomenon is the lymphocytotoxicity technique (14), widely used for the study of HLA antigens and antibodies. The complement-fixation (CF) method can also be applied to a study of this kind. Less frequently used than lymphocytotoxicity, the classical CF method deserves to be more largely employed because of its quantitative properties. In addition, unlike cytotoxicity methods which can be applied only to living cells, CF can be used on a number of antigenic substrates, including subcellular extracts from various sources. It has mainly been applied to blood platelets (PlCF).

The CF method evaluates the amount of complement fixed by antigen-antibody complexes. This implies the need for a reference system to detect or measure complement. It may conveniently be assayed by its hemolytic activity on sheep erythrocytes sensitized by an anti-sheep erythrocyte antibody (hemolysin).

Qualitative CF techniques use a limited amount of complement in the reaction mixture. At the end of the fixation stage, the hemolytic activity of residual complement is checked. The result is said to be positive or negative according to the absence or presence of residual hemolytic activity. Semiquantitative results can be obtained by testing various dilutions of antigens and/or antibodies. Macrotechniques were initially developed; then, because of the saving of reagents (antibodies), microtechniques were devised which made possible the use of CF on a large scale. A standardized international microtechnique was agreed upon (6) and used during the 5th and 6th International Histocompatibility Workshops. Quantitative CF measures the exact number of complement

units fixed by a given substrate (antigen-antibody complexes). When the complexes are formed in the presence of an excess of antibody, the amount of complexes and, consequently, the number of complement units fixed are proportional to the amount of antigen in the reaction mixture. Quantitative CF can thus be used to measure the antigenic content of a substrate. Various techniques have been developed (10, 12), and recently a quantitative form of the international microtechnique was proposed (1).

It has been empirically observed that the use of human serum instead of guinea pig serum as the source of complement gave better results in CF for HLA serology—better sensitivity and reproducibility of the tests, which were less subject to anticomplementarity. No definite explanation was proposed for this phenomenon (3, 12). Nevertheless, complement from both sources can be used, and guinea pig complement is generally more convenient for quantitative CF.

CLINICAL INDICATIONS

Platelet complement fixation

HLA typing by PlCF is efficient and easy. Most of the specificities recognized by lymphocytotoxicity are also defined by PlCF: HLA-A1, 2, 3, 5, 7, 8, 9, 10, 11, 12, 13, W5, W10, W14, W15, W16, W17, W18, W21, W22, W27, W28, W29, W32, Da25 (= W30 + W31), TYT, Fe55, Da34 (= Sabell). Test sera for W23 and W24 (subdivisions of HLA-A9) and for W25 and W26 (subdivisions of HLA-A10) are not yet available for PlCF. Certain immune sera are particularly rare as monospecific reagents: anti-Da25 (W30 + W31), anti-W32. They are more often observed in various mixtures combining some of the subcomponents of W19 (W29, W30, W31, W32). Anti-HLA-A8 sera reaction in PlCF are rare and give a definition of the antigen shorter than the definition given by lymphocytotoxic sera. The same phenomenon is observed for HLA-A10 and HLA-A12. About half the HLA-A12+ individuals are types as HLA-A12− by PlCF.

Quantitative absorption studies showed that the phenomenon could be explained by a weak expression of the antigen HLA-A12 on the platelets of these individuals. It was possible to absorb and/or elute an HLA-A12 antibody from these platelets, but their absorbing activity was 5 to 10 times lower than that of the platelets which reacted directly in the PlCF technique. These results suggest that HLA-A12 specificity is heterogenous (2). On the other hand, the antigens belonging to the Da6 cross-reacting group (HLA-A5, W5, W15, W21) may be defined more clearly by PlCF than by lymphocytotoxicity. The use of these two different but convergent techniques for HLA typing offers a guarantee superior to that when the same groups are typed in duplicate with only one technique. Additionally, this practice increases the accuracy of the typing by using sera from different sources.

Lymphocyte complement fixation

Previous studies have shown that CF may be used for the study of HLA antigens on leukocytes, lymphocytes, and neutrophils (10). Recently, we applied the international CF microtechnique to peripheral lymphocytes. Results showed that the lymphocyte CF (LyCF) microtechnique could be used for large-scale HLA typing as efficiently as PlCF (6).

Lymphocyte suspensions were prepared from defibrinated, heparinized, or disodium ethylenediaminetetraacetate (Na$_2$ EDTA)-treated blood by centrifugation on Ficoll-Isopaque (15). After three washings in saline containing 0.1% N$_3$Na and 2% inactivated (56 C, 30 min) normal human AB serum, the lymphocytes were suspended in the same medium at a concentration of 15,000 μliter. The suspension prepared from defibrinated blood contained virtually no platelets. In other cases, platelets were removed by differential centrifugation during the washings. When kept at 4 C, lymphocyte suspensions retained their antigenic activity for several weeks. The LyCF test was carried out in the same way as the PlCF test with 3 $\times$ 10^4 lymphocytes per test.

HLA typing by LyCF gave essentially the same results as obained with PlCF. The discrepancies between the two techniques concerned only the definitions of HLA-A8, 10, and 12 as mentioned above.

Quantitative complement-fixation microtechnique (1)

The reagents and material used were the same as those described below for the qualitative PlCF. All reagents were used in 2-μliter amounts. The principle of the test was to put the same antigen-antibody mixtures into contact with amounts of complement varying from 1 to 10 H100 (100% hemolytic) units in 10 wells of a microtest plate. Guinea pig serum was used as the source of complement in the quantitative microtechnique, since a complement with a high hemolytic titer was necessary to provide the relatively large amount of complement needed (up to 10 H100 units). Lyophilized guinea pig serum, available commercially, may be used. Guinea pig complement was titrated as described below, and the various dilutions were calculated to make 1 to 10 H100 units per well. The test conditions were the same as those of the qualitative microtechnique. The amount of complement fixed by a given reaction mixture was evaluated as described in Table 1.

To study all the quantitative aspects of the antigen-antibody reactions, several concentrations of antigenic substratum and several concentrations of the same serum should be used. For platelets, a convenient range of dosage would be 2 $\times$ 10^5 to 12 $\times$ 10^5 per test (Fig. 1). The concentration of immune serum should be adjusted to bring about the formation of antigen-antibody complexes with an excess of antibody. Under these conditions, the amount of complement fixed is directly proportional to the amount of antigen, as is the case in Fig. 1, in

TABLE 1. *Example of results of quantitative platelet complement-fixation microtechnique*[a]

Units of complement added to each well	Degree of hemolysis
1	4
2	4
3	4
4	4
5	4
6	1
7	0
8	0
9	0
10	0

[a] Each well of the microtest plate contained 2 μliters of platelet suspension, 2 μliters of anti-HLA immune serum, and 2 μliters of various dilutions of guinea pig complement. Complement dilutions were adjusted so that each successive well contained 1 to 10 H100 units. After 1 h of incubation at 37 C, 2 μliters of sensitized sheep erythrocyte suspension (400,000 cells) was added. After a further incubation for 30 min and centrifugation, the reaction mixture completely inhibited 5 complement units. In the well containing 6 units, an almost complete hemolysis was observed (approximately one of four sheep erythrocytes was left unlysed). The amount of complement fixed by the reaction mixture could then be evaluated at 5.25 units.

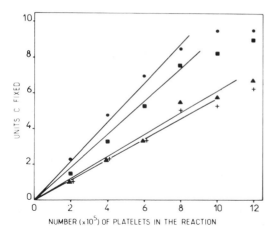

FIG. 1. *Quantitative complement fixation with anti-HLA-A2 and various HLA-A2+ platelets in a family. Anti-HLA-A2 was used at a concentration of 1:10. There was 1 H100 unit of guinea pig complement in 0.01 μliter. The HLA genotypes of the platelet donors were as follows: HLA-A2, 12/HLA-A2, W22 (● and ■); HLA-A2, 12/HLA-A3, 5 (▲); HLA-A2, 12/HLA-A11, − (+). The average amount of complement fixed by 6 × 10⁵ sensitized platelets was 3.5 units for the heterozygous individuals and 6 units for the homozygous individuals.*

which experimental points could be fitted to straight lines in the left-hand part of the curves. The plateau reached in the right half of Fig. 1, especially for HLA-A2 homozygous platelets, indicated that, for these platelet concentrations, the complexes were no longer formed with an excess of antibody.

Quantitative studies show a gene dosage effect for HLA antigens (Fig. 1). Initial studies on HLA-A2 antigens disproved such an effect (10), then further studies (12) showed that it could be clearly demonstrated inside families but that a twofold range of variation in antigenic content existed in a population of unrelated HLA-A2 heterozygous individuals. It now seems that this rather wide individual variation in antigenic content can be explained by cross-reactions between the allelic products of each HLA locus. HLA-A2+, W28 + platelets sensitized by an anti-HL-A2 antibody fix about the same amount of complement as platelets from an HLA-A2 homozygous individual because of the cross-reaction between HLA-A2 and W28 (2, 13). A gene dosage effect was also observed for HLA-A5, 9, and 12. But again, cross-reactions should be taken into account. For instance, HLA-A12+, W21+ or HLA-A12+, W10+ platelets behaved like HLA-A12 homozygous platelets because of the cross-reaction between the antigens. In certain instances, quantitative CF

thus permits the determination of the zygosity of an individual with a "blank" antigen.

Blocking antibodies

Quantitative CF tests enable non-complement-fixing (blocking) anti-HLA antibodies to be studied (10). These antibodies are able to prevent complement-fixing antibodies of the same specificity from combining with the antigen. In consequence, CF is inhibited. Quantitative CF is especially well adapted to this study since it measures the amount of complement fixed by a given reaction mixture containing a known complement-fixing antibody. Two such tests using a complement-fixing serum of known specificity are carried out in parallel. In the experimental test, the antigenic substrate has been preincubated with the serum under investigation before the complement-fixing serum is added. In the control test, preincubation was made with a normal serum. The specificity of the blocking antibody is the same as that of the complement-fixing one. The difference between the amounts of complement fixed in each test measures the blocking effect. A study (4) of 109 patients immunized essentially by blood transfusions showed that in 58 cases (53.2%) the patients' sera contained anti-HLA blocking antibodies. They were either alone or associated with complement-fixing antibodies detected by lymphocytotoxicity and/or PlCF. The blocking was specific as was observed only for one, two, or three of the eight HLA specificities studied (HLA-A1, 2, 3, 5, 7, 9, 10, 12). It was specifically absorbed only on platelets carrying the corresponding antigen. In three sera studied by density gradient centrifugation, the blocking activity was located once in the immunoglobulin M (IgM) and twice in the IgG fractions. These results confirm and enlarge previous observations (10). They show that complement-fixing and non-complement-fixing anti-HLA antibodies are often present in the same immune serum and that they can be distributed among the various immune globulin classes and subclasses, of which some fix complement and others do not. The biological role (enhancement?) of non-complement-fixing antibodies remains to be defined.

Complement fixation on other substrates

Preliminary studies showed that HLA antigens could be studied by the CF microtechnique on lymphoid cell lines. The conservation of these cells was similar to that of peripheral lymphocytes. Their serological reactivity was high. The optimal dose for HLA typing was 1,000 cells per test. The same CF microtechnique was applied to the typing of cultured fibroblasts with the use of 4,000 cells per test. Solubilized HLA antigens cannot be directly used in CF but are able to inhibit CF tests (5).

These results show the versatility of the CF technique, which seems well adapted to the direct comparison of HLA antigen expression on various cell types.

TEST PROCEDURES

Platelet complement-fixation microtechnique

Preparation of platelet suspension. Platelet suspension is prepared from blood drawn in a siliconized or plastic tube, on a 5% Na_2 EDTA solution in saline (1:10 of the blood volume). A 10% sodium citrate solution can also be used as an anticoagulent. All the following centrifugations are made at 4 C. Platelet-rich plasma is obtained by centrifugation at $200 \times g$ for 10 min and pipetted off. The supernatant fluid is then spun at $1,600 \times g$ for 30 min to obtain the platelet button (these centrifugation times and speeds are established for 10- to 20-ml volumes; smaller values are to be used for smaller volumes). Platelets are then washed three times in saline and finally resuspended in saline containing 0.1% N_3Na at a concentration of 2×10^6 platelets per μliter. It is better not to use the suspension at once but only after 1 or 2 days. However, if it is necessary to use it immediately, it is incubated at room temperature for 30 min in a 1% ammonium oxalate solution before centrifugation at the time of the first washing.

Preparation of sensitized sheep erythrocytes. Sheep whole blood is aseptically collected in Alsever's solution, or sodium citrate solution (1:4 of the blood volume), and is kept at 4 C for 1 week before use. The same batch of sheep blood can be used for 4 to 6 weeks. If the supernatant fluid shows hemolysis after the second washing or if an abnormally high titer of complement is observed, the batch must be discarded.

Sheep erythrocytes are washed twice in saline and once in Veronal-buffered saline (VBS, see below), and are finally resuspended in VBS at the concentration of 400,000 cells per μliter. For sensitization, the suspension is incubated for 30 min at 37 C with an equal volume of hemolysin (rabbit antisheep erythrocyte) diluted in VBS to contain 4 minimal hemolytic units. The minimal hemolytic unit was determined under the test conditions by the usual preliminary titration (8). After incubation, sensitized erythrocytes are kept at 4 C until used. They can be used for 1 or 2 days.

VBS, pH 7.3. Dissolve 85.0 g of NaCl and 3.75 g of sodium 5,5-diethyl-barbiturate in 1,400 ml of distilled water. Dissolve 5.75 g of 5,5-diethyl-barbituric acid in 500 ml of hot distilled water. Mix the two solutions and allow to cool at room temperature. Add 5 ml of 1 M $MgCl_2$-0.3 M $CaCl_2$ solution. Adjust the volume to 2,000 ml with distilled water. Keep this stock solution at 4 C. Dilute five times with distilled water for daily use. Add 0.05 g of gelatin/100 ml (Bactogelatin, Difco). The appropriate amount of gelatin is dissolved separately in hot distilled water (8). VBS can also be prepared from commercial Complement Fixation Test Diluent Tablets (Oxoid, Oxo Ltd., London, England).

Preparation and titration of human complement. Human serum used as the source of complement is a pool of at least five sera obtained from AB fasting donors without any history of alloimmunization. The blood is allowed to stand for 1 h at 20 C and then for 2 h at 4 C. It is then centrifuged for 20 min at $2,500 \times g$ at 4 C. The serum is pipetted off and centrifuged again to spin down the few remaining cells. Portions of the pooled sera are kept frozen at -85 C in stoppered tubes. Each portion is used immediately after a quick thawing. It is thawed only once.

Closely spaced serial dilutions (for example, 1:10, 1:15, 1:20, etc., up to 1:90) of complement in VBS are prepared. In each well of a microtest plate (see below), 4 μliters of VBS and 2 μliters of each complement dilution are distributed. After 1 h of incubation in a 37 C incubator, 2 μliters of sensitized sheep erythrocytes is added to each well. After mixing (see below) and a further incubation at 37 C for 30 min, the plate is centrifuged for 3 min at $700 \times g$. Hemolysis is read with the naked eye. The 100% hemolytic unit (H100 unit) is given by the highest dilution of complement producing complete hemolysis. A concentration double this one (2 H100 units) is used for the test.

Test procedure. The test is made in microtest tissue culture plates covered with 6 ml of viscous paraffin oil (Saybolt viscosity 335/350; Merck or Fisher Scientific Co.). Specially ordered, nontreated, i.e., nonwettable, Greiner-Cooke microplates (Greiner, Bischwiller, France), give better results than the standard wettable plates. The reagents are distributed with a microtiter Hamilton syringe, N 710, equipped with a repeating dispenser, PB600 (Hamilton Co., Whittier, Calif.), as shown in Table 2.

Sera are used after heat inactivation (30 min at 56 C). They are stored at -20 C or lower. The dilutions are made with VBS. Sera are tested routinely at a dilution of 1:5. Sera reacting positively are then diluted further. Some weakly reacting sera may be used at higher concentrations (1:3, 1:2), but at those concentrations a nonspecific anticomplementary activity is sometimes observed.

Controls (Table 2) are included in each protocol and are run in parallel with the test. Complete hemolysis must be obtained in all the controls for the test to be valid.

The reagents are mixed with a Vortex mixer. The bottom of the microtest plate is firmly held on the rotating neoprene cup of the mixer for 15 s. The vibrations of the plate cause mixing to occur.

Centrifugation of the plates (3 min at 700 × g) can be done in microtiter centrifuge carriers.

Reading is made under standardized light conditions. The extent of hemolysis is evaluated from the color of the supernatant fluid and from the size of the erythrocyte button. The results are graded according to the degree of hemolysis:

$$0\text{–}20\% = \text{grade } 4$$
$$21\text{–}40\% = \text{grade } 3$$
$$41\text{–}60\% = \text{grade } 2$$
$$61\text{–}80\% = \text{grade } 1$$
$$81\text{–}100\% = \text{grade } 0$$

Histocompatibility typing by platelet complement fixation

Blood platelets were used in CF for practical reasons. Platelet suspensions can easily be prepared in a pure state. They are extremely stable. The separation of platelets from whole blood can be postponed for 4 to 5 days after bleeding on condition that the blood is preserved in a sterile fashion at 4 C. This can be convenient when HLA typing cannot be done on the spot (anthropological studies). One of the peculiarities of platelet surface HLA antigens is that they are not fully active immediately after separation from whole blood in serological reactions. They become completely active after 1 or 2 days. This fact can lead to false-negative reactions when weak immune sera are used. Platelet suspensions keep their activity at 4 C for at least 10 to 12 months (11). It seems that preservation is better in the case of high concentration suspensions (2×10^6 μliter) than when suspensions are diluted (0.5×10^6 μliter).

The extreme stability of platelet suspensions represents a real advantage for serological studies: a reference panel for the identification of new specificities can be kept permanently in the laboratory.

The immune sera which are used for the detection of HLA antigens on platelets are

TABLE 2. *Qualitative platelet complement-fixation microtechnique, test, and controls*[a]

Reagent	Test	Controls for anticomplementary activity of:		Control for complement activity
		Serum	Platelets	
Veronal-buffered saline (VBS)	0	2	2	4
Platelet suspension (0.5 × 10⁶ per ml)	2	0	2	0
Serum dilution in VBS	2	2	0	0
Human complement (2 H100 units in 2 µliters)	2	2	2	2
Mixing, 1 h of incubation at 37 C				
Sensitized sheep erythrocytes (200,000 per µliter)	2	2	2	2
Mixing, 30 min of incubation at 37 C with frequent mixing. Centrifugation and reading.				

[a] The figures in each column of the table indicate the amount in microliters of the various reagents to be distributed successively in four wells of a microtest plate, one for the test and three for the controls.

obtained from the same sources of alloimmunization as those used in the lymphocytotoxicity technique: transfusions, pregnancies, skin grafts, and injections of leukocyte or leukoplatelet suspensions. However, the sensitivities of PlCF and lymphocytotoxicity are different, the latter being about four times more sensitive. Moreover, since the immune sera may be used undiluted in lymphocytotoxicity but not in PlCF, the former technique can detect an anti-HLA immunization 10 or 20 times as weak as that detected by the latter. For this reason, the same immune serum can rarely be used in both techniques in parallel. For instance, the sera of multiparous women, which are generally good lymphocytotoxicity reagents, are often too weak to be used in PlCF. Inversely, sera from polytransfused patients, which are too polyspecific in lymphocytotoxicity, are generally good reagents in PlCF. Though they are polyspecific, these sera often have great differences in titer for the antibiodies of the various specificities which they contain. This means that it is possible to obtain a monospecific reagent by simply diluting the immune serum.

It is also easy to prepare monospecific reagents by absorption and/or elution from multispecific immune sera. Packed cells obtained from the platelet suspension used in PlCF tests are convenient substrata for absorption-elution procedures (7, 9, 10).

CONCLUSION

In conclusion, the CF microtechnique is an efficient method of HLA typing on various substrates: platelets, lymphocytes, and other cell types. Quantitative CF provides a means for the study of histocompatibility antigen-antibody interaction. Together with quantitative absorption, it is a tool for studying variations in antigenic content. Individual variations are related to zygosity, cross-reactions, and possibly other causes. The study of variations from one cell type to another in the same individual could provide information on the histocompatibility antigen distribution on the cell membrane.

LITERATURE CITED

1. Colombani, J., and M. Colombani. 1973. Principle and application of a quantitative complement fixation microtechnique. Symp. Ser. Immunobiol. Stand. **18**:89.
2. Colombani, J., and M. Colombani. 1974. Serological recognition of histocompatibility antigens using complement fixation. Semin. Hematol. **11**:273–280.
3. Colombani, J., M. Colombani, H. Dastot, A. Elias, and J. Dausset. 1968. Utilisation de serum humain comme source de complement dans une reaction de fixation de complement sur plaquettes. Nouv. Rev. Fr. Hematol. **8**:864–868.
4. Colombani, J., M. Colombani, and V. Lepage. 1974. Anticorps anti-HL-A ne fixant pas le complement (bloquants). Nouv. Rev. Fr. Hematol. **14**:518–530.
5. Colombani, J., M. Colombani, D. C. Viza, O. Degani-Bernard, J. Dausset, and D. A. L. Davies. 1970. Separation of HL-A transplantation antigen specificities. Transplant. Proc. **3**:228–239.
6. Colombani, J., J. D'Amaro, B. W. Gabb, G. S. Smith, and A. Svejgaard. 1971. International agreement on a microtechnique of platelet comment fixation. Transplant. Proc. **3**:121–129.
7. Colombani, M., J. Colombani, C. Dehay, and J. Dausset. 1970. A microtechnique of platelet complement fixation. Results obtained with sera and eluates as the source of antibody, p. 553–559. *In* P. I. Terasaki (ed.), Histocompatibility testing 1970. Munksgaard, Copenhagen.
8. Rapp, H. J., and T. Borsos. 1970. Molecular basis of complement action. Appleton-Century Crofts, New York.
9. Rodey, G. F., B. Sturm, and R. H. Aster. 1973. Cross-reactive HL-A antibodies. Separation of multiple HL-A antibody specificities by platelet adsorption and acid elution. Tissue Antigens **3**:63–69.
10. Shulman, N. R., V. J. Marder, M. C. Hiller, and E. M. Collier. 1964. Platelet and leukocyte iso-antigens and their antibodies: Serologic, physiologic and clinical studies. Prog. Hematol. **4**:222–304.
11. Smith, G. S., and R. I. Walford. 1971. Standardization and stability of platelet suspensions in the complement fixation test for HL-A antigens. Tissue Antigens **1**:14–22.
12. Svejgaard, A. 1969. Iso-antigenic systems of human blood platelets. A survey. Ser. Haematol., vol. 2, no. 3.
13. Svejgaard, A., and F. Kissmeyer-Nielsen. 1968. Cross-reactive human HL-A iso-antibodies. Nature (London) **219**:868–869.
14. Terasaki, P. I., and J. D. McCelland. 1964. Micro-droplet assay of human serum cytotoxins. Nature (London) **204**:998–1000.
15. Thorsby, E., and A. Bratlie. 1970. A rapid method for the production of pure lymphocyte suspensions, p. 655–656. *In* P. I. Terasaki (ed.), Histocompatibility testing 1970. Munksgaard, Copenhagen.

Chapter 107

Typing for Specific B Lymphocyte Antigens

LESLIE ABELSON, PIERRE HENKART, AND DEAN MANN

INTRODUCTION

The major human histocompatibility antigens (HLA) can readily be identified on peripheral blood lymphocytes by serological techniques. The importance of these antigens has been clearly demonstrated in clinical organ transplantation. There are, however, situations where histocompatibility antigen matching between donor and recipient is identical, and yet immunological rejection of the transplanted organ occurs. This indicates that cell surface antigens other than HLA participate in the rejection phenomena. Subpopulations of lymphocytes such as T and B cells appear to possess cell surface antigens unique to a particular population. These antigens may play an important role in graft rejection.

Serological identification of these antigens requires separation of the lymphocytes into their various subpopulations, as well as the antisera which will detect these antigens. Currently, limited sera detecting B cell antigens are available. As this field of investigation broadens, more sera will become available. Separation of lymphocytes into the "B" and "T" cell subpopulations is critical for evaluation of their cell surface antigens. B lymphocytes have a unique property in that they possess a receptor for the Fc portion of antibody when that antibody is complexed to an antigen. This is a broad definition for B cells, as it is becoming increasingly apparent that some immunoglobulin-negative cells have Fc receptors. Utilizing this property as a basis for separation, we have developed a technique for typing B lymphocyte cell surface antigens (1–4).

CLINICAL INDICATIONS

As yet, the test procedure we have developed does not have clinical application. However, typing for "B" lymphocyte antigens may be of great benefit in clinical organ transplantation. In addition, these antigens may be associated with certain diseases similar to that described for the HL-A antigens.

TEST PROCEDURE

The technique employs the recognition of antigen-antibody complexes on plastic surfaces by B cell Fc receptors. Basically, peripheral blood lymphocytes may be separated into T and B subpopulations by adding a macrophage-depleted peripheral blood lymphocyte cell suspension to an antigen-antibody treated plastic surface. Fc receptor-bearing cells will adhere to the complex, and nonadherent cells are easily collected by washing. The separated populations can then be used in a modified microcytotoxicity assay. The B cells are tested directly in the microtest wells in which they adhere. Samples of the nonadherent cells are placed in untreated wells for parallel testing.

The microtest plate (Falcon Plastics #3034) is first treated by adding heat-inactivated fetal calf serum to each well. Serum may be dispensed in 10-μliter amounts with Hamilton syringe #750N or with a finely drawn Pasteur pipette. The plates are incubated at 37 C for 20 min; then they are washed by flooding the entire plate three times with distilled water and once with phosphate-buffered saline (PBS), pH 7.4. Subsequently, each well is incubated for 20 min at 37 C with 10 μliters of 10 mM trinitro-benzene-sulfonic acid in PBS, pH 7.4. The plates are washed again as described previously. Finally, 10 μliters of heat-inactivated rabbit anti-DNP-BSA, diluted 1:100 in balanced salt solution-10% fetal calf serum (BSS-FCS), is added to each well. The plates are incubated for at least 20 min at 37 C, or they can be refrigerated for use up to as much as 4 days later. Prior to plating the prepared lymphocytes, the plates are washed by flooding three times with distilled water and once with BSS-FCS.

The T and B cell populations are prepared as follows. Heparinized (20 units/ml) peripheral blood is added to 2.5 ml of Plasmagel (heated to 37 C). The red cells are allowed to sediment in a 37 C water bath for 10 to 15 min. The leukocyte-rich plasma is then transferred to a 50-ml plastic conical tube for the next procedure, macrophage depletion. For each 10 ml of starting material (e.g., peripheral blood), 1 g of carbonyl ion powder is added. The tube is gently vortexed to disperse the filings evenly and is then placed on a Fisher Rotorack at slow speed. The tube should be allowed to tumble gently for 20 min at 37 C, allowing the macrophages to take up as much iron as possible. This procedure may also be carried out in a 250-ml Erlenmeyer flask for a maximum of plasma from 30 ml of blood. The flask is placed in a shaking 37 C water bath for the same time period. In either case, after incubation, the plasma-iron suspension is transferred to a clean 50-ml conical plastic tube, and a large magnet is run down the side of the tube to draw out as much of the excess iron as possible. Finally, the plasma is placed on lymphocyte separation medium (LSM or Ficoll-Hypaque). The plasma is layered over 10 to 15 ml of LSM in a glass or plastic 50-ml tube. The gradients are run at 2,000 rpm for 15 min at 20 C. The cells are harvested, washed twice with PBS and once with BSS-FCS, and adjusted to 2.5×10^6/ml in BSS-FCS. The purified population is free from platelets and contains <3% macrophages.

The purified lymphocytes are separated into T and B populations by placing 10-μliter amounts (2.5×10^4 cells) of the above cell preparation in the antigen-antibody prepared, washed microtest wells. The cells are allowed to settle and adhere for 30 min at 37 C. The entire plate is then filled with 37 C BSS and covered with parafilm so that there are no air pockets. The test plate lid is securely replaced, and the entire plate is turned over for approximately 15 min, allowing the non-Fc receptor-bearing cells to separate from the adherent cell population. The plates are turned right side up, and the entire contents are poured or pipetted into a 50-ml tube. The plates are washed twice with BSS, and the washes are pooled with the original material collected. These nonadherent T cells are adjusted to 2×10^6/ml in BSS and are then transferred with a 705N Hamilton syringe (1 μliter = 2×10^3 cells) into clean untreated test plate wells for parallel testing with B cells. At this point, buffer-saturated filter-paper strips should be placed around the periphery of each plate to keep the atmosphere moist during the microcytotoxicity assay. Prior to the addition of any serum, care should be taken to flick out any excess BSS accumulated in the treated test wells during separation of the two populations.

Depending on the serum to be tested, 1 to 5 μliters is added to each well with the appropriate Hamilton syringe. The cells are allowed to incubate with the serum for 60 min. Each serum-filled well is then washed by adding a small drop of BSS with a finely drawn Pasteur pipette. Care should be taken not to overfill the wells. The cells are allowed to settle for 10 min, and the plates are then "flicked" to remove the serum and BSS wash. A finely drawn Pasteur pipette is again used to dispense rabbit complement, approximately 5 μliters per test. The incubation is carried out for 15 min at room temperature, allowing complement to fix to the antigen-antibody complex on the treated plates. The plates are flicked again, and approximately 5 μliters of fresh rabbit complement is added in the same manner for 45 min at room temperature. The plates are flicked once more, and 5 μliters of 0.3% trypan blue (containing 0.14% ethylenediaminetetraacetate, pH 7.4) is added to each well. The cells are allowed to stain for 10 min, and the plates are then flicked. Each well is filled with BSS. The cells are allowed to resettle for 10 min prior to reading on an inverted phase microscope. The plates may be read immediately or held overnight by saturating the filter-paper collars with 37% formaldehyde. The scoring is as follows: 0 to 14% stained = 1; 15 to 19% = 2; 20 to 29% = 3; 30 to 59% = 4; 60 to 90% = 5; >90% = 6.

REAGENTS

Preparation of treated plastics

Microtest plate, #3034, Falcon Plastics.

2,4,6-Trinitrobenzene sulfonic acid, #29000, Pierce Chemical.

Rabbit anti-DNP-BSA, #61-006, Miles Research.

Phosphate-buffered saline.

Balanced salt solution.

Fetal calf serum, #614, Grand Island Biological Co.

Preparation of lymphocytes

Heparin, #7973, The Upjohn Co.

Plasmagel, Roger Bellon Laboratories, Neuilly, France, or Associate Biomedic Systems, Buffalo, N.Y.

Carbonyl iron powder, #1-1-63800, Grad W, GAF Corp.

Ficoll-Hypaque lymphocyte separation medium, #8410-01, Bionetics.

Fetal calf serum, #614, Grand Island Biological Co.

Fisher Roto-Rack, Fisher Scientific Co.

Modified microcytotoxicity assay

Antisera.

Prepared separated cells.

Rabbit complement, Pel Freeze.

Trypan blue, #525, Grand Island Biological Co.

Hamilton syringes, #750N, 725N, 705N, Lawshe Instrument Co.

LITERATURE CITED

1. Mann, D. L., L. Abelson, S. Harris, and D. B. Amos. 1975. Detection of antigens specific for "B" lymphoid cultured cell lines with human alloantisera. J. Exp. Med. 142:84–89.
2. Mann, D. L., L. Abelson, S. Harris, and D. B.

Amos. 1976. A second genetic locus within the HL-A region for human B cell alloantigens. Nature 259:145–146.

3. Mann, D. L., L. Abelson, P. Henkart, S. Harris, and D. B. Amos. 1975. Serologic detection of B lymphocyte antigens. Proceedings of the Sixth International Histocompatibility Work-shop Conference, p. 705–707.

4. Mann, D. L., L. Abelson, P. Henkart, S. D. Harris, and D. B. Amos. 1975. Specific human B lymphocyte alloantigens (L-B) linked to HL-A. Proc. Natl. Acad. Sci. U.S.A. 72:5103–5106.

Chapter 108

Antiglobulin Cross-Match for Transplantation

A. H. JOHNSON

INTRODUCTION

Numerous techniques have been described and applied as cross-match procedures for transplantation. All are designed to detect antibodies in the serum of the potential recipient to antigens present on donor tissue. The lymphocyte is the most frequently used target cell since it expresses the major histocompatibility antigens and is easy to obtain. Use of the lymphocyte cross-match to minimize the occurrence of hyperacute rejection in transplantation of solid organ grafts has been substantially documented (13). Lymphocytotoxicity is the most widely used technique because the assays are rapid and reproducible, and they utilize a small volume of serum and a small number of cells. Variations of the lymphocytotoxicity assay are numerous (18): some employ a one-stage incubation (8); some, a two-stage incubation (11); some, a wash step (1); some, extended incubation times (7); and some, fluorochromasia (2).

Ideally, more than one technique should be used in cross-matching, although this may not always be feasible in practice. When selecting the cross-match techniques to be used, one should consider the type of transplant contemplated. If the cross-match is for platelet transfusion, then a procedure which uses platelets as targets should be chosen, for example, platelet complement fixation (4) or platelet aggregation. For kidney transplantation, kidney cells may be used as target cells in the cross-match procedure. Here one may use cytotoxicity (14), immune adherence (15), or mixed antiglobulin (17). Also, techniques which do not require the fixation of complement may be used; examples are leukoagglutination (19, 25) and indirect immunofluorescence (21).

To facilitate detection of low levels of antibodies in potential recipients, sensitive techniques must be used (3, 7, 10, 12, 17, 24). The correlation between hyperacute rejection and the presence of serum antibody against donor tissue is well established (9, 24). Also, cases of irreversible rejection during the first days following transplantation may be delayed expression of a secondary response to donor antigens due to low levels of antibody undetected in the lymphocyte cross-match (10, 12). More sensitive procedures, used retrospectively, have detected antibody missed by the usual cross-match procedure (7, 10, 16, 23).

The antiglobulin microcytotoxicity test is a sensitive method which may be used to supplement other lymphocytotoxicity cross-match procedures. It is from 4- to 64-fold more sensitive than a standard direct test (Fig. 1 and 2), and it detects the presence of cross-reactive antibodies in sera which appear monospecific by direct techniques. In addition, it detects weak or low levels of antibodies to histocompatibility antigens HLA other than the major specificity in the typing sera tested. Non-lytic antigen-antibody interactions observed in cytotoxicity-negative, absorption-positive reactions are converted to lytic reactions in the presence of antiglobulin (3, 5). Experiences in several transplant laboratories indicate that the antiglobulin technique is a useful supplement to other lymphocytotoxicity techniques presently used for monitoring serum antibody levels in prospective transplant recipients and in pretransplant cross-match procedures.

This chapter will be limited to technical considerations in the performance of the antiglobulin microcytotoxicity assay. The technique is highly reproducible and very sensitive, and it uses the same equipment as most other microcytotoxicity assays. It can be incorporated easily into existing laboratory procedures as a supplementary technique.

CLINICAL INDICATIONS

Ideally, the antiglobulin microcytotoxicity assay, in conjunction with at least one other assay, should be used as a cross-match procedure for all prospective donor-recipient pairs to detect preformed serum antibody. In addition, the antiglobulin procedure should be used in frequent monitoring of serum antibody levels of prospective transplant recipients. The antiglobulin procedure is one of the most sensitive complement-dependent assays for serum antibody to cell surface antigens and has been clini-

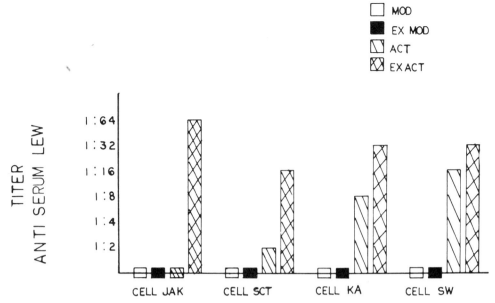

FIG. 1. *Lymphocytotoxic titers of antiserum LEW for four lymphocyte preparations tested by four techniques. MOD = Amos "modified"; EX MOD = Amos "modified" with extended incubation times of 60 min for serum plus cells and 120 min following addition of complement; ACT = antiglobulin microcytotoxicity with 30-min incubation for serum plus cells and 60 min following addition of complement; EX ACT = antiglobulin microcytotoxicity with extended incubation times of 60 min for serum plus cells and 120 min following addition of complement.*

cally important in the detection of sensitization in transplant recipients both retrospectively (7) and prospectively (Yunis, personal communication).

TEST PROCEDURES

Preparation of lymphocytes

Any routine laboratory method that yields purified lymphocytes can be used; however, Ficoll-Hypaque gradient centrifugation is most commonly used (20). When lymphocytes are prepared from a cadaver donor, the lymphocyte preparation is usually better when lymphocytes are prepared from a lymph node or spleen than from peripheral blood. After preparation, resuspend the lymphocytes in tissue culture media (medium 199, minimal essential medium, or McCoy's 5A) or balanced salt solution and adjust to a concentration of 2.5×10^6 lymphocytes/ml. Care should be taken to obtain a lymphocyte preparation with as few dead cells as possible. When there is a background of dead cells, weak reactions with a recipient serum become difficult to determine. Techniques which have been employed to get rid of dead cells are treatment with deoxyribonuclease (6) or separation on a second Ficoll-Hypaque gradi-

ent. The lymphocyte preparation should be free from platelets, red cells, and polymorphonuclear cells, both to facilitate visual score determination and to prohibit antigen excess by the presence of HLA antigens of platelets and polymorphonuclear cells.

Serum samples

Serum samples should be collected and frozen at least bimonthly (preferably once a month) from all transplant candidates. These serum samples should be screened against a reference panel of lymphocytes in which all HLA and W specificities are represented. This screen should be run monthly, and an up-to-date record of antibody levels should be kept on all transplant candidates (Fig. 2). Samples giving positive reactions should be titered in twofold dilutions against lymphocytes from at least three individuals showing positive reactions.

Samples to be used in the pretransplant cross-match vary according to the group of patients. Selection of serum samples from patients on chronic dialysis who have never formed a demonstrable lymphocytotoxic antibody should take into consideration the transfusion history of the patient. Samples drawn after

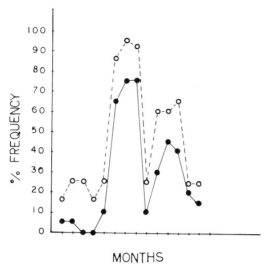

MONTHS

FIG. 2. *Frequency of reactivity of serum collected and tested monthly over a 15-month period from a potential transplant recipient against a 20-person lymphocyte panel. Symbols:* ○, *antiglobulin microcytotoxicity;* ●, *direct cytotoxicity.*

transfusions should be used. For patients who have formed demonstrable lymphocytotoxic antibody, at least two representative serum samples (preferably more) should be chosen to reflect the patient's antibody history. For example, one sample would be taken from each antibody activity peak, including peaks in frequency and/or in titer. For patients studied within 3 months or less of transplant, use all samples. An additional sample collected within 24 h prior to transplantation should be included in every cross-match. Each sample should be tested in at least triplicate and in twofold serial dilutions from 1:1 to 1:64. In addition, each undiluted sample should be tested in 1- and 2-μliter serum volumes.

Preparation of tray

Dispense 1 μliter of each dilution of each serum sample into each well of a microtest plate. (Prepare one plate for each technique to be used.) The serum can be dispensed under 2 μliters of light-weight mineral oil, or, alternatively, a strip of wetted bibulous paper can be placed around the periphery of the plate to prevent evaporation. Each mineral oil lot should be screened for toxicity before use (unpublished data).

Controls

Donor serum in dilutions versus donor cells should be included as a negative control. If donor serum is not available, one should use AB serum from a nontransfused male donor. An autologous control (recipient's serum plus recipient's lymphocytes) should be run if the patient is available. Percent dead cells in the negative controls (background) should be subtracted from the test value.

Each cross-match tray should likewise include a positive control serum, such as antilymphocyte serum, as a 100% cytotoxic antiserum. The positive serum should be diluted out past the point at which it is cytotoxic by direct tests. This serum also serves as a positive control for the antiglobulin reagent.

Each step of the antiglobulin procedure, except the addition of the antiglobulin reagent, should be followed by use of a duplicate tray. These trays serve as controls for the washes, the extended incubation time, and the antiglobulin reagent. Cells prepared from cadaver donors may be particularly fragile, and washing may cause an increase in background lysis.

Antiglobulin microcytotoxicity technique

1. Add 1 μliter of lymphocytes (2.5×10^6 cells/ml) to 1 μliter of antiserum in microtest trays with a Hamilton syringe, taking care not to carry over serum on the tip of the syringe.

2. Gently mix the serum and the cell droplet by placing the tray against a Yankee pipette shaker. Incubate the cells with the sera at room temperature for 60 min.

3. Wash the sensitized cells three times with barbital buffer. To wash, fill wells with buffer using a thinly drawn Pasteur pipette. (Alternately, one may fill wells with 10 μliters of buffer using a Hamilton syringe.) Allow cells to settle for 10 min or centrifuge the microtest trays in carriers for microtiter trays at 800 to 900 × g for 1 min. The buffer is removed by flicking the trays with a quick motion of the wrist or with a suction device as described previously (7).

4. Add 1 μliter of antiglobulin reagent in predetermined appropriate dilution (see below, Technical notes) to each well. Mix by placing the tray against a Yankee pipette shaker and incubate for 1 min at room temperature.

5. Immediately after 1 min of incubation, add 5 μliters of rabbit complement and incubate the mixture for 2 h at room temperature.

6. After 2 h, remove complement by flicking and fill each well with 0.3% trypan blue in ethylenediaminetetraacetate (EDTA), using a thinly drawn Pasteur pipette. Let the tray stand for *at least* 7 min. Remove the trypan blue by flicking. Then fill the wells with barbital buffer and let settle for 10 min before reading.

7. The reactions are read by placing the plate

under a standard or inverted-phase microscope at 150× (10× objective, 15× ocular) and judging for percentage of lysis. If the lymphocyte cell membrane has the corresponding antigenic determinant sites for the antiserum against which it is being tested, antigen-antibody binding will occur and, in turn, bind antiglobulin. The addition of complement to the complex causes lysis of the lymphocyte, and dye will be taken up by the dead cell so that it appears dark blue and two to three times larger than the refractile viable lymphocyte.

Scoring scale:

1 = 0–9% lysis	(0)	
2 = 10–19% lysis	(±)	
3 = 20–35% lysis	(+)	
4 = 36–59% lysis	(++)	
5 = 60–94% lysis	(+++)	
6 = 95–100% lysis	(++++)	
0 = not readable, invalid		

Technical notes

Not all anti-human immunoglobulin G (IgG) reagents will augment the reactivity of alloantisera. In addition, some are more effective than others. Therefore, several antiglobulin reagents must be tested and titered to find one that "works." (For tested lot numbers, see below, Reagents.)

The optimal dilution for the antiglobulin reagent is determined by testing serial dilutions of the antiglobulin against serial dilutions of allogenic sera to determine the highest dilutions of each which give a positive reaction (Table 1). Adding neutral red to the antiglobulin reagent eliminates errors due to skipping a well or row. Prozone is seen when high concentrations of antiglobulin are used.

The optimal incubation time with antiglobulin must be determined for each antiglobulin reagent. With our anti-human IgG, a 1-min incubation at room temperature was sufficient to detect maximal cytotoxic titers. This incubation time is critical. Prolonged incubation with antiglobulin gives less reproducible results.

In washing, wells should be filled to level with the rim. If the wells are overfilled (i.e., convex surface), cells will not settle properly and will be lost during the washing process. Three washes are critical. Using four washes increases the number of antiglobulin-positive, direct cytotoxicity-negative reactions obtained with a panel of antisera and panel of lymphocytes by 10% above the antiglobulin-positive, direct cytotoxicity-negative reactions observed after three washes.

This test works adequately when eosin and

TABLE 1. *Determination of optimal concentration of anti-human IgG*

Serum	Cell	Direct microcytotoxicity[a]		Dilution of anti-human IgG				
		Mod	Ex Mod	1:16	1:128	1:256	1:512	1:1,024
WB	WKS	neg	neg	1:2[b]	*1:4*	*1:4*	1:2	1:1
	KA	neg	neg	*1:2*	*1:2*	*1:2*	*1:2*	1:1
	JeA	1:8	1:16	1:16	1:32	*1:128*	*1:128*	1:64
BSt	WKS	1:4	1:8	1:32	*1:64*	*1:64*	1:32	1:16
	KA	1:2	1:4	*1:32*	*1:32*	*1:321*	*1:32*	*1:32*
	JeA	neg	neg	1:4	*1:8*	1:8	1:4	1:4
RA	WKS	neg	neg	*1:16*	*1:16*	*1:16*	1:8	1:4
	KA	neg	neg	—	—	—	—	—
	JeA	1:4	1:8	1:16	*1:32*	*1:32*	*1:32*	*1:32*
RsS	WKS	neg	1:1±	*1:64*	*1:64*	1:32	1:16	1:4
	KA	1:2	1:4	1:64	1:64	*1:128*	1:64	1:64
	JeA	neg	neg	1:4	*1:8*	*1:8*	*1:8*	1:2

[a] Mod = Amos "modifed" technique; Ex Mod = Amos "modified" technique with extended incubation times; neg = negative.

[b] Results are from the antiglobulin microcytotoxicity text with extended incubation times. The highest dilution of alloantiserum which gave a positive reaction is shown, and the peak titer is in italics.

formalin are used instead of trypan blue, following incubation with complement.

Plates can be stored for several days for subsequent rechecking by adding several drops of formalin to the filter strip or moat and placing the trays at 4 C. For long-term storage, the buffer may be replaced with buffered formaldehyde, pH 7.2, covered with a 2 × 3 inch cover slip, and sealed with Vaseline.

Visually checking that all components are added prevents errors. Skipping a well or jumping a row may be largely eliminated by (i) adding a small amount of dye to serum when setting up the plate, (ii) adding dye (trypan blue or trypan red) to the cell suspension, and (iii) adding dye to the complement. Excess dye, however, is anticomplementary.

REAGENTS AND SUPPLIES

Antiglobulin reagent

Information kindly suppled by Donald Cross, Veterans Administration Hospital, Transplant Laboratory, Kansas City, Kans.

Hyland Anti-Fab
    Goat 8258VOO3A1
    Avg optimal dilution, 1:32
    Avg titer increase, 6.4×

Behring Anti-Fab
  Rabbit 2327Q
    Avg optimal dilution, 1:256
    Avg titer increase, 3.5×
Meloy Anti-K
  Sheep A112
    Avg optimal dilution, 1:32
    Avg titer increase, 4.1×
Behring anti-IgG + IgA + IgM
  Goat 2335H
    Avg optimal dilution, 1:64
    Avg titer increase, 3.2×
Behring anti-IgG + IgA + IgM
  Goat 2500B
    Avg optimal dilution, 1:256
    Avg titer increase, 3.0×

Commercial sources

Barbital buffer: Complement Fixation Diluent Tablets, code BR16, 1 box = 6 bottles (100 tablets/bottle); made by Oxoid, Ltd., London, England, and distributed by Inolex Biomedical Division, Glenwood, Ill.

Bibulous paper: Reeve Angel Co., Clifton, N.J.

EDTA: disodium EDTA, dihydrate (crystal), 1 case = six 1-lb bottles, 1-8993; J. T. Baker Chemical Co., Phillipsburg, N.J.

Hamilton repeating dispenser: PB-600-1; Hamilton Co., Reno, Nev.

Hamilton syringes: model #705 for 1-μliter samples, model #725 for 5-μliter samples; Hamilton Co.

Hanks balanced salt solution: 10× concentrated, without sodium bicarbonate and phenol red; Microbiological Associates, Inc., Bethesda, Md., or Grand Island Biological Co., Grand Island, N.Y.

Liquid petroleum: mineral oil, white, light; Fisher Scientific Co., Silver Spring, Md.

McCoy's 5A medium: Grand Island Biological Co. or Microbiological Associates, Inc.

Microtest plates:
  Microtest plates #3034, 1 case contains 100 plates and covers; Falcon Plastics, Oxnard, Calif.
  Costar Histo-plates, 72 well (#236-72) 60 well (#236-1); Cooke Laboratory.

Pasteur pipettes (9 inch): diSPo pipettes Pasteur type, P 5211-2, 4 packages/case (2½ gross/package); Scientific Products.

Rabbit complement: Pel-Freeze Biologicals, Rogers, Ark. Trypan blue: C.I. No. 23850 (2nd ed.), 25 g/bottle; Harleco, Philadelphia, Pa.

Yankee pipette shaker: B-4110-2, six pipettes; Scientific Products.

Laboratory preparation

Antiglobulin reagent. The antiglobulin reagent can be stored at −90 C at a 1:20 or 1:30 dilution in McCoy's 5A medium plus 30% fetal calf serum dispensed in 50-μliter portions into microtubes by use of a Hamilton syringe. This is the stock solution. Immediately prior to use, enough of the stock solution is removed, thawed, and diluted with McCoy's 5A or barbital buffer to the predetermined optimal working dilution. Any unused working dilution should be discarded.

Complement (rabbit). Each lot number of complement must be titrated to determine the optimal dilution for use in the microlymphocytotoxicity test (see reference 18). Complement is extrememly labile and should be thawed and diluted or reconstituted and diluted immediately prior to use.

Trypan blue (working solution). Combine 3 parts of 1% trypan blue (stock solution) and 7 parts of 2% EDTA in barbital buffer (stock solution) to obtain 10 parts of 0.3% trypan blue in EDTA (working solution). *Note:* Working solution should be prepared immediately before use.

To prepare 1% trypan blue (stock solution), place 1 g of trypan blue powder in a 100-ml volumetric flask and add distilled water to make 100 ml. Filter and store at 4 C. The stock solution should be filtered weekly.

To prepare 2% EDTA in barbital buffer (stock solution), place 2 g of EDTA (disodium EDTA, dihydrate) in a 100-ml volumetric flask and add barbital buffer to make 100 ml. Adjust the pH to 7.2 using concentrated NaOH. Store at 4 C.

INTERPRETATION

Detection of lysis >10% over background should be considered a positive cross-match and indicative of histoincompatibility between that recipient and donor pair. A strong reaction (≥50% cell death) is >98% reproducible. However, reactions giving only 10 to 20% lysis are very sensitive to minor variations from well to well, such as cell number, amount of buffer removed before addition of antiglobulin, etc., and replicates often may not be in agreement. A general rule to follow is: if greater than one-half of the replicates are weakly positive, the reaction is positive. (Minor differences are harder to detect when the cell preparation contains any background of dead cells; thus, care must be exerted to obtain the best preparation possible.)

The antiglobulin microcytotoxicity test primarily detects low levels of anti-HLA antibodies and cross-reactive HLA antibodies. About 5% of the reactions cannot be explained by presently defined HLA specificities. However, these reactions segregate with HLA in families (22). Thus, the increase in sensitivity gained by using this technique to detect low levels of HLA antibodies merits its use as a cross-match procedure.

LITERATURE CITED

1. Amos, D. B., G. Cabrera, W. B. Bias, J. M. MacQueen, S. L. Lancaster, J. G. Southworth, and F. E. Ward. 1970. The inheritance of human leukocyte antigens. III. The organization of specificities, p. 259–276. In P. I. Terasaki (ed.), Histocompatibility testing 1970. Munksgaard, Copenhagen.

2. Bodmer, W., M. Tripp, and J. Bodmer. 1967. Application of a fluorochromatic cytotoxicity assay to human leukocyte typing, p. 341–350. In E. S. Curtoni, P. L. Mattiuz, and R. M. Tosi (ed.), Histocompatibility testing 1967. Munksgaard, Copenhagen.

3. Cannady, W. G., R. P. Reckel, D. Tripodi, S. M. Shaw, D. Baldassari, and L. A. Metz. 1974. Sensitivity of various HL-A typing techniques. Tissue Antigens 4:564–570.

4. Colombani, J., J. D'Amaro, B. Gabb, G. Smith, and A. Svejgaard. 1971. International agreement on a microtechnique of platelet complement fixation (Pl. C Fix). Transplant. Proc. 3:121–126.

5. dos Reis, A. P., H. Betuel, E. G. Reisner, and D. B. Amos. 1973. The utilization of antiglobulin reagents in cytotoxicity testing for HL-A. Transplantation 15:36–41.

6. Dupont, B., C. Jerild, and B. Jakobsen. 1972. Elimination of non-viable cells by DNase treatment prior to lymphocytotoxicity test. Tissue Antigens 2:141–144.

7. Johnson, A. H., R. D. Rossen, and W. T. Butler. 1972. Detection of alloantibodies using a sensitive antiglobulin microcytotoxicity test: identification of low levels of preformed antibodies in accelerated allograft rejection. Tissue Antigens 2:215–226.

8. Kissmeyer-Nielsen, F., and K. E. Kjerbye. 1967. Lymphocytotoxic micro-technique. Purification of lymphocytes by flotation, p. 381–383. In E. S. Curtoni, P. L. Mattiuz, and R. M. Tosi (ed.), Histocompatibility testing 1967. Munksgaard, Copenhagen.

9. Kissmeyer-Nielsen, F., S. Olsen, V. P. Peterson, and O. Fjeldborg. 1966. Hyperacute rejection of kidney allografts associated with pre-existing humoral antibodies against donor cells. Lancet 2:662–665.

10. Lucas, Z. J., N. Coplon, R. Kempson, and R. Cohn. 1970. Early renal transplant failure associated with subliminal sensitization. Transplantation 10:522–529.

11. Mittal, K. K., M. R. Mickey, D. P. Singal, and P. I. Terasaki. 1968. Serotyping for homotransplantation. XVIII. Refinement of microdroplet lymphocyte cytotoxicity test. Transplantation 6:913–927.

12. Patel, R., and W. A. Briggs. 1971. Limitation of the lymphocyte cytotoxicity cross-match test in recipients of kidney transplants having performed anti-leukocyte antibodies. N. Engl. J. Med. 284:1016.

13. Patel, R., and P. I. Terasaki. 1969. Significance of the positive cross-match test in kidney transplantation. N. Engl. J. Med. 280:735–739.

14. Perkins, H. A., K. M. Douglas, K. Cochrum, and S. Kountz. 1970. Direct typing of kidney cells by standard cytotoxic techniques, p. 583–585. In P. I. Terasaki (ed.), Histocompatibility testing 1970. Munksgaard, Copenhagen.

15. Pierce, J. C., and D. M. Hume. 1971. Crossmatching for organ transplantation. I. The use of kidney cells and immune adherence. Transplant. Proc. 3:127–129.

16. Pierce, J. C., and D. W. Smith. 1975. Antibody against donor-specific kidney cells detected by mixed agglutination. Transplant. Proc. 7:621–623.

17. Pierce, J. C., M. Waller, and M. Phibbs. 1975. A mixed antiglobulin test with kidney cells in suspension for IgG antibody in human allograft recipients. Transplantation 19:343–348.

18. Ray, J. G., Jr., D. B. Hare, and D. E. Kayhoe (ed.). July 1973. Manual of tissue typing techniques. Department of Health, Education, and Welfare Publication No. NIH 74-545. NIH, Bethesda, Md.

19. Thompson, J. S., C. D. Severson, A. R. Lavender, M. Forland, and H. P. Russe. 1968. Assay of human leukoagglutinins by capillary migration. Transplantation 6:728–736.

20. Thorsby, E., and A. Bratlie. 1970. A rapid method for preparation of pure lymphocyte suspensions, p. 655–656. In P. I. Terasaki (ed.), Histocompatibility testing 1970. Munksgaard, Copenhagen.

21. Unanue, E. R., and M. J. Karnovsky. 1973. Redistribution and fate of Ig complexes on surface of B lymphocytes: functional implications and mechanisms. Transplant. Rev. 14:184–210.

22. Ward, F. E., J. M. MacQueen, D. B. Amos, Y. Delmas-Marsalet, and A. Johnson. 1975. The antiglobulin microcytotoxicity assay in HL-A genotyped families. Transplantation 19:286–290.

23. Williams, G. M., B. de Planque, R. R. Lower, and D. M. Hume. 1969. Antibodies and human transplant rejection. Ann. Surg. 170:603–616.

24. Williams, G. M., H. M. Lee, R. F. Weymouth, W. R. Harlan, K. A. Holden, C. M. Stanley, G. A. Millington, and D. M. Hume. 1967. Studies in hyperacute and chronic renal homograft rejection in man. Surgery 62:204–212.

25. Zmjewski, C. M., R. L. St. Pierre, J. L. Fletcher, S. F. Wilson, W. Cannady, and H. E. Zmjewski. 1967. A comparison of two micro-leukoagglutination tests, p. 389–395. In E. S. Curtoni, P. L. Mattiuz, and R. M. Tosi (ed.), Histocompatibility testing 1967. Munksgaard, Copenhagen.

Chapter 109

Mixed Lymphocyte Reaction

JAMES O'LEARY, NANCY REINSMOEN, AND EDMOND J. YUNIS

INTRODUCTION

The mixed lymphocyte interaction was first described in 1963 by Bain, Vos, and Lowenstein (Fed. Proc. **22**:428, 1963) and Bach and Hirschhorn (3). They demonstrated that leukocytes from two unrelated individuals when mixed together resulted in the transformation of some of the cells into blasts typical of a proliferative response. Since dividing cell populations synthesize deoxyribonucleic acid (DNA), one measure of this response is the uptake of radiolabeled thymidine, which is specifically incorporated into DNA. Both ^{14}C- and ^{3}H-labeled thymidine can be used and are available commercially. To distinguish the response due to a single individual stimulated by another individual, it is generally necessary to inhibit the DNA synthesis of cells from one individual. The response observed will then be that of the uninhibited cell population. This inhibition is achieved either by mitomycin C treatment (4) of the stimulating cell population or by X-irradiation (17).

There are two basic methods of mixed lymphocyte culture (MLC): the "tube" or macromethod and the micromethod. We have chosen the micromethod for routine MLC because it requires fewer cells and smaller amounts of reagents while retaining reasonable precision (for a review of various technical aspects, see Freiesleben-Sørenson [9]). The MLC microtest was originally developed by Hartzman et al. (11), and except for details of technique the same basic methodology is used by many laboratories. Although we will discuss the merits of some procedural modifications, a good reference for the justification of various aspects of the method can be found in "Reports from an MLC Workshop" (22).

CLINICAL INDICATIONS

One of the primary clinical uses of the MLC has been the selection of compatible donors for transplantation. The literature on this subject is voluminous and the reader is referred to, for example, *Tissue Typing and Organ Transplantation,* edited by Yunis, Gatti, and Amos (31), for detailed information. Briefly, there is a good correlation between graft survival and a lack of response in MLC (24). In particular, a mutually nonstimulatory response in MLC between siblings is critical to avoid graft-versus-host (GVH) reactions in bone marrow transplantation. Although many investigators feel that MLC compatibility is critical to good graft survival, serological testing for HLA antigens is always done before transplantation, along with extensive cross-match procedures. Poor matches are usually not considered, and transplantation in the face of a positive cross-match indicating preformed antibodies of donor specificity is invariably not considered. The primary drawback to MLC testing is the time needed to obtain a meaningful result. For this reason, it has proved to be a useful tool for selecting a donor only in cases when the patient has some family members willing to donate. For transplants using living related donors, MLC testing can only serve as a prognostic indicator of kidney survival and is usually performed to corroborate HLA identity. The use of MLC typing for selection of unrelated donors for skin or kidney transplantation is controversial (12, 19, 20, 31). The apparent correlation of some reports could be explained by genetic linkage disequilibrium between MLC determinants and HLA (6, 28).

As we shall point out, care must be taken in interpreting the results of MLC testing. The degree of stimulation between related individuals is different from that between unrelated individuals. A low or no response in related individuals is usually interpreted as a negative response; however, a low response may be found in MLC between heterozygotes (one haplotype difference). Therefore, the decision as to what constitutes negative response can be difficult (24).

The factors which determine MLC stimulation are apparently carried by genes at the major histocompatibility locus. Much evidence indicates that this region is located on chromosome 6 of humans (13). The factors which control the MLC response are found at loci outside of those which control the HLA-B (FOUR locus HLA) antigens (2, 7, 8, 30, 32). Recently, it has become possible to type for these factors present on leukocytes; these factors are called MLR-S LD, or HLA-D (12). This typing, although still in the development stage, is a topic of increasing interest. It is apparent that there is some relationship between MLC and other HLA determinants, immune responsiveness, and certain diseases. Eventually, MLC and HLA testing may be of clinical value in evaluation of the risk of developing certain diseases. At present, however, the meaning of such relationships is not clearly enough defined to justify their clinical use.

TEST PROCEDURES

Collection of specimen

Sterile technique must be employed throughout the entire procedure. Contaminated cultures can lead to false-positive and false-negative results. Since the culture is liberally dosed with antibiotics, fungi are the major contaminating organisms. (In our laboratories all procedures in which a specimen is open to the air are carried out in a laminar flow hood or isolation cabinet to prevent airborne contamination.) In handling whole blood, serum, cells, etc., it is also critical to keep in mind the possibility of hepatitis. Always treat the material as if it were a microbiological hazard.

Two methods of collection may be used. First, collect the blood in a sterile syringe and transfer to a sterile Erlenmeyer flask. A 50-ml flask will generally be sufficient for most specimens. Add a volume equal to the volume of the specimen of sterile saline, or barbital buffer; put about 30 sterile glass beads (approximately 3 mm in diameter) in the flask and swirl gently for 10 min to complete defibrination of the blood. For the second method of collection, obtain the blood in either a sterile syringe or Vacutainer tube containing 10 IU of heparin/ml of sample. The first technique yields a specimen relatively free from platelets; however, we prefer the second because the ultimate yield of cells is greater and the risk of contamination is smaller. The volume collected depends on the expected yield of cells and the size of the planned culture.

Isolation of lymphocytes

Generally, the specimen should be used on the same day in which it is collected. The isolated cells show deterioration in their ability to respond within 24 to 48 h. The isolation is performed in sterile disposable snap-top culture tubes, 17 × 100 mm (Falcon #2006; Falcon Plastics, Oxnard, Calif.). If the blood was collected by the second method in the preceding section, add an equal volume of the culture medium. Put 3 ml of the separation fluid in each tube used and carefully layer 5 ml of the diluted blood over it. Care must be taken to preserve the integrity of the blood-fluid interface. A greater volume, up to 10 ml, of blood may be used per tube, but contamination of the isolated white cells by erythrocytes may result, and a careful microscopic examination of the cells should be performed before use. Alternatively, to save separation fluid you may first centrifuge the whole blood at low speed (150 × g) for about 10 min and take off the buffy coat layer. Add an equal volume of medium to the buffy coat and use 4 ml of this mixture per 3 ml of separation fluid.

Using care to avoid mixing the layers (note that soon after addition the red cells begin to settle rapidly to the bottom of the tube), place the tube in a centrifuge and spin at 400 × g for 40 min at room temperature. Be sure that the air inside the centrifuge is close to the temperature of room air (20 to 25 C). Even moderate elevation of the temperature will alter the density of the separation fluid enough to contaminate the cells with large numbers of neutrophils, etc.

Pipette 5 ml of culture medium into a snap-top tube. With a sterile pipette carefully remove the lymphocyte-enriched layer, which is the light white ring-shaped layer between the top layer with medium and the layer of clear separation fluid (the red cells are at bottom), and add it to the tube containing medium. Bring the volume up to about 10 ml with medium and mix gently. Mixing can be conveniently performed on a Vortex mixer. Spin at 150 × g for 10 min, discard the supernatant fluid, and resuspend the cell button in 10 ml of medium. Spin and wash in this fashion two more times.

The technique of isolation is based on that of Bøyum (5). Except for minor modifications, most laboratories prefer this technique (22). Cells isolated in this way are also suitable for use with mitogen stimulation. In our hands the typical yield of lymphocytes is about 10^6 to $2 × 10^6$ cells/ml of whole blood. We generally obtain about 95% viability as determined by trypan blue exclusion and 95 to 99% lymphocytes. When setting up a mixed culture system, it would be advisable to check the quality of the separation. If there is difficulty in obtaining a reasonable yield of viable cells, it may be necessary to check the temperature of the centrifuge or to manipulate the specific gravity of the separating fluid as described under Reagents.

Preparation of stimulating cells

The method we have chosen is mitomycin C treatment of the stimulating cell suspension. Irradiation is used by some investigators (27); however, access to a radiation source may be a critical limitation. Irradiation has the advantage that cell recovery is greater and the stimulating cell suspension need not be recounted before use.

After the third wash in the preceding section, resuspend the cells in exactly 4 ml of culture medium. To prepare the stimulating cells, transfer 2 ml of the cell suspension to another tube and add 0.2 ml of mitomycin C (0.25 mg/ml). Incubate at 37 C for 20 min in a CO_2 incubator. After the incubation, resuspend the cells and wash three times as in the preceding section. Up to one-half of the cells may be lost in this procedure. We have found this treatment to be effective in blocking thymidine uptake, while retaining good viability and allowing stimulation. Cells treated in this way still show some response to mitogens, but they will not respond in MLC as measured by [³H]thymidine uptake.

Culture set-up

Count the number of cells per milliliter in both the responding and stimulating cell suspensions. This may be done in an ordinary hemacytometer. If available, a Coulter counter may be used; however, the increase in precision does not significantly improve the precision of the results. This type of instrument can speed the counting of multiple samples.

The next step is to adjust the final cell concentration in both suspensions to 10^6 cells/ml by the addition of an appropriate amount of medium. Then add pooled human serum (PHS) and medium so that the final concentration of PHS is 20% and the cell concentration is 5×10^5 cells/ml. This concentration of PHS has been found to be optimal for cell growth in MLC (1).

The culture is set up in sterile round-bottomed plates with lids. We used Microtiter U plates (Cooke Laboratory Products, Alexandria, Va.). A wide variety of plates of various volumes and geometry are available from various manufacturers (e.g., Linbro, New Haven, Conn., or Falcon Plastics, Oxnard, Calif.). The plates we use have 96 wells of sufficient volume for the procedure outlined here. Numerous volumes and cell concentrations are used by various investigators (22). We recommend the round-bottomed geometry, since it makes it possible to culture fewer cells. In Table 1 are shown the results of one control experiment comparing round- and flat-bottomed plates at

TABLE 1. *Comparison of mean response of six stimulator-responder combinations with the use of plates of two different geometries but identical well volume*

| Cells/ml | | PHS^a (%) | Plates | |
Stimulator	Responder		Round-bottom	Flat-bottomed
0.5×10^6	0.5×10^6	15	39,380	24,663
		20	48,331	31,210
0.5×10^6	1.0×10^6	15	48,979	45,793
		20	47,487	51,601
1.0×10^6	1.0×10^6	15	67,446	76,884
		20	60,912	77,338

^{a} Pooled human serum.

two different concentrations of PHS. We generally obtain good results with a concentration of 5×10^5 cells/ml in round-bottomed plates.

Each stimulator-responder combination is set up in triplicate. To each well are added 100 μliters of the appropriate responder and 100 μliters of the appropriate stimulator. There will be 5×10^4 responders and 5×10^4 stimulators per well in 200 μliters per well. Pipetting is best done with a dispenser with disposable autoclavable plastic tips, e.g., an Eppendorf pipetter. To prevent carry-over, a different sterile tip should be used for each cell suspension. A typical plate is shown schematically in Fig. 1. The responders are usually designated by a letter code and the stimulators are subscribed with the letter m to designate mitomycin treatment. This simple coding facilitates marking the lids with a waterproof marker showing the stimulator-responder matrix, the date, and the technician. A Xerox copy of the lid is a convenient method of keeping a record of the experiment. Note that autologous as well as allogeneic combinations are set up for each responder.

The completed plate is then placed in a CO_2 incubator for 5 days. The incubator should be maintained at 37 C with 100% humidity and 5% CO_2. Periodic checks of culture wells with an inverted microscope are helpful in determining whether the incubator or cultures have become contaminated. In our experience the thymidine uptake of the cultures peaks at about 6 days and begins to decline at longer incubation times (Fig. 2). At 5 days, the cultures are still growing exponentially, and this time point is chosen as the optimum for estimating the degree of response.

Labeling procedure

After 5 days (120 h), the plates are removed from the incubator, and 50 μliters of [³H]thymi-

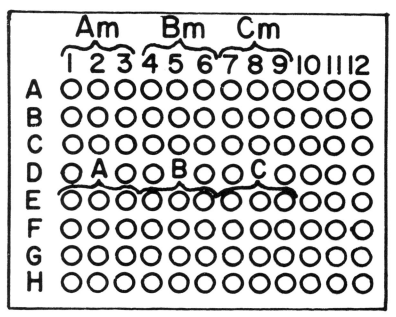

FIG. 1. *Schematic drawing of a mixed culture plate. All combinations are done in triplicate. Unstimulated responder cells and stimulator cells are also done.*

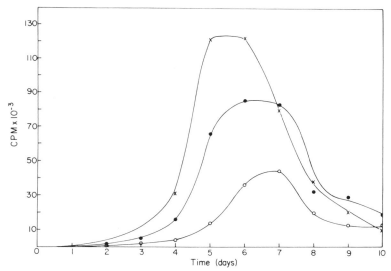

FIG. 2. *Results of MLC tests for three allogenic cell mixtures. The uptake is plotted in counts per minute as a function of time.*

dine in culture medium is added. For routine cultures a specific activity of 6.7 Ci/mmol and a dose of 0.5 μCi are adequate. The plates are returned to the incubator for 18 h. They are then removed and covered with a pressure-sensitive plastic film (Falcon Plastics); they may be harvested immediately or placed in an ordinary refrigerator at 4 C until harvested. We have successfully harvested plates stored in this way for up to 30 days after termination of the incubation.

The labeling time of 18 h seems to be optimal, as shown in Fig. 3. The ratio of the response to the autologous background is also small at this time. For experiments in which it is desirable to estimate the number of cells synthesizing DNA, it would be better to choose a labeling time in the linear portion of the uptake curve. The [³H]thymidine uptake will then be a linear function of the number of cells synthesizing

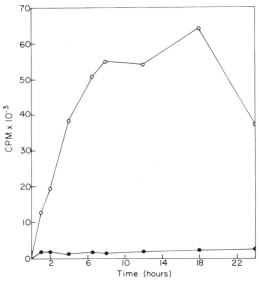

FIG. 3. *Mean uptake of six allogenic cell stimulations plotted versus the length of time in culture with [³H]thymidine (specific activity = 6.7 Ci/mmol at 0.5 μCi per well). Background is mean of three autologous cell combinations.*

DNA during the labeling period. The mean effects of increasing dose and specific activity are shown in Fig. 4; 6.7 Ci/mmol seems to be adequate at 18 h. We have arbitrarily chosen a dose of 0.5 μCi. This dose is consistent with reasonable economy in the use of the isotope, and a statistical analysis shows that precision is no better at higher doses.

Harvesting procedure

After incubation with the labeled thymidine, the tritiated cellular material is generally recovered by either trichloroacetic acid precipitation (26) or filtration on glass-fiber filters. The former method recovers only the cellular DNA, and no unincorporated thymidine in the cells, though this quantity is generally small relative to the incorporated thymidine in the DNA. Another advantage of this technique is that elaborate cell harvesters are not necessary. For large-scale MLC testing, however, multiple harvesting on glass-fiber filters is preferred. The principal advantage is rapid and efficient recovery of the cells. The cells and media are removed by suction from the wells, and simultaneously the wells are thoroughly flushed and the filters are washed of any unbound [³H]thymidine. The cellular material is apparently bound to the filter by ionic interaction. We generally use Whatman GF/C glass-fiber filters in a semiautomated multiple cell harvester (Skatron, Lierbylen, Norway). A number of such devices are available (e.g., Biomedical

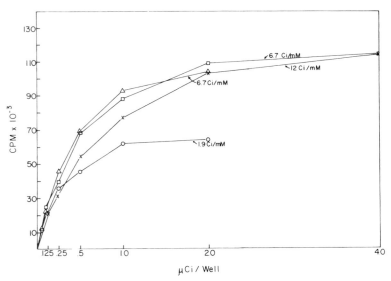

FIG. 4. *Effects of varying dose and specific activity of [³H]thymidine (pulse time, 18 h). Each point is the mean uptake of six allogenic cell mixtures. Source of [³H]thymine: 1.9 Ci/mmol, Schwarz Bioresearch; 6.7 Ci/mmol, New England Nuclear Corp.; 12 Ci/mmol, ICN.*

Research Institute, Rockville, Md.; ADAPS Inc., Deeham, Mass.; Spectroderm International, Fairfax, Va.) at a variety of prices. Before purchasing a particular instrument, however, it would be wise to check into the triplicate variation of the machine, since variations due to unevenness of flow, for example, can be a major source of error.

Scintillation counting

Before the scintillation cocktail is added, the glass-fiber filters should be thoroughly air-dried. A small amount of water can result in serious quenching of the fluorescence of the cocktail and lead to low counts. A 7-ml amount of scintillation cocktail is placed over the filter in a 15-ml glass scintillation vial. Plastic vials may expand and jam the counter with the toluene-based cocktail recommended here. The precise quantity of cocktail needed to get maximal accuracy and precision will depend on the counter used. Any scintillation counter of reasonable efficiency can be used provided the discrimination is properly set for ^{3}H.

REAGENTS

Heparin

Sodium heparin USP (Beef Lung; The Upjohn Co., Kalamazoo, Mich.) or a comparable product may be used. If a collected sample is to be left unseparated for a few hours preservative-free (without benzyl alcohol or other agents), heparin is recommended. The preservatives can kill the lymphocytes after a period of storage.

Separation fluid

The lymphocyte purification is based on the slightly lower density of lymphocytes versus most of the other cells in whole blood. Two reagents may be used: Ficoll-Isopaque or Ficoll-Hypaque. To make Ficoll-Isopaque, first make solutions of 9% Ficoll in distilled water and 33.56% Isopaque (Nyegaard, Oslo, Norway) in distilled water. Mix 24 parts Isopaque solution to 10 parts Ficoll, and adjust the specific gravity to 1.078 with a hydrometer. For Ficoll-Hypaque use 24 parts 9% Ficoll to 10 parts 33.9% Hypaque (Winthrop Laboratories, New York, N.Y.), and adjust the specific gravity to 1.075 to 1.076. For both solutions the specific gravity is raised by adding the Isopaque or Hypaque solution and lowered by the addition of more Ficoll solution. As noted in the Test Procedures section, yields may sometimes be improved by changing the specific gravity slightly from that recommended here. The final solution is steri-lized prior to use by vacuum filtration (0.45-μm grid membrane).

Culture media

Various standard tissue culture formulations can be used. Medium 199, RPMI 1640, and MEM (minimal essential medium) with Earle's salts are commonly used. The media should be supplied without L-glutamine and should be a formulation designed for suspension culture. In our laboratory we use MEM with Earle's salts for suspension culture (catalog #138, Grand Island Biological Co., Grand Island, N.Y.). Just prior to use, the medium is supplemented with 1.0 ml of 200 mM L-glutamine/100 ml and 100 IU of penicillin and 100 μg of streptomycin/ml. The L-glutamine and penicillin-streptomycin solutions are available from Grand Island Biological Co. and can be conveniently stored frozen in small portions prior to use.

Mitomycin C

Mitomycin C (Sigma Chemical Co., St. Louis, Mo.) is diluted to 0.25 mg/ml in distilled water. Since mitomycin C is sensitive to light, it should be wrapped in aluminum foil and refrigerated for storage.

Pooled human serum

Ten or more untransfused normal males are needed for donors. This number is necessary to maintain uniformity of the product. Normal females or transfused donors may have cytotoxic antibodies or inhibitory factors. Whole blood is collected, and the serum is isolated from the clotted blood by centrifugation. The sera are pooled in a sterile flask or bag and then divided into portions and stored at −20 C until used. ABO antibody testing is generally unnecessary.

[^{3}H]thymidine

As noted in the Test Procedures section, [^{3}H]-thymidine at 6.7 Ci/mmol (New England Nuclear Corp., Boston, Mass.) is recommended. A stock solution can be made by diluting 1 part thymidine to 24 parts sterile distilled water. Prior to labeling the culture, the stock is diluted 1:4 with the culture medium. The solution is dispensed in 50-μliter amounts per well. The total dose is 0.5 μCi/well. The labeling solution may be conveniently dispensed with a Hamilton repeating dispenser (Hamilton Co., Reno, Nev.) and a 2.5-ml Hamilton syringe.

Scintillation cocktail

We have chosen a toluene-based cocktail. To 1 gallon (3.8 liters) of toluene, add 157 ml of

Liquifluor (New England Nuclear Corp.). The choice of cocktail is not critical, and others may be substituted.

Miscellaneous materials

Sources of most of the materials needed have been noted above. Serological disposable pipettes of 1-, 5-, and 10-ml capacity are available from Corning Glassworks, McGraw Park, Ill. Glass-fiber filters can be obtained from Gelman Instruments, Ann Arbor, Mich. (Type A), and Whatman glass-fiber filters are available from W & R Balston Ltd., England, or Whatman Inc., Clifton, N.J. Sterilizing filters are catalog #245, Nalgene Labware Div., Nalge, Rochester, N.Y.

INTERPRETATION

Presentation and treatment of data

The results of a family MLC are presented in Table 2. The data presented are in counts per minute taken over a 1-min period. It is conventional to present the data in tabular form with the stimulators along the top and the responders as rows along the side. The values of the triplicates should be averaged as shown. In literature reports of MLC data, the standard error of the counts per minute and the coefficient of variation (standard error/mean counts per minute × 100%) are helpful in interpreting the results.

It is evident that occasionally one value in a triplicate seems to be quite far from the other two. A convenient method of determining whether such a value represents a statistical "outlier," which cannot be accounted for by the degree of randomness in the data, is taken from Lieblen (21). For each triplicate calculate $y = (x' - x''/x_3 - x_1)$, where $x' - x''$ is the difference between the two closest values and $x_3 - x_1$ is the range from the highest to the lowest values. The value of this ratio can be used to determine the probability that y does not exceed a certain value (see Table 7B.3 of Lieblen [21]). With an arbitrary value of $P = 0.25$, if the value of y is less than 0.14128 we then take the median value of the triplicate (i.e., only 25% of all values of y lie outside this value). In Table 2 the triplicates for which the ratio was less than the value 0.14128 are marked with an asterisk. Note that the use of this technique demands that it be applied in every case regardless of the "appearance" of the data or it should not be applied at all. As an example, in Table 2, for the combination A × Dm the values for the triplicate are 23,563, 28,346, and 28,621. The difference between the two closest values ($x' -$

x'') is 275. The difference between the highest and the lowest values ($x_1 - x_3$) is 5,058. The value of the ratio $y = (x' - x''/x_1 - x_3)$ is 0.0544. This ratio is less than the critical value, and therefore the median of the three values is chosen as most closely approximating the true mean of the triplicate.

The averaged triplicate data can be expressed in a number of fashions, as shown in Table 3. The methods of calculation and the usefulness of the various expressions are discussed below. Since none of them unambiguously distinguishes a negative from a positive result in all cases, it should be possible for a reader to calculate the counts per minute from the data presented.

The first method of expression is simply the average counts per minute. The primary drawback here is that it fails to take into account the autologous control. It can be difficult to distinguish a low response from no response when the control is of comparable magnitude. The data may also be expressed as some form of "increment," where some control value is subtracted from the test value. One difficulty here is deciding which value to use as the control, i.e., the unstimulated responder, the unstimulated stimulator, or the autologous value. In Table 3 the "increment" is the test value minus the autologous value for the particular responder. From the data in Tables 2 and 3, it can be seen that the combinations A × Cm, B × Cm, B × Dm, and C × Dm appear to be low compared with the other combinations. The distinction is clearly not unambiguous.

A second general method is to express the response of a particular individual as a "stimulation ratio" (SR). The SR is the test value divided by the autologous control for the responding individual. SR values are strongly biased by the control value. The control is inherently imprecise as a result of the inability of a scintillation counter to give precise counting of low values in short time intervals. As shown in Table 3, the SR may be also expressed as the natural logarithm of the SR. One can see that the SR does not offer much improvement in the interpretation of this MLC.

The third method is to determine some reference value for a given responding cell population to which a test response can be compared. This reference should reflect the "inherent" responsiveness of the cell in question. There are three methods used to find a reference value. First, the maximal response given to a stimulator panel in a particular MLC can be used. Unfortunately, the maximal response is randomly distributed and may be a statistical outlier. Second, the median response to a panel of

TABLE 2. *Results of Sc family MLC (counts per minute over a 1-min period)*[a]

Subject	Am	Mean SE CV	Bm	Mean SE CV	Cm	Mean SE CV	Dm	Mean SE CV	Em	Mean SE CV	Fm	Mean SE CV	Gm	Mean SE CV
A. Mother Sc	13,237	1,171	49,765	39,943	4,707	7,243	23,563	28,356*	67,070	76,019	78,072	79,142	74,758	84,126
2-7/9-W5	402	105	33,628	8,621	6,526	2,960	28,346		63,483	3,511	80,685	1,369	95,753	10,668
	1,789	(60%)	36,436	(22%)	10,496	(41%)	28,621		70,505	(5%)	78,669	(17%)	81,838	(13%)
B. Father Sc	53,787	44,881	1,229	888	9,654	9,999*	9,449	7,076	28,648	34,823	56,008	54,872	40,972	43,336
3-7/-W5	36,285	8,756	868	332	4,260		4,290	2,604	32,168	8,326	61,468	7,231	40,972	6,059
	44,572	(20%)	566	(37%)	4,997		7,488	(37%)	44,152	(24%)	47,140	(13%)	38,816	(14%)
C. MS, Daught.	44,950	40,345	19,107	17,536*	14,097	1,288	7,846	13,800	47,827	45,196	54,332	60,704	46,920	45,891
3-7/2-7	36,489	9,280	17,341		15,896	377	13,860	5,925	41,915	3,009	62,780	5,628	42,636	2,881
	39,595	(10.6%)	17,536		865	(29%)	19,695	(43%)	45,847	(6.7%)	64,999	(9.2%)	48,116	(6.3%)
D. MAL	80,805	69,251	20,872	28,833	11,055	7,330	1,984	2,624	52,392	53,541	81,209	81,205	73,038	75,212
1-7/3-W15	67,300	10,713	28,341	9,218	4,779	3,299	3,410	724	55,186	1,462	81,440	237	82,915	6,878
	59,647	(15%)	37,285	(28.5%)	6,156	(45%)	2,477	(28%)	53,045	(2.7%)	80,966	(0.5%)	69,684	(9%)
E. JY	63,246	57,480	22,575	29,721	28,310	27,160	38,972	37,126*	2,325	2,298	54,286	49,884	48,776	44,811
9,W19,W15	57,158	5,611	36,054	6,776	32,232	5,734	26,129		3,117	832	45,416	4,435	40,133	4,365
	52,036	(19.8%)	30,533	(23%)	20,938	(21%)	37,126		1,453	(36%)	49,950	(8.9%)	45,524	(9.7%)
F. JD	63,119	63,697	48,957	48,957*	61,355	61,355*	88,986	83,412	76,545	98,427	2,434	2,266	86,597	86,597*
1,W19,8,W15	59,699	4,319	47,944		61,436		78,914	5,036	64,543	6,305	1,741	465	86,669	
	68,278	(6.8%)					83,836	(6.0)	67,192	(9.1%)	2,624	(21%)	74,208	
G. RE	88,343	82,050	46,207	47,320	54,154	54,407	63,457	73,320	68,653	67,746	81,521	76,646*	672	1,536
3,W5,W10	74,684	6,892	57,669	9,840	54,294	325	70,014	11,866	72,639	5,404	76,646		426	125
	83,123	(8.4%)	38,084	(21%)	54,773	(0.6%)	86,488	(16%)	61,946	(8.0%)	43,615		511	(8.1%)
Stimulator × 20%	358	358*	633	321*	643	606	430	426*	150	276	456	801*	338	653
PHS-MEM	326		321		426	165	426		311	113			554	375
	728		285		749	(27%)	129		368	(41%)	801		068	(57%)
Responder × 20%	869	960*	886	857	976	1,158	1,603	1,568	1,904	1,908*	5,082	5,647	798	1,539
PHS-MEM	1,518		1,081	271	1,064	244	1,617	725	1,908		6,019	478	2,019	651
	960		545	(32%)	1,435	(21%)	1,485	(4.2%)				(8.5%)	1,800	(92.3%)
PHS, 20%														568
														367
														(6.7%)

[a] Values of each triplicate are shown. SE = standard error; CV = coefficient of variation. Asterisks indicate that the median value of the triplicate, $y = (x' - x''/x_1 - x_3)$, was less than 0.14128 (see text).

TABLE 3. *Various expressions of MLC data in Sc family, calculated from Table 2*

Expression[a]	Am	Bm	Cm	Dm	Em	Fm	Gm
A	1,171	39,943	7,243	28,346	67,019	79,142	84,126
Inc		38,772	6,072	27,175			
SI		37.6	6.7	26.6			
ln SI		3.63	1.90	3.28			
RR_{med}		49.7	7.8	34.9			
RR_{max}		46.7	7.3	32.8			
B	44,881	888	4,997	7,076	34,824	54,872	43,336
Inc	43,993		4,109	6,188			
SI	57.7		6.30	8.97			
ln SI	4.1		1.84	2.19			
RR_{med}	104		9.7	14.6			
RR_{max}	81.4		7.6	11.5			
C	40,345	17,536	1,288	13,800	45,196	60,704	45,891
Inc	39,057	16,248		12,512			
SI	34.2	14.8		11.6			
ln SI	3.53	2.70		2.45			
RR_{med}	87.6	36.4		28.1			
RR_{max}	65.7	27.3		21.1			
D	69,251	28,833	7,330	2,624	53,541	81,205	75,212
Inc	66,627	26,209	4,706				
SI	27.5	11.4	2.87				
ln SI	3.32	2.44	1.06				
RR_{med}	91.8	36.1	6.5				
RR_{max}	84.8	33.4	6.0				

[a] Inc = increment; SI = stimulation index; ln SI = log of stimulation index; RR_{med} = relative response to median of three unrelated controls; RR_{max} = relative response to maximum of three unrelated controls.

unrelated donors may be used (14–16). We find that a minimum of five unrelated donors gives a median of reasonable precision. Third, the response to a pool of unrelated donor cells can be used (22). The difficulty here is that the response may be greater than that for an ordinary stimulator-responder combination (23). In Table 3 the relative responses to a panel of three unrelated donors have been calculated, Em, Fm, and Gm. Dm was not used to calculate the relative response (RR), because this cell was part of the test situation as explained below. The formulas for the relative responses are RR_{med} = test − autologous control/median response − autologous control × 100; RR_{max} = test − autologous control/maximal response − autologous control × 100.

As we have pointed out, the variability inherent in the MLC response makes precise interpretation difficult. Jørgensen and Lamm (14) have performed a detailed statistical comparison of the three basic methods for expression of MLC data. They found that the RR_{med} had a smaller coefficient of variation than SR with autologous control, and SR was slightly smaller than the raw counts per minute. Use of the RR, furthermore, gives good correlation between repeat MLCs performed on different days (15). Jørgensen and Lamm (14) performed a further statistical analysis of MLC data. It appears that the majority of the variance in MLC data is due to the biological component and not to technical error. The relative response versus the median control response is the best method to express the results of MLC response, especially when using homozygous HLA-D cells for HLA-D pheno- or genotyping (10, 14, 22, 25).

Clinical and genetic interpretation of mixed lymphocyte cultures

In using MLC data in transplant programs, the clinician must keep in mind the problems illustrated above. The expression of results, interpretation of the response, and in vivo meaning of MLC are subjects of great controversy at the present time. In some situations, the presence or absence of a response may be relatively unambiguous. In these cases, the results of an MLC may serve as a useful adjunct to planning therapy or choosing a favorable donor for a recipient. In particular, a clear negative response seems necessary for planning bone marrow transplantation.

The genetics of MLC determinants are currently being studied in many laboratories. Because of the difficulty in discriminating one and two allele differences and because of the variability of most MLC data, attempts are being made to find "homozygous" stimulator cells. The family shown in Table 2 illustrates the behavior of a homozygous cell. Individual MS, the daughter designated as C, shows a vigorous to moderate response to cells from both parents, but when her lymphocytes are used as stimulators both parents fail to respond. Negative or weak response by lymphocytes stimulated in MLC, where the response to some unrelated controls is strong, is taken to indicate that the responding cell "sees" no determinants different from those it possesses. In this case the cell MS must have received two identical determinants for MLC from each parent. Thus, the parents' cells do not respond, since they do not recognize any foreign determinants on MS. That MS and MAL are only weakly stimulatory for one another relative to other unrelated combinations is presumptive evidence that MAL is also a "homozygous" cell.

With the determination that a particular cell bears only a single major MLC determinant, it should be possible to look for the presence of this determinant in the general population. The MLC determinants have previously been named MLR-S or LD. At the Sixth Histocompatibility Workshop Conference (Aarhus, Denmark, 1975), the MLC locus was named HLA-D and the determinants are named by use of the prefix W. Thus, a negative or weak response to a cell, which appears to be homozygous at the HLA-D locus, indicates that one or both of the D determinants of the responding cell are identical to the determinant of the stimulating, "typing," cell.

Several difficulties are involved in this procedure. Sharing of one HLA-D determinant between a homozygous stimulating cell and a heterozygous responding cell, as revealed by family studies, seldom results in a completely negative MLC response. A weak to moderate response is usually observed, such as that between MS and her parents in the example shown above. This may be due to genetic disparity at nearby loci (8, 10, 25), release of blastogenic factors ("back stimulation") from the mitomycin-inhibited, but metabolically active, stimulator cells recognizing the foreign determinant on the responder cells (29), or disparity of a responder determinant (MLR-R) on the responding cells.

The cell MS (designated in workshop reports Sc) and others like it have been studied in several different laboratories. It has become apparent that the HLA-D typing will become an important tool in histocompatibility testing, studies of disease associations, and genetic mapping in humans. Therefore, part of the Sixth Histocompatibility Workshop was devoted to the exchange and comparison of cells from the various laboratories. These comparisons have resulted in the identification of six HLA-D determinants designated: Dw_1, Dw_2, Dw_3, Dw_4, Dw_5, and Dw_6.

As we noted above, the identification of HLA-D determinants is complicated by the fact that weak to moderate responses are generally observed between homozygous stimulator cells and heterozygous responder cells sharing the homozygotes' HLA-D determinant. The main problem, then, is to determine what characterizes a "typing" response. Clearly, to be useful as a typing cell, the homozygous cell should be able to divide the responses of a panel of cells into two distinct groups: those who "respond" and therefore do not possess the determinant and those whose response indicates that they in fact have the same determinant as the typing cell. Figure 5 shows the results of two experiments with homozygous cells Sc and JH. Each cell was used to stimulate a random panel of responder cells. The frequency of second locus HLA antigens in this panel is: HLA-B7 = 26%, HLA-B8 = 29%, HLA-B13 = 7% and HLA-Bw$_{16}$ = 2.5%. The relative responses versus the median control response to JH can be separated into two groups: 0 to 50% and 83 to 137% in one experiment and 0 to 49% and 64 to 114% in the second experiment. The first experiment shows a clear separation at the 95% confidence level, but the second experiment had two responses at an intermediate level, and the separation is not significant. Cell Sc shows relative responses of 13 to 48% and 84 to 160% in the first experiment and 23 to 54% and 66 to 107% in the second. A complete separation at the 95% confidence level is observed in the first experiment, and some overlap at this level is seen in the second experiment. For the cell JH the 99% confidence interval for the high responder group of the combined experiments gives an upper limit for a typing response in a single determination of 35% with a mean for the high responders of 97%. For typing cell Sc the mean of the high responder group is 99% and the low value for this group at the 99% confidence interval is 42%. The results of these experiments indicate that for values of the RR_{med} between 0 and 35% versus *unrelated* responding cells, we can be 99% sure that the response belongs to the low group and can call this a typing response. It should be borne in mind that the significance of a moderate response among heterozygotes is not understood and such re-

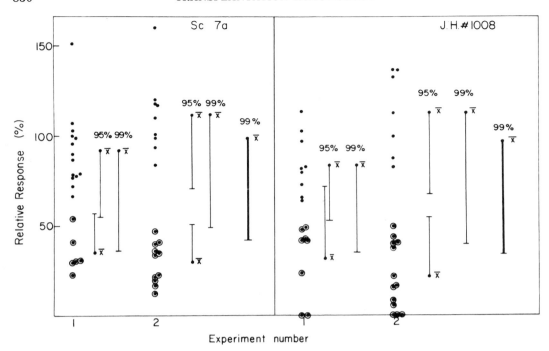

FIG. 5. *Relative responses of a responder cell panel to homozygous cells Sc and JH. The 99 and 95% confidence intervals (one-sided) have been plotted.*

sponses are not to be interpreted as typing responses.

In addition to defining HLA-D specificities, the participants in the Sixth Histocompatibility Workshop also considered the HLA serological specificities of the typing and responding cells. This was done because HLA-B and HLA-D are closely linked at the major histocompatibility region of humans (30). The HLA-B typing of the cells that determined the specificity Dw_1 was HLA-B W_{35} and HLA-B W_{27}. Among the responding cells that showed typing responses for Dw_1, a greater number had HLA-B W_{35} than would be expected by chance. This phenomenon has been dubbed "linkage disequilibrium" and has yet to be adequately explained. The determinant Dw_2 was identified by cells that were HLA-B7 or HLA-B12, and linkage disequilibrium was observed with HLA-B7. Dw_3 was identified by cells that were HLA-B8, and linkage disequilibrium was found with B8. Dw_4 was identified by cells that were typed as HLA-B7, HLA-B12, or HLA-BW$_{15}$, but linkage disequilibrium was found only in association with the third locus specificity, HLA-Cw$_3$. The determinant Dw_5 was established by cells typed as HLA-Bw$_{35}$, Bw$_{16}$, or B18, and the determinant Dw_6 was typed by cells that were HLA-B12, Bw$_{16}$, B8, or Bw$_{15}$. Dw_5 and Dw_6 were not found

in linkage disequilibrium with any of the HLA-A, -B, or -C specificities. It is interesting to note that the majority of typing cells are also homozygous at the FOUR or second locus of HLA (HLA-B). In our example (cf. Table 2) the typing cell Sc (MS) is heterozygous at the first locus and homozygous for HLA-B7 at the second locus. This is consistent with the finding of Yunis and Amos (30) that MLC determinants are located outside of the region which determines the serological specificities but are closely linked to the HLA-B (FOUR) locus.

Despite the excellent progress made in determining the HLA-D specificities, one further difficulty deserves mention. Some HLA-D typing cells when used against a random responder panel produce anomalous patterns. That is, two typing cells which are negative in response to each other and presumably determine the same HLA-D haplotype may not generate an identical pattern of response in the random panel. Also, two homozygous cells for an HLA-D determinant may give weak to moderate responses to each other or in one or two directions (10, 18). This may be due to something like the "inclusion" phenomena of HLA serology with the existence of long or short antigens, interference by non-HLA-D determinants, or technical inadequacy. Alternatively, this may also be explained by the existence of two or more loci that control allogeneic stimulation.

With the use of the HLA-D typing, it should be possible to predict the outcome of MLC tests between unrelated individuals. Jørgensen, Lamm, and Kissmeyer-Nielsen have shown that this can be accomplished by using the patterns of response to three typing cells (16). This predictive value is good for a multiple screen, but equivocal for the individual case. Again, a large part of the problem is the fact that "identical" individuals produce a weak but distinct reaction in MLC. Thus, the predictive value has only a statistical reliability.

In conclusion, we have emphasized the genetic aspects of MLC typing, because they are of current interest in the field of human genetics. In illustrating them, we hope to have created the impression that the use of MLC as a clinical tool in transplantation is limited by the variability of the response. In many family studies, however, the MLC response can provide useful information for the selection of a donor. With the establishment of specific HLA-D determinants and the availability of frozen typing cells and typing cells that have been established in culture, it is hoped that further characterization of the major histocompatibility region of humans will be possible. Finally, it would be expected that, as in the mouse system (H-2), this region may be associated with possible Ir genes, which determine the immunological status of the individual. It is hoped that the advent of MLC typing will aid in the clinical investigation of immunological disorders.

ACKNOWLEDGMENTS

This work was supported by Efficacy of Tissue Typing Contract AI 22530 and Public Health Service Grant HL-06314.

LITERATURE CITED

1. Alexander, P., and R. Powles. 1972. The possible occurrence in vivo of the autostimulating factor for lymphocytes. Birth Defects, Orig. Artic. Ser. 9:111–128.

2. Bach, F. H., and D. B. Amos. 1967. Hu-1: major histocompatibility locus in man. Science 156:1506–1508.

3. Bach, F. H., and K. Hirschhorn. 1964. Lymphocyte interaction: a potential histocompatibility test in vitro. Science 143:813–814.

4. Bach, F. H., and N. K. Voynow. 1966. One-way stimulation in mixed leucocyte cultures. Science 153:545–547.

5. Bøyum, A. 1968. Separation of leucocytes from blood and bone marrow. Scand. J. Clin. Lab. Invest. 21(Suppl. 97):1–108.

6. Cochrum, K. C., H. A. Perkins, R. O. Payne, S. L. Kountz, and F. O. Belzer. 1973. The corre-

7. Dupont, B., R. A. Good, G. S. Hansen, C. Jersild, L. S. Nielsen, B. H. Park, A. Svejgaard, M. Thomsen, and E. J. Yunis. 1974. Two separate genes controlling stimulation in mixed lymphocyte reaction in man. Proc. Natl. Acad. Sci. U.S.A. 71:52–56.

8. Dupont, B., E. J. Yunis, J. A. Hansen, N. Reinsmoen, N. Sucia-Foca, E. Mickelson, and D. B. Amos. 1975. Evidence for three genes involved in the expression of the LD determinants in mixed lymphocyte culture reaction. VI International Histocompatibility Workshop Conference (1975), Aarhus, Denmark. Histocompatibility testing 1975, p. 547–551. Munksgaard, Copenhagen.

9. Freiesleben-Sørensen, S. 1972. The mixed lymphocyte culture interaction: techniques and immunogenetics. Acta Pathol. Microbiol. Scand., Sect. B, Suppl. 230.

10. Hansen, J. A., B. Dupont, P. Rubinstein, N. Sucia-Foca, S. M. Fu, E. Mickelson, C. Whitsett, C. Jersild, H. G. Kunkel, N. K. Day, R. A. Good, E. D. Thomas, K. Reempsma, F. H. Allen, Jr., and M. Fotino. 1975. MLC determinants in the North American (New York City) caucasian population as defined by MLC homozygous test cells. VI International Histocompatibility Workshop Conference (1975), Aarhus, Denmark. Histocompatibility testing 1975, p. 470–478. Munksgaard, Copenhagen.

11. Hartzman, R. J., M. Segall, M. L. Bach, and F. H. Bach. 1971. Histocompatibility matching. VI. Miniaturization of the mixed leucocyte culture test: a preliminary report. Transplantation 11:268–273.

12. International Histocompatibility Workshop. 1975. Proceedings of VI International Histocompatibility Workshop Conference, Aarhus, Denmark. Histocompatibility Testing 1975. Munksgaard, Copenhagen.

13. Jongsma, A., H. van Someren, A. Westerveld, A. Hagemeijer, and P. Pearson. 1973. Localization of genes on human chromosomes by studies of human-Chinese hamster somatic cell hybrids: assignment of PGM_3 to chromosome C6 and regional mapping of the PGD, PGM_1, and PEP-C genes on chromosome A1. Humangenetik 20:195–202.

14. Jørgensen, F., and L. U. Lamm. 1974. MLC—a micromodification of the mixed leucocyte culture technique. In Reports from an MLC workshop. Tissue Antigens 4:482–494.

15. Jørgensen, F., L. U. Lamm, and F. Kissmeyer-Nielsen. 1974. Three LD (MLC) determinants. A Danish population study. Tissue Antigens 4:419–428.

16. Jørgensen, F., L. U. Lamm, and F. Kissmeyer-Nielsen. 1975. MLC results among unrelated can be predicted. Tissue Antigens 5:262–265.

17. Kasakura, S., and L. Lowenstein. 1965. The effect of irradiation in vitro on mixed leukocyte cultures and on leukocyte cultures with phytohaemagglutinin, p. 211–212. In Histo-

compatibility Testing (1965), Proceedings of Conference and Workshop on Histocompatibility Testing, Leyden, 1965. The Williams & Williams Co., Baltimore.

18. Keuning, J. J., A. Termijtelen, A. Blusse, T. G. van oud Alblas, T. G. van den Tweel, J. Schrevder, and J. J. van Rood. 1975. Typing for MLC (LD). Transplant. Proc., in press.

19. Koch, C. T., E. Fredericks, V. P. Eijsvoogel, and J. J. van Rood. 1971. Mixed-lymphocyte-culture and skin-graft data in unrelated HL-A identical individuals. Lancet 2:1334–1336.

20. Koch, C. T., J. P. van Hooff, A. van Leeuwen, J. G. van den Tweel, E. Fredericks, G. J. van der Steon, H. M. A. Schippers, and J. J. van Rood. 1973. The relative importance of matching for the MLC versus the HL-A loci in organ transplantation, p. 521–524. In J. Dausset and J. Colombani (ed.), Histocompatibility testing 1972. V Conference and Workshop on Histocompatibility Testing, Evian-les-Bains, France, 1972. Munksgaard, Copenhagen.

21. Lieblen, J. 1962. The closest two out of three observations, p. 129–135. In A. E. Sarhan and B. G. Greenberg (ed.), Contributions to order statistics. John Wiley & Sons, Inc., New York.

22. MLC Workshop. 1974. Reports from an MLC Workshop. Tissue Antigens 4:454–525.

23. Osoba, D., and K. J. Falk. 1974. The mixed leucocyte culture in man: effects of pools of stimulating cells selected on the basis of crossreacting HL-A specificities. Cell. Immunol. 10:117–135.

24. Park, B. H., and R. A. Good. 1973. The meaning and use of the mixed leukocyte culture test in transplantation, p. 71–92. In E. J. Yunis, R. A. Gatti, and D. B. Amos (ed.), Tissue typing and organ transplantation. Academic Press Inc., New York.

25. Reinsmoen, H., M. Stewart, L. Emme, L. R. Hanrahan, B. Dupont, J. A. Hansen, P. Friend, D. B. Amos, and E. J. Yunis. 1975. Definition of several MLR-S (MLC) homozygous cells and the typing for these determinants in the North American caucasian population (Minnesota). VI International Histocompatibility Workshop Conference (1975), Aarhus, Denmark. Histocompatibility testing 1975, p. 459–463. Munksgaard, Copenhagen.

26. Sengar, D. P. S., and P. I. Terasaki. 1971. A semimicro mixed leucocyte culture test. Transplantation 3:260–267.

27. Thomsen, M., G. S. Hansen, A. Svejgaard, C. Jersild, J. A. Hansen, R. A. Good, and B. Dupont. 1974. Mixed lymphocyte culture technique standardization of a test-system with 10^5 responding and 10^5 stimulating lymphocytes per 1 ml. In Reports from a Mixed Lymphocyte Culture Workshop. Tissue Antigens 4:495–506.

28. van Rood, J. J., C. T. Koch, J. P. van Hooff, A. van Leeuwen, J. G. van den Tweel, E. Fredericks, H. M. A. Schippers, G. Hendricks, and G. J. van der Steon. 1973. Graft survival in unrelated donor-recipient pairs matched for MLC and HLA. Transplant. Proc. 5:409–414.

29. von Boehmer, H. 1974. Separation of T and B lymphocytes and their role in the mixed lymphocyte reaction. J. Immunol. 112:70–78.

30. Yunis, E. J., and D. B. Amos. 1971. Three closely linked genetic systems relevant to transplantation. Proc. Natl. Acad. Sci. U.S.A. 68:3031–3035.

31. Yunis, E. J., R. A. Gatti, and D. B. Amos (ed.). 1973. Tissue typing and organ transplantation. Academic Press Inc., New York.

32. Yunis, E. J., J. M. Plate, F. E. Ward, and D. B. Amos. 1971. Anomalous MLR responsiveness among siblings. Transplant. Proc. 3:118.

Chapter 110

Cryopreservation of Lymphocytes

MICHAEL A. S. JEWETT, JOHN A. HANSEN, AND BO DUPONT

INTRODUCTION

Cryopreservation of the function as well as the structure of fowl spermatozoa was reported by Polge, Smith, and Parkes in 1949 (16). Success was achieved by mixing glycerol with the spermatozoa, which protected them from injury. The technique of adding a protective agent, or cryoprotectant, was applied to human red blood cells by Lovelock in 1953 (12), and since then a great variety of normal and neoplastic plant and mammalian cells have been cryopreserved, including lymphocytes and hematopoietic stem cells. Although cryopreservation is an established technique of value, there are still major unsolved problems that limit its practical application and make many aspects of the procedure empirical. In this chapter, we shall outline the theory of cryopreservation and describe our technique of cryopreservation of human peripheral blood lymphocytes.

Early in the history of cryopreservation, it was generally held that the cause of injury was simply the formation of intracellular ice which physically disrupted and killed frozen cells. Ultrastructural studies have confirmed that the formation of crystalline intracellular ice is almost always associated with cell death and that by avoiding this cells can survive. However, the mechanism of injury is more complex, and studies with red blood cells, yeast, and other cells show that they shrink with freezing as a result of dehydration of the intracellular space (20). At least two forces produce the flow of water from the intracellular to the extracellular space. As the cell suspension is cooled to and below its freezing temperature, the intracellular water remains liquid, generating a vapor pressure difference. Secondly, the extracellular space becomes hypertonic as ice forms, producing an osmotic gradient. The reduction in volume may change the spatial relationship of macromolecules in the cell, producing abnormal chemical bonds (11).

Lovelock has emphasized the changes in the electrolyte concentration with the shift of water rather than cell shrinkage per se. He attributed the damage to the direct or indirect surface effects of these changes (12). This could explain why too slow cooling, which prolongs exposure to these abnormal solute concentrations, is deleterious. Recent work supports this, and it is now generally agreed that the primary site of injury is the cell membrane and that other changes and damage are secondary.

It would appear that study of the action of cryoprotectants should shed light on the mechanisms and the sites of injury. Cryoprotectants have been divided into two categories: those that penetrate the cell membrane and those that do not. Agents that penetrate, e.g., glycerol and dimethyl sulfoxide (Me_2SO), provide better protection, presumably on a colligative basis, than those that do not, e.g., sucrose and polyvinyl pyrollidine, although these nonpenetrating substances definitely produce better results than no cryoprotectant at all. This is evidence for the importance of protecting the cell membrane which, if damaged, is more permeable.

By changing various parameters during cell freezing, a number of important empirical observations have been made and must be considered when undertaking cryopreservation:

1. *Optimal rates of cooling* vary between cell types. Generally, 1 C per min of cooling is recommended for mammalian cells, but it has been repeatedly shown that there is wide variation. Varying the rate of cooling shows that there is a biphasic effect on cell survival. This means that cells can be cooled too slowly and too quickly, with a peak survival occurring at an intermediate rate. Too slow cooling prolongs exposure to abnormal concentrations of solute, whereas too rapid cooling causes intracellular crystallization of water. Also, an activated cell may require a different rate from the same cell type in a resting state. It is generally agreed that rapid warming is the best method of thawing the cells.

2. *The rate of cryoprotectant removal* by dilution after thawing must be extremely slow, particularly with lymphocytes, to produce optimal survival (8).

3. *The presence of serum* in the freezing and thawing medium gives additional protection from injury.

CRYOPRESERVATION OF HUMAN LYMPHOCYTES

A variety of techniques have been employed successfully to cryopreserve functional human peripheral blood lymphocytes. Purified cells are suspended in medium containing serum and a cryoprotectant, usually Me_2SO, and are chilled before freezing. The procedures for freezing can be considered as noncontrolled and controlled.

Noncontrolled freezing

The simplest method of cryopreservation is to place the specimen in a mechanical low-temperature freezer with subsequent storage in the same freezer or in liquid nitrogen. By trial and error, each laboratory will determine the shape of container and position in the freezer that is optimal. Satisfactory in vitro lymphocyte transformation to mitogens and antigens and function in mixed lymphocyte cultures, by use of cells frozen in this manner, have been described (15, 18, 22). In general, however, sensitive in vitro lymphocyte functions such as the ability to respond in mixed lymphocyte cultures and to specific antigens are better preserved by controlled-rate freezing (2). A modification of this approach by suspending the sample in a predetermined position over liquid nitrogen is also satisfactory (e.g., Lunde BF-S).

Controlled freezing

A number of freezers are available that can be programmed to lower the temperature of the sample at an adjustable rate by cooling a chamber with vaporized liquid nitrogen. Each piece of equipment varies in the details of instrumentation, but the principle of operation is the same. The starting and finishing temperatures, as well as the rate of cooling, are controlled. Some machines have the additional feature of compensating for the heat of effusion, which is the release of heat by the sample at the temperature of crystallization (Fig. 1). This is usually below 0 C because of supercooling, and causes a sudden and often large rise in the sample temperature. An immediate jet of nitrogen can prevent this rise and maintain the gradual cooling rate that had been programmed. The best results with freezing have been obtained in experienced laboratories that use this type of equipment, but the value of this feature has not been specifically demonstrated.

Although the freezers that can be programmed are more expensive, they ensure consistent and automated freezing that generally gives reproducible results.

INDICATIONS

The capacity of cryopreserved lymphocytes to function in the in vitro lymphocyte transforma-tion assays to mitogens and antigens and in mixed lymphocyte culture is maintained (3, 9, 19). Also, cytotoxic "killer cell" function and the capacity of lymphocytes to release mediator molecules (e.g., migration inhibitory factor) are preserved. We have demonstrated that the use of cryopreserved peripheral blood lymphocytes gives improved results in longitudinal studies by reducing nonbiological day-to-day laboratory variation (9). Lymphocyte subpopulations, as determined by surface markers, appear to be altered with a decrease in non-T cells, but this does not significantly influence functional studies. We are increasing our reliance on cryopreservation for in vitro assessment of a patient's immune function.

Histocompatibility testing is readily performed with cryopreserved lymphocytes. Histocompatibility locus A serotyping does not require as careful cryopreservation techniques as other assays. The capacity to stimulate in mixed lymphocyte cultures is similarly preserved, but the ability of cryopreserved lymphocytes to respond in mixed lymphocyte cultures to the same degree as fresh cells is only maintained by careful controlled-rate freezing. Cell-mediated lympholysis techniques can also be performed with cryopreserved cells.

The special advantages and possibilities of cryopreservation include:

1. Improved standardization of all cellular functional assays by the use of the same stored control cells and target cells.

2. Shipping of cells from one laboratory to another for comparative studies.

3. Possible selection of cell populations, most notably bone marrow cells, but also peripheral blood lymphocytes, by varying the rate of cooling during freezing. The optimal rate for one type of cell in a mixture can be selected, thereby purifying for that population.

4. Possible use of immune lymphocytes for tumor immunotherapy, as suggested by animal experiments but as yet untried in humans.

Despite the many advantages of cryopreservation, there are significant gaps in our knowledge of mechanisms in cryodamage to cells. The 30% net loss of cell which occurs with freezing, thawing, and washing, despite the use of cryoprotectant substances and careful technique, still presents a problem. Other disadvantages of cryopreservation are the capital investment necessary for equipment and possible changes in lymphocyte subpopulations.

PROCEDURE FOR CONTROLLED FREEZING

Any recipe for cryopreservation must be empirical and must be customized to the individual laboratory. The following is the method used in our laboratory. This technique is suitable for the functional in vitro lymphocyte assays generally in use in clinical immunology. Individual investigators should, however, be prepared to modify various steps as suggested in the literature if the results of the in vitro assays are changed considerably by using cryopreserved cells.

Preparation of cell suspension

The technique used for the separation of lymphocytes from peripheral blood does not appear to influence the results of cryopreservation. The Ficoll-Hypaque or Lymphoprep method is fast and adequate (16). As the optimal rate of cooling differs for various cell types, the freezing procedure followed here tends to reduce the number of contaminating nonlymphocyte cells that may be present after purification of the fresh specimen when it is frozen and thawed. The concentration of cells should be 12×10^6 to 40×10^6/ml, as they are diluted 1:1 with the cryoprotectant to produce a final concentration of 6×10^6 to 20×10^6/ml. The cells are suspended in a complete medium such as RPMI 1640 (Herpes buffer) with penicillin (20,000 U/500 ml), streptomycin (20,000 μg/500 ml), L-glutamine (120 mg/500 ml), and 20% (vol/vol) fetal calf or pooled human serum.

Preparation of the cryoprotectant (dimethyl sulfoxide)

An equal volume of Me_2SO solution is added to the cell suspension before freezing (1:1 dilution). This solution is prepared by adding Me_2SO (commercial stock) to the above 20% serum in medium solution to produce a final concentration of 20% Me_2SO (vol/vol). This will in effect reduce the serum concentration to 16% in the Me_2SO solution and 18% in the final freezing preparation. The stock Me_2SO may be sterilized by filtration, but it has not been a recognized source of contamination without filtration.

Selection and preparation of sample containers

Glass or plastic ampoules are commercially available for freezing cells. We use labeled screw-top polypropylene 2-ml tubes, which are convenient and do not burst. However, for small volumes, the sealable glass ampoules may be easier and certainly do not allow the liquid nitrogen to leak into the sample, as we occasionally see with screw-top containers. We freeze in 1-ml amounts.

Preparation of freezing apparatus

Prior to diluting the cell suspension with Me_2SO, the freezing apparatus must be prepared and cooled to 4 C. The exact procedure depends on the type of freezing equipment used, but in the case of the Planer R201 Programmed Freezer this involves pumping up the liquid nitrogen reservoir and precooling the chamber. This preparation reduces the period of Me_2SO-cell contact before freezing, which is injurious to the cells.

Mixing of cell suspension and cryoprotectant

The cell suspension and cryoprotectant should be combined *slowly* with constant gentle mixing to allow time for the Me_2SO to penetrate the cells. It is convenient to mix the cell suspension with one Pasteur pipette while adding the Me_2SO solution drop by drop with a second pipette. The final suspension is placed on ice and pipetted as soon as possible (in measured 1-ml volumes) into the waiting ampoules.

Freezing

It is essential that one ampoule containing the same cell and medium concentration be used as the control sample to monitor the freezing if a programmed freezer is used. This is placed in the chamber, with a thermocouple in it, and the system is stabilized again at 4 C. The samples should be arranged in a rack which allows uniform circulation of the coolant, and they should be immediately adjacent to the control sample to insure similar conditions. The program is begun by cooling the samples at 1 C/min to -40 C; then they are rapidly cooled to -100 C before transferral to the storage container. Figure 1 depicts two temperature curves measured during freezing of lymphocytes at 6×10^6/ml; the recorder or sample curve reflects the temperature of the specimen. This demonstrates the heat of effusion (crystallization), which is rapidly compensated for by the automatic controller, whose temperature curve reflects the temperature in the chamber. Without cells in the control sample, this initial supercooling and sudden rise in temperature with crystallization will not be recorded or compensated for by the freezer, which may reduce ultimate cell survival. The detailed technique of freezer operation will be followed from the respective manual. If the equipment used is not programmed, a satisfactory cooling curve may be obtained by trial and error with a recording thermocouple, refrigerator, and freezer.

Storage

The frozen cells should be stored at as cold a temperature as possible. Liquid nitrogen or a

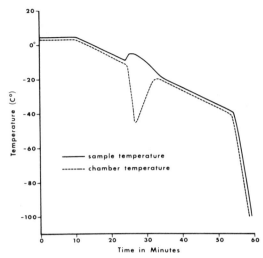

FIG. 1. *Schematic representation of a typical recording of the temperature during controlled-rate freezing of lymphocytes in 10% dimethyl sulfoxide and 20% serum. The curve from the recorder thermocouple reflects the temperature within the sample and shows the sharp rise due to the heat of effusion at the crystallization point. This rise is diminished by an additional burst of coolant which in fact has to reduce the chamber temperature temporarily, as represented by the controller tracing, which is a thermocouple adjacent to the sample but free in the chamber.*

vapor-phase liquid nitrogen refrigerator, which will keep the cells at at least -100 C, are ideal. A mechanical freezer can also be used, but probably the cell survival decreases with time.

Thawing and dilution of cryoprotectant

The cells are quick-thawed in a 37 C water bath. As soon as the specimen is liquid, it is diluted 10:1 with 20% medium prepared as above. This dilution must be done extremely slowly and continuously over 5 to 10 min at room temperature, and upon completion the cells should be washed in Hanks or other balanced salt solution. With low cell numbers, one wash will reduce cell loss and seems to be adequate for cell function. It cannot be emphasized too much how important it is to dilute the cell suspension slowly. After washing, the cells are resuspended at the concentration and in the media desired for testing.

Testing viability

A number of techniques are used to determine viable cell recovery after thawing, but the only true test of survival is cellular function in the assay system for which it was preserved. Trypan blue dye exclusion is the simplest

method of assessing viability, and the above technique yields an average of 70% viable cell recovery. This is called not viable recovery and means that 70% of the living cells which are frozen are recovered alive after thawing and washing. A portion of the loss takes place during washing and therefore is not directly the result of freezing and thawing. Base-line data must be obtained for frozen cells compared with fresh cells in any assay system to insure that their function is indeed preserved.

EQUIPMENT AND SUPPLIES

Major equipment

There are a number of freezers available and new ones being developed. Information may be obtained from the following partial list of manufacturers:

Union Carbide Corp., Linde Division, New York, N.Y. 10017. Phone: (212) 551-3752.
G. V. Planer Ltd., Sunbury-on-Thames, Middlesex, England. Phone: Sunbury-on-Thames (STD Code 09327) 86262.
Cryosan Technisch Laboratorium, Middenbeemster, Holland.
Cryo-Med, Mt. Clemens, Mich. 48043. Phone: (313) 949-4507.
Vertis Co. Inc., Gardiner, N.Y. 12525. Phone: (914) 255-5000.

Supplies

Dimethyl sulfoxide: grade 1, 100-ml bottle; Sigma Chemical Co., catalog no. D5879. Not sterile, which is satisfactory for lymphocytes used in short-term culture, but it should be filtered before use with cells for long-term culture or for infusion in patients.
Freezing vials: A/S Nunc serum tube, 38 × 12.5 mm, with marking area, screw cap, silicone washer, 2 ml.
Each laboratory will devise its own best method of cooling the racks containing the samples prior to freezing and the use of sterile mixing tubes, pipettes, etc. These supplies are generally available.

INTERPRETATION

Effect of cryopreservation on in vitro lymphocyte function

Most in vitro functional properties of lymphocytes have now been shown to be preserved with freezing and thawing. Many of these in vitro assays are subject to considerable day-today variation, which may make interpretation difficult, especially when changes are minimal. Some of the variation is eliminated by testing consecutively cryopreserved cell samples and performing the tests simultaneously on one occasion. For example, with lymphocyte transformation to mitogens and antigens, Fig. 2a represents the five dose-response curves to decreasing concentrations of phytohemagglutinin (PHA), expressed as counts per minute, obtained with fresh cells collected on five separate occasions from one normal donor and demonstrates the wide variation in peak responses from experiment to experiment. This interexperimental variation also causes a shift in the dose-response curve so that the peak response does not always occur at the same dose of PHA. At the time each of these specimens was collected, a sample of each was frozen. The sets of five frozen samples from each donor were studied together subsequently on a single occasion (Fig. 2b). The results demonstrate a significant decrease in the variation of response for each individual. Figure 2c compares the means of the five fresh and five frozen curves ±1 standard deviation. The curves for the average of five tests are almost identical, but the standard deviation is markedly reduced by the use of five different samples of cryopreserved cells in a

single experiment. Plotting the peak responses for each of the five determinations on fresh or frozen cells shows that the frozen cell responses are very consistent, as compared with wide fluctuation in the responses of the same samples of fresh cells (Fig. 2d). During the period of time that these blood samples were collected, the normal donor was apparently well. Similar data were obtained with concanavalin A (Con A) and poke weed mitogen (PWM).

With transformation to the antigens, the results were somewhat different. Figure 3 represents the mean stimulation ±1 standard deviation of samples of fresh and frozen cells collected on the five different occasions. Again, the variation is markedly reduced when five different samples of frozen cells are tested in a single experiment, although the level of response is sometimes less with the frozen cells.

To demonstrate that the reduced variability in the in vitro responses of frozen cells was due to technical and not biological phenomena, a large stock of cells from one donor was frozen on a single occasion, and samples of this stock were thawed and tested on five subsequent days. The results were compared with the responses of fresh cells obtained from the same donor on each of these days. Figure 4 shows the peak PHA, Con A, and PWM responses on each

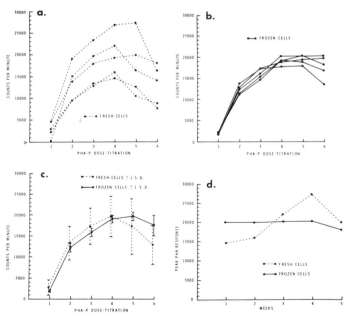

FIG. 2. *Dose-response curves to decreasing concentrations of PHA-P as expressed in counts per minute. The curves obtained with fresh cells collected at weekly intervals (a) show large week-to-week variation which is reduced by studying cells from the same samples simultaneously after freezing, storage, and thawing. The means of the curves for the fresh and the frozen cells are similar (c). Plotted differently, the peak response for each sample shows little variation with frozen cells but larger variation with fresh cells (d).*

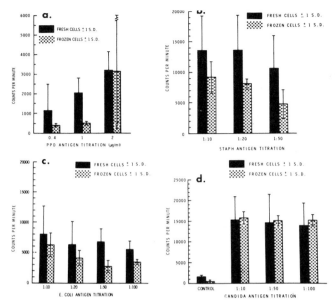

FIG. 3. *Mean stimulation ± 1 standard deviation of peripheral blood lymphocytes by titrated doses of antigens expressed in counts per minute for samples of fresh and frozen cells collected on five different occasions. The variation is reduced when the different samples of frozen cells are tested on a single occasion.*

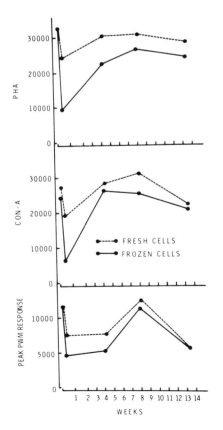

of five different test days for the fresh compared with the frozen cells. As these frozen cells were all obtained from a single collection, one would expect that each sample would respond in the same way; however, they vary considerably in parallel to the responses of the fresh cells.

Cytotoxic function of cryopreserved lymphocytes is maintained or slightly reduced compared with fresh cells, but sequential control studies have not been reported.

In mixed lymphocyte culture, frozen cells provide almost the same responses although usually slightly lower. Figure 5 illustrates the results of two experiments in which fresh responder lymphocytes from the same 20 donors were stimulated by fresh and frozen DW2 homozygous typing cells. The relative responses of the cultures stimulated by the fresh typing cells are plotted against those stimulated by the same but frozen typing cells. This was repeated in a second experiment performed in the same way but at a different time. The slope of the regression lines generated by the two sets of data is slightly less than 1 (0.84 and

FIG. 4. *Peak PHA, Con A, and PWM responses to counts per minute on each of five different days for fresh compared with frozen cells. The frozen cells were obtained on the same day prior to the test, and samples were thawed on each test day when a fresh sample was obtained from the donor. Both samples were then studied simultaneously.*

0.77, respectively), which is the expected value if the fresh and frozen cells give equal stimulation. However, the coefficients of determination ($r^2 = 0.86$ and 0.97, respectively) are very high so that the data are equally reproducible whether fresh or frozen stimulators are used. Similar data for responders show that actual counts per minute are slightly lower, but the responses expressed as relative responses are approximately the same for frozen and fresh cells.

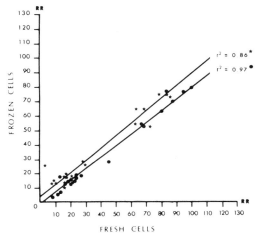

FIG. 5. *Comparison of mixed lymphocyte culture responses obtained with fresh responder leukocytes from 20 donors stimulated by fresh and frozen DW2 homozygous typing cells. The data are from two independent experiments; the first is shown as dots and the second as stars. The coefficient of determination ($r^2 = 0.86$ and 0.92) for the linear regression line of each experiment indicates the "goodness of fit." The figure demonstrates that mixed lymphocyte culture responses obtained with the same fresh and frozen stimulating cells are comparable, although the frozen cells produce slightly lower responses.*

Effects of cryopreservation on lymphocyte subpopulations

Previous reports of the effects of cryopreservation on lymphocyte subpopulations suggest that there are no significant changes. The methodology for enumeration of subpopulations varies so much in different laboratories at this time that it is difficult to compare results. Table 1 is a comparison of a number of markers on fresh and frozen lymphocytes from seven normal donors. The sample of fresh cells was divided, and half was frozen and tested subsequently for each donor. Storage time varied from 3 to 8 weeks, but this did not influence results. The percentage of E rosettes increases ($P < 0.05$), whereas all the markers of non-T cells decrease.

The significant decrease in B lymphocyte recovery as defined by surface immunoglobulin M receptors (9% → 3.5%) was constantly observed. The decrease in the non-T, non-B lymphocyte subpopulation defined by Ripley rosette formation was not as profound in a subsequent, more elaborate experiment (15.8% → 12.7%, $n = 3$), so it is possible that the recovery of surface markers from freeze-thawing varies for different lymphocyte membrane receptors. Incubation of the thawed cells for 24 h prior to testing did not increase the non-T cell recovery, which might have been expected if damage to the cell surface was interfering with the tests, producing a false low. However, irreversible damage of the metabolic pathways for the production of some surface receptors may account for the result. Studies with purified subpopulations and established cell lines may answer these questions.

Cryopreservation of peripheral lymphocytes is a useful technique for both experimental and clinical immunological studies. It is convenient

TABLE 1. *Enumeration of lymphocyte subpopulation of seven normal donors compared with the subpopulations recovered from the same samples when frozen, stored, and thawed*[a]

| Subjects | T cells | | Non-T cells | | | | | | | | | |
| | (E rosettes) | | SmIg | | SmIgM | | Fc | | Ripley rosette | | M rosette | |
	Fresh	Frozen	Fresh	Frozen	Fresh	Frozen	Fresh	Frozen	Fresh	Frozen	Fresh	Frozen
1	85	96.5	14.5	4	11.5	2	24	5.5	23	8.5	4	3
2	89.5	91	19.5	5	6	3	25	7	15	1.5	5	1
3	87.5	93	6.7	6	4	5	10.6	9	—	—	—	—
4	77.5	91	28	2.5	11	1.5	27.5	1	12.5	—	3	2
5	86	87	—	—	7.5	—	—	—	—	—	2.5	0
6	89	89	28	7	6	5	29.5	2.5	—	8	2	0
7	61	93	33.5	13	17	7	35	3.5	10	—	7	0
Means	82.2	91.5	21.7	6.3	9	3.5	25.3	4.8	15	6	3.9	1

[a] E rosettes, Sheep red blood cell rosettes; SmIg, surface membrane immunoglobulin; SmIgM, surface membrane immunoglobulin M; Fc, Fc receptor; M rosette, mouse red blood cell rosette, expressed as percentage of total peripheral blood lymphocytes counted.

and can be performed with a minimum of equipment. The resulting standardization of in vitro studies and the ease of cell handling will undoubtedly lead to increased utilization of this technique.

ACKNOWLEDGMENTS

This work was supported by Public Health Service grants CA17404-01 and CA08748 from the National Cancer Institute and by the Special Fund for the Advanced Study of Cancer. M.A.S.J. was the recipient of an Ontario Ministry of Health Fellowship.

LITERATURE CITED

1. Boyum, A. 1968. Separation of leucocytes from blood and bone marrow. Scand. J. Clin. Lab. Invest. 21(Suppl. 97):1–109.
2. Eijsvoogel, V. P., R. du Bois, and P. T. A. Schellekens. 1974. The use of frozen lymphocytes in MCL tests, p. 512–514. In Reports from a mixed lymphocyte culture workshop. Tissue Antigens 4:453–525.
3. Eijsvoogel, V. P., M. J. G. J. du Bois, P. T. A. Schellekens, and D. R. Huismans. 1973. Cryopreserved lymphocytes: functional properties in vitro. Colloque de l'I.N.S.E.R.M.: Cryopreservation of normal and neoplastic cells, p. 101–106.
4. Farrant, J., S. C. Knight, and G. J. Morris. 1973. Use of cryobiological techniques in cell separation. Colloque de l'I.N.S.E.R.M.: Cryopreservation of normal and neoplastic cells, p. 27–39.
5. Fotino, M., E. J. Merson, P. Benoit, A. W. Rowe, and F. H. Allen, Jr. 1967. Lymphocyte typing by simplified microcytotoxicity using frozen and thawed cells, p. 429–432. In Histocompatibility testing, Munksgaard.
6. Goldman, J. M., and K. H. Think. 1973. The functional capacity of frozen mouse and human bone marrow cells. Colloque de l'I.N.S.E.R.M.: Cryopreservation of normal and neoplastic cells, p. 71–80.
7. Golub, S. H., H. L. Sulit, and D. L. Morton. 1975. The use of viable frozen lymphocytes for studies in human tumor immunology. Transplantation 19:195–202.
8. Greene, A. E., J. J. Manduka, and L. L. Coriell. 1975. Viability of cell cultures stored up to 12 years in liquid nitrogen. Cryobiology, in press.
9. Jewett, M. A. S., J. A. Hansen, S. Gupta, S. Cunningham-Rundles, F. P. Siegal, R. A. Good, and B. Dupont. 1975. The use of cryopreserved lymphocytes to standardize longitudinal studies of immune function in normal controls and patients. Cryobiology, in press.
10. Leguit, P., Jr., A. Meinesa, W. P. Zeijlemaker, P. T. A. Schellekens and V. P. Eijsvoogel. 1973. Immunological studies in burn patients lymphocyte transformation in vitro. Int. Arch. Allergy 44:101–121.
11. Levitt, J. 1962. A sulfhydryl-disulfide hypothesis of frost injury and resistance in plants. J. Theor. Biol. 3:355–391.
12. Lovelock, J. E. 1953. The mechanism of the protective action of glycerol against haemolysis by freezing and thawing. Biochim. Biophys. Acta 11:28–36.
13. Meryman, H. T. 1968. Modified model for the mechanism of freezing injury in erythrocytes. Nature (London) 218:333–336.
14. Meryman, H. T. 1970. The exceeding of a minimum tolerable cell volume in hypertonic suspension as a cause of freezing injury, p. 51–64. In G. E. W. Wolstenholme and M. O'Connor (ed.), The frozen cell. J. and A. Churchill, London.
15. Netzel, B., H. Grosse-Wilde, P. Bauman, and W. Mempel. 1975. LD typing in man using cells frozen and stored in microtiter plates. Tissue Antigens 6:8–14.
16. Polge, G., A. L. L. Smith, and A. S. Parkes. 1949. Revival of spermatozoa after vitrification and dehydration at low temperatures. Nature (London) 164:666.
17. Schaefer, U. W., and K. A. Dicke. 1973. Preservation of haemopoietic stem cells. Transplantation potential and CFU-C activity of frozen marrow tested in mice, monkeys and man. Colloque de l'I.N.S.E.R.M.: Cryopreservation of normal and neoplastic cells, p. 63–69.
18. Simon, J. D., M. M. Albalag, and L. J. Flinton. 1975. Recovery of T and B lymphocytes at −80°C. J. Cryobiol., in press.
19. Strong, D. M., J. N. Woody, M. A. Factor, A. Ahmed, and K. W. Sell. 1975. Immunological responsiveness of frozen-thawed human lymphocytes. Clin. Exp. Immunol. 21:442–445.
20. Walter, C. A., S. C. Knight, and J. Farrant. 1975. Ultrastructural appearance of free-substituted lymphocytes frozen by interrupted rapid cooling with a period at −26°C. Cryobiology 12:103–109.
21. Weiner, R. S., J. Breard, and C. O. O'Brein. 1973. Cryopreserved lymphocytes in sequential studies of human responsiveness: problems and prospects. Colloque de l'I.N.S.E.R.M.: Cryopreservation of normal and neoplastic cells, p. 117–131.
22. Wood, N., H. Bashir, J. Greally, D. B. Amos, and E. J. Yunis. 1972. A simple method of freezing and storing live lymphocytes. Tissue Antigens 2:27–31.

Chapter 111

HLA and Disease

ARNE SVEJGAARD

INTRODUCTION

A variety of human diseases have been found to arise more often in individuals carrying certain histocompatibility locus A (HLA) antigens than in those lacking them. The associations between HLA and disease have been the subject of several recent reviews (5, 7, 14), and in general they are much stronger than those which have been found between various other blood groups and diseases (16). This new field of immunogenetic research is likely to be fruitfully continued for some time yet, as the existence of such associations may provide insight not only into the genetics but also into the etiology of the HLA-associated disorders (12).

The purpose of this report is to outline how such studies may be performed, in the hope of enabling the clinical immunologist to plan and perform them and to evaluate critically data reported by other investigators.

It should be stressed that the list of references primarily includes surveys which should be consulted for further detail in case detailed data are needed.

METHODS

Since a simple survey about the HLA system has recently appeared (10) and the techniques for HLA typing have been discussed elsewhere in this *Manual*, only the problems which relate to the study of HLA in disease will be treated here. In particular, the pitfalls inherent in such studies will be stressed.

Either or both of the following two approaches may be used when attempts are made to establish whether or not the HLA system is involved in the susceptibility, or resistance, to a disease: population studies and family studies. In general, population studies are easier to perform, but in some cases a relationship can only be established by family studies.

Population studies

Population studies require a group of unrelated patients and a group of unrelated healthy control individuals. The selection of these individuals, sources of typing errors, and the statistical treatment of the results are discussed below.

Selection of patients and controls. Although it may not be of great importance in a preliminary study, it is worth keeping in mind that the patients who are HLA typed often represent selected groups: in most cases, we are dealing with patients who attend or have attended hospital clinics, and such patients are likely to be more severely affected than those who have never been admitted to a hospital. Moreover, it is likely that the patients who are most troubled by their disease are more likely to cooperate. Thus, it seems likely that the psoriatic patients who have been HLA typed so far are biased towards being more severely affected. This problem is less for diseases which are inevitably treated in hospitals, but here another source of bias may arise: in retrospective studies of lethal diseases, patients who died early in the course obviously "escape" HLA typing, and accordingly, there will be a bias towards too many long-term survivors in the group of patients who are HLA typed. If an HLA antigen is more frequent in such patients than in controls, the possibility should be kept in mind that this HLA antigen confers resistance to death rather than susceptibility to the disease. Such a relationship can only be unraveled by a prospective study of all newly diagnosed patients.

Concerning "unrelatedness" of the patients, it is usually sufficient to ask the patients whether they have affected relatives and then to make sure that these are not included in the study. However, for very rare recessive disorders, it is striking how often individuals do not know that they are related. In this context, it should be kept in mind that patients with such rare recessive disorders often are inbred (e.g., offspring of first cousins or even of incest) and thus homozygous on more loci (including HLA) than outbred individuals. Obviously, patients belonging to the same isolate often share many genes (e.g., HLA genes and disease genes not linked to HLA), which may cause spurious associations between HLA and a disease.

Special problems arise when studying mixed populations which have not yet reached equilibrium (stratification), and it may be difficult to find good control groups for such patients. For example, it is well known that the degree of Caucasian admixture varies among American Blacks, and American Blacks developing a "Caucasian" disease are more likely to have more "Caucasian" genes (including HLA) than others. This may lead to a spurious association between "Caucasian" HLA antigens and a "Caucasian" disease in these patients. On the other hand, an association, for example, between a "Caucasian" disease and an "African" HLA antigen may be meaningful.

The selection of a control group may thus be difficult when we are dealing with mixed populations, and it is worth mentioning that HLA antigen frequencies also vary considerably within the same racial group. However, quite large amounts of normal materials are now available from different countries, and it may be worthwhile to compare the control groups with some of these.

The control groups often consist predominantly of blood donors, and so far it has not been possible to show that these differ from the normal population; if there are differences, they would appear to be small. Moreover, the HLA antigen frequencies do not seem to differ between different age groups or between sexes. Accordingly, blood donors constitute in general a satisfying control group provided ethnic differences are taken into account. Unrelated individuals involved in paternity testing and other healthy randomly selected individuals may also be included.

Serological pitfalls. Serological pitfalls are discussed elsewhere in this *Manual,* but it seems worth mentioning that in some disorders, e.g., systemic lupus erythematosus, the lymphocytes are more susceptible to the action of antibody and complement, which may cause false-positive reactions due to weak unknown extra antibodies in the typing sera. Chronic lymphocytic leukemia is a special case because most of the circulating leukocytes are B lymphocytes which may react with unknown anti-B cell antibodies in the typing sera.

On the other hand, it has also been found that treatment of patients with chloramphenicol may cause a disappearance of detectable HLA antigens on lymphocytes, and it is not known whether other drugs have similar properties.

The best way of excluding such typing errors is to type the healthy relatives and see whether the HLA antigens of the patients are inherited.

Statistical treatment of the results. The comparison between patients and controls is usually done by 2 × 2 tables (Table 1) for each of the antigens studied. Distinction should be

made between the *strength* of an association and its *statistical significance* (1, 11).

The *strength* is usually estimated by the *relative risk* (= relative incidence ratio [17]), which is simply the cross-product ratio of the four entries in the 2 × 2 table (Table 1). This risk indicates how many times more often the disease occurs in individuals having the antigen as compared with those lacking it. A relative risk above one is seen when the antigen is more frequent in patients than in controls and indicates increased risk, whereas decreased frequency of an antigen in the patient group gives a risk below one, i.e., a decreased risk. When there is no difference between patients and controls, the risk is one. The absolute number of patients and controls in the 2 × 2 table is not necessary to estimate the relative risk, as it can also be obtained from the frequencies of the antigens in patients (h_p) and in controls (h_c) by the formula $x = \dfrac{h_p(1 - h_c)}{h_c(1 - h_p)}$, but these numbers — or the total numbers of patients and controls — should always be given, because they are needed for significance testing and for combining various sources of data (cf. below).

If an antigen is present in or absent from all patients, the relative risk becomes indefinite or zero, respectively. This is inconvenient for several reasons, and in these cases Haldane's modification (Table 1) can be used.

TABLE 1a. *The 2 × 2 table*[a]

Group	No. of individuals		
	HLA-A8-positive	HLA-A8-negative	Total
Patients ...	a	b	$a + b$
Controls ...	c	d	$c + d$
Total	$a + c$	$b + d$	$N = a + b + c + d$

[a] Relative risk (strength):

$$\text{Woolf } x = \frac{ad}{bc}$$

$$\text{Haldane } x = \frac{(a + \frac{1}{2})(d + \frac{1}{2})}{(b + \frac{1}{2})(c + \frac{1}{2})}$$

Significance:

Fisher's exact test (one-sided)

$$P = \frac{a!b!c!d!N!}{(a + b)!(c + d)!(a + c)!(b + d)!}$$
$$+ \text{ more extreme } P\text{'s}$$

Chi square (one degree of freedom)

$$\chi^2 = \frac{(ad - bc)^2 N}{(a + b)(c + d)(a + c)(b + d)}$$

TABLE 1b. *Example of the 2 × 2 table*[a]

Group	No. of individuals		
	HLA-A8-positive	HLA-A8-negative	Total
Patients ...	20	10	30
Controls ...	467	1,500	1,967
Total	487	1,510	1,997

[a] Relative risk:

$$\text{Woolf } x = \frac{20 \times 1,500}{467 \times 10} = 6.42$$

$$\text{Haldane } x = \frac{(20 + \frac{1}{2})(1,500 + \frac{1}{2})}{(467 + \frac{1}{2})(10 + \frac{1}{2})} = 6.27$$

Fisher's exact test:

$$P = \frac{20!10!467!1,500!1,997!}{487!1,510!30!1,967!} + \text{more extreme } P\text{'s}$$
$$= 8.3 \times 10^{-7} + 1.4 \times 10^{-7} = 9.7 \times 10^{-7}$$

Chi square

$$\frac{(20 \times 1,500 - 10 \times 467)^2 \times 1,997}{487 \times 1,510 \times 30 \times 1,967} = 29.53$$

which for one degree of freedom gives
$P = 2.8 \times 10^{-8}$ one-sided.

The "more extreme P's" in Fisher's test are derived by stepwise changing the entries in the 2 × 2 table (keeping the marginals constant) in more extreme directions. For example, the "next" P value in this case would be:

$$P = \frac{21!9!466!1,501!}{487!1,510!30!1,967!} = 1.2 \times 10^{-7}$$

This procedure is continued until one of the entries is zero ($0! = 1$) and all the P values are then added.

The statistical significance of an association can be evaluated by Fisher's exact test or by various approximate tests, e.g., a chi square test. Fisher's test gives the exact probability (P) of finding differences as extreme as or more extreme than that observed. This test is the only reliable one when one or more of the expected numbers in the 2 × 2 table is less than five, but it can also be applied to large samples by means of computers. It is a one-sided test, and thus the P value should be multiplied by two if there is no a priori assumption that an antigen has either decreased or increased frequency. When the expected numbers in the 2 × 2 table are above five, the approximation of the chi square test to the exact test is usually good, and this value is easier to compute (Table 1). Occasionally, Yate's correction for discontinuity is used by substituting $(|ad - bc| - N/2)^2 N$ for the denominator in Table 1. Note that Yate's correction is not a correction for small numbers. When several chi square values are

to be added, Yate's correction must not be used. In addition to the classical chi square test shown in Table 1, an extension of the relative risks may also be used to create chi square values as shown in Table 3.

The main reason to stress the distinction between the strength and the statistical significance is that a relative risk may well be high but insignificant (when the number of patients and/or controls is low), and, conversely, a risk differing only slightly from unity may do so in a statistically highly significant way when large numbers of individuals have been studied.

The deviation of the risk from unity tells something about the *biological* significance of the association: the more it deviates, the more important it is.

It is sometimes assumed that the number of controls should equal that of patients. This is a misunderstanding, but it derives from the fact that, if a difference is to be established by investigating the smallest possible number of individuals (patients plus controls), this is done by investigating equal numbers in the two groups. Usually, however, it is convenient to have a large control group, because this gives more accurate estimates of the normal antigen frequencies and because it increases the statistical significance of an association. In this relation, it is worth noting that even with a large amount of control material it is more difficult to establish a decreased than an increased frequency of an antigen with a frequency below 50% in controls. In the former case, more patients need to be studied.

The level of significance is somewhat complicated in these studies because a considerable number of antigen frequencies are usually compared between patients and controls. Usually, 20 or more antigens are studied, and on an average one of these will differ "significantly" at the 5% probability level by chance alone, i.e., if there is no true difference. This phenomenon (type I or alpha error) may be taken into account by multiplying the P values by the number of antigens studied. Although this yields a conservative measure, I would still recommend that the P values *after* multiplication be evaluated by the scheme: $0.05 > P > 0.01$ is probably significant; $0.01 > P > 0.001$ is significant; and $P < 0.001$ is highly significant. A P value of 0.05 indicates that the observed difference will be found in one of 20 random investigations if there is no difference, and "one-in-twenty" is not a rare occurrence. Obviously, multiplication times the number of antigens studied is not necessary in a second study showing deviation of the same antigen in the same disease. In fact, such subsequent studies are the best way to prove or disprove an association.

One problem yet to be solved derives from the fact that the antigens are not independent: an increase of one antigen inevitably is accompanied by a decrease of one or more of the other antigens belonging to the same segregant series. However, until this is worked out, it seems reasonable to treat each antigen separately.

Table 2 shows an analysis of the HLA antigen frequencies in 85 patients with juvenile diabetes compared with 1,967 controls (14). It appears that only the P values for HLA-A7 and 8 can stand the test of being multiplied times 2 (for one-sidedness) and 23 (for the number of antigens investigated). The increase of HLA-A15 remains probably significant after this procedure, whereas all other P values are insignificant. The increase of HLA-A15 has been found by other workers, and, accordingly, I believe that we are dealing with primary increases of HLA-A8 and 15 followed by a secondary decrease in HLA-A7.

Combination of data from various sources cannot be done by simply adding the entries in the 2 × 2 tables, as this may give spurious values both of the risk and of the significance. A procedure which can be used was developed by Woolf (17), and a worked out example is shown in Table 3 for HLA-A8 in myasthenia

TABLE 2. *HLA antigen frequencies (percent) in juvenile diabetes and controls*[a]

Antigen	Controls (N = 1,967)	Patients (N = 85)	Relative risk	Fisher's P	P × 2 × 23
HLA-A1 ..	31.1	32.9	1.09	0.40	
HLA-A2 ..	53.6	64.7	1.58	0.03	1.4
HLA-A3 ..	26.9	25.9	0.95	0.47	
HLA-A9 ...	17.3	27.1	1.78	0.02	0.92
HLA-A10 ..	9.6	5.9	0.59	0.17	
HLA-A11 ..	10.1	7.1	0.68	0.24	
HLA-A28 ..	10.0	7.1	0.69	0.25	
W19	17.8	7.1	0.35	0.004	0.18
HLA-A5 ...	10.6	7.1	0.64	0.19	
HLA-A7 ...	26.8	10.6	0.32	0.0003	0.01
HLA-A8 ...	23.7	44.7	2.60	0.00003	0.001
HLA-A12 ..	25.2	16.5	0.57	0.03	1.4
HLA-A13 ..	4.3	4.5	1.06	0.54	
HLA-A14 ..	4.5	0.0	0.00	0.02	0.92
HLA-A15 ..	17.9	32.9	2.25	0.0008	0.04
HLA-A16 ..	5.4	10.6	2.08	0.04	1.84
HLA-A17 ..	7.7	4.7	0.59	0.22	
HLA-A18 ..	7.1	9.4	1.36	0.26	
HLA-A21 ..	3.5	2.4	0.68	0.44	
HLA-A22 ..	3.8	2.4	0.61	0.37	
HLA-A27 ..	8.6	14.1	1.74	0.07	
W5	13.1	10.6	0.79	0.32	
W10	17.9	18.8	1.06	0.47	

[a] Data from Thomsen et al. (13).

gravis. This example shows also how standard deviations (SD) and 95% confidence limits can be estimated. Figure 1 gives the relative risks ± SD for the five sources of data in Table 3 and for the combined estimate.

Family studies

When an association has been established in unrelated individuals, it is usually worthwhile to perform family studies to see whether non-HLA genes are also involved in the pathogenesis. On the other hand, diseases not associated with known HLA factors may still be controlled by unknown HLA factors not associated with known ones. This relationship can only be clarified by family studies.

Diseases with known HLA association. The simplest form of family study consists of questioning the propositi of a possible family history, keeping in mind that the patients are not always informed on whether their relatives are affected or not. The relevant figure concerns the frequency of the disease among first-degree relatives: parents, siblings, and children. These groups should be treated separately until it is seen that there are no differences between them; e.g., the incidence in children is usually lower than those in parents and siblings if the disease does not have an early onset. Note that it is not sufficient to know that there are one or two affected sibs or children; the total numbers of sibs and children must be known. By comparing the frequency of the disease in first-degree relatives of patients carrying the disease-associated HLA factor with the corresponding frequency for the remaining patients, it may, for example, be found that the former patients have more affected relatives, which indicates that if other HLA factors are involved then they are not as important.

A more laborious kind of family study is the typing of kindreds with more than one affected member to see whether the disease is always inherited together with the disease-associated HLA antigen. For all diseases studied so far, exceptions to this rule have been found, and these are best explained by assuming that non-HLA factors may also be involved in the development of the disease: we are dealing with *polygenic* disorders. One important pitfall in such family studies is the biased ascertainment of the families as they are selected because they contain two or more affected members. Accordingly, they are likely to possess more disease-liability genes than families with isolated cases.

Perhaps the worst difficulty in family studies derives from the fact that most diseases have varying degrees of penetrance and age-at-onset

TABLE 3. *Calculation of combined relative risk of myasthenia gravis in HLA-A8-positive individuals*[a]

Study (ref. no.)[b]	No. of patients		No. of controls		Relative risk ($x = ad/bc$)	$y = \ln \cdot x$	Variance of y ($V = 1/a + 1/b + 1/c + 1/d$)	Wt ($W = 1/V$)	yw	$\chi^2 = y^2w$
	HLA-A8-positive (a)	HLA-A8-negative (b)	HLA-A8-positive (c)	HLA-A8-negative (d)						
1 (2)	17	9	186	411	4.17	1.428	0.1777	5.63	8.04	11.48
2 (8)	20	23	18	77	3.72	1.314	0.1620	6.17	8.11	10.65
3 (3)	59	41	103	430	6.01	1.793	0.0534	18.73	33.58	60.21
4 (4)	21	35	16	74	2.78	1.022	0.1522	6.57	6.71	6.86
5 (6)	17	18	59	267	4.27	1.452	0.1351	7.40	10.74	15.60
Total								44.50	67.18	104.80

[a] Combined estimate: $Y = \Sigma wy/\Sigma w = 67.18/44.50 = 1.510$. Relative risk: $X = \text{antilog}_e Y = 4.53$.
Standard deviation of Y: SD $= 1/\sqrt{\epsilon w} = 1/\sqrt{44.50} = 0.150$.
The 95% limits of Y: $1.510 \pm 1.96 \times 0.150 = 1.216$ and 1.804.
The 95% limits of X: $\text{antilog}_e 1.216$ and $\text{antilog}_e 1.804 = 3.37$ and 6.07.
The χ^2 for significance that $Y \neq$ from 0 ($X \neq 1$): $Y^2 \chi \Sigma w = (1.510)^2 \times 44.50 = 101.46$, for 1 degree of freedom $P \ll 10^{-11}$.
The χ^2 for significance that $Y \neq$ from 0 ($X \neq 1$):$Y^2 \chi \Sigma w = (1.510)^2 \times 44.50 = 101.46$, for 1 degree of freedom 3.34, for $5 - 1 = 4$ degrees of freedom $P = 0.5$.
[b] These references can be found in Ryder et al. (7).

because environment plays a role in their manifestations (i.e., they are multifactorial). Hence, the absence of psoriasis in an HLA-A17-positive relative of an HLA-A17-positive psoriatic is noninformative, as the disease may become manifest at a later time. Phrased more directly: only affected relatives are really informative. Nevertheless, when the ages are taken into account, such family studies may provide important information as to the risk of developing the disease for relatives with various HLA phenotypes.

Diseases not associated with known HLA factors. It is, of course, possible that a disease may largely be controlled by HLA genes (e.g., immune response [Ir] genes) not associated with known HLA factors. This relationship would go entirely undetected by ordinary HLA typing but could be discovered by typing of families with more than one affected member. It should be stressed, however, that such studies are likely to be very laborious and the results often difficult to interpret. Only affected relatives are truly informative, although it is often necessary to type other relatives to establish the genotypes. These studies are often termed linkage studies, and it is worth noting that one affected parent and one affected child do not provide information, as they always share an HLA haplotype. Probably the most straightforward way of doing such studies is to type affected sib pairs (or triplets) to see whether such affected pairs share a haplotype more often than expected; i.e., significantly more than 75% of the pairs must share a haplotype before proof is obtained. The minimal

number of sib pairs required to obtain significance at the 1% level is 20. In this relation, it should be kept in mind that two siblings with the phenotypes of, say, HLA-A1,2,7,8 and HLA-A1,9,8,12 need not share the same HL-A1,8 haplotype; the parents should also be typed if possible.

ASSOCIATIONS

Table 4 lists most of the diseases which have so far been investigated with respect to HLA. There are two major groups which show association: the HLA-A27-associated arthropathies (ankylosing spondylitis, reactive arthritis, and acute anterior uveitis), and the HLA-A8-associated "immunopathic disorders" (myasthenia gravis, coeliac disease, dermatitis herpetiformis, Addison's and Graves' diseases, and juvenile diabetes mellitus). Diabetes mellitus is also associated with HLA-A15. In addition, multiple sclerosis is associated with the MLC determinant LD-7a, and psoriasis vulgaris is associated with at least three SECOND series antigens: HLA-A13, 17, and TY.

The malignant disease studied so far have shown no or only weak associations. In both Hodgkin's disease and acute lymphatic leukemia, the associations have mostly been found in retrospective studies, and thus the associated HLA antigens seem primarily to confer increased survival value (i.e., resistance) once these conditions have developed.

Which markers are primarily involved?

The question of which markers are primarily involved is, of course, difficult to answer as long

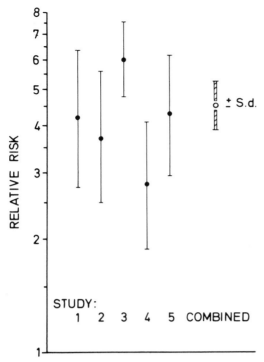

FIG. 1. *Relative risks, with standard deviations, of myasthenia gravis for HLA-A8-positive individuals for the five different studies quoted in Table 3. The combined estimate from these five sources of data is shown to the right.*

as we do not know all HLA markers, in particular not the immune response (Ir) determinants. However, it is possible to investigate whether we are dealing primarily with an increase of FIRST, SECOND, THIRD, or MLC series antigens, although this may occasionally be difficult. For example, it was for some time difficult to decide whether the HLA-A8-associated diseases involved an isolated increase of the *HLA-A1,8* haplotype because an increase of HLA-A8 inevitably leads to surplus of HLA-A1 positives, too. It now appears that all haplotypes carrying HLA-A8 are about equally increased in these disorders. The question now is whether the MLC determinant LD-8a is the one primarily increased, which may be the case for diabetes, Addison's disease, Graves' disease, and dermatitis herpetiformis, but perhaps not for myasthenia gravis. One way of solving these problems is to compare the relative risks for the two factors in question to see whether one is significantly higher than the other, i.e., whether there is significant heterogeneity between them. This has been done for multiple sclerosis, and here the risk for LD-7a

positives is significantly higher than for HLA-A7 positives. However, quite large amounts of material are often needed to obtain significance by this method, and instead it may be worthwhile to make "simulations" with the control material to see what happens with one of the factors (e.g., HLA-A8) when there is a primary increase of the other (e.g., LD-8a).

One still unsolved question is whether the increase of HLA-A13, 17, and TY in psoriasis is due to a primary increase of the THIRD series antigen, T7, which is almost always present in HLA-A13-, 17-, and TY-positive individuals.

Finally, it should be stressed again that still unknown HLA determinants may be primarily involved. None of the associations observed so far has been absolute, and, if we are dealing with monogenic disorders (which we do not know for all diseases), this would indicate the involvement of yet unknown HLA factors.

Dominance versus recessivity, susceptibility versus resistance

If the factors which we have found associated with a disease were in fact those primarily responsible for the associations, then it would be quite easy to decide whether the susceptibility was dominant or recessive (11, 12). In ankylosing spondylitis, for example, most of the patients would possess HLA-A27 as the only SECOND series antigen if the susceptibility was recessive. However, most HLA-A27-positive patients are not homozygous, and thus the susceptibility is dominant. Even if this association is due to an unknown HLA factor strongly associated with HLA-A27, we would expect a much higher frequency of HLA-A27-homozygous patients. In general, it may be stated that if such an unknown factor causes recessive susceptibility, then there will be a considerable excess of patients homozygous for the detectable associated factor. It seems likely that we are dealing with dominant susceptibility for all of the diseases listed in Table 4. It is worth noting that an excess of, say, HLA-A7 homozygotes in multiple sclerosis may reflect a primary association with an MLC determinant (LD-7a in multiple sclerosis): HLA-A7 homozygotes have about twice the chance of being LD-7a positive as HLA-A7 heterozygotes; still, the susceptibility conferred by LD-7a may be simple dominant.

For nonlethal diseases, resistance to a disease should be reflected in decreased frequencies for one or more antigens (relative risks below one) with small increases of those remaining. This has not yet been observed, and one reason may be that decreased frequencies are more difficult to demonstrate. However, the

TABLE 4. *Associations between HLA and disease*[a]

Disease	Antigen	Frequency (%) of antigen		Relative risk	Significance (P)	No. of studies	No. of patients investigated
		Controls	Patients				
Arthropathies							
Ankylosing spondylitis	HLA-A27	8.6	88	80	$<10^{-6}$	6	
Reiter's syndrome	HLA-A27	8.6	79	40	$<10^{-6}$	4	116
Reactive arthritis	HLA-A27 increased in *Yersinia* and *Salmonella* arthritis, but not in meningococcal arthritis						
Psoriatic arthritis	HLA-A27	8.6	31	4.7	$<10^{-5}$	1	44
Juvenile arthritis	HLA-A27 apparently increased when the spine is involved						
Rheumatoid arthritis	No definite associations					5	313
Gout	No deviations						66
Eye diseases							
Acute anterior uveitis	HLA-A27	8.6	74	30.7	$<10^{-6}$	2	61
Chronic anterior uveitis	No deviations					1	13
Skin diseases							
Psoriasis vulgaris	HLA-A13	4.3	16.2	4.3	$<10^{-6}$	8	820
	HLA-A17	7.7	28.6	4.8	$<10^{-6}$	8	820
	TY	1.2	9.3	8.4	$<10^{-6}$	>1	220
Pustular psoriasis	No deviations					>1	31
Pemphigus	HLA-A10 perhaps increased in Jewish patients					3	61
Dermatitis herpetiformis	HLA-A8	23.7	57	4.3	$<10^{-6}$	3	89
Intestinal diseases							
Coeliac disease	HLA-A8	23.7	75	9.5	$<10^{-6}$	5	248
Ulcerative colitis	No deviations					4	111
Crohn's disease	No deviations					5	139
Liver diseases							
Chronic autoimmune hepatitis	HLA-A8	23.7	53	3.6	$<10^{-6}$	3	170
Acute hepatitis, chronic persistent hepatitis, liver cirrhosis, healthy Au-carriers: no deviations							
"Systemic" diseases							
Myasthenia gravis	HLA-A8	23.7	58	4.4	$<10^{-6}$	5	260
Sarcoidosis	No deviations					3	262
Systemic lupus erythematosus	No deviations					4	64
Cystic fibrosis	No deviations					1	24
Chronic glomerulonephritis	HLA-A2	53.6	63	1.5	10^{-3}	>1	485
Endocrine diseases							
Insulin-dependent diabetes mellitus	HLA-A8	23.7	39	2.1	10^{-4}	3	156
	HLA-A15	17.9	40	3.0	$<10^{-6}$	3	156
Non-insulin-dependent diabetes mellitus	No deviations					>2	100
Graves' disease	HLA-A8	23.7	53	3.6	10^{-6}	>1	48
Idiopathic Addison's disease	HLA-A8	23.7	67	6.4	10^{-5}	1	30
Neurological diseases							
Multiple sclerosis	HLA-A7	26.8	35.4	1.5	10^{-4}	5	>1,000
	LD-7a	18.2	53	5.0	$<10^{-6}$	3	95
Paralytic polio	Discordant results					2	136
Allergy							
Childhood asthma	No definite deviations					2	71
Atopic dermatitis	No deviations					2	88
Ragweek hayfever	No deviations but perhaps linkage in family studies					3	
Infections							
Leprosy						1	39
Tuberculosis						1	119

TABLE 4—*Continued*

Disease	Antigen	Frequency (%) of antigen		Relative risk	Significance (P)	No. of studies	No. of patients investigated
		Controls	Patients				
Haemophilus influenza	Definite no deviations					1	65
Infectious mononucleosis						1	40
Malignant diseases							
Hodgkin's disease	HLA-A1	31.1	39	1.4	$<10^{-6}$	17	1,508
	HLA-A5	10.6	16	1.6	$<10^{-6}$	17	1,508
	HLA-A8	23.7	29	1.3	10^{-4}	17	1,508
	HLA-A18	7.1	13	1.9	$<10^{-6}$	12	1,165
Acute lymphatic leukemia	HLA-A2	53.6	60	1.3	$<10^{-2}$	10	527
	HLA-A8	23.7	29	1.3	<0.05	10	527
	HLA-A12	25.2	29	1.2	0.05	10	527
Mammary carcinoma	No deviations					4	593
Malignant melanoma	No deviations					5	349

[a] The above data are collected from the literature and surveyed in references 2, 3, and 6. The frequencies in controls are from a Danish population sample of 1,967 unrelated individuals (Staub Nielsen et al., 1975). The frequencies in patients were estimated from these control frequencies (h_c) and the relative risk by the formula h_p (frequency in patients) = $xh_c/[1 + h_c (x - 1)]$.

abnormal antigen frequencies in the retrospective studies of Hodgkin's disease and in acute lymphatic leukemia may reflect resistance to the progression of these disorders.

CLINICAL IMPLICATIONS

Associations between HLA and disease may be relevant in the relation to the genetics, diagnosis, etiology, and subdivision of various clinical entities.

Genetics of diseases

Table 5 lists the various modes of inheritance for a disease or condition. The fact that most disorders do not show complete (100%) concordance in monozygotic twins demonstrates that environment plays a role in addition to genetic factors: we are dealing with *multifactorial* diseases. As discussed above, no complete association between HLA and a disease has been observed, and this cannot come as a surprise to geneticists, who for many years have been working with *polygenic* models for disease susceptibility. In these models, it is assumed that the hereditary element of a disease is due to several—if not many—usually nonlinked genes. Each of these genes acts by decreasing the threshold below which the disease is likely to occur in the relevant environment. Even for the strongly HLA-associated ankylosing spondylitis, there is good evidence from family studies that non-HLA genes are involved.

Diagnosis

Only in one condition can HLA typing be considered of diagnostic value: in doubtful cases of ankylosing spondylitis, typing for HLA-A27 may be considered a diagnostic test with about 8% false-positive results (the normal frequency of HLA-A27) and about 10% false-negative results (the frequency of HLA-A27 negatives in the disease). If there is an a priori chance of about 50% that an individual has this disorder, this chance will increase to about $(1 - 0.1) \times 0.5/[(1 - 0.1) \times 0.5 + 0.08 (1 - 0.5)] = 0.92 = 92\%$ if he is HLA-A27-positive, whereas it is only about $0.1 \times 0.5/[0.1 \times 0.5 + (1 - 0.08) (1 - 0.5)] = 0.10 = 10\%$ if he does not have this antigen. Note that the a priori chance—in our case 0.5—greatly influences these a posteriori probabilities. Thus, if the a priori chance of the disease is 10%, the a posteriori chances are 56 and 1% for HLA-A27-positive and -negative individuals, respectively.

For most other diseases associated with HLA, HLA typing would not appear to be of great help in the diagnosis.

Finally, I wish to warn strongly against typing for only one HLA antigen (e.g., HLA-A27), because lymphocytes from some patients may give abnormal reactions which are only disclosed when a full HLA typing is performed.

Etiology or pathogenesis

Little can as yet be said about the possible contribution of an HLA association to the understanding of the pathogenesis of a disease. However, it seems fair to state that infections and/or autoimmune phenomena may be involved in several of the diseases listed in Table 4, and the mere demonstration of an association for a disease with unknown etiology may give

TABLE 5. *Modes of inheritance for a disease or condition*

| Relevant genetic make-up in: | Modes of inheritance[a] | | | | |
| | Monogenic | | | Oligogenic | Polygenic |
	Dominant	Intermediate	Recessive		
General population	A	A	A	A, B, C	A, B, C, D, ...
High-risk individuals	A/A or A/O	A/A	A/A	A, B, C	Many of the genes in any combination
Medium-risk individuals		A/O		A, B, or A, C, or B, C	Fewer of the genes in any combination
Low-risk individuals				A, B, or C	Few of the genes in any combination

[a] The letters refer to nonlinked genes responsible for increased disease susceptibility.

hints in that direction. In multiple sclerosis, for example, the HLA association gave rise to immunological investigations showing that these patients have an abnormal reaction to measles virus. In analogy, it may be indicated to look for infectious agents in other HLA-associated disorders.

When an association has been found for a disease with autoimmune phenomena, it is worthwhile to investigate whether these are more frequent in patients carrying the associated antigen. For example, in primary Addison's disease, anti-adrenal autoantibodies are significantly more frequent in HLA-A8-positive than in HLA-A8-negative patients, which supports the concept that HLA-A8-associated autoimmunity is an important factor in the development of that disease. The same may be true of HLA-A8 in juvenile diabetes and Graves' disease. It is of interest to note that HLA-A8/W15 heterozygotes have about twice the risk of developing disease as individuals carrying only one of these antigens; this indicates that HLA-A8 and W15 act differently and that there is an interaction between the two.

For some disorders, we are, however, still entirely left with speculations. It is likely that this is going to change when more becomes known on the nature of the HLA system, in particular about the interaction between this system and virus.

Subdivisions of diseases

In line with the above discussion, HLA associations may be used to distinguish or confirm the distinction between various clinical forms

of a disease entity. For example, only the common form of psoriasis is associated with HLA; the pustular form is not. Moreover, HLA-associated psoriasis is characterized by early onset. This is true also of myasthenia gravis, in which disorder the association is also much more pronounced in females than in males. In analogy, the fact that HLA only shows association with juvenile and not with maturity-onset diabetes mellitus strengthens the concept that these are two different diseases.

On the other hand, associations between various diseases and the same HLA antigen may indicate a common pathogenic pathway, e.g., in the HLA-A27-associated arthropathies.

MECHANISMS WHICH CAN EXPLAIN THE ASSOCIATIONS

It is outside the scope of this chapter to go into the details of the mechanisms which explain the associations, but I should like to mention those which have been suggested most often (5, 10, 12, 14, 15).

1. The fact that most of the associations seem primarily to involve SECOND series or MLC series antigens has been used as evidence that the associations are due to the action of specific *immune-response (Ir)* genes closely linked to and in linkage disequilibrium with factors from these series. Obviously, Ir genes must be of great biological importance as a defense mechanism against microbial invasions, and the lack of an adequate Ir determinant could give rise to a recessive (as these Ir characters are dominant) susceptibility to certain infections. Conversely, an "autoaggressive" Ir determinant

could give rise to dominant susceptibility to autoimmune phenomena (15).

2. In *molecular mimicry* it is assumed that the antigens of certain microorganisms resemble some HLA antigen(s) which would cause a dominant susceptibility to severe infection for individuals carrying these HLA antigens. However, it is also possible that such antigenic resemblance could lead to break-down of self-tolerance, and thus to a dominant susceptibility, e.g., to virus-induced autoimmunity.

3. Cell surface structures such as HLA factors could serve as *receptors* for certain virus, which would also cause dominant susceptibility to infection. Some HLA factors could also interfere with the interaction between hormones – or other ligands – and the corresponding receptors in the cell surface; in this way, the HL-A system might influence endocrine function or the interaction between cells.

4. Abnormalities of a complement factor controlled by the HLA system (such as C2 or Bf) could cause susceptibility to infections or give rise to autoimmune phenomena.

Still other mechanisms are possible, but the above seem most likely at the present time.

ACKNOWLEDGMENTS

This study was aided by grants from the Danish Medical Research Council, the Danish Blood Donor Foundation, the Nordic Insulin Foundation, and the Danish Arthritis Society. My thanks are due to L. P. Ryder and N. Morling for critical comments during the preparation of the manuscript.

LITERATURE CITED

1. Armitage, P. 1971. Statistical methods in medical research. Blackwell Scientific Publications, Oxford.
2. Behan, P. O., J. A. Simpson, and H. Dick. 1973. Immune response genes in myasthenia gravis? Lancet ii:1033–1033.
3. Feltkamp, T. E. W., P. M. van der Berg-Loonen, L. E. Nijenhuis, C. P. Engelfriet, A. L. van Rossum, J. J. van Loghem, and H. J. G. H. Oosterhuis. 1974. Myasthenia gravis, autoantibodies and HLA antigens. Br. Med. J. 1:131–133.
4. Fritze, D., C. Hermann, F. Naeim, G. S. Smith, and R. L. Walford. 1974. HLA antigens in myasthenia gravis. Lancet i:240–242.
5. McDevitt, H. O., and W. F. Bodmer. 1974. HLA, immune response genes and disease. Lancet i: 1269–1275.
6. Pirskanen, R., A. Tiilikainen, and E. Hokkanen. 1972. Histocompatibility (HLA) antigens associated with myasthenia gravis. Ann. Clin. Res. 4:304–306.
7. Ryder, L. P., L. Staub Nielsen, and A. Svejgaard. 1974. Associations between HLA histocompatibility antigens and non-malignant diseases. Humangenetik 25:251–264.
8. Säfwenberg, J., J. B. Lindblom, and P. O. Osterman. 1973. HLA frequencies in patients with myasthenia gravis. Tissue Antigens 3:465–469.
9. Staub Nielsen, L., C. Jersild, L. P. Ryder, and A. Svejgaard. 1975. HLA antigen, gene, and haplotype frequencies in Denmark. Tissue Antigens 6:70–76.
10. Svejgaard, A., M. Hauge, C. Jersild, P. Platz, L. P. Ryder, L. Staub Nielsen, and M. Thomsen. 1975. The HLA system – an introductory survey. Monogr. Human Genet., vol. 7.
11. Svejgaard, A., C. Jersild, L. Staub Nielsen, and W. F. Bodmer. 1974. HLA antigens and disease. Statistical and genetical considerations. Tissue Antigens 4:95–105.
12. Svejgaard, A., P. Platz, L. P. Ryder, L. Staub Nielsen, and M. Thomsen. 1975. HL-A and disease associations – a survey. Transplant. Rev. 22:3–43.
13. Thomsen, M., P. Platz, O. Ortved Andersen, M. Christy, J. Lyngsøe, J. Nerup, K. Rasmussen, L. P. Ryder, L. Staub Nielsen, and A. Svejgaard. 1975. MLC typing in juvenile diabetes mellitus and idiopathic Addison's disease. Transplant. Rev. 22:125–147.
14. Transplantation Reviews, vol. 22, 1975. HLA and disease. Munksgaard, Copenhagen.
15. Vladutin, A. O., and N. R. Rose. 1974. HLA antigens and susceptibility to disease. Immunogenetics 1:305–328.
16. Vogel, F., and W. Helmbold. 1972. Blutgruppen–Populationsgenetik und Statistik. *In* Humangenetik. Ein kurzes Handbuch in Fünf Bänden. Georg Thieme Verlag, Stuttgart.
17. Woolf, B. 1955. On estimating the relation between blood group and disease. Ann. Hum. Genet. 19:251–253.

Chapter 112

Use of the Cell-Mediated Lympholysis Test in Transplantation Immunity

JAMES LIGHTBODY

INTRODUCTION

Cell-mediated immunity is of primary importance in allograft rejection (5). In this process, lymphocytes participate directly by cell-cell interaction rather than indirectly through the production of humoral antibodies. The afferent or recognition phase of graft rejection occurs when lymphocytes of the recipient come in contact with the foreign histocompatibility antigens of the donor. A small percentage of these lymphocytes which have receptors for the foreign antigens respond by differentiation and proliferation. The second or effector phase involves destruction of the allograft by the sensitized lymphocytes.

The in vitro equivalent of the recognition phase occurs when lymphoid cells are placed in tissue culture with allogenic lymphocytes—the mixed leukocyte culture (MLC; 4). (The reader is referred to chapter 109 of this *Manual* for a more detailed explanation of the MLC.) Numerous in vitro systems have been devised to investigate the effector or destructive phase of graft rejection (33). It was originally demonstrated by Govaerts (15) in the dog that lymphocytes sensitized in vivo are cytotoxic to allogenic target cells in vitro. These studies were further extended by the work of Brunner et al. in the mouse (6). Ginsburg and Sachs, using a xenogenic model, were the first to demonstrate that lymphocytes sensitized in vitro were cytotoxic to target cells syngenic to the sensitized cells (14). In an allogenic system, Hayry and Defendi produced evidence in the mouse that MLC-generated effector cells were cytotoxic to mastocytoma cells derived from the same strain as the sensitizing cells (17). Similar results were obtained by Hardy et al. in humans (16).

For in vitro models to be used as indicators of allograft rejection, convincing evidence must be obtained of a significant correlation between the in vitro parameters measured and the in vivo situation. To show such a correlation in humans with the above model systems would require establishment of either fibroblast or lympho-blast cell lines to be used as targets. The demonstration by Lightbody et al. (20) that normal human peripheral blood lymphocytes when stimulated with phytohemagglutinin (PHA) became sensitive targets for effector cells generated in MLC alleviated this problem. This process has become known as cell-mediated lympholysis (CML), and a schematic representation is presented in Fig. 1. The lymphocytes from individual A are used as responders and those from individual B are used as stimulators in MLC. During the 6 days in culture, the lymphocytes of A are transformed into effector cells with specificity directed against the histocompatibility antigens of B. On day 0, other lymphocytes from B are put into tissue culture to be used as targets. These lymphocytes are stimulated on day 3 with PHA, and on day 6 they are labeled with ^{51}Cr and used as targets. The effector lymphocytes and target cells are incubated together for 4 h. The amount of ^{51}Cr released during this time indicates the degree of effector activity generated during the MLC. If target lymphocytes other than B are to be utilized, they are treated in a manner identical to the B targets. (For further references, see 3, 18, 19, and 23.)

CLINICAL APPLICATIONS

Transplantation

Cell-mediated immunity plays a major role in allograft rejection. The ability to predict accurately the degree of immune response of the recipient to the donor is a major goal of transplantation immunologists. One approach toward achieving this goal is to develop in vitro models which, it is hoped, will mimic the in vivo response. At the present time, the MLC appears to be the best model for investigating the afferent or sensitization phase of allograft rejection. Complementary to this, the CML represents the efferent or destructive phase of allograft rejection.

It was originally thought that allelic differences at histocompatibility locus A (HL A), i.e.,

851

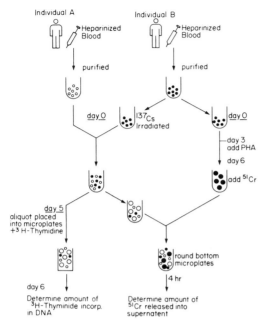

FIG. 1. *Schematic representation of MLC and CML.*

differences at the LA or first series and the FOUR or second series, resulted in MLC stimulation. It was clear in related individuals that identical HLA alleles usually resulted in no MLC stimulation (2), prolonged skin grafts (10), longer survival of kidneys (30), and better functioning bone marrow grafts (7). Yunis and Amos, however, using families in which genetic recombination had taken place at HLA, demonstrated that MLC stimulation was due to differences at a genetic locus or loci separate from but closely linked to HLA (34). The successful bone marrow transplant between individuals who differed at HLA but were MLC unreactive provided further evidence for the importance of MLC locus antigens in graft rejection (13).

To generate effector cells in CML, it was originally suggested by the work of Eijsvoogel et al. (12), who used recombinant families, that differences at the MLC locus initiated the reaction, but the effector cells generated showed specificity toward the HLA antigens. However, subsequent work has provided evidence that HLA identical unrelated individuals usually stimulate in MLC and give positive but weak CML activity. Such individuals would no doubt demonstrate strong graft rejection. These results suggest that, in the face of a positive MLC, strong effector activity is generated toward the HLA antigens, but in addition weaker activity

is generated toward other as yet unknown antigens.

Over the past few years, work from numerous laboratories has revealed the area of the major histocompatibility locus in the mouse, and the same is no doubt true in humans, to be a multigene complex associated with recognition. The future will probably bring forth many as yet unrecognized loci, some of which will be associated with histocompatibility. As has been suggested by Yunis and Amos (34), a separate locus responsible for CML will probably be demonstrated. This is supported by experiments in which a nondetectable MLC was obtained between related individuals which differed at HLA and gave a positive CML (25).

The usefulness of in vitro assays for measuring histocompatibility depends upon their ability to predict graft survival. Although it is agreed that among related donor-recipient pairs transplantation between sibs who are identical at HLA have the best graft survival, the predictive value of HLA typing with unrelated individuals is still under discussion (29). Skin graft experiments using HLA-nonidentical MLC-nonstimulatory unrelated combinations have suggested that compatibility at MLC is more important than HLA if no prior immunization is involved (31). If the recipient has been immunized, the HLA antigens appear to be of greater importance (32). In view of the previously discussed reports suggesting the possibility of a positive CML without a detectable MLC, the CML assay may prove to be an additional parameter for measuring incompatibility. This is supported by the occasional report of kidney rejection between HLA-identical MLC-unreactive sibs (24). In addition, skin grafts between HLA-identical sibs, although they function longer, are ultimately rejected. Descamps et al. (11) have also reported a case of hyperacute rejection between identical MLC-unreactive related individuals.

Immunodeficiency patients

The MLC-CML model may also prove useful in the study of the afferent and efferent phases of cellular immunity in patients thought to be defective in these areas. This type of investigation has been conducted on the family of a patient with both a severe combined immunodeficiency disease and absent adenosine deaminase (9). In several members of the family, including the mother and father, abnormal to absent CML was observed despite adequate MLC stimulation and disparity at the HLA loci. Mawas et al. (25) studied 18 immunodeficient patients and found that 4 were unable to generate CML activity despite a normal MLC response. Reports from several laboratories have suggested that subpopulations of lymphocytes may be responsible for various cellular immune functions (8, 26). Evidence has suggested that a separate cell population may be responsible for MLC and CML activities (1). The studies on immunodeficiency are also compatible with this concept. An alternative explanation is that several lymphocyte populations cooperate to obtain CML and that the immunodeficient patients are lacking helper cell activity. These results suggest that the CML assay may also be useful in detecting defects in the efferent phase of cellular immunity and may prove helpful in analyzing and categorizing the various types of immune deficiency syndromes. In addition, the ability to detect this defect in parents of the combined immunodeficient patient suggests that it may be useful in detecting the heterozygote carriers of such diseases.

TEST PROCEDURES

Leukocyte preparation

Method a—For small volumes of blood (10 ml or less). Heparinized peripheral blood is diluted two times with tissue culture medium RPMI (10 ml of blood is diluted to 30 ml). The 30 ml of diluted blood is then layered on 12 ml of Ficoll-Hypaque in a 50-ml conical centrifuge tube (20 × 130 mm). The tube is centrifuged at 400 × g (at interface) for 40 min at 20 C. The leukocytes are collected from the interface, diluted with an equal volume of RPMI, and centrifuged at 300 × g for 10 min. The resulting pellet is resuspended in 1 ml of RPMI and counted on a hemacytometer.

Method b—For volumes greater than 10 ml or if plasma is to be conserved. Heparinized peripheral blood is centrifuged at 320 × g at 20 C for 10 min. The plasma and top layer of cells (buffy coat) are removed and recentrifuged at 170 × g for 10 min. The resulting cell pellet containing the leukocytes with contaminating erythrocytes is resuspended in 20 ml of RPMI. The leukocytes are then layered on Ficoll-Hypaque as described under Method a. The buffy coat from a maximum of 50 ml of blood is used for 50 ml tube for gradient centrifugation.

Sensitization procedure

Inhibition of stimulating cells. The one-way MLC is utilized to generate effector cells (28). Two methods can be used to inhibit the stimulating cells from dividing.

Method a. The cells to be used as stimulators are resuspended at a concentration of 10^7 lymphocytes/ml in RPMI. To these cells, 25 μg of mitomycin C/ml is added, and the mixture is incubated for 20 min in a 37 C water bath. The cells are subsequently washed two times in RPMI.

Method b. The stimulator cells are resuspended at a concentration of 10^7 small lymphocytes/ml. An irradiating source such as an X-ray machine or ^{137}Cs irradiator is utilized to deliver radiation at the rate of 140 rads/min for 10 min (21).

Mixed leukocyte culture

Method a—When small numbers of effector cells are required. The MLC is conducted in 16 × 100 mm round-bottom glass tubes with 1.5 × 10^6 responder lymphocytes and 1.5 × 10^6 stimulator cells in a total volume of 2 ml of RPMI with 20% plasma (RPMI-20). The cells are incubated at 37 C in an atmosphere of 95% air and 5% CO_2 for 6 days. To determine the degree of proliferation, on day 5, 0.2-ml samples are removed from the tube and put into Linbro microculture plates with 2 μCi of tritiated thymidine (0.05 ml). After 12 h, the cells are put on glass-fiber filters by use of a multiple sample harvester (MSH), washed with 0.9% saline, and dried at 150 C for 2 h. The radioactive filter is placed into a scintillation vial, and 3.0 ml of scintillation fluid is added to each vial. The vials are subsequently counted on a liquid scintillation spectrometer. In the event that an MSH is unavailable, the lymphocytes may be removed from the wells by a Pasteur pipette and placed on a filter apparatus containing a glass-fiber filter. The filter is subsequently washed with 0.9% saline and dried as previously described. The cells remaining in the tubes on day 6 are utilized as effector cells in CML.

Method b—When large quantities of effector cells are required. The MLC is conducted in Falcon 3013 tissue culture flasks with 10^7 responder lymphocytes and 10^7 stimulator cells in a total volume of 10 ml of RPMI-20. The bottle is incubated at 37 C in an atmosphere of 95% air and 5% CO_2. On days 2 and 4, 5 ml of fresh RPMI-20 is added to the flask. On day 5, 2 × 10^5 viable cells are removed from the flask ($\approx$ 0.2 ml), centrifuged (300 × g, 10 min), and resuspended in the used media at 2 × 10^6 viable cells/ml. To determine the degree of proliferation, 0.2 ml is added to Linbro microculture plates and treated as in Method a. The cells remaining in the flask are used on day 6 as effector cells in CML.

Target cell preparation for cell-mediated lympholysis

Two types of target lymphocytes may be utilized. Lymphocytes stimulated with PHA appear to be more susceptible to cell destruction [20] and also take up more ^{51}Cr. These advantages are offset by the fact that it is difficult to remove the PHA completely, which sometimes results in nonspecific killing. In this case, fresh lymphocytes or lymphocytes put into tissue culture unstimulated may also be utilized as targets [22].

Method a—PHA-stimulated target cells. Lymphocytes to be used as target cells are taken from the donor at the same time as the sensitizing cells and are purified as described above. The target cells are resuspended in RPMI-20 and put into plastic bottles (Falcon Plastics 3040) at a concentration of 10^6/ml (8-ml total volume). On the 3rd day, they are stimulated with PHA (1:150 final dilution). On day 6, the PHA-stimulated lymphocytes are centrifuged ($200 \times g$) for 10 min and resuspended in 0.3 ml of RPMI-20; 250 μCi of sodium chromate ^{51}Cr is then added. The cells are incubated for 1 h, washed twice in RPMI-20 in the cold, and diluted to 10^5 cells/ml.

Method b—Non-PHA-stimulated target. Lymphocytes to be used as target cells are taken from the donor on the same days as the CML assay is to be performed. They are purified and labeled with ^{51}Cr as described above. Alternatively, they may be taken from the donor on day 0, put into tissue culture flasks under the same concentration and conditions described under Method a, but without PHA, and utilized on day 6.

Cell-mediated lympholysis procedure

On day 6, lymphocytes from the MLC are centrifuged for 10 min ($200 \times g$), suspended in RPMI-20 at a concentration of 10^7 viable cells/ml, and added to wells of round-bottom Linbro microculture plates (10^6 cells/0.1 ml) already containing 10^4 labeled target cells in 0.1 ml. The mixture is then incubated for 4 h at 37 C in an atmosphere of 95% air and 5% CO_2. After incubation, 0.05 ml of cold RPMI is added to each well with a Hamilton syringe, the plate is centrifuged ($1,000 \times g$) for 5 min, and a sample of the supernatant fluid is counted to determine the amount of ^{51}Cr released. The spontaneous release is measured by incubating target cells alone in an equal volume. The maximal release is determined by freeze-thawing a portion of the cells, centrifuging them, and counting a sample of the supernatant fluid.

Removal of sample from microplates. Several methods may be utilized to remove a sample from the well of the microplate. The method which I have developed is presented in Fig. 2. After the addition of 0.05 ml of cold RPMI and centrifugation, the cells have formed a small pellet at the bottom of the well. An 18-gauge needle is inserted in the well. The bevel of the needle has been cut off and squeezed together, and a small hole has been placed 1 mm above the bottom of the needle. The hole can be made simply by using a jeweler's file. The needle is attached to a glass counting tube by means of a small-diameter tubing. The whole system is placed under suction, and the supernatant fluid is removed from the well. The needle is washed with 1 ml of water, the counting tube is removed, and the process is repeated with the use of a new counting tube for the next well. This provides a rapid and reproducible method for removing a sample from the wells of the microplate.

Calculation of results

Several methods have been used to calculate ^{51}Cr release. The method which I use involves the following formula:

$$\% \text{ CML} = \frac{\bar{x} \text{ experimental value} - \bar{x} \text{ spontaneous release}}{\bar{x} \text{ frozen thawed} - \bar{x} \text{ spontaneous release}} \times 100$$

where $\bar{x}$ is the mean of ^{51}Cr values.

An alternative equation which is frequently used is

$$\% \text{ CML} = \frac{\bar{x} \text{ experimental value} - \bar{x} \text{ spontaneous release}}{\bar{x} \text{ frozen thawed}} \times 100$$

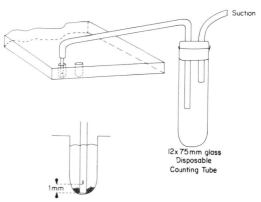

FIG. 2. *Method of removing supernatant fluid from microplate wells.*

If the spontaneous release is a significant percentage of the entire ^{51}Cr taken up by the target cells, the % CML value obtained with the first equation would be much higher than when the second equation is used. In general, whenever presenting data involving ^{51}Cr release, the raw data of a representative experiment should be given. For a more detailed analysis the reader is referred to Stulting and Berke (28).

Plasma used for mixed leukocyte culture and cell-mediated lympholysis

In the process of purifying the lymphocytes by the buffy coat method, the plasma is removed, heated to 56 C for 0.5 h, and subsequently frozen at −70 C. When approximately 1 liter has accumulated, all the plasma is thawed, combined, divided into small portions, and refrozen. One of the portions is tested for its ability to support MLC stimulation and CML activity. Plasma from females who have been pregnant or individuals who were ever transfused are eliminated from the pool.

REAGENTS

Ficoll-Hypaque:
(A) 38.2 g of Ficoll (Sigma Chemical Co., St. Louis, Mo.; catalog #F-4375) is dissolved in 424 ml of distilled water.
(B) 50.0 g of sodium diatrizoate (Winthrop Laboratories, New York, N.Y.) is dissolved in 120 ml of distilled water.
   Mix A and B together. Adjust density to 1.077 ± 0.001 by adding distilled water if density is too high or Hypaque if the density is too low.
Medium RPMI-1640 with 25 mM N-2-hydroxyethylpiperazine-N'-2-ethanesulfonic acid buffer: Grand Island Biological Co., Grand Island, N.Y.; catalog #240 with sodium bicarbonate and glutamine.
Linbro microculture plates: Linbro Scientific, Inc., New Haven, Conn.; catalog #IS-MRC-96-TC (round bottom) or #IS-FB-96-TC (flat bottom).
Sodium chromate-51: New England Nuclear Corp., Boston, Mass.; 5 mCi/ml in sterile saline. I do not use ^{51}Cr which has gone through more than 0.75 half-life.
Repeating dispenser: catalog #PB600-10, 50-μ-liter; Hamilton Co., Reno, Nev.
2,5-Diphenyloxazole and 1,4-bis-(5-phenyloxazolyl)benzene: scintillation grade; Packard Instrument Co.
IEC refrigerated centrifuge, model PR-J: International Equipment Co., Needham Hts., Mass.

Micro-Mixer: Cooke Engineering Co., Alexandria, Va.
Centrifuge carriers for microculture plates: Cooke Engineering Co.
Searle automatic gamma counter: Searle Analytic Inc.
Counting tubes for ^{51}Cr: 16 × 100 mm glass disposable tubes, catalog #99455; Corning Glass, Corning, N.Y. Mitomycin C, 2 μg/ampoule; Nutritional Biochemicals Corp.
Penicillin-streptomycin, Grand Island Biological Co.; catalog #5141.
Glass-fiber filters: 1 × 28 inches, grade 934AH; Reeve-Angel Co., Clifton, N. J.
Automated microsample harvester: Otto Hiller, Madison, Wis.
Phytohemagglutinin M, final dilution 1:150: catalog #0528-57; Difco Laboratories, Detroit, Mich.
Scintillation vials: Research products, International Corp., Elk Grove Valley, Ill.
Bottles for culturing target cells or effector cells when large quantities are needed: Falcon culture flask, catalog #3013; Falcon Plastics, Oxford, Calif.

TEST RESULTS AND INTERPRETATION

The results of a typical experiment are presented in Table 1. A, B, and C represent normal unrelated individuals. The first column represents the different MLC combinations with the stimulator cells (denoted by X) ^{137}Cs-irradiated. The second column represents the amount of [^{3}H]thymidine incorporation. Targets are stimulated with PHA and usually incorporate 2,000 to 4,000 counts per min per 10^4 lymphocytes. If the cells are not stimulated with PHA, the values range from 800 to 15,000 counts per min per 10^4 cells. After 4 h of incubation, approximately 10 to 15% of the ^{51}Cr is released spontaneously. The freeze-thaw value for maximal release is about 80% of the total ^{51}Cr taken up. If the value is significantly less, new ^{51}Cr should be obtained. ^{51}Cr which has gone through more than one half-life should not be used, as cytotoxic products begin to accumulate. With PHA-stimulated targets, the effector cells generated in the MLC sometimes destroy targets in a nonspecific manner (auto-killing). To determine the extent of auto-killing, target cells autologous to the responder cells are used. This is demonstrated in Table 1 by AB_x/A and AC_x/A. Under the experimental conditions described, auto-killing is observed in about 10% of the experiments. Non-PHA-stimulated targets do not appear to be a problem. When the target

TABLE 1. *Cell-mediated lympholysis*

| Responder/ stimulator | MLC (counts/min ± SD) | Target | ^{51}Cr released (counts/min) | | | Percent ^{51}Cr released |
			Expt[a] value	Spontaneous release	Freeze-thawed	
AAₓ	1,563 ± 251	B	337	351	3,864	−0.4
ABₓ	35,627 ± 1,549	B	1,641	351	3,864	36.7
ACₓ	27,184 ± 956	B	863	351	3,864	14.6
AAₓ	1,563 ± 251	A	651	626	4,175	0.7
ABₓ	35,627 ± 1,549	A	701	626	4,175	2.1
ACₓ	27,184 ± 956	A	636	626	4,175	0.3
AAₓ	1,563 ± 251	C	341	389	2,998	−1.8
ABₓ	35,627 ± 1,549	C	751	389	2,998	13.9
ACₓ	27,184 ± 956	C	1,629	389	2,998	47.5

[a] All experiments are done in triplicate, and the values presented represent the mean value. Triplicates are within 10% of the mean.

is allogenic to the stimulator cell (AB_x/C or AC_x/B), significant CML is often observed, although it is almost always less than the autologous combination (AB_x/B or AC_xC). This has been attributed to cross-reactivity among the antigens responsible for CML. Values of under 10% are considered insignificant and are in the range observed when responder and stimulator are autologous (AA/B). Values from 10 to 20% ^{51}Cr releases are considered significant but weak. Normal values of CML range between 20 and 50% with the experimental protocol described. When no effector activity is observed, negative values are frequently recorded and result when the experimental value is less than the spontaneous release. This is due presumably to some kind of a protective effect mediated by the large number of extra cells. A more appropriate control would be to add an equivalent number of unlabeled target cells. This is difficult to do when lymphocytes from the donor are at a premium, and in addition the negative values are always small and do not significantly alter the results.

When conducting experiments to determine whether a patient can generate effector cell activity in CML, another control must be performed in addition to those already mentioned. If the individual does not demonstrate effector cell activity, it must be determined that the target cells utilized can be destroyed by other effector cells. An example of this is shown in Table 2 where we have investigated the MLC and CML activity of the father of a child with combined immune deficiency disease. The father (F) was unable to generate CML activity against the PHA blasts from normal individuals N_1 and N_2 despite a normal MLC response. To determine that these results were not associated

TABLE 2. *MLC and CML of father of child with combined immune deficiency disease[a]*

| Responder/ stimulator | MLC (counts/ min ± SD) | Target | ^{51}Cr released | |
			Expt value (counts/ min)	Percent
FFₓ	931 ± 15	N_1	877	−4.1
FFₓ	931 ± 15	N_2	1,048	1.3
FN₁ₓ	10,932 ± 671	N_1	1,187	11.6
FN₂ₓ	22,172 ± 3,760	N_2	1,054	6.4
FN₁ₓ	10,932 ± 671	F	1,178	5.3
FN₂ₓ	22,172 ± 3,760	F	1,058	1.6
N_1N_{2x} ...	38,570 ± 5,159	N_2	1,695	37.8
N_2N_{1x} ...	25,906 ± 137	N_1	1,545	24.5

[a] F = father; N_1 and N_2 = normal unrelated individuals. Spontaneous release: N_1 = 865; N_2 = 923; F = 1,007. Freeze-thawed: N_1 = 3,642; N_2 = 2,964; F = 4,172.

with the target cells, an MLC was performed with a normal individual as responder, and in this case a normal CML reaction was obtained (N_1N_2/N_2, N_2N_1/N_1).

LITERATURE CITED

1. Bach, F. H., M. Segall, K. S. Zier, P. M. Sondel, B. J. Alter, and M. L. Bach. 1973. Cell mediated immunity: separation of cells involved in recognitive and destructive phases. Science **180**:403–406.
2. Bach, F. H., and N. K. Voynow. 1966. One way stimulation in mixed leukocyte cultures. Science **153**:545–547.
3. Bach, M. L., B. J. Alter, J. J. Lightbody, and F. H. Bach. 1972. Abrogation of cytotoxicity of mixed leukocyte cultures. Transplant. Proc. **4**:169–172.
4. Bain, B., M. R. Vas, and L. Lowenstein. 1964. The development of large immature mononu-

clear cells in mixed leukocyte cultures. Blood **23**:108–115.

5. Brent, L., J. Brown, and P. B. Medawar. 1958. Skin transplantation immunity in relations to hypersensitivity. Lancet **2**:561–564.

6. Brunner, R. T., V. Mauel, H. Rudolf, and B. Chapius. 1970. Studies of allograft immunity in mice. Immunology **18**:501–515.

7. Buckley, R. H. 1971. Reconstitution: grafting of bone marrow and thymus, p. 1061–1080. *In* D. B. Amos (ed.), Progress in immunology. Academic Press Inc., New York.

8. Cantor, H. and R. Asofsky. 1972. Synergy among lymphoid cells mediating the graft vs. host response. J. Exp. Med. **135**:764–779.

9. Cohen, F., and J. J. Lightbody. 1975. Effector phase abnormalities of cell mediated immunity in family members of a child with hereditary T cell immunodeficiency and absent adenosine deaminase, p. 201–212. *In* H. Meuwissen, R. Pickering, B. Pollara, and I. Porter (ed.), Combined immunodeficiency disease and adenosine deaminase deficiency, a molecular defect. Academic Press Inc., New York.

10. Dausset, J., F. T. Rapaport, P. Ivanyi, and J. Colombani. 1965. Tissue alloantigens and transplantation, p. 63–71. *In* H. Balner and F. J. Cleton (ed.), Histocompatibility testing. Munksgaard, Copenhagen.

11. Descamps, B., N. Hinglais, and J. Crosnier. 1973. Renal transplantation between 33 HL-A-identical siblings. Transplant. Proc. **5**:231–236.

12. Eijsvoogel, V. P., R. du Bois, C. J. M. Melief, W. P. Zeylemaker, L. Raat-Koning, and L. de Groat-Kooy. 1973. Lymphocyte activations and destruction *in vitro* in relation to MLC and HL-A. Transplant. Proc. **5**:415–420.

13. Gatti, R. A., H. J. Meuwissen, P. J. Terasaki, and R. A. Good. 1971. Recombination within the HL-A locus. Tissue Antigens **1**:239–241.

14. Ginsburg, H., and L. Sachs. 1965. Destruction of mouse and rat embryo cells in tissue culture by lymph node cells from unsensitized rats. J. Cell. Comp. Physiol. **66**:199–219.

15. Govaerts, A. 1960. Cellular antibodies in kidney homotransplantation. J. Immunol. **85**:516–522.

16. Hardy, D. A., N. R. Ling, J. M. Wallin, and T. Aviet. 1970. Destruction of lymphoid cells by activated human lymphocytes. Nature (London) **227**:723–725.

17. Hayry, P., and V. Defendi. 1970. Mixed lymphocyte cultures produce effector cells: model *in vitro* for allograft rejection. Science **168**:133–135.

18. Lightbody, J. J., and F. H. Bach. 1973. Cell mediated lympholysis: effect of papain on effector and target cells. Ann. Immunol. (Paris) **124C**:311–319.

19. Lightbody, J. J., and F. H. Bach. 1972. Specificity of destruction by lymphocytes activated in mixed leukocyte culture. Transplant. Proc. **4**:307–310.

20. Lightbody, J. J., O. Bernoco, V. C. Miggiano, and R. Ceppellini. 1971. Cell mediated lympholysis in man after sensitization of effector lymphocytes through mixed leukocyte cultures. G. Batteriol. Immunol. **64**:273–289.

21. Lightbody, J. J., and Y. C. Kong. 1974. Comparison of ^{137}Cs irradiation and mitomycin C treatment of stimulator cells in the mixed lymphocyte culture reaction. Cell. Immunol. **13**:326–330.

22. Lightbody, J. J., and J. C. Rosenberg. 1974. Antibody-dependent cell-mediated cytotoxicity in prospective kidney transplant recipients. J. Immunol. **112**:890–896.

23. Lightbody, J. J., L. Urbani, and M. D. Poulik. 1974. Effect of B$_2$ microglobulin antibody on effector function of T-cell mediated cytotoxicity. Nature (London) **250**:227–228.

24. Lundgren, G., G. Magnusson, E. Moller, H. Nordenstar, R. Werner, and G. Westberg. 1972. Rejection of an HL-A identical renal transplant. Tissue Antigens **2**:32–40.

25. Mawas, C., M. Sasportes, and Y. Christen. 1975. Reproducible exceptions in the cell-mediated-lympholysis (CML) system. Transplant. Proc. **7**(Suppl. 1):53–55.

26. Raff, M., and H. Cantor. 1971. Subpopulations of thymus cells and thymus-derived, p. 83–96. *In* D. B. Amos (ed.), Progress in immunology. Academic Press Inc., New York.

27. Schapira, M., C. Legendre, and M. Jeannet. 1975. HL-A system and cell-mediated lympholysis in unrelated individuals. Transplant. Proc. **7**:259–261.

28. Stulting, R. D., and G. Berke. 1973. The use of ^{51}Cr release as a measure of lymphocyte mediated cytolysis *in vitro*. Cell. Immunol. **9**:474–476.

29. Terasaki, P. I., and M. R. Mickey. 1971. Histocompatibility transplant correlations, reproducibility and new matching methods. Transplant. Proc. **3**:1057–1064.

30. Terasaki, P. I., G. Opelz, and A. Ting. 1973. Tissue typing in human kidney transplantation, p. 92–111. *In* R. Calne (ed.), Immunological aspects of transplantation surgery. John Wiley & Sons, Inc., New York.

31. van Rood, J. J., A. Blusse van Ond Alblas, J. J. Keuning, E. Frederiks, A. Termijtelen, J. P. van Hoaff, A. S. Pena, and A. van Leeuwen. 1975. Histocompatibility genes and transplantation antigens. Transplant. Proc. **7**(Suppl. 1):25–30.

32. von Hoaff, J. P., H. M. A. Schippers, and G. J. van der Steen. 1972. Efficacy of HL-A matching in Eurotransplant. Lancet **2**:1385–1388.

33. Wagner, H., M. Rollinghoff, and G. J. V. Nossal. 1973. T-cell mediated immune responses induced in vitro: a probe for allograft and tumor immunity. Transplant. Rev. **17**:3–36.

34. Yunis, E. J., and D. B. Amos. 1971. Three closely linked genetic systems relevant to transplantation. Proc. Natl. Acad. Sci. U.S.A. **68**:3031–3035.

Chapter 113

Reactions Involving Cytolytic Antibody and Normal Lymphocytes

EURIPIDES FERREIRA

INTRODUCTION

This chapter describes techniques for measuring lymphocyte-dependent antibody-mediated lysis (LDA). These procedures can detect antibodies not recognized by the complement-dependent lysis assays.

Role of lymphocyte in immune function

Two main populations of lymphocytes are effective in the immune response: T lymphocytes, arising from the stem cells in the bone marrow and maturing in the thymus, are primarily involved in the cellular immune response; B cells, also arising from stem cells in the bone marrow but maturing elsewhere, are responsible for humoral immunity (46). There are six major differences between these two populations of lymphocytes: function (46), distribution among lymphoid organs (16), ability to form spontaneous rosettes with sheep erythrocytes (51), ability to respond to specific antigens and mitogens (2, 46), life-span (12), and the amount of immunoglobulin detectable on their membrane surface (3). The interaction between these two populations in immune responses has been demonstrated in animals (2, 10) and has been indicated in humans (10).

There are also two major categories of immune response:

1. The cellular immune response involves the direct lysis of target cells by "sensitized" lymphocytes. The in vitro determination of cellular immunity is measured by exposing appropriate target cells to cells obtained from immunized donors (cells sensitized in vivo) or cells that have been sensitized in vitro. This mechanism has been regarded as a function of immune T lymphocytes (10, 39).

2. The other type of immune response is a humoral response. Target cell lysis can be brought about by antibody, which is produced by immune B lymphocytes or plasma cells (46) in the presence of complement (37). This antibody-directed, complement-mediated cytotoxicity (AMC) is a rapid and efficient process in

vitro. Immunity can also be passively transferred in vivo by the simple administration of immune serum. This protective or neutralizing effect of immune serum is generally assumed to be through AMC.

Lymphocyte-dependent antibody

There exists, however, at least one additional effector system, that resulting from the interaction between antibody and unsensitized lymphoid cells, leading to destruction of target cells (34, 39, 42, 56, 58). It is known that this method of antibody-mediated cytotoxic killing by lymphoid cells in the absence of complement is extremely efficient in vitro. Studies in mice (21) have indicated that this process is operative in vivo as well. If so, conclusions drawn from experiments in which immunity was transferred by lymphocytes or by antibody will need reinterpretation. The process has been variously designated. Terms used include: lymphocyte-dependent antibody-mediated lysis (LDA; 61), antibody-induced cell-mediated cytotoxicity (AIC; 14); and lymphocyte-antibody-lymphocytolytic interaction (LALI; 56).

Experimentally, LDA activity is measured directly or indirectly. In direct LDA, antibody directed against the target cells is added to a target cell suspension. Excess antibody may be removed by washing, or may be left in the assay mixture (39, 56, 61). The indirect test consists of the inhibition of LDA by antibody directed against the effector cell (19).

In LDA, then, there are three distinct components: target cells, antibody, and effector cells.

Target cells. Numerous cell types have been used as target cells. These include chicken erythrocytes (42), burro erythrocytes (57), duck erythrocytes (8), human erythrocytes (61), fibroblasts (36), cultured human liver cells (4), fresh human lymphocytes (22), phytohemagglutinin (PHA)-transformed human lymphocytes (56), and tumor cells (6, 14). The sensitivity of target cells to lysis is dependent upon the assay system used. The effector to target ratio is also important in obtaining optimal lysis (6,

34). Figure 1 shows the lysis obtained with varying effector to target ratios when antibodies and fresh human peripheral blood lymphocytes were employed.

Effector cells. A non-thymus-dependent lymphoid cell has been demonstrated to be responsible for target cell lysis in LDA in a variety of systems, using different sources of target cells, antibody, and effector cells (7, 14, 17, 23, 36, 42, 43, 57, 58). In support of this conclusion is the demonstration of the inability of purified T cells to induce lysis (20, 59).

The presence of an Fc receptor has been shown to be a necessary component of the effector cells (42). Monocytes, macrophages, neutrophils, and B lymphocytes have all been shown to have an Fc receptor; T cells do not (3, 26).

Although the effector cell in LDA is not a T lymphocyte, its identity is far from clear. It has been claimed to be, again in a variety of systems, a macrophage (23, 50), a B cell (14, 36, 42, 57, 59), or a cell that is nonadherent and neither T nor B (17, 44, 60). It is thus probable that several types of cells may be effective at killing in LDA. In my hands, it appeared that B cells were required for effective killing of allogeneic lymphoid cells. Mononuclear leukocytes, depleted of B cells by using an anti-B cell serum (11) and complement, followed by Ficoll-

Hypaque sedimentation to remove killed cells, were not able to kill human lymphocytes coated with anti-HLA antibody, as shown in Table 1. A good correlation was found between the percentage of cells staining with fluorescein conjugated to anti-immunoglobulin and LDA activity before and after treatment with anti-B cell serum and complement. Similarly, passage of a lymphoid population over an anti-immuno-globulin-coated column eliminated the ability of that population to induce target cell lysis (40, 42).

B cell lines maintained in long-term culture, however, were not able to kill lymphocytes coated with anti-HLA antibody (Table 2). This failure to kill may be a consequence of culturing; storage for 24 h at 37 C of freshly prepared human lymphocytes decreased their ability to kill (56). Similarly, mouse spleen cells stimulated in vitro with mitogens were reported to act as effectors 24 h after stimulation; however, by 48 to 72 h, they had lost this capability (14).

Results indicating that the effector may not be a B cell are somewhat confusing. Mononuclear leukocytes lacking cell surface immunoglobulins, from patients with severe hypogammaglobulinemia, were able to kill chicken erythrocytes but not human lymphocytes, coated with anti-chicken erythrocyte antibody and anti-HLA antibody, respectively (A. V. Muchmore et al., Fed. Proc. **34**:824, 1975).

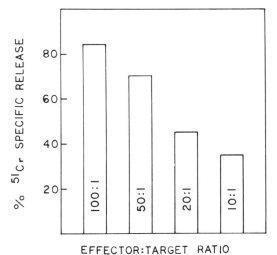

FIG. 1. *Variation of effector to target ratio in LDA. Effectors were human peripheral blood lymphocytes, isolated on Ficoll-Hypaque gradients. Targets were also human peripheral blood lymphocytes, isolated in the same manner, and were coated with anti-HLA antibody. The assay was performed as described in Assay procedure.*

TABLE 1. *Treatment with anti-B cell serum[a]*

Target	Effector			
	Immuno-globulin bearing cells (%)	[51]Cr specific release (%)	Immuno-globulin bearing cells (%)	[51]Cr specific release (%)
1	28	42	3	8
2	26	43	2.5	3
3	31	54	3	7

[a] Human peripheral blood lymphocytes isolated on Ficoll-Hypaque gradients were employed as effector cells against anti-HLA antibody-coated target lymphocytes isolated in the same manner. A sample of the effector cell suspension was also labeled with a fluorescein conjugate of goat anti-human immunoglobulin serum by incubation for 15 min at 4 C, and the percentage of stained cells was determined by comparison of cell counts under bright-field and fluorescent illumination. Additional samples were treated with rabbit anti-human B cell serum (32) and complement in a cytotoxicity test; remaining viable cells were adjusted to the proper concentration and used as effectors in LDA and stained as above for surface immunoglobulin.

TABLE 2. *Inability of cultured B cell lines to act as effectors in LDA[a]*

Target	Effector		
	Normal	IM-1[b]	SB[b]
T₁	78[c]	7	3
T₂	60	5	4
T₃	57	6	8

[a] Freshly isolated human peripheral blood lymphocytes and two cultured human B cell lines, IM-1 and SB, were used as effectors against three different anti-HLA antibody-coated human peripheral blood lymphocyte targets. The tests were performed as described in Assay procedures.

[b] IM-1 is a cultured B cell line isolated from human lymphoma; SB is also a cultured B cell line, isolated from B cell leukemia. Both secrete immunoglobulin and have high concentrations of surface immunoglobulin. These cell lines were provided by Dean L. Mann, National Cancer Institute.

[c] Specific ^{51}Cr-release (percent).

When normal human mononuclear cells were employed as effector cells against chicken erythrocytes and human erythrocytes, they were able to kill both target cells in the presence of the appropriate antibody. However, when these mononuclear cells were depleted of monocytes by an iron filing magnetic separation, they were able to kill only chicken erythrocytes (D. G. Poplack, G. D. Bonnard, and R. M. Blaese, Fed. Proc. **34**:823, 1975).

There is also documentation of variations in the efficiency of effector cells from different individuals or on different days (27). These variations may be caused by differences in age and physical health of the adult donors (27).

The above conflicting results may be due to different sources of target cells, antibody, and effector cells, and to the purification methods employed for the effector cells. The principal source of agreement is that the effector cells in LDA have an Fc receptor and are not T cells.

Antibody. The antibody involved in LDA belongs to the immunoglobulin G (IgG) class; IgA and IgM are not able to induce lysis of target cells (39, 48, 63). When aggregated normal and myeloma IgG preparations of all four subclasses were used to block LDA, the results indicated that the effector cell used in the various systems could not discriminate between the IgG subclasses, with the exception of IgG₄, which failed to block (10, 34, 42, 60).

Antibody molecules with intact Fc portions were necessary to promote lysis of targets (31, 34, 36). Antibody digested by pepsin lacked the ability to promote lysis (31, 36): F(ab')₂ or Fab

fragments, which are able to block the reaction of intact antibodies, are not themselves able to induce lysis (31, 36). In addition, 2-mercaptoethanol, which reportedly cleaves the inter-H-chain disulfide bonds in the Fc portions of the IgG molecules, decreased the ability of the molecule to fix complement (47) and eliminated its ability to induce LDA (13).

Antibody not cytotoxic to human lymphocytes in the presence of complement (22, 30, 33, 53, 55), when measured by either a direct (1) or an indirect assay (25), was able to initiate LDA, as shown in Table 3. Some investigators have found that antibody directed against HLA antigens promotes LDA (22, 30, 56). Others have found that the target antigen is clearly not the HLA molecule proper (62). It has been postulated that the target in these instances is the mixed lymphocyte culture locus product (28, 29).

In LDA, a very small amount of antibody is required (42, 56). When anti-HLA antibodies were used in both complement-dependent cytotoxicity and LDA, the maximal dilution of antisera that promoted lysis was 10- to 100-fold higher for LDA than for AMC (22, 56). When the antibody used is directed against antigens shared by effector and target, killing is less efficient than when the effector lacking the antigen is used (22).

Other factors. Complement is thought not to participate in LDA (41, 58). Sera are routinely heat-treated to eliminate complement activity. Although this in itself is inconclusive, sera treated with complement inhibitors were active in LDA (58). Animals genetically deficient in complement components were also able to provide mononuclear effectors which, in combination with complement-depleted sera, were ac-

TABLE 3. *LDA activity of an AMC-inactive serum[a]*

Target	Assay		
	AMC	A'Glob	LDA
Related; 1-8	0/2[b]	0/2	2/2
Related; not 1-8	0/2	0/2	0/2
Unrelated; 1-8	0/5	0/5	1/5
Unrelated; not 1-8	0/3	0/3	0/3

[a] The serum RHB was tested against a variety of cell types for activity in three assays: complement-dependent lysis (AMC), indirect cytotoxicity antiglobulin (A'Glob), and LDA. Targets were from donors related or unrelated to the serum donor, who did or did not share antigens HLA 1-8 with her husband.

[b] Number of positive results/number of targets tested.

tive in LDA, indicating that complement components possibly provided by the effector cells are not essential for LDA activity (58). In addition, in vivo depletion of complement had no effect on antitumor activity of LDA antibody (21).

Soluble toxic factors do not mediate lysis (36, 40, 42). In fact, close contact between antibody-coated target cells and effector cells is required in LDA (4, 42). Cytological observations of antibody-coated target monolayer and effector cells demonstrate this close contact (4). There is no evidence of cytopathomorphological alteration, although uropod formation was observed, indicating mobility of effector cells (4). This close contact occurs early in the interaction; the addition of free hapten 10 min after combination of antibody-coated target cells and effectors cannot block the reaction (49).

In LDA, effector cells treated with mitomycin were able to kill (14); thus no protein or deoxyribonucleic acid (DNA) synthesis was required (36, 39, 42). Killing was, however, energy dependent (39, 42). Experiments employing cytochalasins and microtubule disruptive agents suggested that, in LDA, cytotoxicity is a surface membrane-initiated process (15).

Assay procedures

All LDA test procedures are designed to expose target cells to a designated antibody in the absence of added complement, and then to determine the extent of target cell damage after addition of normal mononuclear leukocytes. Different methods have been used to demonstrate LDA.

Counting method. In this procedure, a predetermined number of target cells are transferred to tubes, petri dishes, or microplates to which antibody and effector cells are added. After incubation, the cells are stained and the number of viable target cells remaining is determined. This procedure is laborious, the incubation times are lengthy, and the variability is so great that several replicates are required. The evaluation of results is, of course, subjective. The procedure can most effectively be used when target and effector cells are morphologically different (39).

Monolayers. Monolayers to which antibody and effector cells are added have been used to show the close contact between antibody-coated target and effector cells. The positive reactions are determined by monolayer destruction after detachment of target cells. However, nonspecific detachment has been found to induce error in results and interpretation (4, 35).

Inhibition of colony formation. This method is applicable only to cells that have the ability to attach to glass and to develop colonies by multiplication. Targets alone are incubated in petri dishes for 24 h to allow attachment; antiserum and effector cells are added, and after 3 to 4 days of further incubation colonies are counted. A decrease in the number of colonies compared with controls indicates activity (39).

Release of isotope. Radioactive markers are widely used to measure target cell lysis. The DNA precursor thymidine, either ^3H or ^{14}C, has the advantage of stability and can be employed for long incubation times (39). Release will occur only when damaged cells are completely disintegrated (39). The reutilization of released isotope by cells synthesizing DNA can be partially avoided by the addition of cold thymidine (39). Labeled amino acids, [^{32}P]phosphate, and [^{125}I]iododeoxyuridine have all been used to label target cells (14, 39). The use of these markers is limited by the long incubation time necessary, the spontaneous release of labeled amino acids by some cell types, and the difficulty in preventing reutilization of labeled amino acids and [^{32}P]phosphate (39).

Chromium-51 has been used in several systems (39); it binds noncovalently to proteins and other cell constituents, is reduced during the binding, and is then not reutilized (39). It has a relatively low spontaneous release during a 4-h incubation and is almost totally released from dead cells (39). Release can be measured within a few hours of the addition of effector cells (39). Because chromium labeling is precise, simple, sensitive, quantitative, and reproducible, it has been chosen to demonstrate LDA activity in the system described below. This technique is derived from that of Trinchieri et al. (56) and is optimized for the use of human material. Microplates are used because they allow the use of small numbers of cells, close contact between target, antibody, and effectors, and a relative degree of safety from contamination with radioactive material.

CLINICAL INDICATIONS

Studies of organ transplantation, tumor immunity, and autoimmune disease have indicated that the LDA activity detectable in vitro may have an important counterpart in vivo.

Alloantibodies from Campbell ducks, able to promote rejection of tolerated Peking duck skin grafts on Campbell ducks, are also able to promote the lysis of Peking duck erythrocytes in vitro by normal Campbell duck lymphocytes. A good correlation was reported between the LDA activity of antibodies in vitro and their ability to promote graft rejection in vivo (8).

In humans it is generally accepted that hyperacute rejection occurs because the kidney graft recipient has preformed antibodies cytotoxic (in the presence of complement) to donor antigens (24, 52). In the usual crossmatch, serum from the recipient is exposed to lymphocytes of the donor in the presence of complement. However, hyperacute rejection occurs even if this classical crossmatch is negative; LDA-active antibodies have been demonstrated in such patients (53, 55). Similarly, sera from multiparous women or from patients on hemodialysis, which were negative by complement-dependent cytotoxicity, were positive when the LDA assay was employed (30, 33, 55). LDA may be an important prognostic tool and kidney donor selection should be on the basis of an LDA assay as well as the classical crossmatch (for suggested crossmatch scheme, see below, Interpretation).

LDA assays have also been used in studies of autoimmune disorders. In the presence of normal human lymphoid cells, serum from patients with Hashimoto's thyroiditis induces lysis of thyroglobulin-coated chicken erythrocytes (9).

Spleen cells from normal guinea pig also lyse chicken erythrocytes coated with anti-thyroglobulin antibodies (45). This assay may prove to be a powerful clinical tool in the diagnosis of autoimmune disorders involving the presence of IgG antibodies.

It has also been reported that patients with cancer provide less efficient effector cells than normal individuals (54), suggesting that lack of LDA may play an important role in the progression of cancer. Hyperimmune plasma, obtained by planned immunization of a healthy donor with normal lymphocytes, was reported to promote temporary remission in patients with chronic lymphocytic leukemia (32). Rabbit antiserum to mouse ovarian carcinoma was able to prolong the survival of tumor-bearing mice (38). Xenogeneic antisera to rat lymphomas were able to promote LDA in vitro and to have a protective effect in vivo (21). Further experiments done in vitro showed that nonlymphoid cells were able to kill tumor target cells coated with an appropriate antibody (43). Thus, in the future, LDA may be important in indicating appropriate immunotherapy of cancer.

TEST PROCEDURE (see Fig. 2)

Preparation of target cells

1. A 10-ml amount of whole blood, heparinized (The Upjohn Co., Kalamazoo, Mich.) with 25 IU/ml, is dripped slowly (1 drop/s) through a nylon column (see below, Reagents) to remove platelets and adherent cells (18).

2. The recovered blood is diluted 1:3 in phosphate-buffered saline (PBS), and about 8 ml is layered over 2 ml of Ficoll-Hypaque in a 10-ml tube. The tube is spun at $800 \times g$ for 10 min in a clinical centrifuge (5).

3. The interface layer containing the mononuclear leukocytes is harvested with a Pasteur pipette. An equal amount of PBS is added to the harvested cells to disrupt the density gradient, and the cells are spun at $350 \times g$ for 5 min. The resulting supernatant fluid is discarded.

4. If red cells are visible in the pellet, 2 ml of Tris-NH_4Cl is added, the pellet is gently resuspended, and the suspension is incubated at 37 C for 5 min.

5. After two washes with PBS (spinning at $200 \times g$ for 5 min), 6×10^6 target cells are resuspended in 0.5 ml of medium and incubated with 100 μCi of sodium chromate (Na_2CrO_4; Amersham-Searle, Arlington Heights, Ill.), added in a volume of less than 0.2 ml, for 2 h at 37 C with frequent shaking in a humidified 5% CO_2 atmosphere.

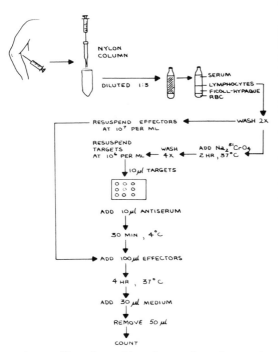

FIG. 2. Flow chart of lymphocyte-dependent antibody assay.

6. The labeled cells are then washed four times in 5 to 10 ml of cold PBS, spinning at 200 × *g* for 5 min each time, and finally are resuspended at 10^6 cells/ml in medium. Target cell suspensions should be kept on ice until use to decrease spontaneous release of the label.

Preparation of effector cells

1. To test one serum sample in triplicate with controls, mononuclear leukocytes from 20 ml of whole blood are required. These mononuclear leukocytes are isolated as above (steps 1–3) and are resuspended to a concentration of 10^7 cells/ml in medium after the second wash. They should be retained at room temperature until use. Effector cells must not be treated with Tris-NH$_4$Cl to remove red cells, as this treatment abolishes killing.

Sera

All sera used in LDA are decomplemented by heat inactivation at 56 C for 30 min, and are stored in small portions at −70 C. Serum samples should not be frozen and thawed more than four times before use. The dilution of antiserum must be empirically determined for each sample; sera that are inactive in LDA at a low dilution may be active at a higher dilution.

Assay procedure

1. Add 10 μliters of serum or serum diluted in PBS to each well of a round-bottom Linbro plate (Linbro Scientific Co., New Haven, Conn.; model IS-MRC 96 and cover 55) with a Hamilton syringe (Hamilton Co., Reno, Nev.). (See also Controls, below.)

2. Add 10 μliters of ^{51}Cr-labeled target cell suspension (total 10^4 cells/well) in the same manner.

3. Incubate the mixture for 30 min at 4 C.

4. Add 100 μliters of the effector cell suspension (total 10^6 cells/well) with a disposable pipette graduated in 0.01 ml (#7506; Falcon Plastics, Oxnard, Calif.).

5. Incubate the plates for 4 h at 37 C in a humidified 5% CO$_2$ atmosphere.

6. Add 30 μliters of medium or PBS at 4 C with a Hamilton syringe.

7. Centrifuge the plates at 400 × *g* for 10 min at 4 C in a 13 × 9 cm carrier (Microtiter; Cooke Engineering Co., Alexandria, Va.) in an International PR-6 centrifuge with a 4-place head (#277), or equivalent apparatus.

8. Carefully remove 50 μliters of the supernatant fluid from the side of each well with an Eppendorf pipette and disposable tip (Brinkmann Instruments Inc., Westbury, N.Y.) to a 10 × 75 mm glass tube, and count for chromium release in an automatic gamma counting system (Nuclear-Chicago Corp., Chicago, Ill.).

Controls

Total incorporation. Place 10 μliters of target cell suspension in a 10 × 75 mm tube, and count for total ^{51}Cr incorporation, in triplicate.

Maximal releasable chromium. Add 20 μliters of 0.5% sodium deoxycholate (DOC) to the above samples. After 4 h of incubation at room temperature, add 720 μliters of cold medium or PBS, spin the tubes at 400 × *g* for 10 min at 4 C, and count 250 μliters of the resulting supernatant fluid.

Spontaneous release. In triplicate Linbro plate wells, add each of the following, in 100-μliter amounts, at the appropriate time:

	Target	Antibody	Effector
Control 1	targets	medium	medium
Control 2	targets	serum	medium
Control 3	targets	medium	effectors

Controls 1 and 2 are necessary to determine that the antibody alone is not cytotoxic. Control 3 is used as the spontaneous release in the calculation of results.

Calculations

1. Multiply the counts per minute (minus machine background) for each well by 3 to yield total counts per minute released per well.

2. Calculate the mean, standard deviation, and standard error.

3. Calculate the percent specific release (%SR) or percent chromium released (%^{51}Cr):

$$\%SR = \frac{E - S}{DOC} \times 100$$

$$\%^{51}Cr = \frac{E}{DOC} \times 100$$

where E is the experimental counts per minute released, S is the spontaneous counts per minute released (control 3 under Spontaneous release), and DOC is the maximal releasable chromium.

4. When %SR is greater than 10, the reaction is positive; %SR greater than 20 is considered to be reliable.

REAGENTS

Medium

Prepare RPMI 1640 medium (H-18, Grand Island Biological Co., Grand Island, N.Y.) by diluting 104.3 g of powdered medium in 10 liters of double-distilled water and sterilize by filtration. Add 250 ml of 1 M sterile HEPES buffer (N-2-hydroxyethylpiperazine-N'-2-ethanesulfonic acid buffer) (Sigma Chemical Co., St. Louis, Mo.). The medium is supplemented with 20% heat-inactivated fetal calf serum (#614, Grand Island Biological Co.), 100 IU of penicillin G/ml (Pfizer, Inc., New York, N.Y.), and 100 μg of streptomycin/ml (Eli Lilly & Co., Indianapolis, Ind.). Medium is stored at 4 C.

Phosphate-buffered saline

Dissolve 96 g of PBS (K-13, Dulbecco's; Grand Island Biological Co.) in 10 liters of distilled water. After thorough mixing, add 1.3 g of calcium chloride (supplied by the manufacturer in a separate package). When the calcium chloride has dissolved, adjust the pH to 7.2. PBS is also stored at 4 C; shelf life is approximately 1 month.

Tris-NH₄Cl (Tris buffer)

Prepare Tris buffer by mixing 1 part of solution A with 9 parts of solution $B;$ adjust the pH to 7.2. Solution A consists of 2.06 g of Trizma base (Sigma Chemical Co.) diluted to a volume of 100 ml; the pH was adjusted to 7.2 to 7.4 by the addition of concentrated HCl. Solution B is made by dissolving 8.3 g of NH₄Cl in 1,000 ml of distilled water. All solutions are stored at 4 C until use; shelf life is 3 months.

Sodium deoxycholate

DOC (0.5%) is prepared by dissolving 0.5 g of DOC (Fisher Scientific Co., Fairlawn, N.J.) in 100 ml of distilled water. The DOC solution is also stored at 4 C; shelf life is approximately 1 month.

Nylon column

1. Heat together for 30 min at 65 to 70 C: 250 g of nylon (semidull, ½'', 30 deriver,

type 200, #67030, E. I. Dupont de Nemours & Co., Inc., Wilmington, Del.); 4 liters of water; 40 ml of Duponal (#241900 Dupont).
2. Rinse overnight in tap water.
3. Rinse thoroughly in distilled water.
4. Air-dry.
5. Use comb and brush to separate fibers.
6. Pack 0.7 g firmly into a 6-inch Pasteur pipette, and cap with a 5-mm rubber serum stopper (Arthur Thomas, 8753-022).

Ficoll-Hypaque

Ficoll-Hypaque can be purchased as sterile LSM solution (#8410-01) from Bionetics, Kensington, Md., or can be prepared as follows.

Mix 24 ml of 9% (9 g in 100 ml) Ficoll (type 400, #F4375, Sigma Chemical Co.) in distilled water with 10 ml of 34% (34 g in 100 ml) Hypaque (Hypaque Sodium 50%, Winthrop Laboratories, New York, N.Y.). The specific gravity must be adjusted to 1.078 to 1.080. The solution is stored at 4 C; shelf life is approximately 2 months.

INTERPRETATION

There are no standard normal values for LDA assay. Because effector cell sources, antibody, and target cell sources all vary from laboratory to laboratory, normal values will also vary. Different effector cells will lyse different targets coated with the same antibody to varying extents. Distinction should not, therefore, be made on the basis of small differences within a single assay or between determinations made on different days, without appropriate controls. The HLA specificities of effector cell and target influence the result.

A suggested protocol for an LDA transplant crossmatch is given in Table 4. As suggested

TABLE 4. *Suggested LDA crossmatch*

Effector source	Antibody source	Target source	Purpose
Transplant recipient	Transplant recipient	Transplant donor	Experimental detection of LDA antibody
Transplant recipient	None	Transplant donor	Possible indication of cell-mediated immunity
Transplant recipient	Directed against unrelated target	Unrelated[a]	Measure of ability of recipient to act as effector in LDA
Normal	Transplant recipient	Transplant donor	May detect LDA antibody in recipient with deficient effector population
Normal	None	Transplant donor	Negative control
Normal	Directed against unrelated target	Unrelated	Positive control

[a] Unrelated cell type should share no HLA antigens with either donor or recipient.

in Test procedures, a specific release (that is, with background subtracted) of 20% or greater should be considered a positive reaction. Specific release between 10 and 20% is probably significant. In such instances, the test should be repeated.

ACKNOWLEDGMENTS

I am grateful to Ann Berger for her assistance in the preparation of this manuscript and also to D. Bernard Amos for discussion and critical review.

LITERATURE CITED

1. Amos, D. B., H. Bashir, N. Boyle, M. MacQueen, and A. Tiilikainen. 1969. A simple microcytotoxicity test. Transplantation 7:220–223.
2. Andersson, J., O. Sjöberg, and G. Möller. 1972. Mitogens as probes for immunocyte activation and cellular cooperation. Transplant. Rev. 11:131–177.
3. Bianco, C., R. Patrick, and V. Nussenzweig. 1970. A population of lymphocytes bearing a membrane receptor for antigen-antibody-complement complexes. I. Separation and characterization. J. Exp. Med. 132:702–720.
4. Biberfeld, P., G. Biberfeld, P. Perlmann, and G. Holm. 1973. Cytological observations on the cytotoxic interaction between lymphocytes and antibody-coated monolayer cells. Cell. Immunol. 7:60–72.
5. Bøyum, A. 1968. Separation of lymphocytes from blood and bone marrow. Scand. J. Clin. Lab. Invest. 21(Suppl.):97.
6. Britton, S., and J. Forman. 1974. Some characteristics of the antibody-induced cell-mediated cytotoxicity against leukemia cells. Transplantation 17:180–187.
7. Britton, S., H. Perlmann, and P. Perlmann. 1973. Thymus-dependent and thymus-independent effector functions of mouse lymphoid cells. Comparison of cytotoxicity and primary antibody formation in vitro. Cell. Immunol. 8:420–434.
8. Bubeník, J., P. Perlmann, and M. Hašek. 1970. Induction of cytotoxicity of lymphocytes from tolerant donors by antibodies to target cell alloantigens. Transplantation 10:290–296.
9. Calder, E. A., W. J. Penhale, D. McLeman, E. W. Barnes, and W. J. Irvine. 1973. Lymphocyte-dependent antibody-mediated cytotoxicity in Hashimoto thyroiditis. Clin. Exp. Immunol. 14:153–158.
10. Cerottini, J.-C., and K. T. Brunner. 1974. Cell-mediated cytotoxicity, allograft rejection, and tumor immunity. Adv. Immunol. 18:67–132.
11. Cresswell, P., and S. Geier. 1975. Antisera to human B lymphocyte membrane glycoproteins block stimulation in mixed lymphocyte culture. Nature 270:147.
12. Davies, A. J. S. 1969. The thymus and the cellular basis of immunity. Transplant. Rev. 1:43–91.
13. Denk, H., H. Stemberger, G. Wiedermann, R. Eckerstorfer, and G. Tappeiner. 1974. The influence of 2-mercaptoethanol (2-ME) treatment of IgG antibody on its ability to induce cytotoxicity in nonsensitized lymphocytes. Cell. Immunol. 13:489–492.
14. Forman, J., and G. Möller. 1973. The effector cell in antibody-induced cell mediated immunity. Transplant. Rev. 17:108–149.
15. Gelfand, E. W., S. A. Morris, and K. Resch. 1975. Antibody-dependent cytotoxicity: modulation by the cytocholasins and microtubule disruptive agents. J. Immunol. 114:919.
16. Good, R. A., A. P. Dalmasso, C. Martinez, O. Archer, J. C. Pierre, and B. W. Papermaster. 1962. The role of the thymus in development of immunologic capacity in rabbits and mice. J. Exp. Med. 116:773–795.
17. Greenberg, A. H., L. Shew, and I. M. Roitt. 1973. Characterization of the antibody-dependent cytotoxic cell. A non-phagocytic monocyte? Clin. Exp. Immunol. 15:251–259.
18. Greenwalt, T. J., M. Gajewski, and J. L. Mackenna. 1962. A new method for preparing buffy-coat-poor blood. Transfusion 2:221–229.
19. Halloran, P., V. Schirrmacher, and H. Festenstein. 1974. A new sensitive assay for antibody against cell surface antigens based on inhibition of cell-dependent antibody-mediated cytotoxicity. I. Specificity and sensitivity. J. Exp. Med. 140:1348–1363.
20. Harding, B., D. J. Pudifin, F. Gotch, and I. C. M. MacLennan. 1971. Cytotoxic lymphocytes from rats depleted of thymus processed cells. Nature (London) New Biol. 232:80–82.
21. Hersey, P. 1973. A new look at antiserum therapy of leukemia. Nature (London) New Biol. 224:22–24.
22. Hersey, P., P. Cullen, and I. C. M. MacLennan. 1973. Lymphocyte-dependent cytotoxic antibody activity against human transplantation antigens. Transplantation 16:9–16.
23. Holm, G., E. Engwall, S. Hammstrom, and J. B. Natvig. 1974. Antibody-induced hemolytic activity of human blood monocytes. Scand. J. Immunol. 3:173–180.
24. Jeannet, M., V. W. Pinn, M. H. Flax, H. J. Winn, and P. S. Russel. 1970. Humoral antibodies in renal allotransplantation in man. N. Engl. J. Med. 282:111–117.
25. Johnson, A. H., R. D. Rossen, and W. T. Butler. 1972. Detection of alloantibodies using a sensitive antiglobulin microcytotoxicity test: identification of low levels of pre-formed antibodies in accelerated allograft rejection. Tissue Antigens 2:215–226.
26. Kerbel, R. S., and A. J. S. Davies. 1974. The possible biological significance of Fc receptors on mammalian lymphocytes and tumor cells. Cell 3:105–112.
27. Kovithavongs, T., W. C. Hottmann, and J. B. Dossetor. 1974. Effector cell activity in antibody-mediated cell-dependent immune lympholysis. I. Normal individuals. J. Immunol.

113:1178–1183.

28. Kovithavongs, T., L. Hyshka, P. R. McConnachie, and J. B. Dossetor. 1974. Serological detection of mixed lymphocyte culture identity between cells that differ by one HL-A haplotype. Science 186:1124.

29. Kovithavongs, T., L. Hyshka, P. R. McConnachie, and J. B. Dossetor. 1975. Serotyping for MLC gene products. I. Presumptive evidence that ABCIL may detect MLC factors. Tissue Antigens 5:165–172.

30. Kovithavongs, T., P. R. McConnachie, and J. B. Dossetor. 1974. Immunity to tissue sensitisation, HL-A and non-HL-A, as detected by the ABCIL system. I. Parous women. Transplantation 17:453–461.

31. Larsson, A., and P. Perlman. 1972. Study of Fab and F(ab')₂ from rabbit IgG and capacity to induce lymphocyte-mediated target cell destruction in vitro. Int. Arch. Allergy 43:80–88.

32. Laszlo, J., C. E. Buckley, III, and D. B. Amos. 1968. Infusion of isologous immune plasma in chronic lymphocytic leukemia. Blood 31:104–110.

33. Lightbody, J. J., and J. C. Rosenberg. 1974. Antibody-dependent cell-mediated cytotoxicity in prospective kidney transplant recipients. J. Immunol. 112:890–896.

34. MacLennan, I. C. M. 1972. Antibody in the induction and inhibition of lymphocyte cytotoxicity. Transplant. Rev. 13:67–90.

35. Moller, G., V. Beckmann, and G. Lundgren. 1966. In vitro destruction of human fibroblasts by non-immune lymphoid cells. Nature (London) 212:1203–1207.

36. Möller, G., and S.-E. Svehag. 1972. Specificity of lymphocyte-mediated cytotoxicity induced by in vitro antibody-coated target cells. Cell. Immunol. 4:1–19.

37. Müller-Eberhard, H. J. 1968. Chemistry and reaction mechanisms of complement. Adv. Immunol. 8:1–80.

38. Order, S. E., V. Donahue, and R. Knapp. 1973. Immunotherapy of ovarian carcinoma. An experimental model. Cancer 32:573–579.

39. Perlmann, P., and G. Holm. 1969. Cytotoxic effects of lymphoid cells in vitro. Adv. Immunol. 11:117–193.

40. Perlmann, P., H. Perlmann, and P. Biberfeld. 1972. Specifically cytotoxic lymphocytes produced by preincubation with antibody-complexed target cells. J. Immunol. 108:558–561.

41. Perlmann, P., H. Perlmann, and H. J. Müller-Eberhard. 1975. Cytolytic lymphocytic cells with complement receptor in human blood. Induction of cytolysis by IgG antibody but not by target cell-bound C3. J. Exp. Med. 141:287–296.

42. Perlmann, P., H. Perlmann, and H. Wigzell. 1972. Lymphocyte mediated cytotoxicity in vitro. Induction and inhibition by humoral antibody and nature of effector cells. Transplant. Rev. 13:91–114.

43. Pollack, S. B., K. Nelson, and J. D. Grausz. 1975.

Killer cells from murine spleen: effectors of antibody-dependent cellular cytotoxicity. Transplant. Proc. 7:477.

44. Pudifin, D. J., B. Harding, and I. C. M. MacLennan. 1971. The differential effect of radiation on the sensitizing and effector stages of antibody-dependent lymphocyte-mediated cytotoxicity. Immunology 21:853–860.

45. Ringertz, B., J. Wasserman, T. H. Packalen, and P. Perlmann. 1971. Cellular and humoral immune responses in experimental autoimmune thyroiditis. Int. Arch. Allergy 40:917–927.

46. Roitt, I. M., M. F. Greaves, G. Torrigiani, J. Brostoff, and J. H. L. Playfair. 1969. The cellular basis of immunological response. A synthesis of some current views. Lancet 2:367–371.

47. Schur, P. H., and G. Christian. 1964. The role of disulphide bonds in the complement-fixing and precipitating properties of 7S rabbit and sheep antibodies. J. Exp. Med. 120:531–545.

48. Scornik, J. C., H. Cosenza, W. Lee, H. Köhler, and D. A. Rowley. 1974. Antibody-dependent cell-mediated cytotoxicity. I. Differentiation from antibody-independent cytotoxicity by "normal" IgG. J. Immunol. 113:1510–1518.

49. Scornik, J. C. 1974. Antibody-dependent cell-mediated cytotoxicity. II. Early interactions between effector and target cells. J. Immunol. 113:1519–1526.

50. Scornik, J. C., and H. Cosenza. 1974. Antibody-dependent cell-mediated cytotoxicity. III. Two functionally different effector cells. J. Immunol. 113:1527–1532.

51. Silveira, N. P. A., N. F. Mendes, and M. E. A. Tolnai. 1972. Tissue localization of two populations of human lymphocytes distinguished by membrane receptors. J. Immunol. 108:1456–1460.

52. Terasaki, P. I., D. L. Trasher, and T. H. Hauber. 1968. Serotyping for homotransplantation. XIII. Immediate kidney transplant rejection and associated preformed antibodies, p. 225. In J. Dausset, J. Hamburger, and G. Mathe (ed.), Advances in transplantation. Munksgaard, Copenhagen.

53. Ting, A., and P. I. Terasaki. 1974. Influence of lymphocyte-dependent antibodies on human kidney transplants. Transplantation 18:371–373.

54. Ting, A., and P. I. Terasaki. 1974. Depressed lymphocyte-mediated killing of sensitized targets in cancer patients. Cancer Res. 34:2694–2698.

55. Ting, A., and P. I. Terasaki. 1975. Lymphocyte-dependent antibody crossmatching for transplant patients. Lancet 1:304.

56. Trinchieri, G., M. deMarchi, W. Mayr, M. Savi, and R. Ceppellini. 1973. Lymphocyte antibody lymphocytolytic interaction (LALI) with special emphasis on HL-A. Transplant. Proc. 5:1631–1646.

57. Van Boxel, J. A., W. E. Paul, M. M. Frank, and I. Green. 1973. Antibody-dependent lymphoid

cell-mediated cytotoxicity: role of lymphocytes bearing a receptor for complement. J. Immunol. **110**:1027–1036.

58. Van Boxel, J. A., W. E. Paul, I. Green, and M. M. Frank. 1974. Antibody-dependent lymphoid cell-mediated cytotoxicity: role of complement. J. Immunol. **112**:398–403.

59. Van Boxel, J. A., J. D. Stobo, W. E. Paul, and I. Green. 1972. Antibody-dependent lymphoic cell-mediated cytotoxicity: no requirement for thymus-derived lymphocytes. Science **175**:194.

60. Wisløff, F., and S. S. Frøland. 1973. Antibody-dependent lymphocyte-mediated cytotoxicity in man: no requirement for lymphocytes with membrane-bound immunoglobulin. Scand. J. Immunol. **2**:151–157.

61. Wunderlich, J. R., E. B. Rosenberg, and J. M. Connoly. 1971. Human lymphocyte-dependent cytotoxic antibody and mechanisms of target cell destruction in vitro., p. 473–482. *In* B. Amos (ed.), Progesss in immunology. Academic Press Inc., New York.

62. Yust, I., J. Wunderlich, D. L. Mann, G. N. Rogentine, Jr., B. Leventhal, R. Yankee, and R. Graw. 1974. Human lymphocyte-dependent antibody mediated cytotoxicity and direct lymphocyte cytotoxicity against non-HL-A antigens. Nature (London) **249**:263–265.

63. Yust, I., J. R. Wunderlich, D. L. Mann, and W. D. Terry. 1971. Identification of lymphocyte-dependent antibody in sera from multiply transfused patients. Transplantation **18**:99–107.

Chapter 114

Antileukocyte Capillary Agglutinating Antibody in Pre- and Post-Transplantation Sera

JOHN S. THOMPSON

INTRODUCTION

Capillary agglutination is a sensitive assay system that detects agglutinin-like antibodies by their capacity to prevent dissociation of sensitized cells from a centrifuged pellet in capillary tubes held at a 45° angle (9, 13, 14).

Microscopic observation has revealed that cells detach from the pellet at a rate inversely proportional to antibody concentration, fall to the trough of the capillary tube, and stream down the fluid-filled column. Therefore, antibody concentration may be measured by comparing its effect on streamer length as compared with a simultaneously performed control. This assay can be utilized to detect histocompatibility locus HLA, the specific neutrophil, and 5b leukocyte antigens (9, 15), as well as a large number of uncategorized non-HLA specificities (12, 13, 15).

Previous reports have detailed many of the factors influencing the capillary agglutination assay system. Several of these factors, including a low concentration of ethylenediaminetetraacetic acid (EDTA) in the basic buffer, high calcium concentration, capillary tube size, assay temperature, and prolonged in vitro storage of cells, were shown to influence the results substantially (9).

CLINICAL INDICATIONS

Although capillary agglutination is more difficult to perform than standard lymphocytotoxicity and agglutination procedures, it detects antibodies that may not be revealed by the other methods (8, 12, 13). For example, Olson et al. (8) compared 505 parous sera by the three techniques and found that 40% of the positive reactions were not detected by lymphocytotoxicity and at least one capillary agglutination-positive, lymphocytotoxicity-negative reaction was correlated with anti-HLA-B7. In a survey of 211 multiparous sera selected on the basis of four or more pregnancies at least 4 years prior to donation, lymphocytotoxicity reactions occurred with a total of 11.4% of the sera (10.4% of which were associated with capillary agglutin-

ation responses) and 30.3% were demonstrated by capillary agglutination alone (12). Furthermore, as will be discussed below, this frequency probably does not reflect capillary agglutination reactions with isolated lymphocytes since these were rarely correlated with whole leukocyte reactions.

Another feature distinguishing capillary agglutination pertains to its ability to react with immunoglobulin G (IgG) complement-independent antibodies. The IgG fraction of HLA, neutrophil, postpartum, and transplant sera was isolated by G-200 chromatography and demonstrated no loss in capillary agglutinating antibody activity as compared with whole sera. Stiller et al. (10) also demonstrated that capillary agglutination detects IgG complement-independent as well as IgM agglutinating antibodies and suggested that their frequent detection in prerenal transplant sera of patients with successful grafts may be an indication of an enhancing role.

Finally, the observation that capillary agglutination may be performed with isolated pure lymphocytes or neutrophils (9) further separates it from the standard agglutination assays that require an admixture of both cells to develop detectable agglutination (17).

Recently, I have studied pre- and post-transplant sera obtained from 23 living related and 75 cadaveric renal grafted patients. The development of both lymphocytotoxic and capillary agglutinating antibody with whole leukocytes in preoperatively negative patients generally heralded graft failure, yet the stimulation of capillary agglutination alone correlated with excellent survival. Capillary agglutination reactions accompanying lymphocytotoxic responses commonly correlated with HLA specificities, but those not associated usually did not correlate. The preoperative detection of only capillary agglutinating antibody, however, failed to predict outcome, and 6 of 13 patients went on to elaborate lymphocytotoxic and capillary agglutinating HLA specific antibody postoperatively and rejected their transplants. This reconfirmed a problem with the capillary agglutination assay that had been apparent for some time; i.e., the broad range of response encompassed too much, and non-HLA reactions were commonly obscured by HLA specific antibody responses in the same serum. Vice versa, HLA specific reactions were frequently blurred by additional non-HLA directed antibodies.

To achieve greater antigen-antibody discrimination, I have modified the capillary agglutination assay, taking advantage of its capability to react with purified peripheral blood cellular components. This chapter describes techniques for isolating neutrophils, lymphocytes, and platelets 98 to 100% free from other contaminating cells, demonstrates characteristic capillary agglutination reaction patterns with these components, and briefly illustrates how the results of these assays correlate with clinical renal allograft function.

TEST PROCEDURE

Capillary agglutination

The basic methods employed in the performance of capillary agglutination have been described (9). The standard assay was modified to test isolated peripheral blood neutrophils and lymphocytes as well as whole leukocytes. A 1-μliter amount of antiserum and cells is mixed in microtest plates, incubated for 10 min, and aspirated into 1-μliter capillary pipettes (specially cut, 32 mm long, Drummond Capillary Pipettes, Drummond Scientific Co., Broomall, Pa.). After centrifugation for 30 s at 11,500 rpm, in a microcapillary centrifuge (model MB, International Equipment Co., Needham Heights, Mass.), the tubes are held at a 45° angle with the cell pellet uppermost until the cells dissociate from the pellet to form measurable streamers in control AB sera. The length of the streamers developing with experimental antiserum in sextuplicate is measured and compared with the same number of controls by use of a measuring reticle in the eyepiece of a dissecting microscope, 7× magnification. Since antibody activity is inversely related to the rate of cell dissociation and subsequent streamer length, the percentage of experimental to control streamer is calculated and scored: 40 to 50% of control = 1, 30 to 39% = 2, 20 to 29% = 3, and less than 19% = 4.

Isolation of peripheral blood cells

A 10-ml amount of heparinized blood is centrifuged at 500 × g in a clinical centrifuge for 10 min (Fig. 1). Platelets are isolated from the plasma by centrifugation for 10 min at 1,200 ×

g. The plasma is saved for elution later in the procedure, and the platelet pellet is resuspended and washed two times in 0.1% gelatin, 0.3% EDTA, and 154 mM KCl (GEK; see below, Reagents). The blood cells are diluted with saline to a hematocrit of 20%, divided into three portions, and underlayered with approximately 2.0 ml of Hypaque-Ficoll (10 volumes of 34% Hypaque and 24 volumes of 9% Ficoll; density, 1.077 g/ml). After centrifugation for 40 min at 80 × g, the dense cloudy ring containing lymphocytes is aspirated; then the remaining neutrophil-rich layer is collected.

The red cell-contaminated, neutrophil-rich layer is diluted to 10.0 ml with GEK, and 2.0 ml of 2.0% methyl cellulose-15 in saline is added. After mixing, the red cells are allowed to sediment at a 45° angle for 20 min. The neutrophils and remaining red cells in the supernatant fluid are centrifuged to a pellet at 80 × g for 5 min. The pellet is suspended in 12.0 to 15.0 ml of 0.8% NH$_4$Cl-0.1% EDTA-Na$_3$, pH 7.0, for 10 min at room temperature to shock-lyse the residual erythrocytes. The neutrophils are reconcentrated and washed twice in GEK at 550 × g for 5 min.

The gradient-isolated lymphocytes are freed from contaminating erythrocytes when necessary by shock-lysis, resuspended in 2.0 to 3.0 ml of heparinized autologous plasma, and layered on a 3.5-inch (8.9-cm), 0.5-g washed nylon column. After elution with Barbitone buffer, the lymphocytes are collected and washed twice in GEK buffer at 550 × g for 5 min.

For the assay, the neutrophils and lymphocytes are diluted to a concentration of 20 × 10^6/ml in GEK containing a 1:10 dilution of human AB serum. Volumes of 1 μliter of the cell suspensions are added to microtest wells under oil to prevent evaporation. Samples of each preparation are smeared and stained with Wrights' stain to examine for contamination. Only prep-

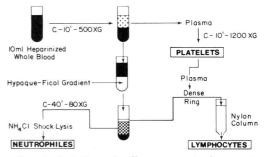

FIG. 1. *Isolation of cell components for use in capillary agglutination assay system. Sufficient numbers of all three cells for assay may be isolated from the same 10.0 ml of heparinized blood.*

arations exceeding 98% purity should be utilized.

The use of the GEK buffer appears to be a critical variable as determined in our studies. As published (9), quite reproducible results were consistently obtained employing the standard conditions with whole leukocytes, but it quickly became evident that isolated lymphocytes failed to form uniform streamers, and very thin irregular streamers frequently prevented accurate measurement. Purified neutrophils, on the other hand, performed as well as whole leukocytes but also suffered from the fate that in vitro storage for a few hours destroyed reproducibility. It was found that potassium concentration in the buffer was a critical determinant, and excellent lymphocyte as well as neutrophil streamers may be regularly achieved with the gelatin-EDTA buffer containing 154 mM KCl (see below, Reagents). Furthermore, cells stored in the cold for at least 24 h may be utilized after two or three washings in this buffer.

Serum

Experimental sera may be obtained from multiparous, renal transplant, platelet and granulocyte transfusion, and whole blood subjects. They are titered by capillary agglutination with whole leukocytes or the appropriate component, and the last dilution giving a maximally strong reaction is utilized. In each microtest plate, negative AB and positive heat-inactivated rabbit antihuman lymphocyte sera are included as controls. In addition, antineutrophil specific sera, i.e., anti-NA_1, -NA_2, -NB_1, etc., are frequently compared in addition to known HLA antiserum.

As a part of routine preoperative or precomponent transfusion screening, sera are obtained at approximately 2- to 3-month intervals or after known antigen challenge and are tested for lymphocytotoxic and capillary agglutinating antibody against a stable cell panel. Although we formerly utilized whole leukocytes as the capillary agglutination target cell, as indicated below, more information may be obtained by testing both isolated neutrophils and platelets. When a final cross-match is performed, not only the most current but also the earlier sera are retested against donor cells.

Postallograft specimens may also be obtained at regular intervals as well as during rejection and after transplant nephrectomy. Pre- and postoperative serological results may be compared with graft success, and we accept a stable serum creatinine of less than 2.0 mg/100 ml as evidence of good renal function.

Absorption of serum

Quantitative absorptions of some experimental and control antisera may be required to explore further the specificity of the reactions. Isolated neutrophils, lymphocytes, or platelets are incubated with heat-inactivated antisera at 37 C for 1 h, after which the sera are clarified by centrifugation at 10,000 $\times$ g for 5 min in a Fisher centrifuge, model 59. Generally, we absorb samples of control and experimental sera with three concentrations of lymphocytes and neutrophils, i.e., 6×10^6/ml, 3.3×10^6/ml, and 0.6×10^6/ml, and with 10×10^9 platelets/ml. Cells known to give both positive and negative reactions should be utilized for absorption, and test sera should be compared with unabsorbed negative control, undiluted experimental samples, and experimental samples diluted 1:2 to compensate for the maximal dilutional loss during absorption.

REAGENTS

The principal buffer utilized in the cell preparations (GEK) is prepared as follows. A 10-fold concentrate is prepared with 3.0 g of ethylenedinitrilotetraacetic acid-trisodium (EDTA-Na_3), 0.3 g of potassium phosphate (KH_2PO_4), 12.5 g of potassium chloride (KCl), and distilled water to 100 ml. The pH is adjusted to 7.0. Ten percent calf-skin gelatin (Eastman Organic Chemicals, Rochester, N.Y.) is prepared in distilled water and neutralized to pH 7.0 with potassium hydroxide (KOH). Prior to use, the concentrated buffer is diluted 10-fold, and 1:100 (vol/vol) of the 10% gelatin is added to yield a final concentration of 0.1% gelatin, 0.3% EDTA-Na_3, and 154 mM KCl.

Barbitone buffer is commercially available from Consolidated Laboratories, Chicago Heights, Ill.

The shock-lysis solution is prepared by adding 8.0 g of ammonium chloride (NH_4Cl), 1.0 g of EDTA-Na_3, and 0.1 g of KH_2PO_4 to 1.0 liter of distilled water. The pH is adjusted to 7.0 with KOH.

INTERPRETATION

Three and perhaps four characteristic patterns of capillary agglutination response to neutrophils and lymphocytes in conjunction with lymphocytotoxic reactions performed by the method of Amos et al. (1) have been observed.

First, positive responses with all capillary tests usually depict HLA reactions whether or not lymphocytotoxicity reactions are also positive (Table 1). Analysis of the specificity of these tests commonly may be correlated with

TABLE 1. *Comparison of the lymphocytotoxic and capillary agglutination responses with a "monospecific" HLA-A2 antiserum (FEH) and an unknown serum (HAU)*

Cell donor HLA	Antiserum							
	FEH (HLA-A2)				HAU (pretransplant)			
	CA[a]			CY[c]	CA[a]			CY[c]
	Le[b]	Ne[b]	Ly[b]		Le[b]	Ne[b]	Ly[b]	
2,3,7,15	4	4	4	8	4	4	4	—
2,1,7,17	3	4	4	8	4	4	4	—
2,11,7,5	3	4	4	8	4	4	4	—
2,3,7,12	3	4	4	8	4	3	4	—
2,19,W-10	4	4	4	8	4	3	4	—
2,11,12,18	4	4	4	8	3	4	4	—
2,9,W-5	2	4	4	8	1	1	4	—
2,28,8,W-5	4	4	4	8	4	4	4	—
19,7,12	—	—	—	—	—	—	—	—
3,28,7,27	—	—	—	—	—	—	—	—
19,14,15	—	—	—	—	—	—	4	—
3,28,7,27	—	—	—	—	—	—	—	—
19,14,15	—	—	—	—	—	—	—	—
9,10,5	—	—	—	—	—	—	—	—
9,8,12	—	—	—	—	—	—	—	—
28,29,12,7	—	—	4	—	—	—	—	—
1,9,8,5	2	—	4	—	—	—	—	—
9,10,18	—	—	4	—	—	—	—	—
1,28,12	—	—	4	—	—	—	—	—

[a] CA = capillary agglutination: 4 = no streamer, 100% agglutination; 3 = less than 10% of control; 2 = less than 25% of control; 1 = less than 50% of control.

[b] Le = CA with whole leukocytes; Ne = CA with isolated neutrophils; Ly = CA with isolated lymphocytes.

[c] CY = lymphocytotoxic test: 8 = 90 to 100% cells killed.

antigens of the first or second segregant series. The clinical importance of the neutrophil and lymphocyte capillary agglutination-positive, lymphocytotoxicity-negative reactions is suggested by their association with decreased renal transplant survival when detected in preoperative recipient sera. In this example an unknown pretransplant serum, HAU, that had been consistently negative in lymphocytotoxic tests and FEH, an excellent monospecific typing serum, reacted by capillary agglutination with whole leukocytes, neutrophils, and lymphocytes from every HLA-A2 cell donor. Subsequently, HAU received a graft mismatched for HLA-28, developed anti-HLA-A2 lymphocytotoxin as well as the capillary agglutinating antibody, and rejected the transplant within 21 days. Nearly all HLA antisera tested have demonstrated a similar pattern of reactivity. Furthermore, both capillary and cytotoxic reactions of these types of sera may be absorbed with neutrophils, lymphocytes, or platelets, a characteristic of the wide distribution of HLA antigens (Table 2).

Second, whole leukocyte and/or neutrophil capillary agglutination assays in conjunction with negative lymphocyte capillary or cytotoxic responses appear to distinguish neutrophil-specific non-HLA specificities. Table 3 illustrates characteristic reactions of two neutrophil-specific sera, PARKER and DeR. In view of the fact that only a few neutrophil agglutinating sera have been described (6, 7), and these were associated with isoimmune congenital neutropenia or febrile transfusion reactions, it was surprising to find this pattern so frequently in surveys of postpartum (8.4%) and pretransplant (22.4%) sera. We have begun to investigate several of these sera and find no correlation with the known neutrophil or HLA antigens when compared with unrelated cell panels or in family segregation studies. Absorption studies, however, indicate that platelets do not absorb the activity, but neutrophils completely absorb the activity, similar to neutrophil typing re-

TABLE 2. *Absorption of a monospecific typing serum with platelets, lymphocytes, and neutrophils from a positive donor*

Absorptions	Cell donors							
	CA[a]			CY[c]	CA[a]			CY[c]
	Le[b]	Ne[b]	Ly[b]		Le[b]	Ne[b]	Ly[b]	
Native serum	2	3	4	8	2	2	4	6
Native serum 1:2	2	3	4	2	2	4	4	6
Native serum 1:4	1	2	—	—	2	2	4	—
Native serum 1:8	—	—	—	—	—	—	—	—
Absorbed with 10 × 10⁹ platelets	2	—	—	—	2	—	—	—
6.0 × 10⁶ lymphocytes	—	—	—	—	2	—	—	—
6.0 × 10⁶ neutrophils	—	—	—	—	—	—	—	—

[a] CA = capillary agglutination: 4 = no streamer, 100% agglutination; 3 = less than 10% of control; 2 = less than 25% of control; 1 = less than 50% of control.

[b] Le = CA with whole leukocytes; Ne = CA with isolated neutrophils; Ly = CA with isolated lymphocytes.

[c] CY = lymphocytotoxic test: 8 = 90 to 100% cells killed; 6 = 60 to 90% killed; 2 = 20 to 30% killed.

TABLE 3. *Comparison of lymphocytotoxic and capillary agglutination responses with two neutrophil antisera*

Cell donor HLA	PARKER (NB1)				DeR (NA1)			
	CA[a]			CY[c]	CA[a]			CY[c]
	Le[b]	Ne[b]	Ly[b]		Le[b]	Ne[b]	Ly[b]	
9,10,5	4	4	−	−	4	4	−	−
2,1,7,17	3	4	−	−	2	4	−	−
2,9,W-5	3	4	−	−	1	4	−	−
1,28,12	4	4	−	−	2	4	−	−
3,28,7,27	3	3	−	−	4	4	−	−
2,3,7,12	3	3	−	−	4	4	−	−
19,14,15	−	3	−	−	−	3	−	−
28,29,12,27	−	−	−	−	2	4	−	−
2,19,W-10	4	4	−	−	4	4	2	−
2,11,12,18	3	3	−	−	4	4	4	−
9,10,18	−	−	−	−	4	4	4	−
1,9,8,5	4	2	−	−	−	−	−	−
19,7,12	1	4	−	−	−	−	−	−
2,11,5,7	3	4	−	−	−	−	−	−
2,3,7,15	4	4	−	−	−	−	−	−
9,8,12	4	2	−	−	−	−	−	−
2,28,8,W-5	−	−	−	−	−	−	−	−

[a] CA = capillary agglutination: 4 = no streamer, 100% agglutination; 3 = less than 10% of control; 2 = less than 25% of control; 1 = less than 50% of control.

[b] Le = CA with whole leukocytes; Ne = CA with isolated neutrophils; Ly = CA with isolated lymphocytes.

[c] CY = lymphocytotoxic test: 8 = 90 to 100% cells killed.

agents. We do not have any information at this time as to whether this emerging group of specificities detected by capillary agglutination will correspond to those recently demonstrated by granulocyte cytotoxicity (4). Although our data are clearly preliminary, capillary agglutinating neutrophil antibodies may or may not be associated with renal allograft failure, and their high incidence in pretransplant sera appears to be related to whole blood immunization.

Third, positive tests with isolated lymphocytes in the absence of any other reactions occur rather commonly, and many are correlated with HLA. The importance of identifying these reactions is demonstrated by WES (Table 4) and other similar observations correlating positive lymphocyte capillary responses with HLA, as in this case HLA-A1 and possibly W-24. This specimen was obtained after WES had rejected a kidney mismatched for HLA-A1 and B8, yet this and several subsequent samples failed to exhibit lymphocytotoxic reactions. Confirmation has been further provided by the fact that lymphocyte capillary agglutinating activity

may be absorbed by neutrophils, lymphocytes, or platelets comparable with HLA (2), but we have also observed reactions that do not correlate and are not absorbed by cells bearing known HLA antigens of the first and second segregant series. The incidence of the lymphocyte capillary agglutinating pattern was similar in the surveys of postpartum (11.6%) and pretransplant (12.2%) specimens, and it is important to note that these sera were otherwise negative by both lymphocytotoxicity and capillary agglutination with neutrophils or whole leukocytes.

The fourth pattern encompassing non-HLA lymphocytotoxicity-negative, capillary agglutination neutrophil- and lymphocyte-positive reactions has been observed with both transplant and postpartum sera as well as a 5b antiserum (16). A limited number of absorptions have been done, and the fact that neutrophils, lymphocytes, and platelets completely absorb the activity suggests that these sera may contain either polyspecific HLA or unrecognized non-HLA leukocyte antigens also present on the three cell types.

Therefore, on the basis of these collected observations, I believe that capillary agglutination with isolated cells may be a very useful cross-matching procedure prior to renal transplantation and an excellent tool for identifying neutrophil and other non-HLA antigens. These latter applications would appear to be of potentially great importance to matching for granulocyte transfusions (3, 5) and bone-marrow transplantation (11) and for the investiga-

TABLE 4. *Comparison of the lymphocytotoxic and capillary responses of a postrenal transplant serum*

Cell donor HLA	Antiserum WES[a]		
	CA[b]		CY[d]
	Ne[c]	Ly[c]	
1,26,13,W-10	−	4	−
1,19,8,14	−	4	−
1,11,12,y	−	4	−
1,11,5,12	−	4	−
1,3,5,y	−	4	−
1,31,8,W-10	−	4	−
1,30,15,W-10	4	4	−
9 (24), 7	1	4	−
9 (24),10,16,W-5	−	2	−
16 other donors[e]	−	−	−

[a] WES, serum donor HLA type: 3 + 7/x + W-10.

[b] CA = capillary agglutination: 4 = no streamer, 100% agglutination; 3 = less than 10% of control; 2 = less than 25% of control; 1 = less than 50% of control.

[c] Ne = CA with isolated neutrophils; Ly = CA with isolated lymphocytes.

[d] CY = lymphocytotoxicity.

tion and prevention of febrile transfusion reactions (12).

ACKNOWLEDGMENTS

This work was supported by the Veterans Administration and by Public Health Service grant AI 10593 from the National Institute of Allergy and Infectious Diseases.

LITERATURE CITED

1. Amos, D. B., H. Bashir, W. Boyle, M. MacQueen, and A. Tiilikainen. 1969. A simple microcytotoxicity test. Transplantation 7:220–223.
2. Cook, K. M. 1974. Distribution of HL-A antigens on blood cells. Tissue Antigens 4:202–209.
3. Graw, R. G., Jr., G. Hersiq, S. Peery, and E. S. Henderson. 1972. Normal granulocyte transfusion therapy: treatment of septicemia due to gram-negative bacteria. N. Engl. J. Med. 287:367–371.
4. Hasegawa, T., O. J. Bergh, R. R. Mickey, and P. I. Terasaki. 1975. Preliminary human granulocyte specificities. Transplant. Proc. 7:75–80.
5. Higby, D. J., J. W. Yates, E. S. Henderson, and J. F. Holland. 1975. Filtration leukopheresis for granulocyte transfusion therapy. N. Engl. J. Med. 292:761–766.
6. Lalezari, P., and G. E. Bernard. 1966. An isologous antigen-antibody reaction with human neutrophils, related to neonatal neutropenia. J. Clin. Invest. 45:1741–1750.
7. Lalezari, P., and E. Radel. 1974. Neutrophil-specific antigens: immunology and clinical significance. Semin. Hematol. 11:281–290.
8. Olson, L., J. Schleut, C. R. Stiller, and J. B. Dossetor. 1974. Comparison of cytotoxic and agglutinating antibodies in the sera of parous women. Transplantation 17:249–253.
9. Severson, C. D., N. A. Greazel, and J. S. Thompson. 1974. Micro-capillary agglutina-
tion. J. Immunol. Methods 4:369–380.
10. Stiller, C. R., L. Olson, J. Haystead, and J. B. Dossetor. 1972. The absence of early rejection crises in human renal allografts as predicted by capillary agglutinating antibodies. Transplantation 14:521–523.
11. Thomas, E. D., R. Storb, R. A. Clift, A. Fefer, F. L. Johnson, P. E. Neiman, K. G. Leiner, H. Glucksberg, and C. D. Buckner. 1975. Bone marrow transplantation. N. Engl. J. Med. 292:832–843, 895–902.
12. Thompson, J. S., D. Jackson, N. A. Greazel, M. J. Parmely, and C. D. Severson. 1976. Antileukocyte antibody in post partum and renal transplant subjects: a comparison of capillary agglutination and lymphocytotoxicity reactions. Transplantation 21:85–93.
13. Thompson, J. S., C. D. Severson, L. W. Coppleson, and G. Stokes. 1970. Leukocyte capillary agglutination: demonstration of additional leukocyte antibodies in cytotoxically "monospecific" antisera, p. 587–593. In P. I. Terasaki (ed.), Histocompatibility testing. Munksgaard, Copenhagen.
14. Thompson, J. S., C. D. Severson, A. R. Lavender, M. Forland, and H. P. Russe. 1968. Assay of human leukoagglutinins by capillary migration. Transplantation 6:728–736.
15. Thompson, J. S., C. D. Severson, M. J. Parmely, B. J. Marmorstein, and A. Simmons. 1971. Pulmonary "hypersensitivity" reactions induced by transfusion of non HL-A leukoagglutinins. N. Engl. J. Med. 284:1120–1125.
16. van Leeuwen, A., J. G. Eernise, and J. J. van Rood. 1964. A new leucocyte group with 2 alleles, leucocyte group 5. Vox Sang. 9:431–446.
17. Zmijewski, C. M. 1965. A critical analysis of the leukocyte agglutination reaction as applied to histocompatibility testing for human renal transplantation, p. 193–202. In D. B. Amos and J. J. van Rood (ed.), Histocompatibility testing. Munksgaard, Copenhagen.

Chapter 115

Prospective Immunodiagnosis of Allograft Rejection in Humans

BALDWIN H. TOM

INTRODUCTION

Assessment of the immune reactivity in humans to alloantigens is usually accomplished through in vitro testing. All of the commonly applied techniques were developed in experimental animal models (2) where the in vitro findings have correlated well with the clinical status of the animal host. In humans, unlike experimental systems, concordance between in vivo and in vitro results is often variable (3, 6, 20). The blastogenic, the cytotoxic. and the macrophage migration inhibition tests have been employed most often in the immunodiagnosis of renal allografted patients.

Of the three methods, the blastogenic test has been the least reliable. A proliferative response, signaled by an increased cellular incorporation of radiolabeled precursors, in the recipient's lymphocytes can be elicited by both specific and nonspecific antigens (5, 18). In practice, the stimulatory effects obtained in this manner have not been useful in evaluating the development of rejection crises. In fact, not only was spontaneous deoxyribonucleic acid synthesis often present in such lymphocyte populations (10) but also blastogenic activation derived from microbial infection (1).

Direct lymphocyte-dependent target cell cytotoxicity assays have been more successful. Cytotoxicity tests have been capable of detecting prior presensitization of cells in patients on dialysis to potential donor tissue (8). Cell-mediated cytotoxic tests have detected alloantigenic reactivities not detected by serological histocompatibility typing (26). Although some investigators have found that the cytotoxic action is directed against the serologically determined HLA antigens of the LA and FOUR series (9), evidence is available that immune events dictated by undefined regions outside of these loci also occur (14). Furthermore, many of these cytotoxic systems utilize lymphoid target cells which are readily susceptible to lysis, instead of the appropriate target type. When fibroblasts (15) and/or kidney cells (the relevant target in renal transplants) are employed, however, lymphocyte-mediated cytotoxicity is more difficult to demonstrate (unpublished data), requiring at least a 20-h reaction time.

The most widely applied in vitro technique and the most successful in humans has been the macrophage migration inhibition system. Interactions between immune lymphocytes and the sensitizing donor antigens generate the release of lymphokinetic mediators (lymphokines) from the blood cells. One of these moieties, migration inhibition factor (MIF), has the capacity to inhibit the egress of macrophages and other leukocytes from capillary tubes. The presence of immune cells in kidney transplant recipients demonstrated by the MIF assay preceded by several days overt clinical rejection (7, 25). In addition, MIF reactivity was found in the rejection of kidney isografts between HLA-identical siblings (24). Although this technique is capable of detecting sensitized lymphocytes in the recipient, its sensitivity to the loading and rejection therapy doses of immunosuppressive drugs creates a potential drawback to its immunodiagnostic worth.

Additional considerations dealing with the applicability of cell-mediated assays for clinical assessment of immunity have recently been reviewed (20).

CLINICAL INDICATIONS

Choice of an assay

The in vitro expression of cell-mediated immunities can be viewed as a dynamic continuum exhibiting at least three distinct facets (Table 1): recognition, activation, and performance. One of the primary considerations in selecting an in vitro assay for clinical use should be the time required for its performance. For optimal applicability in patient management, results should be available within a working day. Adding to the importance of using a short assay is the knowledge that, following immune cell *recognition* and adherence to the relevant target cell antigen(s), both specific and nonspecific factors are generated by the *activated* cell, causing ultimately an involvement of nonspecific cellular elements in the measured result

TABLE 1. *In vitro expression of cell-mediated immunity*[a]

Parameter	Recognition	Activation	Performance
Assessment	Adherence	Metabolic precursors	Cytodestruction
Temporal requirement	Minutes-hours	Hours-days	Days-days
Technique	Leukocyte aggregation	Blastogenesis	Cytotoxicity, MIF

[a] Following *recognition* and adherence of an immune cell to its eliciting antigen, the cell responds by increasing its synthetic processes (*activation*). This activated cell subsequently proceeds to *perform* its immunological duties in producing altered target cell function (macrophage migration inhibition, MIF) and in the cytodestruction of relevant targets. The specificity of reaction along this pathway decreases as the length of time required for expression of each event increases.

(*performance*). Virtually all of the available cell-mediated immune assays, including those described above, fall into the "activation" or "performance" categories. Thus, the recognition phase provides a logical focus for developing a new assay which is (i) rapidly performed, (ii) technically simple, (iii) immunologically specific, (iv) capable of reflecting serum effects on cellular immunity, and (v) conservative of patient materials.

The rationale for developing the leukocyte aggregation test (LAT) with the above characteristics has been discussed (13, 21, 22, 23) and was based on studies by investigators employing animal systems describing the necessity of specific immune cell contact and adhesion to target monolayers for subsequent target cell destruction. In previous reports (21, 23) the characteristics of the LAT, the cells involved, its proposed molecular mechanism, and its potential applications were described. This assay reflects recognition events initiated primarily by immune thymus-derived (T) lymphocytes with support from bone marrow-derived (B) lymphocytes. The result of these events is the discrete, focal production of leukocyte clusters (aggregates) possibly generated by: (i) the release of lymphokines from immune cells which cause the non-committed leukocytes to adhere; (ii) the local release of anti-target cell antibody, inducing leukocyte clumping; (iii) an induction by immune cells of a nucleation process (4) on target cells, conferring upon them an increased adhesive capacity for other cells; (iv) some other undefined cell surface change, following specific adherence, leading to the aggregation phenomenon; or (v) a combination of the above possibilities. The immune cells require physiological temperature, protein, and ribonucleic acid synthesis to function. This test utilizes donor-specific kidney targets cells, is insensitive to base line immunosuppression, and is amenable to serial immunodiagnostic testing.

The main difficulty in applying the LAT is the necessity for tissue culture methodology with its attendant problems. For example:

1. A library of kidney or skin fibroblast cells must be generated to provide panels of known HLA-bearing targets.

2. Since microbial cross-reactivities with HLA antigens exist, constant vigilance in aseptic handling of the cultured cells is required. Otherwise, in what would normally be a negative in vitro test finding, contaminating bacterial elements, co-mingled with target cells, may serve as reaction catalysts in interactions with immune cells or sera, thus engendering false-positive results. Routine maintenance doses of antimicrobial agents are recommended.

3. Finally, it is well established that prolonged maintenance of neoplastic cells in culture can produce antigenic changes resulting in cells differing in their tumorigenic and immunogenic capacities when retransplanted into the origin animal host. Although some experimental evidence suggests that human diploid cells retain their complement of HLA antigens throughout their in vitro lifespan, the possibility of undetectable, but relevant, antigenic alterations effected by extended in vitro cultivation could create difficulties in interpreting results. Therefore, only exponentially growing, early-passaged cells, rather than cells extensively passaged and approaching senescence, should be utilized.

Applications of the leukocyte aggregation test

In spite of any reservations concerning the employment of cultured target cells in this assay, the LAT has been demonstrated to be useful: (i) as a prospective indicator of rejection by detecting developing immune cell reactivity in the absence of any clinical or chemical signs of impending rejection (22); (ii) in differentiating between rejection and other causes of graft failure (13); (iii) in depicting the modulating effects of humoral factors on cellular reactivity (21); (iv) in detecting patient presensitization by identifying the HLA specificities with a battery of kidney targets; and (v) in predicting a patient's response to bolus methylprednisolone therapy (12). It should be noted that LAT results have not been used to dictate clinical practice, but only to clarify complex situations.

TEST PROCEDURES

Establishment of target cells

Kidney biopsy tissues are obtained as fresh surgical specimens, usually at time of transplant. Larger amounts of tissue may be obtained after nephrectomy of transplant or of recipient's nonfunctional kidney. Although the yield will be reduced, biopsy-sized tissue will still contain culturable cells after storage in culture medium at 4 C for 48 h.

The kidney capsule is removed with scissors and forceps and discarded; the tissue is minced into 2- to 3-mm³ pieces and rinsed free from serum three times by gravity sedimentation in minimal essential medium (MEM) without serum. After a final 5-min centrifugation (100 × g; all procedures are performed at ambient temperature) to collect the pieces, they are resuspended in 0.25% trypsin-Hanks balanced salt solution (HBSS) in a stirred trypsinizing flask (usually with two magnets for stirring) for at least five sequential treatments (20 to 30 min, 37 C), or until all the tissue pieces have been completely digested. The best cell yields have usually been from the later trypsinizations. Kidney cells dispersed at each interval are collected in centrifuge tubes by decanting the cell suspension through a double layer of sterile gauze to hold back tissue debris, adding fetal calf serum (10 or 20%) to neutralize trypsin, and recovering cells by centrifugation (270 × g, 5 min). The cells are suspended in MEM 20 (MEM with 20% fetal calf serum) and cultured in 30- or 250-ml plastic culture flasks, depending on the amount of tissue cells obtained. When in doubt, it is better to overseed than underseed a flask. The flasks are incubated at 37 C in 5% CO_2 with humidified air. At 24 h, nonadherent cells from all flasks are pooled, collected, and reseeded with MEM 20 into a new 250-ml flask. The original flasks are refed with fresh MEM at 24 and 48 h to remove debris, and thereafter with 2/3 fresh MEM 20 when necessary. MEM 10 is used after the kidney cells have become established. Cell monolayers are trypsinized for passage, as described below. Although cells can be used in an assay as early as 48 h after initiation of the culture, this procedure will deplete the cells from one flask and, unless several starter flasks were prepared, may sacrifice the entire stock.

Skin fibroblast cultures are obtained by the outgrowth of cells from skin pieces adhering to the surface of plastic culture flasks. Skin biopsies are cleared of subcutaneous tissue, minced into 1- to 3-mm³ pieces, and planted onto the wetted surface of a 30-ml flask. Excess media are removed from around the skin pieces, and the tightly capped flasks are incubated standing on end for 6 to 20 h at 37 C to permit firm adherence. MEM 20 is then added, and the flasks are returned for incubation in the normal position. The culture is refed with 2/3 fresh MEM 20 as needed. After about 3 weeks, the emerging fibroblast cells are ready for use.

Frozen storage of cultured cells

Cultured cells are obtained for frozen storage by treating exponentially growing monolayers (approaching confluency) with an initial rinse and then with 0.1% trypsin diluted in 0.02% ethylenediaminetetraacetic acid (EDTA) for 15 min at 37 C. For passage, a 1:2 or 1:3 split is made from each flask, i.e., seeding into two or three new flasks. The original flask is often used or retained as a backup since some cells will remain in this flask after trypsinization. Detached cells are collected in MEM 20 by centrifugation (270 × g, 10 min), resuspended in a cold freeze preservative consisting of 10% dimethylsulfoxide in MEM 20 (about 2 × 10⁶ cells in 1 ml), and dispensed into 2-ml plastic screw-cap vials. Since greater than 1% dimethylsulfoxide is toxic to cells, all processing is performed with cold reagents and the vials are kept on ice. The cell suspensions are frozen at a rate of 1 C per min to −50 C and then are stored under liquid nitrogen (Linde LR-30 refrigerator). Cells are recovered from the frozen state by rapid thawing in a 37 C water bath, suspended to 15 ml with cold MEM 20, and centrifuged at ambient temperature (300 × g for 10 min). The cells from one vial are resuspended in MEM 20, counted with trypan blue, and seeded into a 30-ml flask for culturing.

Preparation of target monolayers in microtiter trays

Exponentially growing cells are collected by trypsinization, counted, and seeded into microtiter wells. Routinely, 8,000 kidney or 3,000 skin target cells are plated in 0.2 ml of MEM 20, sufficient to establish a 75% confluent monolayer at 24 h. To prepare desired target monolayers for other time periods, alter the inocula (details in 22). In the complete test, five cell targets are used: (i) from the kidney donor, (ii) from another patient possessing the same incompatible HLA antigens as between donor and recipient, (iii) from an individual with cell antigens serologically cross-reactive with the disparate antigens (16, 17), (iv) from an HLA unrelated individual, and (v) from the allograft recipient.

The initial test, employing only two targets (donor and non-cross-reactive), is usually performed between 7 and 10 days post-transplant to detect possible early evidence of cellular immune activity, such as signaling of an impending accelerated-type rejection. If this first test is negative, further serial screening tests are performed with cells from other individuals (rather than the donor) bearing the disparate antigens in order to conserve donor cells. Once evidence of cellular reactivity is presented, then the complete battery of targets, including the donor, is employed.

Preparation of leukocytes and sera for test

Peripheral blood is obtained by venipuncture from test individuals. A minimum of 5 ml of heparinized blood (for leukocytes, 10 units of heparin/ml) and 5 ml of nonheparinized blood (for sera) is drawn. Serum is heated at 56 C for 30 min before use. Leukocytes are obtained by sedimenting erythrocytes in plasmagel, mixing 10 to 15% (vol/vol) plasmagel in blood, and incubating for 30 to 45 min at 37 C. This sedimentation is best accomplished in an upright 10-ml syringe taped to the inside of an incubator. After incubation, the upper gradient of leukocyte-rich plasma can be directly expressed through a clean bent 18-gauge needle (3.8 cm) into a centrifuge tube. Gross erythrocyte contamination will block leukocyte contact with the kidney cell target. Therefore, it is better to sacrifice leukocyte yields by longer sedimentation of erythrocytes in the plasmagel than to rush the collection. Although ammonium chloride lysis of red cells did not appear to affect the leukocytes, we have routinely avoided this step for fear of producing subtle surface changes altering leukocyte reactivity. Leukocytes are washed twice in MEM 10, counted, and diluted in MEM 10 to 400,000 cells/0.2 ml. When Roswell Park Memorial Institute 1640 was substituted as the incubation medium in the assay, large numbers of nonspecific leukocyte clusters appeared. No other media have been tested.

Assay and evaluation of results

Target cell monolayers are drained and rinsed free from nonadherent cells. Whenever available, kidney cells are utilized in preference over skin fibroblasts. Test leukocytes (400,000 cells in 0.2 ml of MEM 10) are added to the drained target wells and allowed to react at 37 C for 5 h in a humidified CO_2 incubator. Effects of serum factors are determined by preincubation of 0.05 ml of heat-inactivated serum directly on the target monolayers for 15 min at 37 C. Test leukocytes are then added and co-incubated for the 5-h reaction period. Spontaneous aggregation of leukocytes with or without serum is evaluated by adding them directly to empty wells. All experimental and control combinations are performed in duplicate. After incubation, wells are rinsed free from nonadherent leukocytes with warmed MEM. Rinsing is accomplished by flipping media out of the wells and then running MEM into the wells through a 5-ml pipette three to five times, or until no cells are seen floating in the leukocyte control wells. After the final rinse, a small amount (about 0.1 ml) of fresh medium is added to each well.

The results are visualized under $150\times$ magnification on an inverted microscope with the use of bright-field objectives (Fig. 1). Aggregates viewed under phase microscopy do not appear as distinct. Scoring is based on the total number of $150\times$ fields exhibiting more than 5 leukocyte-target aggregates, each of which contains at least 10 adherent leukocytes in the cluster. For example, if it requires viewing 10 fields to completely evaluate a microtiter well, then the presence of 5 positive fields (i.e., each field exhibiting at least 5 leukocyte-target aggregates) is scored as 50% aggregation. The reactions are evaluated and scored in the following order: (i) target cells alone, to be certain that the targets have not become toxic or dislodged during the various manipulations; (ii) leukocyte and leukocyte plus serum controls; (iii) test leukocytes on targets; and (iv) serum plus leukocytes on targets. Two or three individuals independently score each test. Spontaneous aggregation scores are subtracted from the experimental values. Each pair of results is averaged, as are the results of each individual scorer.

MATERIALS AND EQUIPMENT

Culturing target cells

Kidney tissue: biopsy, $1 \times 0.5 \times 0.5$ cm
Skin tissue: biopsy, 0.2×1.0 cm

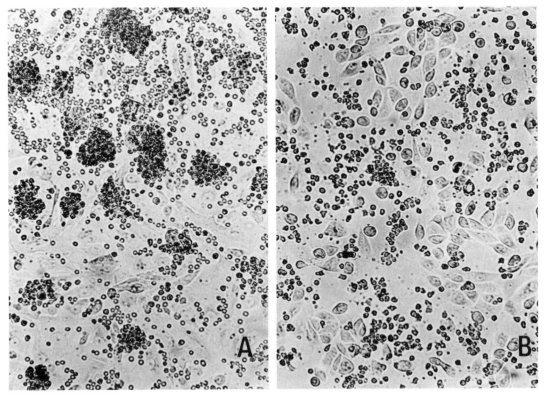

FIG. 1. *Leukocyte aggregation results.* (A) *Immune leukocytes form characteristic aggregates of cells in reaction on targets with donor-specific antigens;* (B) *in a negative reaction, immune leukocytes are evenly dispersed over nonspecific target control cells and form infrequent aggregates. From Tom et al. (22).*

Scissors: 5.5 or 4 inch, straight or curved (Signet)

Forceps: splinter forceps (Signet)

Petri dishes: 100 × 15 mm, plastic, disposable (Falcon #1029)

Centrifuge tubes: conical, heavy duty, screw cap, Pyrex brand, 40-ml size (Corning #8122)

Pasteur pipettes: 9-inch length (Scientific Products diSPo transfer pipettes)

Culture medium: MEM, pH 7.3 (Grand Island Biological Co.); minimal essential medium (Eagle) with Hanks salts (with glutamine and nonessential amino acids, and sodium bicarbonate), plus 100 units of penicillin/ml, 50 μg of streptomycin/ml, and 10 or 20% heat-inactivated (56 C for 30 min) fetal calf serum (MEM 10 = 10%; MEM 20 = 20%)

Trypsin: Grand Island Biological Co. stock 2.5% (1:250) in normal saline; diluted 1:10 (0.25%) in HBSS (Grand Island Biological Co.) for primary culture or 1:25 (0.1%) in EDTA solution (0.02%, wt/vol) for dispersing established monolayers

For 1 liter of 10× EDTA buffer solution:

NaCl . . . . 80.0 g

KCl . . . . 4.5 g

EDTA, $Na_2C_{10}H_{14}N_2O_8 \cdot 2H_2O$ (diaminoethanetetraacetic acid, disodium salt) . . . . 2.0 g

Dissolve ingredients in distilled water to 1 liter. Adjust pH to 7.3 with 7.5% $NaHCO_3$ (about 5 ml of bicarbonate for each 100 ml). Thus 10× EDTA can be sterilized by filtration through a Nalge #120 disposable filter unit (0.20-μm plain membrane, Sybron Corp., Rochester, N.Y.), or a 1× solution can be sterilized by autoclaving.

Trypsinizing flasks: 35, 75, or 150 ml (Bellco #1994)

Stirring bars, magnetic: 0.5 to 1 inch in length (Bellco #1975)

Magnetic stirrer, nonheating: Bellco #7760-06003

Tissue culture flasks: 30 or 250 ml, plastic (Falcon #3013 or #3024)

Frozen storage of target cells

Culture medium: MEM 20

Preservative: dimethylsulfoxide (Fisher D-128), 10% in MEM with 20% fetal calf serum

Pasteur pipettes

Storage vials: plastic, 2-ml serum tubes (38 × 12.5 mm, Vangard International #1076-01, Nunc tubes, Red Bank, N.J., or Microbiological Associates, Pro-Vial #18-351)

Canes for holding vials: aluminum canes for holding six ampoules (1.0 ml); Shur-Bend Mfg. Co., Inc. #A, North Minneapolis, Minn.

Liquid nitrogen refrigerator: Union Carbide #LR-30; liquid nitrogen controlled freezing cone, Linde #BF 5 (Union Carbide), or the Linde BF-4 automatic temperature controlled biological freezing system

Seeding targets on microtiter plate

Trypsin/EDTA: 0.1% trypsin/0.02% EDTA

Pipettes: serological pipettes (Bellco #1210)

Hemacytometer: Spot Lite hemacytometer counting chamber (Scientific Products #B3175)

Inverted microscope: Nikon model MS

Microtest II/Tissue Culture Plate, Falcon #3040; lid for plate, Falcon #3041

Humidified CO_2 incubator

Obtaining leukocytes and sera

Venipuncture materials: B-D Plastikpak disposable syringe, 10 cc (American Hospital Supply #15268-OOX); multiple sample needles, 20G × 1.5 inch (Scientific Products #B3033-2); Bandquet tourniquet, adult (Scientific Products #B3060-1); Vacutainer, red, 10 ml (Scientific Products #B2985-4A); alcohol swabs (Scientific Products #B3062); holder, Vacutainer (Scientific Products #B3023-110); B-D Yale disposable needles, 18G × 1.5 inch (Scientific Products #16274-18J)

Heparin: Sodium Heparin USP aqueous Lipo-Hepin, 1,000 units/ml with 0.9% benzoyl alcohol preservative (Riker Laboratories, Northridge, Calif.)

Plasmagel: Associated Biomedic Systems, Buffalo, N.Y.

Centrifuge tubes, serological pipettes

Addition of leukocytes to plated targets

Serological pipettes: 1 ml

Medium: MEM 10

White blood cell diluting pipettes: Tri-Lyne Accupette pipettes (Scientific Products #B4030-2)

Trypan blue stain: 0.4%, Grand Island Biological Co. #525

Observation of results

Culture media for rinsing plate, serological pipette, inverted microscope

INTERPRETATION

In the evaluation of 1,124 LAT results from 55 patients (manuscript in preparation), the range of false-positive results was between 3 and 10% aggregation; false-negative results were about 35% in patients experiencing chronic or acute rejection and 73% in patients with accelerated rejection. The latter results may reflect an inability of the test to detect immune cell activity in what is considered to be effected predominantly by an antibody-mediated mechanism. Since in vitro assays can become negative during rejection episodes, as discussed below, establishing a meaningful value for false-negative results may not be possible. The ability of the LAT to detect immunological activity is illustrated in the results from seven patients (Table 2). Positive immune cell activity was revealed by the LAT as early as 15 days preceding a clinical rejection. Immunological evidence for rejection in patients 183, 190, and 195 might have been obtained sooner had the tests been performed at earlier times preceding the crises. The specificity of the assay is retained in each host-target combination, except in patients 183 and 195. As described below, nonspecific reactivity may occur during the period of clinical rejection and may become apparent within 2 days preceding rejection, as exhibited in these two patients.

In the event of a rejection episode, distinct patterns of LAT emerge (Fig. 2). The development of immune cells after transplantation can be detected by this assay. Although discrimination of allograft immunity in the acute rather than the hyperacute, accelerated, or chronic rejection setting is most readily revealed by the LAT, LAT results seem to correlate with the response of the patient to bolus therapy rather than type of rejection (12). Generally, LAT reactivity toward donor-specific target cells occurs first, followed by reactivity onto other targets bearing disparate antigens or those cross-reactive with the disparate ones. At peak rejection, LAT activity directed toward donor targets is reduced, or abolished, whereas reactions on targets with disparate and/or cross-reactive antigens persist. In addition, nonspecific reactivity is demonstrated during this period, indicating a significant amount of cellu-

TABLE 2. *Cellular immunity preceding clinical rejection*[a]

Days before rejection	Patient no.	Patient HLA	Donor HLA	Target	Percent aggregation
15	189	A1, A11; B7, B8	A1, *A9*; B8, —[b]	Donor	31
				A9, A11; B7, BW5	0
				A11, —; BW35, B14	0
				A1, A2; B12, —	0
12	199	A2, A9; B7, B12	2, —; 12, *W27*	Donor	50
				A3, A11; B12, BW40	0
				A1, A2; BW17, —	0
				A2, A3; B7, BW15	0
				A2, —; B5, B7	0
8	185	A2, A3; BW40, BW15	*3, 9; 7, 8*	Donor	67
				A2, AW32; *B8*, BW27	50
				A2, A11; BW35, BW15	0
				A2, A3; BW40, BW15	0
6	194	A2, A3; B12, B13	*1*, 2; *8, W18*	Donor	31
				A3, **A9**; B7, *B8*	10
				A3, A11; BW40, B12	0
				A2, A3; B12, B13	0
4[c]	190	A2, A9; B12, BW22	*1*, 2; 12, —	Donor	50
				A1, B9; B8, —	46
				A11, —; BW35, BW14	0
2[c]	183	A2, AW28; BW17, BW18	2, W28; *W14* *W27*	A1, AW30; *B14*, —	50
				A2, AW32; B8, *B27*	25
				A2, A11; BW35, BW15	75
				A9, A10; BW35, BW15	50
				A11, AW19; BW35, —	0
2[c]	195	A2, —; B7, B12	2, *W19; W10*, —	Donor	67
				A1, A2; B8, B18	25
				A1, A2; B13, B18	0
				A2, A3; B12, B13	0

[a] Table adapted from Kahan et al. (13).

[b] The italicized antigens were disparate between donor and host; the boldface antigens are those that cross-react with disparate antigens. According to the 1975 WHO Committee on leukocyte nomenclature (P. I. Terasaki, personal communication), the designation for the previous first locus LA antigens will be locus A and written A1, A2, etc., whereas the second, or FOUR, locus will be locus B, with antigen specificities B5, B7, etc. The third locus will now be called locus C, and the former LD, MLC-1 locus will be called locus D. HLA without the hyphen will now refer to the entire histocompatibility antigen complex.

[c] Tests had not been done before this date.

lar activation associated with graft rejection which appears nonimmunological. Immediately following the reversal of rejection by drugs and local irradiation of the graft, existing LAT values remain positive and cellular reactivity on donor targets reappears. As renal function improves and returns to pre-rejection levels, LAT reactions fall to zero. These same patterns of differential cellular immune activity as revealed by the LAT assay and associated with rejection have also been described with the mixed lym-

phocyte culture (MLC) technique (11, 24). This loss of donor-specific cells from the peripheral circulation during rejection crises has been explained by the sequestering of the reactive cells in the rejecting kidney (11). Direct evidence supporting this hypothesis comes from the recovery of cytotoxic (19), MLC (11), and lymphokine-releasing (11) cells from the rejected organ. In one study (19), the cells recovered were identified as T cells and non-T cells bearing Fc receptors. The finding that at

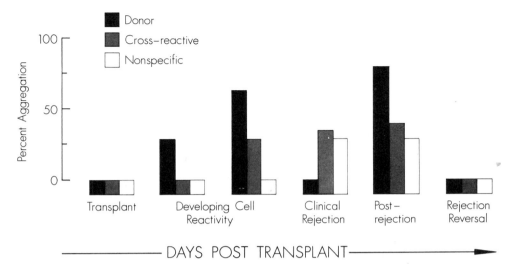

FIG. 2. *Leukocyte aggregation test (LAT) reactions produced during the course of a rejection episode exhibit at least five patterns. Following transplantation, no cellular activity is detectable. In the event of a developing rejection, cellular immune activity increases. During rejection, LAT results on donor targets become negative, and nonspecific leukocyte aggregation is also exhibited. After reversal of rejection, LAT results are positive for all targets but eventually return to zero.*

least 50% of the cells were Fc-bearing suggested that a large number of the recovered cells may be cytotoxic through an antibody-dependent mechanism. This possibility is supported by studies in the LAT system where 50% of LAT reactivity could be reduced by pretreating the immune cell population with goat antihuman immunoglobulin plus complement, indicating that a large population of immunoglobulin-bearing cells contributes to the test results (21).

Although the nature and mechanism by which antibodies modulate cell reactivity in the transplant recipient is not known, the LAT assay has provided data illustrating a differential suppressive or augmenting effect of serum on the in vitro cellular reactions (Fig. 3). During the period following transplantation when kidney function is improving, the addition of autologous serum to the LAT decreases any cellular activity. This antagonistic effect of serum was never associated with rejection, even when the leukocytes alone displayed marked reactions. Contrarily, host serum which possessed positive synergism with immune leukocytes always forecasted a reduction in renal capacity, often leading to clinical rejection. During periods of stable renal function, serum had no effect on the LAT. It is thus important to perform tests in the presence of host serum, especially when the patient is extensively presensitized.

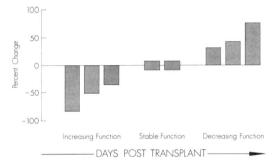

FIG. 3. *Effect of autologous serum on the leukocyte aggregation test (LAT) in engrafted host. Addition of autologous serum to the LAT either decreases the percent LAT activity during the period when kidney function is improving or increases the LAT values when kidney function exhibits deterioration, when compared with reactions by cells alone. Serum has no effect on the LAT when kidney function is stable.*

In summary, the LAT provides a useful adjunct to the prospective immunodiagnosis of allograft rejection in humans. Not only does the LAT detect specific immune activation of host cells, but also it discriminates between rejection and other causes of graft failure. The capacity of the LAT to detect cellular reactivity in the face of uneventful kidney function, coupled with its ability to reflect modulating effects of serum factors, provides the chemotherapist a potentially powerful tool for developing efficacious applications of immunosuppressive drugs. However, given the complexities and dynamics of the immune system operating in the altered environment of the immunosuppressed host, it would be naive to suppose that a single technique could be capable of detecting all the relevant in vivo factors attending allograft rejection. Therefore, additional in vitro tests, such as the macrophage migration inhibition assay and some others described in this *Manual*, should be included to provide a battery of immunological tests. In this manner, definitive prospective diagnoses of allograft rejection may be obtained.

ACKNOWLEDGMENTS

I acknowledge the support of Barry D. Kahan during the course of these studies, including his introducing me to the problems attending surgical immunology, and of Kamal K. Mittal, who provided the HLA evaluations. The excellent technical assistance of Milda M. Jakstys, Li O. Huang, and Ae Za Lee, and the secretarial assistance of Dorothy Shelangoski are also duly noted.

LITERATURE CITED

1. Barnes, R. M. R., G. P. Pegrum, G. B. Williams, E. M. Gordon, and H. D. deWardener. 1974. Assessment of human renal transplantation. Lancet 2:1040–1044.
2. Bloom, B. R., and P. Glade (ed.). 1971. *In vitro* methods in cell-mediated immunity. Academic Press Inc., New York.
3. Bloom, B. R., M. Landy, and H. S. Lawrence. 1973. *In vitro* methods in cell-mediated immunity: a progress report. Cell. Immunol. 6:331–347.
4. Chipowsky, S., Y. C. Lee, and S. Roseman. 1973. Adhesion of cultured fibroblasts to insoluble analogues of cell-surface carbohydrates. Proc. Natl. Acad. Sci. U.S.A. 70:2309–2312.
5. Copeland, D., A. Rashid, T. Steward, and J. Harris. 1974. The use of *in vitro* lymphocyte responsiveness to specific mitogenic agents in the immunological monitoring of human renal allograft recipients. Tissue Antigens 4:106–114.
6. David, J. R. 1973. Lymphocyte mediators and cellular hypersensitivity. N. Engl. J. Med. 288:143–149.
7. Falk, R. E., R. D. Guttman, J. A. Falk, J. G. Beaudoin, G. Deveber, D. D. Morehouse, and D. R. Wilson. 1973. Assessment of the cellular immune response to HL-A antigens in human renal allograft recipients. Clin. Exp. Immunol. 14:47–56.
8. Garovoy, M. R., D. Zschaeck, T. B. Strom, V. Franco, C. B. Carpenter, and J. P. Merrill. 1973. Direct lymphocyte-mediated cytotoxicity as an assay of presensitisation. Lancet 1:573–576.
9. Grunnet, N., T. Kristenson, F. Jørgensen, and F.

10. Hall, J. G. 1969. Spontaneous lymphocyte blastogenesis after transplantation. Lancet 1:25–28.
11. Hattler, B. G., Jr., R. E. Rocklin, P. A. Ward, and F. R. Rickles. 1973. Functional features of lymphocytes recovered from a human renal allograft. Cell. Immunol. 9:289–296.
12. Kahan, B. D., F. Krumlovsky, P. Ivanovitch, J. Greenwald, C. Firlit, J. Bergan, and B. H. Tom. 1975. The leukocyte aggregation test: immunodiagnostic applications and immunotherapeutic implications for clinical renal transplantation. Arch. Surg. (Chicago) 110:984–990.
13. Kahan, B. D., K. K. Mittal, B. H. Tom, and J. J. Bergan. 1974. Immunodiagnostic test for transplant rejection. Lancet 1:37–42.
14. Kristenson, T., N. Grunnet, and F. Kissmeyer-Nielsen. 1974. Cell-mediated lympholysis in man. Occurrence of unexpected, HL-A (LA and FOUR) irrelevant lympholysis. Tissue Antigens 4:378–382.
15. Lundgren, G., E. Möller, and E. Thorsby. 1970. *In vitro* cytotoxicity by human lymphocytes from individuals immunized against histocompatibility antigens. Clin. Exp. Immunol. 6:671–680.
16. Mittal, K. K., and P. I. Terasaki. 1974. Crossreactivity in the HL-A system. Tissue Antigens 2:94–104.
17. Mittal, K. K., and P. I. Terasaki. 1974. Serological cross-reactivity in the HL-A system. Tissue Antigens 4:146–156.
18. Sengar, D. P. S., A. Rashid, and J. E. Harris. 1974. *In vitro* cellular immunity and *in vivo* delayed hypersensitivity in uremic patients maintained on hemodialysis. Int. Arch. Allergy 47:829–838.
19. Strom, T. B., N. L. Tilney, C. B. Carpenter, and G. J. Busch. 1975. Identity and cytotoxic capacity of cells infiltrating renal allografts. N. Engl. J. Med. 292:1257–1263.
20. Tom, B. H. 1975. Cell-mediated immunity: mechanisms, assays and clinical considerations, p. 3–31. *In* A. Mathieu and B. D. Kahan (ed.), Immunological aspects of anesthetic and surgical practice. Grune and Stratton, Inc., New York.
21. Tom, B. H., L. O. Huang, M. M. Jakstys, and B. D. Kahan. 1975. Characteristics of the leukocyte aggregation assay for cell-mediated immunity. Clin. Exp. Immunol. 20:131–141.
22. Tom, B. H., M. M. Jakstys, and B. D. Kahan. 1974. Leukocyte aggregation: an *in vitro* assay for cell-mediated immunity. J. Immunol. 113:1288–1295.
23. Tom, B. H., and B. D. Kahan. 1976. Leukocyte aggregation test for evaluating cell-mediated immunity. Clin. Immunobiol., in press.
24. Turnipseed, W. D., M. R. Folger, and J. Cerilli. 1974. A study of cellular immune response in

HL-A identical renal transplant recipients. Transplantation 17:341–345.

25. Wood, R. F. M., A. C. Gray, J. D. Briggs, and P. R. F. Bell. 1973. The prediction of acute rejection in human renal transplantation using the leukocyte migration test. Transplantation 17:41–45.

26. Wunderlich, J. R., G. N. Rogentine, Jr., and R. A. Yankee. 1972. Rapid *in vitro* detection of cellular immunity in man against freshly explanted allogeneic cells. Transplantation 13:31–37.

Chapter 116

An Interpretation of the Major Histocompatibility Complex

D. B. AMOS

In the various chapters of this section are assembled detailed accounts of a number of procedures that have been found useful in histocompatibility testing. Note that certain tests have not been included, not because they are unimportant, but because they are not applicable to routine testing or because they are too new to have received an adequate evaluation for their specificity. It is the purpose of this chapter to review the various components of the HLA genetic complex and to attempt to interpret the way in which they contribute to immunogenicity and immune responsiveness.

From skin grafts between family members differing at neither, one, or both haplotypes, we know that the HLA complex includes the components of a very potent transplantation system. We know also that HLA differences stimulate lymphocyte proliferation in vitro and in vivo, result in the formation of antibodies against HLA and against bone marrow-derived (B) and thymus-derived (T) lymphocytes as well as those antibodies best detected in lymphocyte-dependent antibody-mediated cytotoxicity (LDA) or in mixed lymphocyte reaction (MLR) blocking, and may also lead to the production of cytotoxic lymphocytes. However, we still do not know how immunity is induced in the transplant recipient. Immunization could, for example, result from the release of subcellular fractions from the transplant following damage during ischemia, or it could result from an efflux of passenger lymphocytes and macrophages or even from detached vascular epithelial cells; alternatively, host macrophages and helper lymphocytes entering the graft could be activated. Better knowledge of the initiating events could perhaps aid the pharmacologist and the immunogist in their attempts to reduce the intensity of the initial response.

Similarly, we know that some of the components of the major histocompatibility complex are highly immunogenic, but we do not know which of them contributes most to the response. A measure of the variability in immunogenicity is provided by skin graft survival across a single haplotype barrier. Some single haplotype differences are associated with rejection times as short as 7 days; other grafts differing at a well-identified haplotype may persist for as long as 30 days (35). The differences do not appear to be correlated with any particular HLA specificity and, although there is still some controversy on this point, do not have a simple correlation with the degree of MLR stimulation. A similar situation has recently been reported in the dog. Rapaport and his collegaues have observed that transplants between dogs of the Cooperstown colony, having the same DLA phenotype, are sometimes accepted and sometimes rejected (26). By tracing the pedigrees back to the 17 founder dogs, they could assign haplotypes to common or to different ancestry. Some of the original haplotypes were histocompatible, others, though they carried the same DLA markers, were histoincompatible. Rapaport ascribed the difference to a locus, detectable only by transplantation, which he called DhR, to denote a similarity to the HDR locus postulated by Yunis and Amos (37). HDR and DhR appear to be genetic loci responsible for the stimulation of strong cytotoxic responses.

A similar locus appears to lie near the K region in the mouse H-2 complex. First noted in the mutant H-2ab haplotype detected by Bailey (2), the mutant differs from the original C57 haplotype in inducing skin graft rejection, stimulation in MLR, especially in presensitized animals, and in the generation of cytotoxic lymphocytes (8). Any serological difference appears to be quantitative rather than qualitative (17). The locus appears to be hypermutable, as no less than eight independent mutations appear to map in the same position (18).

As in the Cooperstown dogs, exactly identical haplotypes appear to be present in the random Caucasian population. Although the majority of unrelated pairs stimulate in MLR regardless of their HLA types, occasional pairs who are phenotypically identical are MLR negative and also give prolonged skin graft survival in the absence of known consanguinity (19). In the mouse, Hammerberg and Klein have found phenotypically identical haplotypes in several stocks descended from wild progenitors (13). These animals are remarkable in two respects.

They carry antigens absent from laboratory stocks, and haplotypes carrying the same H-2 markers fall into the same T locus complementation groups, suggesting that a very long segment of the chromosome is constant. The T complex, which is some 17 crossover units from H-2, is involved in embryonic and fetal development (5). Many forms of T locus mutant found in the wild are deleterious and may be lethal or semilethal in the homozygous form. The finding of the same rare H-2 specificity in conjunction with the same T configuration in animals trapped as far apart as Denmark and the United States and at considerable time separation is very striking and suggests that the components of the haplotype form an interacting unit important in development and in biological defense (4). The mouse data imply extreme linkage disequilibrium. The T and H-2 genes are so far apart on the chromosome that they should be separated from each other and enter into new combinations within a few generations. One can infer that they have remained in a stable configuration for at least several hundred generations. Linkage disequilibrium is very common within the HLA region. However, the maintenance of linkage disequilibrium may be different in the two situations. Amos et al. found that recombination was very frequent between HLA-A1 and B-8, two antigens in linkage disequilibrium in all northern Caucasians (1), whereas recombination between T and H-2 is suppressed by many t^w alleles (16). The possible selective advantage of certain HLA (and H-2) haplotypes remains a subject for intensive investigation.

I shall now review the individual components of the system and give an indication of what their biological role may be. The most conspicuous elements of the HLA system are the HLA and HLA-B determinants. The antigenic product is probably a dipeptide since it contains two disulfide bonds. The molecule carries specific sites for the subtypic antibodies such as HLA-A1 or HLA-B8; it also appears to carry sites for supertypic sites such as 4a. Sequencing of the molecule is in progress, and 3 amino acids of the first 19 at the N terminal end are known to be variable between the A and B locus products; of the remaining amino acids, 14 are constant and 2 have not been resolved at the time of writing (31). From earlier studies, the hydrophilic portion of the H-2 or HLA molecule, as released by proteolytic enzymes or hydrolysis, does not appear to be very immunogenic, but there is little information on detergent-solubilized material and no information as to how the tertiary or quarternary structure of

the molecule, when on the living cell, affects immunogenicity.

We still do not know the nature of the target site on the cell for cytotoxic lymphocytes, whether it is HLA alone, or HLA plus other surface features controlled by HLA region-genes, or whether HLA is largely irrelevant and the activities of genes such as HDR are primarily involved in controlling the target site. However, the HLA or H-2 antigen does appear to be intimately involved in cellular reactions against the target tissue cell. Anti-β_2-microglobulin and anti-HLA antibodies all block many cellular reactions, as do many sera directed against B cell antigens—i.e., antibodies not directed at the HLA molecule itself. Further, the target function or the ability to stimulate in MLR is lost when the cell dies, even though HLA or H-2 antigenicity (in terms of the ability of the antibody to bind) remains. Thus, either the structure of the HLA or H-2 molecule confers its biological activity on the living cell, or HLA or H-2 forms part of a biologically active macromolecular complex which would then appear to be the cell surface feature we associate with HDR.

From genetic studies, the HLA-D locus is known to be separate from the HLA-A and HLA-B loci (25). The evidence for the genetic separation is fairly sound and rests upon studies in several large families. For the site of the recombinational event to be mapped, the families must contain at least two pairs of HLA-identical sibs differing by one haplotype, e.g., two sites with the AC haplotype (sibs 1 and 2) and two with the AD haplotype (sibs 3 and 4). In such families three of the sibs fail to stimulate in any combination in MLR; thus, sibs 1, 3, and 4 might be mutually nonstimulatory, but sib 2 would stimulate the other 3 sibs. This result would occur if the HLA-D locus of sib 1 was recombinant, so that sib 1 was HLA-D identical to sibs 3 and 4. Sib 2 being the normal sib would, of course, stimulate both AD sibs and the recombinant sib 2 (38). Families in which two HLA-identical sibs stimulate are much more common (32). It is believed that these represent recombinants, but they could include an unknown proportion of mutants and do not contribute to the mapping of HLA. The possible contribution of alleles other than HLA-D to MLR must also be considered.

Whereas the products of the HLA-A and -B loci can be purified and characterized, the products of the HLA-D and also the HLA-C loci are elusive. HLA-D is probably expressed on Fc receptor cells or B-type lymphocytes (9). Antisera reacting with B but not T cells are quite readily available (22). Several of these sera react with haplotypes carrying designated HLA-D specificities and may be reacting with the HLA-D product. However, in most instances, the correlation, although close, is not absolute (33). The incongruities would suggest the existence of two genes in close linkage disequilibrium and hence, probably, closely linked, one for an Fc receptor cell differentiation antigen and the other for an HLA-D allele. If the two do prove to be identical, chemical resolution should be rapid, as purified xenoantibodies to B cells are available for precipitation and eventual characterization of the antigen. The possibility exists, however, that the B cell antigen and HLA-D are quite distant and that HLA-D is a property of the B cell rather than a cell surface antigen. It could, for example, be involved in the transfer of adenyl cyclase.

Reasons for the slow resolution of the HLA-C product are quite different and are largely technological. For the preparation of a cell surface antigen, high-titered antisera reacting only against antigens of the locus involved are essential. Most of the sera defining HLA-C are weak and also contaminated with antibodies to HLA-B. Indeed, HLA-B and HLA-C are in such close linkage disequilibrium that the identification of HLA-C specificities is proceeding quite slowly. Thus, little is known of the biological properties of HLA-C or of its chemistry.

Not yet mapped on the haplotype are the differentiation antigens of Fc receptor cells. These appear to be analogous to the Ia antigens of H-2 both in their physical properties and in their distribution. The Ia antigens of the mouse are coded for by the IA and IC regions of H-2 and are mapped between the K and D loci. There are many recombinants between IC and D and few between K and IA, implying that the I region is close to K. There are at least two Fc receptor (B cell) antigens associated with HLA, and these have been separated by recombination (21). One B cell locus was associated with HL A-A and one with HLA-B. Fine structure mapping to further define the position of these loci in relation to the A and B loci of HLA has not yet been reported.

Two antigenic peaks have been identified in the soluble product from B cell membranes; it is therefore possible that there are only two antigens (11). If so, each carries several antigenic sites since two or more sera recognized each specificity in a recombinant and up to six anti-B cell area of varying specificity can react with a single haplotype (21). The molecule is unlikely to show close sequence homology with the HLA-A and HLA-B products as there is no cross-reactivity between the xenoantibodies prepared against different products (11). In contrast, HLA-A and HLA-B have considerable sequence homology, and cross-reactivity can be detected between them (10, 20, 31).

The HLA region also appears to include determinants which are only detected in LDA. These are clearly different from B cell specificities since they are expressed on the majority of lymphocytes. Sera with no detectable anti-HLA activity even in the sensitive antiglobulin cytotoxicity test may give strong LDA activity (see chapter 113). Again, from the study of a recombinant, there appear to be two LDA loci, one associated with HLA-A and one with HLA-B. One gains the impression of not just gene duplication in the HLA region but of duplication of a complex of genes. These may be referred to as the HLA-A and the HLA-B genetic clusters. From skin grafting within families which include a recombinant and from an analysis of skin graft rejection times of haploidentical family members who also share one additional HLA specificity, it is clear that neither the HLA-A cluster nor the HLA-B cluster is exclusively responsible for skin graft rejection (F. E. Ward et al., Abstr. Transplant. Soc., p. 122, 1974). From this analysis of many families by Ward et al., it seems likely that each region plays a part; this is confirmed from studies by skin grafts in recombinant families (34).

The analysis of the part played by HLA in graft rejection is likely to require considerably more research. However, insofar as it is practicable, the effort to match cadaveric donor with most pheotypically similar recipient appears to be justified. Recent reports from England and from Eurotransplant both document the higher success rate for kidneys matched for four HLA antigens (24, 28). Matching also appears to influence corneal transplants when the recipient site is moderately inflamed at the time of grafting (12). When the recipient cornea is not vascularized rejection is rarely a problem, and when it is seriously compromised a poor result cannot be compensated for by the modest degree of matching achieved to date. As mentioned earlier, increased skin graft survival can also be found when unrelated donor and recipient are matched. To what extent the increased transplantability of HLA matched tissues is due to similarity at HLA and to what extent it derives from similarities at other loci in linkage disequilibrium remains to be solved.

No description of HLA would be complete without a discussion of the relationship between HLA and disease. The first association reported, that of antigens of the 4c complex and Hodgkin's disease, has not proved to be a very constant one, being significant in some series and not in others (15). There is a degree of association between certain HLA specificities and a wide variety of diseases; best known are the associations between HLA-B8 and gluten sensitive enteropathy (GSE) or juvenile diabetes (30) and between HLA-B27 and certain rheumatoid diseases, especially ankylosing spondylitis (AS) and Reiter's syndrome (7, 29). The B27-AS association is a very close one and has been substantiated in several series and in family studies, indicating true linkage. There are two fascinating new aspects to the association of specificities of the HLA complex and GSE; one is with HLA-DW3 (33), and the other is with the Br specificity found on B cells and appears different from DW3 (23). The strongest association in these new findings is between the B cell markers and the disease rather than between HLA and disease. Thus, further studies will undoubtedly exploit the presence of additional markers on the HLA haplotype. The eventual outcome of these studies is likely to be momentous and should lead to a better understanding, as well as to a better diagnosis, of many autoimmune disease.

Whatever the advantages to be gained from a knowledge of the histocompatibility complex, other practical aspects of transplantation also demand attention. The form and intensity of the response will depend upon a great many variables, some of which have received relatively little attention. The first is the physiological state of the transplant. The controversy as to whether pulsatile perfusion aids or hinders transplantability is being resolved, but there are many opportunities for changing the perfusate and the method of perfusion. To what extent does soluble antigen released from the graft contribute to or interfere with the induction of immunity? Which features of the transplant are most immunogenic—the lymphocytes or macrophages in the graft tissue, the vascular endothelium, or various parendymal structures? From the universally disappointing results of intestinal and lung transplants with their high load of lymphoid cells to the frequently successful transplantation of liver, kidney, and heart, there does appear to be a gradient of success which correlates with the passenger lymphocyte load.

Another unanswered question concerns storage. It is unfortunate that the misdirected efforts of one individual should have obstructed research on short-term preservation of tissues. There is a certain body of data from both the Russian and Western literature to support the possibility that stored tissues are more readily transplantable than are fresh tissues. For example, Georgiade, in an early study with skin stored at refrigerator temperatures in glycerol, found no loss of transplantability and possible improvement in survival (14); Rose found that cytotoxic lymphocytes could attach freshly cultivated thyroid but not thyroid maintained in culture for a few days (27); and Wells found improved transplantabilities of cultured parathyroid glands (36). The optimal methods for storage for many tissues are unknown, and cultivation may increase susceptibility to other processes such as LDA. Lymphatic drainage and lymphatic connections are also extremely important. The skin pedicle and cheek pouch experiments of Billingham and his colleagues (3, 6) are substantiated by other experiments in which ablation of the draining node greatly increased survival.

Species differences and differences in basal state of recipient immunity contribute greatly to the outcome of a transplant. Permanent acceptance of kidneys in rats or kidneys and hearts in mice may require no immunosuppression, even where the graft and host differ at the major histocompatibility complex of those species, and the acceptance of liver grafts in pigs is now legendary. Needless to say, similar findings are rare in other species, such as humans or dogs. Thus, although the major histocomptability complex of most species appears to be very similar, conclusions drawn from one species cannot be directly applied to another.

In conclusion, the HLA region comprises one of the most complex and fascinating genetic systems. It appears to be a true system in that it contains a variety of genes of diverse function having relevance to differentiation, to disease, and possibly to natural selection. Among its many attributes are its effects on transplantation. The complex probably includes immune response genes that regulate the ability of the host to respond to transplant antigens as well as determining the transplantation antigens themselves. This section details many of the methods used in tissue typing. It is hoped that this concluding chapter will stimulate the reader to consider the broader aspects of the biophysiology of HLA.

LITERATURE CITED

1. Amos, D. B., A. H. Johnson, R. J. Ruderman, N. R. Mendell, and E. J. Yunis. 1975. New concepts of the human HL-1 system including HLA, MLR-S, HDR and Ir loci and the relationship of HL-1 to other attributes of the

same autosome, p. 103–117. *In* Immunological concepts of neoplasia. The Williams & Wilkins Co., Baltimore.

2. Bailey, D. W., G. D. Snell, and M. Cherry. 1971. Complement and serologic analysis of an H-2 mutant, p. 155–162. *In* A. Lengerova and M. Voijtiskova (ed.), Immunogenetics of the H-2 system. Karger, Basel.

3. Barber, C. F., and R. Billingham. 1967. The role of regional lymphatics in the skin homograft response. Transplantation 5:962–966.

4. Bennett, D., E. A. Boyse, and L. J. Old. 1972. Cell surface immunogenetics in the study of morphogenesis, p. 247–263. *In* L. G. Silvestri (ed.), Cell interactions. American Elsevier, New York.

5. Bennett, D., and L. C. Dunn. 1970. Transmission ratio distorting genes on chromosome IX and their interactions, p. 90–103. *In* A. Lengerova and M. Voitjiskova (ed.), Immunogenetics of the H-2 system. Karger, Basel.

6. Billingham, R. E., L. W. Ferrigan, and W. K. Silvers. 1961. A possible new assay method for transplantation antigens, depending upon ability to procure homograft destruction. Transplant. Bull. 27:142.

7. Brewerton, D. A., M. Caffrey, F. D. Hart, D. C. O. James, A. Nicholls, and R. D. Sturrock. 1971. Ankylosing spondylitis and HLA-A 27. Lancet 1:904–907.

8. Chauvenet, P. H., and D. B. Amos. 1975. The mechanism of immunoresistance of H(zl) mice to C57Bl/6 tumors. Cell. Immunol. 17:477–486.

9. Cohrmann, H. P., L. Novikovs, and R. G. Graws, Jr. 1974. Stimulating capacity of human T and B lymphocytes in the mixed leukocyte culture. Nature (London) 125:144–146.

10. Cresswell, P., and J. Ayres. 1976. HLA antigens: rabbit antisera reacting with all A series or all B series specifities. Eur. J. Immunol., in press.

11. Cresswell, P., and S. Geier. 1975. Antisera to human B-lymphocyte membrane glycoproteins block stimulation in mixed lymphocyte culture. Nature (London) 257:147–149.

12. Gibbs., D. C., J. R. Batchelor, A. Werb, W. Schlesinger, and T. A. Casey. 1974. The influence of tissue-type compatibility on the fate of full-thickness corneal grafts. Trans. Opthalmol. Soc. U.K. 94:101–126.

13. Hammerberg, C., and J. Klein. 1975. Linkage disequilibrium between H-2 and t complexes in chromosome 17 of the mouse. Nature (London) 258:296–299.

14. Kepes, J., N. Georgiade, A. Eiring, and K. Pickrell. 1958. Evaluation of post mortem survival of skin by tissue culture methods. Plast. Reconstr. Surg. 21:483–486.

15. Kissmeyer-Nielsen, F., K. E. Kjerbye, and L. U. Lamm. 1975. HL-A in Hodgkin's disease. III. A prospective study. Transplant. Rev. 22:186–174.

16. Klein, J. 1975. Biology of the mouse histocompatibility-2 complex, p. 269. Springer-Verlag, New York.

17. Klein, J., M. Hauptfield, and V. Hauptfield. 1974. Serological distinction of mutants B6.C H(zl) and B6 M505 from strain C57Bl/6. J. Exp. Med. 140:1127–1132.

18. Klein, J., R. W. Melvold, and H. I. Kohn, quoted by J. Klein. 1975. Biology of the mouse histocompatibility-2 complex, p. 22. Springer-Verlag, New York.

19. Koch, C. T., J. P. van Hooff, A. van Leeuwen, J. G. van den Tweel, E. Fredricks, G. J. van der Steen, H. M. Schippers, and J. van Rood. 1972. The relation importance of matching for the MLC versus the HL-A loci in organ transplantation, p. 521–524. *In* J. Dausset and J. Colombani (ed.), Histocompatibility testing 1972. Munksgaard, Copenhagen.

20. Legrand, L., and J. Dausset. 1975. The complexity of the HL-A gene product. II. Possible evidence for a "public" determinant common to the first and second HL-A series. Transplantation 19:177–180.

21. Mann, D. L., L. Abelson, S. Harris, and D. B. Amos. 1976. Evidence for several genes controlling expression of B cell alloantigens: a second genetic locus within the HLA region for human B cell alloantigens. Nature (London), in press.

22. Mann, D. L., L. Abelson, P. Henkart, S. Harris, and D. B. Amos. 1976. Serologic detection of B lymphocyte antigens. *In* F. Kissimeyer-Nielson (ed.), Histocompatibility testing 1975. Munksgaard, Copenhagen.

23. Mann, D. L., W. Strober, S. I. Katz, S. Shia, and D. B. Amos. 1976. Br and Wh. B cell antigens in gluten sensitive enteropathy and dermatitis herpetiformis. *In* B. Benacerraf (ed.), Role of products of the histocompatibility gene complex in immune responses. Brook Lodge, Nov. 1975, in press.

24. Oliver, R. D. T., J. A. Sachs, and H. Festenstein. 1973. A collaborative scheme for tissue typing and matching in renal transplantation. VI. Clinical relevance of HL-A matching in 349 cadaver renal transplants. Transplant. Proc. 5:245–251.

25. Plate, J. M., F. E. Ward, and D. B. Amos. 1970. The mixed leukocyte culture response between HL-A identical siblings, p. 531–535. *In* P. I. Terasaki (ed.), Histocompatibility testing 1970. Munksgaard, Copenhagen.

26. Rapaport, F. 1976. Immunogenetic studies of bone marrow transplantation in the canine species. Transplant. Proc., in press.

27. Rose, N., J. H. Kite, Jr., T. K. Doebbler, and R. C. Brown. 1963. In vitro reactions of lymphoid cells with thyroid tissue, p. 19–31. *In* B. Amos and H. Koprowski (ed.), Cell-bound antibodies. Wistar, Philadelphia.

28. Scandiatransplant Report. 1975. HL-A matching and kidney-graft survival. Lancet 1:240–247.

29. Schlosstein, L., P. I. Terasaki, R. Bluestone, and C. M. Pearson. 1973. High association of an HLA antigen, W27, with ankylosing spondylitis. N. Engl. J. Med. 288:704–706.

30. Stokes, P. L., T. Asquith, F. K. T. Holmes, P.

McIntosh, and W. T. Cooke. 1972. Histocompatibility antigens associated with coeliac disease. Lancet **2**:162–164.

31. Strominger, J. L., L. Chess, R. E. Humphries, D. Mann, P. Parham, R. Robb, S. Schlossman, T. Springer, and C. Terhorst. 1976. Isolation and structure of the human histocompatibility gene complex. *In* B. Benacerraf (ed.), Role of products of the histocompatibility gene complex in immune responses. Brook Lodge, Nov. 1975, in press.

32. Svejgaard, A., A. Bratlie, P. J. Hedin, C. Högman, C. Jersild, F. Kissmeyer-Nielsen, B. Lindblom, A. Lindholm, B. Low, L. Messeter, E. Möller, L. Sandberg, L. Staub-Nielsen, and E. Thorsby. 1971. The recombination fraction of the HL-A system. Tissue Antigens **1**:18–88.

33. van Rood, J. J., A. Van Leeuwen, A. Termijtelen, and J. J. Keuning. 1976. The genetics of the major histocompatibility complex in man, HLA. *In* B. Benacerraf (ed.), Role of products of the histocompatibility gene complex in immune responses. Brook Lodge, Nov., 1975, in press.

34. Ward, F. E. and H. F. Seigler. 1973. Mixed lymphocyte reactions and skin graft survival in an HL-A recombinant family. Transplant. Proc. **5**:359–362.

35. Ward, F. E., H. F. Seigler, J. G. Southworth, C. H. Andrus, and D. B. Amos. 1970. Immunogenicity of HLA antigens, p. 399–410. *In* P. T. Terasaki (ed.), Histocompatibility testing 1970. Munksgaard, Cophenhagen.

36. Wells, S. A., and C. Christiansen. 1974. The transplanted parathyroid gland: evaluation of cryopreservation and other environmental factors which affect its fuction. Surgery **75**:49–55.

37. Yunis, E. J., and D. B. Amos. 1971. Three closely linked genetic systems relevant to transplantation. Proc. Natl. Acad. Sci. U.S.A. **68**:3031–3035.

38. Yunis, E. J., J. M. Plate, F. E. Ward, H. F. Seigler, and D. B. Amos. 1971. Anomalous MLC responsiveness among siblings. Transplant. Proc. **3**:118–120.

Chapter 117

Introduction

DAN F. PALMER

The various chapters in this section reflect an exciting era in the evolution of immunology. Emerging from its status as a rapidly growing infant science, immunology is becoming a mature discipline and, as such, must continue to be constrained directionally to conform with accepted scientific philosophy. The use of the scientific method, with its attendant control measures and reference standards, is, of course, an imperative of science. The chapters "Some Concepts of Quality Control in Immunoserology" and "Standardization of Reagents and Methodology in Immunology" are included in this section to provide some of the control measures that form the conceptual framework by which the immunologist may orient himself in transferring technology from research-derived developments to practical application in the laboratory. In addition to the subjects covered in these two chapters, many of the control measures recommended for use in specific test procedures are designated in appropriate chapters elsewhere in this *Manual*.

As the discipline of clinical immunology develops and its technology is applied in the form of services rendered to those directly concerned with patient care, it becomes obvious that this new clinical science must be organized functionally for its most efficient application. Confounding its functional organization is the fact that it transcends many of the traditional bounds that classically compartmentalize the field of medicine, necessitating innovative approaches to the creation of organizational entities designed to integrate its activities.

The chapter entitled "Organization of the Clinical Immunology Laboratory" offers a cogent, practical approach to the organization of laboratory services which are now scattered throughout several different laboratories in the medical complex but are in need of consolidation because they are of primary concern to the immunologist.

Further organizational considerations are found in the chapter entitled "Clinical Immunology: a New Specialty Based in the Laboratory and Clinical Departments." This chapter contains a convincing discussion of the functions of a clinical immunology unit as an ampli-

fied, clinically based entity; the supervision of the clinical immunology laboratory is mentioned as one of its several responsibilities.

It is important to realize, however, that the viewpoints expressed by the authors of these chapters on organization represent but two of several existing viewpoints on this somewhat controversial subject.

Regardless of the organizational structure of the clinical immunology laboratory, much of its activity will probably be regulated by some government agency. That agency's mission will be similar, in relation to the quality of laboratory work, to that of any conscientious laboratorian, i.e., to insure that adequate safeguards and control measures are taken in the laboratory so that results of diagnostic tests have a high level of credibility.

The role of the government in this regard is discussed philosophically in the chapter "Legal Requirements and Compliance Measures." The authors of this chapter trace the Federal Government's gradual assumption of more regulatory power in health care delivery from the Hill-Burton program of 1946 up to the Clinical Laboratories Improvement Act of 1975 (the latter not yet enacted into law at the time of this writing). They also explain, in a very general way, how a laboratory can comply with the regulations under which it is operating.

More specific details concerning the state's role in implementing the licensure of laboratories are presented in the chapter entitled "State and Federal Regulations Governing the Licensure of Laboratories." Although it is impractical to list each state's regulations, a table in this chapter lists those states that currently regulate licensure of clinical laboratories and those that do not.

It is interesting to note that the authors of both of the last two chapters point to the probability of eventual government regulation of all clinical laboratories in this country. Regardless of the extent of future government control, however, it is incumbent upon the clinical immunology laboratorian to provide credible, objective results supported by an adequate quality control program.

Chapter 118

Organization of the Clinical Immunology Laboratory

SHARAD D. DEODHAR

INTRODUCTION

During the past decade, the field of immunology has progressed by leaps and bounds, and major advances have been made, not only in the theoretical aspects of immunology but also in its practical applications to various subspecialties in clinical medicine. It is now abundantly clear that immunology can no longer be considered an "ivory tower" science; rather, it is a discipline which has important implications and applications in the practice of medicine. With the rapid advances in communication systems, the gap between research and development on the one hand and practical clinical application on the other is rapidly being narrowed, and no field reflects this more clearly than immunology. Historically, the applications of immunology to laboratory medicine were primarily in the areas of infectious disease, serology, and, later, in blood banking. In recent years, the scope of this field has widened greatly, and its practical applications now extend to various areas, such as rheumatology, dermatology, nephrology, allergy and hypersensitivity diseases, cardiology, neurology, pediatrics, gastroenterology, and, finally, two other major fields — transplantation and cancer immunology. The clinical or health-oriented laboratories are now faced with an ever-growing problem of providing service in all or many of the areas mentioned. In many institutions around the country, this problem has been partly resolved by some of the existing departments in a clinical laboratory complex, such as hematology, blood banking, clinical chemistry, microbiology, or a serology laboratory, undertaking one or more of the appropriate immunological tests. As a result, these tests are often performed in many different departments, often physically, administratively, and functionally separated, and this has created problems in integrating all the efforts in the immunology area. The time has now come to recognize this field as a distinct branch of laboratory medicine with an important clinical service function and to start thinking in terms of organizing clinical service activities in this area into a single departmental or laboratory unit for the purpose of achieving maximal efficiency in terms of time, effort, and cost.

The purpose of this chapter is to provide some general guidelines for organization of a clinical immunology laboratory unit. Under consideration will be a unit in a large hospital setting (500 beds or more) where the demands for laboratory services can be expected to come from a wide variety of medical specialties, as mentioned before. The approach suggested here is not the only way, nor the ideal way, but rather one which was adopted at The Cleveland Clinic Foundation and one which has evolved as a result of our experience over the past several years (1). A recent report by the Committee on Hospital-Based Laboratory and Clinical Immunology of the American Association of Immunologists also provides several helpful guidelines (2). Ideally, the clinical immunology laboratory unit should be able to perform a wide range of immunological tests for patient service while at the same time integrating activities in the areas of research and development and teaching at various levels. Since many of the immunological test procedures are still in a state of dynamic evolution, awareness of research and developmental activity in this regard becomes very important. The tests generally considered to be in the realm of the clinical immunology laboratory unit may include various immunoprecipitation techniques, immunomicroscopy, agglutination techniques, tests for serum proteins (including complement components), histocompatibility testing or tissue typing, tests for cellular immunology, and radioimmunoassay procedures. Admittedly, there has always been, and there will always be, a great deal of overlap between the activities of such a unit and those of other areas in laboratory medicine, such as blood banking, microbiology, hematology, and clinical chemistry. Problems regarding such overlap have to be resolved at the level of each individual institution or laboratory medicine department.

PROPOSED ORGANIZATION OF A CLINICAL IMMUNOLOGY LABORATORY UNIT

The laboratory components of such a unit may be divided as follows:

1. General immunology laboratory
2. Cellular immunology laboratory
3. Histocompatibility testing or tissue typing laboratory
4. Radioimmunoassay laboratory

An attempt will be made here to discuss briefly the range of activities of each of these laboratory components and some of the basic requirements.

General immunology section

The general immunology unit should be designed to perform tests such as those in the category of immunoprecipitation techniques, immunomicroscopy (involving fluorescent and enzyme-labeled reagents), serum protein analyses, including those for complement components, agglutination tests, and related procedures. To perform these tests this laboratory must have standard equipment, such as refrigerator-freezer, balance, pH meter, water bath, table-top centrifuges, and light microscopes; in addition, it must have special equipment items such as an electrophoretic cell, a fluorescence microscope in an appropriate darkened room, and a cryostat for sectioning of frozen tissue for immunofluorescence studies.

Various serological tests in the diagnosis of infectious diseases can be performed in this laboratory also. In the detection of circulating antibodies in various autoimmune diseases, the indirect immunofluorescence tests are performed. These include tests for antinuclear antibody, mitochondrial antibodies, antibodies localizing in the intercellular regions and in the basement membrane of the skin in certain bullous lesions, and various other autoantibodies such as those against skeletal muscle, smooth muscle, parietal cells, adrenal cortical cells, renal tubular basement membrane, reticulin, thyroid epithelial cell cytoplasm, salivary gland ductal cell cytoplasm, and several others. Of these, the test for antinuclear antibodies is probably the most popular one, since it is thought to be the best screening test for all diseases of the autoimmune or connective tissue disease group. The other antibody tests mentioned have specific applications in certain diseases thought to have autoimmune etiology. The direct immunofluorescence tests are useful primarily in the study of biopsy specimens, such as those from patients with renal disease, liver disease, and various skin diseases. The significance of all of these fluorescence test procedures in the diagnosis and management of patients with immunological diseases is well known and need not be emphasized here. The immunoprecipitation techniques include those for immunoglobulin (Ig) determination, complement component determination, ceruloplasmin levels, and alpha antitrypsin levels; in recent years, other serum components have been added to this list of procedures. Immunoelectrophoretic procedures are performed primarily for the characterization of myeloma proteins, and, in certain other situations, for identification of rare cases of heavy-chain disease and IgD and IgE myelomas. A prototype for the agglutination techniques is the tanned red cell agglutination test for thyroglobulin antibodies and the test for detecting colonic mucosal antibodies. The former test is useful in evaluation of patients with Hashimoto's or autoimmune thyroiditis, and the latter is requested primarily in the study of patients with various inflammatory diseases of the small and large bowel.

Cellular immunology (tissue culture unit)

The cellular immunology laboratory should be designed for the purpose of performing various tests for cellular immunity. These include the lymphocyte blast transformation test with mitogens and with appropriate antigens, the migration inhibition factor test, quantitation of T and B cells in peripheral blood and in lymphoid tissue, in vitro tests for studying lymphocyte cytotoxicity against various target cells, and general procedures required for short- and long-term culturing of cells. The cellular immunology laboratory is best arranged in two parts: (i) a sterile room for actual tissue culture work, and (ii) an adjacent work area for preparation and processing of test materials. The design and organization of the sterile room are extremely important since most of the procedures call for handling of living cells for various periods of time, and sterility has to be observed in these procedures as rigidly as possible. This room is best located in an area where traffic will be at a minimum. To minimize danger of contamination, one should resort to various devices such as the use of overhead, ultraviolet light, use of positive air pressure (filtered system), and use of laminar flow hoods, as well as observing some of the standard laboratory precautions. This laboratory should also be equipped with tissue culture CO_2 incubator, maintained at 37 C, a table-top centrifuge, a regular light microscope, an inverted stereomicroscope for studying tissue culture flasks, and other standard laboratory items for performing tissue culture operations.

The adjacent room should be designed for performing various procedures in cellular immunology which do not require rigid sterility. These are the procedures in handling of the test samples after the tissue culture period is over. Ideally, this area should have a refrigerator-freezer for storage of materials, a scintillation counter for counting of radioactivity, bench space for radioactive work, a light microscope, and space for staining of slides, preparation of nonsterile reagents, reading of test slides, etc. Study of cellular immunity is becoming increasingly important in evaluation of patients with various immune-deficiency syndromes (primary or secondary), patients with autoimmune diseases of cell-mediated mechanisms, patients with delayed hypersensitivity reactions, and in patients with various malignant diseases.

Histocompatibility testing or tissue typing unit

Histocompatibility testing is a specialized type of service which becomes absolutely essential if a given institution is involved in clinical transplant programs. In most areas around the country, such units provide regional service in that they perform histocompatibility testing for all transplants done in that given area. Thus, the histocompatibility laboratory at Cleveland Clinic performs tissue typing on all donors and recipients in the clinical transplant programs in the Northeastern Ohio region. The techniques most commonly employed involve lymphocyte microcytotoxicity and mixed lymphocyte cultures. Therefore, such a laboratory must be equipped with standard laboratory equipment plus certain special items such as a phase microscope for reading of lymphocyte microcytotoxicity tests, a -70 C freezer for storage of cells and tissues, a tissue culture hood for mixed lymphocyte reactions, and other items necessary for short-term tissue culture work. In addition to the obvious need for histocompatibility testing in clinical transplant programs, this procedure is also assuming increasing importance in other areas, such as for platelet transfusions and also in evaluation of certain diseases where there is a high degree of association of certain histocompatibility antigens.

Radioimmunoassay unit

Radioimmunoassays for various hormones and other substances such as IgE, digoxin, carcinoembryonic antigen, alpha fetoprotein, and many others represent probably the fastest growing area in laboratory medicine. Because these techniques are reproducible, highly sensitive, and specific, and because they lend themselves to the performance of large numbers of tests, they are rapidly replacing the formerly employed bioassay procedures. In most institutions around the country, these techniques are performed by various clinical laboratory departments, including endocrinology, clinical chemistry, or radiology; however, the procedures are essentially immunological, involving antigen-antibody reactions; therefore, one can consider them as one integral part of the clinical immunology laboratory's activities. Knowledge of various considerations in the production of antibodies or antisera and antigen-antibody reactions is very helpful and often essential in performing these techniques. Radioimmunoassay techniques are now commonly used to determine levels of most of the hormones, including growth hormone, insulin, thyroid stimulating hormone, follicle stimulating hormone, luteinizing hormone, testosterone, gastrin, parathormone, T4 and T3, human chorionic gonadotrophin, and others, as well as in the determination of nonhormonal agents mentioned before. By performing all radioimmunoassay or competitive binding type analyses in one laboratory unit, one can offer efficient service with respect to time, effort, and cost. The radioimmunoassay laboratory should be a completely self-sufficient functioning unit, again with all the standard laboratory equipment together with appropriate gamma counter, refrigerated centrifuge, microbalance, various automatic micropipetting devices, programmable calculator or computer, and related items.

PERSONNEL

In any clinical service-type laboratory the technical personnel probably represent the single most important item. For the type of immunological activities described here, the technical individual should have as background education a Bachelor's degree in one of the biological sciences or a Medical Technologist Certification, such as that given by the American Society of Clinical Pathologists. In addition, previous experience in an immunology laboratory is very helpful, but this is not essential for employment in a clinical immunology laboratory. Certain national organizations are already offering or in the process of offering a special certification in clinical immunology for those individuals who, by virtue of previous experience and by successfully completing certain examinations, can demonstrate their proficiency. The quality of the personnel in clinical immunology laboratories is bound to improve through such programs.

OTHER CONSIDERATIONS

Research and development and educational activities at various levels are also additional important items in any clinical immunology laboratory. A well-rounded department can be developed only through integration of activities in all of these areas. Other important items for consideration include external and internal quality control, standardization of reagents and methodology, proficiency testing, and cost accounting; these are discussed in detail in other chapters. Careful attention must also be directed toward planning for space requirements to allow for the inevitable growth of these activities. For anyone interested in clinical immunology, the past few years have provided a very exciting and rewarding experience, and it is now clear that immunology is not just a "passing fad" but that it has important bearing in the practice of clinical laboratory medicine.

LITERATURE CITED

1. Bloch, K. J. 1975. Clinical immunology: meeting report of the committee on hospital-based laboratory and clinical immunology of the American Association of Immunologists. J. Immunol. 115:609–610.
2. Deodhar, S. D. 1973. Anatomy of a clinical immunology center. Lab. Manage. 11:20–24.

Chapter 119

Legal Requirements and Compliance Measures

CARL BLANK AND ARNOLD HICKS

Health has been defined as a state of soundness and well-being, both physical and mental. Public health is an extension of the doctrine of personal hygiene and health and is concerned with the welfare of communities. For the protection of the public and for general control of health matters, a planned health administration must exist and this must be backed by necessary law. In the United States there is no central government department responsible for the health of the nation, nor is there a health officer in the President's Cabinet. Here the individual state is the sovereign, and it is looked to for nearly all health administration. The Federal Government, however, does have much to do with planning, direction, and research connected with public health throughout the United States (4). The following paragraphs give some of the federal and state legal requirements as those requirements relate to clinical laboratories and their personnel.

LEGAL REQUIREMENTS

For the purposes of this chapter, "Legal Requirements and Compliance Measures" refer to State and Federal external control and not internal day-to-day controls imposed by laboratory directors. The "external" controls referred to are governmental: these controls, such as licensure, are exercised by governmental regulatory agencies to protect the public health (3).

In attempting to understand and seek guidance as to what legal requirements and compliance measures clinical laboratories and personnel must contend with, it is important to bear in mind several governmental principles which are applicable and will continue to be applicable unless we change our system of government. One basic governmental principle is that a Constitution, both State and Federal, is the fundamental or basic law to which all others must conform. Its function is to establish the framework and general principles of government and an objective standard of conduct by which all departments of the government shall be bound. The Federal Constitution is the supreme law of the land. It is a compact established by the people of the United States and not by the states in their sovereign capacity. It

is a grant of power and should not be considered as a detailed statute, but rather a working set of practical principles (16 Corpus Juris Secundum [C.J.S.] Constitutional Law, section 3).

The constitution of a state, like that of the nation, is the supreme law within the realm and sphere of its authority, but is a limitation on the power of the legislature, binding on the several departments of state government, and the people themselves, subject to the restraints of the Federal Constitution (16 C.J.S. Constitutional Law, section 3). Therefore, the Constitution of the United States is primarily a grant or delegation of power from the people, and in turn the Federal Government possesses only powers that are conferred by the Constitution either expressly or by implication (16 C.J.S. Constitutional Law, section 68). All other powers are reserved to the people, or are considered inherent governmental powers reserved as the right of the states.

RESERVED POWER

There is one reserved power, the police power, that is of particular interest to clinical laboratory personnel. It is the power inherent in a government to enact laws, within constitutional limits, to promote the order, safety, health, morals, and general welfare of society. "Thus, the 50 states are separate repositories of police power, while the national government, which, in its origins, is a government of delegated power, does not possess the police power, at least not in its usual broad sense" (2). "Yet the Federal Government obviously exercises vast powers in the field of public health and has become the leader in many enforcement and service activities. It has done so mainly through the exercise of two delegated powers, namely through its power to regulate interstate commerce, and through its power to tax—and to spend money—for the general welfare. The Federal Government's regulatory activities— such as, for instance, in the regulation of food, drugs, and cosmetics, or in the labeling of hazardous substances or economic poisons—are commonly derived from the power to regulate interstate commerce, while many of its service programs frequently operating through assistance to the states, are based on its power to tax and spend money. The impact of federal law and regulation on state and local public health enforcement is, of course, considerable . . . " (2).

ADMINISTRATIVE AGENCIES

Since state government's power to protect the public health is an inherent power, state administrative agencies, such as state health departments, derive their powers from the state legislature, which enacts the law, the legislators being representatives of and having been elected by the people. Once a health statute has been approved as law, state health departments, as a member of the Executive branch of government, put the law into effect and have public accountability for administering the law within its legislative intent. With this power to enforce certain statutes also comes the duty to do so. State health departments are responsible for administering the statutes for the purposes intended.

These departments are broken down into administrative agencies with rule-making and decision-making powers (3), but they cannot transfer, surrender, or abridge their powers and duties which under the law are entrusted to them. Although they may delegate ministerial functions, they cannot delegate powers and functions which are discretionary or quasi-judicial in character or which require the exercise of judgment (73 C.J.S. Public Administrative Bodies and Procedures, section 57).

The above gives us some understanding of governmental interest, responsibilities, and basis for some of the legal requirements that have been applied to date.

ROLE OF FEDERAL GOVERNMENT INVOLVEMENT IN HEALTH CARE DELIVERY

There is and has been since 1946 a trend toward more involvement of the Federal Government in health care delivery. Congressional interest in effective health planning and resources development began with the enactment of the Hill-Burton program in 1946. The Hill-Burton program provided funds for the construction of needed new hospitals, but it clearly contemplated that the states which received those funds would use them in accordance with a planning process to determine their need for an existing supply of medical facilities. Little change in this federal effort occurred until 1964 when the Hill-Burton Act was modified by the addition of legislative authority for the funding of regional, or areawide, voluntary health facilities planning agencies (1974 U.S. Code Congressional and Administrative News 7845).

The 89th Congress in 1965 and 1966 provided for further expansion of health legislation. The enactment of Medicare and Medicaid provided for the first time for extensive federal participation in health insurance for the aged and indigent population. Providers of medical or other health services were required to meet specific conditions.

Diagnostic laboratory tests were included within the Medicare definition of "medical and other health services" (1965 U.S. Code Cong. & Ad. News 345). This meant that no diagnostic test performed in any laboratory other than those located in an excluded physician's office or an excluded hospital would be eligible for Medicare reimbursement unless the laboratory and personnel met certain conditions. One of the conditions to be met required the laboratories to be licensed by the state if the laboratory was situated in a state having such requirements. In 1965, very few states had laboratory licensing laws although many states had laboratory approval laws for certain tests such as syphilis serology, water, and milk.

Another Medicare requirement was for the laboratory to meet other health and safety conditions for the protection of the patient as determined by the Secretary of Health, Education, and Welfare (1965 U.S. Code Cong. & Ad. News 2125).

The Secretary subsequently established a series of standards as criteria for determining compliance. The law made provision for the designation of state health agencies, or other state agencies, to assist the Secretary in determining whether laboratories are in compliance with the conditions for coverage of laboratory services. The designated state agencies certify to the Secretary those laboratories which they find meet conditions such as: (i) conforms with all applicable state and local laws; (ii) is under the direction and supervision of qualified persons; (iii) performs only those laboratory tests and procedures that are within the specialties in which the laboratory director and supervisors are qualified; (iv) has a sufficient number of properly qualified personnel for the volume and diversity of tests performed; and (v) maintains records, equipment, and facilities which are adequate and appropriate for the services offered (Code of Federal Regulations, Title 20, Chapter III, Subpart M, Part 405).

Shortly after the enactment of Medicare in 1965, Congress passed and the President signed into law the Partnership for Health Amendments of 1967, 5 December 1967 (Public Law 90-174, Section 5(a), 81 Statute 536), which included the "Clinical Laboratories Improvement Act of 1967." This Act authorized the Secretary of Health, Education, and Welfare to regulate, by licensing, clinical laboratories which operate in interstate commerce. The basic method of regulation contemplated was an objective system of proficiency testing to assure consistent performance of accurate procedures and services. The Secretary was authorized to set standards for quality control programs, records, equipment, facilities, and qualification of the laboratory director and supervisory personnel.

Congress believed at this time that in the long run the improvement of clinical laboratories and their performance was a job for state governments since the Act authorized the Secretary to exercise his functions through state and local agencies. The Act also provided for licensure of clinical laboratories accredited by a nationally recognized accreditation body approved by the Secretary, but only if the accreditation standards are equal to or more stringent than those established by the Secretary.

Trends

In recent years, we have seen the Federal Government enact health programs such as Hill-Burton, Medicare, Comprehensive Health Planning, Health Manpower, and, more recently, Health Maintenance Organizations, Health Planning and Resources Development, and Clinical Laboratory Licensing, and some kind of comprehensive National Health Insurance looms in the near future as the bottom line.

Even though many of the federal legislative proposals, including the Clinical Laboratories Improvement Act of 1975, have not been enacted into law, these proposals do indicate the trend toward greater federal involvement in the quality of health care, the cost of health care, and the qualifications of health care personnel. Indications are that the Federal Government will develop broad national health priorities within which state and local health plans and priorities must conform. There is already a tremendous amount of federal involvement and federal program funding which has caused state legislatures to enact many new health program laws to take advantage of federal assistance.

It is important to note, however, that, although vast federal tax funds are being spent to promote the health and general welfare of the people, the Federal Government does seem to recognize that the states still have certain inherent powers and the basic responsibility to protect the public health. However, where federal funds are being spent, federal standards must be met by the health care providers to be eligible for reimbursement. Certification that health care providers meet the standards will be performed by the states through a designated state agency as is being done under the present Medicare program. The designated state agency has not always been the state health department.

Under the new National Health Planning and Resources Development Act of 1974 (approved 4 January 1975, Public Law 93-641; 88 Statute 2225), a nonprofit private organization, a unit of local government, or a public regional planning body will be designated as the health systems agency for each local area to develop area health plans and priorities which must conform to an overall state plan and federal health priorities. However, the local health system agency will have the power to review the need for new institutional health services and will exercise control over federal funds.

"No matter what our sentiments might be, whether we welcome or oppose the expanding federal role in health, we can scarcely be unconcerned by it. For beyond any doubt, the health-care system of the United States is in a process of change no less sweeping and no less profound than that experienced over the past several decades in virtually all the other advanced nations of the world. And the federal government is the principal instrument of that change" (1).

COMPLIANCE MEASURES

What does all this mean to the operating laboratory? Is the regulation of laboratories really necessary? How does a laboratory comply with regulations? Although specific licensure and certification requirements will be discussed in chapter 120 and detailed quality control practices for diagnostic immunology will be described in chapter 121, a general response to these questions is needed.

Basically, the concept of regulation of their profession is repugnant to most laboratory scientists, but let us consider why we have regulations governing the operation of laboratories. One of the most fundamental reasons has to do with the fact that laboratories are not operated solely as scientific services, but are essentially a business. This applies to hospital laboratory services as well as independent laboratories. Traditionally, income from the laboratory in nonprofit institutions has helped to subsidize money-losing activities in other parts of the hospital.

Only recently, with growing concern for medical care costs, have cost accounting and cost analysis concepts been applied to laboratory procedures in hospitals. Hospital administrators are now having to justify cost of laboratory services before payment will be made.

The business, or profit motivation, if you will, has caused scientists who know the theories and reasons for good quality control practices to adopt and apply practices in their laboratories which actually subvert the principles of good laboratory practice. Although the need to control test procedures has been taught in the most basic laboratory courses since the time of Pasteur and other historically renowned scientists, it has only been in the past 6 to 10 years that there has been a concerted effort, in a substantial part of the laboratory community, to practice quality control as it was intended to be practiced in the day-to-day operation of a laboratory. Unfortunately, this concern came about, not out of any altruistic motivation, but because of the pressures of Federal legislation.

Subjective as this observation may appear to be, there is substantial circumstantial evidence to indicate its validity.

The increased concern for quality control can be measured directly with adoption of the Medicare Act of 1965 (Social Security Amendments of 1965, 30 July 1965; Public Law 89-97; 79 Statute 286) and the Clinical Laboratories Improvement Act of 1967 (Partnership for Health Amendments of 1967, 5 December 1967; Public Law 90-174, Section 5(a); 81 Statute 536). There is nothing required in these laws and their implementing regulations which is contrary to good laboratory practice. In fact, the regulations establish an absolute minimum standard for good laboratory performance. Most "good" laboratories would impose more stringent requirements of quality control for their laboratory services.

Now we can answer the question, "How do I comply with the regulations?"

First, hire personnel, from director to technologist, who are qualified to perform laboratory services. Without competent, conscientious laboratory personnel, there can be no hope for good quality laboratory services. Paper qualifications do not guarantee competence, but unqualified personnel do not have the basic knowledge necessary to perform their jobs satisfactorily. They are not capable of solving a problem or, even worse, do not even recognize a problem when it exists. In addition, unqualified personnel are less likely to recognize their own limitations.

Second, establish written guidelines for all laboratory procedures including the calibration requirements for instrumentation and the quality control requirements for each method in use. Then insist that these methods be followed precisely by every member of the laboratory staff.

Third, keep records concurrently with the work.

Fourth, process each specimen as if it were your own and your life and well-being depended on the result.

If every laboratorian followed these practices, we might not need regulation of diagnostic immunology or any other laboratory discipline.

To answer specific questions about meeting state and Federal regulations, you should contact the laboratory director of your state health department. He or a member of his staff should be able to provide you with the latest information pertaining to both State and Federal requirements for the operation of a laboratory. If not able to provide this information directly, they can provide reference sources.

LITERATURE CITED

1. Edwards, C. C. 1975. The federal involvement in health. N. Engl. J. Med. 292:559–562.
2. Grad, F. P. 1970. Public health law manual, 2nd printing. American Public Health Association, Washington, D.C.
3. Hicks, H. A. 1973. Philosophy of laboratory control. Health Lab. Sci. 10:268–270.
4. Jones, H. W. 1959. Public health, p. 758–763. In Encyclopedia Americana, vol. 22. Grolier Inc., New York, N.Y.

Chapter 120

State and Federal Regulations Governing the Licensure of Laboratories

WILLIAM KAUFMANN

Immunology is both a clinical specialty and a clinical laboratory entity. When viewed in the context of clinical medicine, clinical immunology is obviously an integral part of the practice of medicine and therefore subject to the laws regulating the profession of the healing arts. In other words, individuals practicing clinical immunology must hold a license to practice medicine in the state in which they work. When applied to laboratory practice, the situation is much more complex.

Wherever laboratory practice or laboratory medicine is considered the practice of medicine, as for example in Texas or New Hampshire, no individual except a licensed physician may perform laboratory tests, including immunological tests. Some states have legislation which rigidly outlines the responsibilities of individuals who may direct or perform in clinical laboratories, whereas in other states no legal regulations exist, and laboratory testing, including that used in immunology, is under no legal control.

To complicate matters further, the Federal Goverment in 1967 promulgated the Clinical Laboratories Improvement Act (CLIA) of 1967 which became operative in 1969 (Title 42 – Public Health. Chapter 1 – Public Health Service; Department of Health, Education and Welfare. Subchapter F – Quarantine, Inspection, Licensing. Part 74 – Clinical Laboratories). It delineates in detail the requisites for the operation of independent clinical laboratories engaged in interstate commerce; it establishes rules and regulations for the operation of clinical laboratories; and it extends the regulations to personnel (from director to supervisor and medical technologist), to physical facilities, to internal and external quality control (the latter requiring participation in a proficiency testing program approved by the Secretary of Health, Education and Welfare [HEW]), and to equipment, reagents, and safety measures. Penalties for noncompliance are outlined in the act, and responsibility for their enforcement is delegated to the Center for Disease Control in Atlanta, Ga.

In 1975, Senators Jacob K. Javits and Edward M. Kennedy introduced a bill into the U.S. Senate known as S.1737 and cited as the Clinical Laboratories Improvement Act of 1975 (Senate 1737, 74th Congress, 1st Session, 14 May 1975). This act defines the term "laboratory" or "clinical laboratory" as "a facility for the biological, microbiological, serological, chemical, immuno-hematological, hematological, biophysical, cytological, pathological, or other examination of materials derived from the human body for the purpose of providing information for the diagnosis, prevention, or treatment of any disease or impairment of, or the assessment of the health of, man, or a facility for the collection, processing, and transmission of such materials for such purposes." In contrast to the CLIA of 1967, which is restricted to laboratories engaged in interstate commerce, this act would include all clinical laboratories, both inter- and intrastate, and both hospital and independent. Not yet clear is whether or not laboratories operated by physicians and/or groups of physicians who test specimens on their own patients solely, for the purpose of aiding in the diagnosis and treatment of disease, are excluded from the act. The act specifically, among other requirements, stipulates "participation in a proficiency testing program and on-site inspection program acceptable to the Secretary," and it establishes within the Department of Health, Education and Welfare an Office of Clinical Laboratories.

The Office of Clinical Laboratories, after consultation with a newly formed Advisory Council to the Secretary, "shall establish, within thirteen months after the date of enactment of this Act, a uniform set of testing, quality control, personnel, proficiency testing, and other necessary guidelines for clinical laboratories that will assure quality performance and otherwise serve the purposes of this section as well as the purposes of other programs within the Department of Health, Education and Welfare. The Office of Clinical Laboratories shall report annually to the Congress through the Secretary concerning its activities under this section together with such findings and recommendations as it deems necessary."

The above-mentioned Advisory Council on

clinical laboratories shall "advise, consult with, and make recommendations to the Office of Clinical Laboratories." The Council's functions and responsibilities are meticulously detailed, and its composition is regulated. A further extension of the CLIA of 1967 would be a "Model Certification for Technical Laboratory Personnel."

The act offers to states which presently operate clinical laboratory improvement programs of their own the opportunity to have the authority to issue licenses delegated to the appropriate health authority of the state, subject to the determination that the state has enacted a law and adopted regulations applicable to clinical laboratories, which laws and regulations meet or exceed the standards established under the federal regulations, and provided the state "is enforcing the provisions of such laws and regulations with respect to all clinical laboratories within its jurisdiction in a manner which does not discriminate against any type or class of such laboratories."

Presently, 18 states have enacted and are operating under laws regulating clinical laboratories, albeit with a wide range of stringency (Table 1). Other states periodically introduce in their legislatures bills to regulate clinical laboratories, and therefore this number is undoubtedly going to increase over the years. One state, New York, has since 1965 been operating under a state CLIA (Article 5, Title V, of the Public Health Law), which grew out of a New York City Sanitary Code regulation promulgated in 1960 and which is at this writing the most all-encompassing state-mandated and -operated laboratory improvement act in the nation. In 1971, the Secretary of HEW approved the New York State act as equal to or more stringent than the federal CLIA of 1967, thereby offering laboratories in New York State and engaged in interstate commerce the opportunity to obtain a letter of exemption from his office.

The New York State CLIA through its rules and regulations requires that all directors of clinical laboratories (independent and hospital alike) must hold a certificate of qualification issued by the State Department of Health. It limits such certificates to individuals holding a doctor's degree (either M.D. or Ph.D.) and specifically outlines the training and experience subsequent to graduation required for the issuance of a certificate of qualification. It limits an individual to directorships in no more than two clinical laboratories or blood banks. Specific personnel requirements are outlined for clinical laboratory supervisors and medical technologists. These in general coincide with those required by the Social Security Act under Title 20

(Federal Health Insurance for the Aged. Conditions for Coverage of Services of Independent Laboratories. Code of Federal Regulations. Title 20, Chapter III, Part 405). Certificates of qualification are issued to the director on the basis of educational qualifications in the following categories: (i) microbiology or one or more of the subspecialties of bacteriology, serology, virology, mycology, and parasitology; (ii) hematology; (iii) transfusion services, blood grouping, and Rh typing; (iv) clinical chemistry; (v) tissue pathology and/or exfoliative cytology; (vi) biophysics (radiobioassay); and (vii) other specific categories, procedures, or specialties designated by the department.

Interpretation of the extent of these specialties (or categories, as they are frequently called) has presented difficulties on the state and federal level at times, especially as new test procedures become available in the clinical laboratory. For example, with the advent of radioimmunoassays as tests in many laboratory specialties, definition of the relevant terms became essential. Thus, under Subpart M, Part 405, Chapter III, of Title 20 of the Social Security Act, the definition of radiobioassay reads as follows: "(1) an examination to identify radionuclides or determine and quantitate body levels of radionuclides which are taken in by chronic or acute absorption, ingestion, or inhalation; and (2) following the administration of a radioactive material to a patient, the subsequent analysis of a body fluid, or excreta, in order to evaluate body function." On the basis of this definition, it is evident that radiobioassay is a distinct specialty area in the practice of medicine and requires a license to practice medicine.

Procedures other than those defined above as radiobioassays but which utilize radioisotopes as an in vitro tool for the quantitative and qualitative measurement of specific substances (radioimmunoassays, displacement or competitive binding techniques, etc.), whether in the category of chemical, seroimmunological, microbiological, or hematological determinations, are considered integral to the appropriate subspecialty. Under this definition, therefore, radioimmunoassays such as the determination of Australia antigen fall under the category of immunohematology, and the use of radionuclides for digoxin quantitation comes under clinical chemistry.

In addition to the state and federal regulation, the Joint Accreditation Commission of the American Hospital and American Medical Associations has assumed responsibility for the supervision of hospital clinical laboratories under its prerogatives to accredit hospitals

TABLE 1. *Regulation of clinical laboratories under state laws (as of 1 August 1975)*

State	Requirement			Offers participation in voluntary proficiency testing
	Licensure of laboratories	Licensure of directors	Proficiency evaluation	
Alabama	No	No	No	No
Alaska	No	No	No	No
Arizona	Yes	Yes	Yes[a]	No
Arkansas	No	No	No	No
California	Yes	Yes	Yes	Yes
Colorado	No	No	No	No
Connecticut	Yes	Yes	Yes[a]	No
Delaware	No	No	Yes	Yes
Florida	Yes	No	Yes	Yes
Georgia	Yes	No	Yes[a]	Yes
Hawaii	Yes	Yes	Yes	Yes
Idaho	No	No	No	No
Illinois	Yes	Yes	Yes	Yes
Indiana	No	No	No	No
Iowa	No	No	No	No
Kansas	No	No	No	No
Kentucky	No	No	No	No
Louisiana	No	No	No	No
Maine	No	No	No	No
Maryland	Yes	Yes	Yes[a]	Yes
Massachusetts	No	No	No	No
Michigan	Yes	Yes	Yes[a]	Yes
Minnesota	No	Yes	Yes[a]	Yes
Mississippi	No	No	No	No
Missouri	No	No	No	No
Montana	No	No	No	No
Nebraska	No	No	No	No
Nevada	Yes	Yes	Yes	Yes
New Hampshire	No	No	No	Yes
New Jersey	No	Yes	Yes[a]	No
New Mexico	No	No	No	No
New York	Yes	Yes	Yes[a]	No
North Carolina	No	No	No	No
North Dakota	No	No	No	No
Ohio	No	No	No	No
Oklahoma	No	No	No	No
Oregon	Yes	Yes	Yes	Yes
Pennsylvania	Yes	No	Yes[a]	No
Rhode Island	Yes	Yes	Yes	Yes
South Carolina	No	No	No	No
South Dakota	No	No	No	No
Tennessee	Yes	Yes	Yes	Yes
Texas	No	No	No	No
Utah	No	No	No	Yes
Vermont	No	No	No	No
Virginia	No	No	No	No
Washington	No	No	No	No
West Virginia	No	No	No	No
Wisconsin	Yes[b]	No	No	Yes
Wyoming	No	No	No	No
Guam	No	No	No	No
Puerto Rico	Yes	Yes	Yes[a]	No
Virgin Islands	No	No	Yes	Yes
New York City[c]	Yes	Yes	Yes[a]	No

TABLE 1—*Continued*

[a] Requires participation in its own proficiency testing program.

[b] Applies to hospital laboratories only.

[c] Permitted under New York State law to operate its own laboratory improvement program.

throughout the nation. The standards for such accreditation are rather vague and in no way approach those stipulated by governmental agencies or even those established by the College of American Pathologists. Attempts by the College of American Pathologists to have the Joint Accreditation Commission fully accept the College's inspection and accreditation program as its accreditation program for hospitals have so far not been successful.

The growth of laboratory practice during the past decade has resulted in the development of large interstate clinical laboratories, frequently operated by drug companies or hospital supply firms, whose avowed purpose is accurate, precise testing of large numbers of samples in order to reduce the cost of laboratory medicine. Although this is the principal purpose of this type of endeavor, the fact that it is also a business venture is not denied by its proponents. It is a definite growth industry, which is avowedly willing and anxious to submit to governmental regulation in order to demonstrate its total reliability. Not only individual physicians or physician groups but hospitals and scientific institutions alike are making increasing use of these facilities, which therefore seem to be fulfilling a demonstrated need. This voluntary and businesslike centralization and regionalization program in one field of medical endeavor has yet to demonstrate its viability, but its vitality is not in doubt and may well be a sign of the future.

One may ask why governmental regulation became necessary and appears to be growing. Professional organizations such as the College of American Pathologists and the American Association of Bioanalysts have for a considerable time — in fact, long before governmental regulations were instituted — conducted proficiency testing programs of clinical laboratories and unquestionably have contributed to the improvement of clinical laboratory practice. However, such professional organizations lack legal authority to enforce their programs and depend entirely on voluntary participation. Improvement therefore may be demonstrable in laboratories which are desirous of improvement and would have shown it without participation in any program, whereas those which showed deficiencies might or might not institute remedial action. Nonparticipation in any inspection and accreditation program or proficiency testing program cannot be challenged under the voluntary approach. Presently there is no argument over the necessity of accreditation and proficiency testing programs, regardless of whether they are voluntary or governmentally controlled. Sufficient evidence exists that such programs have improved performance and thereby benefit the public.

Title 20 of the Social Security Act (Medicare) has had an additional impact on governmental regulation of clinical laboratories since 1967. This act gives detailed requirements for independent clinical laboratories participating in the medical reimbursement of services rendered under the act. Although originally the regulations stipulated under the CLIA of 1967 differed to some extent from those promulgated under Title 20 of the Social Security Act, attempts have recently been made by the Secretary of HEW to overcome these divergencies and to promote uniformity of application. Thus, the educational, training, and experience requirements of both acts were brought in line, and requirements for participation in proficiency testing programs approved by the Secretary of HEW were made uniform. A recent, widely felt change in the Medicare regulations, especially applicable to independent laboratories, reads in part as follows (Subpart S, 405.1909):

(c) Independent laboratories previously found in compliance, but which have had their approval revoked in total or in a specialty or subspecialty because of unsatisfactory

performance in proficiency testing, may subsequently be certified by the State agency and determined by the Secretary to be in compliance with the conditions where:
(1) After a 6-month period, an appraisal of the laboratory's performance in a proficiency testing program as defined in 405.1310 (c) reflects satisfactory results on at least two sets of specimens, or
(2) After a 3-month period, the State agency's assessment of the laboratory's performance in examining proficiency test samples analyzed during at least two State agency on-site visits, establishes the laboratory's competency.

This change in the Medicare regulations does not extend to hospital laboratories and thereby may be considered discriminatory against one group of laboratories – namely, independent ones – since it may interfere with a laboratory's or an individual's right to "earn a living." The constitutionality of this requirement remains to be tested.

It is apparent that at the time of this writing a multitude of regulations, both state and federal, exist throughout the land. Many attempts to produce means for states to reciprocate with one another have failed so far because there is no uniformity in legislation. The introduction of the Javits-Kennedy bill in the U.S. Senate and the likely introduction of another similar bill by Congressman Paul G. Rogers of Florida in the House of Representatives are attempts to bring order out of chaos. It is unlikely that less stringent regulations will be the end result, especially if and when a program of national health insurance should ultimately be enacted.

Chapter 121

Some Concepts of Quality Control in Immunoserology

DAN F. PALMER AND JOSEPH J. CAVALLARO

INTRODUCTION

Over the past few years, many new immunological methods have been developed which now provide the clinical laboratory with a large array of potentially valuable diagnostic tools. However, it is incumbent upon the immunologist to utilize only those methods designed to provide appropriate data which permit objective analysis leading to valid inferences. This requirement may be met if the validity of data is assured by a system of sound experimental design to detect errors in experimentation, observation, or measurement; to detect variation in experimental material; and to monitor combined effects of all other factors not singled out for individual analysis.

These concepts apply to all diagnostic methods used by the immunologist and are currently referred to collectively under the terms "quality control" or "quality assurance." These terms encompass not only those activities directly associated with the conduct of a particular procedure, but also such considerations as the educational background of the laboratory personnel, bookkeeping and specimen labeling, washing of glassware, and calibration of volumetric ware. The latter topics are covered adequately elsewhere (1, 2, 4), so in the limited space available discussion will center on some of the major criteria involved in establishing the validity of diagnostic laboratory procedures through the use of reference or control materials.

Each performance of an immunological procedure on a patient or a patient's specimen is a unique instance requiring a rigorous scientific approach and objectivity. Assuming that the procedure is chosen so that information collected is relevant to the problems presented, attention is required to insure that levels of precision, accuracy, sensitivity, and specificity are adequate.

These four terms refer to the dimensions by which the credibility of an immunological procedure is measured. They are cursorily defined here so that each concept may be understood relative to the others when it is discussed in detail.

"Precision" refers to the magnitude of the differences among quantitative results obtained with repeated assays on the same specimen without reference to the true value of the substance measured. The smaller the differences among results obtained with repeated assays, the greater the precision of the procedure is. Obviously, a procedure may be precise without being accurate and, occasionally, accurate without being precise. "Accuracy," on the other hand, refers to the magnitude of the discrepancy between a quantitative test result and the true quantity of the substance being measured. The greater the difference between the value obtained for a substance and its true value, the less accurate is the procedure used to measure it.

Immunologists customarily consider the "sensitivity" of a procedure to be a measure of its ability to signal the presence of a low concentration of a component of interest. The smaller the quantity of a substance that is detected by a procedure, the more sensitive the procedure is. In contrast, "specificity" refers to the ability of a procedure to yield a negative result when the true state of the specimen is negative.

All four terms, as used in quality control, are interrelated to some extent, are often misunderstood, and are subject to interpretational discrepancies.

In the following sections each will be discussed as a separate entity, but they all must be considered together when establishing a properly controlled laboratory procedure.

PRECISION

The precision of a test is a reference to its reproducibility, or repeatability. It is the degree to which results from repeated assays on the same specimen agree with one another. The terms "precision," "reproducibility," and "repeatability" are commonly used interchangeably, but some authorities prefer to use the term "reproducibility" to denote the deviation of results when a given procedure is performed on the same specimen by different technicians over a period of time and the term "repeatability" to denote the deviation of results when replicates of a specimen are tested by a given procedure at one time. Recently, Dybkaer (3) suggested that "dispersion of the disturbance distribution" is more descriptive of the set of repetitive data from which inferences are made concerning how well a procedure can reproduce results. However, until standardized terminology can be adopted officially, the term "precision" should be used as it has been in the past.

Because precision describes a particular characteristic of quantitative data, mathematical expressions must be applied which convey, numerically, the concepts set forth in the preceding paragraph. The most common expression used for describing the scatter of replicate measurements is the standard deviation (SD). Its estimate requires that a mean be computed for all of the replicate measurements and that the square root be taken of the average of the squared deviations of the measurements from their mean:

$$SD = \sqrt{\frac{\Sigma(x - \bar{x})^2}{n - 1}}$$

Frequently, comparisons must be made in studying the relative variability of different types of data. In such cases, it is not meaningful to simply compare the magnitudes of the different standard deviations, since the units of measurements are different. The coefficients of variation should then be used because this facilitates the comparisons by expressing standard deviations as percentages of the means:

$$\text{coefficient of variation} = \frac{SD}{\bar{x}}(100)$$

On the basis of the results of quality control programs in several clinical laboratories, we recommend that one of the first steps in considering the adoption of a procedure is to estimate its precision. This should involve an evaluation of both "within-run" and "between-run" variation.

The within-run precision of a procedure can be estimated by performing 30 or more replicate determinations on samples of the same specimen and calculating the mean and standard deviation of the test results. Alternately, within-run precision may be measured by testing routine specimens in duplicate until 30 or more duplicate results are accumulated. To reduce bias, the duplicates must be randomly distributed in the run rather than tested consecutively. Use the following equation for computing the standard deviation when employing the latter method:

$$SD = \sqrt{\frac{(\Sigma d^2)}{2n}}$$

where d is the difference between duplicate results, and n is the total number of pairs.

Between-run variation is usually of more value in estimating the precision of a procedure. It is determined by assaying the same specimen in each of at least 30 tests run over a period of time and computing the mean and standard deviation of the test values. Between-run precision is generally poorer than that obtained within-run, but the former is a more realistic appraisal of a method's precision because it provides an estimate of the variation due to the many factors caused by day-to-day differences in the laboratory.

The precision of a method often varies with the concentration of the substance being assayed. In general, relative precision is poorest at extremely low or extremely high concentrations, so variation should be measured at low, normal, and high levels for a thorough characterization of the method being evaluated.

Obviously, variation of results from replicate assays of a given specimen is a manifestation of the cumulated experimental error to which the method used is subject. The magnitude of the error depends upon factors such as the type of equipment used, the technique of the person performing the test, and the purity of reagents. Further, the errors may be categorized into systematic and random types.

A systematic error is the consequence of a method's tendency to yield results which deviate, on the average, in a given direction and usually of a certain magnitude from the true value. This type of error may be detected by comparing a sufficient number of results obtained from a test method with results on the same specimens obtained from a base-line or reference method. If bias is present, as indicated by a tendency for test method results to vary in one direction, a systematic error is said to be present.

Further, within the category of systematic error are uncontrolled trends manifested over a period of time. These trends may be caused by gradual deterioration of reagents, fading of a color standard, or other similar occurrences in the test system. This type of error is best detected by consistently monitoring reference or control reagents of known titer and plotting results of repeated testing on a "quality control chart." Trends can often be visually identified by this method.

Random errors are those resulting from intrinsic variable properties of the test procedure.

They are not characterized by deviation in a given direction nor are they of consistent magnitude. They do, however, fall within a predictable range and, since they ordinarily follow Gaussian distribution, they may be measured by computing the standard deviation of test results, as explained in a preceding paragraph. In this sense, the standard deviation is a measure of how large the predictable error is (an index of the test's precision).

Currently, there are no established universally *accepted allowable limits of error* (ALE) for most of the procedures performed in the clinical immunology laboratory. These limits are generally set by individual laboratories after the variations obtained with their reagents and equipment and their technicians have been measured. Obviously, when designing a quality control program in the laboratory, one must not demand more precision than that actually required for practical diagnostic purposes or that attainable under actual working conditions.

Tonks (5) has proposed a rule of thumb for establishing the ALE for a given procedure. The rule is predicated on the requirement that the ALE (expressed as a percentage of concentration) must not be greater than 100 times one-fourth the length of the normal range divided by the midpoint of the normal range; expressed mathematically:

$$\text{ALE } (\%) = \frac{\frac{1}{4} \text{ length of normal range}}{\text{midpoint of normal range}} \times 100$$

The use of this equation is exemplified by the following:

Example. One of the recommended normal ranges for serum immunoglobulin G (IgG) in adult Caucasian males = 77 to 171 IU/ml as determined by radial immunodiffusion and a specified set of commercial reagents. The mean of this range is 124 IU; therefore

$$\text{ALE } = \frac{\frac{1}{4} (171 - 77)}{124} \times 100 = 18.95\%$$

The ALE for a procedure purporting to measure IgG under the conditions set forth in this example are therefore the value obtained for a determination ±18.95% of that value, according to Tonk's equation.

The conditions set forth in the foregoing equation were meant primarily for procedures performed in clinical chemistry laboratories and are too restrictive for many immunoserological tests at the present time. Nevertheless, it is an interesting approach to setting precision requirements for laboratory tests.

ACCURACY

Once the precision of a method has been estimated, its accuracy should be determined. Generally, the accuracy of immunoserological methods can only be estimated, since the absolute values of immune substances in reference or control specimens available to most clinical laboratories are seldom established. Nevertheless, some degree of confidence about a method's accuracy can be developed in several ways. One of the most successful ways is by recovery studies in which specimens containing known amounts of carefully measured, purified preparation of the substance of interest are tested by the particular method in question. Assessment of the method's accuracy is then based on how close its results can come to indicating the concentration of the substance added. Most of the national and international standards facilitate this kind of study.

Another approach, currently employed by many laboratories, is the use of specimens which have been assayed by many different authoritative laboratories. These specimens are usually aliquants of those sent to a large number of participating laboratories in a proficiency testing program and are characterized by a summary analysis of test results. The assumption is made that the mean of all results reported for a given specimen by the best participating laboratories is the best estimate of the concentration or titer of the substance being assayed. The laboratory then adopts the specimen as a "standard," and a method's accuracy is determined by comparing the value obtained for the specimen to that assumed to be the true value.

Different laboratories variously employ several other ways of estimating the accuracy of a method. Results from a new or modified method may be compared with results on the same specimen obtained with a recognized reference method, if such exists. Likewise, results from a method being evaluated may be compared with results from the same method performed in another laboratory known to produce good results. Finally, a method's accuracy may be assessed by comparing the range of normal values determined by the test method with the range of normal values accepted by the scientific community as the true one.

SENSITIVITY

In immunoserology, the term "sensitivity" denotes the ability of a procedure to detect very low concentrations of a substance.

This concept may be more descriptively conceived in relation to "limits of detection"; the more "sensitive" procedures are capable of detecting lower concentrations of a component and thus have a lower limit of detection than the less "sensitive" ones.

The ideally sensitive test method is one which signals a positive result when the true state of the specimen is positive. If the test is occasionally negative when the true state of the specimen is positive (as is more often the case), false negatives are said to occur (see Table 1). A crude measure of the test's sensitivity may be calculated by taking into account the number of false negatives that occur, as follows:

Index of sensitivity =

$$\frac{\text{true positives} - \text{false negatives}}{\text{true positives}} \times 100$$

The number of true positives may be estimated on the basis of clinical criteria, i.e., the number of patients exhibiting the appropriate symptoms and other laboratory findings.

Of course, in many immunological assays, there is a finite component concentration below which there is no relevance to the patient's clinical status. In such a case, there is no need to seek a procedure with a limit of detection lower than that needed for clinical relevancy. One can then establish a "threshold of significance" (i.e., concentration of a component below which there is no clinical relevance) for the component of interest. Since the lower limit of detection of a procedure varies from one time to the next, the extent of that variation must be monitored, especially if the threshold of significance is close to the lower limit of detection for that procedure. The appropriate quality control measure to institute at this step is the inclusion in the procedure of a "comparison material" (3) containing the component at a concentration equivalent to that at the threshold of significance. If the comparison material is treated in the same way as the patient's specimen and if it closely resembles the patient's specimen in every way except that the concentration of the component of interest is known, a positive result affords one the assumption that the procedure is "sensitive" enough to detect the component in the patient's specimens at the lowest meaningful concentration.

The concept of sensitivity of a procedure is more classically concerned with the ability to measure small differences in concentration of a component in a series of specimens. This is of great importance to the immunologist or serologist seeking to demonstrate changes in the concentration of immune substances as a function of time. A "sensitive" procedure in this respect is typically one in which small changes in concentration of a component being assayed are manifested by gross, readily measurable changes in the property which varies as a function of the component's concentration. In other words, the procedure is "sensitive" to small changes in the component's concentration. Before the immunologist adopts a procedure for use in diagnostic work, he or she must have some knowledge of the magnitude of measurement variation obtained over repeated tests on the same specimens. By applying appropriate statistical tests on accumulated data, he or she can then be prepared to make probability statements concerning whether two or more specimens yielding different levels of reaction contain the same component concentration. Having characterized the procedure in these terms, one should then employ quality control specimens in the test to monitor the extent of measurement variation at different component concentration levels and determine whether the variation is within the assumed bounds.

SPECIFICITY

In the immunologist's domain, the concept of specificity is characterized by two major distinctions. The first is the characteristic of an immunological procedure that determines its ability to yield a negative test result when the true state of the specimen is negative. As shown in Table 1, specimens that are negative in their true state but react positively by the immunological procedure are designated false positives. A measure of the procedure's specificity in this sense, then, may be calculated in a manner similar to that used for obtaining an index of sensitivity, except that the number of false positives is placed in the numerator and the number of true negatives is placed in the denominator:

$$\frac{\text{true negatives} - \text{false positives}}{\text{true negatives}}$$

$$\times 100 = \text{index of specificity}$$

Implicit in this concept of specificity is the assumption that any false positives that occur do not contain the component being assayed for. Instead, these false-positive specimens react to give positive results as a result of the action of out-of-control variables, such as pH

TABLE 1. *Determination of test sensitivity*

Test result	True state of the specimens	
	Positive	Negative
Positive	Correct reaction	False positive
Negative	False negative	Correct reaction

and ionicity, or because of the presence of components in the test reagents or patients' sera which can confound the indicator system. Quality control measures to determine whether false-positive reactions occur in this scheme are often inadequate. A true negative control specimen is ordinarily included in the test to detect the action of out-of-control variables operating to produce false-positive results, but this comparison material cannot act as a control for variation of components in patients' sera which might react with the indicator system to produce false-positive results. The latter is most often monitored by individual patient's serum control specimens, which are simply mixtures of the patient's serum with components of the test indicator system, omitting the antigen (if testing for antibodies) or antiserum (if testing for antigen). If a positive reaction occurs in a patient's serum control, then the significance of the positive reaction in that same patient's test sequence is in doubt, and the confounding substance must be eliminated via processing.

The second distinction which characterizes the concept of specificity is concerned with the presence of so-called "cross-reacting" immune substances in the patient's specimen. These immune substances may be reacting specifically with the reference antigen or antibody employed in a test, but the immunologist views them as nonspecific in that they may have arisen as a result of a different disease process or, indeed, they may have been elicited by a different pathogenic organism altogether. There appear to be many instances of similar antigenic determinants shared by different pathogens (such as *Histoplasma* spp. and *Blastomyces* spp., or *Brucella* and *Francisella*) which elicit antibodies that react to some degree with all of the organisms sharing the determinants. In this case, the antigen-antibody reaction may be specific, at least in some sequential or configurational aspect, although antibodies present as

a consequence of infection with one organism are reacting with a reference antigen prepared from another organism. Quality control of this aspect of specificity involves testing the patient's serum specimen with reference antigens prepared from all of the pathogens known to share antigenic determinants with the pathogen of interest. Generally, but not in all cases, the antigen which is specifically involved will react with the patient's serum specimen to give the highest antibody titer or show the greatest rise in antibody titer in sequential specimens taken early in the disease.

The concepts discussed comprise but a fraction of the considerations for a comprehensive quality control program. However, a thorough understanding of the precepts construed under each section, along with a comparable search into the reason and nature of all other variables affecting the results of the immunologist's scientific inquiry, will most certainly facilitate development of an adequate system of control.

LITERATURE CITED

1. Bartlett, R. C. 1974. Medical microbiology: quality, cost, and clinical reference. Wiley-Interscience, New York.
2. Bartlett, R. C., W. R. Irving, Jr., and C. Rutz. 1968. Quality control in clinical microbiology. Committee on Continuing Education, American Society of Clinical Pathologists, Chicago, Ill.
3. Dybkaer, R. 1973. Problems in terminology. Proceedings: international conference on standardization of diagnostic materials.
4. Russell, R. L. 1974. Quality control in the microbiology laboratory, p. 862–870. *In* E. H. Lennette, E. H. Spaulding, and J. P. Truant (ed.), Manual of clinical microbiology, 2nd ed. American Society for Microbiology, Washington, D.C.
5. Tonks, D. B. 1972. Quality control in clinical laboratories. Warner-Chilcott Laboratories Co., Ltd., Scarborough, Ontario.

Chapter 122

Standardization of Reagents and Methodology in Immunology

IRENE BATTY AND G. TORRIGIANI

INTRODUCTION

In recent years, there has been increasing emphasis on the importance of the standardization of the reagents used in the clinical immunology laboratory (14). The primary aim of such standardization is to improve the quality of laboratory results and to provide a means to ensure uniformity in the designation of the concentration of clinically important substances in body fluids which cannot be adequately characterized by chemical and physical means.

Although immunology is a relatively young discipline, the time has long since passed, at least in the major areas, when comparability and uniformity of results could be ensured by the interchange of materials between interested workers. It is also no longer the case that most of the test systems and techniques are controlled by competent involved laboratory immunologists; many tests are in routine use and performed by technicians who, although technically competent, have little intimate knowledge of the immunological basis of the tests.

It might be thought that reagents which are used by scientists for in vitro tests in the laboratory, where expense, time, and inclination are virtually the only factors which determine how well the performance of the test and the reagents are controlled, was the area least in need of standardization. This might be true if each test result could be regarded in isolation and there was no need to communicate results to others or to compare results obtained in different laboratories or even in one laboratory at different times.

EARLY WORK ON STANDARDIZATION

This point becomes clearer if we consider the history of biological standardization which started in the late 1880s after Roux and Yersin Behring and Kitasato had shown that certain bacterial species produce toxins and that animals receiving repeated doses of such toxins produce substances which specifically neutralize these toxins. It almost immediately became clear to these early workers that, if these phenomena were to be studied in anything more than the most superficial manner and have any practical application, it was necessary to quantify the interaction of these substances. By 1897, therefore, Ehrlich had produced his classical work on the standardization of diphtheria toxin, and Kraus had shown that when homologous antiserum and soluble antigen meet a visible precipitate is produced; that is, the foundation of immunological standardization was laid.

ELEMENTS OF STANDARDIZATION

Units

The first stage in any attempt at quantification is the definition of units by which activity is to be measured. Units in the immunological context are analogous to the international and national physical units of length and mass in that they are defined by reference to the activity of a given weight or, more rarely, volume of an arbitrarily designated standard preparation.

Originally, Erhlich measured the potency of diphtheria toxin in terms of the least volume which, when injected by a stated route, would kill an animal of a designated species and weight within a certain time, that is, in terms of its minimal lethal dose (MLD). This parameter measures the toxicity of a toxin and, although it is independent of its ability to combine with antitoxin, it has the grave disadvantage that such measurements are particularly sensitive to changes in the indicator systems. The apparent toxicity of a toxin has been found to vary with the diet of the indicator animal and even the season of the year, as this affects its susceptibility. Such tests show poor reproducibility either within a single laboratory at different times or between laboratories at the same time. A further problem was that toxins were also found to lose toxicity both on storage or following treatment with a variety of chemical reagents without any diminution in ability to combine with antitoxin. Therefore, although

Erhlich originally defined the unit of antitoxin as the smallest amount of antiserum which would neutralize 100 MLD of toxin, a unit of antiserum is now defined as that amount of an antiserum which has the same ability to combine with a volume of toxin, some of which may be toxoid, as had the arbitrary unit of antitoxin in the original serum laid down by Erhlich, that is, as a certain weight of his dried standard preparation of antitoxin. In this example one international unit of diphtheria antitoxin has the same combining, neutralizing activity as 0.0638 mg of the international standard.

Size of units. Although the weight of the standard preparation to which unit activity is assigned may have been originally related to a particular degree of biological activity, it is not necessarily related to other activities of the antibody. It happens, therefore, that some units appear small for certain purposes and large by other criteria. For instance, a therapeutic dose of tetanus antitoxin contains thousands of units, whereas a reasonable level of circulating tetanus antitoxin in an immune animal is only a fraction of a unit.

Comparability of units. There is no relationship between the unit of one specific antibody and the unit of a second different antibody; for example, a unit of immunoglobulin G (IgG) will not precipitate the same mass of specific Ig as a unit of IgE. In the early days of standardization, antibodies were almost always used as the standard materials because they tended to be more stable. Nowadays, it is the custom to choose a standard on the basis of the precision with which it can be characterized and the ease with which a sufficiently large homogenous batch of material can be accurately divided into small portions and lyophilized.

Reagents under consideration

A very high proportion of tests used in diagnostic laboratories, particularly in the fields of microbiology and hematology, depend on reactions between antigens and antibodies, i.e., are immunologically based. However, many reagents used in such tests, for example, blood grouping antisera, agglutinating sera, etc., are properly outside the scope of this chapter. The discussion will be confined to those reagents which are used for detection and quantitation in an immunological context.

There are two other major facets to the problem of standardizing the reagents and methods for immunological tests which govern attempts at achieving a solution.

Complexity

The first is the complexity of the materials being considered. It is now possible to obtain many of the antigens under consideration in a relatively pure form, but, however pure the antigen, the antibodies raised against it will be heterologous, differing at least in specificity, class, and avidity. The choice of materials for an antibody standard is therefore extremely difficult.

Many of the antigens used in clinical immunology are still complex; for example, the crude extract of *Candida albicans* used to detect immune deficiencies may have at least 70 antigenic components, all capable of eliciting antibody responses. If such antigens are purified, the result is commonly an unstable material unsuitable for use as a standard.

Functional activity

The second problem is the importance to the user of functional activity. It would be slightly simpler if it were sufficient to quantitate the number of molecules of the designated substance present in the biological fluid, but it is sometimes more important to be able to estimate the functional activity of the material present. In complement, for example, it may be desirable to know both the hemolytic and chemotactic properties. For certain antigens it may be necessary to estimate both the antibody binding and immunogenic capacity.

Standard reference materials

The first step in producing standard reference materials is the writing of the specification, which should be the combined effort of a group of experts in the field drawn from all countries where clinical immunology backed by laboratory work of a high standard is practiced on a large scale. This way, it is likely that a reasonably unequivocal specification can be written for a standard material which will be satisfactory when used under many different circumstances. Such a group of experts is best sponsored by the appropriate international scientific society, for example the International Union of Immunological Societies (IUIS), working in conjunction with the World Health Organization (WHO). Appendix I gives the specification of an anti-human IgM conjugate prepared in such a way.

The WHO, which has many years of experience in the standardization of biological substances, in particular vaccines and antisera for prophylactic and therapeutic use, has written the specifications for freeze-drying (lyophilizing) such materials (13). These methods have not been superseded, although such methods should always be considered critically whenever the standardization of a different antigen or antibody or of an antigen or antibody for use in a different situation is being undertaken. It is conceivable that changes take place during freeze-drying that without necessarily affecting potency do affect suitability for a particular purpose. An instance of this is the present International Standard for Immunoglobulins G, M, and A which, though highly satisfactory for radial immunodiffusion, reconstitutes to give a slightly turbid solution unsatisfactory for nephelometric measurement by automated techniques, as it gives too high a blank reading.

The second step is the procurement of material to meet the specifications. This may come from a hospital or research laboratory or from a commercial undertaking. It is important to prepare a large batch, sufficient for at least 4,000 ampoules, as replacement necessitates a further collaborative comparative assay and is time- and labor-consuming.

The third step is the international collaborative assay of the material. Again, this is undertaken by acknowledged experts drawn from as many countries as possible, so that it is tested under many different conditions. The design of the protocol of such a collaborative assay is best done in consultation with a statistician.

Methods

It should be appreciated that it is counterproductive to insist that a standard methodology be used in all clinical immunology laboratories even if any regulatory authority were in a position to do this. It is generally agreed that what is required is a reference method which, if followed closely, should give the correct value within the agreed limits to the standard material and by inference to other similar materials. Given this, the user can both control his own method and set up his own laboratory standard for day to day use. By this, it is implied that any reference method correctly applied will enable the user to obtain results which he/she can confidently state are inside or outside the agreed normal ranges for the population under consideration.

IMMUNOGLOBULINS

Methods of test

The most commonly used methods for measuring the Ig's are:

Radial immunodiffusion (6)

Electroimmunoassay (5)
Automated immunoprecipitation (4)
Radioimmunoassay (2)
Radioallergosorbent test (RAST) for IgE (3, 11)

Radial immunoassay (6). Of the methods listed, radial immunoassay has the longest history and the most complete documentation. The method is given in more or less detail in most recent textbooks of immunological methods, and the Association of Clinical Pathologists has issued one of its methods broadsheets which sets out the method in great detail. The points in the method which are critical if results are to be precise (i.e., reproducible) and accurate (i.e., in the case of the standard, close to the agreed value) are emphasized. Examples of such critical points are the importance of the uniformity of the depth of the agar, the need for freshly cut wells and with precise dimensions not distorted by contraction or rounded by time, and the accuracy with which the wells should be filled. The sensitivity of the method (10), which depends upon the ability to detect, visually, antigen/antibody precipitates in gels, can be increased if after the reaction has been allowed to run to completion the plate is washed and then treated by applying a second antiserum which contains radioactive antibody to the antibody Ig in the precipitate; e.g., if the serum used in the plate was goat, then a radioactive antibody to goat Ig would be used. The area of the ring shows a linear relationship to the initial concentration of antigen in the well.

Electroimmunoassay (rockets; 5). Electroimmunoassay is increasingly being used where previously radial immunoassay would have been used. It has the slight advantage over the radial immunoassay technique that it is easier to measure accurately a peak height rather than the area of a circle and can give a result in less time. For a given antibody concentration the relationship between the distance traveled by the precipitate and the antigen concentration is linear. In both methods the use of a standard antigen of known potency is virtually obligatory. For Ig's there are international reference preparations for G, M, and A (9) and research standards for D (10) and E (11) against which laboratory standards (pools of healthy adult sera held in small portions at −70 C or lower) should be calibrated.

Automated immunoprecipitation. Automated immunoprecipitation is based on a nephelometric approach (4) to antigen-antibody combination. An admixture of suitably diluted monospecific antiserum with a microvolume of the sample is passed through delay and mixing coils. The binding of antigen to soluble antibody is observed by the increase in light scattering of a beam of incident light. The intensity of light scattered is proportional to the molecular weight and concentration of particles. This method has the advantage that it has been automated and as many as 50 to 100 determinations can be made in 1 h, but it is important that the samples and standards tested have minimal initial turbidity, and the quality of the results depends to a large extent on the quality of the antibodies used.

Radioimmunoassay (2). As a method of quantitating proteins, although it is more cumbersome and needs a higher degree of skill and more expensive equipment than the two methods already discussed, radioimmunoassay has the advantage that by this means it is relatively simple to measure picogram amounts of specific protein. There are several methods available for separating bound and free antigens, the double antibody and solid phase being the most common. Which method is used is less important than that it be controlled by the use of appropriate standards, although it is important to determine that the efficiency of the separation is such that no labeled antigen is found in the "bound" fraction in the absence of antibody and all the labeled antigen is found in the "bound" fraction in the presence of excess antibody.

Radioallergosorbent test (3, 11). The RAST is virtually limited in its use to allergologists, as it is used to measure IgE reagins which appear to react as functionally monovalent molecules. The allergen is conjugated with an insoluble substrate and added to the serum under test. After allowing time for the allergen-specific antibodies to react, the insoluble complex is washed, and radioactively labeled anti-IgE antibodies are added. After further washing, the concentration of label is determined by counting, and the IgE reagin content of the serum is thus established. The problems of standardization in this test system are mainly dependent on the resolution of the problems of standardizing the allergen preparations used. The IUIS and the International Union of Allergologists are currently working on the standardization of the RAST technique and of reference preparations of some of the most commonly occurring allergens, e.g. ragweed, cocksfoot.

Serum proteins

The methods given for measuring Ig (other than the RAST) have also in recent years been used for the measurement of other serum proteins, and, as with the Ig's, the quality of the results obtained depends largely on the quality of the antibodies used in the test system. The most important qualities of these antisera are that they should be monospecific, at least so far as the sensitivity of the test system is capable of detecting any contaminating antibodies, and should be of high avidity so that antigen binding is firm and does not readily dissociate. Here again, it would be valuable to have an international standard antigen against which commercially available standards and laboratory standards could be calibrated. Such a preparation is not at present available, although the IUIS/WHO and the International Federation of Clinical Chemists are currently working toward one.

AUTO-ANTIBODIES

Methods of test

The following are the most commonly used:
Immunofluorescence tests
Enzyme-labeled antibody tests
Hemagglutination tests

Immunofluorescence. With the immunofluorescence technique, one is faced not only with the inherent variability of the immunological reagents because of the inhomogeneity of antibodies, but also with differences in labeling efficiencies, differences in substrates, and differences in the optical systems, including the light sources and type of illumination used.

However, that being said, there is no doubt as to the crucial importance of the conjugate in any attempt to obtain reproducible results both within and between laboratories. To have a conjugate which in the quantitation of auto-antibodies gives good strong specific staining at the recommended working dilution without any nonspecific or unwanted staining of the substrate, so that a sharp end point is achieved, it is essential to start with a high-titered anti-human globulin serum. Ideally, such a serum is best raised by using as antigen purified Ig from a pool composed of bleedings from a large number of donors so that the reagent will recognize all classes of Ig's equally. Where monospecific conjugates are required, it is not sufficient to show that the starting serum is monospecific by gel diffusion techniques or even after conjugation of the globulins by its ability to stain or not stain monoclonal bone marrow smears. Rather, it should be shown to be monospecific in an indirect immunofluorescence test in which one uses in the sandwich patient's sera of known reactivity of particular class specificities against the substrate. That is, the monospecificity of the conjugate must be established by using the most sensitive test system in which it may be used.

It has also been found that the fluorochrome used can adversely affect the performance of the conjugate. Fluorescein isothiocyanate (FITC) has the highest emission intensity of those commonly used, but even with FITC it is essential to use preparations of the highest purity. Impurities give rise to variability in performance and make the calculation of the fluorochrome to protein ratio, on which the sensitivity of the test depends, invalid. Impurities are a common cause of nonspecific staining. A standard test for the labeling efficiency of FITC has been promulgated by the U.S. National Committee for Clinical Laboratory Standards, and a document outlining the parameters which govern the production of good conjugates has been issued by the Medical Research Council of Great Britain's working party on the use of antisera to Ig's (7).

Standardization of immunofluorescent materials and techniques is still far from perfect, but the report of a joint IUIS/WHO Consultation produced recommended methods for the fluorescent-antibody test for antinuclear factor, *Treponema pallidum* antibodies (FTA-ABS), and *Toxoplasma* antibodies (Appendix III). A group under the auspices of WHO, the New York Academy of Sciences, IUIS, and other interested parties has now met five times, and a study of the reports of these meetings will give the reader a deeper insight into the problems involved (1).

Enzyme (e.g., peroxidase)-labeled antibody tests and hemagglutination tests. These test systems for quantitating auto-antibodies have not been the subject of much study from the point of view of their standardization. Workers in this field rely on the use of WHO- designated expert reference centers to help them to resolve problems of method and to confirm comparability of results.

The necessity for standardization and quality control of immunological reagents is not as readily appreciated as is that for drugs. In the past, methods used in the diagnosis of pathological conditions were relatively insensitive and it was comparatively easy to distinguish between normal and abnormal states, but the highly sensitive techniques now used have shown that in most circumstances these differences in level are quantitative rather than qualitative. It is clear, therefore, that the precision and accuracy of test methods and the standardization and quality control of reagents should no longer be neglected.

APPENDIX I

Anti-IgM conjugate specification

1. *Specificity*
   1.1 It must be class specific for human IgM in the definitive fluorescent-labeled antibody (FLA) tests for syphilis, toxoplasma, rubella, etc.
   1.2 It must not react with other Ig classes, light chains, or complement components, or exhibit other inappropriate reactions in the definitive FLA test systems.
   1.3 It must be free from immune complexes and all other human serum components.
   1.4 Insolubilized absorbents should be used.
2. *Potency*
   2.1 It must have a plateau titer of at least 1:8 in a congenital syphilis system.
   2.2 It must not show nonspecific staining at a concentration less than four times the endpoint titer.
3. *Immunogen*
   Purified IgM from a pool of monoclonal sera or from normal human sera.
4. *Filling and freeze-drying*
   This should be according to the recommendations WHO/BS/773/65 pages 7–12.
5. Adequate stability data must be provided.
6. Information on the material as laid down at the 1968 London meeting on Standardization of Immunofluorescence and by the Medical Research Council working party (Immunology, vol. 20, no. 1, January 1975) should be provided:
   6.1 The name and address of the manufacturer.
   6.2 The proper name of the product and its batch or lot number.
   6.3 The manufacturer's recommended expiration date.
   6.4 The type of fluorochrome used to label the antibodies.
   6.5 (a) If a standard is available the potency in relation to the standard, or
       (b) If a standard is not available the intended working dilution (with range), as found in a specified test.
   6.6 The ratio of optical densities before the addition of any stabilizers.
   6.7 Any special information about processing, including additions and absorptions.
   6.8 Any known cross-reactivity, especially to Ig of other species.
   6.9 The type and concentration of preservative present, if any.

APPENDIX II

List of substances to be estimated

Immunoglobulins: IgG, IgM, IgA, IgD, IgE
Other serum proteins: in particular pre-albumin, albumin, alpha$_2$-macroglobulin, alpha$_1$-glycoprotein, hemopexin, transferrin, haptoglobin, ceruloplasmin, alpha$_1$-antitrypsin, beta-lipoprotein
Auto-antibodies: against adrenal gland, gastric parietal mucosa, glomerular basement membrane,

intrinsic factor mitochondria, parathyroid gland, parotic duct cells, skin, smooth muscle, striated muscle, sperm, thyroglobulin, thyroid microsomes, and single- and double-stranded deoxyribonucleic acid.

APPENDIX III

Provisional Recommended Methods of Test

Antinuclear factor (ANF) test

Reagents – minimum
1. Fluorescein-labeled antihuman IgG
2. Phosphate-buffered saline (PBS), pH 7.6

NaCl	8.5 g
Na$_2$HPO$_4$	1.28 g
NaH$_2$PO$_4 \cdot$2H$_2$O	0.156 g
Distilled water to	1 liter

3. Mounting fluid, pH 9 (buffered glycerol)

NaHCO$_3$	0.0715 g
Na$_2$CO$_3$	0.016 g
Distilled water to	10 ml
Glycerol to	100 ml

4. Cryostat sections of rat liver
5. WHO International Standard human ANF serum

Method – commonly accepted – note:
1. All dilutions should be made in PBS.
2. Standard ANF serum is allowed to react with substrate for 30 min at room temperature (20 to 25 C) in a humid chamber.
3. Wash for 30 min in at least two changes of PBS with gentle agitation.
4. Drain and remove excess moisture from around edges with lint-free absorbent.
5. Dilutions of conjugate in PBS are allowed to react for 30 min at room temperature in a humid chamber.
6. Wash for 30 min in at least three changes of PBS.
7. Drain slides, rinse distilled water, drain, mount in mounting fluid given above.

Results
Plateau of ANF = ANF titer obtained with at least three twofold titer steps of conjugate.
Plateau end point = last dilution of conjugate giving the ANF plateau.
Where possible the emission should be measured.

Toxoplasma test

Reagents – minimum
1. Fluorescein-labeled antihuman IgG
2. Phosphate-buffered saline (PBS), pH 7.6

NaCl	8.5 g
Na$_2$HPO$_4$	1.28 g
NaH$_2$PO$_4 \cdot$2H$_2$O	0.156 g
Distilled water to	1 liter

3. Mounting fluid, pH 9 (buffered glycerol)

NaHCO$_3$	0.0715 g
Na$_2$CO$_3$	0.016 g
Distilled water to	10 ml
Glycerol to	100 ml

4. *Toxoplasma gondii* RH strain
5. Methyl alcohol (absolute) or dry acetone
6. WHO International Standard *Toxoplasma* serum
7. Evans Blue, 0.5 g in 50 ml of PBS

Method – commonly accepted – note:
1. Air-dry antigen smear and fix for 10 min in absolute alcohol or dry acetone.
2. Wash for 5 min in PBS.
3. Allow serum to react with antigen for 30 min at room temperature (20 to 25 C) in a humid chamber.
4. Wash for 30 min with at least three changes of PBS with gentle agitation.
5. Allow dilutions of conjugate to react with preparation for 30 min at room temperature in a humid chamber.
6. Wash for 1 h in at least four changes of PBS.
7. Rinse with distilled water, blot, and mount in mounting fluid given above.
8. All conjugate dilutions should be made so that a final concentration of 0.2% Evans Blue is attained.

N.B. It is appreciated that the use of Evans Blue reduces the sensitivity of the test.

Results
Plateau of *Toxoplasma* = *Toxoplasma* titer obtained with at least three twofold titer steps of conjugate.
Plateau end point = last dilution of conjugate giving the toxoplasma plateau.
Where possible the emission should be measured.

FTA-ABS test

Reagents – minimum
1. Fluorescein-labeled anti-IgG
2. Phosphate-buffered saline (PBS), pH 7.6

NaCl	8.5 g
Na$_2$HPO$_4$	1.28 g
NaH$_2$PO$_4 \cdot$2H$_2$O	0.156 g
Distilled water to	1 liter

3. Mounting fluid, pH 9 (buffered glycerol)

NaHCO$_3$	0.0715 g
Na$_2$CO$_3$	0.016 g
Distilled water to	10 ml
Glycerol to	100 ml

4. *Treponema pallidum*, well washed
5. WHO International Standard Positive Syphilitic Serum
6. Sorbent
7. Dry acetone

Method – commonly accepted – note:
1. All dilutions to be made in PBS.
2. Ensure even distribution of treponemes; if necessary, break up clumps by repeated aspiration into a syringe with a 25-gauge needle.
3. Fix in *dry* acetone for 10 min.
4. Inactivate serum at 56 C for 30 min.
5. Prepare serum/sorbent mixtures not more than 30 min before using.

6. React serum with treponemes on slide for 30 min at 37 C in a humid chamber.
7. Wash in four changes of PBS for 20 min room temperature.
8. Allow conjugate to react with preparation for 30 min at 37 C in a humid chamber.
9. Wash in four changes of PBS for 20 min, rinse in distilled water, blot gently.
10. Mount in mounting fluid as given above.

Results

Plateau of FTA-ABS = FTA-ABS titer obtained with at least three twofold titer steps of conjugate.

Plateau end point = last dilution of conjugate giving the FTA-ABS plateau.

Where possible, the emission should be measured.

LITERATURE CITED

1. Hijmans, W., and M. Schaeffer. 1975. The 5th International Conference on Immunofluorescence and the Related Staining Techniques. Ann. N.Y. Acad. Sci. 254:21–172.
2. International Atomic Energy Agency. 1974. Radio immunoassay and related procedures. Standardization and control of reagents and procedures. Medicine 1:3–87.
3. Johansson, S. G. O., H. Bennich, and T. Berg. 1971. *In vitro* diagnosis of atopic allergy. III. Quantitative estimation of circulating IgE antibodies by the radio allergosorbent test. Int. Arch. Allergy 41:443–451.
4. Larson, C., P. Orenstein, and R. F. Ritchie. 1971. Automated nephelometric determination of antigen antibody interaction: theory and application. Advances in automated analysis, p. 101. Mediad Inc., Tarrytown, N.Y.
5. Laurell, C. B. 1966. Quantitative estimation of proteins by electrophoresis in agarose gel containing antibodies. Anal. Biochem. 15:45–52.
6. Mancini, G., A. O. Carbonara, and J. F. Heremans. 1965. Immunochemical quantitation of antigens by single radial immunodiffusion. Immunochemistry 2:235–254.
7. MRC Working Party. 1971. Recommendations on the characterization of antisera as reagents. Immunology 20:1–10.
8. Rowe, D. S. 1969. Radioactive single radial diffusion. A method of increasing the sensitivity of immunochemical quantification of proteins in agar gel. Bull. WHO 40:613–616.
9. Rowe, D. S., S. G. Anderson, and B. Grab. 1970. A research standard for human serum immunoglobulins IgG, IgA and IgM. Bull. WHO 42:535–552.
10. Rowe, D. S., S. G. Anderson, and L. Tackett. 1970. A research standard for human serum immunoglobulin D. Bull. WHO 43:607–609.
11. Rowe, D. S., L. Tackett, H. Bennich, K. Ishizaka, S. G. O. Johansson, and S. G. Anderson. 1970. A research standard for human serum immunoglobulin E. Bull. WHO 43:609–611.
12. Wide, L., H. Bennich, and S. G. O. Johansson. 1967. Diagnosis of allergy by an *in vitro* test for allergen antibodies. Lancet 2:1105–1107.
13. World Health Organization. 1965. Notes on the preparation of materials to serve as international biological standards reference preparations and reference reagents, p. 1–13. WHO/BS/773/65. World Health Organization, Geneva.
14. World Health Organization. 1972. 24th Report of the WHO Expert Committee on Biological Standardization. WHO Tech. Rep. Ser. No. 486, p. 7.

Chapter 123

Proficiency Testing and Clinical Laboratory Immunology

PIERRE W. KEITGES

The technical nature of laboratory tests in clinical immunology and the data generated therefrom create unique problems for a proficiency testing system. The problems are of such a degree that one might validly question the validity of proficiency testing in this area with the present state of the art. However, because of the continued development of legislation and regulations requiring proficiency testing as one of the measures of quality of performance in a clinical laboratory, it is clear that proficiency testing must be carried out. Systems must be designed which will attempt to meet regulatory needs, define specific problems with regard to state of the art, and yet be flexible and sensitive to the problems which will be discussed in this chapter.

At the Second National Conference on Proficiency Testing conducted by the National Council on Health Laboratory Services, some of the characteristics of clinical laboratory immunology which directly affect proficiency testing were delineated. These included:

1. Significant lack of physical and performance standards for most of the tests in this field.

2. The fact that much of the data generated by these tests is qualitative and nondimensional.

3. The marked need for education with regard to understanding and applying the data generated by these tests, especially with regard to clinical relevance.

4. The wide range of diversity in this area extending from serological tests for syphilis to B and T cell function studies.

For purposes of clarity I shall discuss proficiency testing with regard to the immunological tests for infectious diseases and the immunological tests for cellular immunity, subdividing these two groups into those which are well established and those which are developmental.

All existing proficiency testing systems in clinical immunology have certain generic features in common. These systems include those conducted by the Center for Disease Control, The College of American Pathologists Surveys, the American Association of Bioanalysts, and many State Public Health Departments, especially in the area of serological testing for syphilis. These generic features include the fact that at specified times throughout the year, usually quarterly, a given set of samples are sent to the participant who is asked to perform a battery of immunological procedures. Information is generated via the reporting questionnaire, which includes not only the result obtained but also the method used and the manner in which results are reported. These latter features constitute a valuable mechanism, by which one obtains information concerning the "state of the art." Proficiency testing data which are needed to satisfy regulatory requirements are then scored and evaluated on the basis of accuracy and precision. Data generated which are not needed for a regulatory purpose are used primarily to identify problems which it is hoped will then be resolved through the educational arm of the program.

The immunology of infectious disease contains the most established and defined test procedures. First are the serological tests for syphilis. At this point, credit must be given to the outstanding contribution made by the Venereal Disease Research Laboratory. The efforts of this group not only markedly improved the quality of performance in the area of serological testing for syphilis but also set many principles and models for proficiency testing in this entire area. The *Manual of Tests for Syphilis 1969* should be used as the reference publication. However, the important need for a new edition is obvious, since several procedures including the automated reagin test, quantitative rapid plasma reagin test, automated fluorescent treponemal antibody test, and microhemagglutination test for treponemal antibodies are now accepted but are not in the 1969 edition. In the interim, it still has value, and procedures used in clinical laboratories should conform to this manual. The Center for Disease Control should be contacted if the procedure and technique being considered in your laboratory are not included in the manual.

Much study has been given to the mechanics of proficiency testing in syphilis serology. Most recently, it has been determined that significant data can be generated and the value of proficiency testing in this area can be preserved by using fewer samples for this purpose! As a result, the same goal can be reached through decreased cost and time expenditure by the individual laboratory. Percentages of agreement and reproducibility are achievable at very high levels (85 to 95%) in the existing systems. Since qualitative nondimensional values are in a large share the mode of reporting for these tests, the proficiency testing samples become extremely important with regard to reflecting these variations, i.e., specimens having weakly reactive and borderline activity. There has been a definite burden placed on industry to supply these systems with these difficult specimens. It should be remembered that the most important point clinically is that a given laboratory will not miss a case of syphilis, i.e., the false negative. In addition, quantitation of all positive results must be done and proficiency must be tested as well. Currently, all proficiency testing systems for this procedure include 10 to 60 specimens per year, which include duplicates as well as negative, weakly reactive, borderline, and reactive samples having reactivity from 1 to 32 dilutions. Both percent agreement and percent reproducibility are evaluated, and for the most part the performance of clinical laboratories in the field is exemplary.

This type of model has been extended now to include other immunological procedures dealing with infectious disease or inflammation. Antistreptolysin O titer, rheumatoid factor, cold agglutinins, febrile agglutinins, and tests for infectious mononucleosis are included in most systems. In addition, most of the laboratories involved in basic immunological procedures include immunological tests for pregnancy, which can be effectively included. Certain specific comments should be made with regard to the current state of proficiency testing in each of these parameters.

It seems reasonable from survey results to evaluate separately the tests for the antistreptolysin O titer which are quantitative and those which are qualitative. In addition, it is most beneficial if the qualitative tests are evaluated simply as being positive or negative for recent or current streptococcal infection. The problem with the variation and dilution schemes for the antistreptolysin O quantitative tests cannot be resolved until a dependable and reliable standard is universally available. The World Health Organization standard for the antistreptolysin O titer should be more widely used in this regard; however, the World Health Organization standard is not always readily available.

Commercially prepared antistreptolysin O standards do exist; however, most are diluted 1:100 and therefore, applicable only to (Rantz and Randall) modification of the Todd dilution scheme. Proficiency testing has pointed out the need for proper handling of the streptolysin O reagent in that it should be handled carefully with no vigorous shaking, reconstituted with cold distilled water, and added to the test within 5 min (maximum, 10 min) after reconstitution.

Rheumatoid factor tests do show differences in sensitivity between slide and tube tests and, hence, most proficiency testing systems evaluate these separately. In this area proficiency testing has shown that manufacturers' directions should be followed implicitly. This is especially true with regard to the sample size and the speed and time of centrifugation, which seem to effect the titer markedly.

With regard to the immunological tests for infectious mononucleosis, it is well recognized that false positives do occur. Here again, strict observance of the manufacturers' directions, especially with regard to interpretation of positive results, is mandatory. It is proper to state that the ox cell hemolysin test certainly is valuable as a confirmatory test and may in certain instances, especially in problematic cases, be preferable. There are fewer naturally occurring hemolysins to beef red cells than there are hemagglutinins to sheep or horse red blood cells.

Proficiency testing has shown in the area of immunological tests for pregnancy that the manufacturers designated sensitivity levels with regard to human chorionic gonadotropin are quite valid, and these tests perform very well in the field when the user acknowledges the differences in the sensitivity levels of the various kits as well as the differences in response when using diluted or undiluted specimens. Most of the tests have eliminated a large amount of the problem encountered with blood; however, a specimen grossly contaminated with blood, of course, should not be tested. Most of the tests are still sensitive to high levels of protein in the urine, and the importance of dealing with a concentrated specimen as indicated by the specific gravity is obvious.

To date, proficiency testing has proved of little value in solving the problems concerning the tests for the febrile and cold agglutinins.

Proficiency testing data generated by these relatively well-established tests in the area of basic laboratory clinical immunology can be used not only to meet regulatory requirements but also to serve as a valuable tool for education. Under no circumstances should proficiency testing be considered the single tool to determine quality of laboratory performance. Other systems that must be considered are laboratory inspection and accreditation, documentation of internal daily quality control data, and documentation of personnel qualifications and their continuing education.

Currently, those proficiency testing samples directed at testing the so-called "gray zones" in these constituents should be looked upon as developmental. These are often expressed in the most qualitative and nondimensional way; therefore, this aspect of a proficiency testing program could be looked upon to improve the state of the art and establish performance standards, especially with regard to the sensitivity and specificity of kit tests.

The second general area concerns cellular immunology. Here the need for the development of primary physical and performance standards is most evident, and the introduction of secondary physical standards into the laboratory itself seems imperative. The first group of tests in this area are relatively well established and clinically oriented. These include the quantitation of immunoglobulins, tests for antinuclear antibodies and other autoantibodies, and lupus erythematosus cell preparations.

The need for a uniform, reliable, and readily available international protein standard as well as a national standard for the quantitation of immunoglobulins is paramount. Currently, most manufacturers rely on their own internal standards to calibrate the reagents used for quantitating human immunoglobulins. These products are well prepared, well studied, and excellent. However, each applies only to the products manufactured by that given supplier, and, hence, similar results often cannot be obtained if one uses a different manufacturer's material. Meaningful evaluation and comparison of results obtained from the quantitation of immunoglobulins will not be possible until some uniform, generally applicable standard is available.

Other tests involving the area of cellular immunology are in themselves developmental; hence, proficiency testing in these areas has not been initiated or is developmental at best. This concerns the determination of total complement and certain of its components, primarily C4 and C3; tests dealing with immunofluorescence in general; and tests dealing with B and T cell identification and their function, including phagocytic activity. It would seem appropriate to design proficiency testing system to define the ability of laboratories doing immunofluorescence to determine fluorescein-protein ratios. Also, a similar need for standards exists in the area of complement determination.

The entire area of proficiency testing of radioimmune assays is a separate topic and will not be considered in this chapter.

It would be appropriate, in summary, to state some of the conclusions drawn by the Second National Conference on Proficiency Testing. The committee recommended that the currently existing systems, private and governmental, be encouraged and allowed to grow and develop. However, to implement the entire group of established and developmental programs as indicated above, it would be ideal if a "Joint Board" consisting of representatives from federal and state governments, professional societies, and industry would meet regularly to monitor and in some cases arbitrarily decide which changes in systems will be necessary on a continuing basis to keep current with the discipline. This would include redefinition of test classifications and criteria of evaluation. Within this system, private and governmental programs could function efficiently. The programs should meet the goals of proficiency testing, especially with regard to the detection of unacceptable performance, to meet legislative requirements at one end while permitting continued development to define the state of the art, identify problems, and educate at the other. The Second National Conference stressed that it is imperative for these comprehensive programs described to place scientific knowledge and patient care ahead of the legislative process, so that the legislative process would respond appropriately to these needs rather than dictate them.

Chapter 124

Clinical Immunology: a New Specialty Based in the Laboratory and Clinical Departments

INTRODUCTION

During the past 20 years, there has been tremendous growth in immunology. From a discipline concerned with immunity to infectious diseases, immunology has developed into a science concerned with the characteristics and effects of the immune response per se. The science of immunology has been rapidly applied to problems in human biology and pathology, and, as a consequence, applied immunology has had a significant impact on all aspects of medical practice. This impact has taken several forms. Modern immunology has defined new areas of medical practice as in the immunodeficiency diseases, has lent major strength to development of other areas such as transplantation, has provided new understanding of the etiology and pathogenesis of certain diseases, and has provided new investigative approaches and laboratory tools for the study of diseases.

Despite the rapid growth of the science of immunology and its recognized impact on other disciplines, universities and medical schools have been slow to accord formal recognition to these developments through the creation of Departments of Immunology. The function of such departments would include the training of undergraduates, as well as M.D. and Ph.D. immunologists. At present, there is movement in many institutions to create Departments, Committees, or Centers for Immunology. These administrative entities will serve as a nucleus for activities in immunology, as well as providing training in immunology at the undergraduate and graduate levels.

Several references are available on clinical immunology and the organization of Clinical Immunology Units (1–4).

CREATION OF CLINICAL IMMUNOLOGY UNITS

Within the framework of established Departments of Immunology, it will become easier to define clinical immunology as the application of the science of immunology to problems of human disease. In turn, the clinical immunologist

may be defined as a physician who applies immunological theories, principles, and techniques in the diagnoses, treatment, and evaluation of disease. The Ph.D. immunologist can participate in many, but not all, of the activities of the clinical or medical immunologist. It is anticipated that Clinical Immunology Units will be staffed by a number of individuals, some of whom may be Ph.D. immunologists. Ideally, the teachers and practitioners of clinical immunology should constitute one part of a Department or Committee of Immunology at a medical school. In some institutions, however, the Clinical Immunology Unit may be a part of a different department of the university or medical school, or it may be based in a large community hospital. In such instances, close ties between the basic science Department or Committee of Immunology and the Clinical Immunology Unit should be maintained by combined conferences and joint responsibility for the training of students and fellows.

Functions of Clinical Immunology Units

1. To create and maintain a community of interest in immunology within the hospital setting.

2. To serve as a repository of knowledge of immunological concepts, principles, and techniques related to human disease, and to maintain close contacts with basic immunology in order to facilitate the exploitation of new discoveries for the benefit of patients.

3. To teach clinical immunology to medical students, house staff, fellows, attending staff, and other medical and paramedical personnel; to conduct research in clinical immunology; and to develop new procedures and tests related to that discipline.

4. To direct and supervise special laboratories concerned with clinical immunology.

5. To engage in direct patient care and/or consultative activities.

Content of clinical immunology

Although clinical immunology is undergoing continuous and rapid development, it is possi-

921

ble to outline the body of knowledge comprising this new specialty. This knowledge includes:

1. The principles involved in assessing the humoral and cellular immune competence of patients, and in diagnosing and treating the various inherited and acquired immunodeficiency diseases.

2. The amplification mechanisms of inflammation including the complement systems, vasoactive amines, kinins, clotting factors, lymphokines, and prostaglandin, as well as the diverse cell types involved in inflammation and the control proteins influencing the action of soluble mediators or cellular components of the inflammatory response.

3. Immunological abnormalities of the skin, endocrine organs, gastrointestinal tract, nervous system, eyes, reproductive organs, the hematological system, the kidneys, and the lungs.

4. The immunology of infectious and parasitic diseases, including streptococcal diseases, tuberculosis, leprosy, histoplasmosis, and chronic fungal diseases, and the influence of bacterial and viral infections on the immune response.

5. Transplantation immunology, including the histocompatibility locus A (HLA) system and principles involved in serological typing and cellular recognition systems.

6. Cancer, including tumor antigens, immunotherapy of cancer, and immunological aspects of multiple myeloma and related plasma cell dyscrasias, lymphoma, Hodgkin's disease, and leukemia.

7. Connective tissue diseases in which immunological mechanisms are presumed to have an etiological or contributory role, including rheumatoid arthritis, systemic lupus erythematosus, polymyositis, Sjögren's syndrome, and systemic vasculitis.

8. Immediate hypersensitivity diseases including allergic rhinitis, allergic asthma, and urticaria.

9. Immunology of drug reactions.

10. Immunotherapy, including specific immunotherapy as in the administration of allergenic extract, adjunctive therapy as in the administration of BCG, and the use of drugs to manipulate immune response.

11. Immunogenetics, including the relationship of HLA antigens to disease and the role of immune response genes.

Activities of the clinical immunology laboratory

The practice of clinical immunology is highly dependent upon certain specialized laboratory procedures. The laboratory procedures of spe-cial concern to the clinical immunologist include the following:

1. Quantitation of immunoglobulins, including radioimmunodiffusion, rocket immunoelectrophoresis, nephelometric procedures, and radioimmunoassay for trace proteins such as immunoglobulin E (IgE) in serum or IgG in cerebrospinal fluid. Detection and identification of M components, including Bence-Jones proteins, by immunoelectrophoresis. Determination of serum viscosity.

2. Determination of the concentration and activity of total serum complement, and of components of the classical and alternative complement system.

3. Immunofluorescence as applied in the indirect method to the detection of antibodies to nuclear, microsomal, thyroid, gastric parietal cell, smooth and striated muscle, skin, and other antigens, and as applied in the direct method to the detection of immunoglobulin, complement, or other antigens in tissues including the skin, kidney and vascular structures.

4. Serological procedures including hemagglutination, complement fixation, and other procedures employed in the diagnosis of infectious diseases, including parasitic diseases.

5. Assessment of the function of cells involved in host defense. Assays of phagocytic cell activity including the activities of polymorphonuclear leukocyte and macrophage, and detection of defects in the functions of these cells. Identification and enumeration of T, B, and null cells. Measurement of the response of T and B cells to mitogens and antigens. Detection and measurement of lymphokines. Performance and interpretation of tests involved in cell-mediated responses; assessment of cytotoxic T cells and of antibody-mediated cytotoxicity.

6. Blood and tissue typing including the Coombs' test procedures, detection of warm and cold anti-erythrocyte antibodies; HLA typing of lymphocytes, mixed lymphocyte reaction, and cell-mediated lympholysis; control of Rh immunization.

7. Tests involved in the evaluation of allergic patients including prick tests, intradermal tests, passive transfer techniques, and radioallergosorbent procedures.

8. Quantitation of tumor antigens including α-fetoprotein, carcinoembryonic antigen, and others.

9. Radioimmunoassay, including principles and practices related to the detection and measurement of trace proteins, allergens, tumor antigens, bacterial antigens, and viral antigens, as in the detection of the hepatitis B surface antigen.

In the capacity of director of the Clinical Immunology Laboratory, the clinical immunologist will also be expected to be aware of the principles of laboratory organization and management, including the requirements of quality control and to have knowledge of the requirements of different regulatory agencies concerned with laboratory management.

In view of the large number of laboratory procedures to be performed, it is expected that the Clinical Immunology Laboratory will consist of several modules. Each module will have a supervisor and one or more technicians who will be specifically trained in immunological techniques and procedures. The Clinical Immunology Laboratory will have a director, who may also serve as the director of the entire Clinical Immunology Unit. It is recognized that in some institutions the clinical immunology laboratories constitute part of a larger Department of Laboratory Medicine. Under such circumstances, it is of great importance that the individual in charge of the clinical immunology section of such a large department have a very close relationship to the Clinical Immunology Unit.

RELATIONSHIP OF THE CLINICAL IMMUNOLOGY UNIT TO PATIENT CARE

The relationship of the Clinical Immunology Unit to patient care may take one of two major forms. In some Clinical Immunology Units, the relationship to patients will be limited to consultations only, and other units may engage in the direct care of patients in addition to offering consultation services. The former type of unit does not require a unique patient base, whereas the latter unit requires that certain patients be identified for short- or long-term care by the clinical immunologist. At present, some Clinical Immunology Units have their patient base in a conventional allergy, rheumatology, or hematology section. It is expected that, in the future, other combinations of conventional specialty groups will serve as the patient base of certain Clinical Immunology Units. These combinations may include allergy and rheumatology groups, or oncology, transplantation, and hematology groups, or allergy, pulmonary disease, and dermatology groups. In some centers,

the patient base may be even larger and may include the patient population presently cared for by allergy and rheumatology units, patients with immunodeficiency diseases, patients with organ or tissue transplants, and some oncology patients. The guiding principle behind such reorganization of conventional practices is that certain patients may be identified in whom immunological principles and techniques provide a major contribution to an understanding of the pathogenesis, treatment, and evaluation of their disease. One of the major reasons for providing direct patient care in large Clinical Immunology Units is to assure access to the large numbers of patients required for the training of future generations of clinical immunologists. An important aspect of that training involves the interpretation of the clinical immunology laboratory tests in the context of the clinical presentation of patients. Considerable experience is required to preclude both the over- and under-interpretation of the laboratory test results during the evolution of this new specialty.

ACKNOWLEDGMENTS

Although I assume full responsibility for the preparation of this chapter, I should like to acknowledge that many of the concepts presented were developed during the discussions of the Committee on Hospital-based Laboratory and Clinical Immunology of the American Association of Immunologists.

Preparation of this chapter was supported by Public Health Service grants AM-03564 and AM-05067 from the National Institute of Arthritis, Metabolism, and Digestive Diseases and by grants from the Massachusetts Chapter, Arthritis Foundation, and the L. H. Bendit Foundation.

Publication No. 683 of the Robert W. Lovett Memorial Group for the Study of Diseases Causing Deformities, Massachusetts General Hospital, Boston, Mass.

LITERATURE CITED

1. Natvig, J. B., and H. H. Fudenberg. 1975. Clinical immunology, present and future. Vox Sang. 28:329–336.
2. Vaughan, J. 1972. The emerging concept of clinical immunology. J. Allergy Clin. Immunol. 50:294–304.
3. Whittingham, S., and I. R. MacKay. 1971. Design and functions of department of clinical immunology. Clin. Exp. Immunol. 8: 857–861.
4. World Health Organization. 1972. Clinical immunology. WHO Tech. Rep. Ser. No. 496.

AUTHOR INDEX

Abelson, Leslie, 811
Adkinson, N. Franklin, Jr., 590
Agnello, Vincent, 669
Albritton, William L., 318
Alexander, A. D., 352
Amos, D. Bernard, 797, 884
Andiman, Warren A., 428
Artenstein, Malcolm S., 274
Balows, A., 280
Barker, Lewellys F., 481
Bartlett, Ann, 506
Batty, Irene, 911
Bellanti, Joseph A., 155
Bidwell, Dennis, 506
Bigazzi, P. E., 682
Black, Francis L., 444
Blank, Carl, 898
Blatt, Philip M., 542
Bloch, Kurt J., 921
Brandt, Brenda L., 276
Braun, W. E., 790
Brunell, Philip A., 421
Cavallaro, Joseph J., 906
Chernesky, Max A., 452
Chess, Leonard, 77
Clausen, Jens E., 101
Cline, Martin J., 142
Collins, R. D., 718
Colombani, Monique, 805
Colombani, J., 805
Craig, John P., 324
Dausset, Jean, 787
David, Hugo L., 332
Davis, Neil C., 4
Demetriou, J. A., 242
Deodhar, Sharad D., 206, 894
DeWitt, Wallis E., 289
Dienstag, Jules L., 467
Dimond, Richard C., 197
Dixon, F. J., 676
Dowdle, Walter R., 433
Dumonde, D. C., 129
Dupont, Bo, 833
Epstein, Lois B., 120
Fahey, John L., 3
Fair, Daryl S., 110
Feeley, John C., 289
Ferreira, Euripides, 858
Fink, Jordan N., 616
Flexner, J. M., 718
Freter, Rolf, 285
Fudenberg, H. Hugh, 515, 562
Gewurz, Henry, 36
Gill, Thomas J., III, 169
Gleich, Gerald J., 575
Glick, A. D., 718
Golde, David W., 142
Golub, Sidney H., 770
Gordon, Morris A., 338
Granger, Gale A., 110
Greenberg, L. J., 783

Haber, Edgar, 190
Hambie, Edith A., 315
Hansen, John A., 833
Henkart, Pierre, 811
Herrmann, Kenneth L., 416
Hicks, Arnold, 898
Ho, Monto, 4
Hong, Richard, 620
Inami, Y. H., 656
Jewett, Michael A. S., 833
Johnson, A. H., 814
Jones, Wallis L., 315
Jordon, Robert, 701
Josimovich, J. B., 213
Kagan, I. G., 382
Kapikian, Albert Z., 467
Kaufman, Leo, 363
Kaufmann, William, 902
Kayhoe, D. E., 790
Keitges, Pierre W., 918
Kellogg, D. S., 280
Kenny, George E., 357
Klein, George C., 264
Kochwa, Shaul, 17
Koistinen, Jukka, 562
Kumar, Manjula S., 206
Kupchik, Herbert Z., 753
Kyle, Robert A., 734
Larsen, P. Reed, 222
Larsen, Sandra A., 318
Leech, J. H., 718
Levine, Bernard B., 83
Levitt, M. J., 172, 213
Lewis, John E., 110
Lichtenstein, Lawrence M., 573
Lightbody, James, 851
Lundak, Robert L., 110
McCullough, Norman B., 304
McGuigan, James E., 182
McIntire, K. R., 765
Mackenzie, Ross, 239
Mahgoub, El Sheikh, 338
Maini, R. N., 129
Manclark, Charles R., 312
Mann, Dean, 811
Miller, George, 428
Monath, Thomas P., 456
Mufson, Maurice A., 438
Murphy, Frederick A., 463
Nakamura, R. M., 656
Nankin, Howard R., 248
Neter, Erwin, 263
Norman, L., 382
Norman, Philip S., 585
O'Leary, James, 820
Oppenheim, Joost J., 81
Palmer, Dan F., 893, 906
Peebles, C., 660
Peters, Stephen M., 155
Petz, Lawrence D., 527
Pilch, Yosef H., 770
Pillarisetty, Rao, 652

Pollack, William, 559
Pool, Pamela, 797
Poulsen, Knud, 190
Prieur, Anne-Marie, 110
Purcell, Robert H., 467, 481
Rabin, Bruce S., 256
Rawls, William E., 452
Reinsmoen, Nancy, 820
Reiss, Alice M., 559
Reynoso, Gustavo, 231
Roberts, Harold R., 542
Rocklin, Ross E., 51, 95
Rola-Pleszczynski, Marek, 155
Rose, N. R., 682
Rosenfield, Richard E., 516
Ross, G., 64
Rothfield, Naomi F., 647
Russell, Philip K., 413
Schachter, Julius, 494
Schecter, Bilha, 81
Schlossman, Stuart F., 77
Schmidt, Nathalie J., 488
Schmitt, K. W., 172
Schwartz, Robert S., 717
Selin, Merle J., 232
Shulman, Sidney, 710
Siraganian, Reuben P., 603
Snyder, Merrill J., 302
Spitler, Lynn E., 53
Stewart, John A., 416, 423
Stossel, Thomas P., 148
Suyehira, Lisbeth A., 36
Svejgaard, Arne, 841
Talal, Norman, 652
Tan, Eng M., 645, 660
Taylor, Marilyn, 148
Territo, Mary C., 142
Theofilopoulos, A. N., 676
Thompson, John S., 868
Tom, Baldwin H., 874
Top, Franklin H., Jr., 448
Torrigiani, G., 911
Tramont, Edmund C., 274
Troen, Philip, 248
Vinson, J. William, 500
Voller, Alistair, 506
Waldmann, T. A., 765
Waldron, J. A., 718
Waner, J. L., 423
Ward, Peter A., 106
Weller, T. H., 423
Wiggins, Geraldine L., 318
Wilson, Curtis B., 692
Winblad, Sten, 296
Winchester, Robert J., 64, 665
Wolstencroft, R. A., 129
Wood, Ronald M., 341
Yunginger, John W., 575
Yunis, Edmond J., 783, 820
Zamcheck, Norman, 753
Zollinger, Wendell D., 274

924

SUBJECT INDEX